# The GALE ENCYCLOPEDIA of GENETIC DISORDERS

## THIRD EDITION

### VOLUME

**2**

M–Z
APPENDIX
GLOSSARY
INDEX

LAURIE J. FUNDUKIAN, EDITOR

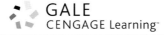

GALE
CENGAGE Learning·

Detroit • New York • San Francisco • New Haven, Conn • Waterville, Maine • London

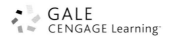
## GALE
### CENGAGE Learning™

**Gale Encyclopedia of Genetic Disorders, Third Edition**

Project Editor: Laurie J. Fundukian

Editorial: Kristin Key

Product Manager: Kate Hanley

Editorial Support Services: Andrea Lopeman

Indexing Services: Factiva, a Dow Jones Company

Rights Acquisition and Management: Barb McNeil and Susan Rudoloph

Composition: Evi Abou-El-Seoud

Manufacturing: Wendy Blurton

Imaging: John Watkins

Product Design: Pam Galbreath

For product information and technology assistance, contact us at **Gale Customer Support, 1-800-877-4253.**
For permission to use material from this text or product, submit all requests online at **www.cengage.com/permissions.**
Further permissions questions can be emailed to **permissionrequest@cengage.com**

While every effort has been made to ensure the reliability of the information presented in this publication, Gale, a part of Cengage Learning, does not guarantee the accuracy of the data contained herein. Gale accepts no payment for listing; and inclusion in the publication of any organization, agency, institution, publication, service, or individual does not imply endorsement of the editors or publisher. Errors brought to the attention of the publisher and verified to the satisfaction of the publisher will be corrected in future editions.

**Library of Congress Cataloging-in-Publication Data**

Gale encyclopedia of genetic disorders, 3rd ed. / edited by Laurie J. Fundukian, editor.
   p. cm. --
   Other title: Encyclopedia of genetic disorders
   Other title: Genetic disorders
   Includes bibliographical references and index.
   ISBN-13: 978-1-4144-7602-5 (set) -- ISBN-13: 978-1-4144-7603-2 (vol. 1) --
ISBN-13: 978-1-4144-7604-9 (vol. 2) -- ISBN-10: 1-4144-7602-7 (set) -- [etc.]
   1. Medical genetics–Encyclopedias. 2. Genetic disorders–Encyclopedias. I. Fundukian, Laurie J., 1970- II. Title: Encyclopedia of genetic disorders. III. Title: Genetic disorders.
   [DNLM: 1. Genetics, Medical–Encyclopedias–English. 2. Genetic Diseases, Inborn–Encyclopedias–English. 3. Genetic Predisposition to Disease–Encyclopedias–English. QZ 13 G1517 2011]

RB155.5.G35 2011
616′.04203–dc22                                                          2010002222

Gale
27500 Drake Rd.
Farmington Hills, MI, 48331-3535

ISBN-13: 978-1-4144-7602-5 (set)          ISBN-10: 1-4144-7602-7 (set)
ISBN-13: 978-1-4144-7603-2 (vol. 1)       ISBN-10: 1-4144-7603-5 (vol. 1)
ISBN-13: 978-1-4144-7604-9 (vol. 2)       ISBN-10: 1-4144-7604-3 (vol. 2)

This title is also available as an e-book.
ISBN-13: 978-1-4144-7605-6  ISBN-10: 1-4144-7605-1
Contact your Gale, a part of Cengage Learning sales representative for ordering information.

Printed in China by China Translation & Printing Services Limited
1 2 3 4 5 6 7 14 13 12 11 10

# CONTENTS

# LIST OF ENTRIES

# H

Haim-Munk syndrome
Hair loss syndromes
Hallermann-Streiff syndrome
Hand-foot-uterus syndrome
Harlequin fetus
Hemifacial microsomia
Hemihypertrophy
  (Hemihyperplasia)
Hemochromatosis
Hemolytic-uremic syndrome
Hemophilia
Hepatocellular carcinoma
Herceptin
Hereditary angioneurotic edema
Hereditary colorectal cancer
Hereditary Coproporphyria
Hereditary desmoid disease
Hereditary hearing loss
  and deafness
Hereditary multiple exostoses
Hereditary Nonpolyposis
  Colorectal Cancer
Hereditary pancreatitis
Hereditary spastic paraplegia
Hereditary spherocytosis
Hermansky-Pudlak syndrome
Hermaphroditism
Hirschsprung disease
Holoprosencephaly
Holt-Oram syndrome
Homocystinuria
Human Genome Project
Huntington disease
Hydrocephalus
Hydrolethalus syndrome
Hydrops fetalis
Hyperlipoproteinemia
Hyperoxaluria
Hyperphenylalaninemia
Hypochondrogenesis
Hypochondroplasia
Hypophosphatasia
Hypophosphatemia
Hypospadias and epispadias

# I

Ichthyosis
Imprinting
Incontinentia pigmenti
Infantile refsum disease
Inheritance

# J

Jackson-Weiss syndrome
Jacobsen syndrome
Jervell and Lange-Nielsen
  syndrome
Joubert syndrome

# K

Kabuki syndrome
Kallmann syndrome
Kartagener syndrome
Karyotype
Kennedy disease
Klinefelter syndrome
Klippel–Feil syndrome
Klippel-Trenaunay-Weber
  syndrome
Kniest dysplasia
Krabbe disease

# L

Langer-Saldino achondrogenesis
Larsen syndrome
Laterality sequence
Leber congenital amaurosis
Lebers hereditary optic atrophy
Leigh syndrome
Lesch-Nyhan syndrome
Leukodystrophy
Li-Fraumeni syndrome
Limb-girdle muscular dystrophy
Lipoprotein lipase deficiency
Lissencephaly

Long QT syndrome
Lowe oculocerebrorenal
  syndrome

# M

Machado-Joseph disease
Macular degeneration—age-related
Major histocompatibility complex
Malignant hyperthermia
Mannosidosis
Marfan syndrome
Marshall syndrome
Marshall-Smith syndrome
MCAD deficiency
McCune–Albright syndrome
McKusick-Kaufman syndrome
Meckel's diverticulum
Meckel-Gruber syndrome
Menkes syndrome
Metaphyseal dysplasia
Methylmalonic acidemia
Methylmalonicaciduria due to
  methylmalonic CoA mutase
  deficiency
Micro Syndrome
Microcephaly (childhood)
Microphthalmia with linear skin
  defects (MLS)
Miller-Dieker syndrome
Moebius syndrome
Monosomy 1p36 syndrome
Mowat-Wilson Syndrome
Moyamoya
Mucolipidosis
Mucopolysaccharides
Mucopolysaccharidosis type I
Mucopolysaccharidosis type II
Muir-Torre syndrome
Multifactorial inheritance
Multiple endocrine neoplasias
Multiple epiphyseal dysplasia
Multiple lentigenes syndrome
Multiple sclerosis
Multiplex ligation-dependent
  probe amplification

Sjögren-Larsson syndrome
Skeletal dysplasia
Smith–Fineman–Myers syndrome
Smith-Lemli-Opitz syndrome
Smith-Magenis syndrome
Sotos syndrome
Spastic cerebral palsy
Spina bifida
Spinal muscular atrophy
Spinocerebellar ataxia
Spondyloepiphyseal dysplasia
Spondyloepiphyseal dysplasia
 congenita
SRY (sex determining region Y)
Stargardt disease
Stickler syndrome
Sturge-Weber syndrome
Sutherland-Haan syndrome

## T

Tangier disease
TAR syndrome
Tay–Sachs disease
Teratogen
Thalassemia
Thalidomide embryopathy
Thanatophoric dysplasia
Thrombasthenia of Glanzmann
 and Naegeli
Tomaculous neuropathy
Tourette syndrome
Treacher Collins syndrome

Trichorhinophalangeal syndrome
Triose phosphate isomerase
 deficiency
Triple X syndrome
Triploidy
Trismus-pseudocamptodactyly
 syndrome
Trisomy 13
Trisomy 18
Trisomy 8 mosaicism syndrome
Tuberous sclerosis complex
Turner syndrome

## U

Urea cycle disorders
Urogenital adysplasia syndrome
Usher Syndrome

## V

Van der Woude syndrome
Vater association
Von Hippel-Lindau syndrome
von Recklinghausen's
 neurofibromatosis
von Willebrand disease

## W

Waardenburg syndrome
Walker-Warburg syndrome

Weaver syndrome
Weissenbacher-Zweymuller
 syndrome
Werner syndrome
Williams syndrome
Wilson disease
Wiskott-Aldrich syndrome
Wolf-Hirschhorn syndrome
Wolman disease

## X

X-linked hydrocephaly
X-linked mental
 retardation
X-linked severe combined
 immunodeficiency
Xeroderma pigmentosum
XX male syndrome
XXXX Syndrome
XXXXX syndrome
XYY syndrome

## Y

YY syndrome

## Z

Zellweger syndrome
Zygote

# PLEASE READ—IMPORTANT INFORMATION

The *Gale Encyclopedia of Genetic Disorders, Third Edition* is a health reference product designed to inform and educate readers about a wide variety of diseases, disorders and conditions, treatments and dignostic tests, as well as other issues associated with genetic disorders. Gale, Cengage Learning believes the product to be comprehensive, but not necessarily definitive. It is intended to supplement, not replace, consultation with a physician or other healthcare practitioners. While Gale, Cengage Learning has made substantial efforts to provide information that is accurate, comprehensive, and up-to-date, Gale, Cengage Learning makes no representations or warranties of any kind, including without limitation, warranties of merchantability or fitness for a particular purpose, nor does it guarantee the accuracy, comprehensiveness, or timeliness of the information contained in this product. Readers should be aware that the universe of medical knowledge is constantly growing and changing, and that differences of opinion exist among authorities. Readers are also advised to seek professional diagnosis and treatment for any medical condition, and to discuss information obtained from this book with their healthcare provider.

# INTRODUCTION

The *Gale Encyclopedia of Genetic Disorders* is a unique and invaluable source for information regarding diseases and conditions of a genetic origin. This collection of nearly 500 entries provides in-depth coverage of disorders ranging from exceedingly rare to very well-known. In addition, several non-disorder entries have been included to facilitate understanding of common genetic concepts and practices such as Chromosomes, Genetic counseling, and Genetic testing.

This encyclopedia avoids medical jargon and uses language that laypersons can understand, while still providing thorough coverage of each disorder medical professionals will find beneficial as well. The *Gale Encyclopedia of Genetic Disorders* fills a gap between basic consumer health resources, such as single-volume family medical guides, and highly technical professional materials.

Each entry discussing a particular disorder follows a standardized format that provides information at a glance. The rubric used includes:

• Definition

• Description

• Genetic profile

• Demographics

• Signs and symptoms

• Diagnosis

• Treatment and management

• Prognosis

• Resources

• Key terms

### Inclusion criteria

A preliminary list of diseases and disorders was compiled from a wide variety of sources, including professional medical guides and textbooks, as well as consumer guides and encyclopedias. The advisory board, made up of medical and genetic experts, evaluated the topics and made suggestions for inclusion. Final selection of topics to include was made by the advisory board in conjunction with Gale, Cengage Learning editors.

### About the contributors

The essays were compiled by experienced medical writers, primarily genetic counselors, physicians, and other health care professionals. The advisors reviewed the completed essays to insure they are appropriate, up-to-date, and medically accurate.

### How to use this book

The *Gale Encyclopedia of Genetic Disorders* has been designed with ready reference in mind.

• Straight **alphabetical arrangement** of topics allows users to locate information quickly.

• **Bold-faced terms** direct the reader to related articles.

• **Cross-references** placed throughout the encyclopedia point readers to where information on subjects without entries may be found.

• A list of **key terms** are provided where appropriate to define unfamiliar terms or concepts. Additional terms may be found in the **glossary** at the back of volume 2.

• The **Resources** section directs readers to additional sources of medical information on a topic.

• Many entries contain "Questions to Ask Your Doctor" sidebars, which enable a patient or caregiver to be armed with questions for their medicial professionals that pertain to the disease or disorder they need to discuss.

• Valuable **contact information** for organizations and support groups is included with each entry. The appendix contains an extensive list of organizations arranged in alphabetical order.

• A comprehensive **general index** guides readers to all topics and persons mentioned in the text.

## Graphics

The *Gale Encyclopedia of Genetic Disorders* contains more than 200 full color illustrations, including photos and pedigree charts. A complete **symbol guide** for the pedigree charts can be found in the appendix.

# ADVISORY BOARD

An advisory board comprised of genetic specialists from a variety of backgrounds provided invaluable assistance in the formulation of this encyclopedia. This advisory board performed a myriad of duties, from defining the scope of coverage to reviewing individual entries for accuracy and accessibility. We would therefore like to express our sincere thanks and appreciation for all of their contributions.

# CONTRIBUTORS

**Christine Adamec**
*Medical Writer*
Palm Bay, FL

**William Adkins**
*Medical Writer*
Pekin, IL

**Margaret Alic, PhD**
*Science Writer*
Eastsound, WA

**Lisa Andres, MS, CGC**
*Certified Genetic Counselor*
*Medical Writer*
San Jose, CA

**Greg Annussek**
*Medical Writer/Editor*
New York, NY

**Sharon Aufox, MS, CGC**
*Genetic Counselor*
Rockford Memorial Hospital
Rockford, IL

**Deepti Babu, MS, CGC**
*Genetic Counselor*
Edmonton, Alberta, Canada

**Kristin Baker Niendorf, MS, CGC**
*Genetic Counselor*
Massachusetts General Hospital
Boston, MA

**Maria Basile, PhD**
*Neuropharmacologist*
Newark, NJ

**Carin Lea Beltz, MS, CGC**
*Genetic Counselor and Program Director*
The Center for Genetic Counseling
Indianapolis, IN

**Abdel Hakim Ben Nasr, PhD**
*Medical Writer Dept. of Genetics*
Yale University School of Medicine
New Haven, CT

**Tanya Bivins, BS**
*Nursing Student*
Madonna University
Livonia, MI

**Bethanne Black**
*Medical Writer*
Atlanta, GA

**Jennifer Bojanowski, MS, CGC**
*Genetic Counselor*
Children's Hospital Oakland
Oakland, CA

**Shelly Q. Bosworth, MS, CGC**
*Genetic Counselor*
Eugene, OR

**Michelle L. Brandt**
*Medical Writer*
San Francisco, CA

**Ray Brogan, PhD**
*Medical Writer*
Falls Church, VA

**Dawn Cardeiro, MS, CGC**
*Genetic Counselor*
Fairfield, PA

**Suzanne M. Carter, MS, CGC**
*Senior Genetic Counselor*
Division of Reproductive Genetics
Montefiore Medical Center
Bronx, NY

**Rhonda Cloos, R.N.**
*Medical Writer*
Austin, TX

**Pamela E. Cohen, MS, CGC**
*Genetic Counselor*
San Francisco, CA

**Randy Colby, MD**
*Senior Medical Genetics Fellow*
Greenwood Genetic Center
Greenwood, SC

**Sonja Eubanks, MS, CGC**
*Genetic Counselor*
Genetic Counseling Program
University of North Carolina at Greensboro
Greensboro, NC

**David B. Everman, MD**
*Clinical Geneticist*
Greenwood Genetic Center
Greenwood, SC

**L. Fleming Fallon, Jr., MD, DrPH**
*Associate Professor of Public Health*
Bowling Green State University
Bowling Green, OH

**Antonio Farina, MD, PhD**
*Medical Writer*
Dept. of Embryology
University of Bologna
Italy

**Kathleen Fergus, MS, CGC**
*Genetic Counselor*
Kaiser Permanente
San Francisco, CA

**Lisa Fratt**
*Medical Writer*
Ashland, WI

**Sallie B. Freeman, PhD**
*Assistant Professor*
Dept. of Genetics Emory University
Atlanta, GA

**Mary E. Freivogel, MS, CGC**
*Genetic Counselor*
Denver, CO

**Rebecca Frey, PhD**
*Consulting Editor*
East Rock Institute
Yale University
New Haven, CT

**Sandra Galeotti, MS**
*Medical Writer*
Sau Paulo, Brazil

**Avis L. Gibons**
*Genetic Counseling Intern*
UCI Medical Center
Orange, CA

**Taria Greenberg, MHS**
*Medical Writer*
Houston, TX

**David E. Greenberg, MD**
*Medicine Resident*
Baylor College of Medicine
Houston, TX

**Benjamin M. Greenberg**
*Medical Student*
Baylor College of Medicine
Houston, TX

**Farris Farid Gulli, MD**
*Plastic and Reconstructive Surgery*
Farmington Hills, MI

**Judy C. Hawkins, MS**
*Certified Genetic Counselor*
Department of Pediatrics
University of Texas Medical Branch
Galveston, TX

**David Helwig**
*Medical Writer*
London, ON, Canada

**Edward J. Hollox, PhD**
*Medical Writer*
Institute of Genetics, Queen's
    Medical Center
University of Nottingham
Nottingham, England

**Katherine S. Hunt, MS**
*Genetic Counselor*
University of New Mexico Health
    Sciences Center
Albuquerque, NM

**Cindy Hunter, MS, CGC**
*Genetic Counselor*
Medical Genetics Department
Indiana University School of Medicine
Indianapolis, IN

**Kevin Hwang, MD**
*Medical Writer*
Morristown, NJ

**Holly A. Ishmael, MS, CGC**
*Genetic Counselor*
The Children's Mercy Hospital
Kansas City, MO

**Dawn A. Jacob, MS**
*Genetic Counselor*
Obstetrix Medical Group of Texas
Fort Worth, TX

**Paul A. Johnson**
*Medical Writer*
San Diego, CA

**Melissa Knopper**
*Medical Writer*
Chicago, IL

**Terri A. Knutel, MS, CGC**
*Genetic Counselor*
Chicago, IL

**Karen Krajewski, MS, CGC**
*Genetic Counselor*
Assistant Professor of Neurology
Wayne State University
Detroit, MI

**Sonya Kunkle**
*Medical Writer*
Baltimore, MD

**Dawn Jacob Laney, MS, CGC**
*Genetic Counselor*
Department of Human Genetics
Emory University
Atlanta, GA

**Renée Laux, MS**
*Certified Genetic Counselor*
Eastern Virginia Medical School
Norfolk, VA

**Marshall Letcher, MA**
*Science Writer*
Vancouver, BC

**Christian L. Lorson, PhD**
*Assistant Professor*
Dept. of Biology

Arizona State University
Tempe, AZ

**Maureen Mahon, BSc, MFS**
*Medical Writer*
Calgary, AB

**Nicole Mallory, MS**
*Medical Student*
Wayne State University
Detroit, MI

**Sajid Merchant, BSc, MS, CGC**
*Genetic Counselor*
Department of Medical Genetics
University of Alberta Hospital
Edmonton, Alberta, Canada

**Leslie Mertz, PhD**
*Medical Writer*
Kalkaska, MI

**Ron C. Michaelis, PhD, FACMG**
*Research Scientist*
Greenwood Genetic Center
Greenwood, SC

**Bilal Nasser, MSc**
*Senior Medical Student*
Universidad Iberoamericana
Santo Domingo, Domincan
    Republic

**Jennifer E. Neil, MS, CGC**
*Genetic Counselor*
Long Island, NY

**David E. Newton, PhD**
*Medical Writer*
Ashland, OR

**Deborah L. Nurmi, MS**
*Public Health Researcher*
Atlanta, GA

**Pamela J. Nutting, MS, CGC**
*Senior Genetic Counselor*
Phoenix Genetics Program
University of Arizona
Phoenix, AZ

**Theresa Odle, ELS**
*Medical Writer*
Albuquerque, NM

**Marianne F. O'Connor, MT
    (ASCP), MPH**
*Medical Writer*
Farmington Hills, MI

**Barbara Pettersen, MS, CGC**
*Genetic Counselor*
Genetic Counseling of Central Oregon
Bend, OR

**Toni Pollin, MS, CGC**
*Research Analyst*
Division of Endocrinology,
    Diabetes, and Nutrition
University of Maryland School
    of Medicine
Baltimore, MD

**Scott J. Polzin, MS, CGC**
*Medical Writer Certified
    Genetics Counselor*
Buffalo Grove, IL

**Nada Quercia, Msc, CCGC, CGC**
*Genetic Counselor*
Division of Clinical
    and Metabolic Genetics
The Hospital for Sick Children
Toronto, ON, Canada

**Cristi Radford, BS(s)**
*Medical Writer
Genetic Counseling Student*
University of South Carolina
Columbia, SC

**Robert Ramirez, BS**
*Medical Student*
University of Medicine &
    Dentistry of New Jersey
Stratford, NJ

**Julianne Remington**
*Medical Writer*
Portland, OR

**Jennifer Roggenbuck, MS, CGC**
*Genetic Counselor*
Hennepin County Medical Center
Minneapolis, MN

**Edward R. Rosick, DO, MPH, MS**
*University Physician/Clinical
    Assistant Professor*
The Pennsylvania State University
University Park, PA

**Judyth Sassoon, ARCS, PhD**
*Medical Writer*
Dept. of Chemistry
    and Biochemistry

University of Bern
Bern, Switzerland

**Jason S. Schliesser, DC**
*Chiropractor*
Holland Chiropractic, Inc.
Holland, OH

**Charles E. Schwartz, PhD**
*Director of Center for Molecular
    Studies*
JC Self Research Center
Greenwood Genetic Center
Greenwood, SC

**Laurie H. Seaver, MD**
*Clinical Geneticist*
Greenwood Genetic Center
Greenwood, SC

**Nina B. Sherak, MS, CHES**
*Health Educator/Medical Writer*
Wilmington, DE

**Judith Sims, MS, Public Health**
*Medical Writer*
Utah Water Research Laboratory
*Research Associate Professor*
Logon, UT

**Genevieve Slomski, PhD**
*Freelance writer/editor*
New Britain, CT

**Java O. Solis, MS**
*Medical Writer*
Decatur, GA

**Amie Stanley, MS**
*Genetic Counselor*
University of Florida
Gainesville, FL

**Constance K. Stein, PhD**
*Director of Cytogenetics*
Assistant Director of Molecular
    Diagnostics
SUNY Upstate Medical University
Syracuse, NY

**Kevin M. Sweet, MS, CGC**
*Cancer Genetic Counselor*
James Cancer Hospital
Ohio State University
Columbus, OH

**Catherine Tesla, MS, CGC**
*Senior Associate, Faculty*
Dept. of Pediatrics, Division
    of Medical Genetics
Emory University School of Medicine
Atlanta, GA

**Oren Traub, MD, PhD**
*Resident Physician*
Dept. of Internal Medicine
University of Washington
    Affiliated Hospitals
Seattle, WA

**Amy Vance, MS, CGC**
*Genetic Counselor*
GeneSage, Inc.
San Francisco, CA

**Brian Veillette, BS**
*Medical Writer*
Auburn Hills, MI

**Chitra Venkatasubramanian,
    MBBS, MD**
*Fellow in Stroke/Neurocritical
    Care*
Stanford Stroke Center
Stanford University
Palo Alto, CA

**Linnea E. Wahl, MS**
*Medical Writer*
Berkeley, CA

**Ken R. Wells**
*Freelance Writer*
Laguna Hills, CA

**Barbara Wexler, MPH**
*Medical Writer*
Portland, OR

**Jennifer F. Wilson, MS**
*Science Writer*
Haddonfield, NJ

**Philip J. Young, PhD**
*Research Fellow*
Dept. of Biology
Arizona State University
Tempe, AZ

**Michael V. Zuck, PhD**
*Medical Writer*
Boulder, CO

# SYMBOL GUIDE FOR PEDIGREE CHARTS

Pedigree charts are visual tools for documenting biological relationships in families and the presence of disorders. Using these charts, medical professionals such as geneticists and genetic counselors can analyze the genetic risk in a family for a particular trait or condition by tracking which individuals have the disorder and determining how it is inherited.

A standard set of symbols has been established for use in creating pedigree charts. Those found within the body of several entries in the encyclopedia follow the symbol guide explained on the next page. The exact style and amount of information presented on the chart varies for each family and depends on the trait or condition under investigation. Typically, only data that is directly related to the disorder being analyzed will be included. For more information, see the "Pedigree analysis" entry in the second volume.

# Symbol Guide for Pedigree Charts

☐ Male

○ Female

■ Affected male

● Affected female

⊡ Carrier male

⊙ Carrier female

⧄ Deceased male

⊘ Deceased female

Male adopted into a family

Female adopted into a family

◇ Gender not specified

⬧P Pregnancy

4 Four males

3 Three females

⊿ Miscarriage

Pregnancy terminated due to affected condition

Elective termination of pregnancy

Female with no children by choice

Female with no children due to medical infertility

Identical twin females

Fraternal twin females

Consanguineous relationship

Relationship no longer exists

? Unknown family history

d.79y    Died at 79 years

dx.41y    Diagnosed at 41 years

Relationship line
Line of descent
Sibship line
Individual line

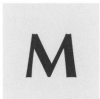

# Machado-Joseph disease

## Definition

Machado-Joseph Disease (MJD), also known as **spinocerebellar ataxia** Type 3 (SCA 3), is a rare hereditary disorder affecting the central nervous system, especially the areas responsible for movement coordination of limbs, facial muscles, and eyes. The disease involves the slow and progressive degeneration of brain areas involved in motor coordination, such as the cerebellar, extrapyramidal, pyramidal, and motor areas. Ultimately, MJD leads to paralysis or a crippling condition, although intellectual functions usually remain normal. Other names of MJD are Portuguese-Azorean disease, Joseph disease, and **Azorean disease**.

## Description

Machado-Joseph disease was first described in 1972 among the descendants of Portuguese-Azorean immigrants to the United States, including the family of William Machado. In spite of differences in symptoms and degrees of neurological degeneration and movement impairment among the affected individuals, it was suggested by investigators that in at least four studied families the same **gene** mutation was present. In early 1976, investigators went to the Azores Archipelago to study an existing neurodegenerative disease in the islands of Flores and São Miguel. In a group of 15 families, they found 40 people with neurological disorders with a variety of different symptoms among the affected individuals.

Another research team in 1976 reported an inherited neurological disorder of the motor system in Portuguese families, which they named Joseph disease. During the same year, the two groups of scientists both published independent evidence suggesting that the same disease was the primary cause for the variety of symptoms observed. When additional reports from other countries and ethnic groups were associated with the same inherited disorder, it was initially thought that Portuguese-Azorean sailors had been the probable disseminators of MJD to other populations around the world during the sixteenth century period of Portuguese colonial explorations and commerce. Presently, MJD is found in Brazil, United States, Portugal, Macau, Finland, Canada, Mexico, Israel, Syria, Turkey, Angola, India, United Kingdom, Australia, Japan, and China. Because MJD continues to be diagnosed in a variety of countries and ethnic groups, there are current doubts about its exclusive Portuguese-Azorean origin.

## Causes and symptoms

The gene responsible for the MJD appears at **chromosome** 14, and the first symptoms usually appear in early adolescence. **Dystonia** (spasticity or involuntary and repetitive movements) or gait ataxia is usually the initial symptom in children. Gait ataxia is characterized by unstable walk and standing, which slowly progresses with the appearance of some of the other symptoms, such as hand dysmetria, involuntary eye movements, loss of hand and superior limbs coordination, and facial dystonia (abnormal muscle tone). Another characteristic of MJD is clinical anticipation, which means that in most families the onset of the disease occurs progressively earlier from one generation to the next. Among members of one same family, some patients may show a predominance of muscle tone disorders, others may present loss of coordination, some may have bulging eyes, and yet another sibling may be free of symptoms during his/her entire life. In the late stages of MJD, some people may experience delirium or **dementia**.

According to the affected brain area, MJD is classified as Type I, with extrapyramidal insufficiency; Type II, with cerebellar, pyramidal, end extrapyramidal insufficiency; and Type III, with cerebellar insufficiency. Extrapyramidal tracts are networks of uncrossed motor nerve fibers that function as relays between the motor

## KEY TERMS

**Autosomal**—Relating to any chromosome besides the X and Y sex chromosomes. Human cells contain 22 pairs of autosomes and one pair of sex chromosomes.

**Cerebellar**—Involving the part of the brain (cerebellum) that controls walking, balance, and coordination.

**Dysarthria**—Slurred speech.

**Dystonia**—Painful involuntary muscle cramps or spasms.

**Extrapyramidal**—Refers to brain structures located outside the pyramidal tracts of the central nervous system.

**Genotype**—The genetic makeup of an organism or a set of organisms.

**Mutation**—A permanent change in the genetic material that may alter a trait or characteristic of an individual, or manifest as disease. This change can be transmitted to offspring.

**Penetrance**—The degree to which individuals possessing a particular genetic mutation express the trait that this mutation causes. One hundred percent penetrance is expected to be observed in truly dominant traits.

**Phenotype**—The physical expression of an individual's genes.

**Spasticity**—Increased mucle tone, or stiffness, which leads to uncontrolled, awkward movements.

**Trinucleotide**—A sequence of three nucleotides.

areas and corresponding areas of the brain. The pyramidal tract consists of groups of crossed nerves located in the white matter of the spinal cord that conduct motor impulses originated in the opposite area of the brain to the arms and legs. Pyramidal tract nerves regulate both voluntary and reflex muscle movements. However, as the disease progresses, both motor systems tracks will eventually suffer degeneration.

### Diagnosis

Diagnosis depends mainly on the clinical history of the family. Genetic screening for the specific mutation that causes MJD can be useful in cases of persons at risk or when the family history is not known or a person has symptoms that raise suspicion of MJD. Initial diagnosis may be difficult, as people present symptoms easily mistaken for other neurological disorders such as Parkinson and Huntington diseases, or even **Multiple sclerosis**.

### Treatment and management

Although there is no cure for Machado-Joseph disease, some symptoms can be relieved, The medication Levodopa or L-dopa often succeeds in lessening muscle rigidity and tremors, and is often given in conjunction with the drug Carbidopa. However, as the disease progresses and the number of neurons decreases, this palliative (given for comfort) treatment becomes less effective. Antispasmodic drugs such as baclofen are also prescribed to reduce spasticity. Dysarthria, or difficulty to speak, and dysphagia, difficulty to swallow, can be treated with proper medication and speech therapy. Physical therapy can help patients with unsteady gait, and walkers and wheelchairs may be needed as the disease progresses. Other symptoms also require palliative treatment, such as muscle cramps, urinary disorders, and sleep problems.

### Clinical Trials

Further basic research is needed before clinical trials become a possibility for MJD. Ongoing genetic and molecular research on the mechanisms involved in the genetic mutations responsible for the disease will eventually yield enough data to provide for future development and design of experimental gene therapies and drugs specific to treat those with MJD.

### Prognosis

The frequency with which such genetic mutations trigger the clinical onset of disease is known as penetrance. Machado-Joseph disease presents a 94.5% penetrance, which means that 94.5% of the mutation carriers will develop the symptoms during their lives, and less than 5% will remain free of symptoms. Because the intensity and range of symptoms are highly variable among the affected individuals, it is difficult to determine the prognosis for a given individual. As MJD progresses slowly, most patients survive until middle age or older.

**Resources**

**BOOKS**

Fenichel, Gerald M. *Clinical Pediatric Neurology: A Signs and Symptoms Approach,* 4th ed. Philadelphia: W. B. Saunders Company, 2001.

**OTHER**

National Institute of Neurological Disorders and Stroke. *Machado-Joseph Disease Fact Sheet.* May 5, 2003.

http://www.ninds.nih.gov/health_and_medical/pubs/
machado-joseph.htm (June 7, 2004).

**ORGANIZATIONS**

International Machado-Joseph Disease Foundation, Inc.
P.O. Box 994268, Redding, CA 96099-4268. Phone:
(530) 246-4722. Email: MJD@ijdf.net. http://
www.ijdf.net.

National Ataxia Foundation (NAF). 2600 Fernbrook Lane
North, Suite 119, Minneapolis, MN 55447-4752.
Phone: (763) 553-0020. Fax: (763) 553-0167. Email:
naf@ ataxia.org. http://www.ataxia.org.

National Organization for Rare Disorders (NORD). P.O.
Box 1968 (55 Kenosia Avenue), Danbury, CT 06813-
1968. Phone: (203) 744-0100. Fax: (203) 798-2291. Toll-
free phone: (800) 999-NORD (6673). Email: orphan@
rarediseases.org. http://www.rarediseases.org.

Dystonia Medical Research Foundation. 1 East Wacker
Drive, Suite 2810, Chicago, IL 60601-1905. Phone:
(312) 755-0198. Fax: (312) 803-0138. Email: dystonia
@dystonia-foundation.org. http://www. dystonia-
foundation.org.

Worldwide Education & Awareness for Movement Disorders (WE MOVE). 204 West 84th Street, New York,
NY 10024. Phone: (212) 875-8312. Fax: (212) 875-8389.
Tollfree phone: (800) 437-MOV2 (6682). Email:
wemove@wemove.org. http://www.wemove.org.

Sandra Author Galeotti

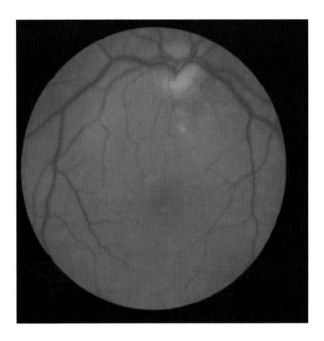

**A retinal photograph showing macular degeneration.**
*(Custom Medical Stock Photo, Inc.)*

# Macular degeneration— age-related

## Definition

Age-related macular degeneration (AMD) is one
of the most common causes of vision loss among
adults over age 55 living in developed countries. It is
caused by the breakdown of the macula, the central
part of the retina located in the back of the eye. The
macula allows people to see objects directly in front of
them (called central vision), as well as fine visual
details. People with AMD usually have blurred central
vision, difficulty seeing details and colors, and they
may notice distortion of straight lines.

## Description

The normal function of the macula and AMD is
best understood accompanying a description of normal eye function. The eye is made up of many layers of
different types of cells that all work together to send
images from the environment to the brain, similar to

the way a camera records images. When light enters the
eye, it passes through the lens and lands on the retina, a
very thin tissue, which lines the inside of the eye. The
retina is made up of 10 different layers of specialized
cells, which allow it to function similarly to film in a
camera, by recording images. The macula is a small,
yellow-pigmented area located in the center of the back
of the eye on the retina. The macula contains blood
vessels and nerve fibers. The retina contains many specialized cells called photoreceptors that sense light coming into the eye, convert light into electrical messages,
and send them to the brain through the optic nerve.
They allow the brain to perceive the environment.

The retina contains two types of photoreceptor
cells: rod and cones. The rods are located primarily
outside of the macula and they allow for peripheral
(side) and night vision. Most of the photoreceptor cells
inside the macula are the cone cells, which are responsible for perceiving color and viewing objects directly
in front of the eye (central vision). If the macula is
diseased, as in AMD, color and central vision are
altered. There are two different types of AMD: dry
AMD and wet AMD.

### Dry AMD

Approximately 90% of individuals with AMD
have the dry form. This condition is sometimes referred
to as nonexudative, atrophic, or drusenoid macular

## KEY TERMS

**Central vision**—The ability to see objects located directly in front of the eye; necessary for reading and other activities that require people to focus on objects directly in front of them.

**Choroid**—A vascular membrane that covers the back of the eye between the retina and the sclera and serves to nourish the retina and absorb scattered light.

**Drusen**—Fatty deposits that can accumulate underneath the retina and macula, and sometimes lead to age-related macular degeneration (AMD). Drusen formation can disrupt the photoreceptor cells, which causes central and color vision problems for people with dry AMD.

**Exudate**—Fluid that accumulates and penetrates the walls of vessels, leaking into the surrounding tissue.

**Genetic heterogeneity**—The occurrence of the same or similar disease, caused by different genes among different families.

**Macula**—A small spot located in the back of the eye that provides central vision and allows people to see colors and fine visual details.

**Multifactorial inheritance**—A type of inheritance pattern where many factors, both genetic and environmental, contribute to the cause.

**Optic nerve**—A bundle of nerve fibers that carries visual messages from the retina in the form of electrical signals to the brain.

**Peripheral vision**—The ability to see objects that are not located directly in front of the eye; allows people to see objects located on the side or edge of their field of vision.

**Photoreceptors**—Specialized cells, rod cells and cone cells, lining the innermost layer of the eye that convert light into electrical messages so that the brain can perceive the environment; rod cells allow for peripheral and night vision, while cone cells are responsible for perceiving color and for central vision.

**Retina**—The light-sensitive layer of tissue in the back of the eye that receives and transmits visual signals to the brain through the optic nerve.

**Visual acuity**—The ability to distinguish details and shapes of objects.

degeneration. In dry AMD, some of the layers of retinal cells (called retinal pigment epithelium, or RPE cells) near the macula begin to degenerate. The RPE is the insulating layer between the retinal and choroid layer, which contains blood vessels. The RPE acts as a protective shield against damaging chemicals and a filter for the nutrients that reach the retina from the choroid blood vessels. The RPE cells normally help remove waste products from the rods and cones. When the RPE cells are no longer able to provide this function, fatty deposits called drusen begin to accumulate, enlarge, and increase in number underneath the macula. The drusen formation can disrupt the cones and rods in the macula, causing them to degenerate, or atrophy (die). This usually leads to central and color vision defects for people with dry AMD. However, some people with drusen deposits have minimal or no vision loss, and require regular eye examinations to check for AMD. Dry AMD is sometimes called nonexudative, because even though fatty drusen deposits form in the eye, people do not have leakage of blood or other fluid (often called exudate) in the eye. Dry AMD symptoms remain stable or worsen slowly from early stages to intermediate or advanced stages of dry AMD. Advanced stages of AMD may result in vision loss. In addition,

approximately 10% of people with dry AMD eventually develop wet AMD, the advanced stage of AMD.

### Wet AMD

Approximately 10% of patients with AMD have wet AMD that progressed from some stage of the dry form. This form of AMD is also called subretinal neovascularization, choroidal neovascularization, exudative form, or disciform degeneration. Wet AMD is caused by leakage of fluid and the formation of abnormal blood vessels (called neovascularization) in the choroid layer of the eye. The choroid is located underneath the retina and the macula, and it normally supplies them with nutrients and oxygen. When new, delicate blood vessels form, blood and fluid can leak from them. The formation of abnormal blood vessels underneath the macula leaks enough fluid to raise the macula up and away from the back of the eye and damages it. This causes central vision loss and distortion as the macula is pushed away from nearby retinal cells. Eventually a scar (called a disciform scar) can develop underneath the macula, resulting in severe and irreversible vision loss. Wet AMD does not have early or intermediate stages. It is considered advanced AMD and is more severe than dry AMD.

## Genetic profile

AMD is considered a complex disorder, caused by a combination of genetic and environmental factors. AMD exhibits **multifactorial inheritance**, and the many factors interact with one another and cause the condition. The aging process is one of the strongest risk factors for developing AMD. There is also genetic heterogeneity among different families with AMD, meaning that different genes can lead to the same or similar disease among different families. Overall, it has been estimated that siblings of individuals with AMD have four times the risk of developing AMD, compared to other individuals.

In 1998, a family in which a unique form of AMD was passed from one generation to the next was discovered. Although most families with AMD do not display an obvious **inheritance** pattern, this particular family's pedigree showed an autosomal dominant form of AMD. Autosomal dominant refers to a specific type of inheritance in which only one allele (one copy of a gene pair) needs to have a mutation for the disease to develop. An affected person with an autosomal dominant condition thus has one allele with a mutation and one allele that functions properly. There is a 50% chance for this individual to pass on the allele with the mutation and a 50% chance to pass on the normal allele to each offspring. **Genetic testing** revealed that the autosomal dominant gene was located on **chromosome** 1q25-q31, in a locus now known as the ARMD1 gene locus. In 2004, possible AMD linkage evidence was discovered in four chromosomal regions: 1q31, 9p13, 10q26, and 17q25. In 1997, mutations in the gene for the retinal ATP-binding cassette transporter, also on chromosome one, were found in individuals diagnosed with AMD. However, it is clear that the retinal ABCR gene is not a major susceptibility gene for AMD.

In March 2005, the National Eye Institute (NEI) described the discovery of a gene for AMD in Caucasians. The genomes from AMD patients were screened by three separate research groups. All three groups discovered a commonly inherited variant of the same gene, called complement factor H (CFH). The CFH gene encodes a protein that regulates inflammation in the portion of the immune system that disposes of diseased and damaged cells. In some individuals with AMD, eye inflammation may trigger a biological process leading to AMD. This variation is in a region of CFH that binds the C-reactive protein involved in inflammation. CFH functions as a brake on the immune system. The variation in CFH found in AMD causes the brake to be defective. The CFH gene is located on chromosome 1q25-31 in the ARMD1 locus that is repeatedly linked to AMD in family-based studies. Individuals with the variant gene have two to seven times the risk of macular degeneration, with the greatest risk in individuals with two copies of the variation. The CFH gene variation may account for a large percentage of risk for AMD, but is not an absolute determinant. Not all individuals with AMD have the CFH variant, and not all those with the variant have AMD. However, there is accumulating evidence that macular degeneration, much like atherosclerosis, is at least partly caused by inflammation.

It is also possible that although one particular gene may be the main cause of susceptibility for AMD, other genes or environmental factors may help alter the age of onset of symptoms or eye defects. Studies have revealed numerous risk factors for AMD, including:

- obesity
- heart disease
- high blood pressure
- cataracts
- farsightedness
- light skin and eye color
- cigarette use
- high fat/high cholesterol diet
- ultraviolet (UV) exposure (sunlight)
- low levels of dietary antioxidant vitamins and minerals
- female gender

The exact amount of risk associated with many of these factors is still undetermined, though studies have consistently found a strong association between AMD and smoking. Risk factors in combination with a family history of AMD place an individual at highest risk.

## Demographics

Among adults aged 55 and older, AMD is the leading cause of vision loss in developed countries. The risk of developing AMD increases with age, and is most commonly seen in adults in the sixth and seventh decade. However, AMD has been reported in adults in the fourth decade. In developed countries, approximately one in 2,000 individuals is affected by AMD. By the age of 75, approximately 15% of people have early or mild forms of AMD, and approximately 7% have an advanced form of AMD. Although AMD occurs in both sexes, it is slightly more common in women.

The number of people affected with AMD is different in regions of the world and between ethnic groups.

AMD is generally considered more common in Caucasians than in African Americans. Studies done in Japanese and other Asian populations have shown an increasing number of affected individuals.

The dry form of AMD is more common than the wet form of AMD. More than 85% of all intermediate and advanced cases of AMD have the dry form. Within the category of advanced AMD about two-thirds of AMD cases are the wet form. Almost all AMD-related vision loss results from advanced AMD, therefore the wet, advanced form of AMD leads to significantly more vision loss than the dry form, which has varying stages of development. Individuals who have advanced AMD in one eye are at very high risk of developing advanced AMD in the other eye.

### Signs and symptoms

AMD causes no pain. In some cases, AMD advances so slowly that affected individuals may not notice much change in their vision. In other cases, the disease progresses fast and may lead to a loss of vision in both eyes. One of the most common signs of early AMD is drusen, which is yellow deposits under the retina, most common in individuals over the age of 60. Drusen can be detected during a comprehensive dilated eye exam. Individuals with early AMD have several small drusen to a few medium-sized drusen. At this stage, there are no other symptoms and no vision loss. Individuals with intermediate AMD have many medium-sized drusen to one or more large drusen. The most common symptom at this stage is a blurred area in the central field of vision. Increased light may be necessary for reading and other tasks. Individuals with advanced AMD have drusen along with a degeneration of light-sensitive cells and supporting tissue in the central retinal area. A blurred spot in the central field of vision gets larger and darker over time. There is difficulty reading and recognizing objects from afar. As the AMD progresses, functional vision may be entirely lost in both eyes. AMD may also cause decreased color vision. Vision loss from dry AMD in only one eye may make it harder to notice changes in overall vision, as the other eye compensates.

While the majority of people with AMD maintain their peripheral vision, the severity of symptoms is dependent on the type of AMD. Wet AMD and advanced dry AMD are associated with the most symptoms. Wet AMD may cause straight lines to have a wavy appearance. The degree of change of visual acuity and other symptoms that can be seen by an eye exam increases over time. Individuals with dry AMD usually develop decreased visual acuity very slowly over a period of many years. Detectable changes are small from year to year, and central vision is partially retained.

However, individuals with wet AMD usually have symptoms that precipitate quickly and have a greater risk of developing severe central vision loss in as little as a two-month period. Individuals with dry AMD may suddenly develop wet AMD without undergoing progressive stages of dry AMD.

### Diagnosis

A variety of tests is used to diagnose AMD. The visual acuity test measures the smallest letters an individual can read with one eye on a standardized chart at a distance of 20 ft (6 m). The refraction test involves the same standardized eye chart, but requires the patient to focus through a refraction lens to determine the amount of correction needed for optimum visual acuity. The pupillary reflex test examines the ability of the pupil to constrict or dilate in the presence or absence of bright light. The slit lamp examination is also known as biomicroscopy. A high-intensity light source is focused to shine as a slit on the anterior portion of the eye. The eyes are examined with a microscope designed for the eye called a biomicroscope. The eyes may be temporarily stained with an orange-colored dye called fluorescein to help visualize the structures of the eye. Examination of the posterior portion of the eye involves dilating the pupils with specialized eye drops before examination. Retinal photography can then be performed. Fluorescein angiography, or retinal photography, uses fluorescein dye injected into a vein of the arm and a special camera to analyze and photograph the retina, choroid, and associated blood vessels. This examination can be used to visualize the changes in vasculature associated with wet AMD. Tonometry measures the pressure levels inside the eye. Color testing assesses the functioning of the cone cells in recognizing colors. Standardized pictures made up of dots of different colors are arranged in specific patterns and used to determine color recognition. The Amsler grid test uses a printed paper grid to test for decreased central vision, distorted vision, or blind spots.

Genetic testing for genes associated with AMD is not recommended. The utility of such tests would be minimal at best, because there is no information available on how to interpret test results as applies to an individual's likelihood of developing AMD. Individuals with AMD are encouraged to monitor changes in their own vision through the use of an Amsler grid.

### Treatment and management

There is no universal cure for either type of AMD. Some individuals with wet AMD can prevent further progression of damage with laser photocoagulation therapy. Light rays are focused by a thermal laser to burn off abnormal blood vessels forming beneath the macula, preventing further leakage of blood and fluid. Some normal tissue is also affected. Previously lost vision is not restored with this treatment. Only a small percentage of wet AMD cases can be treated with laser surgery. Laser surgery is most effective if the abnormal blood vessels have developed away from the fovea, the central part of the macula. Laser photocoagulation treatments do not prevent future abnormal blood vessels from forming, and are not effective for dry AMD. In 2000, the FDA approved the use of a light-activated drug called Visudyne (verteporfin). Visudyne is injected into the bloodstream via a vein in the arm. It circulates through the body to the eyes, specifically attaching to the abnormal AMD blood vessels present under the macula. When light rays from a non-thermal laser hit these blood vessels, the Visudyne is activated to produce a chemical reaction that destroys the abnormal vessels, causing very little damage to nearby healthy tissues. If the abnormal blood vessels regrow, the procedure is repeated. While this therapy does not cure AMD, it is useful in managing specific problem areas and reducing further vision loss.

There is no specific treatment for dry macular degeneration; laser therapy is not useful. Once dry AMD reaches the advanced stage, no form of treatment can prevent vision loss. The National Eye Institute's Age-Related Eye Disease Study (AREDS) reported that taking a high-dose antioxidant and zinc supplement significantly reduced the risk of advanced AMD and vision loss. The specific daily quantities reported were 500 mg vitamin C, 400 I.U. vitamin E, 15 mg beta-carotene (equivalent to 25,000 I.U. vitamin A), and 80 mg zinc oxide. Two milligrams of copper in the form of cupric oxide was added to the formulation to prevent a condition called copper deficiency anemia, associated with high levels of zinc intake. Supplementation is indicated in individuals with intermediate AMD in one or both eyes, or advanced AMD in one, but not the other eye. The AREDS reported that supplementation did not keep individuals with early AMD from progressing to an intermediate stage.

In December 2004, the FDA approved Macugen drug treatment. This treatment attacks a growth factor protein involved in abnormal blood vessel growth in the eye. Macugen was developed by Eyetech Pharmaceuticals and Pfizer, and is administered through injections directly into the eye every six weeks. In previous clinical trials with Macugen, some patients experienced slower rates of vision loss, or restored vision. There are other drugs currently in clinical trials that have not yet been approved by the FDA. Avastin has a mechanism of action similar to Macugen, but is administered by intravenous injection into a vein in the arm. In 2005, Avastin had FDA approval for treatment of colorectal **cancer**, but not for macular degeneration. The FDA has issued a caution that Avastin has been shown to increase the risk of stroke and heart attack. Another drug in clinical trials is Retaane, which attacks enzymes involved in abnormal blood vessel growth. Retaane would not be administered with a needle and treatments would be every six months. In October 2000, it was reported that a medication called Iloprost, over a six-month time period, caused improvements in visual acuity, daily living activities, and overall quality of life for individuals with dry AMD. Follow-up research is being done to investigate the safety and usefulness of these medications.

Multiple future therapies are being investigated. Radiation treatment to destroy abnormal blood vessels and implantable telescopes to improve vision are being tested. Japan developed a method of blood filtration called rheopheresis to remove harmful proteins and fatty acids to treat the dry form of AMD. This technique has not been approved by the FDA in the United States, but is being used in Canada and Europe.

Low-vision devices are available to help improve AMD vision difficulties by using magnifying lenses and bright lights. Some low-vision aids shift images to the periphery for clearer vision. There are many different types of low-vision devices that can help to overcome vision impairment and live independently.

### Prognosis

Most individuals with mild dry macular degeneration never develop disabling central vision loss. However, there is no current method of predicting which individuals will progress to an advanced stage of AMD. AMD can cause the loss of central vision only and cannot cause peripheral vision loss. Loss of central vision may interfere with many activities of daily life and significantly impact its quality. An individual with advanced AMD may become functionally blind, so that reading, driving, recognizing faces, and many other common activities become impossible. The prognosis depends on the stage of the disease and type. Mild forms of dry AMD have a better prognosis than advanced dry or wet AMD. As symptoms progress, individuals with AMD become at higher risk for psychological distress due to decreasing quality of life and independence. The prognosis improves if low-vision devices and support groups are utilized to improve the quality of life.

## Resources

### BOOKS

D'Amato, Robert, and Joan Snyder. *Macular Degeneration: The Latest Scientific Discoveries and Treatments for Preserving Your Sight.* New York: Walker & Co., 2000.

Solomon, Yale, and Jonathan D. Solomon. *Overcoming Macular Degeneration: A Guide to Seeing Beyond the Clouds.* New York: Morrow/Avon, 2000.

### PERIODICALS

Bressler, Neil M., and James P. Gills. "Age-related Macular Degeneration." *British Medical Journal* 321, no. 7274 (December 2000): 1425–1427.

Fong, Donald S. "Age-Related Macular Degeneration: Update for Primary Care." *American Family Physician* 61, no. 10 (May 2000): 3035–3042.

"Macular Degeneration." *Harvard Women's Health Watch* 6, no. 2 (October 1998): 2–3.

"Researchers Set Sights on Vision Disease." *Harvard Health Letter* 23, no.10 (August 1998):4–5.

"Self-test for Macular Degeneration." *Consumer Reports on Health* 12, no.12 (December 2000): 2.

### WEBSITES

*Medline.* (April 6, 2005.) http://www.nlm.nih.gov/medline plus.gov/.

*National Eye Institute AMD.* (April 6, 2005.) http://www. nei.nih.gov/health/maculardegen/armd_facts.asp#1.

*National Eye Institute News and Events.* (April 6, 2005.) http://www.nei.nih.gov/news/statements/genes_amd. asp.

*Recent Research and Publications AMD.* (April 6, 2005.) http://www.chg.mc.duke.edu/research/amdx.html.

### ORGANIZATIONS

AMD Alliance International. PO Box 550385, Atlanta, GA 30355. (877) 263-7171. http://www. amdalliance.org.

American Macular Degeneration Foundation. PO Box 515, Northampton, MA 01061-0515. (413) 268-7660. http:// www.macular.org.

Foundation Fighting Blindness. 11435 Cronhill Dr., Owings Mills, MD 21117. (410) 568-0150. http://www. blindness.org.

Macular Degeneration Foundation. PO Box 531313, Henderson, NV 89053. (888) 633-3937. http://www. eyesight.org.

Retina International. Ausstellungsstrasse 36, Zürich, CH-8005. Switzerland (+41 1 444 10 77). http:// www.retina-international.org.

Maria Basile, PhD
Pamela J. Nutting, MS, CGC

Madelung deformity *see* **Leri-Weill dyschondrosteosis**

Maffuci disease *see* **Chondrosarcoma**

# Major histocompatibility complex

## Definition

In humans, the proteins coded by the genes of the major histocompatibility complex (MHC) include human leukocyte antigens (HLA), as well as other proteins. HLA proteins are present on the surface of most of the body's cells and are important in helping the immune system distinguish "self" from "non-self."

## Description

The function and importance of MHC is best understood in the context of a basic understanding of the function of the immune system. The immune system is responsible for distinguishing "self" from "non-self," primarily with the goal of eliminating foreign organisms and other invaders that can result in disease. There are several levels of defense characterized by the various stages and types of immune response.

### Natural immunity

When a foreign organism enters the body, it is encountered by the components of the body's natural immunity. Natural immunity is the non-specific first-line of defense carried out by phagocytes, natural killer cells, and components of the complement system. Phagocytes are specialized white blood cells

### HLA disease associations

| Disease | MHC allele | Approximate relative risk |
|---|---|---|
| Ankylosing spondylitis | B27 | 77–90 |
| Celiac disease | DR3 1 DR7 | 5–10 |
| Diabetes, Type 1 | DR3 | 5 |
| Diabetes, Type 1 | DR4 | 5–7 |
| Diabetes, Type 1 | DR3 1 DR4 | 20–40 |
| Graves disease | DR3 | 5 |
| Hemochromatosis | A3 | 6–20 |
| Lupus | DR3 | 1–3 |
| Multiple sclerosis | DR2 | 2–4 |
| Myasthenia gravis | B8 | 2.5–4 |
| Psoriasis vulgaris | Cw6 | 8 |
| Rheumatoid arthritis | DR4 | 3–6 |

The relative risks indicated in this table refer to the increased chance of a patient with an MCH allele to develop a disorder as compared to an individual without one. For example, a patient with DR4 is three to six times more likely to have rheumatoid arthritis and five to seven times more likely to develop type 1 diabetes than an individual without the DR4 allele.

*(Table by GGS Creative Resources. Reproduced by permission of Gale, a part of Cengage Learning.)*

capable of engulfing and killing an organism. Natural killer cells are also specialized white blood cells that respond to **cancer** cells and certain viral infections. The complement system is a group of proteins called the class III MHC that attack antigens. Antigens consist of any molecule capable of triggering an immune response. Although this list is not exhaustive, antigens can be derived from toxins, protein, carbohydrates, **DNA**, or other molecules from viruses, bacteria, cellular parasites, or cancer cells.

### Acquired immunity

The natural immune response holds an infection at bay as the next line of defense mobilizes through acquired, or specific immunity. This specialized type of immunity is usually needed to eliminate an infection and is dependent on the role of the proteins of the major histocompatibility complex. There are two types of acquired immunity. Humoral immunity is important in fighting infections outside the body's cells, such as those caused by bacteria and certain viruses. Other types of viruses and parasites that invade the cells are better fought by cellular immunity. The major players in acquired immunity are the antigen-presenting cells (APCs), B-cells, their secreted antibodies, and the T-cells.

### Humoral immunity

In humoral immunity, antigen-presenting cells, including some B-cells, engulf and break down foreign organisms. Antigens from these foreign organisms are then brought to the outside surface of the antigen-presenting cells and presented in conjunction with class II MHC proteins. The helper T-cells recognize the antigen presented in this way and release cytokines, proteins that signal B-cells to take further action. B-cells are specialized white blood cells that mature in the bone marrow. Through the process of maturation, each B-cell develops the ability to recognize and respond to a specific antigen. Helper T-cells aid in stimulating the few B-cells that can recognize a particular foreign antigen. B-cells that are stimulated in this way develop into plasma cells, which secrete antibodies specific to the recognized antigen. Antibodies are proteins that are present in the circulation, as well as being bound to the surface of B-cells. They can destroy the foreign organism from which the antigen came. Destruction occurs either directly, or by "tagging" the organism, which is then more easily recognized and targeted by phagocytes and complement proteins. Some of the stimulated B-cells go on to become memory cells, which are able to mount an even faster response if the antigen is encountered a second time.

### Cellular immunity

Another type of acquired immunity involves killer T-cells and is termed celluar immunity. T-cells go through a process of maturation in the organ called the thymus, in which T-cells that recognize "self" antigens are eliminated. Each remaining T-cell has the ability to recognize a single, specific, "non-self" antigen that the body may encounter. Although the names are similar, killer T-cells are unlike the non-specific natural killer cells in that they are specific in their action. Some viruses and parasites quickly invade the body's cells, where they are "hidden" from antibodies. Small pieces of proteins from these invading viruses or parasites are presented on the surface of infected cells in conjunction with class I MHC proteins, which are present on the surface of most all of the body's cells. Killer T-cells can recognize antigen bound to class I MHC in this way, and they are prompted to release chemicals that act directly to kill the infected cell. There is also a role for helper T-cells and antigen-presenting cells in cellular immunity. Helper T-cells release cytokines, as in the humoral response, and the cytokines stimulate killer T-cells to multiply. Antigen-presenting cells carry foreign antigen to places in the body where additional killer T-cells can be alerted and recruited.

The major histocompatibility complex clearly performs an important role in functioning of the immune system. Related to this role in disease immunity, MHC is also important in organ and tissue transplantation, as well as playing a role in susceptibility to certain diseases. HLA typing can provide important information in parentage, forensic, and anthropologic studies.

## Genetic profile

Present on **chromosome** 6, the major histocompatibility complex consists of more than 70 genes, classified into class I, II, and III MHC. There are multiple alleles, or forms, of each HLA gene. These alleles are expressed as proteins on the surface of various cells in a co-dominant manner. This diversity is important in maintaining an effective system of specific immunity. Altogether, the MHC genes span a region that is four million base pairs in length. Although this is a large region, 99% of the time these closely-linked genes are transmitted to the next generation as a unit of MHC alleles on each chromosome 6. This unit is called a haplotype.

**Acquired immunity**—Also called specific immunity, refers to immune reaction mediated by B-cells and/or T-cells. Includes humoral and cellular immunity.

**Allele**—One of two or more alternate forms of a gene.

**Antibody**—A protein produced by the mature B cells of the immune system that attach to invading microorganisms and target them for destruction by other immune system cells.

**Antigen**—A substance or organism that is foreign to the body and stimulates a response from the immune system.

**Antigen presenting cell**—Cells that are able to present foreign antigen in conjunction with MHC proteins to the immune system.

**Autoimmune**—Referring to an immune reaction erroneously directed toward "self" tissues.

**Bcell**—Specialized type of white blood cell that is capable of secreting infection-fighting antibodies.

**Base pairs**—Building blocks of DNA, the chemical that genes are made of.

**Beta-2 microglobulin**—A component protein of class I MHC.

**Bone marrow**—A spongy tissue located in the hollow centers of certain bones, such as the skull and hip bones. Bone marrow is the site of blood cell generation.

**Cellular immunity**—A type of acquired immunity mediated by killer T-cells; important in fighting "hidden" infections, such as those caused by cellular parasites and some viruses.

**Class I MHC**—Includes HLA-A, HLA-B, and HLA-C. Important in cellular immunity.

**Class II MHC**—HLA-DP, HLA-DQ, and HLA-DR. Important in humoral immunity.

**Class III MHC**—Includes the complement system.

**Co-dominant**—Describes the state when two alleles of the same gene are both expressed when inherited together.

**Complement system**—Class III MHC (major histocompatibility complex) proteins capable of destroying invading organisms directly via natural immunity, as well as indirectly through an interaction with other components of the immune system.

### Class I

Class I MHC genes include HLA-A, HLA-B, and HLA-C. Class I MHC are expressed on the surface of almost all cells. They are important for displaying antigen from viruses or parasites to killer T-cells in cellular immunity. Class I MHC is particularly important in organ and tissue rejection following transplantation. In addition to the portion of class I MHC coded by the genes on chromosome 6, each class I MHC protein also contains a small, non-variable protein component called beta-2 microglobulin coded by a gene on chromosome 15. Class I HLA genes are highly polymorphic, meaning there are multiple forms, or alleles, of each gene. There are at least 57 HLA-A alleles, 111 HLA-B alleles, and 34 HLA-C alleles.

### Class II

Class II MHC genes include HLA-DP, HLA-DQ, and HLA-DR. Class II MHC are particularly important in humoral immunity. They present foreign antigen to helper T-cells, which stimulate B-cells to elicit an antibody response. Class II MHC is only present on antigen presenting cells, including phagocytes and B-cells. Like class I MHC, there are hundreds of alleles that make up the class II HLA **gene pool**.

### Class III

Class III MHC genes include the complement system (i.e., C2, C4a, C4b, Bf). Complement proteins help to activate and maintain the inflammatory process of an immune response.

### Demographics

There is significant variability of the frequencies of HLA alleles among ethnic groups. This is reflected in anthropologic studies attempting to use HLA-types to determine patterns of migration and evolutionary relationships of peoples of various ethnicity. Ethnic variation is also reflected in studies of HLA-associated diseases. Generally speaking, populations that have been subject to significant patterns of migration and assimilation with other populations tend to have a more diverse HLA gene pool. For example, it is unlikely that two unrelated individuals of African ancestry would have matched HLA types. Conversely,

**Cytokines**—Proteins released by helper T-cells stimulate and support immune responses mediated by B-cells and killer T-cells.

**Graft-versus-host disease**—In bone marrow transplantation, the complication that occurs when the donor's cells attack the recipient's tissues, in part due to non-identical donor-recipient HLA types.

**Haplotype**—A set of alleles that are inherited together as a unit on a single chromosome because of their close proximity.

**Helper T-cell**—Specialized white blood cell that assists in humoral and cellular immunity.

**Human leukocyte antigens (HLA)**—Proteins that help the immune system function, in part by helping it to distinguish "self" from "non-self."

**Humoral immunity**—A type of acquired immunity mediated by B-cells and their secreted antibodies; important in fighting bacterial and some viral infections.

**Major histocompatibility complex (MHC)**—Includes HLA, as well as other components of the immune system. Helps the immune system function, in part by helping it to distinguish "self" from "non-self."

**Memory cells**—B-cells whose antibodies recognized antigens from a previous infection; able to mount a quick, efficient response upon a second infection by the same organism.

**Naturalimmunity**—First line immune response that is non-specific. Includes action of phagocytes, natural killer cells, and complement cells.

**Natural killer cells**—Specialized white blood cells involved in natural immunity. Can kill some viruses and cancer cells.

**Phagocyte**—White blood cells capable of engulfing and destroying foreign antigen or organisms in the fluids of the body.

**Plasma cells**—Antibody-secreting B-cells.

**Polymorphic**—Describes a gene for which there exist multiple forms, or alleles.

**Thymus gland**—An endocrine gland located in the front of the neck that houses and transports T cells, which help to fight infection.

populations that have been isolated due to geography, cultural practices, and other historical influences may display a less diverse pool of HLA types, making it more likely for two unrelated individuals to be HLA-matched.

### Testing

#### Organ and tissue transplantation

There is a role for HLA typing of individuals in various settings. Most commonly, HLA typing is used to establish if an organ or tissue donor is appropriately matched to the recipient for key HLA types, so as not to elicit a rejection reaction in which the recipient's immune system attacks the donor tissue. In the special case of bone marrow transplantation, the risk is for graft-versus-host disease (GVHD), as opposed to tissue rejection. Because the bone marrow contains the cells of the immune system, the recipient effectively receives the donor's immune system. If the donor immune system recognizes the recipient's tissues as foreign, it may begin to attack, causing the inflammation and other complications of GVHD. As advances

occur in transplantation medicine, HLA typing for transplantation occurs with increasing frequency and in various settings.

#### Disease susceptibility

There is an established relationship between the **inheritance** of certain HLA types and susceptibility to specific diseases. Most commonly, these are diseases that are thought to be autoimmune in nature. Autoimmune diseases are those characterized by inflammatory reactions that occur as a result of the immune system mistakenly attacking "self" tissues. The basis of the HLA association is not well understood, although there are some hypotheses. Most autoimmune diseases are characterized by the expression of class II MHC on cells of the body that do not normally express these proteins. This may confuse the killer T-cells, which respond inappropriately by attacking these cells. Molecular mimicry is another hypothesis. Certain HLA types may look like antigen from foreign organisms. If an individual is infected by such a foreign virus or bacteria, the immune system mounts a response against the invader. However, there may be a cross-reaction with cells displaying the HLA type that is mistaken for foreign antigen. Whatever the underlying mechanism, certain HLA-types are known factors that increase the relative risk for developing specific autoimmune diseases. For example, individuals who carry the HLA B-27 allele have a relative risk of 77–90 for developing ankylosing spondylitis—meaning such an individual has a 77–90-fold chance of developing this form of spinal and pelvic arthritis, as compared to someone in the general population.

In addition to autoimmune disease, HLA-type less commonly plays a role in susceptibility to other diseases, including cancer, certain infectious diseases, and metabolic diseases. Conversely, some HLA-types confer a protective advantage for certain types of infectious disease. In addition, there are rare immune deficiency diseases that result from inherited mutations of the genes of components of the major histocompatibility complex.

### Parentage

Among other tests, HLA typing can sometimes be used to determine parentage, most commonly paternity, of a child. This type of testing is not generally done for medical reasons, but rather for social or legal reasons.

### Forensics

HLA-typing can provide valuable DNA-based evidence contributing to the determination of identity in criminal cases. This technology has been used in domestic criminal trials. Additionally, it is a technology that has been applied internationally in the human-rights arena. For example, HLA-typing had an application in Argentina following a military dictatorship that ended in 1983. The period under the dictatorship was marked by the murder and disappearance of thousands who were known or suspected of opposing the regime's practices. Children of the disappeared were often "adopted" by military officials and others. HLA-typing was one tool used to determine non-parentage and return children to their biological families.

### Anthropologic studies

HLA-typing has proved to be an invaluable tool in the study of the evolutionary origins of human populations. This information, in turn, contributes to an understanding of cultural and linguistic relationships and practices among and within various ethnic groups.

## Resources

### BOOKS

Abbas, A. K., et al. Cellular and Molecular Immunology. Philadelphia: W. B. Saunders, 1991.

Doherty, D. G., and G. T. Nepom. "The human major histocompatibility complex and disease susceptibility." In Emery and Rimoin's Principles and Practice of Medical Genetics. 3rd ed. Ed. D. L. Rimoin, J. M. Connor, and R. E. Pyeritz, 479–504. New York: Churchill Livingston, 1997.

Jorde L. B., et al. "Immunogenetics." In Medical Genetics. 2nd ed. St. Louis: Moseby, 1999.

### PERIODICALS

Diamond, J. M. "Abducted orphans identified by grand-paternity testing." Nature 327 (1987): 552–53.

Svejgaard, A., et al. "Associations between HLA and disease with notes on additional associations between a 'new' immunogenetic marker and rheumatoid arthritis." HLA and Disease—The Molecular Basis. Alfred Benzon Symposium. 40 (1997): 301–13.

Trachtenberg, E. A., and H. A. Erlich. "DNA-based HLA typing for cord blood stem cell transplantation." Journal of Hematotherapy 5 (1996): 295–300.

### WEBSITES

"Biology of the immune system." The Merck Manual. http://www.merck.com/mmhe/index.html.

Jennifer Denise Bojanowski, MS, CGC

Male turner syndrome *see* **Noonan syndrome**

Malignant fever *see* **Malignant hyperthermia**

Malignant hyperpyrexia *see* **Malignant hyperthermia**

# ▌Malignant hyperthermia

## Definition

Malignant hyperthermia (MH) is a condition that causes a number of physical changes to occur among genetically susceptible individuals when they are exposed to a particular muscle relaxant or certain types of medications used for anesthesia. The changes may include increased rate of breathing, increased heart rate, muscle stiffness, and significantly increased body temperature (i.e., hyperthermia). Although MH can usually be treated successfully, it sometimes leads to long-term physical illness or death. Research has identified a number of genetic regions that may be linked to an increased MH susceptibility.

## Description

Unusual response to anesthesia was first reported in a medical journal during the early 1960s, when physicians described a young man in need of urgent surgery for a serious injury. He was very nervous about exposure to anesthesia, since he had 10 close relatives who died during or just after surgeries that required anesthesia. The patient himself became very ill and developed a high temperature after he was given anesthesia. During the next decade, more cases of similar reactions to anesthesia were reported, and specialists began using the term *malignant hyperthermia* to describe the newly recognized condition. The word hyperthermia was used because people with this condition often develop a very high body temperature rapidly. The word malignant referred to the fact that the majority (70–80%) of affected individuals died. The high death rate in the 1960s occurred because the underlying cause of the condition was not understood, nor was there any known treatment (other than basically trying to cool the person's body with ice).

Increased awareness of malignant hyperthermia and scientific research during the following decades improved medical professionals' knowledge about what causes the condition, how it affects people, and how it should be treated. MH can be thought of as a chain reaction that is triggered when a person with MH susceptibility is exposed to specific drugs commonly used for anesthesia and muscle relaxation.

Triggering drugs that may lead to malignant hyperthermia include:

- halothane
- enflurane
- isoflurane
- sevoflurane
- desflurane
- methoxyflurane
- ether
- succinylcholine

Once an MH susceptible person is exposed to one or more of these anesthesia drugs, they can present with a variety of signs. One of the first clues that a person is susceptible to MH is often seen when they are given a muscle relaxant called succinyl choline. This drug generally causes some stiffness in the masseter (jaw) muscles in most people. However, individuals with MH susceptibility can develop a much more severe form of jaw stiffness called *masseter spasm* when they receive this drug. They may develop muscle stiffness in other parts of their bodies as well. When exposed to any of the trigger drugs (inhalants for anesthesia), people with MH susceptibility can develop an increased rate of metabolism in the cells of their body, resulting in rapid breathing, rapid heartbeat, high body temperature (over 110°F), muscle stiffness, and muscle breakdown. If these signs are not recognized, treated, or able to be controlled, brain damage or death can occur due to internal bleeding, heart failure, or failure of other organs.

The series of events that occur after exposure to trigger drugs is activated by an abnormally high amount of calcium inside muscle cells. This is due to changes in the chemical reactions that control muscle contraction and the production of energy. Calcium is normally stored in an area called the sarcoplasmic reticulum, which is a system of tiny tubes located inside muscle cells. This system of tubes allows muscles to contract (by releasing calcium) and to relax (by storing calcium) in muscle cells. Calcium also plays an important role in the production of energy inside cells (i.e. metabolism). There are at least three important proteins located in (or nearby) the sarcoplasmic reticulum that control how much calcium is released into muscle cells and thus help muscles contract. One of these proteins is a calcium release channel protein that has been named the *ryanodine receptor protein*, or RYR. This protein (as well as the **gene** that tells the body how to make it) has been an important area of research. For some reason, when people with MH susceptibility are exposed to a trigger drug, they can develop very high levels of calcium in their muscle cells. The trigger drugs presumably stimulate the proteins that control the release of calcium, causing them to create very high levels of calcium in muscle cells. This abnormally high calcium level then leads to increased metabolism, muscle stiffness, and the other symptoms of MH.

The amount of time that passes between the exposure to trigger drugs and the appearance of the first symptoms of MH varies between different people. Symptoms begin within 10 minutes for some individuals, although several hours may pass before symptoms appear in others. This means that some people do not show signs of MH until they have left the operating room and are recovering from surgery. In addition, some individuals who inherit MH susceptibility may be exposed to trigger drugs numerous times during multiple surgeries without any complications. However, they still have an increased risk to develop an MH episode during future exposures. This means that people who have an increased risk for MH susceptibility due to their family history cannot presume they are not at risk simply because they previously had successful surgeries. Although MH was frequently a fatal condition in the past, a drug called dantrolene sodium became available in 1979, which greatly decreased the rate of both death and disability.

### Genetic profile

Susceptibility to MH is generally considered to be inherited as an autosomal dominant trait. "Autosomal" means that males and females are equally likely to be affected. "Dominant" refers to a specific type of **inheritance** in which only one copy of a person's gene pair needs to be changed in order for the susceptibility to be present. In this situation, an individual susceptible to MH receives a changed copy of the same gene from one parent (who is also susceptible to MH). This means that a person with MH susceptibility has one copy of the changed gene and one copy of the gene that works well. The chance that a parent with MH susceptibility will have a child who is also susceptible is 50% for each pregnancy. The same parent would also have a 50% chance to have a non-susceptible child with each pregnancy.

It is not unusual for people to not know they inherited a genetic change that causes MH susceptibility. This is because they typically do not show symptoms unless they are exposed to a specific muscle relaxant or certain anesthetics, which may not be needed by every person during his or her lifetime. In addition, people who inherit MH susceptibility do not always develop a reaction to trigger drugs, which means their susceptibility may not be recognized even if they do have one or more surgeries. Once MH susceptibility is diagnosed in an individual, however, it is important for his or her family members to know they too have a risk for MH susceptibility, since it is a dominant condition. This means that anyone with a family member who has MH susceptibility should tell their doctor about their family history. Since MH may go unrecognized, it is important that anyone who has had a close relative die from anesthesia notify the anesthesiologist before any type of surgery is planned. People with a family history of MH susceptibility may choose to meet with a genetic counselor to discuss the significance of their family history as well. In addition, relatives of an affected person may consider having a test to see if they also inherited MH susceptibility.

Although there are many people who have the same symptoms of MH when exposed to trigger drugs, genetic research has shown that there are probably many genes, located on different chromosomes, that can all lead to MH susceptibility. This indicates that there is genetic heterogeneity among different families with MH susceptibility, meaning that different genes can lead to the same or similar disease among different families. Researchers identified six different types of MH susceptibility. Although specific genes have been discovered for some of these types, others have been linked only to specific chromosomal regions.

Genetic classification of malignant hyperthermia includes:

- MHS1—Located on chromosome 19q13.1. Specific gene called RYR1. Gene creates the RYR protein.
- MHS2—Located on chromosome 17q11.2-24. Suspected gene called SCN4A.
- MHS3—Located on chromosome 7q21-22. Suspected gene called CACNA2DI. Gene creates part of the DHPR protein called the alpha 2/delta subunit.
- MHS4—Located on chromosome 3q13.1. Specific gene and protein unknown.
- MHS5—Located on chromosome 1q32. Specific gene called CACNA1S. Gene creates part of the DHPR protein called the alpha 1 subunit.
- MHS6—Located on chromosome 5p. Specific gene and protein unknown.

Over half of all families with MH susceptibility are believed to have MHS1 (i.e., have changes in the RYR1 gene), while the rest have MHS2, MHS3, MHS4, MHS5, or MHS6. Only about 20% of all families tested have specific genetic changes identified in the RYR1 gene. This is because there are many different types of genetic changes in the gene that can all lead to MH susceptibility, and many families have changes that are unique. As a result, **genetic testing** of the RYR1 gene is complicated, time consuming, and often cannot locate all possible genetic changes. In addition, genetic testing for families may become more complex as knowledge about MH grows. Although MH susceptibility has typically been described as an autosomal dominant trait caused by a single gene that is passed from one generation to the next, MH susceptibility may actually depend upon various genetic changes that occur in more than one gene. Further research may clarify this issue.

While specific genes have been identified for some of the MH susceptibility types (i.e., RYR1 and DHPR alpha 1 subunit), not all changes in these genes lead specifically to MH susceptibility. For example, although at least 20 different genetic changes have been identified in the RYR1 gene that can lead to MH susceptibility, some people who have certain types of these changes actually have a different genetic condition that affects the muscles called **central core disease** (CCD). Infants with this autosomal dominant condition typically have very poor muscle tone (i.e., muscle tension) as well as an increased susceptibility to MH. Among families who have CCD, there are some individuals who do not have the typical muscle changes, but have MH susceptibility instead. Future research may help scientists understand why the same genetic change in the RYR1 gene can cause different symptoms among people belonging to the same family.

## Demographics

The exact number of individuals who are born with a genetic change that causes MH susceptibility is not known. Until genetic research and genetic testing improves, this number will likely remain unclear. It is estimated that internationally one in 50,000 people who are exposed to anesthesia develop an MH reaction. Among children, it is estimated that one in 5,000 to one in 15,000 develop MH symptoms when exposed to anesthesia. MH has been seen in many countries, although there are some geographic areas where it occurs more often in the local populations, including parts of Wisconsin, North Carolina, Austria, and Quebec.

## Signs and symptoms

Although the specific symptoms of malignant hyperthermia can vary, the most common findings include:

- stiffness/spasms of jaw muscles and other muscles
- rapid breathing, causing decreased oxygen and increased carbon dioxide in the blood
- rapid or irregular heartbeat
- high body temperature (over 110°F)
- muscle breakdown (may cause dark or cola-colored urine)
- internal bleeding, kidney failure, brain damage, or death (if not treated successfully)

## Diagnosis

The diagnosis of MH susceptibility can be made before or during a reaction to a triggering drug. Ideally, the diagnosis is made before a susceptible individual is exposed and/or develops a reaction. This is possible for people who learn they have an increased chance for MH because they have a relative with MH susceptibility. Testing these individuals requires a surgical procedure called a muscle biopsy, in which a piece of muscle tissue is removed from the body (usually from the thigh). Safe (i.e., non-triggering) anesthetics are used during the procedure. The muscle is taken to a laboratory and is exposed to halothane (a triggering anesthetic) and caffeine, both of which cause any muscle tissue to contract, or tighten. Thus, the test is called the caffeine halothane contracture test (CHCT). Muscle tissue taken from individuals with MH susceptibility is more sensitive to caffeine and halothane, causing it to contract more strongly than normal muscle tissue from non-susceptible people. This type of test is a very accurate way to predict whether a person has MH susceptibility or not. However, the test does require surgery, time to recover (typically three days), and it is expensive (approximately $2,500US). In the United States, many insurance companies will pay for the testing if it is needed. Although the test is not available in every state or country, there are at least 40 medical centers worldwide that can perform the test.

Unfortunately, not all MH susceptible people will learn from their family histories that they have an increased risk for MH before they are exposed to a trigger drug. For these individuals, the diagnosis of MH susceptibility is often made during surgery by the anesthesiologist (a physician specializing in anesthesia) who is providing the anesthesia medications. Other health care specialists also may notice symptoms of MH during or after surgery. Symptoms such as rapid breathing, rapid heart rate, and high body temperature can usually be detected with various machines or devices that examine basic body functions during surgery. Muscle stiffness of the jaw, arms, legs, stomach and chest may be noticed as well. These symptoms may happen during surgery or even several hours later. If the diagnosis is made during or after surgery, immediate treatment is needed to prevent damage to various parts of the body or death. If a person has a suspicious reaction to anesthesia, he or she may undergo a muscle biopsy to confirm MH susceptibility at a later date.

In spite of the fact that a number of important genes and genetic regions associated with MH susceptibility have been identified, testing a person's **DNA** for all of the possible changes that may cause this condition is not easily done for affected individuals and their families. Existing genetic testing identifies some changes that have been seen among families with MHS1 and MHS6. Research studies may provide information for families with MHS2, MHS3, MHS4, and MHS5 as well. Sometimes the testing requires DNA from only one affected person, but in other cases, many samples are needed from a variety of family members. Until genetic technology improves, the contracture test that is done on muscle tissue will likely remain the "gold standard" for diagnosis of MH susceptibility.

## Treatment and management

The early identification of an MH episode allows for immediate treatment with an antidote called dantrolene sodium. This medication prevents the release of calcium from the sarcoplasmic reticulum, which decreases muscle stiffness and energy production in the cells. If hyperthermia develops, the person's body can be cooled with ice. In addition, the anesthesiologist will change the anesthetic from a trigger drug to a non-trigger drug. Immediate treatment is necessary to prevent serious illness and/or death.

Once a person with definite or suspected MH susceptibility is diagnosed (by an MH episode, muscle biopsy, or family history), prevention of an MH episode is possible. There are many types of non-triggering anesthetic drugs and muscle relaxants that can be used during surgical procedures. The important first step in this process is for people with known or suspected MH susceptibility to talk with their doctors before any surgery, so that only non-triggering drugs are used. People with definite or suspected MH susceptibility should always carry some form of medical identification that describes their diagnosis in case emergency surgery is needed. The Malignant Hyperthermia Association of the United States provides wallet-sized emergency medical ID cards for its members.

## Prognosis

Early diagnosis and treatment of MH episodes with dantrolene sodium has dramatically improved the prognosis for people who develop MH during or just after surgery. When the condition was first recognized in the 1960s, no real treatment (other than cooling the person's body) was available, and only 20–30% of people who developed MH survived. When the antidote (dantrolene sodium) became available in 1979, the survival rate increased to 70–80%. However, 5–10% of people who develop MH after exposure to a trigger drug still may die even with proper medication and care. Among those who do survive, some are disabled due to kidney, muscle or brain damage. The best prognosis exists for people with definite or suspected MH susceptibility who are able to prevent exposures to trigger drugs by discussing their history with their doctors. Improved genetic testing in the future may help identify most or all people with inherited MH susceptibility, so they too may prevent exposures that trigger MH episodes.

## Resources

### BOOKS

Hopkins, Philip M., and F. Richard Ellis, eds. *Hyperthermic and Hypermetabolic Disorders: Exertional Heat Stroke, Malignant Hyperthermia and Related Syndromes.* Port Chester, NY: Cambridge University Press, 1996.

Morio, Michio, Haruhiko Kikuchi, and O. Yuge, eds. *Malignant Hyperthermia: Proceedings of the 3rd International Symposium on Malignant Hyperthermia, 1994.* Secaucus, NJ: Springer-Verlag, 1996.

Ohnishi, S. Tsuyoshi, and Tomoko Ohnishi, eds. *Malignant Hyperthermia: A Genetic Membrane Disease.* Boca Raton, FL: CRC Press, 1994.

### PERIODICALS

Denborough, Michael. "Malignant hyperthermia." *The Lancet* 352, no. 9134 (October 1998): 1131–36.

Hopkins, P. M. "Malignant Hyperthermia: Advances in clinical management and diagnosis." *British Journal of Anesthesia* 85, no. 1 (2000): 118–28.

Jurkat-Rott, Karin, Tommie McCarthy, and Frank Lehmann-Horn. "Genetics and Pathogenesis of Malignant Hyperthermia." *Muscle & Nerve* 23 (January 2000): 4–17.

### WEBSITES

Larach, Marilyn Green, MD, FAAP. "Making anesthesia safer: Unraveling the malignant hyperthermia puzzle." *Federation of American Societies for Experimental Biology (FASEB).* http://www.faseb.org.

"Malignant hyperthermia." *UCLA Department of Anesthesiology.* http://www.anes.ucla.edu/dept/mh.html.

ORGANIZATIONS

Malignant Hyperthermia Association of the United States. PO Box 1069, 11East State St., Sherburne, NY 13460. (607) 674.7901. http://www.mhaus.org.

Pamela J. Nutting, MS, CGC

Manic-depressive psychosis *see* **Bipolar disorder**

# Mannosidosis

## Definition

Mannosidosis is a rare inherited disorder, an inborn error of metabolism, that occurs when the body is unable to break down chains of a certain sugar (mannose) properly. As a result, large amounts of sugar-rich compounds build up in the body cells, tissues, and urine, interfering with normal body functions and development of the skeleton.

## Description

Mannosidosis develops in patients whose genes are unable to make an enzyme required by lysosomes (structures within the cell where proteins, sugars, and fats are broken down and then released back into the cell to make other molecules). Lysosomes need the enzyme to break down, or degrade, long chains of sugars. When the enzyme is missing and the sugar chains are not broken down, the sugars build up in the lysosomes. The lysosomes swell and increase in number, damaging the cell. The result is mannosidosis.

The enzyme has two forms: alpha and beta. Similarly, the disorder mannosidosis has two forms: alpha-mannosidosis (which occurs when the alpha form of the enzyme is missing) and beta-mannosidosis (which occurs when the beta form of the enzyme is missing). Production of each form of the enzyme is controlled by a different **gene**.

First described in 1967, alpha-mannosidosis is classified further into two types. Infantile (or Type I) alpha-mannosidosis is a severe disorder that results in mental retardation, physical deformities, and death in childhood. Adult (or Type II) alpha-mannosidosis is a milder disorder in which mental retardation and physical deformities develop much more slowly throughout the childhood and teenage years.

Beta-mannosidosis was identified nearly 20 years later in 1986. Patients with this form of the disorder

are also mentally retarded but over a wide range of severity, from mild to extreme. Beta-mannosidosis is not well understood, in part because it is such a rare disease. It was discovered only because researchers searched for it: a deficiency of the beta form of the enzyme was known to cause disease in animals.

## Genetic profile

The two forms of mannosidosis, alpha and beta, are caused by changes on two different genes. Mutations in the gene MANB, on **chromosome** 19, result in alpha-mannosidosis. This gene is also known as MAN2B1 or LAMAN. Defects in MANB cause alpha-mannosidosis in both infants and adults.

Beta-mannosidosis is caused by mutations in the gene MANB1 (also called MANBA). This gene is on chromosome 4.

Both genes, MANB and MANB1, are inherited as autosomal recessive traits. This means that if a man and woman each carry one defective gene, then 25% of their children are expected to be born with the disorder. Each gene is inherited separately from the other.

## Demographics

Mannosidosis is a rare disorder, occurring in both men and women. The disorder does not affect any particular ethnic group but rather appears in a broad range of people. Alpha-mannosidosis has been studied in Scandinavian, Western and Eastern European, North American, Arabian, African, and Japanese populations. Researchers have identified beta-mannosidosis in European, Hindu, Turkish, Czechoslovakian, Jamaican-Irish, and African families.

### Signs and symptoms

The various forms and types of mannosidosis all have one symptom in common: mental retardation. Other signs and symptoms vary.

Infants with alpha-mannosidosis appear normal at birth, but by the end of their first year, they show signs of mental retardation, which rapidly gets worse. They develop a group of symptoms that includes dwarfism, shortened fingers, and facial changes. In these children, the bridge of the nose is flat, they have a prominent forehead, their ears are large and low set, they have protruding eyebrows, and the jaw juts out. Other symptoms include lack of muscle coordination, enlarged spleen and liver, recurring infections, and cloudiness in the back of the eyeball, which is normally clear. These patients often have empty bubbles in their white blood cells, a sign that sugars are being stored improperly.

The adult form occurs in 10–15% of the cases of alpha-mannosidosis. The symptoms in adults are the same as in infants, but they are milder and develop more slowly. Patients with adult alpha-mannosidosis are often normal as babies and young children, when they develop mentally and physically as expected. In their childhood or teenage years, however, mental retardation and physical symptoms become evident. These patients may also lose their hearing and have pain in their joints.

Beta-mannosidosis is characterized by symptoms that range from mild to severe. In all patients, however, the most frequent signs are mental retardation, lung infections, and hearing loss with speech difficulties. In mild cases, patients have red, wart-like spots on their skin. In severe cases, patients may have multiple seizures, and their arms and legs may be paralyzed. Because the symptoms of beta-mannosidosis vary so greatly, researchers suggest that the disorder may frequently be misdiagnosed.

### Diagnosis

All types of mannosidosis are tested in the same way. In an infant, child, or adult, doctors can check the patient's urine for abnormal types of sugar. They may also test the patient's blood cells to learn if the enzyme is present.

If doctors suspect that a pregnant woman may be carrying a child with mannosidosis, they can test cells in the fluid surrounding the baby for enzyme activity.

### Treatment and management

There is no known treatment for mannosidosis. The symptoms—mental retardation and skeletal abnormalities—are managed by supportive care, depending on the severity. Patients with adult alpha-mannosidosis and beta-mannosidosis may show mild mental retardation or behavior problems (such as **depression** or aggression) and may be mainstreamed into society. Others may require institutionalization. Skeletal abnormalities may require surgery to correct them, and recurring infections are treated with antibiotics.

Research with animals suggests that mannosidosis can be treated by placing healthy cells without defective genes into the animals' bones (bone marrow transplant). Other researchers have successfully treated mannosidosis in animals by inserting healthy genes into the unborn offspring of a pregnant animal. These treatments have not been proven on humans, however.

### Prognosis

The future for patients with mannosidosis varies with the form of their disorder. For infants with alpha-mannosidosis, death is expected between ages three and 12 years. For infants with beta-mannosidosis, death will come earlier, by the time they are 15 months old.

Patients with mild forms of alpha- and beta-mannosidosis often survive into adulthood, but their lives are complicated by mental retardation and physical deterioration. They will generally die in their early or middle years, depending on the severity of their disorder.

**Resources**

**BOOKS**

Thomas, George. "Disorders of Glycoprotein Degradation: Alpha-Mannosidosis, Beta-Mannosidosis, Fucosidosis, and Sialidosis." *The Metabolic and Molecular Bases of Inherited Disease.* Scriver, Charles R., et al., ed. Vol. II, 8th ed. New York: McGraw-Hill, 2001.

**PERIODICALS**

Alkhayat, Aisha H., et al. "Human Beta-Mannosidase cDNA Characterization and First Identification of a Mutation Associated with Human Beta-Mannosidosis." *Human Molecular Genetics* 7, no. 1 (1998): 75–83.

Berg, Thomas, et al. "Spectrum of Mutations in Alpha-Mannosidosis." *American Journal of Human Genetics* 64 (1999): 77–88.

Michalski, Jean-Claude, and Andre Klein. "Glycoprotein Lysosomal Storage Disorders: Alpha- and Beta-Mannosidosis, Glucosidosis, and Alpha-N-Acetylgalactosaminidase Deficiency." *Biochimica et Biophysica Acta: Molecular Basis of Disease* 1455, no. 2–3 (October 8, 1999): 69–84.

**WEBSITES**

Website for Rare Genetic Diseases in Children: Lysosomal Storage Diseases. http://mcrcr2.med.nyu.edu/murphp01/lysosome/lysosome.htm.

**ORGANIZATIONS**

Arc (a National Organization on Mental Retardation). 1010 Wayne Ave., Suite 650, Silver Spring, MD 20910. (800) 433-5255. http://www.thearc.org.

Children Living with Inherited Metabolic Diseases. Climb Building, 176 Nantwich Rd., Crewe, Cheshire, CWZ 6BG UK 127 025 0221. Fax: 0870-7700-327. http://www.climb.org.uk.

International Society for Mannosidosis and Related Diseases. 2922 Decrford St., Lakewood, CA 90712. (410) 254-4903. http://www.mannosidosis.org.

National MPS Society. p.o. box 14686, Durham, nc 27709-4686. (877) MPS-1001 or (919) 806-0101. info@mps society.org. http://www.mpssociety.org.

Linnea E. Wahl, MS

# Marfan syndrome

## Definition

Marfan syndrome is an inherited disorder of the connective tissue that causes abnormalities of the eyes, cardiovascular system, and musculoskeletal system. It is named for the French pediatrician, Antoine Marfan (1858–1942), who first described it in 1896.

## Demographics

The National Marfan Foundation estimates that about one person in every 5,000 has Marfan syndrome including men and women of all races and ethnic groups. Marfan syndrome is one of the more common inheritable disorders.

## Description

Marfan syndrome is sometimes called arachnodactyly, which means "spider–like fingers" in Greek, since one of the characteristic signs of the disease is disproportionately long fingers and toes. Marfan syndrome affects three major organ systems of the body: the heart and circulatory system, the bones and muscles, and the eyes. The genetic mutation responsible for Marfan was discovered in 1991. It affects the body's production of fibrillin, which is a protein that is an important part of connective tissue. Fibrillin is the primary component of the microfibrils that allow tissues to stretch repeatedly without weakening. Because the patient's fibrillin is abnormal, his or her connective tissues are looser than usual, which weakens or damages the support structures of the entire body.

The most common external signs associated with Marfan syndrome include excessively long arms and legs, with the patient's arm span being greater than his or her height. The fingers and toes may be long and slender, with loose joints that can bend beyond their normal limits. This unusual flexibility is called hypermobility. The patient's face may also be long and narrow, and he or she may have a noticeable curvature of the spine. It is important to note that Marfan patients vary widely in the external signs of their disorder and in their severity; even two patients from the same family may look quite different. Most of the external features of Marfan syndrome become more pronounced as the patient gets older, so that diagnosis of the disorder is often easier in adults than in children. In many cases, the patient may have few or very minor outward signs of the disorder, and the diagnosis may be missed until the patient develops vision problems or cardiac symptoms.

Marfan syndrome by itself does not affect a person's intelligence or ability to learn. There is, however, some clinical evidence that children with Marfan have a slightly higher rate of attention–deficit and hyperactivity disorder (ADHD) than the general population. In addition, a child with undiagnosed nearsightedness related to Marfan may have difficulty seeing the blackboard or reading printed materials, and thus do poorly in school.

### Risk factors

People at highest risk for Marfan syndrome are those who have a family history of the condition. If a person has Marfan syndrome, each of offspring has a 50% chance of having the altered **gene** that causes the condition.

## Causes and symptoms

Marfan syndrome is caused by a single gene for fibrillin on **chromosome** 15, which is inherited in most cases from an affected parent. Between 15% and 25% of cases result from spontaneous mutations. Mutations of the fibrillin gene (FBNI) are unique to each family affected by Marfan, which makes rapid genetic

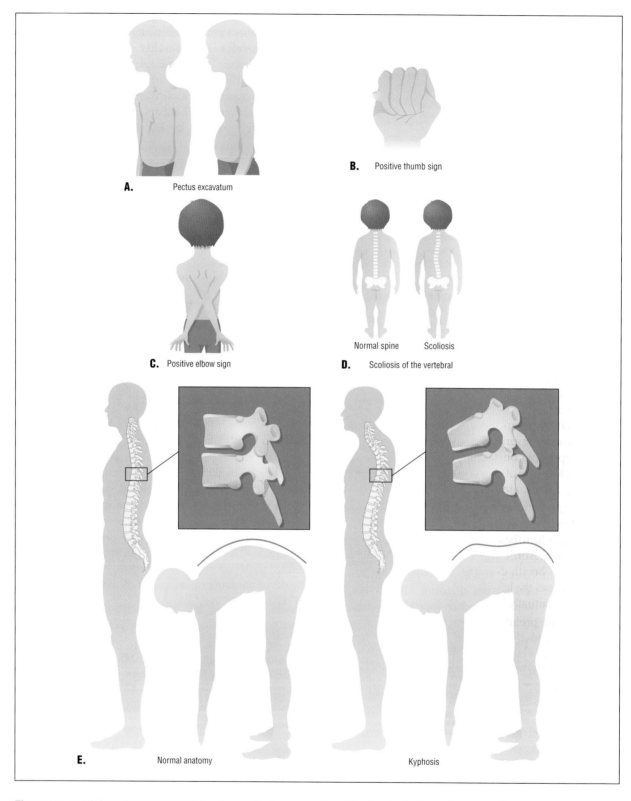

**A.** Pectus excavatum

**B.** Positive thumb sign

**C.** Positive elbow sign

**D.** Scoliosis of the vertebral

Normal spine   Scoliosis

**E.** Normal anatomy

Kyphosis

Five common clinical signs for Marfan syndrome. Pectus excavatum (A) refers to the inward curve of the chest. Positive thumb sign (B) is the appearance of the thumb tip when making a closed fist. Positive elbow sign (C) is the ability to touch one's elbows behind their back. Scoliosis (D) is a marked side-to-side curvature of the spine, and kyphosis (E) is the hunchback form resulting from an outward curvature of the spine. *(Gale, a part of Cengage Learning.)*

diagnosis impossible. The syndrome is an autosomal dominant disorder, which means that someone who has it has a 50% chance of passing it on to any offspring.

Another important genetic characteristic of Marfan syndrome is variable expression. This term means that the mutated fibrillin gene can produce a variety of symptoms of very different degrees of severity, even in members of the same family.

### Cardiac and circulatory abnormalities

The most important complications of Marfan syndrome are those affecting the heart and major blood vessels; some are potentially life–threatening. About 90% of Marfan patients will develop cardiac complications.

- Aortic enlargement. This is the most serious potential complication of Marfan syndrome. Because of the abnormalities of the patient's fibrillin, the walls of the aorta (the large blood vessel that carries blood away from the heart) are weaker than normal and tend to stretch and bulge out of shape. This stretching increases the likelihood of an aortic dissection, which is a tear or separation between the layers of tissue that make up the aorta. An aortic dissection usually causes severe pain in the abdomen, back, or chest, depending on the section of the aorta that is affected. Rupture of the aorta is a medical emergency requiring immediate surgery and medication.
- Aortic regurgitation. A weakened and enlarged aorta may allow some blood to leak back into the heart during each heartbeat; this condition is called aortic regurgitation. Aortic regurgitation occasionally causes shortness of breath during normal activity. In serious cases, it causes the left ventricle of the heart to enlarge and may eventually lead to heart failure.
- Mitral valve prolapse. Between 75% and 85% of patients with Marfan syndrome have loose or "floppy" mitral valves, which are the valves that separate the chambers of the heart. When these valves do not cover the opening between the chambers completely, the condition is called mitral valve prolapse. Complications of mitral valve prolapse include heart murmurs and arrhythmias. In rare cases, mitral valve prolapse can cause sudden death.
- Infective endocarditis. Infective endocarditis is an infection of the endothelium, the tissue that lines the heart. In patients with Marfan syndrome, it is the abnormal mitral valve that is most likely to become infected.
- Other complications. Some patients with Marfan syndrome develop cystic disease of the lungs or recurrent spontaneous pneumothorax, a condition in which air accumulates in the space around the lungs. Many patients eventually develop emphysema.

### Musculoskeletal abnormalities

Marfan syndrome causes an increase in the length of the patient's bones, with decreased support from the ligaments that hold the bones together. As a result, the patient may develop various deformities of the skeleton or disorders related to the relative looseness of the ligaments.

### Disorders of the spine

- Scoliosis. Scoliosis, or curvature of the spine, is a disorder in which the vertebrae that make up the spine twist out of line from side to side into an S–shape or a spiral. It is caused by a combination of the rapid growth of children with Marfan, and the looseness of the ligaments that help the spine to keep its shape.
- Kyphosis is an abnormal outward curvature of the spine, sometimes called hunchback when it occurs in the upper back. Patients with Marfan syndrome may develop kyphosis either in the upper (thoracic) spine or the lower (lumbar) spine.
- Spondylolisthesis. Spondylolisthesis is the medical term for a forward slippage of one vertebra on the one below it. It produces an ache or stiffness in the lower back.
- Dural ectasia. The dura is the tough, fibrous outermost membrane covering the brain and the spinal cord. The weak dura in patients with Marfan syndrome swells or bulges under the pressure of the spinal fluid. This swelling is called ectasia. In most cases, dural ectasia occurs in the lower spine, producing low back ache, a burning feeling, or numbness or weakness in the legs.

### Disorders of the chest and lower body

- Pectus excavatum. Pectus excavatum is a malformation of the chest in which the patient's breastbone, or sternum, is sunken inward. It can cause difficulties in breathing, especially if the heart, spine, and lung have been affected by Marfan. It also usually causes concerns about appearance.
- Pectus carinatum. In other patients with Marfan syndrome the sternum is pushed outward and narrowed. Although pectus carinatum does not cause breathing difficulties, it can cause embarrassment about appearance. A few patients may have a pectus excavatum on one side of their chest and a pectus carinatum on the other.

- Foot disorders. Patients with Marfan syndrome are more likely to develop pes planus (flat feet) or so-called "claw" or "hammer" toes than people in the general population. They are also more likely to have chronic pain in their feet.
- Protrusio acetabulae. The acetabulum is the socket of the hip joint. In patient's with Marfan syndrome, the acetabulum becomes deeper than normal during growth for reasons that are not yet understood. Although protrusio acetabulae does not cause problems during childhood and adolescence, it can lead to a painful form of arthritis in adult life.

### Disorders of the eyes and face

Although the visual problems that are related to Marfan syndrome are rarely life–threatening, they are important in that they may be the patient's first indication of the disorder. Eye disorders related to the syndrome include the following:

- Myopia (nearsightedness). Most patients with Marfan develop nearsightedness, usually in childhood.
- Ectopia lentis. Ectopia lentis is the medical term for dislocation of the lens of the eye. Between 65% and 75% of patients with Marfan syndrome have dislocated lenses. This condition is an important indication for diagnosis of the syndrome because there are relatively few other disorders that produce it.
- Glaucoma. This condition is much more prevalent in patients with Marfan syndrome than in the general population.
- Cataracts. Patients with Marfan are more likely to develop cataracts, and to develop them much earlier in life, sometimes as early as 40 years of age.
- Retinal detachment. Patients with Marfan syndrome are more vulnerable to this disorder because of the weakness of their connective tissues. Untreated retinal detachment can cause blindness. The danger of retinal detachment is an important reason for patients to avoid contact sports or other activities that could cause a blow on the head or being knocked to the ground.
- Other facial problems. Patients with Marfan syndrome sometimes develop dental problems related to crowding of the teeth caused by a high–arched palate and a narrow jaw.

### Other disorders

- Striae. Striae are stretch marks in the skin caused by rapid weight gain or growth; they frequently occur in pregnant women, for example. Patients with Marfan often develop striae over the shoulders, hips, and lower back at an early age because of rapid bone growth. Although the patient may be self–conscious about the striae, they are not a danger to health.
- Obstructive sleep apnea. Obstructive sleep apnea refers to partial obstruction of the airway during sleep, causing irregular breathing and sometimes snoring. In patients with Marfan syndrome, obstructive sleep apnea is caused by the unusual flexibility of the tissues lining the patient's airway. This disturbed breathing pattern increases the risk of aortic dissection.

## Diagnosis

There is no objective diagnostic test for Marfan syndrome, in part because the disorder does not produce any measurable biochemical changes in the patient's blood or body fluids, or cellular changes that could be detected from a tissue sample.

### Examination

The diagnosis is established by taking a family history and a thorough examination of the patient's eyes, heart, and bone structure. The examination includes a slit–lamp eye examination by an ophthalmologist, and a work–up of the patient's spinal column by an orthopedic specialist. The importance of the slit–lamp examination is that it allows the doctor to detect a dislocated lens, which is a significant indication of the syndrome.

### Tests

In terms of the cardiac examination, a standard electrocardiogram (EKG) is not sufficient for diagnosis; only the echocardiogram can detect possible enlargement of the aorta. Other tests include magnetic resonance imaging (MRI) and computed tomography (CT) used to check the heart valves and aorta. These scans also are used to check for dural ectasia, a typical complication of Marfan syndrome.

The symptoms of Marfan syndrome in some patients resemble the symptoms of **homocystinuria**, which is an inherited disorder marked by extremely high levels of homocystine in the patient's blood and urine. This possibility can be excluded by a urine test.

In other cases, the diagnosis remains uncertain because of the mildness of the patient's symptoms, the absence of a family history of the syndrome, and other variables. These borderline conditions are sometimes referred to as marfanoid syndromes.

## Treatment and management

### Traditional

The treatment and management of Marfan syndrome is tailored to the specific symptoms of each patient. Some patients find that the syndrome has little impact on their overall lifestyle; others have found their lives centered on the disorder.

After a person has been diagnosed with Marfan syndrome, he or she should be monitored with an echocardiogram every six months until it is clear that the aorta is not growing larger. After that, the patient should have an echocardiogram once a year. If the echocardiogram does not allow the physician to visualize all portions of the aorta, CT or MRI may be used. In cases involving a possible aortic dissection, the patient may be given a TEE (transesophageal echocardiogram).

Children diagnosed with Marfan syndrome should be checked for **scoliosis** by their pediatricians at each annual physical examination. The doctor simply asks the child to bend forward while the back is examined for changes in the curvature. In addition, the child's spine should be x rayed in order to measure the extent of scoliosis or kyphosis. The curve is measured in degrees by the angle between the vertebrae as seen on the x ray. Curves of 20° or less are not likely to become worse. Curves between 20° and 40° are likely to increase in children or adolescents. Curves of 40° or more are highly likely to worsen, even in an adult, because the spine is so badly imbalanced that the force of gravity will increase the curvature.

Scoliosis between 20° and 40° in children is usually treated with a back brace. The child must wear this appliance about 23 hours a day until growth is complete. If the spinal curvature increases to 40° or 50°, the patient may require surgery in order to prevent lung problems, back pain, and further deformity. Surgical treatment of scoliosis involves straightening the spine with metal rods and fusing the vertebrae in the straightened position.

Spondylolisthesis is treated with a brace in mild cases. If the slippage is more than 30°, the slipped vertebra may require surgical realignment.

Dural ectasia can be distinguished from other causes of back pain on an MRI. Mild cases are usually not treated. Medication or spinal shunting to remove some of the spinal fluid are used to treat severe cases.

Pectus excavatum and pectus carinatum can be treated by surgery. In pectus excavatum, the deformed breastbone and ribs are raised and straightened by a metal bar. After four to six months, the bar is removed in an outpatient procedure.

Protrusio acetabulae may require surgery in adult life to provide the patient with an artificial hip joint, if the arthritic pains are severe.

Patients with Marfan syndrome should consider wearing shoes with low heels, special cushions, or orthotic inserts. Foot surgery is rarely necessary.

### Drugs

A patient may be given drugs called beta–blockers to slow down the rate of aortic enlargement and decrease the risk of dissection by lowering the blood pressure and decreasing the forcefulness of the heartbeat. The most commonly used beta–blockers in patients with Marfan syndrome are propranolol (Inderal) and atenolol (Tenormin). Patients who are allergic to beta–blockers may be given a calcium blocker such as verapamil.

Because patients with Marfan syndrome are at increased risk for infective endocarditis, they must take a prophylactic dose of an antibiotic before having dental work or minor surgery, as these procedures may allow bacteria to enter the bloodstream. Penicillin and amoxicillin are the antibiotics most often used.

Pain in the feet or limbs is usually treated with a mild analgesic such as acetaminophen.

### Alternative

Surgery may be necessary if the width of the patient's aorta increases rapidly or reaches a critical size (about 2 in, 5 cm). The most common surgical treatment involves replacing the patient's aortic valve and several inches of the aorta itself with a composite graft, which is a prosthetic heart valve sewn into one end of a Dacron tube. This surgery has been performed widely since about 1985; most patients who have had a composite graft have not needed additional surgery.

Patients who have had a valve replaced must take an anticoagulant medication, usually warfarin (Coumadin), in order to minimize the possibility of a clot forming on the prosthetic valve.

### Visual and dental concerns

Patients with Marfan syndrome should have a thorough eye examination, including a slit–lamp examination, to test for dislocation of the lens as well as nearsightedness. Dislocation can be treated by a combination of special glasses and daily use of 1% atropine sulfate ophthalmic drops, or by surgery.

Because patients with Marfan syndrome are at increased risk of **glaucoma**, they should have the fluid pressure inside the eye measured every year as part of an eye examination. Glaucoma can be treated with medications or with surgery.

Cataracts are treated with increasing success by implant surgery. It is important to seek treatment at medical centers with eye surgeons familiar with the possible complications of cataract surgery in patients with Marfan syndrome.

All persons with Marfan syndrome should be taught to recognize the signs of retinal detachment (sudden blurring of vision in one eye becoming progressively worse without pain or redness) and to seek professional help immediately.

Children with Marfan syndrome should be evaluated by their dentist at each checkup for crowding of the teeth and possible misalignment, and referred to an orthodontist if necessary.

People with Marfan syndrome should avoid sports or occupations that require heavy weight lifting, rough physical contact, or rapid changes in atmospheric pressure (e.g., scuba diving). Weight lifting increases blood pressure, which in turn may enlarge the aorta. Rough physical contact may cause retinal detachment. Sudden changes in air pressure may produce pneumothorax. Regular noncompetitive physical exercise, however, is beneficial for patients with Marfan syndrome. Good choices include brisk walking, shooting baskets, and slow–paced tennis.

### Social and lifestyle issues

Smoking is particularly harmful for patients with Marfan because it increases their risk of emphysema.

In the past, women with Marfan syndrome were advised to avoid pregnancy because of the risk of aortic enlargement or dissection. The development of beta–blockers and echocardiograms, however, allows doctors now to monitor patients throughout pregnancy. It is recommended that patients have an echocardiogram during each of the three trimesters of pregnancy. Normal, vaginal delivery is not necessarily more stressful than a Caesarian section, but patients in prolonged labor may have a Caesarian birth to reduce strain on the heart. A pregnant woman with Marfan syndrome should also receive **genetic counseling** regarding the 50% risk of having a child with the syndrome.

## QUESTIONS TO ASK YOUR DOCTOR

- How do you plan to treat my Marfan syndrome?
- Are there treatment options?
- Is surgery required?
- What is the expected outcome?
- How do people inherit Marfan syndrome?

Children and adolescents with Marfan syndrome may benefit from supportive counseling regarding appearance, particularly if their symptoms are severe and causing them to withdraw from social activities. In addition, families may wish to seek counseling regarding the effects of the syndrome on relationships within the family. Many people respond with guilt, fear, or blame when a genetic disorder is diagnosed in the family, or they may overprotect the affected member. Support groups are often good sources of information about Marfan syndrome; they can offer helpful suggestions about living with it as well as emotional support.

### Prognosis

The prognosis for patient's with Marfan syndrome has improved markedly. The life expectancy of people with the syndrome had increased to 72 years; up from 48 years in 1972. This dramatic improvement is attributed to new surgical techniques, improved diagnosis, and new techniques of medical treatment.

The most important single factor in improving the patient's prognosis is early diagnosis. The earlier that a patient can benefit from the new techniques and lifestyle modifications, the more likely he or she is to have a longer life expectancy.

### Prevention

Marfan syndrome that occurs because of spontaneous new mutations (15-25% of the cases) cannot be prevented. However, for prospective parents with a family history of Marfan syndrome, genetic counseling is recommended. Also, older fathers are more likely to have new mutations appear in chromosome 15.

### Resources

**BOOKS**

Parker, Philip. *Marfan Syndrome —A Bibliography and Dictionary for Physicians, Patients, and Genome*

*Researchers.* San Diego, CA: ICON Health Publications, 2007.

Parker, Philip, and James Parker, editors. *The Official Patient's Sourcebook on Marfan Syndrome.* San Diego, CA: ICON Health Publications, 2002.

## PERIODICALS

Goland, S., et al. "Pregnancy in Marfan syndrome: maternal and fetal risk and recommendations for patient assessment and management." *Cardiology in Review* 17, no. 6 (November–December 2009): 253–262.

Hung, C. C., et al. "Mutation spectrum of the fibrillin–1 (FBN1) gene in Taiwanese patients with Marfan syndrome." *Annals of Human Genetics* 73, pt. 6 (November 2009): 559–567.

Shirley, E. D., and P. D. Sponseller. "Marfan syndrome." *Journal of the American Academy of Orthopaedic Surgeons* 17, no. 9 (September 2009): 572–581.

Sponseller, P. D., et al. "Growing rods for infantile scoliosis in Marfan syndrome." *Spine* 34, no. 16 (July 2009): 1711–1715.

Stout, M. "The Marfan syndrome: implications for athletes and their echocardiographic assessment." *Echocardiography* 26, no. 9 (October 2009): 1075–1081.

Voermans, N., et al. "Neuromuscular features in Marfan syndrome." *Clinical Genetics* 76, no. 11 (July 2009): 25–37.

## OTHER

"About Marfan Syndrome." *National Marfan Foundation.* Information Page. http://www.marfan.org/marfan/ 2280/About-Marfan-Syndrome (accessed October 24, 2009).

"Arachnodactyly." *Medline Plus.* Encyclopedia. http:// www.nlm.nih.gov/medlineplus/ency/article/003288.htm (accessed October 24, 2009).

"Marfan Syndrome." *Medline Plus.* Health Topics. http:// www.nlm.nih.gov/medlineplus/marfansyndrome.html (accessed October 24, 2009).

"Marfan Syndrome." *Genetics Home Reference.* Health Topics. http://ghr.nlm.nih.gov/condition= marfansyndrome (accessed October 24, 2009).

"Marfan Syndrome." *Nemours Kids Health.* Information Page. http://kidshealth.org/kid/health_problems/ birth_defect/marfan.html (accessed October 24, 2009).

"What is Marfan Syndrome?" *Canadian Marfan Association.* Information Page. http://www.marfan.ca/content/ view/65/29/ (accessed October 24, 2009).

"What is Marfan Syndrome?" *NHLBI.* Information Page. http://www.nhlbi.nih.gov/health/dci/Diseases/mar/ mar_whatis.html (accessed October 24, 2009).

## ORGANIZATIONS

Canadian Marfan Association. Centre Plaza Postal Outlet. 128 Queen Street S., P.O. Box 42257, Mississauga, ON, Canada, L5M 4Z0. (905) 826-3223 (866) 722-1722. info@marfan.ca. http://www.marfan.ca.

National Marfan Foundation. 22 Manhasset Avenue. Port Washington, NY, 11050. (516) 883-8712 (800) 8-MARFAN. FAX:(516) 883-8040. mary@magicfoundation.org. http://www.marfan.org.

Stanford University Center for Marfan Syndrome and Aortic Disorders. 300 Pasteur Drive, Room H2157, Stanford, CA, 94305-5233. (650) 725-8246. (650) 724-4034. http://marfan.stanford.edu.

Rebecca J. Frey, PhD

Judith Sims, MS

Marie-Strumpell spondylitis bechterew syndrome *see* **Ankylosing spondylitis**

Maroteaux-Lamy syndrome (MPS VI) *see* **Mucopolysaccharidosis (MPS)**

# Marshall syndrome

## Definition

Marshall syndrome is a very rare genetic disorder with an autosomal dominant pattern that equally affects males and females. It is caused by an abnormality in collagen, which is a key part of connective tissue.

## Description

Marshall syndrome was first described by Dr. D. Marshall in 1958 and it has been studied periodically by researchers since then. The disease is most apparent in the facial features of those affected, which include an upturned nose, eyes spaced widely apart, making them appear larger than normal, and a flat nasal bridge. This facial formation gives subjects a childlike appearance. The upper part of the skull is unusually thick, and deposits of calcium may appear in the cranium. Patients may also have palate abnormalities. In addition, they may experience early **osteoarthritis**, particularly in the knees.

**Myopia** (nearsightedness), cataracts and **glaucoma** are common in Marshall syndrome. Moderate to severe hearing loss is often preceded by many incidents of otitis media (middle ear infection) and can occur in children as young as age three. Some patients have osteoarthritis, particularly of the knees.

In the 40 years following Dr. Marshall's discovery, some physicians have argued that Marshall syndrome is actually a subset of **Stickler syndrome**, a more common genetic disorder. Individuals with

## KEY TERMS

**Cataract**—A clouding of the eye lens or its surrounding membrane that obstructs the passage of light resulting in blurry vision. Surgery may be performed to remove the cataract.

**Collagen**—The main supportive protein of cartilage, connective tissue, tendon, skin, and bone.

**Glaucoma**—An increase in the fluid eye pressure, eventually leading to damage of the optic nerve and ongoing visual loss.

**Myopia**—Nearsightedness. Difficulty seeing objects that are far away.

**Osteoarthritis**—A degenerative joint disease that causes pain and stiffness.

**Saddle nose**—A sunken nasal bridge.

both syndromes have similar facial features and symptoms. Other experts have argued against this view, stating that Marshall syndrome is a distinct disorder on its own. For example, most patients with Stickler syndrome have cataracts, while this problem is less common among those with Marshall syndrome. In addition, most subjects with Marshall syndrome have moderate to severe hearing loss, which rarely occurs among those with Stickler syndrome, who have normal hearing.

Genetic research performed in 1998 and 1999 revealed that both sides were right. There are clear genetic differences between the two syndromes. There are also patients who have apparent overlaps of both syndromes.

In 1998, a study used **genetic testing** to establish that a collagen genetic mutation on COL11A1 caused Marshall syndrome and that a change on COL2A1 caused Stickler syndrome. It also found that other types of mutations could cause overlaps of both syndromes.

A study in 1999 described a genetic study of 30 patients from Europe and the United States, all of whom were suspected to have either Marshall or Stickler syndrome. These genetic findings confirmed those of the previous (1998) study. Twenty-three novel mutations of COL11A1 and COL2A1 were found among the subjects. Some patients had genetic overlaps of both Marshall and Stickler syndromes.

Physical differences were also noted between the two syndromes. For example, all the patients with Marshall syndrome had moderate to severe hearing loss, while none of the patients with Stickler syndrome had hearing loss. About half the patients with overlapping disorders of both diseases had hearing loss. All the patients with Marshall syndrome had short noses, compared to about 75% of the patients with Stickler syndrome. Palate abnormalities occur in all patients with Stickler syndrome, compared to only about 80% of those with Marshall syndrome. Also, about a third of the Stickler patients had dental abnormalities, compared to 11% of the patients with Marshall syndrome. Those with Stickler (71%) had a higher percentage of cataracts than those with Marshall syndrome (40%). Patients with Marshall syndrome were much more likely to have short stature than those with Stickler syndrome.

### Genetic profile

The **gene** name for Marshall syndrome is Collagen, Type XI, alpha 1. The gene symbol is COL11A1. The chromosomal location is 1p21. Marshall syndrome is an autosomal dominant genetic trait and the risk of an affected parent transmitting the gene to the child is 50%. Human traits are the product of the interaction of two genes from that condition, one received from the father and one from the mother. In dominant disorders, a single copy of the abnormal gene (received from either parent) dominates the normal gene and results in the appearance of the disease. The risk of transmitting the disorder from affected parent to offspring is 50% for each pregnancy regardless of the sex of the resulting child.

### Demographics

Because of the rarity of this disease, very little demographic data is available. Less than 100 cases of individuals with this syndrome have been reported worldwide in medical literature. Some cases are probably undiagnosed because of the high expense of genetic testing. It is known that Marshall syndrome presents in infancy or early childhood and severe symptoms such as hearing loss and cataracts manifest before the age of 10 years. Adults with the syndrome retain the facial traits that are characteristic of this disease, such as flat nose, large nasal bridge and widely spaced eyes. Among those with Stickler syndrome, in contrast, these distinctive facial characteristics diminish in adulthood.

### Signs and symptoms

Characteristic features of this disease are short upturned nose with a flat nasal bridge. Some patients also have glaucoma, crossed eyes, detached retinas, and protruding upper teeth. Patients often have short stature compared to other family members without the disease.

### Diagnosis

Individuals are diagnosed by their features as well as by the very early onset of serious eye and ear disease. Because Marshall syndrome is an autosomal dominant hereditary disease, physicians can also note the characteristic appearance of the biological parent of the child. Genetic testing is costly, thus, it is not ordered for most people. As a result, people may be diagnosed as possible Marshall syndrome or possible Stickler syndrome, based on their symptoms and appearance.

### Treatment and management

Marshall syndrome cannot be cured; however, the symptoms caused by the disease should be treated. Children with Marshall syndrome should have annual eye and ear checkups because of the risk for cataracts and hearing loss. Cataract surgery is needed if cataracts develop. At present, the only treatment for the progressive hearing loss is a hearing aid. The flat "saddle nose" can be altered with cosmetic surgery. If a child with Marshall syndrome has osteoarthritis, doctors may advise against contact sports.

### Prognosis

As they age, vision and hearing problems generally worsen for patients with Marshall syndrome. Many also develop osteoarthritis at an earlier age than for patients without Marshall syndrome, such as in the teens or twenties. Because there are so few identified cases, the life expectancy is afflicted individuals is unknown.

### Resources

**PERIODICALS**

Annunen, Susanna, et al. "Splicing mutations of 54-bp exons in the COL11A1 gene cause Marshall syndrome, but other mutations cause overlapping Marshall/Stickler phenotypes." *American Journal of Human Genetics* 64 (1999).

Griffith, Andrew J., et al. "Marshall syndrome associated with a splicing defect at the COL11A1 locus." *American Journal of Human Genetics* 62, no. 4 (1998).

**WEBSITES**

Annunen, Susanna. "From rare syndromes to a common disease: Mutations in minor cartilage collagen genes cause Marshall and Stickler syndromes and intervertebral disc disease." Academic dissertation, *Oulu University Library*, Oulu, Finland. http:/herkules. oulu.fi/isbn9514254139/. (1999).

"Entry 120280: Collagen, Type XI, Alpha-1; COL11A1." *OMIM—Online Mendelian Inheritance in Man.* http:// www.ncbi.nlm.nih.gov/entrez/omim/ dispomim.cgi?id=120280.

**ORGANIZATIONS**

National Organization for Rare Disorders (NORD). 55 Kenosia Ave., PO Box 1968, Danbury. CT 06813-1968. (203) 744-0100 or (800) 999-6673. Fax: (203) 746-6481. http://www.rarediseases.org.

Stickler Involved People. 15 Angelina, Augusta, KS 67010. (316) 259-2194. http://www.sticklers.org/sip.

Christine Adamec

Martin-Bell syndrome *see* **Fragile X syndrome**

MASA syndrome *see* **X-linked hydrocephaly**

# Marshall-Smith syndrome

## Definition

Marshall-Smith syndrome is a childhood condition involving specific facial characteristics, bone maturation that is advanced for the individual's age, failure to grow and gain weight appropriate for the individual's age, and severe respiratory (breathing) problems.

## Description

Marshall-Smith syndrome (MSS) was first described in two males seen in 1971 by Drs. Marshall, Graham, Scott, and Smith. They noticed changes in the skeletal system of these patients. Bones normally mature through several stages, naturally progressing through these stages with time. Specifically, a young child's bones have more

## KEY TERMS

**Cartilage**—Supportive connective tissue which cushions bone at the joints or which connects muscle to bone.

**Corpus callosum**—A thick bundle of nerve fibers deep in the center of the forebrain that provides communications between the right and left cerebral hemispheres.

**Gastrostomy**—The construction of an artificial opening from the stomach through the abdominal wall to permit the intake of food.

**Hirsuitism**—The presence of coarse hair on the face, chest, upper back, or abdomen in a female as a result of excessive androgen production.

**Larynx**—The voice box, or organ that contains the vocal cords.

**Phalanges**—Long bones of the fingers and toes, divided by cartilage around the knuckles.

**Trachea**—Long tube connecting from the larynx down into the lungs, responsible for passing air.

**Tracheostomy**—An opening surgically created in the trachea (windpipe) through the neck to improve breathing.

**Umbilical hernia**—Protrusion of the bowels through the abdominal wall, underneath the navel.

---

cartilage and less calcium deposits than an adult's bones. A child's bones appear less "dense" on an x ray than an adult's bones. A constant feature of MSS is skeletal maturation that is advanced for age. For example, in 1993 a newborn child with MSS was found to have the bone age of a three year-old child.

Specific facial features in MSS include a wide and prominent forehead, protruding and widely spaced eyes, a very small chin, and a small, upturned nose. Because individuals may not gain weight or grow well, they are often smaller than other children of the same age. There are often problems with structures in the respiratory tract (such as the larynx and trachea) and this can lead to difficulty with breathing. Pneumonia, or a lung infection, is common and can occur several times.

Significant mental and physical delays are almost always expected in MSS. Since children with MSS are often hospitalized for long periods of time to help treat respiratory problems, they may be slower to do physical things like crawling or walking.

No two patients with MSS have the exact same symptoms, as there is some variability with the condition. There are no alternate names for Marshall-Smith syndrome, though it is sometimes incorrectly referred to as **Weaver syndrome**, a separate condition with similar symptoms.

Families with MSS can be put under a great deal of stress, because long-term hospitalizations in the intensive care unit are common for children with MSS.

### Genetic profile

The vast majority of people with MSS are unique in their family; there is usually no family history of the condition. Because of this, MSS is thought to be a random, sporadic event when it occurs. No specific **gene** has been associated with MSS, and other genetic background is still largely unknown. Standard **genetic testing**, such as **chromosome** analysis and metabolic studies, typically are normal for patients with MSS.

In 1999, a group in Saudi Arabia reported a young girl with features of MSS who had a chromosome abnormality. She was found to have some duplication of the material on a region of chromosome 2. This has led researchers to believe that the gene for MSS may actually be on chromosome 2. This is the only individual with MSS found to have a chromosome abnormality. Current research is under way to determine the exact genetic cause for MSS.

### Demographics

Marshall-Smith syndrome is very rare in the general population. In fact, no statistical rates are available for the condition. It appears to be present across the world, affecting males and females equally.

### Signs and symptoms

The most medically serious complication in MSS is the associated respiratory problems. Structures in the respiratory system, such as the larynx and trachea, may not function properly because they can be "floppy," soft, and less muscular than usual. Because of this, airways can become plugged or clogged, since air does not move through to clear them like usual. Mucus may start collecting, causing an increased amount of bacteria that can lead to pneumonia. Ear infections are common, because the bacteria can spread to the ears as well. Internal nasal passages may be narrower in people with MSS, which can pose difficulty with breathing.

Children with MSS may have problems with eating, due to similar reasons that they may have difficulty breathing. Additionally, they may have a weak "suck" and "swallowing" reflex, normally controlled by muscular movements. As mentioned earlier, another feature of MSS is lack of proper growth and weight gain. This can be in part due to the difficulty in feeding for these individuals, though they are often very small even at birth.

Advanced bone age is present in all people with MSS. In particular, the bones of someone with MSS appear more dense on an x ray than they should, according to their age. While x rays of their hands and wrists often determine a person's "bone age," people with MSS often have a generalized advanced bone age within their entire skeleton. They may also have broad middle phalanges of the hand, which can be seen on an x ray.

Facial characteristics of people with MSS include those mentioned earlier, but other features may also occasionally be present. These can be blue-tinged sclerae (the white sections of the eyes), a large head circumference (measurement around the head), and a small, triangle-shaped face (with the point of the triangle being at the chin).

Occasionally, creases in the hands are deeper than usual in people with MSS. The first (big) toe can be longer and bigger than usual. Additional features include hirsuitism and an umbilical hernia. Hearing loss can sometimes occur. Ears may be larger, have a crumpled appearance, or be lower on the head than usual.

Changes in the brain can occur in MSS. An individual was reported in 1997 to have a smaller optic nerve (the nerve the connects the eyes to the brain) than usual, and had some vision problems as a result. Some children may be missing the corpus callosum, a structure in the brain. Mental and physical delays are commonly present in MSS, and are usually quite significant. These may in part be due to the brain abnormalities that are sometimes seen. There may be partial to complete lack of speech for individuals with MSS, another sign of the mental delays.

### Diagnosis

Because there is no genetic testing available for Marshall-Smith syndrome, all individuals have been diagnosed through a careful physical examination and study of their medical history.

Advanced skeletal age can be seen on x rays of the patient's hands and wrists, since this is the typical way to assess bone age. A full x ray survey of the body is a good way to assess age of other bones as well. Advanced bone age is always seen in Marshall-

Smith syndrome, but it may also be present in other genetic syndromes. **Sotos syndrome** involves similar skeletal findings, but individuals are generally larger than usual and can have mental delays. Weaver syndrome includes advanced skeletal maturation, but individuals are often larger than usual and have other specific facial characteristics (such as very narrow, small eyes). These and other conditions can be ruled out if the respiratory complications and facial characteristics seen in MSS are not present.

### Treatment and management

As mentioned earlier, long hospitalizations are common for people with MSS. Most of these involve treating severe respiratory complications of MSS. These types of complications often necessitate placing a tracheotomy to assist with breathing. Manual removal of the mucus buildup by suctioning near the tracheotomy is common. Frequent pneumonia is common, and intravenous antibiotics are often the treatment, as in people without MSS. There is no specific treatment for the advanced bone age.

Because feeding can be difficult for children with MSS, a gastrostomy is often needed, and feeding is done directly through the gastrostomy tube. It is a challenge to make sure children with MSS maintain proper growth, and sometimes a gastrostomy is the only way to achieve this.

### Prognosis

Marshall-Smith syndrome is considered a childhood condition because affected individuals do not typically survive past childhood. There is no long-term research on the disease due to it being rare and not typically present in adults.

Most children with MSS die in early infancy, often by three years of age, largely due to severe respiratory complications, and infections that may result from them. There have been reports of children surviving until age seven or eight, but these children did not have severe respiratory problems. These children give hope that the condition is variable, and not every person diagnosed with the condition will have a severely shortened life span.

## Resources

### WEBSITES

"Marshall-Smith syndrome." *Health Library*. http://www.marchallsmith.org.

### ORGANIZATIONS

Arc (a National Organization on Mental Retardation). 1010 Wayne Ave., Suite 650, Silver Spring, MD 20910. (800) 433-5255. Fax: (301) 565-5342, Info@thearc.org, http://www.thear.org.

Human Growth Foundation. 997 Glen Cove Ave., Glen Head, NY 11545. (800) 451-6434 or (516) 671-4041. Fax: (516) 671-4055. hgfound@erols.com. http://www.hgfound.org.

Little People of America, Inc. National Headquarters, 250 EL Camino Real. Suite 201 Tustin, CA 92780. (888) LPA. 2001, (714) 368.3689, Fax: (718) 368.3867. lpadatabase@ juno.com, http://www.lpaonline.org.

MAGIC Foundation for Children's Growth. 6645 W North Ave., Harlem Ave., Oak Park, IL 60302. (800) 362-4423 or (708) 383-0808. Fax: (708) 383-0899. mary@magicfoundation.org. http://www.magicfoundation.org.

Deepti Babu, MS, CGC

# MCAD deficiency

## Definition

Medium chain acyl-CoA dehydrogenase (MCAD) deficiency is a rare genetic disorder characterized by a deficiency of the MCAD enzyme. This enzyme is responsible for the breakdown of certain fatty acids into chemical forms that are useable by the human body. MCAD deficiency accounts for approximately one to three of every 100 cases of sudden infant death syndrome (SIDS). MCAD deficiency is transmitted through a non-sex linked (autosomal) recessive trait. The first recognized cases of MCAD deficiency were reported in 1982.

## Description

MCAD is one of four enzymes in the mitochondria of the cells that is responsible for the breakdown of medium chain fatty acids into acetyl-CoA. Medium chain fatty acids are defined as fatty acids containing between four and 14 carbon atoms. Acetyl-CoA, the desired product of the breakdown of these fatty acids, is a two-carbon molecule. MCAD is the enzyme responsible for the breakdown of straight-chain fatty acids with four to 14 carbons. There are two other enzymes that are responsible for the breakdown of short straight-chain (less than four carbons) fatty acids, and long straight-chain (more than 14 carbons) fatty acids. These other two enzymes are not able to take over the function of MCAD when MCAD is deficient.

Individuals affected with MCAD deficiency produce a form of the MCAD enzyme that is not nearly as efficient as the normal form of MCAD. This lack of efficiency results in a greatly diminished, but still functional, capability to break down medium chain fatty acids.

## Genetic profile

The **gene** that is responsible for the production of MCAD is located on **chromosome** 1 at 1p31. Twenty-six different mutations of this gene have been identified as causing MCAD deficiency; however, 95–98% of all cases are the result of a single point mutation. In this mutation, adenosine is substituted for guanine in base 985 (G985A), which causes a substitution of lysine (AAA) by glutamic acid (GAA) in residue 329 of the MCAD protein.

MCAD deficiency is a recessive disorder. This means that in order for a person to be affected with MCAD deficiency, he or she must carry two abnormal copies of the MCAD gene. In a population of individuals known to be affected with the G985A mutation, 81% were found to be homozygous for this mutation (two chromosomes, each with the same mutation). The remaining 19% were found to be heterozygous for the G985A mutation (only one chromosome carried the G985A mutation), but their other chromosomes carried one of the other MCAD **gene mutations**.

## Demographics

MCAD deficiency is estimated to occur in approximately one out of every 13,000 to 20,000 live births. This estimate is confounded to a certain degree by the fact that up to 25% of all individuals affected with MCAD deficiency die the first time they exhibit any symptoms of the disease. Many of these children are often misdiagnosed with either sudden infant death

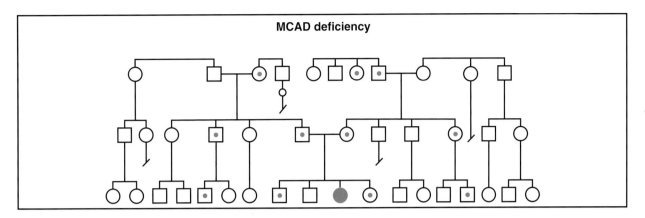

**MCAD deficiency**

(Gale, a part of Cengage Learning.)

syndrome (SIDS) or Reye syndrome. Unless an autopsy is performed, MCAD generally goes undetected in these individuals; and, even then, unless the physician performing the autopsy is familiar with MCAD deficiency, the cause of death may still be misreported.

MCAD deficiency is seen almost exclusively in Caucasians of Northern European descent (this includes people from every European country not bordering the Mediterranean Sea). Approximately 80% of the Caucasian population of the United States can be considered to be a part of this subpopulation. In this subpopulation, it is estimated that one in every 40 to 100 people is a carrier of the G985A mutation, and one in every 6,500 to 20,000 people is homozygous in this mutation. Homozygous individuals (carriers of two sets of the G985A mutation) should be affected with MCAD deficiency; however, the incidence rate of MCAD deficiency is lower than that predicted from the carrier populations. There are two possible reasons for the lower number of observed cases of MCAD deficiency than the carrier data suggests should occur. First, many individuals with MCAD deficiency may be misdiagnosed. Secondly, there may be a significant number of homozygous people who for unknown reasons remain unaffected (asymptomatic).

As a comparison, one in every 29 Caucasians is a carrier for **cystic fibrosis**, but only one in every 3,300 people in this subpopulation develop the disease.

The high frequency of a single mutation leading to MCAD deficiency, combined with the extreme similarity of the other known mutations to this mutation, and the high concentration of MCAD deficiency within a single subpopulation, suggests a founder effect from a single person in a Germanic tribe.

Because MCAD deficiency is a recessive disease, both parents must be carriers of this trait in order for their children to be affected. If both parents carry a copy of the mutated gene, there is a 25% likelihood that their child will be homozygous for MCAD deficiency. Genetically, the probability that an affected person will have a sibling who is also affected is also 25%. In population studies of known MCAD deficient individuals, it has been observed that an average of 32% of these individuals have at least one sibling either known to be affected with MCAD deficiency or to have died with a misdiagnosis of SIDS.

### Signs and symptoms

There is no classic set of symptoms that characterize MCAD deficiency. The severity of symptoms observed in individuals affected with MCAD deficiency ranges from no symptoms at all (asymptomatic) to the occurrence of death upon the first onset of symptoms. The first symptoms of MCAD deficiency generally occur within the first three years of life. The average age of onset of the first symptoms is one year of age. Some individuals become symptomatic prior to birth. The onset of symptoms in adults is extremely rare.

Lethargy and persistent vomiting are the most typical symptoms of MCAD deficiency. The first episode of symptoms is generally preceded by a 12 to 16 hour period of stress. Most affected individuals show intermittent periods of low blood sugar (hypoglycemia) and higher than normal amounts of ammonia in the blood (hyperammonemia). An abnormally large liver (hepatomegaly) is also associated with MCAD deficiency.

Approximately half of all individuals showing symptoms of MCAD deficiency for the first time experience respiratory arrest, cardiac arrest, and/or sudden infant death. Between 20% and 25% of all MCAD deficiency affected infants die during their first episodes of symptoms.

Some individuals affected with MCAD deficiency are affected with a degenerative disease of the brain and

## KEY TERMS

**Apnea**—An irregular breathing pattern characterized by abnormally long periods of the complete cessation of breathing.

**Carnitine**—An amino acid necessary for metabolism of the long-chain fatty acid portion of lipids. Also called vitamin $B_7$.

**Enzyme efficiency**—The rate at which an enzyme can perform the chemical transformation it is expected to accomplish. This is also called turnover rate.

**Founder effect**—Increased frequency of a gene mutation in a population that was founded by a small ancestral group of people, at least one of whom was a carrier of the gene mutation.

**Hepatomegaly**—An abnormally large liver.

**Hyperammonemia**—An excess of ammonia in the blood.

**Hypoglycemia**—An abnormally low glucose (blood sugar) concentration in the blood.

**Medium chain acyl-CoA dehydrogenase**—Abbreviated MCAD, this is the enzyme responsible for the breakdown of medium chain fatty acids in humans. People affected with MCAD deficiency produce a form of MCAD that is not as efficient as the normal form of MCAD.

**Medium chain fatty acids**—Fatty acids containing between four and 14 carbon atoms.

central nervous system (encephalopathy). Seizures, coma, and periods of halted breathing (apnea) have also been seen in people with MCAD deficiencies.

Long-term symptoms of MCAD deficiency may include: attention deficit disorder (ADD), **cerebral palsy**, mental retardation, and/or developmental delays.

The severity of the symptoms associated this MCAD deficiency is linked to the age of the person when the symptoms first happen. The risk of dying from an onset of the disease is slightly higher in individuals who show the first symptoms after the age of one year. The highest risk ages are the ages of 15 to 26 months. Seizures and encephalopathy are most frequently seen in affected individuals between the ages of 12 and 18 months. Seizures at these ages are often associated with future death during a symptomatic episode, recurrent seizures throughout life, the development of cerebral palsy, and/or the development of speech disabilities.

### Diagnosis

The Departments of Health in Massachusetts and North Carolina require mandatory newborn screening for MCAD deficiency. California has a voluntary newborn screening policy. Additionally, Neo Gen Screening offers voluntary newborn screening at birthing centers throughout the Northeastern United States. In September 2000, Iowa also began a pilot program to screen all newborns in that state.

These newborn screening methods employ either a recently developed (1999) tandem mass spectrometry (MS/MS) blood test method or a PCR/FRET analysis. The MS/MS test discovers the presence of the G985A mutation in the MCAD gene by the difference in molecular weight in this gene versus the molecular weight of the normal MCAD gene.

In the PCR/FRET test, a sample of blood is drawn and the **DNA** is extracted. This DNA is then reproduced multiple times by the polymerase chain reaction (PCR amplification). Once enough sample has been made, the sample is labeled with a fluorescent chemical that binds specifically to the region of chromosome 1 that contains the MCAD gene. How this fluorescent chemical binds to the MCAD gene region containing the G985A mutation allows the identification of homozygous G985A, heterozygous G985A, and normal (no G985A mutations) MCAD genes (FRET analysis).

An older method for the detection of MCAD deficiency is a urine test that checks for elevated levels of the chemicals hexanoylgylcine and phenylpropionylgylcine.

Prenatal testing for MCAD deficiency is available using a test similar to the PCR/FRET blood test. In this case, the DNA to be studied is extracted from the amniotic fluid rather than from blood. Another prenatal test involves studying the ability of cultured amniotic cells to breakdown added octanoate, an 8-carbon molecule that requires MCAD to break it down.

Because MCAD deficiency is generally treatable if it is recognized prior to the onset of symptoms, most parents of a potentially affected child choose to wait until birth to have their children tested.

### Treatment and management

Because individuals affected with MCAD deficiency can still break down short chain and long chain fatty acids at a normal rate and most have a diminished, but functional, ability to break down medium chain fatty acids, a precipitating condition must be present in order for symptoms of MCAD deficiency to develop. The most common precipitators of MCAD deficiency symptoms are stress caused by fasting or by infection. At these times, the body requires a higher than normal breakdown of medium chain fatty acids. MCAD deficient individuals often cannot meet these increased metabolic demands.

The main treatments for MCAD deficiency are designed to control or avoid precipitating factors. Persons affected with MCAD deficiency should never fast for more than 10 to 12 hours and they should strictly adhere to a low-fat diet. Blood sugar monitoring should be undertaken to control episodes of hypoglycemia. During acute episodes, it is usually necessary to administer glucose and supplement the diet with carbohydrates and high calorie supplements.

Many individuals affected with MCAD deficiency benefit from daily doses of vitamin $B_7$ (L-carnitine). This vitamin is responsible for transporting long chain fatty acids across the inner mitchondrial membrane. Elevated levels of L-carnitine ensure that these individuals breakdown long chain fatty acids in preference to medium chain fatty acids, which helps prevent acute symptomatic episodes of MCAD deficiency. Additionally, L-carnitine helps remove toxic wastes from the bloodstream to the urine, so it is also pivotal in controlling hyperammonemia.

Some individuals affected with MCAD deficiency present symptoms for the first time when they receive the diphtheria-pertussis-tetanus (DTP) vaccine. It is important that any person suspected to be affected with MCAD deficiency should receive treatment for hypoglycemia in connection with the administration of this vaccine. Chicken pox and middle ear infections (otitis media) have also been shown to initiate symptoms of MCAD deficiency.

### Prognosis

MCAD deficiency has a mortality rate of 20–25% during the first episode of symptoms. If an affected individual survives this first attack, the prognosis is excellent for this individual to have a normal quality of life as long as appropriate medical treatment is sought and followed.

### Resources

#### PERIODICALS

Berberich, S. "New developments in Iowa's newborn screening program." *The University of Iowa Hygienic Library Hotline* (September 2000): 1-2.

Chace, D., Hillman, S., J. Van Hove, and E. Naylor. "Rapid diagnosis of MCAD deficiency: Quantitative analysis of octanoylcarnitine and other acylcarnitines in newborn blood spots by tandem mass spectrometry." *Clinical Chemistry* (November 1997): 2106-2113.

Yokota, I. et al. "Molecular survey of a prevalent mutation, 985A-to-G transition, and identification of five infrequent mutations in the medium-chain Acyl-CoA dehydrogenase (MCAD) gene in 55 patients with MCAD deficiency." *American Journal of Human Genetics* (December 1991): 1280-91.

#### WEBSITES

Matern, D., P. Rinaldo, N. Robin. "Medium-chain acyl-coenzyme: A dehydrogenase deficiency." *GeneClinics*. http://www.geneclinics.org/profiles/mcad/details.html.

*OMIM—Online Mendelian Inheritance in Man.* http://www.ncbi.nlm./omim/

*Pediatric Database (PEDBASE) Homepage.* http://www.icondata.com/health/pedbase/files/MCADDEF1.htm.

#### ORGANIZATIONS

Fatty Oxidation Disorders (FOD) Family Support Group. 2041 Tomahank. Ovemos, MI 48864. (517) 381-1940. fodgroup@aol.com. http://www.fodsupport.org/welcome.htm.

National Organization for Rare Disorders (NORD). 55 Kenosia Ave PO Box 1968, Danbury, CT 06813 1968. (203) 744-0100 or (800) 999-6673. Fax: (203) 746-6481. http://www.rarediseases.org.

Organic Acidemia Association. PO Box 1008, Pinole, CA 94564. (510) 672.2974. Fax: (866) 539.4060. http://www.oaanews.org.

Sudden Infant Death Syndrome Network. PO Box 520, Ledyard, CT 06339. http://sids-network.org.

Paul A. Johnson

# McCune–Albright syndrome

## Definition

A disorder characterized by abnormalities in bone development, skin pigmentation, and endocrine gland function.

## Description

The McCune–Albright syndrome (MAS) is an uncommon disorder in which a mutation distributed across various cell populations results in a wide variety of clinical features. The most notable features are abnormal bone development, pigmented skin spots, and endocrine gland dysfunction.

## Genetic profile

The McCune–Albright syndrome is not hereditary but scientists have identified a specific genetic defect that causes MAS. The defect is a mutation in the *GNAS1* gene, which is associated with a type of G protein. These proteins are present in a wide variety of cells in the body. G proteins are part of the system of

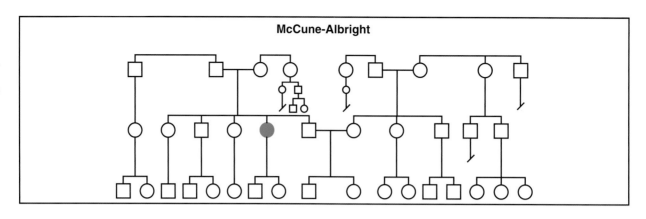

**McCune-Albright**

(Gale, a part of Cengage Learning.)

proteins and enzymes that regulate communication between cells and various agents such as hormones and the nervous system. If a cell's G protein is abnormal, this sets off a chain reaction that causes the cell to multiply inappropriately and the subsequent cells produce too much hormone. The mutation first occurs in a single cell during the early stages of formation of the embryo. This cell multiplies into many other cells that eventually become part of the bones, skin, and endocrine glands. The severity of the syndrome is dependent on the percentage of cells involved. The earlier the mutation occurs, the more cells are affected. There is some evidence that a second mutation must occur before the clinical manifestations become evident.

## Demographics

McCune–Albright syndrome is a rare genetic disorder with unknown incidence. It occurs equally in all races. Precocious puberty is far more common in affected girls than in boys, while other manifestations of the syndrome are believed to occur equally in both sexes. MAS had an estimated worldwide prevalence of between 1 in 100,000 and 1 in 1,000,000.

## Signs and symptoms

The McCune–Albright syndrome is classically characterized by three main features.

### Abnormal bone development

Pockets of abnormal fibrous tissue develop within the bone, which may cause deformity, fractures, and nerve entrapment. Most of these lesions appear during the first decade of life. The pelvis and femur, or thigh bone, are the most commonly involved areas of the skeleton. Bony abnormalities in the skull can cause blindness or **deafness**. The majority of patients with

MAS have many of these lesions, hence the name polyostotic fibrous dysplasia.

In addition to these fibrous lesions, some patients develop **osteosarcoma**, which is a malignant tumor of the bone. Although it has not been proven, these tumors may originate from the fibrous lesions within the bone.

### Pigmented skin spots

Patients with MAS typically have pigmented skin lesions called *café au lait* spots. These are flat areas of discoloration of the skin that may be associated with a variety of conditions. Those that are found in MAS have irregular borders. They are located on one side of the body, usually on the buttocks or lower back. Sometimes these lesions are present at birth.

### Endocrine gland dysfunction

The McCune–Albright syndrome is striking for its association with a number of endocrine abnormalities. Endocrine glands are those that secrete hormones directly into the bloodstream to be transported to other tissues of the body. In MAS, one or more of these glands secrete abnormally high amounts of hormone.

The most common endocrine abnormality in MAS is excessive function of the gonads, which are ovaries in females and testicles in males. The ovaries secrete estrogen and the testicles secrete testosterone. When these organs secrete too much estrogen or testosterone in children, the result is early puberty. Females are more commonly affected than males. In fact, early puberty in a girl is the hallmark sign of MAS. Typically, these girls develop secondary sexual characteristics, such as breasts and pubic hair, before the age of nine. Menses also begins early. Sometimes the normal sequence of development is disrupted, in

## KEY TERMS

**Dysplasia**—The abnormal growth or development of a tissue or organ.

**Pituitary gland**—A small gland at the base of the brain responsible for releasing many hormones, including luteinizing hormone (LH) and follicle–stimulating hormone (FSH).

that affected girls might have menses before breast or pubic hair development.

Hyperfunction of the pituitary gland also occurs in MAS, resulting in excess production of growth hormone and/or prolactin. Excess growth hormone leads to **acromegaly**, or marked overgrowth of certain bones and tissues, especially in the face and extremities. Some people with acromegaly grow to very tall stature. Acromegaly in MAS affects boys and girls equally. If too much prolactin is produced, then breast tissue will secrete milk inappropriately, both in boys and girls. This is called galactorrhea. In some patients, the pituitary gland dysfunction is caused by a tumor.

Other endocrine glands that may be hyperactive are the thyroid and adrenal glands. The thyroid gland produces thyroid hormones, which help regulate the body's metabolism. If excess thyroid hormones are produced, i.e. hyperthyroidism, then patients may have diarrhea, weight loss, nervousness, tremor, and rapid heartbeat. In some patients, the hyperthyroidism is caused by thyroid nodules. The adrenal gland produces several hormones in the steroid hormone class, such as cortisol, aldosterone, and testosterone. Cortisol is most commonly over–produced. Similar to the pituitary gland, hyperfunction of the adrenal gland in MAS is sometimes caused by tumors.

Another feature of McCune–Albright syndrome is phosphate deficiency caused by excess excretion of phosphate in the urine. Since phosphate is a vital mineral for bone formation, this results in soft bones and some degree of pain. This condition is called rickets in children and osteomalacia in adults. There are two theories that have been proposed to explain the loss of phosphate in the urine. First of all, it is thought that the fibrous bone lesions may produce an agent that circulates through the blood stream to the kidneys that makes the kidneys unable to retain phosphate. Secondly, perhaps the kidneys are intrinsically unable to retain the appropriate amount of phosphate.

It is important to emphasize the variability of clinical features among patients with MAS. Not every patient has the three features of bony lesions, pigmented skin spots, and endocrine abnormalities. Each patient is affected differently. There are rare subtypes of the syndrome in which patients have hepatitis, cardiac arrythmias, or intestinal polyps.

### Diagnosis

There is no single test that is diagnostic for MAS. Certain clinical features can be easily observed, such as skin pigmentation and early puberty. The bony abnormalities can be confirmed by x ray. Blood tests for hormone levels can detect endocrine gland dysfunction.

### Treatment and management

There is no specific treatment that cures the disease. Testalactone, a drug that inhibits estrogen production, has been successful in the short term treatment of girls with early puberty, but long term treatment has not been very effective. Patients with pituitary tumors may benefit from drugs to reduce tumor size, or surgery to remove the tumors. Thyroid nodules can be treated by surgical removal or destruction with radioactive iodine. In addition, adrenal tumors can be removed by surgery.

#### Clinical trials

A few clinical trials on MAS and related conditions are sponsored by the National Institutes of Health (NIH) and other agencies. As of 2009, NIH was reporting 11 on–going and completed studies.

Examples include:

- The evaluation of the effectiveness of alendronate in treating the bone abnormality in MAS. (NCT00001728)
- A study to determine the natural history of MAS in a group of patients. (NCT00001727)
- The evaluation of the histamine response in patients with MAS. (NCT00318097)

Clinical trial information is constantly updated by NIH and the most recent information on MAS trials can be found at: http://www.clinicaltrials.gov.

### Prognosis

The life span in patients with McCune–Albright syndrome is essentially normal. Women who experienced early puberty as girls are generally fertile.

### Resources

**BOOKS**

Hsu, C. Y., and Scott A. Rivkees. *Congenital Adrenal Hyperplasia: A Parents' Guide.* Bloomington, IN: AuthorHouse, 2005.

Parker, James N. *The Official Parent's Sourcebook on McCune–Albright Syndrome.* San Diego, CA: ICON Health Publications, 2002.

### PERIODICALS

Bajpai, A., et al. "Platelet dysfunction and increased bleeding tendency in McCune–Albright syndrome." *Journal of Pediatrics* 153, no. 2 (August 2008): 287–289.

Congedo, V., and F. S. Cell. "Thyroid disease in patients with McCune–Albright syndrome." *Pediatric Endocrinology Reviews* 4, suppl. 4 (August 2007): 429–433.

Dumitrescu, C. E., and M. T. Collins. "McCune–Albright syndrome." *Orphanet Journal of Rare Diseases* 3 (May 2008): 12.

Lietman, S. A., et al. "Genetic and molecular aspects of McCune–Albright syndrome." *Pediatric Endocrinology Reviews* 4, suppl. 4 (August 2007): 380–385.

Rivkees, S. A. "McCune–Albright syndrome: 70 years of fascination and discovery." *Journal of Pediatric Endocrinology & Metabolism* 20, no. 8 (August 2007): 849–851.

Wagoner, H. A., et al. "GNAS mutation detection is related to disease severity in girls with McCune–Albright syndrome and precocious puberty." *Pediatric Endocrinology Reviews* 4, suppl. 4 (August 2007): 395–400.

### WEBSITES

*McCune–Albright Syndrome.* Medical Encyclopedia. Medline Plus, August 11, 2006 (February 12, 2009). http://www.nlm.nih.gov/medlineplus/ency/article/001217.htm.

*McCune–Albright Syndrome.* Information Page. NICHD, February 19, 2007 (February 12, 2009). http://www.nichd.nih.gov/health/topics/McCune_Albright_Syndrome.cfm.

*McCune–Albright Syndrome.* Information Page. Madisons Foundation, November 16, 2004 (February 12, 2009). http://www.madisonsfoundation.org/index.php/component/option,com_mpower/Itemid,49/diseaseID,548.

*McCune–Albright Syndrome.* Information Page. Genetics Home Reference, January 2009 (February 12, 2009). http://ghr.nlm.nih.gov/condition=mccunealbright syndrome.

### ORGANIZATIONS

MAGIC Foundation. 6645 W. North Avenue, Oak Park, Illinois 60302. (708) 383-0808 or (800) 3MAGIC3 or (800) 362-4423. Fax: (708) 383-0899. http://www.magicfoundation.org.

National Institute of Arthritis and Musculoskeletal and Skin Diseases (NIAMS). 1 AMS Circle, Bethesda, MD 20892-3675. (301) 495-4484 or (877) 22-NIAMS (226-4267). Fax: (301) 718-6366. Email: NIAMSinfo@mail.nih.gov. http://www.niams.nih.gov.

National Institute of Child Health and Human Development (NICHD). P.O. Box 3006, Rockville, MD 20847. (800) 370-2943. Fax: (866) 760-5947. Email: NICHD InformationResourceCenter@mail.nih.gov. http://www.nichd.nih.gov.

National Organization for Rare Disorders (NORD). 55 Kenosia Avenue, PO Box 1968, Danbury, CT 06813-1968. (203) 744-0100 or (800) 999-6673. Fax: (203) 798-2291. http://www.rarediseases.org.

Kevin Osbert Hwang, MD

# McKusick-Kaufman syndrome

## Definition

The McKusick-Kaufman syndrome (MKS) is a developmental disorder characterized by a group of conditions that include **congenital heart disease**, buildup of fluid in the female reproductive tract and extra toes and fingers.

## Description

McKusick reported the first case of a disorder which he called hydrometrocolpos syndrome in 1964. Shortly thereafter, Kaufman described another individual with a very similar group of abnormalities. Subsequent writers combined these syndromes into one, calling it the McKusick-Kaufman syndrome and characterizing its wide range of features.

MKS is the first human disorder to be attributed to a mutation occurring in a **gene** and affecting a type of molecule called a chaperonin. Chaperonins are sometimes called "protein cages" in that they protect cells by capturing and refolding misshapen proteins that could otherwise interfere with normal cellular functions.

## Genetic profile

MKS is inherited in an autosomal recessive pattern, meaning that a child must inherit two altered genes, one from each parent, to be affected. An altered gene responsible for a rare developmental syndrome found predominantly among the Old Order Amish population has been identified. Mutations in the gene responsible for MKS have been identified on **chromosome** 20p12 in an Amish family. Scientists have isolated the McKusick-Kaufman syndrome gene by positional cloning.

Based on an earlier genetic analysis of the Old Order Amish population, a research group looked at a region of chromosome 20 thought to contain the gene responsible for the syndrome. A technique called sample sequencing was then used to find candidate genes in that region. One of those genes, dubbed MKS, was altered in a sample from an Amish person as well as in a sample from a non-Amish person

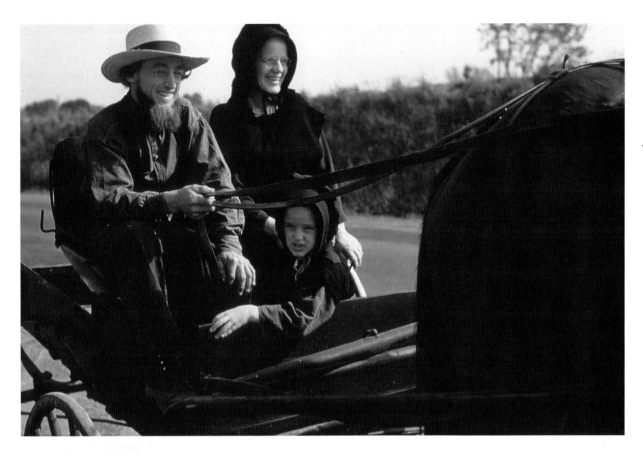

**McKusick-Kaufman syndrome has a high incidence among Amish families.** *(Photo Researchers, Inc.)*

diagnosed with MKS. In both people, errors or "misspellings" in the genetic code were found that would disturb the function of the MKS gene. It was observed that the chemical building blocks (amino acids) coded by the MKS gene appeared to be very similar to those that make up the chaperonins. Although the function of the protein made by the MKS gene is unclear, it appears to be involved in the production of proteins associated with the development of limbs, the heart, and the reproductive system.

In 2000, researchers identified a gene mutation that causes Bardet-Biedel syndrome (BBS), a rare genetic disorder that is related to MKS. BBS is believed to be due to a complete absence of the gene responsible for MKS.

## Demographics

Between 1% and 3% of the Amish people of Lancaster County, Pennsylvania, are believed to be carriers of the disease, having just one copy of the altered gene. The related Bardet-Biedel syndrome is estimated to occur between one in 125,000 and one in 160,000 people. Among an isolated community in Newfoundland, Canada, the prevalence is estimated to be ten times higher.

## Signs and symptoms

Many abnormalities associated with MKS are visible in a physical exam. They include the following abnormalities:

- Limbs: polydactyly (extra fingers or toes)
- Genitourinary system in females: hydrometrocolpos (accumulation of fluids in the uterus and vagina), transverse vaginal membrane, vaginal atresia (absence of a vagina)
- Genitourinary system in males: hypospadias (abnormal opening of the urinary tract), prominent scrotal raphe (ridges), micropenis, cryptorchidism (undescended testicles)
- Cardiac: congenital heart defects
- Head: pituitary dysplasia (abnormal development of the pituitary gland), choanal atresia (bony or membranous blockage of the passageway between the nose and pharynx), retinitis pigmentosa (overactive cells in the retina of the eye leading to blindness),

tracheo-esophageal fistula (abnormal passage in the throat region)
- Skeleton: vertebral anomalies
- Abdomen: distension, peritoneal cysts, Hirschsprung megacolon (enlarged and poorly functioning large intestine)
- Other: nonimmune hydrops fetalis (massive build-up of fluids in a fetus or newborn)

### Diagnosis

A diagnosis of McKusick-Kaufman syndrome is usually made at birth when a newborn is given a post-natal physical exam. The diagnosis is made by noting physical abnormalities such as: **polydactyly**, hydrometrocolpos, a transverse vaginal membrane, vaginal atresia, **hypospadias**, prominent scrotal raphe, micropenis,

cryptorchidism, congenital heart defects, pituitary **dysplasia**, choanal atresia, tracheo-esophageal fistula, vertebral anomalies, abdominal distension, peritoneal cysts, Hirschsprung megacolon, or nonimmune **hydrops fetalis**. The probability of a correct diagnosis increases with each additional abnormality present. A diagnosis may sometimes be confirmed with a chromosomal analysis. Abnormal development of the pituitary gland (pituitary dysplasia) and vertebral abnormalities are visible in a CT or MRI scan. Peritoneal cysts are commonly diagnosed by ultrasonography.

### Treatment and management

Treatment of MKS is limited to surgical correction of defects. Timing is often important. Many abnormalities, if uncorrected, can quickly become life threatening. For example, hydrops fetalis is often fatal. **Genetic counseling** before marriage is recommended for persons who are possible carriers of MKS. Affected rural and Amish girls should be delivered in settings that allow rapid surgical intervention and correction of abnormalities. Such actions could be life saving.

### Prognosis

With appropriate genetic counseling and complete family histories, individuals born with MKS can receive prompt treatment. With rapid initial surgical intervention, most of these persons can live relatively normal lives. Some abnormalities, such as hypospadias, vaginal atresia, choanal atresia, tracheo-esophageal fistula, or Hirschsprung megacolon, may require multiple operations. Due to the risk of **retinitis pigmentosa**, vision should be monitored closely.

## Resources

### BOOKS

Duckett, John W. "Hypospadias." In *Campbell's Urology.* Walsh, P. C. et al., eds W. B. Saunders, Philadelphia, 1998.

McKusick, Victor A. *Mendelian Inheritance in Man: A Catalog of Human Genes and Genetic Disorders,* 12th ed. Johns Hopkins University Press, Baltimore, 1998.

Nelson, Waldo E., et al., eds. "Anomalies of the penis and urethra." In *Nelson Textbook of Pediatrics.* W. B. Saunders, Philadelphia, 2000.

### PERIODICALS

David, A., et al. "Hydrometrocolpos and polydactyly: A common neonatal presentation of Bardet-Biedel and McKusick-Kaufman syndromes." *Journal of Medical Genetics* 36 (1999):599-603

Slavotinek, A. M., and L. G. Biesecker. "Phenotypic overlap of McKusick-Kaufman syndrome with Bardet-Biedel syndrome: A literature review." *American Journal of Medical Genetics* 95 (2000): 208-215

### WEBSITES

"Hypospadias." *Atlas of Congenital Deformities of the External Genitalia.* http://www.atlasperovic.com/contents/9.htm.

"Hypospadias." *The Penis.com.* http://www.the-penis.com/hypospadias.html.

*Society for Pediatric Urology.* http://www.spu.org/.

### ORGANIZATIONS

Hypospadias Association of America. 4950 S. Yosemite Street, Box F2-156, Greenwood Village, CO 80111. hypospadiasassn@yahoo.com. http://www.hypospadias.net.

National Institutes of Health, Office of Rare Diseases. 31 Center Dr., Bldg. 31, Room 1B-19, MSC 2084, Bethesda, MD 20892-2084. (301) 402-4336. Fax: (301) 480-9655. hh70f@nih.gov. http://rarediseases.info.nih.gov.

Support for Parents with Hypospadias Boys. http://clubs.yahoo.com/clubs/mumswithhypospadiaskids.

L. Fleming Fallon. Jr., MD, PhD, DrPH

# Meckel-Gruber syndrome

## Definition

Meckel-Gruber syndrome (MGS) is an inherited condition that causes skull abnormality, enlarged cystic kidneys, liver damage, and extra fingers and toes. Findings vary between affected infants (even in the same family), as well as between ethnic groups. Infants with MGS are usually stillborn or die shortly after birth.

---

## KEY TERMS

**Bile duct**—A passageway that carries bile (fluid secreted by the liver involved in fat absorption) from the liver to the gallbladder to the small intestine.

**Clubfoot**—Abnormal permanent bending of the ankle and foot. Also called *talipes equinovarus.*

**Trimester**—A three-month period. Human pregnancies are normally divided into three trimesters: first (conception to week 12), second (week 13 to week 24), and third (week 25 until delivery).

---

## Description

The first reports of MGS were published in 1822 by Johann Friedrich Meckel. G. B. Gruber also published reports of MGS patients in 1934 and gave it the name dysencephalia splanchnocystica. MGS is also known as Meckel syndrome and Gruber syndrome.

MGS affects many different organ systems including the central nervous system (brain and spinal cord), face, kidneys, liver, fingers and toes, and occasionally the bones of the arms and legs. Some researchers believe that abnormal development and differentiation of the embryonic mesoderm (the early tissue layer that contributes to the formation of the bones, cartilage, muscles, reproductive system, blood cells, heart, and kidneys) is related to MGS. The cells of the mesoderm must divide, migrate, associate, and specialize in a precise manner to form these body parts. Any problem in any step of the process can lead to multiple abnormalities in various organ systems.

Since MGS causes severe birth defects and death in the newborn period, it can be devastating for families. Extensive examination and autopsy is often needed to confirm a diagnosis of MGS, delaying the family's answers regarding their child's death. Most parents do not know they are at risk until they have a child with MGS. This can cause feelings of anger, disbelief, and guilt.

## Genetic profile

The autosomal recessive **inheritance** pattern in MGS is well-documented. MGS affects males and females equally. Parents of affected children are assumed to be carriers and have a 25% chance of MGS recurrence in each pregnancy. A healthy brother or sister of an affected child has a two-thirds chance of being an MGS carrier.

Research involving families in Finland (where MGS is more common) led to the first MGS **gene** being mapped (localized) to the short arm of **chromosome** 17. This means that the gene location has been narrowed down to a small potential area, but the exact location and precise details about the gene are still unknown. Non-Finnish families did not show evidence of a causative gene linked to chromosome 17. This led to the search for a second MGS gene. Studies of Northern African and Middle Eastern families resulted in the second MGS gene being mapped to the short arm of chromosome 11. More research is being performed to learn more about the precise location of both MGS genes, gene changes that cause MGS, and the role of the genes in early development.

## Demographics

MGS has an estimated incidence between one in 13,000 births and one in 140,000 births. This means that between one person per 50 and one person per 180 is an MGS carrier. The incidence varies among ethnic groups. Several ethnic populations have an increased incidence of MGS. The incidence in Finland is one in 9,000 births (one person in 50 is a carrier). The incidence is also higher among Belgians and Bedouins in Kuwait with one affected birth in 3,500 (one person in 30 is a carrier). The highest incidence is reported in the Gujarati Indians with one affected birth per 1,300 (one person in 18 is a carrier). The incidence among Jews in Israel is one in 50,000 (one person in 112 is a carrier). Cases of MGS have been reported in North America, Europe, Israel, Indonesia, India, Kuwait, and Japan.

## Signs and symptoms

The three hallmark features of MGS are **encephalocele**, polycystic kidneys, and **polydactyly**. Approximately 90% of infants with MGS have an encephalocele. This is an opening in the skull that allows brain tissue to grow outside of the skull. Virtually 100% of infants with MGS have enlarged kidneys with cysts. Polydactyly (extra fingers and/or toes) is present in about 80% of affected children. The polydactyly is usually postaxial (the extra fingers/toes are on the same side of the hand/foot as the smallest finger/toe). In MGS, the polydactyly usually affects both the hands and feet. There may also be webbing of the fingers and toes—the skin between the fingers or toes fails to separate—leaving the digits attached to each other.

Internal examination of babies with MGS revealed that virtually 100% have liver abnormalities. This can include halted development of the bile ducts,

extra bile ducts, enlarged bile ducts, and loss of blood vessels. The liver is also usually enlarged. These liver changes are now considered by most to be another hallmark feature of MGS.

Babies with MGS often have similar facial features. Some reported features are eyes that are closer together or farther apart than usual, broad and flat nose, broad cheeks, and a wide mouth with full lips. Other features are commonly seen in MGS and are thought to be caused by a low amount of amniotic fluid surrounding the baby before birth. These features are sloping forehead, small jaw, low-set ears, and short, webbed neck. Low fluid prior to birth also frequently causes **clubfoot** in the newborn.

Other common features of MGS are abnormalities of the genitalia and **cleft palate**. The external (visible) genitalia are often small or ambiguous (not clearly male or female). There have also been reports of babies with MGS having both male and female reproductive parts (hermaphrodite). Cleft palate is seen in about 45% of babies with MGS. **Cleft lip** is less common but has been reported.

The symptoms of MGS are variable. Not all infants with MGS show the same signs and the characteristic signs range in severity. Some features have been described in some babies with MGS but are not as common. These include heart defects, enlarged spleen, extra spleen, hydrocephaly (extra water in the brain), absence or underdevelopment of other brain structures, and arm and leg bones that are shortened, thickened, and bowed.

## Diagnosis

Some of the features of MGS can be detected on **prenatal ultrasound** early in the second trimester. At that time, an encephalocele can often be seen as well as other brain abnormalities. Enlarged kidneys can also be detected at this time. As the pregnancy continues, a low amount of amniotic fluid becomes apparent. Enlarged kidneys make the abdomen appear and measure larger than usual. Cysts make the kidneys appear bright or white on an ultrasound instead of the usual gray color.

Measurement of the alpha-fetoprotein (AFP) level from either maternal blood or amniotic fluid may help to detect an encephalocele (although most encephaloceles are closed and do not elevate AFP levels). AFP can be measured in amniotic fluid after about 12 weeks of pregnancy and in maternal blood after about 15 weeks of pregnancy. AFP elevation in either test increases the chance of an encephalocele or other abnormality in the baby's skull or spine.

When signs of MGS are seen on prenatal ultrasound in the absence of a family history, MGS is often suspected but not confirmed until after birth and autopsy. A chromosome test can be performed before birth to rule out chromosome abnormalities such as **trisomy 13**. However, autopsy is usually needed to distinguish MGS from other syndromes with similar features. Every organ system of the baby is carefully examined for abnormal development.

Families at risk for recurrence of MGS can combine early ultrasound with either maternal blood AFP or amniotic fluid AFP for early detection. If early ultrasound reveals no signs of MGS, later scans are still recommended because of the variability in expression and severity. No routine genetic tests are available to these families.

### Treatment and management

There is no effective treatment or cure for MGS. Babies with MGS have extensive birth defects that require many surgeries to repair. Encephaloceles can be repaired by surgery after birth. Surgeries are most successful for infants with small skull abnormalities. Encephaloceles put infants at high risk for infection. The abnormalities seen in the kidneys and liver often leave the organs nonfunctional. There is often no way to repair the organs other than transplant. Even if all of these problems could be solved, infants with MGS often have underdeveloped lungs that cannot support life after birth. The lungs are underdeveloped because of the low amount of amniotic fluid prior to birth. Due to the extensive birth defects, the extensive surgeries needed to correct them, and the poor prognosis, babies born with MGS are given minimum care for comfort and warmth.

When MGS is suspected in an unborn baby, parents should be given information about the range of symptoms of MGS and the poor prognosis. Parents should also be cautioned that a diagnosis of MGS often cannot be confirmed until after birth. Prognosis can vary if the baby has atypical signs of MGS or if the baby has a different syndrome. Elective termination of affected pregnancies may be an option for some couples.

### Prognosis

The prognosis for MGS is quite poor. Many infants with MGS are stillborn. Those that are born living usually die shortly after birth in the first hours, days, or weeks of life. Death is usually due to inability to breathe (underdeveloped lungs), infection (opening in the skull), or organ failure (decreased function of kidneys and liver). MGS is variable and there have been a

couple reports of infants with milder symptoms living longer. One infant with MGS lived until four months of age. Another lived to seven months of age after surgical repair of a small encephalocele. At birth he had cystic kidneys but normal kidney function. These two case reports show that longer survival is rare but possible because of the variable expression of MGS.

### Resources

#### PERIODICALS

Salonen, R. and P. Paavola. "Meckel Syndrome." *Journal of Medical Genetics* 35 (1998): 497–502.

#### ORGANIZATIONS

Meckel-Gruber Syndrome Foundation. http://www. meckel-gruber.org.

Amie Stanley, MS

Meckel syndrome *see* **Meckel-Gruber syndrome**

# Meckel's diverticulum

### Definition

Meckel's diverticulum is a congenital pouch (diverticulum) approximately 2 in (4 cm) in length and located at the lower (distal) end of the small intestine. It was named for Johann F. Meckel, a German anatomist who first described the structure.

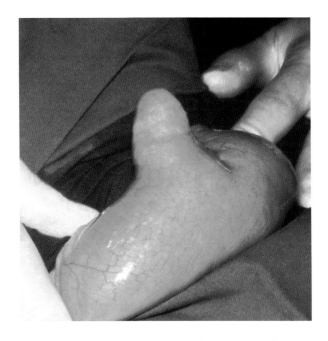

**A patient with Meckel diverticulum.** *(Custom Medical Stock Photo, Inc.)*

## Description

The diverticulum is most easily described as a blind pouch that is a remnant of the omphalomesenteric duct or yolk sac that nourished the early embryo. It contains all layers of the intestine and may have ectopic tissue present from either the pancreas or stomach.

The rule of 2's is the classical description. It is located about 2 ft from the end of the small intestine, is often about 2 in in length, occurs in about 2% of the population, is twice as common in males as females, and can contain two types of ectopic tissue—stomach or pancreas. Many people who have a Meckel's diverticulum never have trouble, but those that do present in the first two decades of life and often in the first two years.

There are three major complications that may result from the development of Meckel's diverticulum. The most common problem is inflammation or infection that mimics appendicitis. This diagnosis is defined at the time of surgery for suspected appendicitis. Bleeding caused by ectopic stomach tissue that results in a bleeding ulcer is the second most frequent problem. Bleeding may be brisk or massive. The third potential complication is obstruction due to intussusception, or a twist around a persistent connection to the abdominal wall. This problem presents as a small bowel obstruction, however, the true cause is identified at the time of surgical exploration.

## Genetic profile

Meckel's diverticulum is not hereditary. It is a vestigial remnant of the omphalomesenteric duct, an embryonic structure that becomes the intestine. As such, there is no genetic defect or abnormality.

## Demographics

Meckel's diverticulum is a developmental abnormality that is present in about 2% of people, but does not always cause symptoms. Meckel's diverticula (plural of diverticulum) are found twice as frequently in men as in women. Complications occur three to five times more frequently in males.

## Signs and symptoms

Symptoms usually occur in children under 10 years of age. There may be bleeding from the rectum, pain and vomiting, or simply tiredness and weakness from unnoticed blood loss. It is common for a Meckel's diverticulum to be mistaken for the much more common disease appendicitis. If there is obstruction, the abdomen will distend and there will be cramping pain and vomiting.

## KEY TERMS

**Catecholamines**—Biologically active compounds involved in the regulation of the nervous and cardiovascular systems, rate of metabolism, body temperature, and smooth muscle.

**Connective tissue**—A group of tissues responsible for support throughout the body; includes cartilage, bone, fat, tissue underlying skin, and tissues that support organs, blood vessels, and nerves throughout the body.

**Diverticulae**—Sacs or pouches in the walls of a canal or organ. They do not normally occur, but may be acquired or present from birth. Plural form of diverticula.

**Enzyme**—A protein that catalyzes a biochemical reaction or change without changing its own structure or function.

**Jaundice**—Yellowing of the skin or eyes due to excess of bilirubin in the blood.

**Linkage analysis**—A method of finding mutations based on their proximity to previously identified genetic landmarks.

**Tortuous**—Having many twists or turns.

### Diagnosis

The situation may be so acute that surgery is needed on an emergency basis. This is often the case with bowel obstruction. With heavy bleeding or severe pain, whatever the cause, surgery is required. The finer points of diagnosis can be accomplished when the abdomen is open for inspection during a surgical procedure. This situation is called an acute abdomen.

If there is more time (not an emergency situation), the best way to diagnose Meckel's diverticulum is with a nuclear scan. A radioactive isotope injected into the bloodstream accumulates at sites of bleeding or in stomach tissue. If a piece of stomach tissue or a pool of blood shows up in the lower intestine, Meckel's diverticulum is indicated.

### Treatment and management

A Meckel's diverticulum that is causing discomfort, bleeding, or obstruction must be surgically removed. This procedure is very similar to an appendectomy.

### Prognosis

The outcome after surgery is usually excellent. The source of bleeding, pain, or obstruction is removed so the symptoms also disappear. A Meckel's diverticulum will not return.

### Resources

#### BOOKS

Aspinall, Richard J., and Simon T. Taylor-Robinson. *Mosby's Color Atlas & Text of Gastroenterology*. St. Louis: Mosby-Year Book, 2001.

Cousins, Claire, and Ralph Boulton. *A Color Handbook of Gastroenterology*. New York: McGraw-Hill, 1999.

Isselbacher, Kurt J., and Alan Epstein. "Diverticular, Vascular, and Other Disorders of the Intestine and Peritoneum." In *Harrison's Principals of Internal Medicine*. New York: McGraw-Hill, pp. 1648-1655, 1998.

Lipsky, Martin S., and Richard Sadovsky. *Gastrointestinal Problems*. Philadelphia: Lippincott Williams & Wilkins Publishers, 2000.

Sanderson, Ian R., and W. Allan Walker. *Development of the Gastrointestinal Tract*. Hamilton, Ontario, Canada: B. C. Decker, 1999.

Stringer, David A., and Paul S. Babyn. *Pediatric Gastrointestinal Imaging and Intervention*, 2nd edition. Hamilton, Ontario, Canada: B. C. Decker, 2000.

#### PERIODICALS

al Mahmeed, T., J. K. MacFarlane, and D. Filipenko. "Ischemic Meckel's diverticulum and acute appendicitis." *Canadian Journal of Surgery* 43, no. 2 (2000): 146-47.

Arnio, P., and I. S. Salonen. "Abdominal disorders arising from 71 Meckel's diverticulum." *Annals of Surgery and Gynecology* 89, no. 4 (2000): 281-84.

Heider, R., D. M. Warshauer, and K. E. Behrns. "Inverted Meckel's diverticulum as a source of chronic gastrointestinal blood loss." *Surgery* 128, no. 1 (2000): 107-08.

Martin, J. P., P. D. Connor, and K. Charles. "Meckel's diverticulum." *American Family Physician* 61, no. 4 (2000): 1037-42.

Nagler, J., J. L. Clarke, and S. A. Albert. "Meckel's diverticulitis in an elderly man diagnosed by computed tomography." *Journal of Clinical Gastroenterology* 30, no. (2000): 87-88.

#### WEBSITES

*American Academy of Family Physicians.* http://www.aafp.org/afp/20000215/1037.html.

"Gastroenterology: Meckel's Diverticulum." *Vanderbilt University Medical Center*, 1998. http://www.mc.vanderbilt.edu/peds/pidl/gi/meckel.htm.

"Meckel's Diverticulum." *Merck Manual*. http://www.merck.com/pubs/mmanual/section19/chapter268/268d.htm.

ORGANIZATIONS

American Academy of Family Physicians. 11400 Tomahawk Creek Parkway, Leawood, KS 66211-2680. (913) 906-6000. http://www.aafp.org/, fp@aafp.org.

American Academy of Pediatrics. 141 Northwest Point Boulevard, Elk Grove Village, IL 60007-1098. (847) 434-4000. Fax: (847) 434-8000. kidsdoc@aap.org. http://www.aap.org.

American College of Gastroenterology. PO Box 342260, Bethesda, MD 20827.2260. (301) 263.9000. http://www.gi.org.

American College of Surgeons. 633 North St. Clair St., Chicago, IL 60611-32311. (312) 202-5000. Fax: (312) 202-5001. postmaster@facs.org. http://www.facs.org/.

American Medical Association. 515 N. State Street, Chicago, IL 60654 (800) 621-8335. http://www.ama-assn.org/.

L. Fleming Fallon, Jr., MD, DrPH

Mediterranean anemia *see* **Beta-thalassemia**

Medium-chain acyl-coenzyme A *see* **MCAD deficiency**

Melnick-Fraser syndrome *see* **Branchiootorenal syndrome**

# Menkes syndrome

## Definition

Menkes syndrome is a sex-linked recessive condition characterized by seizures and neurological deterioration, abnormalities of connective tissue, and coarse, kinky hair. Affected males are often diagnosed within the first few months of life and die in early childhood.

## Description

Menkes syndrome is also known as Menkes disease and kinky hair syndrome. It was originally described in 1962 based on a family of English and Irish descent who had five male infants with a distinctive syndrome of progressive neurological degeneration, peculiar hair, and failure to thrive. Each of the boys appeared normal at birth but, by the age of several months, developed seizures and began to regress in their physical skills. Each child died at an early age, with the oldest surviving only until three-and-a-half years. In 1972, Menkes syndrome was linked to an inborn copper deficiency. It is now clear that this lack of copper, an essential element for normal growth and development, inhibits the work of specific enzymes in the body. The clinical signs and symptoms of Menkes syndrome are a direct result of these biochemical abnormalities.

Approximately 90–95% of patients with Menkes syndrome have a severe clinical course. This represents classical Menkes syndrome. Males with milder forms of Menkes syndrome have also been described. The mildest presentation is now known as occipital horn syndrome (OHS), which is allelic to Menkes syndrome: both conditions are due to different mutations in the same **gene**. Mutations responsible for OHS primarily cause connective tissue abnormalities and have significantly milder effects on intellectual development. Individuals with OHS live longer than those with classical Menkes syndrome.

## Genetic profile

Menkes syndrome is an X-linked recessive condition. The gene, which was identified in 1992, is located on the long arm of the X **chromosome** at band 13.3 (Xq13.3). It is extremely unusual for a female (with two X chromosomes in her cells) to be affected, although it has been reported. Males, who have only one X chromosome, make up the overwhelming majority of patients.

Approximately one-third of affected males are due to a new mutation in the mother's egg cell. There is usually a negative family history, or no other affected male family members. When the mutation occurs as an isolated, random change, the mother's risk of having another affected son is low.

On the other hand, the remaining two-thirds of affected males are born to carrier mothers. Often, there is a family history of one or more affected male relatives (e.g., uncle, brother, cousin), all of whom are related to one another through the maternal side. Carrier females are normal but face a risk of passing on the gene for Menkes syndrome to their children. A carrier mother has a 25% risk of having an affected son, 25% risk of having an unaffected carrier daughter, 25% risk of having a normal son, and a 25% risk of having a normal, non-carrier daughter. These risks apply to each pregnancy.

The Menkes syndrome gene, also known as MNK or ATP7A, is a large gene known to encode a copper-transporting protein. Individuals with Menkes syndrome have low levels of copper in their blood. Their cells are able to take in copper but the metal is unable to leave the cell and be delivered to crucial enzymes that require copper in order to function normally. As a result, copper accumulates in the body tissues, and clinical abnormalities occur. Most symptoms of Menkes syndrome, such as skeletal changes and abnormal hair, may be explained by the loss of specific enzymes. However, the reasons for the brain degeneration are still not entirely clear.

A variety of mutations that cause Menkes syndrome have been identified in the MNK gene. Unfortunately, almost every family studied has had a unique mutation. This makes **genetic testing** difficult, particularly if the mutation in the family has not yet been determined. OHS is also due to mutations in the MNK gene.

### Demographics

Menkes syndrome is relatively rare, with an estimated incidence of one in 100,000–250,000 male births. Among the 3.5 million infants born annually in the United States, approximately 15–35 males have Menkes syndrome.

### Signs and symptoms

Infants with classical Menkes syndrome appear normal at birth and continue to develop normally for roughly the first eight to ten weeks of life. At approximately two to three months of age, affected infants begin to lose previously attained developmental milestones, such as head control and a social smile. They lose muscle tone and become hypotonic, or floppy, develop seizures, and begin to fail to thrive. Changes in the appearance of their face and hair become more apparent. A diagnosis of Menkes syndrome is often made around this time.

Menkes syndrome has several clinical features.:
Neurologic features include:
- mental deterioration and handicap due to structural and functional brain abnormalities
- seizures
- inability to regulate body temperature (hypothermia)
- feeding and sleeping difficulties
- decreased muscle tone

Connective tissues typically display:
- tortuous blood vessels due to abnormal formation of blood vessel walls
- abnormalities of bone formation, as noted by x ray (skull, long bones, and ribs)
- bladder diverticulae
- loose skin, particularly at the nape of neck, under the arms, and on the trunk
- loose joints

Other clinical features are:

- unusual facial features (jowly, pudgy cheeks, large ears)
- abnormal hair, including the eyelashes and eyebrows
- light, even for family, skin and hair coloring (hypopigmentation)
- delayed eruption of teeth
- impaired vision
- normal hearing

The hair of individuals with Menkes syndrome deserves special discussion, particularly since this condition is sometimes also called kinky hair syndrome. Abnormal hair is not typically evident during the first few months of life. However, around the time that the other physical signs of the disorder become more apparent, the hair takes on an unusual appearance and texture. On magnified inspection, it is short, sparse, coarse, and twisted. It has been likened to the texture of a steel wool cleaning pad. It shows an unusual orientation, referred to as *pili torti*, a 180 degree twist of the hair shaft. It is usually fragile and breaks easily. The hair of all affected individuals shows these characteristic changes; it is likewise present in some women who are known gene carriers.

Death occurs early in males with Menkes syndrome, often by the age of three years in classical disease. longer survival is not unusual and is most likely due to more recent improvements in medical care. Severity of disease and its rate of progression are fairly consistent among untreated males in a single family.

### Diagnosis

An initial diagnosis of Menkes syndrome is usually suspected based on the combination of physical features. As these features are generally subtle in the newborn period, they may be missed, particularly if there is no prior family history of the condition.

A somewhat common prenatal and newborn history has been recognized among affected infants. The histories often include: premature labor and delivery; large bruises on the infant's head after an apparently normal, uncomplicated vaginal birth; hypothermia; low blood sugar (hypoglycemia); and jaundice. Hernias may be present at either the umbilicus or in the groin area. These findings are non-specific and occur in normal pregnancies and unaffected infants. However, their presence may alert a knowledgeable physician that Menkes syndrome should be considered as a possibility, especially when other clinical signs are also present.

A clinical diagnosis is strongly supported by decreased serum levels of copper and ceruloplasmin, a protein in the blood to which the majority of copper is attached. Abnormal results, however, do not confirm the diagnosis since both copper and ceruloplasmin levels may also be low in normal infants during the first few months of life. A definitive diagnosis of Menkes syndrome is possible by either specific biochemical analysis to measure the level of copper accumulation in the cells or by identification of the responsible mutation in the MNK gene. Both types of analysis represent highly specialized testing and are available only through a limited number of laboratories in the world.

Prenatal diagnosis, in the context of a family history of the disorder, is possible. Ideally, a woman's carrier status will have been determined prior to a pregnancy as carrier detection may be difficult and time-consuming. Mutation analysis is the most direct and accurate way to determine carrier status. In order for this to be possible, the MNK mutation in an affected family member must have been previously determined. Linkage analysis is another possibility but requires blood samples from other family members, including the affected relative, to facilitate interpretation of results. If the affected relative is deceased, a stored **DNA** sample may be used.

Other, non-molecular methods of carrier detection include analysis of hair samples to look for areas of pili torti, increased fragility, or hypopigmentation. Skin cells cultured in the laboratory may be used to measure the accumulation of radioactive copper. However, these approaches are not always reliable, even in known carriers.

If a woman is found to be a non-carrier, prenatal testing for Menkes syndrome is generally not necessary in any of her pregnancies. However, in the event that a woman is a confirmed carrier, prenatal testing such as chorionic villus sampling (CVS) or **amniocentesis** may be offered. Ultrasound examinations alone will not assist in making a diagnosis. CVS or amniocentesis will determine the fetal sex: if female, additional testing is usually not recommended since carrier daughters would be expected to be normal. Carrier testing on the daughter may be performed after birth, if desired, or postponed until later in life.

Further testing is offered when a fetus is male. If mutation studies cannot be performed because the mutation in the family is unknown, biochemical analysis may be attempted. Biochemical testing has serious drawbacks, and a correct diagnosis may not always be possible. Tissue obtained during CVS normally has a very low copper content and is very susceptible to contamination by maternal tissue or by outside sources, such as laboratory instruments or containers. As a result, if the copper level exceeds a certain level, an unaffected pregnancy could potentially be falsely identified as affected. Specific handling precautions are necessary to minimize this risk.

Similar concerns exist for a sample obtained by amniocentesis. Ordinarily, the cells obtained from this procedure are cultured and grown in the laboratory. A measurement is taken of the total amount of accumulated copper over a certain period. The timing of amniocentesis in the pregnancy is critical because the amniotic fluid cells do not grow as rapidly after a gestational age of 18 weeks. Problems in cell growth cause significant difficulties in the interpretation of the biochemical results.

Other methods of diagnosis are being investigated. Two that hold some promise are assessment of the concentration of copper in a sample of the placenta (extremely high in affected pregnancies) and the level of catecholamines (low) in a sample of blood from the umbilical cord. Both methods, which are fast, reliable, and performed immediately after delivery, clearly require a high level of suspicion of the disorder. In most cases, this will be based on a history of a previous affected son, abnormal or unclear prenatal testing results, or both. Women who do not have a family history of Menkes syndrome and are therefore not expected to be at-risk, are not offered this testing.

### Treatment and management

The underlying, critical problem for patients with Menkes syndrome is an induced copper deficiency. Copper uptake is normal but the gene abnormality prevents the release of copper to the appropriate enzymes in the cells. Copper accumulates in the intestinal system, and patients are unable to meet their most basic nutritional needs. The most serious effects are apparent during the first year of life when growth of the brain and physical development are occurring most rapidly. Copper is required in order for both of these processes to occur normally.

Treatment of Menkes syndrome has focused on providing patients with an extra source of copper to try to deliver it to the enzymes that need it for normal function. Studies at the National Institutes of Health (NIH) have focused on the use of a copper-histidine compound in affected males. Copper-histidine is normally present in human serum and is most likely the form in which copper is absorbed by the liver. Also, in the laboratory, the presence of histidine in serum has been shown to increase the uptake of copper. Daily injections are the most successful form of treatment to date.

Two conclusions have been drawn from this work: (1) Treatment is more successful when started at an early age. Most, but not all, treated boys have achieved more normal developmental milestones and have had milder mental impairment. (2) Treatment is much less effective if started after the age of several months, or when neurologic symptoms have already begun. While milder improvements in the areas of physical development, personality, and sleeping habits have been reported in boys whose treatment started later, the degree of mental handicap has not been significantly altered.

A separate study in 1998 lent further support to these results. This study followed four affected males with classical Menkes syndrome, all of whom were started on copper-histidine treatment soon after birth. Three of the four males were born into families with other affected relatives; the fourth child was diagnosed at the age of three weeks. All four showed significant improvements in their development and clinical course. None were completely normal but their remaining clinical abnormalities were similar to those seen in patients with occipital horn syndrome. The oldest survivor of the group was 20 years old.

This information strongly supports the importance of nutritional therapy in the care of patients with Menkes syndrome. Early treatment is best but requires early diagnosis. It should also not be seen as a "cure." It has been shown to lessen the severity of the syndrome but not eliminate it. Thus, prenatal diagnosis, and its possible limitations, should continue to be discussed with prospective parents known to be at risk. Mutation studies should be performed, whenever possible, to increase the accuracy of testing results.

## Prognosis

Death often occurs by the age of three years in untreated males with classical Menkes syndrome, although longer-term survivors have been reported. Treatment with supplemental copper has resulted in improved physical development, milder mental handicap, and extended life span in some affected males. However, not all patients have responded to the same extent. Additionally, patients treated after the onset of symptoms have done worse than those treated before symptoms occur. Research is continuing to refine the best dosage of copper-histidine, determine the optimal timing and route of treatment, and develop newer treatment strategies.

## Resources

### BOOKS

Jones, Kenneth L., ed. *Smith's Recognizable Patterns of Human Malformations.* 5th ed. Philadelphia: W. B. Saunders Company, 1997.

### PERIODICALS

Christodoulou, John, David M. Danks, Bibudhendra Sarkar, Kurt E. Baerlocher, Robin Casey, Nina Horn, Zeynup Tumer, and Joe T.R. Clarke. "Early treatment of Menkes disease with parenteral copper-histidine: Long-term follow-up of four treated patients." *American Journal of Medical Genetics* 76, no. 2 (March 5, 1998): 154–64.

Kaler, Stephen G. "Diagnosis and therapy of Menkes syndrome, a genetic form of copper deficiency." *American Journal of Clinical Nutrition* 67 supplement (1998): 1029S–34S.

Kaler, Stephen G., and Zeynup Tumer. "Prenatal diagnosis of Menkes disease." *Prenatal Diagnosis* 18 (1998): 287–89.

Tumer, Zeynup, and Nina Horn. "Menkes disease: Underlying genetic defect and new diagnostic possibilities." *Journal of Inherited Metabolic Disease* 21, no. 5 (August 1998): 604–12.

### WEBSITES

"Menkes syndrome." U.S. National Library of Medicine. National Institutes of Health. http://www.nlm.nih.gov/mesh/jablonski/syndromes/syndrome422.html.

"NINDS Menkes Disease Information Page." National Institute of Neurological Disorders and Stroke. http://www.ninds.nih.gov/health_and_medical/disorders/menkes.htm.

Online Mendelian Inheritance in Man. http://www.ncbi.nlm.nih.gov/omim.

### ORGANIZATIONS

Corporation for Menkes Disease. 5720 Buckfield Court, Fort Wayne, IN 46804. (219) 436-0137.

Terri A. Knutel, MS, CGC

Mental retardation *see* **Smith-Fineman-Myers syndrome**

Mental retardation X-linked, syndrome 3 (MRXS3) *see* **Sutherland Haan X-linked mental retardation syndrome**

Mermaid syndrome *see* **Sirenomelia**

# Metaphyseal dysplasia

## Definition

Metaphyseal **dysplasia** is a very rare disorder in which the outer part of the shafts of long bones is unusually thin with a tendency to fracture. Aside from valgus knee deformities (commonly known as knock-knee), many patients with metaphyseal dysplasia exhibit few or no symptoms. The disorder comes in a variety of forms, some of which cause serious problems including mental retardation, blindness, and **deafness**.

## Description

Metaphyseal dysplasia is frequently mistaken for craniometaphyseal dysplasia, a disorder characterized by the thickening of the bones of the head. Metaphyseal dysplasia is genetically distinct from craniometaphyseal dysplasia and has only mild effects on the skull. In fact, metaphyseal dysplasia is so subtle, often it cannot be detected by clinical observation and is uncovered only when x rays are taken for another purpose. The signs are immediately visible on x rays, particularly the cone-like flaring that occurs on the tubular bones of the leg. This flaring is similar in shape to the Erlenmeyer glass flasks used in laboratories.

Another name for metaphyseal dysplasia is Pyle's disease, after Edwin Pyle (1891-1961), an orthopedic surgeon in Waterbury, CT Connecticut who first described it in 1931.

There are eight varieties of metaphyseal dysplasia. They are classified as: Jansen type, Schmid type, McKusick type, metaphyseal anadysplasia, Shwachman-Diamond metaphyseal dysplasia, adenosine deaminase deficiency, Spahr-type metaphyseal chondrodysplasia, and metaphyseal acroscyphodysplasia.

## Genetic profile

**Inheritance** of metaphyseal dysplasia is autosomal recessive, meaning that both parents are carriers of an abnormal **gene** when a child exhibits symptoms.

Children inheriting the gene from one parent become carriers. When both parents are carriers, each child has a 25% chance of having the disorder and a 50% chance of being a carrier. In the case of Jansen type metaphyseal dysplasia, the chromosomal gene locus is 3p22-p21.1. In Schmid type metaphyseal dysplasia, the locus is 6q21-q22.3. For McKusick type (cartilage-hair hypoplasia), it is 9p13. In adenosine deaminase deficiency, the locus is 20q-13.11. The modes of inheritance for Jansen type, Schmid type, and adenosine deaminase deficiency are all autosomal dominant, meaning that a child may inherit the disorder if just one parent is a carrier. For all other varieties of metaphyseal dysplasia the modes are autosomal recessive, with the possible exception of metaphyseal anadysplasia, which may be X-linked recessive. In that case, whenever one parent is a carrier of the disorder, each child would have a chance of either inheriting it or being a carrier.

## Demographics

This disorder is very rare, and the number of recorded cases is too small to draw firm demographic conclusions. There appears to be no preference based on sex.

## Signs and symptoms

The characteristic sign of metaphyseal dysplasia is splaying of the long bones, more severely than in craniometaphyseal dysplasia. Gross Erlenmeyer flask flaring is seen in the tubular bones of the leg, particularly in the femur. Unlike craniometaphyseal dysplasia, few signs occur in the skull in metaphyseal dysplasia, apart from protrusions over the eye sockets.

Metaphyseal dysplasia is also marked by expanded bones of the rib cage and pelvis, and by changes in the angle of the lower jaw. The humerus bone of the arm tends to be unusually broad. Other signs include **scoliosis** (a sideways curvature of the spine) and **osteoporosis** (a condition that makes bones brittle). Patients may complain of muscle weakness or joint pain.

Dentists may notice malocclusion, an inability of the teeth to properly close. Some spinal changes are possible, associated with the flaring of tubular bones. These may include platyspondyly, a broadening of the vertebrae.

### Jansen type

In addition to the above-mentioned signs, Jansen type metaphyseal chondrodysplasia is characterized by short arms, legs and stature (short-limbed dwarfism), which become apparent during early childhood. Affected children experience a gradual stiffening and swelling of their joints. Often, they develop a characteristic "waddling gait" and a stance that appears as if they were squatting. Some facial abnormalities may be evident at birth. These include prominent, widely spaced eyes, a receding chin, or a highly arched palate. Some affected adults develop unusually hardened bones in the back of the head, which sometimes results in deafness and/or blindness. Abnormal cartilage development may harden into rounded bone masses that may be noticeable on the hands, feet, and elsewhere. Other signs and symptoms associated with Jansen type metaphyseal chondrodysplasia include clubbed fingers, a fifth finger permanently fixed in a bent position, fractured ribs, mental retardation, psychomotor retardation, and high blood levels of calcium. Curvature of the spine in these patients may be front-to-back as well as sideways. Testing the blood and urine for calcium can assist in confirming a diagnosis. Jansen type metaphyseal chondrodysplasia was formerly referred to as metaphyseal dysostosis.

### Schmid type

Like Jansen type metaphyseal chondrodysplasia, Schmid type metaphyseal chondrodysplasia is also characterized by short-limbed dwarfism. Other special features may include an outward flaring of the lower rib cage, bowed legs, leg pain, a normal spine, and a hip deformity that causes the thigh bone to angle toward the body's center. Schmid type metaphyseal chondrodysplasia was first discovered in 1943 in a family of Mormons that had experienced 40 cases of the disorder over four generations. The first affected ancestor was traced back to 1833.

### McKusick type

Like Jansen type and Schmid type, McKusick type metaphyseal chondrodysplasia is marked by short-limb dwarfism. Other features include thin, light-colored hair, loose-jointed fingers, elbows that cannot be fully extended, **Hirschsprung disease** (a birth defect in which the usual nerve network fails to develop around the rectum, and in some cases, the colon), and

abnormalities of the immune system. In the shin, the tibia bone is uncharacteristically shorter than the fibula. Patients are at increased risk of developing cancers, especially of the skin and the lymph nodes. McKusick type metaphyseal chondrodysplasia is also known as cartilage hair hypoplasia syndrome. The disorder was first recognized in 1965 among the Old Order Amish. Billy Barty (1924-2000), the actor who founded the dwarfism advocacy group Little People of America, had McKusick type metaphyseal chondrodysplasia.

### Metaphyseal anadysplasia

First noticed in 1971, metaphyseal anadysplasia is a form of metaphyseal dysplasia that starts early. Instead of appearing after puberty, some signs were found to be present at birth, but disappeared after two years. For example, parts of the long bones were irregular. In the thigh bones of these patients, there was an unusually low level of red blood cell production.

### Shwachman-Diamond syndrome

In addition to the skeletal system, Shwachman-Diamond syndrome also affects the pancreas. It is characterized by inadequate absorption of fats because of abnormal pancreatic development and bone marrow dysfunction. Other unusual symptoms and signs include short stature, liver abnormalities, and low levels of any or all blood cells. Reduced levels of white blood cells may cause these patients to be vulnerable to repeated bouts with pneumonia, otitis media, and other bacterial infections. Shwachman-Diamond syndrome is also referred to as Shwachman-Bodian syndrome, Shwachman-Diamond-Oski syndrome, Shwachman syndrome, and congenital lipomatosis of the pancreas. Some researchers call it pancreatic insufficiency and bone marrow dysfunction.

### Adenosine deaminase deficiency

A deficiency of adenosine deaminase (ADA), an essential, broadly distributed enzyme, causes **severe combined immunodeficiency** disease. This can bring about a wide range of effects, including **asthma**, pneumonia, sinusitis, diarrhea, problems with the liver, kidneys, spleen and skeletal system, and failure to thrive. ADA deficiency is similar to McKusick type metaphyseal chondrodysplasia in that both disorders include skeletal changes and problems with cellular immunity. ADA deficiency earned a special place in **genetics** history in 1990, when, in the first application of **gene therapy** in humans, it was corrected using genetically engineered blood.

### Spahr type metaphyseal chondrodysplasia

This is one of several disorders that used to be called metaphyseal dysostosis. It is extremely rare, and its features include severely bowed legs and short-statured dwarfism. In some cases, the bowing of the knees is so severe as to require surgical correction. Spahr type is very similar to Schmid type metaphyseal chondrodysplasia, except that inheritance is believed to be autosomal recessive in Spahr type, unlike Schmid type, which is autosomal dominant.

### Metaphyseal acroscyphodysplasia

This variety is also referred to as wedge-shaped epiphyses of the knees. Its special features include severely retarded growth, psychomotor retardation, abnormally small arms and legs, extremely short fingers, and curvature of the knees.

## Diagnosis

Diagnosis is usually by x ray, in which the bone deformities of metaphyseal dysplasia are very noticeable, even if not apparent in a normal clinical examination. A medical doctor will look for valgus knee deformities. A radiologist will look for Erlenmeyer-flask shaped femur bones and ensure that any deformities to cranial bones are minor, to rule out craniometaphyseal dysplasia. The radiologist will also watch for abnormally broad humerus, radius and ulna bones.

## Treatment and management

Metaphyseal dysplasia cannot be directly treated, but some individual symptoms, such as osteoporosis or joint problems, may be treated or surgically corrected.

## Prognosis

In many cases, patients with metaphyseal dysplasia may be symptomless and very healthy. Other patients, including those with Jansen type metaphyseal chondro-dysplasia, may have more severe complications including blindness, deafness, or mental retardation.

## Resources

### PERIODICALS

Pyle, E. "Case of unusual bone development." *Journal of Bone and Joint Surgery*: 3 (1931): 874-876.

Raad, M. S., and P. Beighton. "Autosomal recessive inheritance of metaphyseal dysplasia (Pyle disease)." *Clinical Genetics*: 14 (1978) 251-256.

Turra, S., C. Gigante, G. Pavanini, and C. Bardi. "Spinal involvement in Pyle's disease." *Pediatric Radiology* (January 2000) 25-27.

David L. Helwig

# Methylmalonic acidemia

## Definition

Methylmalonic acidemia (MMA) is a group of disorders characterized by the accumulation of methylmalonic acid in the fluids of the affected individual. The first recognized cases of these disorders were described in 1967. All known genetic forms of MMA are non-sex linked (autosomal) and recessive. Some non-genetic cases have been reported in which the affected individuals were vegetarians who had been on prolonged cobalamin (vitamin $B_{12}$) deficient diets.

## Description

Methylmalonic acidemia (MMA) is characterized by an accumulation of methylmalonic acid in the blood stream, which leads to an abnormally low pH (high acidity) in nearly every cell in the body (metabolic acidosis). A higher than normal accumulation of ketones in the blood stream (ketosis) similar to that seen in instances of **diabetes** mellitus is also associated with MMA. If left untreated, metabolic acidosis is often fatal.

Methylmalonic acid is an intermediate in the metabolism of fats and proteins. This chemical accumulates in the bodies of individuals with MMA because of a partial or complete inability of these individuals to convert methylmalonyl-CoA to succinyl-CoA in the tricarboxlic acid (TCA) cycle.

## KEY TERMS

**Apoenzyme**—An enzyme that cannot function without assistance from other chemicals called cofactors.

**ATP**—Adenosine triphosphate. The chemical used by the cells of the body for energy.

**Cofactor**—A substance that is required by an enzyme to perform its function.

**Ketosis**—An abnormal build-up of chemicals called ketones in the blood. This condition usually indicates a problem with blood sugar regulation.

**Metabolic acidosis**—High acidity (low pH) in the body due to abnormal metabolism, excessive acid intake, or retention in the kidneys.

**Methylmalomic acid**—An intermediate product formed when certain substances are broken down in order to create usable energy for the body.

**Sudden infant death syndrome (SIDS)**—The general term given to "crib deaths" of unknown causes.

**TCA cycle**—Formerly know as the Kreb's cycle, this is the process by which glucose and other chemicals are broken down into forms that are directly useable as energy in the cells.

MMA is one of the **genetic disorders** that cause problems with mitochondrial metabolism. The mitochondria are the organelles inside cells that are responsible for energy production and respiration at the cellular level. One of the most important processes in the mitochondria is the TCA cycle (also known as the Krebs cycle). The TCA cycle produces the majority of the ATP (chemical energy) necessary for maintenance (homeostasis) of the cell. When blood sugar (glucose) is broken down in preparation to enter the TCA cycle, it is broken down into a chemical known as acetyl-CoA. It is this acetyl-CoA that is then further broken down in the TCA cycle to yield carbon dioxide, water, and ATP. When some fatty acids and certain amino acids from proteins (specifically isoleucine, valine, threonine, methionine, thymine, and uracil) are broken down in preparation to enter the TCA cycle, they are broken down into propionyl-CoA, rather than acetyl-CoA. This propionyl-CoA is then converted into methylmalonyl-CoA, which is next converted to succinyl-CoA. It is succinyl-CoA that enters the TCA cycle to eventually yield carbon dioxide, water, and the ATP needed by the cells.

The conversion of methylmalonyl-CoA to succinyl-CoA involves the apoenzyme methylmalonyl-CoA mutase. An apoenzyme is an enzyme that cannot function without the aid of other chemicals (cofactors). One of the cofactors for this apoenzyme is cobalamin (vitamin $B_{12}$). Genetic MMA is a result of either a deficiency in the methylmalonyl-CoA mutase apoenzyme or a defect in the mechanism inside the cells that converts dietary vitamin $B_{12}$ into its useable form for this chemical reaction.

An enzyme is a chemical that facilitates (catalyzes) the chemical reaction of another chemical or of other chemicals; it is neither a reactant nor a product in the chemical reaction that it facilitates. As a result, enzymes are not used up in chemical reactions; they are recycled. One molecule of an enzyme may be used to facilitate the same chemical reaction over and over again several hundreds of thousands of times. All the enzymes necessary for catalyzing the various reactions of human life are produced within the body by genes. In the case of the enzyme deficiency that causes MMA, the enzyme consists of a genetically produced apoenzyme and a cofactor (vitamin $B_{12}$) that comes from dietary sources.

### Genetic profile

The **gene** responsible for MMA has been mapped to 6p21.2-p12. At least 30 mutations in this gene have been identified which lead to a broad spectrum of clinical symptoms and severities.

### Demographics

The exact frequency of MMA is not known. It is believed to occur with a frequency of approximately one in every 48,000 live births in the United States. As in all recessive non-sex linked (autosomal) genetic disorders, both parents must carry the gene mutation in order for their child to have the disorder. Therefore, in cases where the parents are related by blood (consanguineous), the occurrence rate is higher than in the rest of the population. Parents with one child affected by MMA have a 25% likelihood that their next child will also be affected with MMA.

No increased likelihood for the disease on the basis of sex or ethnicity has been observed in cases of MMA.

### Signs and symptoms

The abnormally high levels of acid in the blood of individuals affected with MMA can produce drowsiness, seizures, and in severe cases, coma and/or stroke. Prolonged acidemia can cause mental retardation. In the very rare instances of a complete apoenzyme absence, MMA is associated with sudden infant death syndrome (SIDS) and at least one known case of sudden child death at an age of 11 months.

Dehydration and failure to thrive are generally the first signs of MMA. These symptoms are generally accompanied by lethargy, lack of muscle tone (hypotonia), and "floppiness" in newborns.

Developmental delay is typically experienced in all individuals affected with MMA if treatment is not instigated early in life.

Some individuals affected with MMA have facial dysmorphisms. These include a broad nose, a high forehead, a skin fold of the upper eyelid (epicanthal folds), and a lack of the normal groove in the skin between the nose and the upper lip (the philtrum). In a few individuals affected with MMA, skin lesions resulting from yeast infections (candidosis) may be present, particularly in the mouth and facial area.

Occasionally, enlargement of the liver (hepatomegaly) is seen in MMA affected individuals.

Uncoordinated muscle movements (choreoathetosis), disordered muscle tone (**dystonia**), slurred speech (dysarthria), and difficulty swallowing (dysphagia), when observed in individuals with MMA, may be signs of an acidemia-induced stroke.

### Diagnosis

In newborns, a history of poor feeding, increasing lethargy, and vomiting are typical symptoms of MMA. In older infants, an episode of lethargy, often accompanied by seizures, is symptomatic. In children or adolescents, the symptoms may include muscle weakness, loss or diminishment of sensation in the legs, and/or blood clots.

Kidney (renal) disease may be observed in affected individuals with long untreated MMA.

A blood test to detect high levels of MMA is a decisive test for MMA. It may also be detected via a urine test for abnormally high levels of the chemical methylmalonate.

Prenatally, MMA may be diagnosed by measuring the activity of the apoenzyme methylmalonyl-CoA mutase in cultured cells grown from the cells obtained during an **amniocentesis**.

In one MMA-related case, a woman named Patricia Stallings was sentenced to life imprisonment for the presumed poisoning of her infant son with ethylene glycol, an ingredient in antifreeze. It was not until she gave birth in prison to a second son affected with MMA (and properly diagnosed) that forensic investigators discovered that the gas chromatography peak originally assigned to ethylene glycol (and used to convict Ms. Stallings) was, in fact, methylmalonic acid. All charges against Ms. Stallings were dropped and she was released from prison. This is an extreme case, but it certainly shows the importance of proper medical diagnosis of MMA.

Family history is often used to diagnose MMA when there are affected siblings or siblings that died shortly after birth for unclear reasons.

### Treatment and management

Individuals affected with MMA are generally placed on low, or no, protein diets supplemented with carnitine and cobalamin (vitamin $B_{12}$) and alkalinizing agents (such as bicarbonate) to neutralize the excess acid caused by MMA. Intravenous administration of glucose may be necessary during acute attacks. In individuals who do not respond to carnitine and/or cobalamin, the anti-bacterial drug, metronidazole, may be prescribed. This drug kills some of the naturally occurring bacteria in the lower digestive tract and thereby reduces the production of propionate, a precursor chemical to methylmalonic acid.

In cases of severe MMA, kidney and/or liver transplants may be called for.

### Prognosis

With appropriate care and diet, MMA is a controllable disease that offers no threat of death or permanent disability in patients beyond the first year of life. If unchecked, MMA can lead to permanent, irreversible disabilities or conditions, or even death. Some infants affected with extremely severe genetic mutations are stillborn or die prior to an appropriate diagnosis of MMA being made.

### Resources

#### PERIODICALS

Smith, Bill. "Not Guilty: How the System Failed Patricia Stallings." *St. Louis Post-Dispatch International Pediatrics* (October 20, 1991): 1+.

Varvogli, L. G. Repetto, S. Waisbren, and H. Levy. "High cognitive outcome in an adolescent with mut- methylmalonic acidemia." *American Journal of Medical Genetics* (April 2000): 192-5.

#### WEBSITES

"Entry 251000: Methylmalonicaciduria due to methylmalonic CoA mutase deficiency." *OMIM—Online Mendelian Inheritance in Man.* http://www.ncbi.nlm. nih.gov/ entrez/dispomim.cgi? = 251000. (December 10, 2009).

"Methylmalonic acidemia."*eMedicine*. http://www.emedicine.com/ped/topic1438.htm. (February 15, 2001).

**ORGANIZATIONS**

National Organization for Rare Disorders (NORD). 55 Kenosia Ave. PO Box 1968, Danbury, CT 06813. (203) 744-0100 or (800) 999-6673. Fax: (203) 798-2291. http://www.rarediseases.org.

Organic Acidemia Association. PO Box 1008, Pinole, CA 94564. (510) 672-2476, (866) 539-4060. Fax: (863) 694-0017. http://www.oaanews.org.

Paul A. Johnson

# Methylmalonicaciduria due to methylmalonic CoA mutase deficiency

## Definition

Methylmalonicaciduria results from an autosomal recessive inherited genetic defect in methylmalonic CoA mutase (MCM), an enzyme required for the proper metabolism of some protein components, cholesterol, and fatty acids. As a result of a deficiency in MCM, methylmalonic acid accumulates in the bloodstream and urine, causing a severe metabolic disorder that may lead to death. Treatment consists chiefly of diet modification and the administration of several medications that may counteract this process.

## Description

Proteins are important building blocks of the body, serving many different functions. They provide the structure of muscles, tissues and organs, and regulate many functions of the human body. Proteins are made from amino acids obtained through the digestion of proteins (found in meats, dairy products, and other foods in the diet). Excess protein that is not required by the body can be broken down into its individual amino acid components. These amino acids can then be converted into glucose or directly enter metabolic pathways that supply the body with energy.

Each of the approximately 20 amino acids that are used to make human proteins are metabolized by specific biochemical reactions. Several of these amino acids (isoleucine, valine, threonine, methionine), as well as cholesterol and some fatty acids, share a common biochemical reaction in the pathway to conversion to usable energy. Each of these substances is converted to methylmalonic acid (also known as

## KEY TERMS

**Amino acid**—Organic compounds that form the building blocks of protein. There are 20 types of amino acids (eight are "essential amino acids" which the body cannot make and must therefore be obtained from food).

**Antibiotics**—A group of medications that kill or slow the growth of bacteria.

**Autosomal recessive**—A pattern of genetic inheritance where two abnormal genes are needed to display the trait or disease.

**Carrier**—A person who possesses a gene for an abnormal trait without showing signs of the disorder. The person may pass the abnormal gene on to offspring.

**Cofactor**—A substance that is required by an enzyme to perform its function.

**Enzyme**—A protein that catalyzes a biochemical reaction or change without changing its own structure or function.

**Methylmalonic acid**—An intermediate product formed when certain substances are broken down in order to create usable energy for the body.

**Methylmalonic CoA mutase (MCM)**—The enzyme responsible for converting methylmalonic acid to succinic acid, in the pathway to convert certain substances to usable energy.

**Methylmalonicacidemia**—The buildup of high levels of methylmalonic acid in the bloodstream due to an inborn defect in an enzyme.

**Methylmalonicaciduria**—The buildup of high levels of methylmalonic acid in the urine due to an inborn defect in an enzyme.

**Mutation**—A permanent change in the genetic material that may alter a trait or characteristic of an individual, or manifest as disease, and can be transmitted to offspring.

**Protein**—Important building blocks of the body, composed of amino acids, involved in the formation of body structures and controlling the basic functions of the human body.

methylmalonic CoA), an intermediate product on the pathway leading to the production of usable energy.

In the next step of this biochemical pathway, methylmalonic acid is converted to succinic acid (also called succinyl CoA) by the enzyme, methylmalonic CoA mutase (MCM). In order for MCM to function properly, it also requires a vitamin $B_{12}$-derivative called adenosylcobalamin (when an enzyme requires another substance in order to perform its job, the helping substance is known as a coenzyme or cofactor).

When there is a defect or deficiency of MCM, methylmalonic acid cannot be converted into succinic acid and methylmalonic acid accumulates in high levels in the bloodstream (methylmalonicacidemia) and in the urine (methylmalonicaciduria). A deficiency in the cofactor, adenosylcobalamin, renders the MCM enzyme unable to perform its job, and will cause a similar effect. Abnormally high amounts of methylmalonic acid in the bloodstream causes a serious and dangerous metabolic condition that may lead to death.

The condition of methylmalonicacidemia was first described by V. G. Oberholzer in 1967 in infants critically sick with accumulations of methylmalonic acid in their blood and urine. An interesting historical note in respect to this disorder relates to the story of a woman named Patricia Stallings. In 1989, Ms. Stallings brought her son, Ryan, to the emergency room in St. Louis because he was very ill, and Ryan was noted to have high levels of acid in his bloodstream. Poisoning with ethylene glycol (antifreeze) also produces high levels of acid in the bloodstream. When Ryan later died, Ms. Stallings was sentenced to life in prison in January 1991, for the crime of murder by poisoning. While in prison the woman gave birth to a second son, who was diagnosed with the condition, methylmalonicacidemia. After discovering this diagnosis, scientists examined frozen samples of the first son's blood and determined that he, too, had methylmalonicacidemia, which was responsible for his death. All charges against Ms. Stallings were dropped, and she was released from prison in September 1991. This is a dramatic illustration of the critical importance of proper diagnosis of complicated and rare **genetic disorders**.

## Genetic profile

MCM deficiency is a genetic condition and can be inherited or passed on in a family. The genetic defect for the disorder is inherited as an autosomal recessive trait, meaning that two abnormal genes are needed to display the disease. A person who carries one abnormal gene does not display the disease and is called a carrier. A carrier has a 50% chance of transmitting the gene to their children, who must inherit one disease gene from each parent to display the disease.

At least two forms of MCM deficiency have been identified. The disease genes are called, *mut0*, in which there is no detectable enzyme activity, and *mut-*, in which there is some, but greatly reduced, enzyme activity present. The gene for MCM is located on **chromosome** 6 (locus 6p21), and about 30 different mutations in the gene have been reported. Other mutations in pathways that produce the cofactor, adenosylcobalamin, exist and produce a condition similar to MCM deficiency.

## Demographics

The incidence of all the conditions that cause methylmalonicacidemia was reported in a Massachusetts screening program at approximately one in 48,000 births. About half of the reported patients with methylmalonicacidemia have a deficiency of MCM *mut0* or *mut-*), as opposed to problems with the cofactor. Thus, incidence of specific MCM deficiency-related methylmalonicacidemia and aciduria in the general population may be estimated as one in 96,000. The geographical distribution of methylmalonicacidemia is not uniform and may be higher in certain ethnic groups. One report shows that the disorder is more common in the Middle East, probably occurring in one in 1,000 or 2,000 births. MCM deficiency is seen in equal amounts in males and females.

## Signs and symptoms

The symptoms experienced by an infant with MCM deficiency vary with the type of mutation present. Infants born with the *mut0* type MCM deficiency will typically show more severe symptoms that manifest in the first one to two weeks of life, while infants with the *mut-* type MCM deficiency have slightly milder symptoms that begin later in infancy.

Both sets of infants may show poor feeding, vomiting, lethargy, and low muscle tone, as well as a failure to grow at the normal rate. The disorder may first come to medical attention as it escalates into a full scale overwhelming attack, often triggered by intake of large amounts of dietary protein. If the condition has not yet been diagnosed, treatment is often poor, and patients may experience kidney damage, inflammation of the pancreas, or strokes that result in severe paralysis. More severe attacks can lead to seizures, coma and eventually, death. As a result, newborns and infants with MCM deficiency may die early, even before a diagnosis can be reached.

If the infant survives the first attack, similar attacks may occur during an infection or following ingestion of a high-protein diet. Between episodes the patient may appear normal, but often, mild to moderate mental retardation will develop. Some infants with this disorder have characteristic facial features with a broad nose bridge, prominent lower eyelid folds, triangular mouth and high forehead. Other symptoms of the disorder include frequent infections (especially yeast infections of the skin and mouth), enlarged liver, and low amounts of red blood cells. Often a family history is present for affected siblings or siblings that died very early in life for unclear reasons.

A small percentage of people with the MCM deficiency apparently experience no symptoms or complications of the disease. For reasons not yet understood, these patients can tolerate a normal protein intake and accumulate high levels of methylmalonic acid in their body fluids without consequence.

### Diagnosis

When symptoms are encountered in a young infant or newborn, a diagnostic search for MCM deficiency should be considered. A routine blood test performed on almost all people who come to the hospital with severe illness will show high levels of acid in the bloodstream. Other clues to possible MCM deficiency include high levels of other substances in the bloodstream that appear with methylmalonicacidemia such as ketones and ammonia, or the presence of abnormally low amounts of glucose or red blood cells.

After high levels of acid in the bloodstream are noted, and if methylmalonicacidemia is suspected, samples of the urine and the blood are taken and tested for the amount of methylmalonic acid. Abnormally high levels of methylmalonic acid suggest that MCM deficiency may be present. Genetic studies can then be performed to determine if any mutation in the MCM gene is present.

When the disease is diagnosed in a child, research laboratories can test unaffected siblings to determine if they are carriers of the mutant MCM gene. The same technology can be used to diagnose MCM deficiency before the birth of a child, by analyzing fluid or tissue from the sac surrounding the unborn fetus.

### Treatment and management

Current research into a cure for MCM deficiency is focusing on the ability of liver transplantation or **gene therapy** to correct the abnormal MCM gene, however there is no cure for MCM deficiency at this time. The methods of treatment focus on three areas: diet/lifestyle modification, treatment with medications, and support during severe attacks of the disease.

Dietary changes include restriction of the amino acids that are converted to methylmalonic acid: methionine, threonine, valine, and isoleucine. As a result, people with MCM deficiency are limited to a low protein diet that provides the minimum natural protein needed for growth. Calcium and multivitamin supplements should also be taken to correct any nutritional deficiencies that result from avoiding high-protein foods. Activity in children with MCM deficiency need not be restricted.

People with MCM deficiency may benefit from several medications when taken daily. The antibiotic, metronidazole, kills bacteria that live in the intestine which produce substances that are converted to methylmalonic acid. The supplement, L-carnitine, is often used to reduce some of the toxic effects of high levels of methylmalonic acid. Although most reports state that there is no benefit from vitamin $B_{12}$ supplementation, a few reports suggest that a trial of vitamin $B_{12}$ may be reasonable to determine if it will result in improved MCM function. Finally, bicarbonate can be used to counteract low levels of acid that persist in the bloodstream.

All of these medications can be used to aid in treatment of a severe attack of methylmalonicacidemia. In addition, a patient in crisis should be given excessive amounts of intravenous fluids, to help clear methylmalonic acid from the circulation. Special blood filtering machines can be used when levels of methylmalonic acid or ammonia become dangerously high. Stressful situations that may trigger attacks (such as infection) should be treated promptly.

Patients with MCM deficiency should be seen regularly by a team of health care specialists including a primary care provider, a dietician, and a biochemical geneticist who is familiar with the management of the disease. Parents should be educated in the signs and symptoms of impending attacks and how to respond appropriately. Close monitoring of amino acid levels, urinary content of methylmalonic acid, and growth progress is necessary to ensure proper balance in the diet and the success of therapy.

### Prognosis

Prognosis depends on early and accurate diagnosis of the disease and the prompt initiation of diet modification and medications. In those infants who escape early diagnosis, the prognosis is poor as severe attacks lead to complications as extreme as sudden death. In those infants that do survive initial attacks, damage to the developing brain and kidneys may result that leave the child severely incapacitated.

The addition of the medications, L-carnitine and metronidazole, to the management of this disorder has changed the prognosis. Before 1985 most patients died; those diagnosed after 1985, when these drugs were introduced, survived with improved general health. Thus, if detected early and treated appropriately, the lifestyle of a well-managed patient with MCM deficiency can be relatively normal, without mental retardation or growth delay.

### Resources

#### BOOKS

Behrman, R. E., ed. *Nelson Textbook of Pediatrics*. Philadelphia: W. B. Saunders, 2000.

Fauci, A. S., ed. *Harrison's Principles of Internal Medicine*. New York: McGraw-Hill, 1998.

#### PERIODICALS

Ledley, F. D. "Mutations in mut methylmalonic acidemia: clinical and enzymatic correlations." *Human Mutation* 9 (1997): 1–6.

#### WEBSITES

"Methylmalonicaciduria due to MCM Deficiency." Online Mendelian Inheritance in Man. http://www.ncbi.nlm. nih.gov/entrez/dispomim.cgi?id = 251000.

#### ORGANIZATIONS

Support Groups For MMA Organic Acidemia Association. 13210 35th Avenue Plymouth, MN 55441. (763) 559-1797. http://www.oaanews.

Oren Traub, MD, PhD

# Micro syndrome

## Definition

Micro syndrome is a rare genetic disorder. Children born with this condition may experience mental retardation, seizures, visual impairment, difficulty eating, and weakness, numbness, and/or abnormal sensations in the limbs.

Alternate names associated with micro syndrome are Warburg micro syndrome, WARBM, and Warburg Sjo Fledelius syndrome.

## Demographics

Micro syndrome is very rare, and, only a few dozen cases have been reported in the literature since its initial description in 1993.

## Description

Researchers described and named micro syndrome in 1993, but others had reported patients with what was probably the same malady as early as 1949. In the 1993 description, the researchers noted the symptoms of a Pakistani brother and sister and their male cousin. The symptoms included a small head and eyes, cataracts and near blindness, mental retardation, excessive facial hair, decreased muscle tone (hypotonia), and incontinence.

Micro syndrome is an inherited disorder resulting from mutations in a **gene** that carries instructions for a membrane-associated Rab3 protein. This protein is important in the secretion of various substances from cells. These substances include neurotransmitters (chemicals that transmit nerve impulses) and hormones. The mutated gene produces faulty proteins, which in turn inhibit the proper flow of neurotransmitters and/or hormones and can lead to a wide range of symptoms.

## Causes and symptoms

Micro syndrome is an autosomal recessive disorder. It occurs when individuals inherit a mutated RAB3GAP gene from each parent. The parents may not have the condition themselves but may be carriers. Carriers are individuals who do not develop the disorder themselves but may pass the gene for the disorder onto their children. If both parents are carriers, each of their children has a 50% chance of being a carrier and a 25% chance of acquiring the disorder. If both parents have micro syndrome, all of their children will acquire the disorder.

---

**Symptoms of Micro syndrome**

Mental retardation
Seizures
A small head (microcephaly)
Slow development of the external reproductive organs
Abnormally small eyes
Visual impairment
Cloudiness of the eye lenses (cataracts)
Drooping eyelid (ptosis)
Difficulty swallowing and therefore feeding
An undersized jaw (micrognathia)
A beaked nose
Decreased muscle tone (hypotonia)
Weakness and numbness in the limbs
Abnormal sensations in the limbs
Inability of the limbs to fully extend (joint contracture)
Delayed puberty

*(Table by GGS Creative Resources. Reproduced by permission of Gale, a part of Cengage Learning.)*

### Genetic profile

Located on **chromosome** 2, the RAB3GAP gene carries the blueprint for making the Rab3 protein, which actually comes in two forms. This gene is important in several normal functions, which include the following:

- Transmission of signals between nerve cells and between other cells and nerve cells. This function allows nerve impulses to travel properly, so that the body may move and function correctly.
- Release of hormones from cells. Hormones travel in the bloodstream to other areas of the body, where they can have an effect on such body processes as growth and development, sexual function and reproduction, and metabolism.

Mutations in the RAB3GAP gene are believed to lead to defects in both the transmission of nerve impulses and the secretion of hormones from cells.

### Symptoms

Many symptoms of micro syndrome are present at birth, but others will become evident as time goes on. Symptoms may include the following:

- mental retardation
- seizures
- small head (microcephaly)
- hypogenitalism (retarded development of the external reproductive organs)
- abnormally small eyes
- visual impairment
- cloudiness of the eye lenses (cataracts)
- drooping eyelid (ptosis)
- difficulty swallowing and therefore feeding
- undersized jaw (micrognathia)
- beaked nose
- decreased muscle tone (hypotonia)
- weakness and numbness in the limbs
- abnormal sensations in the limbs, such as burning or tingling (paresthesia)
- muscle spasms
- inability of the limbs to fully extend (joint contracture)
- delayed puberty

## Diagnosis

### Examination

Doctors may focus primarily on the eyes to make a preliminary diagnosis of micro syndrome. Individuals with the disorder have congenital cataracts, small eyes,

---

## KEY TERMS

**Agenesis/hypoplasia of the corpus callosum**—Birth defect in which the two halves of the brain are not properly separated.

**Cataracts**—Cloudiness of the eye lenses.

**Hypogenitalism**—Retarded development of the external reproductive organs.

**Hypotonia**—Decreased muscle tone.

**Joint contracture**—Inability of the limbs to fully extend.

**Microcephaly**—Small head.

**Micrognathia**—Undersized jaw.

**Neurotransmitters**—Chemicals that transmit nerve impulses.

**Paresthesia**—Presence of abnormal sensations in the limbs.

**Ptosis**—Drooping eyelid.

---

and visual impairment. The diagnosis is made more solid when the infant also shows other symptoms such as severe mental retardation and movement problems.

### Tests

The doctor may order cell samples be examined for the mutated RAB3GAP gene.

### Procedures

The doctor may order an MRI (magnetic resonance imaging) scan to check the patient for malformations of the brain. Patients with micro syndrome typically show agenesis/hypoplasia of the corpus callosum, in which the two halves of the brain are not properly separated. An MRI can detect this abnormality.

## Treatment and management

No treatment exists for micro syndrome, but some help is available to ease some of the symptoms.

### Traditional

A common treatment for cataracts is surgery to remove or dissolve the affected lens. Doctors often recommend physical therapy to help improve muscle tone, to promote full extension of the limbs, and to counter muscle spasms. They may also suggest occupational therapy and speech therapy.

### Drugs

For recurring seizures, doctors may prescribe anti-seizure medication.

### Prognosis

Individuals with micro syndrome are of normal weight at birth, but soon show signs of slowed growth. Other symptoms such as evidence of mental retardation, decreased muscle tone, and movement impairment may also soon begin appearing. By the first birthday, the baby typically has experienced muscle spasms. Children with this disorder can speak few if any words by the time they are ten years old. Many experience incontinence, and some may be unable to walk or even sit up on their own. Puberty is delayed. Vision may decline over time.

### Prevention

There is no way to prevent micro syndrome. Partners who are both carriers of the mutated RAB3GAP gene should consult with a genetics counselor before considering a pregnancy.

### Resources

#### OTHER

Center for Arab Genomic Studies. "Warburg Micro Syndrome." *The Catalogue for Transmission Genetics in Arabs, CTGA Database*. http://www.cags.org.ae/pdf/600118.pdf.
Derbent, Murat, and Pinar Agras. "Micro Syndrome." *Orphanet*. http://www.orpha.net/data/patho/GB/uk-MicroSyndrome.pdf.
Microsyndrome.com. http://microsyndrome.com/default.aspx.
MakingContact.org. http://www.makingcontact.org/index.php?ci=1711.
National Center for Biotechnology Information. "Warburg Micro Syndrome; WARBM." http://www.ncbi.nlm.nih.gov/entrez/dispomim.cgi?id=600118.

Leslie A. Mertz, PHD

# Microcephaly (childhood)

## Definition

Microcephaly is a condition in which the size of the skull and the brain is abnormally small. According to the American Academy of Neurology, the specific criterion for microcephaly is a head circumference that is more than two standard deviations below mean size. Some researchers classify severe microcephaly as head circumference that is more than three standard deviations below mean size.

## Demographics

It is estimated that microcephaly occurs in one out of 4,000 births. When the cause is **inheritance** through an autosomal recessive pattern (one parent carries the **gene**), the incidence is believed to range from 0.2 to 0.33 out of 10,000 births. In the United States, 25,000 infants are diagnosed with microcephaly each year. Incidence is higher in cultures where marriage of close blood relatives is acceptable.

## Description

Microcephaly is an abnormally small sized skull and brain. The defect can be the result of hundreds of factors — genetic causes, exposure to alcohol or other drugs, maternal illness during pregnancy, and environment issues — that may affect brain development. Researchers now classify microcephaly as either congenital or postnatal.

Congenital microcephaly is also referred to as primary microcephaly. Other forms are sometimes called secondary microcephaly.

Microcephaly is often diagnosed in children with **cerebral palsy**, **epilepsy**, cognitive impairments, and developmental delays.

### Risk factors

Risk factors include maternal exposure to certain illnesses, radiation, or toxins during pregnancy. The condition may also be inherited in an autosomal recessive (carried by both parents) or autosomal dominant (carried by one parent) pattern. This means that a child may inherit it if one or both parents carry the chromosomal defect.

Babies born with syndromes such as **Down syndrome** are at higher risk for microcephaly.

### Causes and symptoms

The specific causes of microcephaly are numerous, including:

- Chromosomal. Trisomies 13, 18, and 21
- Degenerative disorders of the mother. Tay-Sachs
- Familial genetics. Autosomal dominant pattern (only one parent carries the gene defect) or autosomal recessive pattern (both parents carry the gene defect)
- Malformations. Lissencephaly, schizencephaly
- Maternal nervous system infections during pregnancy. Bacterial meningitis (group B Streptococcus) or viral encephalitis, herpes virus
- Maternal infections during pregnancy. TORCH complex of maternal infections. TORCH is an acronym for toxoplasmosis, other infections, rubella, cytomegalovirus (CMV), and herpes simplex virus.
- Metabolic disorders of the mother. Phenylketonuria (PKU), maple syrup urine disease
- Placental insufficiency. Toxemia
- Radiation exposure
- Syndromes. Down (most common syndrome cause of microcephaly; 30% of Down syndrome babies have microcephaly), Rubinstein-Taybi, Angelman
- Toxin exposure. Fetal alcohol syndrome, possibly other drugs, such as anticonvulsant medication

In addition to these factors, scientists believe that congenital microcephaly may be caused by maternal tobacco smoking during pregnancy and uncontrolled or poorly controlled **diabetes**. Older children may develop microcephaly due to lead poisoning or chronic renal failure. It is possible that nearly any chronic disease may contribute to microcephaly.

Symptoms include presence of an abnormally undersized skull and brain, usually accompanied by mental retardation.

### Diagnosis

#### Examination

The head circumference of a baby is measured at birth. Follow-up measurements are performed during the first three to five years of life. If microcephaly is to be

## KEY TERMS

**Circumference**—The length around a circle.

**Encephalitis**—Inflammation of the brain.

**Lissencephaly**—A condition in which the brain lacks folds and is smooth.

**Mean**— The average numerical value, such as size, in a set of numbers.

**Neuroimaging**—Imaging studies of the brain, such as x ray, computed tomography (CT) scans, or magnetic resonance imaging (MRI) scans.

**Schizencephaly**—A rare disorder caused by abnormal slits within the brain.

**Standard deviation**—A statistical term that refers to the spread of data in a numerical distribution.

**Trisomy**—Three chromosomes in each cell, rather than two.

found after birth, most frequently the diagnosis will is made by the time the child is two to three years of age.

Head circumference is measured with a measuring tape that is flexible but cannot be stretched. It is placed tightly around the largest portion of the back of the head (occiput), and gently but firmly wrapped around to the front of the head. If the measurement is two standard deviations below normal for the child's age, the measurement's accuracy should be verified and its plot on the growth chart rechecked.

#### Tests

If microcephaly is found, imaging studies and **genetic testing** are performed to attempt to determine the cause. Since children with microcephaly face higher risk for disorders such as cerebral palsy and epilepsy, testing for these conditions should be performed as well.

#### Procedures

Microcephaly may be diagnosed prior to birth, during a sonography (ultrasound) procedure in the latter stages of pregnancy.

Babies may undergo magnetic resonance imaging (MRI) studies to determine brain size and check for abnormalities in the brain

### Treatment and management

#### Traditional

Treatment is supportive. Neuroimaging is important in treating babies with microcephaly to help determine the extent of the disorder.

### Prognosis

About 20-30% of infants with severe microcephaly will die. Those who survive have a prognosis that includes intellectual deficiency, developmental delays, neurological disorders such as epilepsy, and mental retardation. Treatment is supportive.

**Genetic counseling** is recommended for families who have a case of microcephaly within the family.

### Prevention

Microcephaly may develop if the fetus is exposed to a number of infections or toxic substances. Avoiding alcohol, recreational drugs, and possibly certain medications, as well as maintaining optimum health during pregnancy are steps that a mother can take to lower her chances of giving birth to a child with microcephaly. Infections also play a role, and it is important for the pregnant woman to take steps to minimize her chance of acquiring infection. For example, toxoplasmosis is one potential cause of microcephaly, and may be transmitted in feline feces; therefore, pregnant women should not clean feline litter boxes.

If it is suspected that the gene may be present in either the mother or the father, genetic counseling is recommended.

Proper prenatal health care is essential to ensuring that, if health problems arise, they will be appropriately managed.

### Resources

#### BOOKS

Eliot, Lise. *What's Going on in There? How the Brain and Mind Develop in the First Five Years of Life*. Bantam, 2000.

Fauci, Anthony S., et al. *Harrison's Principles of Internal Medicine*. 17th Edition. New York: McGraw-Hill, 2008.

Gage, Fred, H., and Yves Christian, eds. *Retrotransposition, Diversity and the Brain ( Research and Perspectives in Neurosciences)*. Berlin, Germany: Springer-Verlag, 2008.

Hay, William W., et al. *Current Diagnosis and Treatment: Pediatrics*. 19th edition. New York: McGraw-Hill, 2009.

Tortora, Gerard J., and Derrickson, Bryan. *Principles of Anatomy and Physiology*. 12th Edition. John Wiley & Sons, 2009.

#### PERIODICALS

Ashwal, Stephen. "Practice parameter: evaluation of the child with microcephaly (an evidence-based review): Report of the quality standards subcommittee of the american academy of neurology and the practice committee of the child neurology society." *Neurology* 73: (September 2009) 887–897.

#### ORGANIZATIONS

American Academy of Neurology. 1080 Montreal Avenue, Minneapolis, MN, 55116. (651) 695-2717 (800) 879-1960, Fax: (651) 695-2791. memberservices@aan.com. http://www.aan.com.

Rhonda Cloos, RN

Microcephaly with spastic diplegia selmanona syndrome I *see* **Paine syndrome**

Microcephaly-mental retardation-tracheoesophageal fistual syndrome *see* **Oculo-digito-esophago-duodenal syndrome**

Microcephaly-mesobrachyphalangy-tracheo-esophagael fistula syndrome (MMT) *see* **Oculo-digito-esophago-duodenal syndrome**

# Microphthalmia with linear skin defects (MLS)

## Definition

Microphthalmia with linear skin defects (MLS) is a rare genetic disorder that causes abnormalities of the eyes and skin. This disorder was first recognized as a distinct genetic condition in 1990.

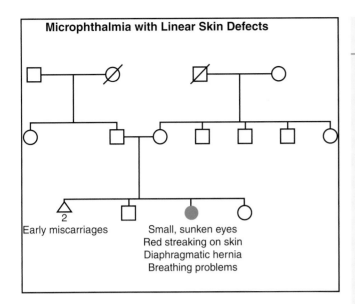

**Microphthalmia with Linear Skin Defects**

2 — Early miscarriages

Small, sunken eyes
Red streaking on skin
Diaphragmatic hernia
Breathing problems

*(Gale, a part of Cengage Learning.)*

## Description

MLS is a rare disorder that is observed only in females because males with the disease do not survive to birth. This disorder is also called MIDAS (Microphthalmia, dermal aplasia, and sclerocornea) syndrome. People affected by MLS have:

- small sunken eyes (microphthalmia)
- irregular red streaks of skin on the head and neck (skin erythema)
- abnormal development of the sclera and cornea of the eye

The eye is composed of three layers: the sclera, the choroid, and the retina. The sclera is the tough white outer coat of the eyeball. As this coat passes over the lens, it normally becomes clear. This clear portion of the sclera is the cornea. Both the sclera and the cornea are affected by MLS.

The choroid is the middle layer of the eye. It serves to nourish the retina and absorb scattered light. The retina is the inner, light-sensitive, layer of the eye. The retina receives the image transmitted by the lens and it contains the rods and cones that are responsible for color vision and vision in dim light. Both the choroid and the retina are unaffected by MLS.

## Genetic profile

The **gene** responsible for MLS has been localized to a portion of the short arm (p) of the X **chromosome** Xp22.3. The specific symptoms of MLS are believed to result from the premature cutoff (terminal deletion) of

the X chromosome at this point. People with MLS do not have the portion of the short arm of the X chromosome beyond the Xp22.2 location.

Nearly all of the cases of MLS are believed to result from *de novo* mutations since parents of affected individuals do not carry the MLS mutation in their chromosomes. A *de novo* mutation is caused by a problem with the chromosomes of the parental egg or sperm cells. The remainder of the chromosomes in the parents are not affected. As the sex cells of one of the parents reproduce, an error occurs. This leads to the transmission of a new mutation from that parent to his or her child. This mutation is expressed for the first time in the child of that parent.

A typical female has two X chromosomes. A typical male has one X chromosome and one Y chromosome. Because no XY male has ever been diagnosed with MLS, it is assumed that MLS is dominant and X-linked with 100% fetal mortality in males. This type of genetic disorder is also called an X-linked male-lethal trait.

There have been a few reported cases of males affected with MLS. These individuals presumably survived because they were XXY males (genetically female with ambiguous or male sex organs), rather than the typical male with XY chromosomes. This condition (XXY) is called **Klinefelter syndrome**.

## Demographics

Approximately 300 individuals, all without a Y chromosome, have been diagnosed with MLS worldwide. MLS is not associated with any particular subpopulations. It appears with equal frequency in all races and across all geographies. Because it is an X-linked male-lethal trait, it is observed exclusively in females or, in a few cases, in XXY males.

## Signs and symptoms

MLS is characterized by:

- small, sunken, eyes (microphthalmia)
- defects of the sclera and cornea portions of the eye
- linear red streaking of the skin on the upper body, primarily the head and neck
- abnormal protrusion of the abdominal contents upward through an opening in the diaphragm (diaphragmatic hernia), which causes difficulty with breathing (respiratory distress)
- a lack of the transparent membrane (septum pellucidum) in the brain that forms a wall between two of the normal cavities (the lateral ventricles) of the brain
- a condition in which the heart is located on the right side, rather than the left side, of the chest (dextrocardia)

In individuals affected with MLS, the bony cavity that contains the eyeball (orbit) often contains small fluid-filled sacs (orbital cysts). The sclera is often not fully or properly formed, and the cornea generally has areas that are opaque rather than transparent. This corneal opacity causes blurring of vision and may result in blindness. Corneal opacities should not be confused with cataracts, which are opacities of the lens of the eye, not of the cornea.

Difficulty in breathing (respiratory distress) is seen at birth in some patients with MLS. This is caused by a hole in the muscle beneath the lungs (diaphragm) that is responsible for the flow of air into and out of the lungs. This condition will rapidly lead to death if it is not surgically repaired.

Seizures and mental retardation have been observed in some MLS patients. It is believed that these individuals do not have a septum pellucidum. The absence of this membrane may allow electrical transmissions between parts of the brain that are usually isolated from each other. These inadvertent electrical signals may cause the seizures and the mental retardation that is sometimes seen in MLS patients.

## Diagnosis

MLS is generally diagnosed by the presence of the characteristic red striping of the skin on the head and neck accompanied by small eyes (microphthalmia) and opaque patches on the corneas.

MLS is differentiated from **Goltz syndrome**, which has a similar gene locus, in that the patient with MLS has skin irregularities only on the upper half of the body, most typically only on the head and neck. Goltz syndrome results in skin irregularities across the entire body. Also, patients with MLS do not have the abnormal fatty tissue deposits seen under the skin of Goltz syndrome patients. Finally, MLS does not have the clefting of the hands or feet (syndactyly) or incomplete formation of certain structures of the eyes (**coloboma**) seen in Goltz syndrome.

Identification of the gene responsible for MLS makes **genetic testing** for this dominant trait potentially possible.

## Treatment and management

The treatment and management of MLS is directed toward the symptoms seen in each patient. All those affected with MLS will need eye care including surgeries to potentially repair damaged areas of the cornea and sclera. Some individuals may require skin care treatments depending on the severity of the skin abnormalities.

In cases of patients with a diaphragmatic hernia, emergency surgery shortly after birth may be necessary to attempt to repair the damaged area. Unfortunately, most cases of this type of hernia cannot be surgically corrected and the patient will die.

In cases of patients with a lack of the septum pellucidum in the brain, anti-seizure medication may be necessary to control the seizures.

## Prognosis

MLS is lethal in males prior to birth. In females, a full life expectancy is possible if the complications are not severe and if medical treatment is followed.

Most problems of the cornea and sclera of the eye associated with MLS can be treated with corrective lenses or potentially surgically repaired with corneal implants or laser surgery.

Seizures, if present, can generally be controlled by anti-seizure medications.

Developmental delays in growth, motor ability, speech, and intellect occur in some, but not all, cases of MLS. The amount of delay that is observed is directly related to the severity of seizure activity in the brain caused by the malformation, or lack, of the septum pellucidum.

### Resources

#### PERIODICALS

Kuno, T., and T. Migita. "Another observation of microphthalmia in an XX male: Microphthalmia with linear skin defects syndrome without linear skin lesions." *Journal of Human Genetics* (1999): 63-8.

#### WEBSITES

"Multiple Congenital Anomaly/Mental Retardation (MCA/MR) Syndromes." *United States National Library of Medicine.* http://www.nlm.nih.gov/mesh/jablonski/syndromes/syndrome453.html. (February 9, 2001).

"Entry 309801: Micropthalmia with linear skin defects; MLS." *OMIM—Online Mendelian Inheritance in Man.* http://www.ncbi.nlm.nih.gov/entrez/dispomim. cgi?id = 309801. (February 9, 2001).

#### ORGANIZATIONS

National Foundation for the Blind. 200 East Wells St. Baltimore, MD 21230. (410) 659-9314. Fax: (410) 685. http://www.nfb. org.

National Organization for Rare Disorders (NORD). 55 Kenosia Ave., PO Box 1968, Danbury, CT 06813. (203) 744-0100 or (800) 999-6673. Fax: (203) 798.2291. http://www.rarediseases.org.

Paul A. Johnson

MIDAS syndrome *see* **Microphthalmia with linear skin defects**

Mild hypophosphatasin *see* **Hypophosphatasia**

# Miller-Dieker syndrome

### Definition

Miller-Dieker, syndrome (MDS) is a rare genetic disorder. Its signs and symptoms include severe abnormalities in brain development as well as characteristic facial features. Additional birth defects may also be present.

### Description

MDS was named for the two physicians, J. Miller and H. Dieker who independently described the condition in the 1960s. The hallmark of MDS is **lissencephaly** (smooth brain), a condition in which the outer layer of the brain, the cerebral cortex, is abnormally thick and lacks the normal convolutions (gyri). In some areas of the brain, gyri are fewer in number but wider than normal (pachygyri). Other areas lack gyri entirely (agyri). Normally, during the third and fourth months of pregnancy, the brain cells in the baby multiply and move to the surface of the brain to form the cortex. Lissencephaly is caused by a failure of this nerve cell migration. MDS is often called Miller-Dieker lissencephaly syndrome.

### Genetic profile

When MDS was first described, geneticists thought it followed an autosomal recessive pattern of **inheritance**. However, in the early 1990s, several patients with MDS were found to be missing a small portion of the short arm of **chromosome** 17 (17p13.3). This is called a partial deletion of chromosome 17. MDS is now classified as a "micro-deletion syndrome" because it is the result of the absence of genes that are normally located in this region of chromosome 17. In 1993, research scientists identified one of the genes in this region. They named it LIS1 for "first lissencephaly gene" because it appeared to be important in normal brain formation. The main evidence for this was that the LIS1 gene was missing in a number of individuals with isolated lissencephaly; that is, lissencephaly without the additional characteristics found in MDS. Researchers then studied a number of patients with MDS and found over 90% of them were missing the LIS1 gene as well as other, as yet unidentified genes, on the short arm of chromosome 17. Geneticists now think that the characteristic facial appearance and other abnormalities seen in MDS are due to the deletion of these other genes. For this reason, MDS has also been described as a contiguous gene syndrome.

Most genes, including all genes on the autosomes (non-sex chromosomes), are normally present in pairs. Individuals with MDS who have a micro-deletion of a small region of the short arm of one copy of their chromosome 17 still have one normal copy of this chromosome region on their other chromosome 17. For this reason, MDS is said to be due to "haploinsufficiency," the term for a genetic condition caused by the lack of function of only one of the two copies of a gene. As with other haploinsufficiency syndromes, MDS has also been described an having an autosomal dominant pattern of inheritance.

Individuals with MDS usually die in infancy. Because they do not live to the age where they can reproduce, they cannot transmit MDS to their offspring. Eighty percent of individuals with MDS have it as the result of a new (*de novo*) deletion of a small part of the short arm of one chromosome 17 in just the

## KEY TERMS

**Amniocentesis**—A procedure performed at 16-18 weeks of pregnancy in which a needle is inserted through a woman's abdomen into her uterus to draw out a small sample of the amniotic fluid from around the fetus. Either the fluid itself or cells from the fluid can be used for a variety of tests to obtain information about genetic disorders and other medical conditions in the fetus.

**Autosomal dominant**—A pattern of genetic inheritance where only one abnormal gene is needed to display the trait or disease.

**Autosomal recessive**—A pattern of genetic inheritance where two abnormal genes are needed to display the trait or disease.

**CAT (CT) scan**—Computerized (axial) tomography. A special x ray technique used to examine various tissues, particularly the brain, in great detail.

**Cerebral cortex**—The outer surface of the cerebrum made up of gray matter and involved in higher thought processes.

**Chorionic villus biopsy**—A procedure used for prenatal diagnosis at 10-12 weeks gestation. Under ultrasound guidance a needle is inserted either through the mother's vagina or abdominal wall and a sample of cells is collected from around the early fetus. These cells are then tested for chromosome abnormalities or other genetic diseases.

**Contiguous gene syndrome**—A genetic syndrome caused by the deletion of two or more genes located next to each other.

**FISH (fluorescence *in situ* hybridization)**—Technique used to detect small deletions or rearrangements in chromosomes by attempting to attach a fluorescent (glowing) piece of a chromosome to a sample of cells obtained from a patient.

**Gastrostomy**—The construction of an artificial opening from the stomach through the abdominal wall to permit the intake of food.

**Haploinsufficiency**—The lack of one of the two normal copies of a gene. Haploinsufficiency can result in a genetic disorder if normal function requires both copies of the gene. Haploinsufficiency is one explanation for a dominant pattern of inheritance.

**Hypotonia**—Reduced or diminished muscle tone.

**Inversion**—A type of chromosomal defect in which a broken segment of a chromosome attaches to the same chromosome, but in reverse position.

**Lissencephaly**—A condition in which the brain has a smooth appearance because the normal convolutions (gyri) failed to develop.

**Magnetic resonance imaging (MRI)**—A technique that employs magnetic fields and radio waves to create detailed images of internal body structures and organs, including the brain.

**Micro-deletion syndrome**—A collection of signs and symptoms caused by a deletion of a gene or genes that is too small to be seen through the microscope.

**Microcephaly**—An abnormally small head.

**Opisthotonos**—An arched position of the body in which only the head and feet touch the floor or bed when the patient is lying on their back.

**Prenatal diagnosis**—The determination of whether a fetus possesses a disease or disorder while it is still in the womb.

**Syndrome**—A group of signs and symptoms that collectively characterize a disease or disorder.

**Translocation**—The transfer of one part of a chromosome to another chromosome during cell division. A balanced translocation occurs when pieces from two different chromosomes exchange places without loss or gain of any chromosome material. An unbalanced translocation involves the unequal loss or gain of genetic information between two chromosomes.

**X-linked**—Located on the X chromosome, one of the sex chromosomes. X-linked genes follow a characteristic pattern of inheritance from one generation to the next.

one egg or sperm that formed that individual. The parents of these affected individuals have normal chromosomes without deletions. This means that their risk of having another child with MDS is very low (probably less than 1%). The other 20% of those with MDS have the syndrome because one of their parents carries a rearrangement of one copy of their own chromosome 17. The rearrangement can be an inversion or a balanced translocation between chromosome 17 and one of the other chromosomes. Since the rearrangement is balanced; that is, all the chromosome material is present but in a rearranged form, the parent is normal. However, when that parent produces an egg or a sperm, the balanced chromosome rearrangement can go through a further rearrangement. This results in a portion of the short arm of chromosome 17 being deleted. The individual who develops from that egg or sperm will have MDS.

## Demographics

MDS is present in fewer than one in 100,000 births. There is no information to suggest that the syndrome is more common in any particular ethnic or racial group.

## Signs and symptoms

Infants with MDS are usually small at birth. Characteristic facial features may include a high forehead with furrows and vertical ridges, indentation of the temples, a small, upturned nose, up-slanting eyes, a small mouth, a thick, broad upper lip with a thin border, low-set ears, and occasionally, a **cleft palate**. Some infants with MDS also have birth defects involving the heart and kidneys. Signs and symptoms can vary among MDS patients. This may relate to the actual size or exact location of the chromosome 17 deletion in that individual.

MDS infants have a very limited capacity for development due to the lissencephaly and associated brain abnormalities. Mental retardation is severe to profound. Infants with MDS may be able to do little more than roll over. Convulsions (seizures) develop within a few weeks of birth and can be severe. Most newborns with MDS have low muscle tone (hypotonia), but later develop stiffness (spasticity) and an arching of the body (opisthotonos). Poor feeding leads to a failure to thrive and increases the risk of pneumonia because the infants can accidentally inhale baby formula into their lungs. Head size is usually in the normal range at birth, but poor brain growth means that, by the age of one year, the children have a smaller-than-normal head size (**microcephaly**).

## Diagnosis

MDS is not the only disorder associated with lissencephaly. Autosomal dominant, autosomal recessive, and X-linked patterns of inheritance have been described among the more than two dozen genetic syndromes featuring this brain abnormality. Less commonly, lissencephaly can be the result of fetal infections such as prenatal cytolomegalovirus (CMV). An accurate diagnosis of MDS is important not only because it can provide a prognosis for the affected child, but because it can give parents an estimate of their risk for having another child with MDS.

MDS may be suspected in the newborn period if an infant has the characteristic facial features along with low muscle tone. Studies of the infant's brain by CAT scan or MRI will show the smooth brain surface. After the diagnosis of MDS is made on the basis of these signs and symptoms, it is very important to study the infant's chromosomes to check for the characteristic chromosome 17 deletion. This is done by sending a small sample of the infant's blood to a cytogenetics laboratory. Trained laboratory personnel (cytogeneticists) first examine the infant's chromosomes through the microscope using traditional techniques. If no deletion or other chromosome rearrangement is detected in this step, newer methods can be used to search for deletions that are too small to see by ordinary means (micro-deletions). A special technique called FISH (**fluorescent in situ hybridization**) can detect chromosome regions where very small pieces of **DNA** are missing. This test is usually done on the same blood sample.

### Carrier detection

When a chromosome deletion is found in an infant, both parents' chromosomes should also be studied to determine if one of them carries a chromosome rearrangement such as a balanced translocation. Although most parents of infants with MDS have normal chromosomes, in approximately 20% of children, one parent will have a chromosome rearrangement, which can increase the risk for having another child with MDS. Other family members should also be offered chromosome studies because these balanced chromosome rearrangements can be passed down through a family undetected, and, thus, other family members may be carriers. The first step in studying other family members is for a geneticist or genetic counselor to obtain a detailed family history and construct a pedigree (family tree) to determine which family members should be offered testing.

### Prenatal diagnosis

If a couple has had one child with MDS, they can be offered prenatal diagnosis in future pregnancies. This option is particularly important for the 20% of MDS families where one parent carries a balanced chromosome rearrangement. The risk for these couples to have another affected child depends on the exact type of chromosome rearrangement present and may be as high as 25-33%. For families in which both parents' chromosomes are normal, the risk of having another child with MDS is low (1% or less). Either chorionic villus sampling (CVS) or **amniocentesis** can be used early in a pregnancy to obtain a small sample of cells from the developing embryo for chromosome studies.

Early prenatal diagnosis by ultrasound is not reliable because the brain is normally smooth until later in pregnancy. Couples who are considering prenatal diagnosis should discuss the risks and benefits of this type of testing with a geneticist or genetic counselor.

### Treatment and management

There is no cure for MDS and treatment is usually directed toward comfort measures. Because of the feeding problems and risk of pneumonia, surgeons often place a tube between the stomach and the outside of the abdomen (gastrostomy tube). Feedings can be made through the tube. Seizures are often difficult to control even with medication.

### Prognosis

Death often occurs in the first three months of life and most infants with MDS die by two years of age, although there have been reports of individuals living for several years.

### Resources

#### BOOKS

Jones, Kenneth Lyons. *Smith's Recognizable Patterns of Human Malformations.* 5th ed. Philadelphia, W. B. Saunders, 1997.

#### WEBSITES

Dobyns, W. B. "Lissencephaly and subcortical band heterotopia (Agyria-pachygyria-band spectrum) Overview." (updated October 4, 1999). *GeneClinics: Clinical genetic information resource.* University of Washington, Seattle. http://www.geneclinics.org.
"Entry 247200: Miller-Dieker Lissencephaly Syndrome." *OMIM—Online Mendelian Inheritance in Man.* http://www.ncbi.nlm.nih.gov/entrez/dispomim.cgi?id=247200.
"Lissencephaly, Information for Parents." http://www.lissencephaly.org/about/lissen.htm.
*The Lissencephaly Network, Inc.* http://www.kumc.edu/gec/support/lissence.html.

#### ORGANIZATIONS

Lissencephaly Network, Inc. 716 Autumn Ridge Lane, Fort Wayne, IN 46804-6402. (219) 432-4310. Fax: (219) 432-4310. lissennet@lissencephaly.org. http://www.lissencephaly.org.

Sallie Boineau Freeman, PhD

Mirhosseini-Holmes-Walton syndrome *see* **Cohen syndrome**

MODY—Maturity-onset diabetes of the young *see* **Diabetes mellitus**

# Moebius syndrome

### Definition

Moebius syndrome is a condition in which the facial nerve is underdeveloped, causing paralysis or weakness of the muscles of the face. Other nerves to the facial structures may also be underdeveloped.

### Demographics

Moebius syndrome is extremely rare and does not seem to affect any particular ethnic group more than others. The families in which genes on chromosomes 3 and 10 were mapped were Dutch.

### Description

Moebius syndrome has been called "life without a smile" because the paralysis of the facial muscles, the most constant feature, leads to the physical inability to form a smile even when happy feelings are experienced. The facial nerve is one of a group of 12 nerves known as the cranial nerves because they originate in the brain. The facial nerve is also known as the seventh cranial nerve. The sixth cranial nerve, also called the abducens, controls blinking and back–and–forth eye movement and is the second most commonly affected cranial nerve in Moebius syndrome. Additional cranial nerves affected in some patients control other eye movements and other functions such as hearing, balance, speech, and feeding.

Individuals with Moebius syndrome may also have abnormalities of their limbs, chest muscles, and tongue. The chance of mental retardation appears to be increased in people with Moebius syndrome, but most people with the disorder have normal intelligence.

### Risk factors

During pregnancy, certain exposures, such as to the drugs misoprostol or thalidomide, appear to increase the risk of Moebius syndrome.

### Causes and symptoms

Most cases of Moebius syndrome are isolated and do not appear to be genetic, but occurrence in multiple individuals within some families indicates that there are multiple genetic forms.

Chromosomes 13, 3, and 10 appear to contain genes causing forms of Moebius syndrome, now named, respectively, types 1, 2, and 3.

One family was reported in which two brothers and their male cousin who were the sons of sisters all had Moebius syndrome along with other physical abnormalities and mental retardation. Boys only have one X **chromosome** and can inherit an X–linked disease from their unaffected mothers, who have two X chromosomes. The pattern of affected children in this family is typical of X–linked **inheritance**, so it is suggested that there may be a **gene** involved in Moebius syndrome on the X chromosome as well. If this is the case, the son of a woman with an altered Moebius gene on one X chromosome would have a 50% chance of inheriting the gene and having the condition. A man with this type of Moebius syndrome would be unlikely to have affected children since his daughters would likely have one normal X chromosome from their mother and his sons would not receive his X chromosome but his Y chromosome. In another family, a brother and sister with unaffected parents had Moebius syndrome, suggesting autosomal recessive inheritance, in which two altered copies of a gene are required to have the disorder. In an autosomal recessive disorder, a couple in which each parents carry one altered copy of the disease gene have a 25% chance of having a child with the condition with each pregnancy.

The first sign of Moebius syndrome in newborns is an inability to suck, sometimes accompanied by excessive drooling and strabismus (crossed eyes). Also seen at birth in some patients are abnormalities of the limbs, tongue, and jaw. Children often have low muscle tone, particularly in the upper body. The lack of facial expression and inability to smile become apparent as children get older.

When cranial nerve palsy is associated with limb reduction abnormalities and the absence of the pectoralis muscles, the condition is known as Poland–Moebius or Möebius–Poland syndrome. Common limb abnormalities are missing or webbed fingers and **clubfoot**.

The prevalence of mental retardation in Moebius syndrome is uncertain. It has been estimated in the past to be between 10% and 50%, but these numbers are thought to be overestimates resulting from the lack of facial expression and drooling seen in people with Moebius syndrome. In one study of familial cases of Moebius syndrome, 3% were reported to be mentally retarded.

### Diagnosis

Diagnosis of Moebius syndrome is made on the basis of clinical symptoms, especially the lack of facial expression. Since exact genes involved in Moebius syndrome have not yet been identified as of 2009, molecular **genetic testing** is not available at this time.

### Treatment and management

The ability to smile has been restored in some cases of Moebius syndrome by surgery that transfers nerve and muscle from the thigh to the face. Other surgeries can be used to treat eye, limb, and jaw problems. In children with feeding problems, special bottles or feeding tubes are used. Physical and speech therapy are used when necessary to improve control over coordination, speech, and eating.

### Prognosis

Moebius syndrome does not appear to affect life span, and individuals who are treated for their symptoms can lead normal lives.

### Prevention

Moebius syndrome cannot be prevented since its cause is unknown. Pregnant women should avoid any kind of illegal drugs, especial cocaine or methamphetamines as well as misoprostol or thalidomide.

## Resources

### BOOKS

ICON Health Publications. *Moebius Syndrome: A Medical Dictionary, Bibliography, and Annotated Research Guide to Internet References.* San Diego, CA: ICON Health Publications, 2004.

### PERIODICALS

Broussard, A. B., and J. G. Borazjani. "The faces of Moebius syndrome: recognition and anticipatory guidance." *American Journal of Maternal Child Nursing* 33, no. 5 (September–October 2008): 272–278.

Lima, L. M., et al. "Moebius syndrome: clinical manifestations in a pediatric patient." *Journal of Clinical Pediatric Dentistry* 31, no. 4 (July–August 2009): 289–293.

Simonsz, H. J. "Historical perspective: first description of the Moebius syndrome." *Strabismus* 16, no. 1 (January–March 2008): 3.

### OTHER

"Moebius Syndrome." *National Craniofacial Association.* Information Page. http://www.faces-cranio.org/Disord/Moebius.htm (accessed October 24, 2009).

"What is Moebius Syndrome?" *Moebius Syndrome Foundation.* Information Page. http://www.ciaccess.com/moebius (accessed October 24, 2009).

### ORGANIZATIONS

Birth Defect Research for Children, Inc.. 800 Celebration Avenue, Suite 225, Celebration, FL, 34747. (407) 566-8304, (407) 566-8341. staff@birthdefects.org. http://www.birthdefects.org.

Moebius Research Trust. 49 Inglis Avenue, Port Seton, East Lothian, Scotland, EH32 0AG. + 44 (01875) 819822. http://www.moebiusresearchtrust.org.

Moebius Syndrome Foundation. PO Box 147, Pilot Grove, MO, 65276. (660) 834-3406. http://www.ciaccess. com/moebius syndrome.com.

National Craniofacial Association FACES. PO Box 11082, Chatta nooga, TN, 37401. (800) 332-2373. faces@faces-cranio.org. http://www.faces-cranio.org.

National Organization for Rare Disorders (NORD). PO Box 1968 55 Kenosia Avenue, Danbury, CT, 06813-1968. (203) 744-0100 (800) 999-NORD, (203) 798-2291. orphan@ rarediseases.org. http://www.rarediseases.org.

Toni I. Pollin, MS, CGC

Mohr syndrome *see* **Oral-facial-digital syndrome (OFD)**

# Monosomy 1p36 syndrome

## Definition

Monosomy 1p36 syndrome is a genetic disorder caused by the deletion of critical **DNA** on the **chromosome** pair 1. Children affected by this disorder have facial abnormalities, mental retardation, and developmental delays. Monosomy refers to the deletion occurring on only one of the chromosomes of the pair. The code 1p36 refers to the exact location on chromosome 1 where the deletion takes place. This location is at the terminal point of the chromosome. A syndrome is a collection of characteristics that tend to occur together in a disorder. Although it is a rare condition, monosomy 1p36 syndrome is the most common terminal deletion disorder.

## Demographics

The estimate of this disorder's occurrence has been accepted the early 2000s as 1 in 10,000. However, research brought the rate of occurrence down to 1 in 5,000. Twice as many females are affected as males. No racial or ethnic ratios have been established.

## Description

Monosomy 1p36 syndrome is a rare disorder. The severity of symptoms is diverse; however, most individuals experiencing this disorder have severe symptoms. The most notable symptoms are the facial features. Almost all children with this disorder have some level of mental retardation. They also experience developmental delays. When they grow into adulthood, most require supportive living such as a group home with special services.

### Risk factors

The cause of this disorder is the terminal deletion on chromosome 1, which is the largest human chromosome. Most cases of monosomy 1p36 syndrome appear to be from a spontaneous mutation. However, most spontaneous mutations take place on genes inherited from the mother. Evidence from research in 2009 suggested that the tendency for the deletion to occur is inherited as an autosomal dominant trait.

The facial characteristics of a person affected by monosomy 1p36 syndrome include deep-set eyes and flat nose bridge. Most individuals have a small head and ears that are disproportionate to one another. Another common characteristic is a pointed chin. Almost 65%t of those affected are born with a **cleft** lip. Almost all children have low muscle tone leading to awkward motor skills.

Those affected with this disorder are born with some form of abnormality in the brain structure. In addition, most experience heart and hearing problems. Delays in language development and structural problems contribute to a lack of verbal communication.

There is no cure for the underlying condition, although genetic research is investigating ways to resolve similar conditions. Most treatment involves solving the individual symptoms and constant monitoring for further complications. Early intervention and life-long education is designed to help the affected person adapt to as independent a lifestyle as possible.

### Causes and symptoms

The cause of this syndrome is a deletion of the continuous DNA on chromosome 1, which is responsible for neurological functioning and normal development. The deletion is usually at the terminal point of the corrupted chromosome; however, in a few cases the deletion takes place in the middle of the strand. The rate of maternal chromosomes affected is slightly higher than paternal chromosomes affected with 60% of affected chromosomes coming from the mother's side. There are no notable differences in characteristics marking the differences in chromosomal differences.

The most observable characteristics are the distinct facial features of an affected person. These include a prominent forehead and an underdeveloped midface. Included in the underdeveloped midface are the characteristics of a flat nose and flat nasal bridge. The eyes are deep set, and the openings are unusually small. Most people affected have **microcephaly** and brachycephaly. Microcephaly is a condition in which the circumference of the head is abnormally small for age and gender. Brachycephaly is a condition contributing to a flat head, in which the head is disproportionately wide but the front to back ratio is abnormally short. The ears are small, low set, and unaligned with each other. People with monosomy 1p36 syndrome have short stature in comparison to others of same age and gender.

Developmental and intellectual disabilities are almost universal among those with this syndrome. Measures of intelligence are often below the standard for moderate mental retardation; although some may be more severe. Language and speech development are often severely delayed. All measures of developmental milestones are later than observed in children from a normal population. Behavioral problems related to these delays are common with a greater than expected rate of self injury.

The most serious and common congenital disorder is the heart malformation. This problem can be manifested as **patent ductus arteriosus** (failure of a prenatal bypass to close at birth) or cardiomyopathy (a congenital weakness of the heart muscle). Other serious congenital problems are associated with brain malformation. The related conditions include cerebral atrophy (loss of brain cells) and cerebral ventricular dilatation (condition where the amount of blood coming into the brain is greater than what can be accommodated by the blood vessels taking blood away from the brain). Other congenital disorders include visual disability to some degree. Many individuals experience problems of the esophagus interfering with normal swallowing. Sensitivity in hearing is reduced to some degree in most affected people due to problems with the ear structure or to the nerve, but complete hearing loss is no greater than in the normal population.

### Diagnosis

Many characteristics of monosomy 1p36 syndrome are observable from birth. Certainly the distinct facial characteristics can be identified as good evidence of the presence of monosomy 1p36 syndrome. There are no known cases of a diagnosis based on the observable features alone.

#### Examination

An examination of the newborn suspected of having this syndrome begins with noting the usual observable features, including a prominent forehead; a flat nose and nasal bridge; deep set eyes; abnormally small, flat head; and small, low set, unaligned ears. In addition to these easily observed features, most children with monosomy 1p36 syndrome have problems with the little finger on one or both hands. This fifth finger may be unusually short or pointed. Oftentimes the fifth finger is either curving toward the other fingers or is inflexible. In newborns, the anterior fontanelle (the soft spot of the head) is either unusually large or is unusually late in closing. Quite a few affected people experience seizures; therefore, it is appropriate to note in the clinical examination whether the child has had seizures.

#### Tests

Tests should be conducted for the expected congenital disorders, including problems of the heart and brain. Tests of reflexes and reaction can be conducted with a newborn to determine intellectual functioning.

In early childhood developmental tests can demonstrate the rate of developmental growth in comparison with normally developing children. However, a diagnosis of monosomy 1p36 syndrome cannot be definite without a test detecting the chromosome 1 deletion.

The main test for recognizing chromosomal disorders is the fluorescence in-situ hybridization (FISH). This method of analyzing the structures of human **genetics** relies on fluorescent probes designed to link to specific genetic particles such as proteins, genes, or chromosomal material. If the correlating probe cannot link to the material for which it is designed, then the result is accepted as an absence of the material. In testing for monosomy 1p36 syndrome, the probes specific to a continuous pattern on the chromosome 1 would be injected into genetic material from the patient. If examination of the probes does not detect a continuous pattern, then it is confirmation that the person has monosomy 1p36 syndrome.

The condition can also be detected prenatally through **amniocentesis**.

### Treatment and management

Treatment is focused on relieving discomfort caused by the secondary characteristics. Depending on what the characteristics are and how severe they are, there may be an effort to reverse the individual symptoms. However, there is little effort to find a cure for the underlying cause of the disorder.

One of the most important sources for treatment for the child diagnosed with monosomy 1p36 syndrome is early intervention for mental retardation. Early intervention can assist the child in overcoming the challenges of developmental delay. As the child grows, the individual will require special services in school and rehabilitative services in adult life. Involving the child in early intervention can assist in making these later services more effective. The agency providing the early intervention can help educate and prepare the parents for the challenges that the child will face over the years. The best intervention is based in a daycare setting with the child living at home, unless the developmental disabilities are too severe. In that case, the child might be recommended to a living facility.

The severity of any congenital physical problems has to be met appropriately from birth. Doing so requires constant observation and medical diagnosis. If the condition is not severe, it may not be dangerous to postpone treatment until later in life; however, diagnosis of the condition and its progress has to be constantly monitored over time.

## QUESTIONS TO ASK YOUR DOCTOR

- What specific congenital disorders does my child have?
- How can we as parents monitor the many conditions of our child?
- What are the chances for my child to grow up to be independent?
- How can we determine what social services are available for our child at all stages of life?
- What can we as parents do to help our child better adapt?
- Where can we find out about trial treatments available now or in the future?

Since most children with monosomy 1p36 syndrome have some level of a hearing disability, lessons in American Sign Language are often recommended. The children often have speech problems; therefore, learning sign language can improve their communication skills. Constant assessment of all symptomatic conditions, including language, intellectual functioning, heart condition, seizures, and hearing, is necessary throughout life.

### Prognosis

There is no cure for monosomy 1p36 syndrome. The prognosis of this syndrome is related to the severity of the condition and the nature of the symptoms. There is a correlation between the extent of the deletion on chromosome 1 and the severity of the conditions of the syndrome. However, the deletion of chromosome 1p36 is never seen as a contributing factor in a fatality. The resulting congenital disorders are more often referred to as contributing to death of a person. Statistics on life expectancy are usually given in relation to those collected for the congenital disorders.

The prognosis for adapting to living conditions and for quality of life is related to the effectiveness and appropriateness of recommended treatments. Family members and advocates have to be constantly aware of the availability of necessary social services for those with developmental disabilities.

### Prevention

There is no prevention for monosomy 1p36 syndrome. **Genetic counseling** and prenatal testing is available but is usually only conducted when one of the parents is suspected of being a carrier. Genetic counseling can help prospective parents recognize the risks of conceiving a child with this syndrome. If the risk is high, the parents might have the option of in vitro fertilization. With in vitro fertilization, the genetic diagnosis, done before implantation, can detect which available **zygote** has the least chance for the syndrome. The advantage of early detection through prenatal testing is that the necessary accommodations and interventions can be ready immediately after birth. The necessary tests for genetic counseling and prenatal assessment are not usually conducted unless there is a known family risk. Therefore, it is important to investigate one's family history. Furthermore, when there is a known risk, it is important to communicate that to all concerned.

## Resources

### BOOKS

Coleman, William B., and Gregory J. Tsongalis. *Molecular Pathology: The Molecular Basis of Human Disease.* Burlington, ME: Academic Press, 2009.

Epstein, Richard. *Human Molecular Biology: An Introduction to the Molecular Basis of Health and Disease.* New York: Cambridge University Press, 2002.

### PERIODICALS

Battaglia, Agatino, et al. "Further Delineation of Deletion 1p36 Syndrome in 60 Patients: A Recognizable Phenotype and Common Cause of Developmental Delay and Mental Retardation." *Pediatrics* 121 (2008): 404-410.

### OTHER

Battaglia, Agatino, and Lisa G Shaffer. *1p36 Deletion Syndrome.* GeneReviews. http://www.ncbi.nlm.nih.gov/bookshelf/br.fcgi?book = gene&part = del1p36.

Slavotinek, Anne. *Chromosome 1p36 Deletions.* Orphanet. http://www.orpha.net/data/patho/GB/uk-1p36.pdf.

### ORGANIZATIONS

American Association on Intellectual and Developmental Disabilities. 501 Third Street NW, Suite 200, Washington, DC, 20001. (202) 387-1968, (203) 746-6481. http://www.aamr.org.

Ray F. Brogan, PhD

## Morquio syndrome (MPS IV) *see* Mucopolysaccharidosis (MPS)

# Mowat-Wilson syndrome

## Definition

Mowat-Wilson syndrome is a rare genetic disorder characterized by moderate to severe mental impairment, distinctive physical features, and a collection of intestinal problems known as Hirschsprung's disease.

An alternate name associated with Mowat-Wilson syndrome is Hirschsprung Disease-Mental Retardation syndrome. A similar condition, called Goldberg-Shprintzen syndrome, is sometimes confused with Mowat-Wilson syndrome, but appears to have a different genetic basis.

## Demographics

Mowat-Wilson syndrome is a rare genetic disorder that affects individuals worldwide and appears to have no preference for gender, ethnicity, or geographic area. Information about its prevalence was not available as of 2009.

## Description

Mowat-Wilson syndrome is named for clinical geneticists David Mowat and Meredith J. Wilson, who with their research team described the disorder in a 1998 issue of the *Journal of Medical Genetics*. In the article, they provided details about six children, five from New South Wales, Australia, and one from Manchester, England. The children were unrelated. Four of the six children had the following combination of primary symptoms:

- distinctive facial appearance, including large, uplifted earlobes
- mental retardation
- small head
- short stature
- severe constipation, intestinal blockage, and enlargement of the colon, a collection of symptoms known as Hirschsprung's disease, which first appeared when these patients were newborns

The remaining two patients had similar symptoms, but one did not develop Hirschsprung's disease until the age of three, and the other did not have Hirschsprung's disease but did experience chronic constipation. The researchers also noted that all six patients had "a generally happy, smiling affect," often with an open-mounted expression.

Mowat and Wilson suggested that the cause of the disorder was a genetic mutation or the loss of a miniscule bit of a **chromosome** (known as a microdeletion). The researchers continued to collect evidence and review other patients with the same suite of symptoms and, in 2003, published their findings that the disorder, by then named Mowat-Wilson syndrome, resulted from the mutation of a specific gene, and this mutation need only affect one of the two copies of the gene in a cell to have an effect.

## Causes and symptoms

Mowat-Wilson syndrome results from a mutation in a gene that carries the instructions for making the protein called zinc finger E-box binding homeobox 2 (ZEB2). When a mutation of this gene, which is generally called the ZEB2 gene, occurs, individuals cannot make a sufficient amount of the functioning ZEB2 protein, and in some cases, they cannot make any at all. This protein is involved in the prenatal development of the nervous, gastrointestinal, cardiovascular, and other systems and tissues in the body, and when it is lacking, a wide range of symptoms can arise

Although this disorder has a genetic component, patients typically do not have a family history of it. Instead, Mowat-Wilson syndrome usually arises spontaneously, which means that it is not passed from one generation to the next, nor is it more likely in brothers or sisters of an affected individual. Mowat-Wilson syndrome is considered an autosomal dominant disorder, because individuals need only have one copy of the mutated gene to develop the disorder.

### Genetic profile

The ZEB2 gene is located on the long arm of chromosome 2. It carries the blueprint for the ZEB2 protein, which is a transcription factor. Transcription factors attach to **DNA** and regulate the expression of genes. In other words, they control whether certain genes' instructions are read. The ZEB2 protein regulates those genes that have roles in early growth and development. In particular, the ZEB2 protein is particularly vital to the development of embryonic tissue called the neural crest, which later transforms into more specific tissues that are critical to a well-functioning nervous system, heart, and other systems and organs, and also to the development of a properly formed face and skull.

Individuals who have the mutated ZEB2 gene cannot make enough properly functioning ZEB2 protein, which causes the neural crest to suffer, and associated organs and tissues do not develop as they should.

Scientists know of more than 100 different mutations in the ZEB2 gene that can lead to Mowat-Wilson syndrome. Usually, the mutation either completely deletes one copy of the gene or affects its instructions such that it makes shortened and nonfunctional ZEB2 protein.

### Symptoms

Individuals with Mowat-Wilson syndrome have a wide range of symptoms, including characteristic facial features, some of which may be evident at birth, and moderate to severe mental impairment. Symptoms may include the following:

- small head (microcephaly)
- heavy eyebrows
- mental impairments that may be severe
- impaired, late-developing speech, or absent speech
- motor-skill delays, including late development of walking
- severe constipation, intestinal blockage, and enlargement of the colon (collectively known as Hirschsprung's disease)
- chronic constipation, even in the absence of Hirschsprung's disease
- short stature
- heart defects
- urinary tract/genital defects, such as the abnormally placed opening of the urethra or undescended testicles among males
- seizures
- improper separation of the two halves of the brain (agenesis/hypoplasia of the corpus callosum)

Facial features common to infants include:

- widely spaced, deep-set, large eyes
- square-shaped face
- broad nasal bridge, and an overall flat, or so-called saddle nose or boxer's nose with a rounded tip
- open, frequently smiling mouth
- full lower lip
- narrow, strongly pointed chin
- cup-shaped ears with large earlobes and a dimple in the middle of each lobe
- thick and horizontal (rather than arched) eyebrows

As the child ages, the facial features typically change in the following ways:

- chin becomes stronger
- rounded tip of the nose becomes more evident
- upper lip becomes narrow at the center point and outer edges, but full elsewhere
- continued smiling, open-mouthed expression
- blue-eyed children with black patches in their irises

Facial features continue to develop into adulthood, and patients generally have a long face with protruding jaw (prognathism); a long, pointed chin;

very thick, horizontal eyebrows; and a long nose that dips down toward the top of the upper lip.

## Diagnosis

### Examination

Facial features (which become more prominent as the affected individual ages), developmental delays, and mental retardation aid in a preliminary diagnosis of Mowat-Wilson syndrome.

### Tests

**Genetic testing** is used to detect ZEB2 **gene mutations** that are indicative of the disorder.

## Treatment and management

No cure is available. Individuals with this disorder are typically treated by a range of specialists that focus on various symptoms.

### Traditional

Depending on the severity of symptoms, the doctor may refer a patient to an orthodontist, ophthalmologist, urologist, cardiologist, or other specialist for additional symptom diagnosis and treatment. For instance, individuals may undergo an electroencephalogram (EEG) or magnetic resonance imaging (MRI) to check for and, if necessary, to initiate treatment of neurologic problems, such as seizures.

### Drugs

A doctor may prescribe anti-epileptic drugs to treat seizures. Additional medication may be of help in treating specific symptoms.

## Prognosis

Initial symptoms, including characteristic facial features, are often seen soon after birth, and mental abilities become evident shortly thereafter. Toddlers generally have poor muscle tone and begin walking late (at about four years of age) or never develop this ability. Seizures may develop in infancy or in later childhood, but in about 10% of patients, seizures do not develop. Nearly one-half of patients develop **congenital heart disease**, and about 60% develop Hirschsprung's disease. Those without Hirschsprung's disease usually have chronic constipation.

## Prevention

There is no way to prevent Mowat-Wilson syndrome. It is a genetic disorder that usually results from a mutation that occurs spontaneously.

## Resources

**PERIODICALS**

Mowat, D. R., M. J. Wilson, M.J., and M. Goossens. "Mowat-Wilson Syndrome." *Journal of Medical Genetics.* 40 (2003):305–310.

Mowat, D. R., et al. "Hirschsprung Disease, Microcephaly, Mental Retardation, and Characteristic Facial Features: Delineation of a New Syndrome and Identification of a Locus at Chromosome 2q22-q23." *Journal of Medical Genetics.* 35 (1996): 617–623.

**OTHER**

Adam, Margaret P., Lora J. H. Bean,, and Vanessa Rangel Miller. *Mowat-Wilson Syndrome.* GeneReviews. http://www.ncbi.nlm.nih.gov/bookshelf/br.fcgi?book = gene&part = mws.

Kugler, Mary. *Mowat-Wilson Syndrome*. About.com: Rare Diseases. http://rarediseases.about.com/od/rarediseases1/a/mowatwilson.htm.

*Mowat-Wilson Syndrome*. MowatWilson.org. http://www.mowatwilson.org/.

National Institutes of Health. *Mowat-Wilson syndrome*. Genetics Home Reference. http://ghr.nlm.nih.gov/condition = mowatwilsonsyndrome.

National Institutes of Health. *ZEB2*. Genetics Home Reference. http://ghr.nlm.nih.gov/gene = zeb2

**ORGANIZATIONS**

Mowat-Wilson Syndrome. davec@mowatwilson.org. http://www.mowatwilson.org.

National Organization for Rare Disorders (NORD). P.O. Box 1968, 55 Kenosia Ave., Danbury, CT, 06813-1968. 203-744-0100. orphan@rarediseases.org. http://www.rarediseases.org.

Leslie A. Mertz, PhD

# Moyamoya

## Definition

Moyamoya is a progressive syndrome characterized by narrowing of the blood vessels in the brain. Moyamoya is the Japanese term for "cloud of smoke drifting in the air."

## Description

The term moyamoya is used to describe how the arteries in the brain look in this syndrome, which was first described in the 1950s. There is no clear cause for this disease. It can be caused genetically, but can also occur as a result of having other diseases. Moyamoya is seen in patients with a variety of diseases, including: **neurofibromatosis**, trisomy 21 (**Down syndrome**), **sickle cell disease**, chronic meningitis, and as a side effect of irradiation.

Moyamoya is a disease of the blood vessels in the brain. The carotid arteries are two of the large arteries that allow blood to flow into the brain. The external carotid artery allows blood to reach areas within the neck, while the internal carotid artery travels to the brain and branches off into smaller vessels to reach all areas of the brain. In patients with moyamoya, there is a symmetric thinning of the width of the internal carotid arteries. The brain responds to this thinning by making the smaller blood vessels bigger, trying to get blood to the areas of the brain that are not getting enough. When dye is injected into the arteries of the brain (a cerebral angiogram), a characteristic pattern is seen. On the angiogram, this looks like a cloud of smoke.

## Genetic profile

The primary form of moyamoya is seen most often in Japan. Studies have found the familial form to account for 7–10% of the cases. A recent study focused on 16 families in order to find the genetic marker for the disease. The gene locus was found to be present on the short arm of **chromosome** 3, specifically 3p26–p24.2. Other studies have found possible involvement of genes on chromosomes 6 and 17 as well.

## Demographics

Although the disease seems to occur most often in Japanese people, patients have been found throughout the world. It is thought that one in a million people are affected each year. The age of onset of the disease has two peaks, the first being in children under 10 years old, and the second in adults in their 20s–40s. Fifty percent of moyamoya cases are found in patients younger than ten years of age. Females seem to have moyamoya more often than males. The female-to-male ratio is 3:2.

## Signs and symptoms

The first signs and symptoms of moyamoya tend to be different in children and adults. Children most often present with a sudden seizure or a stroke. Strokes can cause weakness on one side of the body. These are often brought on with exercise or fast breathing. Less severe strokes, called transient ischemic attacks (TIAs), can occur very often. During these TIAs, the weakness in the body is temporary and will not last more than a few hours. Over a period of years, strokes and TIAs leave patients with permanent weakness on both sides of the body, seizure disorders, and mental retardation. While children will present with seizures or strokes, adults tend to present with intracerebral hemorrhage (bleeding within the brain). Depending on where the bleeding or strokes occur, there can be a variety of chronic symptoms including: speech disturbance, visual disturbance, headaches, difficulties with sensation and involuntary movements (moving parts of the body when you do not intend to).

## Diagnosis

Cerebral angiography is the main method of diagnosis. This is the best way to see the arteries in the brain and to assess their level of occlusion (blockage). Other methods of imaging have been used in an attempt to diagnose moyamoya. High resolution imaging such as computed tomography scans (CT scans) do not show findings specific to this syndrome. However, areas of old strokes or bleeding can be seen. Magnetic resonance imaging (MRI) is also very sensitive at looking for old areas of stroke but cannot show which blood vessels may be blocked as compared with angiography. These non-invasive imaging techniques may however, provide clues for the diagnosis. The doctor would then recommend angiography to confirm the diagnosis.

## Treatment and management

There is no one best treatment for moyamoya. Medical therapy consists of drugs that prevent blood clot formation such as aspirin. Drugs that help dilate the narrowed blood vessels, such as calcium channel blockers, are also used. Calcium channel blockers that have been successful include nicardipine and verapamil. These calcium channel blockers may also help with the headaches that some patients may get during the course of their illness.

Many different surgical approaches have been used to help improve blood flow in these patients. It is not known what the long term outcome of these procedures are. The most popular operations are: encephaloduroanteriosynangiosis (EDAS), encephalomyosynangiosis (EMS), and superficial temporal artery-middle cerebral artery (STA-MCA) anastamosis.

In EDAS, an artery that sits under the scalp called the superficial temporal artery, is separated from the skin. A small opening in the skull is then made. The artery from the scalp is then sewn into the surface of the brain. The piece of skull that was removed is then put back in place to protect the new connection. This procedure has also been termed pial syngiosis.

In the EMS procedure, a muscle overlying the temple region of the forehead, called the temporalis muscle, is detached. Once again, an opening in the skull is made and the muscle is placed on the surface of the brain.

In the STA-MCA operation, the scalp artery is directly connected to an artery in the brain. All of these surgical procedures attempt to provide blood to areas of the brain that are not getting enough. Although symptoms may be improved soon after surgery, it usually takes months for the new blood vessels to form.

## Prognosis

It is unclear what the long-term risk for complications is in people with moyamoya disease. A study published in 2000 looked at 334 patients with moyamoya disease diagnosed between 1976 and 1994. Approximately 60% of the adults who had moyamoya had a cerebral hemorrhage at some point. Approximately 60% of the children who had moyamoya had a stroke or TIA at some point. Cerebral hemorrhage was found to be the most important factor that predicted a poor outcome. The overall effect of medical and surgical treatment on long term outcomes is not well known at this time.

### Resources

#### BOOKS

Aicardi, Jean. *Diseases of the Nervous System in Childhood.* London Mac Keith Press, 1998, pp.554–56.

#### PERIODICALS

Han, D. H., et al. "A co-operative study: clinical characteristics of 334 Korean patients with moyamoya disease treated at neurosurgical institutes (1976-1994)." *Acta Neurochir* 11 (2000): 1263–73.

Hosain, S. A., et al. "Use of a calcium channel blocker (nicardipine HCL) in the treatment of childhood moyamoya disease." *Journal of Child Neurology* 4 (October 1994): 378–80.

Kobayashi, E., et al. "Long-term natural history of hemorrhagic moyamoya disease in 42 patients." *Journal of Neurosurgery* 93 (December 2000): 976–80.

Scott, M. R. "Surgery for Moyamoya Syndrome?: Yes." *Archives of Neurology* 58 (January 2001): 128–30.

Yamauchi, T., et al. "Linkage of familial moyamoya disease (spontaneous occlusion of the circle of Willis) to chromosome 17q25." *Stroke* 31 (April 2000): 930–5.

#### WEBSITES

"Moyamoya Disease." *OMIM—Online Mendelian Inheritance in Man.* http://www.ncbi.nlm.nih.gov/omim/.

"Moya-moya." Pediatric neurosurgery department, Columbia-Presbyterian Medical Center. http://

cpmcnet.columbia.edu/dept/nsg/PNS/moyamoya.
html.
"Moya-Moya Syndrome." Brain Aneurysm/AVM Center,
Massachusetts General Hospital. http://neurosurgery.
mgh.harvard.edu/nvnwin96.htm.

ORGANIZATIONS
Families with Moyamoya Support Network. 4900 McGowen
St. SE, Cedar Rapids, IA 52403.

David E. Greenberg, MD

# Mucolipidosis

## Definition

Mucolipidosis (ML) is a group of rare, inherited
disorders that are characterized by the accumulation of
complex fats, called mucolipids, in the cells of the body.
The symptoms range from skeletal abnormalities and
vision problems to physical and mental retardation.

## Description

### Types of mucolipidosis

There are three major types of mucolipidosis.
Mucolipidosis II (ML II, ML2) or ML disorder type
II, is known as I-cell disease (ICD). Sometimes it is
called Leroy disease, after Jules Leroy who described
the disorder in 1969. ML II is also known as N-
acetylglucosamine-1-phosphotransferase (GNPTA)
deficiency. GNPTA is the enzyme that is defective in
ML II.

Mucolipidosis III (ML III, ML3), or ML disorder
III, is a milder form of ML II. In ML III, the enzyme
GNPTA has reduced activity; whereas it has no activity in ML II. ML III was first described in 1966. It is
often called pseudo-Hurler polydystrophy because its
symptoms resemble a mild form of the mucopolysaccharide disorder known as Hurler syndrome. It is a
polydystrophy because several systems of the body are
affected.

In the past, ML II and ML III were classified as
**mucopolysaccharidoses** (MPS II and MPS III, respectively). MPS is a condition in which complex sugars
called mucopolysaccharides accumulate in the cells
of the body. Although this may occur in ML, excess
amounts of mucopolysaccharides are not excreted in
the urine, as they are in MPS.

Mucolipidosis IV (ML IV, ML4) was first described
in 1974. It also is called ML disorder IV, Berman syndrome, or sialolipidosis.

**Neuraminidase deficiency** originally was classified as mucolipidosis I (ML I). However, neuraminidase deficiency does not involve the accumulation of
mucolipids.

### Lipids

Lipids are large, complex biomolecules that are
very important components of cell membranes. They
also are used to store energy and are present in mucus
secretions.

Lipids are continually broken down and replaced. This breakdown of lipids occurs in a membrane-bound compartment or organelle within cells, called the lysosome. The lysosome contains many enzymes that break down the lipids. These enzymes are produced outside of the lysosome and have to be transported into the organelle. The enzyme GNPTA attaches a signal to these enzymes that directs them to the lysosome.

### Lysosomal storage diseases

MLs are classified as lysosomal storage diseases because the lysosomes accumulate lipids that cannot be broken down. Eventually, the lysosomes become so filled with lipids that the cells form structures called inclusion bodies to contain the lipids. Inclusion bodies give the cells a characteristic appearance. The name "I-cell disease" refers to these inclusion bodies.

Individuals with ML II or ML III have little or no GNPTA enzyme activity. Thus, the lysosomal enzymes cannot reach the lysosome to help break down lipids. ML II and ML III are caused by mutations, or changes, in one of the genes that encodes a part of GNPTA. A disorder called mucolipidosis III, variant form, or complementation group C, is caused by a mutation in a gene that encodes a different part of GNPTA. The symptoms of this form of ML III are very similar to those of the more common type of ML III.

ML IV is caused by a mutation in the gene encoding a protein called mucolipin-1. In ML IV, membrane lipids and mucopolysaccharides accumulate in the lysosomes of cells throughout the body. Apparently, in the absence of mucolipin-1, these substances are transported to the lysosome rather than recycled to the cell membrane.

## Genetic profile

All of the MLs are inherited as autosomal recessive traits. They are autosomal because the genes that are responsible for these disorders are located on autosomal chromosomes, rather than on the X or Y sex chromosomes. The traits are recessive because they are only expressed in individuals who have inherited two copies of the gene that causes the disorder, one copy from each parent.

Individuals with only one copy of a gene that causes ML are called carriers. They usually do not have symptoms of ML. The offspring of two carriers of an ML gene have a 25% chance of inheriting both genes and developing ML.

## Demographics

MLs are very rare disorders that often have been misdiagnosed. Thus, the frequency of ML is not clear. Since MLs are recessive disorders that only develop when both parents are carriers of one of the ML genes, the condition most often occurs in the offspring of closely-related individuals, such as first cousins. These disorders are much more prevalent in small, isolated populations. For example, among French-Canadians in one region of Quebec province, it is estimated that one out of every 39 people carries a gene for ML II and one out of 6,184 infants has the disorder. In contrast, over a 10-year-period, only 35 infants with ML II or ML III were born in Great Britain.

Although ML IV can occur in any nationality or ethnic group, more than 80% of all known cases are Jews of Eastern European descent (Ashkenazim). It is estimated that one out of 50 individuals of Ashkenazi descent is a carrier of ML IV. Worldwide, there are about 100 known cases of the disorder. However, it is thought that there are many more undiagnosed or misdiagnosed cases.

## Signs and symptoms

The symptoms and the age of onset of ML II vary greatly, even within families. Some signs of ML II can be congenital, or present at birth. These may include:

- multiple abnormalities in bone formation, particularly in the hip
- limited mobility of the joints
- multiple abnormalities of the skull and face
- a fold of skin extending from the inner corner of the eyelid, called an epicanthal fold

ML II and ML III are progressive conditions. Infants may show few symptoms of the disorder until lipids begin to accumulate and damage cells. Additional symptoms of ML II may include:

- dwarfism
- delayed mental and physical development
- hearing loss
- heart disease in the aortic valve
- swollen liver and spleen

The symptoms of ML III are similar to those of ML II, but usually less severe. Additional signs of ML III may include:

- acne
- clouding of the cornea, the clear portion of the eye through which light passes
- enlarged tongue

ML IV is characterized by mental and physical retardation and eye disorders. Many individuals with ML IV do not develop beyond the skill level of a one-year-old. However, some individuals with ML IV have very mild symptoms.

Infants with ML IV appear normal at birth. However signs of the disorder usually become apparent during the first year. Often, clouding or opacity of the cornea is the first symptom and vision problems may develop before the age of one. The physical and mental retardation may be mild at first, but often becomes severe as the disorder slowly progresses. Most individuals with ML IV never walk. Other signs of ML IV may include:

- delayed growth
- poor muscle tone
- crossed eyes
- puffy eyelids
- a version to light
- degeneration of the retina, eventually leading to blindness

### Diagnosis

ML II and ML III may be diagnosed by high levels of lysosomal enzymes, called hydrolases, in the blood. The absence of mucopolysaccharides in the urine indicates that the disorder is not a mucopolysaccharidosis. The microscopic examination of various cells reveals inclusion bodies. X rays are used to detect skeletal abnormalities.

The initial diagnosis of ML IV usually results from a biopsy. A small piece from the skin or from the membrane underneath the eyelid is removed and examined under a microscope for the accumulation of lipids and mucopolysaccharides in storage bodies.

### Treatment and management

There is no cure for ML. Management of symptoms, close medical monitoring, and supportive care are the primary treatments.

Surgery can remove the thin layer of cells that causes the corneal cloudiness that is characteristic of ML IV. However, the layer of cells will grow back. Physical, occupational, and speech therapy can improve the functioning of children with ML IV.

### Prognosis

The life expectancy for individuals with ML is not known.

### Resources

#### PERIODICALS

Bargal, R., et al. "Identification of the Gene Causing Mucolipidosis Type IV." *Nature Genetics* 26 (2000): 118-121.

Olkkonen, V. M., and E. Ikonen. "Genetic Defects of Intracellular-Membrane Transport." *New England Journal of Medicine* 343 (2000): 1095-1104.

#### WEBSITES

"Medical Information." *Mucolipidosis IV Foundation.* (April 24, 2001). http://ml4.org/text/medinfo.html.

"Mucolipidosis IV." *National Foundation for Jewish Genetic Diseases, Inc.* (April 24, 2001). http://www.nfjgd.org/FactSheets/mucolipid.htm.

"Mucolipidosis IV." *University of Pittsburgh Department of Human Genetics.* June 1, 2000. (April 24, 2001). http://www.pitt.edu/~edugene/ML4.html.

#### ORGANIZATIONS

Canadian Society for Mucopolysaccharide and Related Diseases. PO Box 30034, RPO Parkgate North Vancocrur. British columbia. Canada (608) 924-5130 or (800) 667-1846. http://www.mpssociety.ca.

Mucolipidosis IV Foundation. 719 East 17th St., Brooklyn, NY 11230. (718) 434-5067. http://www.ml4.org.

National Foundation for Jewish Genetic Diseases, Inc. 250 Park Ave., Suite 1000, New York, NY 10017. (212) 371-1030. http://www.nfjgd.org.

National MPS Society. PO Box , NC 27709.4686, (919)806-0100, (800) MPS–1001. info@ mpssociety.org. http://www.mpssociety.org.

Margaret Alic, PhD

# Mucopolysaccharidoses

## Definition

Mucopolysaccharidosis (MPS) is a general term for a number of inherited diseases that are caused by the accumulation of mucopolysaccharides, resulting in problems with an individual's development. With each condition, mucopolysaccharides accumulate in the cells and tissues of the body because of a deficiency of a specific enzyme. The specific enzyme that is deficient or absent is what distinguishes one type of MPS from another. Before these enzymes were identified, the MPS disorders were diagnosed by the signs and symptoms that an individual expressed. The discovery of these enzymes resulted in a reclassification of some of the MPS disorders. These conditions are often referred to as MPS I, MPS II, MPS III, MPS IV, MPS VI, MPS VII, and MPS IX. These conditions

## KEY TERMS

**Cardiomyopathy**—A thickening of the heart muscle.

**Enzyme**—A protein that catalyzes a biochemical reaction or change without changing its own structure or function.

**Enzyme replacement therapy**—Medical treatment replacing an enzyme in patients in whom that particular enzyme is deficient or absent.

**Joint contractures**—Stiffness of the joints that prevents full extension.

**Kyphosis**—An abnormal outward curvature of the spine, with a hump at the upper back.

**Lysosome**—Membrane–enclosed compartment in cells, containing many hydrolytic enzymes; where large molecules and cellular components are broken down.

**Mucopolysaccharide**—A complex molecule made of smaller sugar molecules strung together to form a chain. Found in mucous secretions and intercellular spaces.

**Recessive gene**—A type of gene that is not expressed as a trait unless inherited by both parents.

**X–linked gene**—A gene carried on the X chromosome, one of the two sex chromosomes.

are also referred to by their original names, which are Hurler, Hurler–Scheie, Scheie (all MPS I), Hunter (MPS II), Sanfilippo (MPS III), Morquio (MPS IV), Maroteaux–Lamy (MPS VI), Sly (MPS VII), and Hyaluronidase deficiency (MPS IX).

### Description

Mucopolysaccharides are long chains of sugar molecules that are essential for building the bones, cartilage, skin, tendons, and other tissues in the body. Normally, the human body continuously breaks down and builds mucopolysaccharides. Another name for mucopolysaccharides is glycosaminoglycans (GAGs). There are many different types of GAGs and specific GAGs are unable to be broken down in each of the MPS conditions. There are several enzymes involved in breaking down each GAG and a deficiency or absence of any of the essential enzymes can cause the GAG to not be broken down completely and results in its accumulation in the tissues and organs in the body. In some MPS conditions, in addition to the GAG being stored in the body, some of the incompletely broken down GAGs can leave the body via the urine. When too

much GAG is stored, organs and tissues can be damaged or not function properly.

### Genetic profile

Except for MPS II, the MPS conditions are inherited in an autosomal recessive manner. MPS conditions occur when both of an individual's genes that produce the specific enzyme contain a mutation, causing them to not work properly. When both genes do not work properly, either none or a reduced amount of the enzyme is produced. An individual with an autosomal recessive condition inherits one non–working gene from each parent. These parents are called carriers of the condition. When two people are known carriers for an autosomal recessive condition, they have a 25% chance with each pregnancy to have a child affected with the disease. Some individuals with MPS do have children of their own. Children of parents who have an autosomal recessive condition are all carriers of that condition. These children are not at risk to develop the condition unless the other parent is a carrier or affected with the same autosomal recessive condition.

Unlike the other MPS conditions, MPS II is inherited in an X–linked recessive manner. This means that the gene causing the condition is located on the X **chromosome**, one of the two sex chromosomes. Since a male has only one X chromosome, he will have the disease if the X chromosome inherited from his mother carries the defective gene. Females will be carriers of the condition if only one of their two X chromosomes has the gene that causes the condition.

### Demographics

The National Institute for Neurological Disorders and Stroke (NINDS) estimates that one in every 25,000 babies born in the United States has some form of the mucopolysaccharidoses. Males and females are affected equally.

### Causes and symptoms

Each type of MPS is caused by a deficiency of one of the enzymes involved in breaking down GAGs. It is the accumulation of the GAGs in the tissues and organs in the body that cause the wide array of symptoms characteristic of the MPS conditions. The accumulating material is stored in cellular structures called lysosomes, and these disorders are also known as lysosomal storage diseases.

## MPS I

MPS I is caused by a deficiency of the enzyme alpha–L–iduronidase. Three conditions, Hurler, Hurler–Scheie, and Scheie syndromes, are all caused by a deficiency of this enzyme. Initially, these three conditions were believed to be separate because each was associated with different physical symptoms and prognoses. Once the underlying cause of these conditions was identified, it was realized that these three conditions were all variants of the same disorder. The gene involved with MPS I is located on chromosome 4p16.3.

**MPS I H (HURLER SYNDROME).** It has been estimated that approximately one baby in 100,000 will be born with Hurler syndrome. Individuals with Hurler syndrome tend to have the most severe form of MPS I. Symptoms of Hurler syndrome are often evident within the first year or two after birth. These infants often begin to develop as expected, but then reach a point where they begin to lose the skills that they have learned. Many of these infants may initially grow faster than expected, but their growth slows and typically stops by age three. Facial features also begin to appear "coarse." They develop a short nose, flatter face, thicker skin, and a protruding tongue. Additionally, their heads become larger and they develop more hair on their bodies with the hair becoming coarser. Their bones are also affected, with these children usually developing joint contractures (stiff joints), kyphosis (a "hunchback" curve of the spine), and broad hands with short fingers. Many of these children experience breathing difficulties, and respiratory infections are common. Other common problems include heart valve dysfunction, thickening of the heart muscle (cardiomyopathy), enlarged spleen and liver, clouding of the cornea, hearing loss, and carpal tunnel syndrome. These children typically do not live past age 12.

**MPS I H/S (HURLER–SCHEIE SYNDROME).** Hurler–Scheie syndrome is felt to be the intermediate form of MPS I, meaning that the symptoms are not as severe as those in individuals who have MPS I H but not as mild as those in MPS I S. Approximately one baby in 115,000 will be born with Hurler–Scheie syndrome. These individuals tend to be shorter than expected, and they can have normal intelligence, however, some individuals with MPS I H/S will experience learning difficulties. These individuals may develop some of the same physical features as those with Hurler syndrome, but usually they are not as severe. The prognosis for children with MPS I H/S is variable with some individuals dying during childhood, while others live to adulthood.

**MPS I S (SCHEIE SYNDROME).** Scheie syndrome is considered the mild form of MPS I. It is estimated that approximately one baby in 500,000 will be born with Scheie syndrome. Individuals with MPS I S usually have normal intelligence, but there have been some reports of individuals with MPS I S developing psychiatric problems. Common physical problems include corneal clouding, heart abnormalities, and orthopedic difficulties involving their hands and back. Individuals with MPS I S do not develop the facial features seen with MPS I H and usually these individuals have a normal life span.

## MPS II (Hunter syndrome)

Hunter syndrome is caused by a deficiency of the enzyme iduronate–2–sulphatase. All individuals with Hunter syndrome are male, because the gene that causes the condition is located on the X chromosome, specifically Xq28. Like many MPS conditions, Hunter syndrome is divided into two groups, mild and severe. It has been estimated that approximately one in 110,000 males are born with Hunter syndrome, with the severe form being three times more common than the mild form. The severe form is felt to be associated with progressive mental retardation and physical disability, with most individuals dying before age 15. In the milder form, most of these individuals live to adulthood and have normal intelligence or only mild mental impairments. Males with the mild form of Hunter syndrome develop physical differences similar to males with the severe form, but not as quickly. Men with mild Hunter syndrome can have a normal life span and some have had children. Most males with Hunter syndrome develop joint stiffness, chronic diarrhea, enlarged liver and spleen, heart valve problems, hearing loss, kyphosis, and tend to be shorter than expected. These symptoms tend to progress at a different rate depending on if an individual has the mild or severe form of MPS II.

## MPS III (Sanfilippo syndrome)

MPS III, like the other MPS conditions, was initially diagnosed by the individual having certain physical characteristics. It was later discovered that the physical symptoms associated with Sanfilippo syndrome could be caused by a deficiency in one of four enzymes. Each type of MPS III is now subdivided into four groups, labeled A–D, based on the specific enzyme that is deficient. All four of these enzymes are involved in breaking down the same GAG, heparan sulfate. Heparan sulfate is mainly found in the central nervous system and accumulates in the brain when it cannot be broken down because one of those four enzymes are deficient or missing.

MPS III is a variable condition with symptoms beginning to appear between ages two and six years of age. Because of the accumulation of heparan sulfate in the central nervous system, the central nervous system is severely affected. In MPS III, signs that the central nervous system is degenerating usually are evident in most individuals between ages six and 10. Many children with MPS III develop seizures, sleeplessness, thicker skin, joint contractures, enlarged tongues, cardiomyopathy, behavior problems, and mental retardation. The life expectancy in MPS III is variable. On average, individuals with MPS III live until they are teenagers, with some living longer and others not that long.

MPS IIIA (SANFILIPPO SYNDROME TYPE A). MPS IIIA is caused by a deficiency of the enzyme heparan N–sulfatase. Type IIIA is felt to be the most severe of the four types, in which symptoms appear and death occurs at an earlier age. A study in British Columbia estimated that one in 324,617 live births are born with MPS IIIA. MPS IIIA is the most common of the four types in Northwestern Europe. The gene that causes MPS IIIA is located on the long arm of chromosome 17 (location 17q25).

MPS IIIB (SANFILIPPO SYNDROME TYPE B). MPS IIIB is due to a deficiency in N–acetyl–alpha–D–glucosaminidase (NAG). This type of MPS III is not felt to be as severe as Type IIIA and the characteristics vary. Type IIIB is the most common of the four in southeastern Europe. The gene associated with MPS IIIB is also located on the long arm of chromosome 17 (location 17q21).

MPS IIIC (SANFILIPPO SYNDROME TYPE C). A deficiency in the enzyme acetyl–CoA–alpha–glucosaminide acetyltransferase causes MPS IIIC. This is considered a rare form of MPS III. The gene involved in MPS IIIC is believed to be located on chromosome 14.

MPS IIID (SANFILIPPO SYNDROME TYPE D). MPS IIID is caused by a deficiency in the enzyme N–acetylglucosamine–6–sulfatase. This form of MPS III is also rare. The gene involved in MPS IIID is located on the long arm of chromosome 12 (location 12q14).

### MPS IV (Morquio syndrome)

As with several of the MPS disorders, Morquio syndrome was diagnosed by the presence of particular signs and symptoms. However, it is now known that the deficiency of two different enzymes can cause the characteristics of MPS IV. These two types of MPS IV are called MPS IV A and MPS IV B. MPS IV is also variable in its severity. The intelligence of individuals with MPS IV is often completely normal. In individuals with a severe form, skeletal abnormalities can be extreme and include dwarfism, kyphosis (outward–curved spine), prominent breastbone, flat feet, and knock–knees. One of the earliest symptoms seen in this condition usually is a difference in the way the child walks. In individuals with a mild form of MPS IV, limb stiffness and joint pain are the primary symptoms. MPS IV is one of the rarest MPS disorders, with approximately one baby in 300,000 born with this condition.

MPS IV A (MORQUIO SYNDROME TYPE A). MPS IV A is the "classic" or the severe form of the condition and is caused by a deficiency in the enzyme galactosamine–6–sulphatase. The gene involved with MPS IV A is located on the long arm of chromosome 16 (location 16q24.3).

MPS IV B (MORQUIO SYNDROME TYPE B). MPS IV B is considered the milder form of the condition. The enzyme, beta–galactosidase, is deficient in MPS IV B. The location of the gene that produces beta–galactosidase is located on the short arm of chromosome 3 (location 3p21).

### MPS VI (Maroteaux–Lamy syndrome)

MPS VI, which is another rare form of MPS, is caused by a deficiency of the enzyme N–acetylglucosamine–4–sulphatase. This condition is also variable; individuals may have a mild or severe form of the condition. Typically, the nervous system or intelligence of an individual with MPS VI is not affected. Individuals with a more severe form of MPS VI can have airway obstruction, develop **hydrocephalus** (extra fluid accumulating in the brain) and have bone changes. Additionally, individuals with a severe form of MPS VI are more likely to die while in their teens. With a milder form of the condition, individuals tend to be shorter than expected for their age, develop corneal clouding, and live longer. The gene involved in MPS VI is believed to be located on the long arm of chromosome 5 (approximate location 5q11–13).

### MPS VII (Sly syndrome)

MPS VII is an extremely rare form of MPS and is caused by a deficiency of the enzyme beta–glucuronidase. It is also highly variable, but symptoms are generally similar to those seen in individuals with Hurler syndrome. The gene that causes MPS VII is located on the long arm of chromosome 7 (location 7q21).

### MPS IX (Hyaluronidase deficiency)

MPS IX is a condition that was first described in 1996 and has been grouped with the other MPS conditions by some researchers. MPS IX is caused by the deficiency of the enzyme hyaluronidase. In the few individuals described with this condition, the symptoms are variable, but some develop soft–tissue masses (growths under the skin). Also, these individuals are shorter than expected for their age. The gene involved in MPS IX is believed to be located on the short arm of chromosome 3 (possibly 3p21.3–21.2)

Many individuals with an MPS condition have problems with airway constriction. This constriction may be so serious as to create significant difficulties in administering general anesthesia. Therefore, it is recommended that surgical procedures be performed under local anesthesia whenever possible.

### Diagnosis

While a diagnosis for each type of MPS can be made on the basis of the physical signs described above, several of the conditions have similar features. Therefore, enzyme analysis is used to determine the specific MPS disorder. Enzyme analysis usually cannot accurately determine if an individual is a carrier for a MPS condition. This is because the enzyme levels in individuals who are not carriers overlaps the enzyme levels seen in those individuals who are carrier for a MPS. With many of the MPS conditions, several mutations have been found in each gene involved that can cause symptoms of each condition. If the specific mutation is known in a family, **DNA** analysis may be possible.

Once a couple has had a child with an MPS condition, prenatal diagnosis is available to them to help determine if a fetus is affected with the same MPS as their other child. This can be accomplished through testing samples using procedures such as an **amniocentesis** or chorionic villus sampling (CVS). Each of these procedures has its own risks, benefits, and limitations.

### Treatment and management

There is no cure for mucopolysaccharidosis, however, several types of experimental therapies are being investigated. Typically, treatment involves trying to relieve some of the symptoms. For MPS I and VI, bone marrow transplantation has been attempted as a treatment option. In those conditions, bone marrow transplantation has sometimes been found to help slow down the progression or reverse some of symptoms of the disorder in some children. The benefits of a bone marrow transplantation are more likely to be noticed when performed on children under two years of age. However, it is not certain that a bone marrow transplant can prevent further damage to certain organs and tissues, including the brain. Furthermore, bone marrow transplantation is not felt to be helpful in some MPS disorders and there are risks, benefits, and limitations with this procedure.

In 2006, the FDA approved the drug idursulfase (Elaprase) for the treatment of MPS II (Hunter syndrome), the first treatment ever shown to have beneficial effects for this syndrome. Enzyme replacement therapies are also currently in use or are being tested. Enzyme replacement therapy has proven useful in reducing non–neurological symptoms and pain.

### Clinical trials

Clinical trials on mucopolysaccharidoses are sponsored by the National Institutes of Health (NIH) and other agencies. As of 2009, NIH was reporting 31 on–going and completed studies.

Examples include:

- The evaluation of the use of enzyme replacement therapy into the spinal fluid for treatment of spinal cord compression in some forms of mucopolysaccharidosis I. (NCT00215527)

- A study to determine whether growth hormone is a safe and effective treatment for short stature in children with Mucopolysaccharidosis type I, II, and VI. (NCT00748969)

- The development of a registry to provide information to better characterize the natural history and progression of MPS I as well as the clinical responses of patients receiving enzyme replacement therapy. (NCT00144794)

Clinical trial information is constantly updated by NIH and the most recent information on mucopolysaccharidoses trials can be found at: http://clinicaltrials. gov.

### Prevention

No specific preventive measures are available for genetic diseases of this type. For some of the MPS diseases, biochemical tests are available that will identify healthy individuals who are carriers of the defective gene, allowing them to make informed reproductive decisions. There is also the availability of prenatal diagnosis for all MPS disease to detect affected fetuses.

## Resources

### BOOKS

ICON Health Publications. *The Official Parent's Sourcebook on Mucopolysaccharidoses: A Revised and Updated Directory for the Internet Age.* San Diego, CA: ICON Health Publications, 2002.

### PERIODICALS

Ashworth, J. L., et al. "Mucopolysaccharidoses and the eye." *Survey of Ophthalmology* 51, no. 1 (January–February 2006): 1–17.

Clarke, L. A. "The mucopolysaccharidoses: a success of molecular medicine." *Expert Reviews in Molecular Medicine* 10 (January 2008): e1.

Coman, D. J., et al. "Enzyme replacement therapy for mucopolysaccharidoses: opinions of patients and families." *Journal of Pediatrics* 152, no. 5 (May 2008): 723–727.

Haves, I. M., et al. "Newborn screening for mucopolysaccharidoses: opinions of patients and their families." *Clinical Genetics* 71, no. 5 (May 2007): 446–450.

Malinowska, M., et al. "Abnormalities in the hair morphology of patients with some but not all types of mucopolysaccharidoses." *European Journal of Pediatrics* 167, no. 2 (February 2008): 203–209.

### WEBSITES

*MPS Disorder Fact Sheet.* Information Page. MPS Society (February 12, 2009). http://www.mpssociety.org/content/4020/MPS_Fact_Sheet/.

*Mucopolysaccharides.* Medical Encyclopedia. Medline Plus, January 29, 2009 (February 12, 2009). http://www.nlm.nih.gov/medlineplus/ency/article/002263.htm.

*Mucopolysaccharidoses Fact Sheet.* Information Page. NINDS, July 28, 2008 (February 12, 2009). http://www.ninds.nih.gov/disorders/mucopolysaccharidoses/detail_mucopolysaccharidoses.htm.

*Mucopolysaccharidoses Information Page.* Information Page. NINDS, July 28, 2008 (February 12, 2009). http://www.ninds.nih.gov/disorders/mucopolysaccharidoses/mucopolysaccharidoses.htm.

### ORGANIZATIONS

Canadian Society for Mucopolysaccharide & Related Diseases. PO Box 30034, RPO Parkgate, North Vancouver, BC V7H 2Y8, Canada. (604) 924-5130 or (800) 667-1846. Fax: (604) 924-5131. Email: info@mpssociety.ca. http://www.mpssociety.ca.

Hide and Seek Foundation for Lysosomal Storage Disease Research. 4123 Lankershim Blvd., Suite 302, N. Hollywood, CA 91602-2828. (818) 762-8621. Fax: (818) 762-2502. Email: info@hideandseek.org. http://www.hideandseek.org.

National MPS Society. PO Box 14686, Durham, NC 27709-4686. (919) 806-0101 or (877) MPD-1001. Fax: (919) 806-2055. http://www.mpssociety.org.

National Organization for Rare Disorders (NORD). 55 Kenosia Avenue, PO Box 1968, Danbury, CT 06813-1968. (203) 744-0100 or (800) 999-6673. Fax: (203) 798-2291. http://www.rarediseases.org.

Society for Mucopolysaccharide Diseases. MPS House, Repton Place, White Lion Rd., Amersham, Buckinghamshire HP7 9LP, UK. +44 0845-389-9901. http://www.mpssociety.co.uk.

Sharon A. Aufox, MS, CGC

---

# Mucopolysaccharidosis type I

## Definition

Mucopolysaccharidosis type I (MPS–I) is a rare lysosomal storage disease belonging to the group of **mucopolysaccharidoses**. There are three variants, differing widely in their severity, with Hurler syndrome (MPS–1H) being the most severe, Scheie syndrome (MPS–IS) the mildest, and Hurler–Scheie syndrome (MPS–I H/S) intermediate. Because there is no clear distinction between these three syndromes, MPS I is currently divided into the severe and attenuated forms. MPS I results when cells cannot break down two by–products of normal metabolism. These by–products, dermatan sulfate and heparan sulfate, build up and disrupt normal cell function, leading to severe disease. The disease affects most body systems, causing progressive deterioration of tissues and organs.

## Description

In the severe form of the disease (Hurler syndrome), skeletal deformities and a delay in motor and intellectual development are the leading symptoms. Though present from conception, Hurler syndrome may be undetectable at birth. The newborn often looks healthy and seems to develop normally for the first few months. However, symptoms begin to appear 6–8 months after birth, when dermatan sulfate and heparan sulfate reach dangerous levels. Other manifestations include corneal clouding, abnormal enlargement of organs (organomegaly), heart disease, short stature, hernias, abnormal facial features (facial dysmorphology), and overabundance of hair (hirsutism). Enlargement of the head (hydrocephaly) can occur after the age of two.

Individuals with MPS–I lack sufficient amounts of the enzyme needed to break down dermatan sulfate and heparan sulfate. This enzyme, alpha–L–iduronidase, is part of a biochemical pathway which splits complex molecules into smaller, recyclable units. Without alpha–L–iduronidase, the complex molecules cannot be eliminated and deposit themselves in cells, tissues, and organs. Deposits in the soft tissues of the

**Alpha–L–iduronidase**—An enzyme that breaks down dermatan sulfate and heparan sulfate. People with Hurler syndrome do not make enough of this enzyme.

**Carpal tunnel syndrome**—Painful disorder caused by compression of a nerve; characterized by discomfort and weakness in the hands and fingers.

**Enzyme replacement therapy (ERT)**—Class of medications that seek to provide people with sufficient quantities of an important enzyme that they cannot fabricate on their own.

**Haematopoietic stem cell transplantation (HSCT)**—Transplantation of blood stem cells derived from the bone marrow or blood.

**Haematopoietic stem cells**—Stem cells that give rise to all the blood cell types.

**Hernia**—A rupture in the wall of a body cavity, through which an organ may protrude.

**Laronidase**—A highly purified protein, also known under its trademark name Aldurazyme, that is identical to a naturally occurring form of the human enzyme

alpha–L–iduronidase. It is used in enzyme replacement therapy.

**Lysosomal storage diseases**—Group of more than 40 human genetic disorders that result from defects in lysosomal function.

**Lysosome**—Membrane–enclosed compartment in cells, containing many hydrolytic enzymes; where large molecules and cellular components are broken down.

**Mucopolysaccharide**—A complex molecule made of smaller sugar molecules strung together to form a chain. Found in mucous secretions and intercellular spaces.

**Mucopolysaccharidosis–IH (MPS–IH)**—Another name for Hurler syndrome.

**Stem cells**—Cells found in multi–cellular organisms. They are characterized by the ability to renew themselves through cell division and differentiating into a diverse range of specialized cell types.

**Tracheostomy**—An opening surgically created in the trachea (windpipe) through the neck to improve breathing.

---

face lead to a typical appearance, causing children with Hurler syndrome to resemble each other more than they resemble their own healthy siblings. The spleen and liver become enlarged early in the course of the disease. Deposits stored in the growth plates of bones lead to dwarfism, **scoliosis**, joint stiffness, and other skeletal abnormalities. Corneal clouding caused by the deposits results in vision damage. Hearing loss usually occurs as well. Deposits in the brain cause loss of skills gained early in life, and severe mental retardation occurs.

The accumulation of dermatan sulfate and heparan sulfate in the airways leads to frequent respiratory tract and ear infections. Deposits also cause coronary artery obstruction and damage to the heart. In fact, respiratory complications and heart failure are the most frequent causes of death in Hurler syndrome patients. Many children with Hurler syndrome die by the age of 12.

Dermatan sulfate and heparan sulfate belong to a class of complex molecules known as mucopolysaccharides, or glycosaminoglycans (GAGs), chains formed by smaller sugar molecules strung together. For this reason, MPS I is classified as a mucopolysaccharidosis, a name meaning, "too many mucopolysaccharides." Besides MPS–I, there are several other mucopolysaccharidoses,

each resulting from absence or deficiency of a different enzyme. Mucopolysaccharidoses are lysosomal storage diseases. Lysosomes are cell parts which normally contain enzymes needed to break down complex molecules. When the enzymes are absent or deficient, the lysosomes store the complex molecules, expand, and eventually destroy the cells from within.

### Genetic profile

Researchers have identified the **gene** responsible for MPS–I and have mapped it to the 4p16.3 site on **chromosome** 4. The gene is named IDUA, for the iduronidase enzyme which it produces when working properly. The IDUA gene provides instructions for producing an enzyme that is involved in the breakdown of GAGs. Mutations in this gene reduce or eliminate the function of the IDUA enzyme, which leads to the accumulation of GAGs within cell lysosomes.

MPS–I is an autosomal recessive disorder. This means that it occurs only when a person inherits two defective copies of the IDUA gene. If one copy is normal and the other has a mutation, the person does not have the disease. However, the person carries the mutated gene and can pass it on to the next generation.

Carriers of IDUA mutations have only one working gene. As a result, these carriers produce less alpha–L–iduronidase enzyme than do people with two normal IDUA genes. Nevertheless, they produce enough enzyme to break down dermatan sulfate and heparan sulfate, so disease does not occur.

## Demographics

Prevalence is estimated at 0.7–1.6/100,000 for the Hurler and Hurler–Scheie syndromes and at 1/500,000 for Scheie syndrome.

Different IDUA **gene mutations** appear more frequently in certain populations. For instance, two specific mutations account for most Hurler syndrome cases among Northern Europeans, while two other mutations appear most often in Japanese patients.

## Signs and symptoms

A child with Hurler syndrome may be born with a hernia. In fact, hernia is often the first sign of this disorder. However, since it can also occur in other conditions or as an isolated event, it does not immediately point to Hurler syndrome.

Other symptoms appear within six to 12 months of birth. Tissue damage in airways leads to breathing difficulties and frequent respiratory and ear infections. The child's face begins to take on the coarse, typical features of Hurler syndrome. The skull appears large and unusually shaped, scalp veins are prominent, and the bridge of the nose is flat. The lips are large and the mouth is frequently open due to an enlarged, protruding tongue. Teeth may be late to emerge and are usually small, short, widely spaced, and somewhat malformed. The earlobes are thick, and the eyelids are full.

Skeletal abnormalities begin to appear. The hands are broad, with short, stubby fingers. Joints are often stiff and may limit the child's movement. The neck is very short; the spine is crooked and bends outward, resulting in a hunchback appearance.

Children under the age of one may already show signs of heart disease. This is usually due to tissue damage in the arteries or valves of the heart, caused by accumulation of dermatan sulfate and heparan sulfate. Accumulation also causes the liver and spleen to become severely enlarged, but these organs continue to function normally.

Hurler syndrome has a devastating effect on mental development. By the age of one or two, developmental delay occurs. The child may make slow progress for a few more years, but then actually begins to lose skills gained earlier. The mental capacity of a person with Hurler syndrome is similar to that of a normal three–year–old. Deterioration of the senses makes this situation worse. Corneal clouding damages vision. Hearing loss, narrowed airways, and enlarged tongue contribute to poor language skills.

Many infants with Hurler syndrome grow quickly during their first few months. However, skeletal abnormalities and progressive tissue damage cause growth to slow down and then to stop before it should. As a result, most people with Hurler syndrome do not grow beyond four feet tall.

Patients with the adult onset form (Scheie syndrome) are of almost normal height and do not show intellectual deficiency. Typical symptoms are stiff joints, corneal opacities, carpal tunnel syndrome and mild skeletal changes. Aortic valve disease can be present. Patients with the intermediate form (Hurler–Scheie syndrome) have normal or almost normal intelligence, but exhibit various degrees of physical impairment.

## Diagnosis

Hurler syndrome shares many symptoms with other mucopolysaccharidoses and with different lysosomal storage diseases. For this reason, laboratory tests are used to confirm Hurler syndrome diagnosis based on a physical exam.

The simplest test available is urine screening. People with MPS–I excrete increased amounts of dermatan sulfate and heparan sulfate in their urine. In addition, a blood test reveals deficiency of alpha–L–iduronidase enzyme. White blood cells and skin cells can be microscopically examined for damage caused by deposits of dermatan sulfate and heparan sulfate.

If MPS–I is present in a family, healthy family members could carry a mutated IDUA gene. Several clinical laboratories offer carrier screening to these individuals. A blood sample is all that is required. Most labs screen for carrier status by measuring the level of the alpha–L–iduronidase enzyme. Levels are lower in carriers than they are in people who have two normal IDUA genes. It is also possible to examine the actual genes to see if a Hurler syndrome mutation appears.

Since MPS–I is a rare disorder, most carriers have children with non–carrier partners. Thus, there is generally no risk of the disease occurring in the children. However, if two carriers have children together, each child has a 25% chance of having the syndrome. Carrier screening provides an opportunity to assess the risk and consider reproductive options before pregnancy occurs.

Each child born to two carriers has a 50% risk of inheriting one mutated gene and one normal gene. This child, like the parents, is a carrier.

Because a rare autosomal recessive gene can be passed for generations before two carriers have a child together, sometimes an affected child is born into a family with no previous history of MPS–I. This is generally an indication that both parents carry a mutated IDUA gene. These parents worry not only about the health of the affected child, but also about the risk to future children.

Prenatal testing is available to find out if a fetus has Hurler syndrome. This can be done by **amniocentesis** or chorionic villus sampling. Amniocentesis involves removal of a small amount of amniotic fluid from the uterus. Chorionic villus sampling involves removal of a small sample of placental tissue. In either case, the cells present in the sample are checked for enzyme deficiency or gene mutations.

### Treatment and management

Currently there is no cure for MPS–I disorders. Treatment of individual symptoms does offer some relief. Surgical repair is available to correct a hernia. Hearing aids sometimes improve hearing and language skills, and eyeglasses may enhance eyesight. Some children with Hurler syndrome improve communication skills by learning sign language.

Skeletal abnormalities require attention, especially if they affect the upper part of the spine and compress the spinal cord. Spinal cord compression and storage of dermatan sulfate and heparan sulfate in the surrounding membranes cause fluid to accumulate in the brain. Brain damage often occurs unless this condition is corrected. A surgeon can implant a shunt in the brain to remove excess fluid. Once present, the mental retardation caused by Hurler syndrome is generally not reversible.

It is important to protect the upper back and neck of a patient with Hurler syndrome. This area should not be manipulated during chiropractic or physical therapy. If the patient undergoes anesthesia for any reason, care should be taken to support the neck and upper back at all times.

Orthopedic treatment can help reduce joint stiffness and its effects on movement.

Several options are available to correct breathing difficulties. Some patients respond well to oxygen treatments. Others require tonsillectomy, adenoidectomy or tracheostomy to remove upper airway obstruction.

Medications are available to treat common respiratory infections.

If heart disease is limited to valve damage, valve replacement may be an option for some patients with Hurler syndrome.

Children with Hurler syndrome are generally easy–going and affectionate. They benefit greatly from safe and caring environments. Community support and social services can improve the quality of life for the entire family unit. The family of a child with Hurler syndrome experiences grief and loss throughout the lifetime and upon the death of the child. **Genetic counseling** is available to offer support, educate families about the disease, and assess the risk to other family members. The National MPS Society provides additional support and information.

Enzyme replacement therapies (ERT) are currently in use or are being tested for reducing non–neurological symptoms and pain.

Bone marrow transplantation (BMT) and umbilical cord blood transplantation (UCBT) have had limited success in treating the mucopolysaccharidoses. Abnormal physical characteristics, except for those affecting the skeleton and eyes, may be improved, but neurologic outcomes have varied. BMT replaces the child's entire blood system with the blood system of a healthy person. The healthy bone marrow contains stem cells, cells from which other cells and tissues arise. These cells produce enough alpha–L–iduronidase to break down dermatan sulfate and heparan sulfate.

BMT is a complicated procedure. If the donated bone marrow is not compatible with the child's own body tissues, the child's immune system will destroy it. BMT is most successful if the donor is a close relative of the patient, since this increases the chance of compatibility between donor and patient bone marrow. To reduce the risk of donor bone marrow rejection, the patient receives drugs and radiation to suppress the immune system, leaving the patient vulnerable to infection.

Studies are evaluating a combination a of ERT and hematopoietic stem cell transplantation (HSTC) as therapy for Hurler syndrome. Some studies have reported psychomotor improvements and reduction of head circumference.

#### Clinical trials

Clinical trials on mucopolysaccharidosis type I are currently sponsored by the National Institutes of Health (NIH) and other agencies. As of 2009, NIH was reporting 23 on–going and completed studies.

Examples include:

- The evaluation of the use of enzyme replacement therapy into the spinal fluid for treatment of spinal cord compression in some forms of mucopolysaccharidosis I. (NCT00215527)
- A study to determine whether growth hormone is a safe and effective treatment for short stature in children with Mucopolysaccharidosis type I, II, and VI. (NCT00748969)
- The evaluation of stem cell transplant infusions of Laronidase prior to transplant for Hurler syndrome patients. (NCT00176891)

Clinical trial information is constantly updated by NIH and the most recent information on MPS–I trials can be found at: http://clinicaltrials.gov.

## Prognosis

As of 2009, research funded by the National Institute of Neurological Disorders and Stroke (NINDS) has shown that viral–delivered **gene therapy** in animal models of the mucopolysaccharidoses can stop the buildup of storage materials in brain cells and improve learning and memory. Additional studies are being planned to understand how gene therapy prompts recovery of mental function in these animal models. However, it may be years before such treatment becomes available to humans. Scientists are also trying to identify all genes associated with the mucopolysaccharidoses and plan to test new therapies in animal models and in humans. Animal models are also being used to investigate therapies that replace the missing or insufficient enzymes needed to break down the sugar chains.

Until these or other therapies become available, patients who cannot undergo BMT can receive treatment for individual symptoms. While treatment provides temporary relief, it cannot prevent the progressive damage caused by accumulation of dermatan sulfate and heparan sulfate. Death due to respiratory complications or heart failure usually occurs by age 12.

## Resources

### BOOKS

ICON Health Publications. *Hurler Syndrome: A Medical Dictionary, Bibliography, And Annotated Research Guide To Internet References*. San Diego, CA: ICON Health Publications, 2004.

ICON Health Publications. *The Official Parent's Sourcebook on Mucopolysaccharidoses: A Revised and Updated Directory for the Internet Age*. San Diego, CA: ICON Health Publications, 2002.

### PERIODICALS

Aldenhoven, M., et al. "The clinical outcome of Hurler syndrome after stem cell transplantation." *Biology of Blood and Marrow Transplantation* 14, no. 5 (May 2008): 485–498.

El Dib, R. P., and G. M. Pastores. "Laronidase for treating mucopolysaccharidosis type I." *Genetics and Molecular Research* 30, no. 6 (September 2007): 667–674.

Moore, D., et al. "The prevalence of and survival in Mucopolysaccharidosis I: Hurler, Hurler–Scheie and Scheie syndromes in the UK." *Orphanet Journal of Rare Diseases* 16, no. 3 (September 2008): 24.

Muenzer, J., et al. "Mucopolysaccharidosis I: management and treatment guidelines." *Pediatrics* 123, no. 1 (January 2009): 19–29.

Taylor, C., et al. "Mobility in Hurler syndrome." *Journal of Pediatric Orthopaedics* 28, no. 2 (March 2008): 163–168.

Tolar, J., et al. "Combination of enzyme replacement and hematopoietic stem cell transplantation as therapy for Hurler syndrome." *Bone Marrow Transplantation* 41, no. 6 (March 2008): 531–535.

### WEBSITES

*Hurler Syndrome*. Medical Encyclopedia. Medline Plus, May 22, 2007 (February 15, 2009). http://www.nlm.nih.gov/medlineplus/ency/article/001204.htm.

*MPS I/Hurler Syndrome*. Information Page. Hide & Seek Foundation (February 15, 2009). http://www.hideandseek.org/index.php?option=com_content&task=view&id=238&Itemid=75.

*Mucopolysaccharides*. Medical Encyclopedia. Medline Plus, January 29, 2009 (February 15, 2009). http://www.nlm.nih.gov/medlineplus/ency/article/002263.htm.

*Mucopolysaccharidosis I (MPS I)*. Information Page. Children's Memorial Hospital, January 29, 2009 (February 15, 2009). http://www.childrensmemorial.org/depts/genetics/mps1.aspx.

*Mucopolysaccharidosis Type I*. Information Page. Genetics Home Reference, December 2008 (February 15, 2009). http://ghr.nlm.nih.gov/condition=mucopolysaccharidosistypei.

*Scheie Syndrome*. Medical Encyclopedia. Medline Plus, January 29, 2009 (February 15, 2009). http://www.nlm.nih.gov/medlineplus/ency/article/001246.htm.

### ORGANIZATIONS

Canadian Society for Mucopolysaccharide & Related Diseases. PO Box 30034, RPO Parkgate, North Vancouver, BC V7H 2Y8, Canada. (604) 924-5130 or (800) 667-1846. Fax: (604) 924-5131. Email: info@mpssociety.ca. http://www.mpssociety.ca.

Hide and Seek Foundation for Lysosomal Storage Disease Research. 4123 Lankershim Blvd., Suite 302, N. Hollywood, CA 91602-2828. (818) 762-8621. Fax: (818) 762-2502. Email: info@hideandseek.org. http://www.hideandseek.org.

National MPS Society. PO Box 14686, Durham, NC 27709-4686. (919) 806-0101 or (877) MPD-1001. Fax: (919) 806-2055. http://www.mpssociety.org.

National Organization for Rare Disorders (NORD). 55 Kenosia Avenue, PO Box 1968, Danbury, CT 06813-1968. (203) 744-0100 or (800) 999-6673. Fax: (203) 798-2291. http://www.rarediseases.org.

Society for Mucopolysaccharide Diseases. MPS House, Repton Place, White Lion Rd., Amersham, Buckinghamshire HP7 9LP, UK. +44 0845-389-9901. http://www.mpssociety.co.uk.

Monique Laberge, PhD
Avis L. Gibons

# Mucopolysaccharidosis type II

## Definition

Mucopolysaccharidosis type II (Hunter syndrome or MPS–II) is a defect in the ability to break down or metabolize a type of molecule known as a mucopolysaccharide. Only males are affected. Short stature, changes in the normal curvature of the spine (kyphosis), a distinctive facial appearance characterized by coarse features, an oversized head (hydrocephaly), thickened lips, and a broad, flat nose characterize the syndrome. The clinical picture ranges from severe (the most frequent form) with early psychomotor regression, to mild.

## Description

Hunter syndrome belongs to a group of diseases called **mucopolysaccharidoses**. It is caused by the deficiency of an enzyme called iduronate–2–sulfatase (I2S) that is required to metabolize or break down mucopolysaccharides (also called glycosaminoglycans). The syndrome is called mucopolysaccharidosis type II (MPS–II) to distinguish it from other similar diseases. The Hunter syndrome involves a defect in the extracellular matrix of connective tissue. One of the components of the extracellular matrix is a molecule called a proteoglycan. Like most molecules in the body, it is regularly replaced. When this occurs, one of the products of the reaction is a class of molecules known as mucopolysaccharides (glycosoaminoglycans or GAGs). Two of these are important in Hunter syndrome: dermatan sulfate and heparan sulfate. These are found in the skin, blood vessels, heart and heart valves (dermatan sulfate) and lungs, arteries and cellular surfaces (heparan sulfate). The partially broken–down molecules are collected by lysosomes and stored in various locations in the body. Over time, these accumulations of partially metabolized

mucopolysaccharides impair the heart, nervous system, connective tissue, and bones.

Both of these molecules require the enzyme iduronate–2–sulfatase (I2S) to be broken down. In people with Hunter syndrome, this enzyme is partially or completely inactive. As a result, unchanged molecules accumulate in cells. These mucopolysaccharides are stored and interfere with normal cellular functions. The rate of accumulation is not the same for all persons with Hunter syndrome. Variability in the age of onset is thought to be due to lingering amounts of activity by this enzyme.

The cells in which mucopolysaccharides are stored determine the symptoms that develop. When mucopolysaccharides are stored in skin, the proportions of the face change (coarser features than normal and an enlarged head). When they are stored in heart valves and walls, cardiac function progressively declines. If intact mucopolysaccharides are stored in airways of the lung, difficulty in breathing develops due to obstruction of the upper airway. Storage of the molecules in joints decreases mobility and dexterity. Storage in bones results in decreased growth and short stature. As mucopolysaccharides are stored in the brain, levels of mental functioning decline.

There are two variants of Hunter syndrome: a severe form (MPS–IIA) and a mild form (MPS–IIB). These can be diagnosed early in life and are distinguished on the basis of mental and behavioral differences. External manifestations of the severe form occur between two and four years of age and the mild form later, up to age 10.

### Genetic profile

Mutations in the iduronate–2–sulfatase (IDS) **gene** cause MPS II. The IDS gene provides instructions for producing the iduronate–2–sulfatase (I2S) enzyme, which is involved in the breakdown of GAGs. The IDS gene is located on the long (q) arm of the X **chromosome** at position 28 (Xq28). Hence, Hunter syndrome is a X–linked disease. The Y chromosome of a male is never affected in Hunter syndrome. Males only have one copy of the IDS gene while females have two. A male who inherits an abnormal IDS gene will develop Hunter syndrome. This can occur in two ways: from a mother who already has the gene (she is a carrier) or from a fresh mutation. Fresh mutations are unusual.

There are four possible genetic configurations. (1) A male can have a normal IDS gene and will be unaffected. (2) A male can have an abnormal IDS gene and will have Hunter syndrome. Should this male reproduce, his sons will not have Hunter syndrome and his daughters will all be carriers. (3) A female can have two normal IDS genes and be unaffected. (4) A female can have one abnormal IDS gene and be a carrier. Should this female reproduce, half of her sons will, on average, have Hunter syndrome. Half of her daughters, on average, will be carriers. It is possible that no sons will have Hunter syndrome or no daughters will be carriers.

### Demographics

In the United States, MPS II occurs in approximately 1 in 100,000 to 1 in 170,000 males. Worldwide, it is present at birth in between one in 72,000 and one in 130,000 males. Because it is carried on the X chromosome, only males can be affected.

### Signs and symptoms

Individuals with Hunter syndrome experience a slowing of growth between one and four years of age. They attain an average height of 4–5 ft (122–152 cm). The facial features of persons with Hunter syndrome are coarser than normal. Their heads tend to be large in proportion to their bodies. Over time, their hands tend to become stiff and assume a claw–like appearance. Their teeth are delayed in erupting. Progressive hearing loss eventually leads to **deafness**. Internal organs such as the liver and spleen are larger than normal. They are quite prone to hernias.

### Diagnosis

Hunter syndrome can be identified early in life and is often initially diagnosed by the presence of an enlarged liver and spleen (hepatosplenomegaly), hernias, or joint stiffness. Skeletal changes can be seen with radiographs. Elevated mucopolysaccharide levels in urine focuses the diagnosis to a group of disorders. The concentration of dermatan sulfate and heparan sulfate is 5–25 times higher than in normal urine. Both are present in approximately the same amounts. The diagnosis of Hunter syndrome is confirmed by measuring iduronate–2–sulfatase activity in white blood cells, serum, or skin fibroblasts. Prenatal diagnosis is widely available by measuring the activity of I2S enzyme in amniotic fluid.

Hunter syndrome has many diagnostic characteristics in common with Hurler syndrome. However, there are some distinct differences between the two syndromes. Individuals with Hunter syndrome have clear corneas and tend to have deposits of mucopolysaccharides in the skin. These are characteristically on the back of the hands and elbows (the extensor surfaces) and on the upper surfaces of the shoulders. All are males. These differences are important in diagnosis.

### Treatment and management

There is no cure for Hunter syndrome. Until recently, general support and treatment of specific symptoms and complications were the only treatment options available. In 2006 the Food and Drug Administration (FDA) approved Elaprase (idursulfase) for the treatment of MPS–II by enzyme replacement therapy (ERT), a treatment aimed at synthetically replacing the deficient enzyme of Hunter Syndrome. Clinical studies seem to demonstrate that idursulfase may be the first successful symptomatic therapy that can benefit patients with MPS II.

#### Clinical trials

Clinical trials on mucopolysaccharidosis type II are currently sponsored by the National Institutes of

Health (NIH) and other agencies. As of 2009, NIH was reporting eight on–going and completed studies.

Examples include:

- The evaluation of the safety and clinical outcomes in Hunter Syndrome patients 5 years of age and younger receiving idursulfase therapy. (NCT00607386)
- A study to determine whether the administration of iduronate–2–sulfatase enzyme in a weekly or every other week therapy frequency is safe and efficient in patients with MPS II. (NCT00069641)
- The evaluation of the safety and feasibility of treating mucopolysaccharidosis II by gene therapy. (NCT00004454)

Clinical trial information is constantly updated by NIH and the most recent information on MPS–II trials can be found at: http://clinicaltrials.gov.

### Prognosis

In the severe form, death usually occurs by age 10–15. Persons with the mild form usually live near–normal lives and have normal intelligence.

### Resources

#### BOOKS

ICON Health Publications. *Hunter Syndrome: A Medical Dictionary, Bibliography, And Annotated Research Guide To Internet References.* San Diego, CA: ICON Health Publications, 2004.

ICON Health Publications. *The Official Parent's Sourcebook on Mucopolysaccharidoses: A Revised and Updated Directory for the Internet Age.* San Diego, CA: ICON Health Publications, 2002.

#### PERIODICALS

Farooq, M. U., et al. "A novel mutation in the iduronate 2 sulfatase gene resulting in mucopolysaccharidosis type II and chorea: case report of two siblings." *Movement Disorders* 23, no. 10 (July 2008): 1487–1488.

Martin, R., et al. "Recognition and diagnosis of mucopolysaccharidosis II (Hunter syndrome)." *Pediatrics* 121, no. 2 (February 2008): e377–e386.

Wraith, J. E. "Enzyme replacement therapy with idursulfase in patients with mucopolysaccharidosis type II." *Acta Paediatrica Supplement* 16, no. 3 (April 2008): 768–78.

Wraith, J. E., et al. "Initial report from the Hunter Outcome Survey." *Genetics in Medicine* 10, no. 7 (July 2008): 508–516.

#### WEBSITES

*Hunter Disease (MPS II).* Information Page. Society for Mucopolysaccharide Diseases (February 15, 2009). http://www.mpssociety.co.uk/index.php?page=hunter-disease.

*Hunter Syndrome.* Medical Encyclopedia. Medline Plus, September 28, 2007 (February 15, 2009). http://www.nlm.nih.gov/medlineplus/ency/article/001203.htm.

*Hunter Syndrome.* Information Page. Madisons Foundation (February 15, 2009). http://www.madisonsfoundation.org/index.php/component/option,com_mpower/Itemid,49/diseaseID,450/.

*MPS II Hunter Syndrome.* Information Page. Hide & Seek Foundation (February 15, 2009). http://www.hideandseek.org/index.php?option=com_content&task=view&id=147&Itemid=75.

*Mucopolysaccharides.* Medical Encyclopedia. Medline Plus, January 29, 2009 (February 15, 2009). http://www.nlm.nih.gov/medlineplus/ency/article/002263.htm.

*Mucopolysaccharidoses Fact Sheet.* Information Page. NINDS, July 28, 2008 (February 15, 2009). http://www.ninds.nih.gov/disorders/mucopolysaccharidoses/detail_mucopolysaccharidoses.htm.

#### ORGANIZATIONS

Canadian Society for Mucopolysaccharide & Related Diseases. PO Box 30034, RPO Parkgate, North Vancouver, BC V7H 2Y8, Canada. (604) 924-5130 or (800) 667-1846. Fax: (604) 924-5131. Email: info@mpssociety.ca. http://www.mpssociety.ca.

Hide and Seek Foundation for Lysosomal Storage Disease Research. 4123 Lankershim Blvd., Suite 302, N. Hollywood, CA 91602-2828. (818) 762-8621. Fax: (818) 762-2502. Email: info@hideandseek.org. http://www.hideandseek.org.

National MPS Society. PO Box 14686, Durham, NC 27709-4686. (919) 806-0101 or (877) MPS-1001. Fax: (919) 806-2055. http://www.mpssociety.org.

National Organization for Rare Disorders (NORD). 55 Kenosia Avenue, PO Box 1968, Danbury, CT 06813-1968. (203) 744-0100 or (800) 999-6673. Fax: (203) 798-2291. http://www.rarediseases.org.

Society for Mucopolysaccharide Diseases. MPS House, Repton Place, White Lion Rd., Amersham, Buckinghamshire HP7 9LP, UK. +44 0845-389-9901. http://www.mpssociety.co.uk.

L. Fleming Fallon, Jr., MD, PhD, DrPH

Mucoxiscidosis *see* **Cystic fibrosis**

# Muir-Torre syndrome

## Definition

A syndrome is a condition in which a certain set of features is regularly seen. In Muir-Torre syndrome, the consistent features are skin tumors (sebaceous neoplasms) and internal organ cancers, most commonly colon **cancer**.

**Screening recommendations for patients with Muir-Torrie syndrome**

| Test/Procedure | Age | Frequency |
|---|---|---|
| Physical exam | 20+ | Every 3 years |
| | 40+ | Annually |
| Digital rectal exam | Any | Annually |
| Gualac of stool for occult blood | Any | Annually |
| Lab work-up | Any | Annually |
|   Carcinoembryonic antigen | | |
|   Complete blood cell count | | |
|     with differential and platelet count | | |
|   Erythrocyte sedimentation rate | | |
|   Serum chemistries (SMA-20) | | |
|   Urinalysis | | |
| Chest roentgenogram | Any | Every 3–5 years |
| Colonoscopy | Any | Every 5 years |
| | If positive for polyps | Every 3 years |

*(Table by GGS Creative Resources. Reproduced by permission of Gale, a part of Cengage Learning.)*

**Additional screening recommendations for females with Muir-Torrie syndrome**

| Test/Procedure | Age | Frequency |
|---|---|---|
| Breast exam | 20240 | Every 3 years |
| | 401 | Annually |
| Pelvic exam | 181 or sexually active | Annually |
| Pap smear | 181 or sexually active | Annually |
| Mammogram | 40149 | Every 1–2 years |
| | 501 | Annually |
| Endometrial biopsy | Menopause | Every 3–5 years after onset |

*(Table by GGS Creative Resources. Reproduced by permission of Gale, a part of Cengage Learning.)*

## Description

Muir-Torre syndrome is named for two authors who provided some of the earliest descriptions of the condition, Muir in 1967 and Torre in 1968. Originally thought to be separate conditions, it is now known that Muir-Torre syndrome and hereditary non-polyposis colon cancer (HNPCC), also known as Lynch syndrome, are due to alterations in the same genes. Some of the features of the conditions are the same including increased risk of colorectal cancer (cancer of the colon and rectum) and cancer of other organs. Both conditions are hereditary cancer predisposition syndromes meaning that the risk of cancer has been linked to an inherited tendency for the disease. A unique feature of Muir-Torre syndrome is the skin tumors. The most common skin tumors associated with Muir-Torre syndrome are benign (non-cancerous) or malignant (cancerous) tumors of the oil-secreting (sebaceous) glands of the skin. Another relatively common skin finding is the presence of growths called keratoacanthomas.

## Genetic profile

HNPCC and Muir-Torre syndrome are allelic meaning that these disorders are due to changes in the same genes. Genes, the units of instruction for the body, can have changes or mutations that develop over time. Certain mutations are repaired by a class of genes known as mismatch repair genes. When these genes are not functioning properly, there is a higher chance of cancer due to the alterations that accumulate in the genetic material. Heritable mutations in at least five mismatch repair genes have been linked to HNPCC although the majority, over 90%, are in the hMLH1 and hMSH2 genes. Mutations in hMLH1 and hMSH2 also have been reported in Muir-Torre syndrome although most have been hMSH2 mutations. The location of the hMLH1 gene is on **chromosome** 3 at 3p21.3 while the location of hMSH2 is chromosome 2, 2p22-p21. **Genetic testing** for hMLH1 and hMSH2 is available but the detection rate for mismatch repair **gene mutations** is less than 100%. Therefore, diagnosis of Muir-Torre syndrome is not based on genetic testing alone but also on the presence of the typical features of the disease.

Muir-Torre syndrome is inherited in an autosomal dominant fashion. Thus, both men and women can have Muir-Torre syndrome and only one gene of the paired genes, needs to be altered to have the syndrome. Children of individuals with Muir-Torre syndrome have a one in two or 50% chance of inheriting the gene alteration. The symptoms of the syndrome are variable and not all individuals with the condition will develop all of the features.

## Demographics

At least 250 cases of Muir-Torre syndrome, specifically, have been reported. It is estimated that between one in 200 to one in 2,000 people in Western countries carry an alteration in the genes associated with HNPCC but the rate of Muir-Torre syndrome itself has not been clarified. More males than females appear to exhibit the features of Muir-Torre syndrome. The average age at time of diagnosis of the syndrome is around 55 years.

## Signs and symptoms

### Skin findings

Sebaceous neoplasms typically appear as yellowish bumps on the skin of the head or neck but can be

## KEY TERMS

**Allelic**—Related to the same gene.

**Benign**—A non-cancerous tumor that does not spread and is not life-threatening.

**Biopsy**—The surgical removal and microscopic examination of living tissue for diagnostic purposes.

**Colectomy**—Surgical removal of the colon.

**Colonoscopy**—Procedure for viewing the large intestine (colon) by inserting an illuminated tube into the rectum and guiding it up the large intestine.

**Colorectal**—Of the colon and/or rectum.

**Gene**—A building block of inheritance, which contains the instructions for the production of a particular protein, and is made up of a molecular sequence found on a section of DNA. Each gene is found on a precise location on a chromosome.

**Genitourinary**—Related to the reproductive and urinary systems of the body.

**Hereditary non-polyposis colon cancer (HNPCC)**—A genetic syndrome causing increased cancer risks, most notably colon cancer. Also called Lynch syndrome.

**hMLH1 and hMSH2**—Genes known to control mismatch repair of genes.

**Keratoacanthoma**—A firm nodule on the skin typically found in areas of sun exposure.

**Lymph node**—A bean-sized mass of tissue that is part of the immune system and is found in different areas of the body.

**Lynch syndrome**—A genetic syndrome causing increased cancer risks, most notably colon cancer. Also called hereditary non-polyposis colon cancer (HNPCC).

**Malignant**—A tumor growth that spreads to another part of the body, usually cancerous.

**Mismatch repair**—Repair of gene alterations due to mismatching.

**Mutation**—A permanent change in the genetic material that may alter a trait or characteristic of an individual, or manifest as disease, and can be transmitted to offspring.

**Polyp**—A mass of tissue bulging out from the normal surface of a mucous membrane.

**Radiation**—High energy rays used in cancer treatment to kill or shrink cancer cells.

**Sebaceous**—Related to the glands of the skin that produce an oily substance.

**Splenic flexure**—The area of the large intestine at which the transverse colon meets the descending colon.

---

found on the trunk and other areas. The classification of the different types of sebaceous neoplasms can be difficult so microscopic evaluation is usually required for the final diagnosis. Keratoacanthomas are skin-colored or reddish, firm skin nodules that are distinct from sebaceous neoplasms upon microscopic examination. The skin findings in Muir-Torre syndrome can either appear before, during, or after the development of the internal cancer.

### Internal findings

Internal organ cancers are common in Muir-Torre syndrome. Several individuals with Muir-Torre syndrome with multiple types of internal cancers have been reported. The most common internal organ cancer is colorectal cancer. Unlike colon cancers in the general population, the tumors due to Muir-Torre syndrome are more frequently seen around or closer to the right side of an area of the colon known as the splenic flexure. This tumor location, the meeting point of the transverse and the descending colon, is different than the usual location of colon cancer in the general population.

Colon polyps, benign growths with the possibility of cancer development, have been reported in individuals with Muir-Torre syndrome; however, the number of polyps typically is limited.

Symptoms of colorectal cancer or polyps may include:

- red blood in stool
- weight loss
- pain or bloating in abdomen
- long-term constipation
- diarrhea
- decrease in stool size

The next most frequent cancer occurrences in Muir-Torre syndrome are those of the genitourinary system including uterine cancer, ovary cancer, and bladder cancer. Other cancers that have been seen with Muir-Torre syndrome include breast cancers, blood cancers, head and neck cancers and cancers of the small intestine.

### Diagnosis

Since not all families with the features of Muir-Torre syndrome have identifiable mismatch repair gene alterations, diagnosis is based mainly on the presence of the physical features of the disease. Muir-Torre syndrome is defined by the presence of certain types of sebaceous neoplasms (sebaceous adenomas, sebaceous epitheliomas, sebaceous carcinomas and keratoacanthomas with sebaceous differentiation) and at least one internal organ cancer in the same individual. Muir-Torre syndrome may also be diagnosed if an individual has multiple keratoacanthomas, multiple internal organ cancers and a family history of Muir-Torre syndrome. Testing of the hMLH1 and hMSH2 genes is available and could be done to confirm a diagnosis or to assist in testing at-risk relatives prior to development of symptoms. Given the complexity of this disorder, **genetic counseling** may be considered before testing.

Screening recommendations have been proposed for individuals with Muir-Torre or at-risk relatives. In addition to regular screening for the skin findings, screening for internal cancers may be considered. The effectiveness of screening for individuals with or at risk for Muir-Torre syndrome has yet to be proven.

### Treatment and management

While it is not possible to cure the genetic abnormality that results in Muir-Torre syndrome, it is possible to prevent and treat the symptoms of the syndrome. The skin tumors are removed by freezing or cutting. If lymph nodes, small bean-sized lumps of tissue that are part of the immune system, are involved, these must be removed also. Radiation, high energy rays, to the affected area can be beneficial. A medication, isotretinoin, may reduce the risk of skin tumors. Internal organ cancers are treated in the standard manner, removal by surgery and possible treatment with radiation or cancer-killing medication (chemotherapy). Removal of the colon, colectomy, before colon cancer develops is an option with HNPCC and may be considered for individuals with Muir-Torre syndrome.

### Prognosis

The cancers associated with Muir-Torre syndrome are usually diagnosed at earlier ages than typically seen. For instance, the average age at diagnosis of colorectal cancer is 10 years earlier than in the general population. Fortunately, the internal organ cancers seen in Muir-Torre syndrome appear less aggressive. So, the prognosis may be better for a person with colon cancer due to Muir-Torre syndrome than colon cancer in the general population.

### Resources

**BOOKS**

Flanders, Tamar, et al. "Cancers of the digestive system." *Inherited Susceptibility: Clinical, predictive and ethical perspectives.* Edited by William D. Foulkes and Shirley V. Hodgson, Cambridge University Press, 1998. pp.181-185.

**WEBSITES**

*M.D. Anderson Cancer Center.* http://www3.mdanderson. org/depts/hcc.

**ORGANIZATIONS**

American Cancer Society. 1599 Clifton Road NE, Atlanta, GA 30329. (800) 227-2345. http://www.cancer.org.
National Cancer Institute. Office of Communications, 31 Center Dr. MSC 2580, Bldg. 1 Room 10A16, Bethesda, MD 20892-2580. (800) 422-6237. http://www.nci.nih.gov.

Kristin Baker Niendorf, MS, CGC

# Multifactorial inheritance

### Definition

Many common congenital malformations and diseases are caused by a combination of genetic and environmental factors. The term multifactorial **inheritance** is used to describe conditions that occur due to these multiple factors. In contrast to dominantly or recessively inherited diseases, multifactorial traits do not follow any particular pattern of inheritance in families. Multifactorial conditions do tend to cluster in families, but **pedigree analysis** does not reveal a specific pattern of affected individuals. Some multifactorial conditions occur because of the interplay of many genetic factors and limited environmental factors. Others occur because of limited genetic factors and significant environmental factors. The number of genetic and environmental factors vary, as does the amount of impact of each factor on the presence or severity of disease. Often there are multiple susceptibility genes involved, each of which has an additive affect on outcome.

Examples of congenital malformations following a multifactorial pattern of inheritance include **cleft lip and palate**, **neural tube defects**, and heart defects. Adult onset diseases that follow multifactorial inheritance include **diabetes**, heart disease, **epilepsy** and affective disorders like **schizophrenia**. Many normal traits in the general population follow multifactorial inheritance. For instance, height, intelligence, and blood pressure are all determined in part by genetic factors, but are influenced by environmental factors.

### Continuous and discontinuous traits

Some multifactorial traits are considered continuous because there is bell shaped distribution of those traits in the population. These are quantitative traits such as height. Other traits are discontinuous because there is a cutoff or threshold of genetic and environmental risk that must be crossed in order for the trait to occur. An example would be a malformation like a **cleft lip**, in which the person is either affected or unaffected. In both cases, the genetic and environmental factors that are involved in the occurrence of the condition are referred to as liability.

#### *Pyloric stenosis*

An example of a discontinuous multifactorial trait that follows the threshold model is **pyloric stenosis**. Pyloric stenosis is a narrowing of the pylorus, the connection between the stomach and the intestine. Symptoms of pyloric stenosis include vomiting, constipation and weight loss. Surgery is often needed for repair. An important genetic factor in the occurrence of pyloric stenosis is a person's sex. The condition is five times more common in males. The liability is higher in women, such that more or stronger genetic and environmental factors are needed to cause the condition in women. Therefore, male first-degree relatives of a female who is affected with pyloric stenosis have a higher risk to be born with the condition than do female first-degree relatives of the same person. This is because the stronger genetic factors present in the family (represented by the affected female) are more likely to cross the lower liability threshold in male family members.

### Recurrence risks

Recurrence risks for multifactorial traits are based on empiric data, or observations from other families with affected individuals. Most multifactorial traits have a recurrence risk to first-degree relatives of 2-5%. However, empiric data for a specific condition may provide a more specific recurrence risk. Some general characteristics about the recurrence risk of multifactorial traits include:

- The recurrence risk to first-degree relatives is increased above the general population risk for the trait, but the risk drops off quickly for more distantly related individuals.

- The recurrence risk increases proportionately to the number of affected individuals in the family. A person with two affected relatives has a higher risk than someone with one affected relative.

- The recurrence risk is higher if the disorder is in the severe range of the possible outcomes. For instance, the risk to a relative of a person with a unilateral cleft lip is lower than if the affected person had bilateral cleft lip and a cleft palate.

- If the condition is more common in one sex, the recurrence risk for relatives is higher in the less affected sex. Pyloric stenosis is an example of this.

- Recurrence risks quoted are averages and the true risk in a specific family may be higher or lower.

It is important to understand that recurrence risks for conditions may vary from one population to another. For instance, North Carolina, South Carolina, and Texas all have a higher incidence of neural tube defects that other states in the United States. Ireland has a higher incidence of neural tube defects than many other countries.

### Examples of multifactorial traits

#### *Neural tube defects*

Neural tube defects are birth defects that result from the failure of part of the spinal column to close approximately 28 days after conception. If the anterior (top) portion of the neural tube fails to close, the most severe type of neural tube defect called **anencephaly** results. Anencephaly is the absence of portions of the skull and brain and is a lethal defect. If a lower area of the spine fails to close, **spina bifida** occurs. People with spina bifida have varying degrees of paralysis, difficulty with bowel and bladder control, and extra fluid in the brain called **hydrocephalus**. The size and location of the neural tube opening determines the severity of symptoms. Surgery is needed to cover or close the open area of the spine. When hydrocephalus is present, surgery is needed for shunt placement.

Neural tube defects are believed to follow a multifactorial pattern of inheritance. Empiric data suggests that the risk to first-degree relatives of a person with a neural tube defect is increased 3-5%. The risk to other more distantly related relatives decreases significantly. In addition, it is known that a form of vitamin B called folic acid can significantly reduce the chance for the occurrence of a neural tube defect. Studies have shown that when folic acid is taken at least three months prior to pregnancy and through the first trimester, the chance for a neural tube defect can be reduced by 50-70%. This data suggests that one environmental factor in the occurrence of neural tube defects is maternal folate levels. However, some women who are not folate deficient have babies with open spine abnormalities. Other women who are folate deficient do not have babies with spinal openings. The exact interplay of genetic and environmental factors in the occurrence of neural tube defects is not yet clear. Studies are currently underway to identify genes involved in the occurrence of neural tube defects.

### Diabetes

There are two general types of diabetes. Type I is the juvenile onset form that often begins in adolescence and requires insulin injections for control of blood sugar levels. Type II is the more common, later onset form that does not usually require insulin therapy. Both are known to be influenced by environmental factors and show familial clustering. Important environmental factors involved in the occurrence of diabetes include diet, viral exposure in childhood and certain drug exposures. It is clear that genetic factors are involved in the occurrence of type I diabetes since empiric data show that 10% of people with the condition have an affected sibling. An important susceptibility gene for type I diabetes has been discovered on **chromosome** 6. The gene is called IDDM1. Another gene on chromosome 11 has also been identified as a susceptibility gene. Studies in mice have indicated that there are probably 12-20 susceptibility genes for insulin dependent diabetes. IDDM1 is believed to have a strong effect and is modified by other susceptibility genes and environmental factors.

## Analysis of multifactorial conditions

Genetic studies of multifactorial traits are usually more difficult than genetic studies of dominant or recessive traits. This is because it is difficult to determine the amount of genetic contribution to the multifactorial trait versus the amount of environmental contribution. For most multifactorial traits, it is not possible to perform a genetic test and determine if a person will be affected. Instead, studies involving multifactorial traits strive to determine the proportion of the **phenotype** due to genetic factors and to identify those genetic factors. The inherited portion of a multifactorial trait is called heritability.

### Disease association studies

One method of studying the heritability of multifactorial traits is to determine if a candidate gene is more common in an affected population than in the general population.

### Sibling pair studies

Another type of study involves gathering many pairs of siblings who are affected with a multifactorial trait. Researchers try to identify polymorphisms common in the sibling pairs. These polymorphisms can then be further analyzed. They can also study candidate genes in these sibling pairs. Studying individuals who are at the extreme end of the affected range and are thought to have a larger heritability for the trait can strengthen this type of study.

### Twin studies

Another approach is to study a trait of interest in twins. Identical twins have 100% of their genes in common. Non-identical twins have 50% of their genes in common, just like any other siblings. In multifactorial traits, identical twins will be concordant for the trait significantly more often than non-identical twins. One way to control for the influence of a similar environment on twins is to study twins who are raised separately. However, situations in which one or both identical twins were adopted out and are available for study are rare.

Linkage analysis and animal studies are also used to study the heritability of conditions, although there are significant limitations to these approaches for multifactorial traits.

## Ethical concerns of testing

One of the goals of studying the genetic factors involved in multifactorial traits is to be able to counsel those at highest genetic risk about ways to alter their environment to minimize risk of symptoms. However, **genetic testing** for multifactorial traits is limited by the lack of understanding about how other genes and environment interact with major susceptibility genes to cause disease. Testing is also limited by genetic heterogeneity for major susceptibility loci. Often the attention of the media to certain genetic tests increases demand for the test, when the limitations of the test are not fully explained. Therefore, it is important for people to receive appropriate pre-test counseling before undergoing genetic testing. Patients should consider the emotional impact of both positive and negative test results. Patients should understand that insurance and employment discrimination might occur due to test results. In addition, there may not be any treatment or lifestyle modification available for many multifactorial traits for which a genetic test is available. The patient should consider the inability to alter their risk when deciding about knowing their susceptibility for the condition. When a person chooses to have testing, it is important to have accurate post-test counseling about the result and its meaning.

### Resources

**BOOKS**

Connor, Michael, and Malcolm Ferguson-Smith. *Medical Genetics,* 5th Edition. Osney Mead, Oxford: Blackwell Science Ltd, 1997.

Gelehrter, Thomas, Francis Collins, and David Ginsburg. *Principles of Medical Genetics,* 2nd Edition. Baltimore, MD: Williams & Wilkins, 1998.

Jorde, Lynn, John Carey, Michael Bamshad, and Raymond White. *Medical Genetics,* 2nd Edition. St. Louis, Missouri: Mosby, Inc. 2000.

Lucassen, Anneke. "Genetics of multifactorial diseases." In *Practical Genetics for Primary Care* by Peter Rose and Anneke Lucassen. Oxford: Oxford University Press 1999, pp.145-165.

Mueller, Robert F., and Ian D. Young. *Emery's Elements of Medical Genetics.* Edinburgh, UK: Churchill Livingstone, 1998.

Sonja Rene Eubanks, MS

Multiple cartilaginous exostoses *see* **Hereditary multiple exostoses**

# Multiple endocrine neoplasias

### Definition

The multiple endocrine neoplasia (MEN) syndromes are four related disorders affecting the thyroid and other hormonal (endocrine) glands of the body. MEN has previously been known as familial endocrine adenomatosis.

The four related disorders are all neuroendocrine tumors. These tumorous cells have something in common, they produce hormones, or regulatory substances for the body's homeostasis. They come from the amine precursor and uptake decarboxylase (APUD) system, and have to do with the cell apparatus and function to make these substances common to the cell line. Neuroendocrine tumors cause syndromes associated with each other by genetic predisposition.

### Description

The four forms of MEN are MEN1 (Wermer syndrome), MEN2A (Sipple syndrome), MEN2B (previously known as MEN3), and familial medullary thyroid carcinoma (FMTC). Each is an autosomal dominant genetic condition, and all except FMTC predisposes to hyperplasia (excessive growth of cells) and tumor formation in a number of endocrine glands. FMTC predisposes only to this type of thyroid **cancer**.

Individuals with MEN1 experience hyperplasia of the parathyroid glands and may develop tumors of several endocrine glands including the pancreas and pituitary. The most frequent symptom of MEN1 is hyperparathyroidism. Hyperparathyroidism results from overgrowth of the parathyroid glands leading to excessive secretion of parathyroid hormone, which in turn leads to elevated blood calcium levels (hypercalcemia), kidney stones, weakened bones, fatigue, and weakness. Almost all individuals with MEN1 show parathyroid symptoms by the age of 50 years with some individuals developing symptoms in childhood.

Tumors of the pancreas, called pancreatic islet cell carcinomas, may develop in individuals with MEN1. These tumors tend to be benign, meaning that they do not spread to other body parts. On occasion these tumors may become malignant or cancerous and thereby a risk of metastasis, or spreading, of the cancer to other body parts becomes a concern. The pancreatic tumors associated with MEN1 may be called nonfunctional tumors as they do not result in an increase in hormone production and consequently, no symptoms are produced. In some cases, extra hormone is produced by the tumor and this results in symptoms; the symptoms depend upon the hormone produced. These symptomatic tumors are referred to as functional tumors. The most common functional tumor is gastrinoma followed by insulinoma. Other less frequent functional tumors are VIPoma and glucagonoma. Gastrinoma results in excessive secretion of gastrin (a hormone secreted into the stomach to aid in digestion), which in turn may cause upper gastrointestinal ulcers; this condition is sometimes referred to as Zollinger-Ellison syndrome. About one in three people with MEN1 develop a gastrinoma. Insulinoma causes an increase in insulin levels, which in turn causes glucose levels to decrease. This tumor causes

**Association of multiple endocrine neoplasias with other conditions**

| Form | Inheritance | Associated diseases/conditions | Affected gene |
|---|---|---|---|
| MEN 1 (Wermer's syndrome) | Autosomal dominant | Parathyroid hyperplasia<br>Pancreatic islet cell carcinomas<br>Pituitary hyperplasia<br>Thymus, adrenal, carcinoid tumors (less common) | MEN 1 |
| MEN 2A (Sipple syndrome) | Autosomal dominant | Medullary thyroid carcinoma<br>Pheochromocytoma<br>Parathyroid hyperplasia | RET |
| MEN 2B | Autosomal dominant | Medullary thyroid carcinoma<br>Pheochromocytoma<br>Parathyroid hyperplasia<br>Swollen lips<br>Tumors of mucous membranes (eyes, mouth, tongue, nasal cavities)<br>Enlarged colon<br>Skeletal problems such as spinal curving | RET |
| Familial medullary thyroid carcinoma | Autosomal dominant | Medullary thyroid carcinoma | RET |

*(Table by GGS Creative Resources. Reproduced by permission of Gale, a part of Cengage Learning.)*

symptoms consistent with low glucose levels (hypoglycemia, low blood sugar), which include anxiety, confusion, tremor, and seizure during periods of fasting. About 40–70% of individuals with MEN1 develop a pancreatic tumor.

The pituitary may also be affected—the consequence being extra production of hormone. The most frequently occurring pituitary tumor is prolactinoma, which results in extra prolactin (affects bone strength and fertility) being produced. Less commonly, the thymus and adrenal glands may also be affected and in rare cases, a tumor called a carcinoid may develop. Unlike MEN2, the thyroid gland is rarely involved in MEN1 symptoms.

Patients with MEN2A experience two main symptoms, medullary thyroid carcinoma (MTC) and a tumor of the adrenal gland known as pheochromocytoma. Medullary thyroid carcinoma is a slow-growing cancer that is preceded by a condition called C-cell hyperplasia. C-cells are a type of cell within the thyroid gland that produce a hormone called calcitonin. About 40–50% of individuals with MEN2A develop C-cell hyperplasia followed by MTC by the time they are 50 years old and 70% will have done so by the time they are 70 years old. In some cases, individuals develop C-cell hyperplasia and MTC in childhood. Medullary thyroid carcinoma tumors are often multifocal and bilateral.

Pheochromocytoma is usually a benign tumor that causes excessive secretion of adrenal hormones, which in turn can cause life-threatening hypertension (high blood pressure) and cardiac arrhythmia (abnormal heart beats). About 40% of people with MEN2A

develop a pheochromocytoma. Individuals with MEN2A also have a tendency for the parathyroid gland to increase in size (hypertrophy) as well as for tumors to develop in the parathyroid gland. About 25–35% of individuals with MEN2A will develop parathyroid involvement.

Individuals with MEN2B also develop MTC and pheochromocytoma. However, the medullary thyroid carcinomas often develop at much younger ages, often before the age of one year, and they tend to be more aggressive tumors. About half of the individuals with MEN2B develop a pheochromocytoma with some cases being diagnosed in childhood. All individuals with MEN2B develop additional conditions, which make it distinct from MEN2A. These extra features include a characteristic facial appearance with swollen lips; tumors of the mucous membranes of the eye, mouth, tongue, and nasal cavity; enlarged colon; and skeletal abnormalities, such as long bones and problems with spinal curving. Hyperparathyroidism is not seen in MEN2B as it is in MEN2A. Unlike the other three MEN syndromes, individuals with MEN2B may not have a family history of MEN2B. In at least half of the cases and perhaps more, the condition is new in the individual affected.

Medullary thyroid carcinoma may also occur in families but family members do not develop the other endocrine conditions seen in MEN2A and MEN2B. This is referred to as familial medullary thyroid carcinoma (FMTC) and it is a subtype of MEN2. Familial medullary thyroid cancer is suggested when other family members have also developed MTC, if the tumor is bilateral, and/or if the tumor is multifocal. In comparison to MEN2A and MEN2B, individuals with FMTC tend to develop MTC at older ages and the disease appears to be more indolent or slow progressing.

About 25% of MTC occurs in individuals who have MEN2A, MEN2B, and FMTC.

## Genetic profile

All four MEN syndromes follow autosomal dominant **inheritance**, meaning that every individual diagnosed with a MEN syndrome has a 50% (1 in 2) chance of passing on the condition to each of his or her children. Additionally, both men and women may inherit and pass on the genetic mutation.

MEN1 results from alterations or mutations in the MEN1 **gene**. Nearly every individual inheriting the MEN1 gene alteration will develop hyperparathyroidism, although the age at which it is diagnosed may differ among family members. Individuals inheriting the familial mutation may also develop one of the other characteristic features of MEN1, however, this often differs among family members as well.

The three subtypes of MEN2 are caused by mutations in another gene known as RET. Every individual who inherits a RET mutation will develop MTC during his or her lifetime, although the age at the time of diagnosis is often different in each family member. Multiple different mutations have been identified in individuals and families that have MEN2A. Likewise, several different mutations have been identified in individuals and families with FMTC. An interesting finding has been that a few families that clearly have MEN2A and a few families that clearly have FMTC have the same mutation. The reason the families have developed different clinical features is not known. In contrast to MEN2A and FMTC, individuals with MEN2B have been found, in more than 90% of cases, to have the same RET mutation. This mutation is located in a part of the gene that has never been affected in individuals and families with MEN2A and FMTC.

## Demographics

MEN syndromes are not common. It has been estimated that MEN1 occurs in 3–20 out of 100,000 people. The incidence of MEN2 has not been published, but it has been reported that MEN2B is about ten-fold less common than MEN2A. MEN syndromes affect both men and women and it occurs worldwide.

## Signs and symptoms

General symptoms of the characteristic features of the MEN syndromes and their causes include:

- Hyperparathyroidism, which may or may not cause symptoms. Symptoms that occur are related to the high levels of calcium in the bloodstream such as kidney stones, fatigue, muscle or bone pain, indigestion, and constipation.

- Medullary thyroid carcinoma may cause diarrhea, flushing, and depression.
- Pheochromocytoma may cause a suddenly high blood pressure and headache, palpitations or pounding of the heart, a fast heart beat, excessive sweating without exertion, and/or development of these symptoms after rising suddenly from bending over.

### Diagnosis

Diagnosis of the MEN syndromes has in the past depended upon clinical features and laboratory test results. Now that the genes responsible for these conditions have been identified, **genetic testing** provides another means of diagnosing individuals and families with these conditions. However, all of these tumors have a higher incidence of sporadic cases. It is important to ask the patient about family members when one of these types of tumor is diagnosed.

MEN1 is typically diagnosed from clinical features and from testing for parathyroid hormone (PTH). An elevated PTH indicates that hyperparathyroidism is present. When an individual develops a MEN1 related symptom or tumor, a complete family history should also be taken. If no family history of MEN1 or related problems such as kidney stones and peptic ulcers exists and close family members, i.e. parents, siblings and children, have normal serum calcium levels, then the person unlikely has MEN1. However, if the individual is found to have a second symptom or tumor characteristic of MEN1, the family history is suggestive of MEN1, and/or close family members have increased serum calcium levels, then MEN1 may be the correct diagnosis.

Genetic testing for the MEN1 gene has helped with evaluating individuals and families for MEN1. If an individual apparently affected by MEN1 is found to have a mutation in the MEN1 gene, then this positive test result confirms the diagnosis. However, genetic testing of the MEN1 gene does not identify all mutations causing MEN1; consequently, a negative test result does not remove or exclude the diagnosis.

MEN2A is typically diagnosed from clinical features and from laboratory testing of calcitonin levels. Elevated calcitonin levels indicate that C-cell hyperplasia and/or MTC is present. When an individual develops a MEN2A related symptom or tumor, a complete family history should be taken. If no family history of related problems exists and close family members, i.e. parents, siblings, and children, have normal calcitonin levels, then the person unlikely has MEN2A. However, if the individual is found to have a second symptom or tumor characteristic of MEN2A, the family history is suggestive of MEN2A, and/or close family members have increased calcitonin levels, then MEN2A may be the correct diagnosis.

Genetic testing for the RET gene has helped with evaluating an individual and/or family for MEN2A. If an individual apparently affected by MEN2A is found to have a mutation in the RET gene, then this positive test result confirms the diagnosis. Genetic testing of the RET gene does not identify all mutations causing MEN2A and FMTC; consequently, a negative test result does not remove or exclude the diagnosis.

Diagnosis of MEN2B can be made by physical examination and a complete medical history.

Diagnosis of FMTC may be made when the family history includes four other family members having developed MTC with no family member having developed a pheochromocytoma or pituitary tumor. Genetic testing of the RET gene may also assist with diagnosis.

Genetic testing of the MEN1 gene and of the RET gene allows individuals to be diagnosed prior to the onset of symptoms; this is often called predictive genetic testing. It is important to note that individuals should not undergo predictive genetic testing prior to the identification of the familial genetic mutation. Genetic testing of a family member clinically affected by the condition needs to be done first in order to identify the familial mutation. If this is not done, a negative result in an asymptomatic individual may not be a true negative test result.

Prenatal diagnosis of unborn babies is now technically possible via **amniocentesis** or chorionic villus sampling (CVS). However, prior to undergoing these procedures, the familial mutation needs to have been identified. An additional issue in prenatal diagnosis is how the test result will be used with regard to continuation of the pregnancy. Individuals considering prenatal diagnosis of MEN1 or MEN2 should confirm its availability prior to conception.

Genetic testing is best done in consultation with a geneticist (a doctor specializing in **genetics**) and/or genetic counselor.

### Treatment and management

No cure or comprehensive treatment is available for the MEN syndromes. However, some of the consequences of the MEN syndromes can be symptomatically treated and complications may be lessened or avoided by early identification.

For individuals affected by MEN1, hyperparathyroidism is often treated by surgery. The parathyroids may be partially or entirely removed. If they are entirely removed, the individual will need to take calcium and vitamin D supplements. The pancreatic tumors that develop may also be removed surgically or pharmacological treatment (medication) may be given to provide relief from symptoms. The Pituitary tumors that develop may not require treatment, but if so, medication has often been effective. Surgery and radiation are used in rare cases.

Children of a parent affected by MEN1 should begin regular medical screening in childhood. It has been suggested that children beginning at five to 10 years of age begin having annual measurements of serum calcium, serum prolactin and of the pancreatic, pituitary, and parathyroid hormones. The child should also undergo radiographic imaging (ultrasound, MRI examination) of the pancreas and pituitary. If the family history includes family members developing symptoms of MEN1 at younger than usual ages, then the children will need to begin medical screening at a younger age as well.

For the three types of MEN2, the greatest concern is the development of medullary thyroid carcinoma. Medullary thyroid carcinoma can be detected by measuring levels of the thyroid hormone, calcitonin.

Treatment of MTC is by surgical removal of the thyroid and the neighboring lymph nodes, although doctors may disagree at what stage to remove the thyroid. After thyroidectomy, the patient will receive normal levels of thyroid hormone orally or by injection. Even when surgery is performed early, metastatic spread of the cancer may have already occurred. Since this cancer is slow growing, metastasis may not be obvious. Metastasis is very serious in MTC because chemotherapy and radiation therapy are not effective in controlling its spread.

In the past, children who had a parent affected by one of the MEN2 syndromes were screened for MTC by annual measurement of calcitonin levels. More recently, it has been determined that MTC can be prevented by prophylactic thyroidectomy, meaning that the thyroid gland is removed without it being obviously affected by cancer. It is not uncommon for a child as young as one year of age, when the family history is of MEN2B, or six years of age, when the family history is of MEN2A or FMTC, to undergo prophylactic thyroidectomy in order to prevent the occurrence of MTC.

Pheochromocytomas that occur in MEN2A and MEN2B can be cured by surgical removal of this slow growing tumor. Pheochromocytomas may be screened for using annual abdominal ultrasound or CT examination and laboratory testing.

For individuals diagnosed with MEN2, it is also recommended that the pituitary be screened by laboratory tests.

In general, each tumor may be approached surgically. Problems occur when the tumors are multiple, when the whole gland is involved (hyperplasia as opposed to tumor), when replacement therapy is difficult (pituitary or adrenal), or when the gland makes multiple hormones (if the gland is removed, hormone replacement therapy becomes necessary).

## Prognosis

Diagnosed early, the prognosis for the MEN conditions is reasonably good, even for MEN2B, the most dangerous of the four forms. Medullary thyroid cancer can be cured when identified early. The availability of genetic testing to identify family members at risk for developing the conditions will hopefully lead to earlier treatment and improved outcomes.

## Resources

### BOOKS

Offit, Kenneth. "Multiple Endocrine Neoplasias." *Clinical Cancer Genetics: Risk Counseling and Management.* New York: John Wiley & Sons, 1998.

### PERIODICALS

Hoff, A. O., G. J. Cote, and R. F. Gagel. "Multiple endocrine neoplasias." (Review). *Annual Review of Physiology* 62 (2000): 377–422.

### WEBSITES

Gagel, Robert F. *Familial Medullary Thyroid Carcinoma: A guide for families.* http://endocrine.mdacc.tmc.edu/educational/mtc.htm.

Gagel, Robert F. "Medullary Thyroid Carcinoma." *M.D. Anderson Cancer Center*, University of Texas. http://endocrine.mdacc.tmc.edu/educational/thyroid.htm.

Marx, Stephen J. "Familial Multiple Endocrine Neoplasia Type 1." *National Institutes of Health.* http://www.niddk.nih.gov/health/endo/pubs/fmen1/fmen1.htm.

National Institute of Diabetes and Digestive and Kidney Diseases. "Hyperparathyroidism." *National Institutes of Health.* http://www.niddk.nih.gov/health/endo/pubs/hyper/hyper.htm.

Wiesner, Georgia L., and Karen Snow. "Multiple Endocrine Neoplasia Type 2." *GeneClinics.* University of Washington, Seattle. http://www.geneclinics.org/.

### ORGANIZATIONS

Canadian Multiple Endocrine Neoplasia Type 1 Society, Inc. (CMEN). PO Box 100, Meota, SK S0M 1X0. Canada. (306) 892-2080.

Genetic Alliance. 4301 Connecticut Ave. NW, #404, Washington, DC 20008-2304. (800) 336-GENE (Helpline) or (202) 966-5557. Fax: (888) 394-3937. info@ geneticalliance. http://www.geneticalliance.org.

National Institute of Diabetes and Digestive and Kidney Diseases. Building 31, Room 9A06, Bethesda, MD 20892-2560. http://www.niddk.nih.gov.

Cindy L. Hunter, MS, CGC

# Multiple epiphyseal dysplasia

## Definition

Multiple epiphyseal **dysplasia** (MED) is a hereditary disorder characterized by abnormal epiphyses (bone extremities) that lead to early-onset joint pain and recurrent inflammation of cartilage and bone. There are five subtypes of MED, each with varying clinical manifestations and **inheritance** patterns.

## Description

Multiple epiphyseal dysplasia (MED) is a hereditary condition characterized by abnormal development of cartilage and bone. The epiphysis is the portion at the end of a long bone where growth occurs. Dysplasia is an abnormality in development leading to alteration in size, shape, and organization of cells. Thus, in MED, the epiphyses of the long bones are dysplastic and, as a result, joint pain and inflammation result. On x ray, the epiphyses appear flattened and irregular. Cartilage in the joints becomes irregular and this leads to early-onset **osteoarthritis**. Patients often have short hands and stubby fingers.

MED can be divided into five subtypes, four of which are inherited in an autosomal dominant fashion (EDM1, EDM2, EDM3, and EDM5) and one of which is inherited in an autosomal recessive fashion (EDM4). All of the subtypes are characterized by early-onset joint pain, most often in the hips and knees. Most individuals with MED have adult heights that are in the low range of normal, although some may have slightly short stature.

### Dominant MED

Dominant MED was initially divided into two forms: a mild form, called Ribbing disease, and a more severe form, called Fairbank disease. Dominant MED has been further classified into four subtypes to accommodate the extreme clinical variability that exists. In addition to hip and knee pain and occasional short stature, individuals with dominant MED may have a waddling gait and their limbs may be relatively short

when compared to the trunk. Joint pain and deformity become worse with age in these patients and early-onset osteoarthritis is often a problem, especially in the large, weight-bearing joints.

### Recessive MED

Recessive MED is also known as EDM4 and rMED. In addition to early-onset joint pain and possible short stature, this disorder is associated with **scoliosis** (curvature of the spine), as well as malformations of the hands, feet, and knees. Some affected individuals may also present with a **clubfoot** or an abnormality of the kneecap, called a double-layered patella. This finding is very suggestive of recessive MED.

## Genetic profile

### Dominant MED

Mutations in five different genes have been associated with dominant MED:

- EDM1 is caused by mutations in the COMP gene, which codes for the cartilage oligomeric matrix protein. This gene is also responsible for the more severe disorder, called pseudoachondroplasia.
- EDM2 and EDM3 result from mutations in two of the three genes that code for the protein chains of type IX collagen. COL9A2 mutations lead to EDM2 and COL9A3 mutations lead to EDM3. Mutations in these genes can also lead to lumbar/intervertebral disk disease (IDD), which is a very common musculoskeletal disorder.

- Defects in the matrilin 3 protein, caused by mutations in the MATN3 gene, lead to a diagnosis of EDM5. Matrilin 3 plays a key role in the cartilage extracellular matrix.

Extreme variability in clinical manifestations can be seen both between and within families with mutations in the various genes responsible for dominant MED.

EDM1, EDM2, EDM3, and EDM5 are all dominant forms of MED and are inherited in an autosomal dominant pattern. Thus, the majority of affected individuals have a parent that is affected as well. However, this is not always the case as there may be a new (de novo) mutation in the affected individual that was not present in either parent. Additionally, there may appear to be a lack of family history due to the affected parent dying at a young age or the failure to recognize symptoms of the disorder in a parent. Asymptomatic parents of affected individuals should be given a careful clinical and radiographic examination to completely rule out any signs of the disorder.

Most often, one parent of the affected individual will have signs of dominant MED and/or a disease-causing mutation. In this case, siblings of the affected individual have a 50% chance of inheriting the same mutation and being affected as well. However, if a mutation is identified in the affected individual and both parents test negative for this mutation, it is likely that the **gene** mutation is de novo and, therefore, recurrence risk to siblings is very low. The prevalence of de novo mutations in dominant MED is unknown.

Another possibility is germline mosaicism. In this case, the gene mutation may be present only in the egg cells of the mother or the sperm cells of the father. Thus, the parent will not show signs of the disorder, since the gene mutation is confined to the sex cells. However, the mutations present in the egg or sperm would leave a significant recurrence risk for future pregnancies.

No matter how the affected individual inherits the gene mutation, each of his or her children has a 50% chance to inherit the disease-causing mutation and, therefore, be affected with dominant MED.

### Recessive MED

Recessive MED is caused by mutations in the SLC26A2 gene, also known as DTDST. Mutations in this gene cause a spectrum of skeletal disorders of which recessive MED is the mildest. SLC26A2 codes for a protein that plays a key role in the normal development of cartilage and its conversion to bone. When the SLC26A2 gene is mutated, cartilage cannot develop properly and, as a result, bones do not form correctly and skeletal problems result.

As implied by its name, recessive MED is inherited in an autosomal recessive manner. This means that an affected individual will have two abnormal copies of the SLC26A2 gene in each cell. Most often, the parents of an affected individual each carry a mutation on one of their two copies of the SLC26A2 gene. Mutation carriers do not show signs or symptoms of recessive MED. Siblings of affected individuals have a 25% chance of being affected with the disorder and a 50% chance of being carriers of the disorder. Offspring of an affected individual will be obligate carriers of an SLC26A2 gene mutation, but will not show signs or symptoms of the disorder.

### Demographics

#### Dominant MED

Dominant MED is thought to present in at least one in 10,000 births. Due to the clinical variability and range of severity associated with the disorder, it is likely that many individuals have yet to be diagnosed. There are no reports of the condition being more common in specific ethnic groups or geographical regions.

#### Recessive MED

The prevalence of recessive MED is currently unknown. There are no reports of the condition being more common in specific ethnic groups or geographical regions. Due to the mild signs and symptoms of the disorder, it is likely that the disease is under-diagnosed and is more common than once thought.

### Signs and symptoms

#### Dominant MED

Dominant MED often presents in early childhood with pain in the hips and/or knees. Affected patients often complain of this pain, accompanied by fatigue, after physical activity. Over time, this pain progressively worsens, joints become deformed, and early osteoarthritis results, most often in the large, weight-bearing joints. In some cases, joint replacement may be necessary.

Individuals with dominant MED may walk with a waddling gait. Restriction in the range of motion in the elbows is apparent in many cases, as is hypermobility in the knee and finger joints. Characteristic radiographic findings of dominant MED include abnormalities of the epiphyses of the long tubular bones, especially in the hips and/or knees. These abnormalities are due to delayed ossification and manifest as small and irregular ossification centers. This finding may be present very early, even before other clinical signs and symptoms are evident. Later, in adulthood, signs of osteoarthritis can be seen on x rays and the tubular bones may be slightly shortened. The spine is generally not involved in dominant MED. Adult height may be slightly shorter than normal and the limbs are often short relative to the trunk. Intelligence is normal.

There are various clinical manifestations that distinguish the subtypes of dominant MED:

- EDM1 is characterized by mild to moderate short stature and the limbs are usually short when compared to the trunk. Individuals with EDM1 may have minor spine irregularities that can be seen on x ray, but nothing as severe as the scoliosis associated with EDM4. The fingers and metacarpals (bones from the wrists to the fingers) are usually shortened. The main complication of this subtype is early arthritis of the hip.
- EDM2 and EDM3 are associated with mild short stature. There is more severe knee involvement in these subtypes and hip problems are often less severe. The courses of EDM2 and EDM3 are milder than EDM1 and EDM4. In EDM2, the hands are somewhat short but in EDM3, they tend to be normal with shortened metacarpals.
- EDM5 is the mildest form of MED. Affected patients usually have normal stature and less severe involvement of joints. Mild abnormalities in the pelvis seem to be more common in this subtype compared to the others.

### Recessive MED

Approximately 50% of individuals affected with recessive MED show signs or symptoms of the disorder at birth. Examples include clubfoot, **cleft palate**, ear swelling, or clinodactyly (a condition where the little finger is curved towards the ring finger). Joint pain in the hips and knees is very common in affected individuals and most often onsets in late childhood. However, this pain may onset at various times in different individuals and is not always present. Individuals affected with recessive MED are of normal stature, although some may be slightly shorter than expected in adulthood. As in dominant MED, intelligence is normal.

Affected individuals tend to have characteristic facial features, such as anteverted nares (nasal passages) and a round, flat face. They may also be myopic (nearsighted). Malformations of the hands, feet, and knees are very common. These may include **brachydactyly** (abnormal shortness) of toes and fingers, small hands/feet, and absent/small fingernails. A double-layered

patella (kneecap) is found in 60% of patients and is very suggestive of recessive MED. This finding seems to be age-dependent and may disappear when the affected individual reaches adulthood. Scoliosis is fairly common in affected individuals as well and this finding distinguishes recessive MED from dominant forms of MED. Occasionally, recessive MED may be associated with sensorineural **deafness**, hip anomalies, wrist anomalies, or delayed bone age.

### Diagnosis

#### Dominant MED

Clinical and radiographic findings of the patient and family members can assist in the diagnosis of dominant MED. Even before the onset of clinical signs and symptoms, x rays often show delayed ossification of the epiphyses of the long tubular bones. This delayed ossification is usually most noticeable in the hips and/or knees. Additionally, the x rays may show slightly shortened long tubular bones. Radiographic diagnosis of MED is often difficult, if not impossible, in adults. Thus, x rays should be completed in childhood, if possible. Due to the autosomal dominant pattern of inheritance, there are usually multiple family members affected with the disorder.

Molecular **genetic testing** can be used to confirm a diagnosis of dominant MED in a patient with characteristic clinical and radiographic features. Sequence analysis is available to analyze all five genes implicated in dominant MED. Mutations are found in the COMP gene in approximately 35% of cases, in the MATN3 gene in approximately 10% of cases, and in the COL9A2 and COL9A3 genes in less than 5% of cases. However, in about 50% of individuals with clinical and radiographic features consistent with dominant MED, no mutation can be found by molecular genetic testing. Thus, it is believed that other unidentified genes are likely responsible for this disorder. However, there are other conditions that can result from mutations in some of these genes (namely, COMP, COL9A2, and COL9A3). The type of disorder that results depends on the type of mutation in the gene. Thus, genetic test results must be interpreted based on clinical and radiographic findings.

Prenatal diagnosis for at-risk pregnancies is possible via molecular genetic testing, but is not commonly requested. Once a disease-causing mutation has been found in a family, fetal cells obtained by chorionic villus sampling (CVS) or **amniocentesis** can be analyzed for this mutation to determine the mutation status of the fetus.

### Recessive MED

A diagnosis of recessive MED is based on clinical and x-ray findings during childhood or early in adult life. The disorder is suspected when an autosomal recessive pattern of inheritance is seen and when characteristic signs and symptoms are noted, such as hip and knee pain, malformations of hands, feet, and knees, and scoliosis. X rays may show flat epiphyses with early arthritis, mild brachydactyly, and the characteristic double-layered patella.

The diagnosis of recessive MED can be confirmed via molecular genetic testing of the SLC26A2 gene. A mutation is found in approximately 70% of patients who are suspected to have the disorder based on clinical and radiographic features. Interestingly, mutations were found in 100% of patients with double-layered patella, which is a very specific sign for recessive MED. There are three common mutations in the SLC26A2 gene that account for approximately 90% of genetically characterized cases of recessive MED. Thus, molecular genetic testing often begins with analysis for these three mutations. It can be followed by full gene sequence analysis if necessary. There are three other autosomal recessive skeletal dysplasias that can result from mutations in the SLC26A2 gene. The type of disorder that results depends on the severity of the genetic mutations in the gene. Thus, genetic test results must be interpreted based on clinical and radiographic findings.

Carrier testing for at-risk family members who do not show any clinical signs of the disorder is available once the SLC26A2 **gene mutations** have been identified in an affected individual. Carrier detection in reproductive partners of SLC26A2 gene carriers is available as well. If a mutation is found in a reproductive partner, details about the severity of that mutation should be provided due to the fact that various SLC26A2 mutations can lead to various genetic conditions.

Prenatal diagnosis for at-risk pregnancies is possible in the same manner as dominant MED.

### Treatment and management

### Dominant MED

The goal for patients with dominant MED is to decrease pain, restrict joint destruction, and prevent the development of osteoarthritis. Pain is often difficult to control in affected individuals, however, analgesics (i.e., nonsteroidal anti-inflammatory drugs) and physiotherapy have been shown to be effective in some cases. An orthopedic surgeon can advise patients on whether surgical procedures (i.e., realignment osteotomy or acetabular osteotomy) might slow the progression of symptoms. In some patients, joint replacement may be necessary. Affected patients should avoid obesity and activities that strain affected joints.

### Recessive MED

Individuals with recessive MED should seen by an orthopedist who can assess the possibility of treatment. This may include physiotherapy for the purpose of strengthening muscles, use of analgesics (i.e., nonsteroidal anti-inflammatory drugs), and the timing of surgery, if necessary. As in dominant MED, affected patients should avoid obesity and activities that strain affected joints.

### Prognosis

Patients with dominant and recessive MED have a normal life expectancy and generally lead productive and healthy adult lives.

### Resources

#### WEBSITES

Briggs, M. D., M. J. Wright, and G. R. Mortier. "Multiple Epiphyseal Dysplasia, Dominant." *Gene Reviews.* April 18, 2007 (December 11, 2009.) http://www.ncbi.nlm. nih.gov/bookshelf/br.fcgi?book = gene&part = edm-ad# edm%2Dad.

Bonafe, L., D. Ballhausen, and A. Superti-Furga. "Multiple Epiphyseal Dysplasia, Recessive." *Gene Reviews.* December 27, 2006 (December 11, 2009). http://www. ncbi.nlm.nih.gov/bookshelf/br.fcgi?book = gene & part = edm# edm.

"Recessive Multiple Epiphyseal Dysplasia." *Genetics Home Reference.* February 2008 (December 11, 2009). http:// ghr.nlm.nih.gov/ condition = recessivemultipleepiphysealdysplasia.

#### ORGANIZATIONS

International Skeletal Dysplasia Registry, Medical Genetics Institute. 8700 Beverly Blvd., West Tower, Suite 665, Los Angeles, CA 90048. (800) 233-2771. http://www. csmc.edu/3805.html.

Little People of America, Inc., 250 EL Camino Real, Suite 201. Tustin, CA 92780. (714) 368-3689 (888) LPA-2001, Fax: (714) 368-3367. http://www.lpaonline. org/index.html.

National Organization for Rare Disorders (NORD). 55 Kenosia Avenue, PO Box 1968, Danbury, CT 06813-1968. (800) 999-6673. http://www.rarediseases.org.

Mary E. Freivogel, MS, CGC

# Multiple lentigines syndrome

## Definition

Multiple lentigines syndrome is a rare genetic condition that causes the affected individual to have many dark brown or black freckle-like spots on the skin, as well as other symptoms.

## Description

Multiple lentigines syndrome is a genetic disorder that results in characteristic marking of the skin, abnormalities in the structure and function of the heart, hearing loss, wide-set eyes, and other symptoms. Other terms for multiple lentigines syndrome include cardiomyopathic lentiginosis and LEOPARD syndrome. LEOPARD syndrome is an acronym for the seven most commonly observed symptoms of the disorder:

- (L)entigenes, or small dark brown and black spots on the skin
- (E)lectrocardiographic conduction defects, or abnormalities of the muscle activity in the heart
- (O)cular hypertelorism, or eyes that are spaced farther apart than normal
- (P)ulmonary stenosis, or narrowing of the lower right ventricle of the heart
- (A)bnormalities of the genitals, such as undescended testicles or missing ovaries
- (R)etarded growth leading to shortness of stature;
- (D)eafness or hearing loss

The lentigines, or skin spots, observed in multiple lentigines syndrome are similar in size and appearance to freckles, but unlike freckles, they are not affected by sun exposure.

## Genetic profile

Multiple lentigines syndrome is inherited as an autosomal dominant trait. Autosomal means that the syndrome is not carried on a sex **chromosome**, while dominant means that only one parent has to pass on the gene mutation in order for the child to be affected with the syndrome.

The specific gene mutation responsible for multiple lentigines syndrome has not been identified.

## Demographics

Multiple lentigines syndrome is extremely rare. Due to the small number of reported cases, demographic trends for the disease have not been established. There does not seem to be any clear ethnic pattern to the

---

disease. Both males and females appear to be affected with the same probability.

### Signs and symptoms

The most characteristic symptom of the disease is the presence of many dark brown or black spots, ranging in size from barely visible to 2.5 in (5 cm) in diameter, all over the face, neck, and chest. They may also be present on the arms and legs, genitalia, palms of the hands, and soles of the feet. The spots appear in infancy or early childhood and become more numerous until the age of puberty. There may also be lighter brown (café au lait) birthmarks on the skin.

Heart defects, such as the pulmonary stenosis and electrocardiographic conduction abnormalities described above, are another hallmark of multiple lentigines syndrome. Other areas of narrowing (stenosis) in different areas of the heart may be present, as well as abnormalities in the atrial septum, the wall between the upper left and right chambers of the heart. There is an increased risk of heart disease and tumors of the heart.

In addition to the feature of widely spaced eyes, other facial abnormalities may include low-set or prominent ears, drooping eyelids, a short neck, or a projecting jaw. In some cases of multiple lentigines syndrome, additional skeletal malformations have been reported, including a sunken breastbone, rib anomalies, curvature of the spine (**scoliosis**), and webbing of the fingers.

**Deafness** or hearing loss is observed in about 25% of the cases of multiple lentigines syndrome. Some people affected with the syndrome also exhibit mild developmental delay. Other reported neurological findings include seizures, eye tics, and abnormal electrical activity in the brain.

People with multiple lentigines syndrome often exhibit genital abnormalities such as undescended testicles or a small penis in men, or missing or underdeveloped ovaries in women. The onset of puberty may be delayed or even absent. Affected individuals are usually under the twenty-fifth percentile in height, although their body weight is in the normal range.

---

### Diagnosis

Diagnosis is usually made based on the observation of multiple lentigines and the presence of two or more of the other symptoms that form the LEOPARD acronym. A family history is also helpful since the syndrome has dominant **inheritance**. There is currently no medical test that can definitively confirm the diagnosis of multiple lentigines syndrome.

### Treatment and management

Treatment is directed toward the specific conditions of the individual. For example, heart conditions can be managed with the use of a pacemaker and appropriate medications, as well as regular medical monitoring. Hearing loss may be improved with the use of hearing aids.

**Genetic counseling** is recommended when there is a family history of freckle-like spotting of the skin and heart defects, as these suggest the possibility of inherited multiple lentigines syndrome.

### Prognosis

The prognosis for people with multiple lentigines syndrome is good provided that the appropriate care for any associated medical conditions is available.

### Resources

#### PERIODICALS

Abdelmalek, Nagla, and M. Alan Menter. "Marked cutaneous freckling and cardiac changes." *Baylor University Medical Center Proceedings* (December 1999): 272-274.

#### WEBSITES

*HealthlinkUSA Forum—LEOPARD Syndrome.* http://www.healthlinkusa.com/forum/709_1.html (April 20, 2001).

*OMIM - Online Mendelian Inheritance in Man.* http://www.ncbi.nlm.nih.gov/omim.

*Yahoo! Groups: Leopard_syndrome.* http://groups.yahoo.com/group/leopard_syndrome (April 20, 2001).

#### ORGANIZATIONS

National Organization for Rare Disorders (NORD). 55 Kenosia Ave., PO Box 1968, Danbury, CT 06813-1968. (203) 744-0100 or (800) 999-6673. Fax: (203) 798-2291. http://www.rarediseases.org.

Paul A. Johnson

# Multiple sclerosis

## Definition

Multiple sclerosis (MS) is a chronic, degenerative disorder affecting the central nervous system (CNS), which is made up of the brain, spinal cord, and optic nerves. A fatty tissue called myelin coats and protects the nerve fibers in the CNS. When myelin is damaged or destroyed in the CNS, either by inflammation, stroke, immune disorders, metabolic disorders, or nutritional deficiencies, scar tissue, or sclerosis, may form in multiple areas of the nerve fibers. As a result, the ability of the nerves to conduct electrical impulses from the brain to the rest of the body is impaired, and a wide variety of symptoms may appear.

## Description

Although the exact cause of multiple sclerosis is not known, researchers believe that an abnormal response by the body's own immune system, called an autoimmune response, triggers the susceptibility to the disease. The reasons for this abnormal autoimmune response are uncertain, but most scientists agree that several triggers are involved, including **genetics**, gender, and the environment (i.e., viruses, trauma, and heavy metals).

Investigators believe that the genes associated with MS are not abnormal, but include some variations that may or may not occur in the general population. In certain combinations, however, these normal genes appear to predispose some people to develop MS after exposure to unidentified environmental factors. People whose close relatives have multiple sclerosis are more susceptible to developing the disease, but there is no evidence to suggest that MS is inherited directly.

The course of the disease is unpredictable. Although MS affects each person differently, the disease generally occurs in one of four patterns or clinical courses, which are sometimes referred to as chronic progressive MS. The four forms of MS are relapsing-remitting, primary-

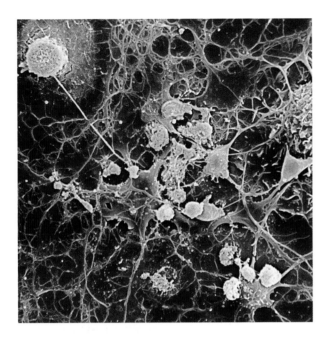

Colored scanning electron micrograph (SEM) of microglial cells (round) ingesting oligodendrocytes (branched). This is the process thought to occur in multiple sclerosis. (© Dr. John Zajicek / Photo Researchers, Inc.)

progressive, secondary-progressive, and progressive-relapsing. Each of these patterns may be mild, moderate, or severe.

At initial diagnosis, the most common form of MS is relapsing-remitting, occurring in approximately 85% of those with the disease. Individuals with this form of MS experience clearly defined flare-ups (also called relapses, attacks, or exacerbations). There are episodes of acute worsening neurologic function, followed by partial or complete periods of recovery (remission) that are free of disease progression.

The primary-progressive form of MS is relatively rare, occurring in approximately 10% of patients. People with this type of MS experience a slow but nearly continuous worsening of their disease from the time of disease onset, and have no clear relapses or remissions. There are, however, variations in rates of progression over time, occasional plateaus, and temporary minor improvements.

About 50% of people with relapsing-remitting MS develop secondary-progressive MS within 10 years of their initial diagnosis and before the introduction of disease-modifying drugs. Long-term data are not yet available to demonstrate if this form of MS is significantly delayed by treatment. People with secondary-progressive MS experience an initial period of relapsing-remitting disease, followed by a steadily worsening disease course that may or may not be

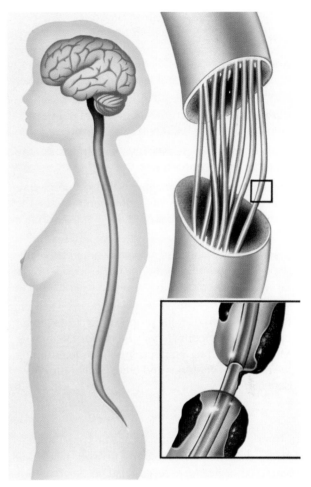

Illustration of the brain and spinal cord of a woman suffering from multiple sclerosis (MS). Upper right is a magnified view of the spinal cord showing individual nerve fibers. Lower right is a magnified view of an axon within one of the nerve fibers which is covered with a protective myelin sheath (grey). In MS, patches of the myelin sheath are destroyed; these patches are known as plaques (black). The affected nerve fibers cannot conduct nerve impulses properly, so body functions such as movement and sensation are lost. (© John Bavosi / Photo Researchers, Inc.)

accompanied by occasional flare-ups, minor remissions, or plateaus.

The progressive-relapsing form of MS is relatively rare, occurring in approximately 5% of patients. People with this form of MS experience a steadily worsening disease from the onset, but also have clear acute relapses, with or without recovery. As opposed to relapsing-remitting MS, the disease continues to progress between periods of relapse.

### Genetic profile

Results from studies indicate that genes not only influence who is at risk for MS but also affect the clinical features of the disease, such as age of symptom onset, severity, progression, and response to drugs. In addition, there is some evidence to suggest that the different forms of MS have different underlying genetic causes. In addition to genes, other components, such as exposure to viruses or environmental factors, play a part in causing MS. For this reason, researchers believe that MS is not inherited directly. Genetic factors, however, determine who is susceptible to the unknown outside trigger.

Epidemiologic studies have determined that a person's risk of developing MS increases several-fold if a close family member, including a first-, second-, or third-degree relative, has the disease. Studies involving twins, for example, have demonstrated that a monozygotic, or identical twin, with MS has a higher risk (estimated at 25–30%) of developing the disease than a dizygotic, or fraternal twin (estimated at 2–5%). Thus, a significant genetic component is involved in transmitting the susceptibility to the disease in families, although the disease is not directly inherited.

Genetically, MS is a complex disease that is neither strictly dominant, recessive, nor sex-linked. Discovering the genes involved in MS requires careful scanning of the entire genome (the entire genetic composition of an organism) of patients and their relatives to identify small chromosomal regions linked to the disease. Once they are discovered, these genomic segments are examined in detail to determine the specific location (locus) and characteristics of the MS-associated genes.

Studies have identified approximately 60 genomic regions that may be involved in MS, with 13 common regions harboring disease susceptibility, supporting the view that multiple genes are involved in this disorder. Seven of those were recently confirmed. This study, in combination with results from teams in Canada, Finland, and England, generated the first MS genetic map. These studies have sparked a global effort to search for the cause of MS susceptibility. A second-generation genome screen is near completion. Further work is needed to identify the complete list of MS loci (locations) and to map the complete set of MS-associated genes.

Thus far, the HLA-DR2 haplotype (a set of closely linked alleles, or alternative forms of genes) within the **major histocompatibility complex** (MHC) on the short arm of **chromosome** 6 is the strongest genetic effect identified in MS. This haplotype has consistently demonstrated both linkage and association in family and case-control studies.

Chromosome 19q13 has been under evaluation since 1993, when the first description of positive linkage was established. Genomic screens have shown some evidence for linkage to this region, which has been identified as the second most significant region after MHC. However, the effect of this locus is rather modest and is estimated to account for only 4–6% of the overall genetic component in MS. Because MS is a complex disease, the data are not entirely consistent; not all studies have shown evidence of linkage.

### Demographics

Multiple sclerosis is one of the most common diseases affecting the CNS. It is estimated that about 300,000 people in North America and more than 2.5 million people worldwide are affected. Peak onset occurs between the ages of 20 and 30. Almost 70% of individuals experience symptoms between the ages of 21 and 40. Although MS rarely occurs in those younger than 10 or older than 60, some cases have been reported. In addition, the disease is two to three times more common in women than men.

Although the reasons for the differences in susceptibility are not known, Caucasians are more than twice as likely as other races to develop MS, and the disease is five times more common in temperate climates, such as the northern United States, Canada, and Europe, than in tropical climates. Native Americans in North America, however, rarely develop the disease. Multiple sclerosis is uncommon in Japan, China, and South America, and is nearly unknown among the indigenous people of equatorial Africa and the native Inuit of Alaska.

### Signs and symptoms

Multiple sclerosis symptoms often progress gradually and vary in intensity and predictability because different areas of myelin are attacked in each person. Each attack produces different symptoms, and new areas of the nervous system are affected. There is usually an increasing progression of symptoms, with episodes lasting days, weeks, or months, alternating with disease-free periods of remission. The disease may progress, however, without any periods of remission.

Early symptoms of MS may include:

- numbness and/or paresthesias (tingling) in the arms or legs
- mono- or paraparesis (partial paralysis affecting one or both of the lower limbs)
- double or blurred vision
- optic neuritis (nerve inflammation)
- ataxia (lack of muscle coordination)
- bowel- or bladder-control problems

Later symptoms of MS may include:

- more prominent upper motor neuron signs, such as increased spasticity (stiff or awkward movements), and increasing para- or quadriparesis
- vertigo (sensation of self or objects moving or spinning)
- lack of coordination (loss of balance) and other cerebellar problems
- depression
- emotional instability
- difficulty walking or gait abnormalities
- dysarthria (impaired speech)
- fatigue
- pain

### Diagnosis

Because there is no definitive test that can identify or rule out MS, and the symptoms of MS mimic a number of other diseases, a combination of tests or procedures is required to diagnose the disease. Moreover, for some people (about 10–15%), a definitive diagnosis is not possible even after thorough testing. In most cases, with time and follow-up clinical examinations in which the condition is monitored closely, diagnosis is possible.

Diagnostic evaluation begins with a complete medical history, which assesses overall health status, including an evaluation of symptoms and time of onset. Physical examination includes an evaluation of nervous system functioning, such as testing of reflexes, balance, coordination, and vision, as well as checking for areas of numbness or weakness.

Diagnostic testing may include:

- Magnetic resonance imaging (MRI): This provides a detailed view of the brain.
- Evoked potential tests: These measure how quickly and accurately the nervous system responds to certain stimulation; the most common of these tests include the visual evoked response test, the brainstem auditory evoked response test, and the sensory evoked response test.
- Lumbar puncture: A sample of cerebrospinal fluid (CSF) is taken from the lumbar area of the spine.
- Electrophoresis: The CSF is analyzed in a laboratory procedure used to evaluate protein levels in the CSF.

The following standard criteria, called the Poser criteria, are often used in diagnosing MS:

- Clinically definite MS is diagnosed with two attacks and clinical evidence of two separate lesions; two attacks, clinical evidence of one lesion and para-clinical (beyond clinical) evidence of another lesion.
- Laboratory-supported definite MS is diagnosed with two attacks, either clinical or para-clinical evidence of one lesion, and CSF immunologic abnormalities; one attack, clinical evidence of two separate lesions, and CSF abnormalities; one attack, clinical evidence of one lesion and para-clinical evidence of another separate lesion, and CSF abnormalities.
- Clinically probable MS is diagnosed with two attacks and clinical evidence of one lesion; one attack and clinical evidence of two separate lesions; one attack, clinical evidence of one lesion, and para-clinical evidence of another separate lesion.
- Laboratory-supported probable MS is diagnosed with two attacks and CSF abnormalities.

### Treatment and management

There is no cure for MS. Nevertheless, there are numerous drug and nondrug therapies available to manage and treat the symptoms of the disease. It is standard practice to wait until a person has experienced two or more MS attacks before initiating drug treatment. Studies, indicate that initiating treatment in the early stages of the disease may lesson damage to the CNS and potentially slow disease progression. The type of treatment a patient receives is based on a wide variety of factors, including the course and severity of disease.

Six disease-modifying drugs have been approved by the U.S. Food and Drug Administration (FDA) for use in people with MS. The drugs approved for relapsing-remitting MS include interferon beta-1a (Avonex, Rebif), interferon beta-1b (Betaseron), and glatiramer acetate (Copaxone).

These drugs, which are injected either under the skin or into the muscle, reduce the number and severity of attacks, and some may slow the onset of disability. Interferons are naturally occurring proteins that fight invading viruses. Although the mechanism of action of these drugs is not fully understood in MS, the drugs appear to protect the CNS from the body's attack of its own immune system. Glatiramer acetate is a synthetic compound made from substances found in myelin, and is thought to help alter the body's immune system.

The most commonly used MS drugs, which have potentially serious adverse side effects, include:

- Natalizumab (Tysabri, formerly known as Antegren), which was voluntarily suspended from marketing by the FDA as of February 28, 2005. This drug, which was approved for the treatment of relapsing forms of MS and was administered by infusion every four weeks, is a monoclonal antibody that prevents certain white blood cells from moving into the CNS, thus decreasing inflammation and potentially allowing the body to repair the damaged myelin. Although generally well-tolerated, the drug was implicated in three cases of progressive multifocal leukoencephalopathy, a usually fatal brain wasting disease, among patients in long-term clinical trials. In March 2006, Tysabri was reevaluated by the FDA, and on June 5, 2006, the FDA approved the marketing of Tysabri under a special restricted distribution program; patients must talk to their doctor, understand the risks and benefits of Tysabri, and agree to all of the instructions in the TOUCH Prescribing Program. For more information see the FDA website: http://www.fda.gov/cder/drug/infopage/natalizumab/default.htm.

- Mitoxantrone (Novantrone) is approved in the treatment of secondary-progressive, progressive-relapsing, and worsening relapsing-remitting MS. The drug has been shown to decrease relapses and slow the progression of disability. Mitoxantrone is administered intravenously. Researchers believe that the drug works by suppressing the immune system; the drug, has many potentially serious side effects, some of which are heart-related.

- Steroids were the gold standard of treatment for patients with MS, until the discovery of the disease-modifying drugs. Although steroids are still prescribed and administered intravenously, primarily to reduce inflammation and manage acute attacks, they produce serious adverse side effects and most often are used for short periods of time. The most commonly prescribed steroids include dexamethasone (Decadron), methylprednisone (Solu-Medrol), and prednisone (Deltasone).

- Copolymer 1 is being investigated in clinical trials and may decrease disease activity. Other drugs are also used to treat the symptoms of the disease, such as fatigue, bladder control problems, and pain.

A nondrug treatment is plasmapheresis (plasma separation or plasma exchange). This is a procedure in which the patient's blood is drawn and the plasma (liquid portion) is replaced with other fluids; an anti-clotting agent (anticoagulant) is given intravenously during the procedure. Plasma contains antibodies; thus, this type of therapy removes antibodies that may attack myelin. The plasma-free blood is then returned to the patient by transfusion. This procedure, which is used to treat other autoimmune diseases, such as **myasthenia gravis**, Lambert-Eaton syndrome, and Guillain-Barré syndrome, has had mixed results in patients with primary- and secondary-progressive forms of MS.

Complementary and alternative therapies include vitamin D and antioxidant vitamin supplementation, as well as diets low in saturated fat and high in omega-3 fatty acids. The efficacy of these treatments, however, has not been determined.

New treatment options include immunotherapy, in which drugs and other procedures are used to suppress the immune system; and manipulating the immune system by destroying or damaging cells that attack myelin.

### Prognosis

Although the average lifespan of those diagnosed with MS is difficult to estimate because the disease pattern and severity vary among individuals, the estimate often given is 25–35 years after diagnosis.

For all MS patients, the chance of walking without assistance in 15 years following disease onset is 50%. About half of all patients require assistance in walking or will be wheelchair bound, while the other 50% of patients will be able to walk without assistance.

Some of the most common causes of death among patients with MS are related to secondary complications associated with immobility, urinary tract infections, swallowing, or breathing. Although the rate of suicide among those with MS is approximately 7.5 times higher than in the general population, the suicide rate does not correlate with disability.

Factors that tend to influence a favorable prognosis include:

- female sex
- low relapse rate
- complete recovery from first attack
- symptoms primarily sensory in nature
- younger age of onset
- low disability at two to five years from disease onset
- later cerebellar involvement
- involvement of only one CNS component at the time of onset

## Resources

### BOOKS

Cook S. D., ed. *Handbook of Multiple Sclerosis (Neurological Disease and Therapy)*, *3rd Edition*. New York: Marcel Dekker, Inc., 2001.

Holland, Nancy J., T. Jock Murray, and Stephen C. Reingold. *Multiple Sclerosis: A Guide for the Newly Diagnosed, 2nd Edition*. New York: Demos Medical Publishing, 2002.

Schapiro, Randall T. *Managing the Symptoms of Multiple Sclerosis, 4th Edition*. New York: Demos Medical Publishing, 2003.

### PERIODICALS

Altmann, D. "Evaluating the Evidence for Multiple Sclerosis as an Autoimmune Disease." *Archives of Neurology* 62, no. 4 (April 2005): 688.

Calabresi, Peter A. "Diagnosis and Management of Multiple Sclerosis." *American Family Physician* 70, no. 10 (November 15, 2004): 1935–1944.

### ORGANIZATIONS

Multiple Sclerosis Association of America. 706 Haddonfield Road, Cherry Hill, NJ 08002. (800) 532-7667. http://www.msaa.com.

Multiple Sclerosis Foundation. 6350 North Andrews Avenue, Ft. Lauderdale, FL 33309-2130. (954) 776-6805, (888) MSFOCUS (673-6287). http://www.msfocus.org.

Multiple Sclerosis International Federation. 3rd Floor Skyline House, 200 Union Street, London SE1 0LX. +44 (0) 20 7620 1911. http://www.msif.org.

National Multiple Sclerosis Society. 733 Third Avenue 6th Floor, New York, NY 10017-3288. (800) 344-4867. http://www.nationalmssociety.org.

Genevieve T. Slomski, PhD

# Multiplex ligation-dependent probe amplification

## Definition

Multiplex ligation-dependent probe amplification (MLPA) is a technique used by laboratories to detect an abnormal number of chromosomes, **gene** deletions, gene duplications, and gene expansions.

## Description

Multiplex ligation-dependent probe amplification (MLPA) was first described by Schouten and his colleagues in 2002. The technique is designed to detect genetic issues ranging from an abnormal number of chromosomes to the location of changes in the "spelling" of genes. The technique is a multiplex assay in that it allows simultaneous testing of multiple genetic sequences.

Chromosomes are the gene-containing structures found in all of the body's cells. In each cell, there are 46 chromosomes that come in 23 pairs. Bodies are so specific that the exact amount of genetic information contained in the 46 chromosomes is required to grow and develop properly; having any more or any less genetic information causes abnormal physical and mental growth and development.

Genes are the blueprints that carry the instructions for making all of the proteins a cell needs and determine traits, such as hair and eye color. Genes contain the inherited information that is passed on from parents to children. Each gene has a specific spelling made of the base pairs, including C, G, A, and T. If the spelling of a gene is changed, or mutated, it can cause abnormalities in the way the gene functions. Missing genetic information from the loss of one normal base pair to the loss of most of a **chromosome** is referred to as a deletion. A copy of genetic information that results in a redundant piece of genetic information is known as a duplication. A gene expansion refers to a genetic abnormality caused by a sequence of base pairs that is repeated too many times in a section of a gene. Detection of **chromosomal abnormalities**, deletions, duplications, and expansions of genetic material is an important part of diagnosing genetic conditions and diseases.

The technique of MLPA uses the spelling of the base pairs to determine if portions of chromosomes or genes are changed or mutated. The technique begins with probes that attach to the base pairs of genes and chromosomes in a specific location. The probes are divided into halves that attach around a specific gene or chromosomal location and then attach to each

## KEY TERMS

**Chromosomes**—The gene-containing structures found in all of the body's cells; in each normal cell, there are 46 chromosomes that come in 23 pairs.

**Deletion**—A mutation resulting in the loss of normal base pair sequence; a deletion may be of any size from one base pair to most of a chromosome.

**Duplication**—Production of one or more copies of any piece of DNA, including a base pair, gene, or entire chromosome.

**Exon**—Segments of a gene that contains instruction for making a protein; in many genes, the exons are separated by intervening segments of DNA, known as introns, which do not code for proteins.

**Expansion**—A genetic abnormality caused by a sequence of nucleotides that is repeated too many times in a section of a gene.

**Genes**—The basic units of heredity that contain the blueprints for the processes crucial to growth and development.

**Multiplex assay**—A procedure that allows the testing of several gene samples simultaneously.

**Polymerase chain reaction (PCR)**—A laboratory process used to make a large number of copies of specific genetic information from small amounts of DNA.

other. This attachment to the area around a gene or chromosome is called hybridization, and the "glue" that attaches the two probe halves to each other is the enzyme ligase. In order to help count the number of probe halves present at the end of the procedure, the probes are made in a series of different lengths. If two probe halves have properly attached to their gene or chromosomal location and each other, they serve as a target for the next step. If the probes are attached to the wrong gene area or a mismatched probe half, they will not participate in the next part of the procedure.

In the next step, a technique called polymerase chain reaction (PCR) is used to make many copies of the correctly paired and attached probe halves. The PCR will not make copies of probes attached or paired incorrectly. Finally, the properly attached and matched probes of each size are separated by size and counted. The amount of each probe size provides the information whether a small area of the gene (called an exon) or the chromosome contains a deletion, duplication, or

expansion. Since there are multiple probe sizes with different gene targets, 40 or more gene exons can be tested for abnormalities at the same time.

### Indications

The technique of MLPA may be indicated when a genetic condition, disease, syndrome, or disorder involving a chromosome abnormality, gene deletion, gene duplication, or gene amplification is suspected. Possible testing options include chromosomal disorders, such as **Down syndrome**, conditions caused by rearrangements of a chromosome, genetic conditions caused by gene deletions and duplications, such as Duchenne's **muscular dystrophy**, certain forms of inherited **cancer** predisposition, and diseases caused by gene amplification, such as **fragile X syndrome**.

### Samples

MLPA can be run on many bodily fluids and tissues, including blood, human embryonic stem cells, amniocytes, chorionic villi, and formalin-fixed paraffin-embedded tissue. The MLPA method requires that **DNA** samples obtained from the fluids and tissues be samples of uniform quality, which reduces false positives.

### Results

The MLPA test can provide information about chromosomal abnormalities and gene duplications, deletions, or expansions. If a chromosome abnormality, gene duplication, deletion, or expansion is found, it may indicate predisposition for, diagnosis of, or carrier status for a specific genetic disorder or condition.

### Benefits

MLPA is a quick technique that requires a smaller amount of DNA than other testing methods. The test exhibits good sensitivity and specificity when probes are made correctly and proper reaction conditions are used. Several genetic locations can be tested in the same procedure and, accordingly, large genes made of many exons can be tested in a quick and efficient manner. Data from the technique are reproducible. DNA degradation to small fragments does not influence results, and thus testing can be done on formalin-fixed paraffin-embedded tissue.

### Limitations

MLPA requires the creation of labor-intensive probes for each new gene or chromosome to be examined before the test can be run. Kits of developed probes are sold, but are not certified by the U.S.

Food and Drug Administration (FDA) for use in diagnostic procedures at this time. The probe kits are labeled for research purposes and to demonstrate the possibilities of the MLPA technique. Accordingly, results detected through MLPA should be verified with an independent method, such as G-banding chromosome analysis or Southern blots. Although MLPA can determine the approximate location of a genetic anomaly within an exon, unless special probes for specific mutations are designed, the test cannot determine the exact mutation of base pair or pairs.

### Alternative tests

There are several testing methods that provide the same information as the MLPA technique. Standard chromosome analysis, comparative genomic hybridization (CGH), **fluorescent in situ hybridization** (FISH), BAC arrays, Southern blots, and loss of heterozygosity (LOH) assays are used to detect chromosomal abnormalities. Some genetic mutations and expansions can be detected with multiplex polymerase chain reaction (PCR) assays, fluorescent in situ hybridization (FISH), and/or Southern blotting.

## Resources

### PERIODICALS

Schouten, J. P., C. J. McElgunn, R. Waaijer, D. Zwijnenburg, F. Diepvens, and G. Pals. "Relative Quantification of 40 Nucleic Acid Sequences by Multiplex Ligation-dependent Probe Amplification." *Nucleic Acids Res.* 30, no. 12 (June 15, 2002): e57.

### WEB SITES

"MLPA Info." MRC-Holland. (April 21, 2005.) http://www.mrc-holland.com/mlpa_info.htm.
National Genetics Reference Laboratories Information on Multiplex Ligation-dependent Probe Amplification. (April 21, 2005.) http://www.ngrl.org.uk/Wessex/mlpa.htm.

Dawn Jacob Laney, MS, CGC

## ▌Muscular dystrophy

### Definition

Muscular dystrophy is the name for a group of inherited disorders in which strength and muscle bulk gradually decline. Nine types of muscular dystrophies are generally recognized.

### Description

The muscular dystrophies include:

- *Duchenne muscular dystrophy (DMD)*: DMD affects young boys, causing progressive muscle weakness, usually beginning in the legs. It is a severe form of muscular dystrophy. DMD occurs in about one in 3,500 male births, and affects approximately 8,000 boys and young men in the United States. A milder form occurs in a very small number of female carriers.

- *Becker muscular dystrophy (BMD)*: BMD affects older boys and young men, following a milder course than DMD. It occurs in about one in 30,000 male births.

- *Emery-Dreifuss muscular dystrophy (EDMD)*: EDMD affects both males and females because it can be inherited as an autosomal dominant or recessive disorder. Symptoms include contractures and weakness in the calves, weakness in the shoulders and upper arms, and problems in the way electrical impulses travel through the heart to make it beat (heart conduction defects). Fewer than 300 cases of EDMD have been reported in the medical literature.

- *Limb-girdle muscular dystrophy (LGMD)*: LGMD begins in late childhood to early adulthood and affects both men and women, causing weakness in the muscles around the hips and shoulders, and weakness in the limbs. It is the most variable of the muscular dystrophies, and there are several different forms of the condition now recognized. Many people with suspected LGMD have probably been misdiagnosed in the past, and therefore, the prevalence of the condition is difficult to estimate. The highest prevalence of LGMD is in a small mountainous Basque province in northern Spain, where the condition affects 69 persons per million.

- *Facioscapulohumeral muscular dystrophy (FSH)*: FSH, also known as Landouzy-Dejerine condition, begins in late childhood to early adulthood and affects both men and women, causing weakness in the muscles of the face, shoulders, and upper arms. The hips and legs may also be affected. FSH occurs in about one out of every 20,000 people, and affects approximately 13,000 people in the United States.

- *Myotonic dystrophy*: Also known as Steinert's disease, it affects both men and women, causing generalized weakness first seen in the face, feet, and hands. It is accompanied by the inability to relax the affected muscles (myotonia). Symptoms may begin from birth through adulthood. It is the most common form of muscular dystrophy, affecting more than 30,000 people in the United States.

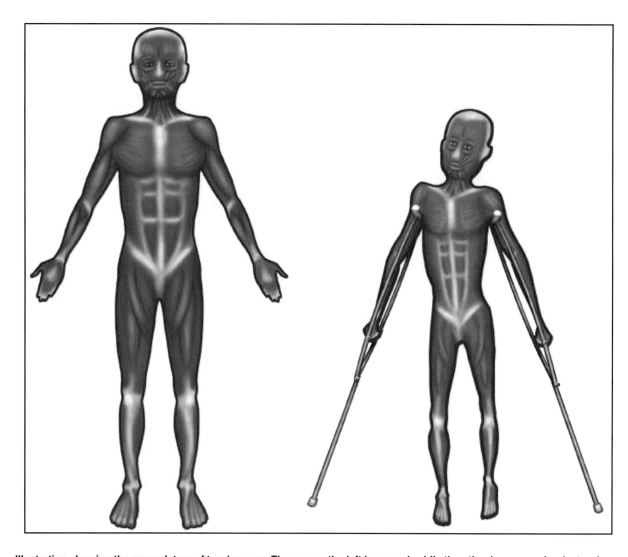

**Illustration showing the musculature of two humans. The one on the left is normal, while the other has muscular dystrophy.**
*(Illustration by Frank Forney. Reproduced by permission of Gale, a part of Cengage Learning.)*

- *Oculopharyngeal muscular dystrophy (OPMD)*: OPMD affects adults of both sexes, causing weakness in the eye muscles and throat. It is most common among French Canadian families in Quebec, and in Spanish-American families in the southwestern United States.

- *Distal muscular dystrophy (DD)*: DD is a group of rare muscle diseases that have weakness and wasting of the distal (farthest from the center) muscles of the forearms, hands, lower legs, and feet in common. In general, the DDs are less severe, progress more slowly, and involve fewer muscles than the other dystrophies. DD usually begins in middle age or later, causing weakness in the muscles of the feet and hands. It is most common in Sweden, and rare in other parts of the world.

- *Congenital muscular dystrophy (CMD)*: CMD is a rare group of muscular dystrophies that have in common the presence of muscle weakness at birth (congenital), and abnormal muscle biopsies. CMD results in generalized weakness, and usually progresses slowly. A subtype, called Fukuyama CMD, also involves mental retardation and is more common in Japan.

## Genetic profile

The muscular dystrophies are genetic conditions, meaning they are caused by alterations in genes. Genes, which are linked together on chromosomes, have two functions; they code for the production of proteins, and they are the material of **inheritance**. Parents pass along genes to their children, providing

**Amniocentesis**—A procedure performed at 16-18 weeks of pregnancy in which a needle is inserted through a woman's abdomen into her uterus to draw out a small sample of the amniotic fluid from around the baby. Either the fluid itself or cells from the fluid can be used for a variety of tests to obtain information about genetic disorders and other medical conditions in the fetus.

**Autosomal dominant**—A pattern of genetic inheritance where only one abnormal gene is needed to display the trait or disease.

**Autosomal recessive**—A pattern of genetic inheritance where two abnormal genes are needed to display the trait or disease.

**Becker muscular dystrophy (BMD)**—A type of muscular dystrophy that affects older boys and men, and usually follows a milder course than Duchenne muscular dystrophy.

**Chorionic villus sampling (CVS)**—A procedure used for prenatal diagnosis at 10-12 weeks gestation. Under ultrasound guidance a needle is inserted either through the mother's vagina or abdominal wall and a sample of cells is collected from around the fetus. These cells are then tested for chromosome abnormalities or other genetic diseases.

**Contracture**—A tightening of muscles that prevents normal movement of the associated limb or other body part.

**Distal muscular dystrophy (DD)**—A form of muscular dystrophy that usually begins in middle age or

later, causing weakness in the muscles of the feet and hands.

**Duchenne muscular dystrophy (DMD)**—The most severe form of muscular dystrophy, DMD usually affects young boys and causes progressive muscle weakness, usually beginning in the legs.

**Dystrophin**—A protein that helps muscle tissue repair itself. Both Duchenne muscular dystrophy and Becker muscular dystrophy are caused by flaws in the gene that instructs the body how to make this protein.

**Facioscapulohumeral muscular dystrophy (FSH)**—This form of muscular dystrophy, also known as Landouzy-Dejerine condition, begins in late childhood to early adulthood and affects both men and women, causing weakness in the muscles of the face, shoulders, and upper arms.

**Limb-girdle muscular dystrophy (LGMD)**—Form of muscular dystrophy that begins in late childhood to early adulthood and affects both men and women, causing weakness in the muscles around the hips and shoulders.

**Myotonic dystrophy**—A form of muscular dystrophy, also known as Steinert's condition, characterized by delay in the ability to relax muscles after forceful contraction, wasting of muscles, as well as other abnormalities.

**Oculopharyngeal muscular dystrophy (OPMD)**—Form of muscular dystrophy affecting adults of both sexes, and causing weakness in the eye muscles and throat.

them with a complete set of instructions for making their own proteins.

Because both parents contribute genetic material to their offspring, each child carries two copies of almost every **gene**, one from each parent. For some conditions to occur, both copies must be altered. Such conditions are called autosomal recessive conditions. Some forms of LGMD and DD exhibit this pattern of inheritance, as does CMD. A person with only one altered copy, called a carrier, will not have the condition, but may pass the altered gene on to his children. When two carriers have children, the chances of having a child with the condition is one in four for each pregnancy.

Other conditions occur when only one altered gene copy is present. Such conditions are called autosomal

dominant conditions. DM, FSH, and OPMD exhibit this pattern of inheritance, as do some forms of DD and LGMD. When a person affected by the condition has a child with someone not affected, the chances of having an affected child is one in two.

Because of chromosomal differences between the sexes, some genes are not present in two copies. The chromosomes that determine whether a person is male or female are called the X and Y chromosomes. A person with two X chromosomes is female, while a person with one X and one Y is male. While the X **chromosome** carries many genes, the Y chromosome carries almost none. Therefore, a male has only one copy of each gene on the X chromosome, and if it is altered, he will have the condition that alteration causes. Such conditions are said to be X-linked. X-linked conditions include DMD, BMD, and EDMD. Women are not usually affected by X-linked conditions, since they will likely have one unaltered copy between the two chromosomes. Some female carriers of DMD have a mild form of the condition, probably because their one unaltered gene copy is shut down in some of their cells.

Women carriers of X-linked conditions have a one in two chance of passing the altered gene on to each child born. Daughters who inherit the altered gene will be carriers. A son born without the altered gene will be free of the condition and cannot pass it on to his children. A son born with the altered gene will have the condition. He will pass the altered gene on to each of his daughters, who will then be carriers, but to none of his sons (because they inherit his Y chromosome).

Not all genetic alterations are inherited. As many as one third of the cases of DMD are due to new mutations that arise during egg formation in the mother. New mutations are less common in other forms of muscular dystrophy.

Several of the muscular dystrophies, including DMD, BMD, CMD, and most forms of LGMD, are due to alterations in the genes for a complex of muscle proteins. This complex spans the muscle cell membrane (a thin sheath that surrounds each muscle cell) to unite a fibrous network on the interior of the cell with a fibrous network on the outside. Theory holds that by linking these two networks, the complex acts as a "shock absorber," redistributing and evening out the forces generated by contraction of the muscle, thereby preventing rupture of the muscle membrane. Alterations in the proteins of the complex lead to deterioration of the muscle during normal contraction and relaxation cycles. Symptoms of these conditions set in as the muscle gradually exhausts its ability to repair itself.

Both DMD and BMD are caused by alterations in the gene for the protein called dystrophin. The alteration leading to DMD prevents the formation of any dystrophin, while that of BMD allows some protein to be made, accounting for the differences in severity and age of onset between the two conditions. Differences among the other muscular dystrophies in terms of the muscles involved and the ages of onset are less easily explained.

A number of genes have been found to cause LGMD. A majority of the more severe autosomal recessive types of LGMD with childhood-onset are caused by alterations in the genes responsible for making proteins called sarcoglycans. The sarcoglycans are a complex of proteins that are normally located in the muscle cell membrane along with dystrophin. Loss of these proteins causes the muscle cell membrane to lose some of its shock absorber qualities. The genes responsible include LGMD2D on chromosome 17, which codes for the alpha-sarcoglycan protein; LGMD2E on chromosome 4, which codes for the beta-sarcoglycan protein; LGMD2C on chromosome 13, which codes for the gamma-sarcoglycan protein; and LGMD2F on chromosome 5, which codes for the delta-sarcoglycan protein. Some cases of autosomal recessive LGMD are caused by an alteration in a gene, LGMD2A, on chromosome 15, which codes for a muscle enzyme, calpain 3. The relationship between this alteration and the symptoms of the condition is unclear. Alterations in a gene called LGMD2B on chromosome 2 that codes for the dysferlin protein, is also responsible for a minority of autosomal recessive LGMD cases. The exact role of dysferlin is not known. Finally, alterations in the LGMD2G gene on chromosome 17 which codes for a protein, telethonin, is responsible for autosomal recessive LGMD in two reported families. The exact role of telethonin is not known. Some families with autosomal recessive LGMD are not accounted for by alterations in any of the above mentioned genes, indicating that there are as yet undiscovered genes which can cause LGMD. The autosomal dominant LGMD genes have mostly been described in single families. These types of LGMD are considered quite rare.

The genes causing these types of LGMD, their chromosomal location, and the proteins they code for (when known) are listed below:

- LGMD1A (chromosome 5): myotilin
- LGMD1B (chromosome 1): laminin
- LGMD1C (chromosome 3): caveolin
- LGMD1D (chromosome 6)
- LGMD1E (chromosome 7)
- COL6A1 (chromosome 21): collagen VI alpha 1
- COL6A2 (chromosome 21): collagen VI alpha 2
- COL6A3 (chromosome 2): collagen VI alpha 3

The causes of the other muscular dystrophies are not as well understood:

- EDMD is due to a alteration in the gene for a protein called emerin, which is found in the membrane of a cell's nucleus, but whose exact function is unknown.
- Myotonic dystrophy is caused by alterations in a gene on chromosome 19 for an enzyme called myotonin protein kinase that may control the flow of

charged particles within muscle cells. This gene alteration is called a triple repeat, meaning it contains extra triplets of DNA code. It is possible that this alteration affects nearby genes as well, and that the widespread symptoms of myotonic dystrophy are due to a range of genetic disruptions.

- The gene for OPMD appears to also be altered with a triple repeat. The function of the affected protein may involve translation of genetic messages in a cell's nucleus.

- The gene(s) for FSH is located on the long arm of chromosome 4 at gene location 4q35. Nearly all cases of FSH are associated with a deletion (missing piece) of genetic material in this region. Researchers are investigating the molecular connection of this deletion and FSH. It is not yet certain whether the deleted material contains an active gene or changes the regulation or activity of a nearby FSH gene. A small number of FSH cases are not linked to chromosome 4. Their linkage to any other chromosome or genetic feature is under investigation.

- The gene(s) responsible for DD have not yet been found.

- About 50% of individuals with CMD have their condition as a result of deficiency in a protein called merosin, which is made by a gene called laminin. The merosin protein usually lies outside muscle cells and links them to the surrounding tissue. When merosin is not produced, the muscle fibers degenerate soon after birth. A second gene called integrin is responsible for CMD in a few individuals but alterations in this gene are a rare cause of CMD. The gene responsible for Fukuyama CMD is FCMD and it is responsible for making a protein called fukutin whose function is not clear.

### Signs and symptoms

All of the muscular dystrophies are marked by muscle weakness as the major symptom. The distribution of symptoms, age of onset, and progression differ significantly. Pain is sometimes a symptom of each, usually due to the effects of weakness on joint position.

**DUCHENNE MUSCULAR DYSTROPHY (DMD).** A boy with **Duchenne muscular dystrophy** usually begins to show symptoms as a pre-schooler. The legs are affected first, making walking difficult and causing balance problems. Most patients walk three to six months later than expected and have difficulty running. Later on, a boy with DMD will push his hands against his knees to rise to a standing position, to compensate for leg weakness. About the same time, his calves will begin to enlarge, though with fibrous tissue rather than with muscle, and feel firm and rubbery; this condition gives DMD one of its alternate names, pseudohypertrophic muscular dystrophy. He will widen his stance to maintain balance, and walk with a waddling gait to advance his weakened legs. Contractures (permanent muscle tightening) usually begin by age five or six, most severely in the calf muscles. This pulls the foot down and back, forcing the boy to walk on tip-toes, and further decreases balance. Climbing stairs and rising unaided may become impossible by age nine or ten, and most boys use a wheelchair for mobility by the age of 12. Weakening of the trunk muscles around this age often leads to **scoliosis** (a side-to-side spine curvature) and kyphosis (a front-to-back curvature).

The most serious weakness of DMD is weakness of the diaphragm, the sheet of muscles at the top of the abdomen that perform the main work of breathing and coughing. Diaphragm weakness leads to reduced energy and stamina, and increased lung infection because of the inability to cough effectively. Young men with DMD often live into their twenties and beyond, provided they have mechanical ventilation assistance and good respiratory hygiene.

Among males with DMD, the incidence of cardiomyopathy (weakness of the heart muscle), increases steadily in teenage years. Almost all patients have cardiomyopathy after 18 years of age. It has also been shown that carrier females are at increased risk for cardiomyopathy and should also be screened.

About one third of males with DMD experience specific learning disabilities, including difficulty learning by ear rather than by sight and difficulty paying attention to long lists of instructions. Individualized educational programs usually compensate well for these disabilities.

**BECKER MUSCULAR DYSTROPHY (BMD).** The symptoms of BMD usually appear in late childhood to early adulthood. Though the progression of symptoms may parallel that of DMD, the symptoms are usually milder and the course more variable. The same pattern of leg weakness, unsteadiness, and contractures occur later for the young man with BMD, often allowing independent walking into the twenties or early thirties. Scoliosis may occur, but is usually milder and progresses more slowly. Cardiomyopathy occurs more commonly in BMD. Problems may include irregular heartbeats (arrhythmias) and congestive heart failure. Symptoms may include fatigue, shortness of breath, chest pain, and dizziness. Respiratory weakness also occurs, and may lead to the need for mechanical ventilation.

**EMERY-DREIFUSS MUSCULAR DYSTROPHY (EDMD).** This type of muscular dystrophy usually begins in early childhood, often with contractures preceding muscle weakness. Weakness affects the shoulder and upper arm initially, along with the calf muscles, leading to foot-drop. Most men with EDMD survive into middle age, although an abnormality in the heart's rhythm (heart block) may be fatal if not treated with a pacemaker.

**LIMB-GIRDLE MUSCULAR DYSTROPHY (LGMD).** While there are several genes that cause the various types of LGMD, two major clinical forms of LGMD are usually recognized. A severe childhood form is similar in appearance to DMD, but is inherited as an autosomal recessive trait. Symptoms of adult-onset LGMD usually appear in a person's teens or twenties, and are marked by progressive weakness and wasting of the muscles closest to the trunk. Contractures may occur, and the ability to walk is usually lost about 20 years after onset. Some people with LGMD develop respiratory weakness that requires use of a ventilator. Life span may be somewhat shortened. Autosomal dominant forms usually occur later in life and progress relatively slowly.

**FACIOSCAPULOHUMERAL MUSCULAR DYSTROPHY (FSH).** FSH varies in its severity and age of onset, even among members of the same family. Symptoms most commonly begin in the teens or early twenties, though infant or childhood onset is possible. Symptoms tend to be more severe in those with earlier onset. The condition is named for the regions of the body most severely affected by the condition: muscles of the face (facio-), shoulders (scapulo-), and upper arms (humeral). Hips and legs may be affected as well. Children with FSH may develop partial or complete **deafness**.

The first symptom noticed is often difficulty lifting objects above the shoulders. The weakness may be greater on one side than the other. Shoulder weakness also causes the shoulder blades to jut backward, called scapular winging. Muscles in the upper arm often lose bulk sooner than those of the forearm, giving a "Popeye" appearance to the arms. Facial weakness may lead to loss of facial expression, difficulty closing the eyes completely, and inability to drink through a straw, blow up a balloon, or whistle. A person with FSH may not be able to wrinkle thier forehead. Contracture of the calf muscles may cause foot-drop, leading to frequent tripping over curbs or rough spots. People with earlier onset often require a wheelchair for mobility, while those with later onset rarely do.

**MYOTONIC DYSTROPHY.** Symptoms of **myotonic dystrophy** include facial weakness and a slack jaw, drooping eyelids (ptosis), and muscle wasting in the forearms and calves. A person with myotonic dystrophy has difficulty relaxing his grasp, especially if the object is cold. Myotonic dystrophy affects heart muscle, causing arrhythmias and heart block, and the muscles of the digestive system, leading to motility disorders and constipation. Other body systems are affected as well; myotonic dystrophy may cause cataracts, retinal degeneration, mental deficiency, frontal balding, skin disorders, testicular atrophy, sleep apnea, and insulin resistance. An increased need or desire for sleep is common, as is diminished motivation. The condition is extremely variable; some individuals show profound weakness as a newborn (congenital myotonic dystrophy), others show mental retardation in childhood, many show characteristic facial features and muscle wasting in adulthood, while the most mildly affected individuals show only cataracts in middle age with no other symptoms. Individuals with a severe form of mytonic dystropy typically have severe disabilities within 20 years of onset, although most do not require a wheelchair even late in life.

**OCULOPHARYNGEAL MUSCULAR DYSTROPHY (OPMD).** OPMD usually begins in a person's thirties or forties, with weakness in the muscles controlling the eyes and throat. Symptoms include drooping eyelids and difficulty swallowing (dysphagia). Weakness progresses to other muscles of the face, neck, and occasionally the upper limbs. Swallowing difficulty may cause aspiration, or the introduction of food or saliva into the airways. Pneumonia may follow.

**DISTAL MUSCULAR DYSTROPHY (DD).** DD usually begins in the twenties or thirties, with weakness in the hands, forearms, and lower legs. Difficulty with fine movements such as typing or fastening buttons may be the first symptoms. Symptoms progress slowly, and the condition usually does not affect life span.

**CONGENITAL MUSCULAR DYSTROPHY (CMD).** CMD is marked by severe muscle weakness from birth, with infants displaying "floppiness," very poor muscle tone, and they often have trouble moving their limbs or head against gravity. Mental function is normal but some are never able to walk. They may live into young adulthood or beyond. In contrast, children with Fukuyama CMD are rarely able to walk, and have severe mental retardation. Most children with this type of CMD die in childhood.

## Diagnosis

The diagnosis of muscular dystrophy involves a careful medical history and a thorough physical exam to determine the distribution of symptoms and to rule out other causes. Family history may give important clues, since all the muscular dystrophies are genetic conditions (though no family history will be evident in the event of new mutations; in autosomal recessive inheritance, the family history may also be negative).

Lab tests may include:

- Blood level of the muscle enzyme creatine kinase (CK). CK levels rise in the blood due to muscle damage, and may be seen in some conditions even before symptoms appear.

- Muscle biopsy, in which a small piece of muscle tissue is removed for microscopic examination. Changes in the structure of muscle cells and presence of fibrous tissue or other aberrant structures are characteristic of different forms of muscular dystrophy. The muscle tissue can also be stained to detect the presence or absence of particular proteins, including dystrophin.

- Electromyogram (EMG). This electrical test is used to examine the response of the muscles to stimulation. Decreased response is seen in muscular dystrophy. Other characteristic changes are seen in DM.

- Genetic tests. Several of the muscular dystrophies can be positively identified by testing for the presence of the altered gene involved. Accurate genetic tests are available for DMD, BMD, DM, several forms of LGMD, and EDMD. Genetic testing for some of these conditions in future pregnancies of an affected individual or parents of an affected individual can be done before birth through amniocentesis or chorionic villus sampling. Prenatal testing can only be undertaken after the diagnosis in the affected individual has been genetically confirmed and the couple has been counseled regarding the risks of recurrence.

- Other specific tests as necessary. For EDMD, DMD and BMD, for example, an electrocardiogram may be needed to test heart function, and hearing tests are performed for children with FSH.

For most forms of muscular dystrophy, accurate diagnosis is not difficult when done by someone familiar with the range of conditions. There are exceptions, however. Even with a muscle biopsy, it may be difficult to distinguish between FSH and another muscle condition, polymyositis. Childhood-onset LGMD is often mistaken for the much more common DMD, especially when it occurs in boys. BMD with an early onset appears very similar to DMD, and a genetic test may be needed to accurately distinguish them.

The muscular dystrophies may be confused with conditions involving the motor neurons, such as **spinal muscular atrophy**; conditions of the neuromuscular junction, such as **myasthenia gravis**; and other muscle conditions, as all involve generalized weakness of varying distribution.

Prenatal diagnosis (testing of the baby while in the womb) can be done for those types of muscular dystrophy where the specific disease-causing gene alteration has been identified in a previously affected family member. Prenatal diagnosis can be done utilizing **DNA** extracted from tissue obtained by chorionic villus sampling or **amniocentesis**.

## Treatment and management

### Drugs

There are no cures for any of the muscular dystrophies. Prednisone, a corticosteroid, has been shown to delay the progression of DMD somewhat, for reasons that are still unclear. Some have reported improvement in strength and function in patients treated with a single dose. Improvement begins within ten days and plateaus after three months. Long-term benefit has not been demonstrated. Prednisone is also prescribed for BMD, though no controlled studies have tested its benefit. A study is under way in the use of gentamicin, an antibiotic that may slow down the symptoms of DMD in a small number of cases. No other drugs are currently known to have an effect on the course of any other muscular dystrophy.

Treatment of muscular dystrophy is mainly directed at preventing the complications of weakness, including decreased mobility and dexterity, contractures, scoliosis, heart alterations, and respiratory insufficiency.

### Physical therapy

Physical therapy, regular stretching in particular, is used to maintain the range of motion of affected muscles and to prevent or delay contractures. Braces are used as well, especially on the ankles and feet to prevent tip-toeing. Full-leg braces may be used in children with DMD to prolong the period of independent walking. Strengthening other muscle groups to compensate for weakness may be possible if the affected muscles are few and isolated, as in the earlier stages of the milder muscular dystrophies. Regular, nonstrenuous exercise helps maintain general good health. Strenuous exercise is usually not recommended, since it may damage muscles further.

### Surgery

When contractures become more pronounced, tenotomy surgery may be performed. In this operation, the tendon of the contractured muscle is cut, and the limb is braced in its normal resting position while the tendon regrows. In FSH, surgical fixation of the scapula can help compensate for shoulder weakness. For a person with OPMD, surgical lifting of the eyelids may help compensate for weakened muscular control. For a person with DM, sleep apnea may be treated surgically to maintain an open airway. Scoliosis surgery is often needed in boys with DMD, but much less often in other muscular dystrophies. Surgery is recommended at a much lower degree of curvature for DMD than for scoliosis due to other conditions, since the decline in respiratory function in DMD makes surgery at a later time dangerous. In this surgery, the vertebrae are fused together to maintain the spine in the upright position. Steel rods are inserted at the time of operation to keep the spine rigid while the bones grow together.

When any type of surgery is performed in patients with muscular dystrophy, anesthesia must be carefully selected. People with MD are susceptible to a severe reaction, known as **malignant hyperthermia**, when given halothane anesthetic.

### Occupational therapy

The occupational therapist suggests techniques and tools to compensate for the loss of strength and dexterity. Strategies may include modifications in the home, adaptive utensils and dressing aids, compensatory movements and positioning, wheelchair accessories, or communication aids.

### Nutrition

Good nutrition helps to promote general health in all the muscular dystrophies. No special diet or supplement has been shown to be of use in any of the conditions. The weakness in the throat muscles seen especially in OPMD and later DMD may necessitate the use of a gastrostomy tube, inserted in the stomach to provide nutrition directly.

### Cardiac care

The arrhythmias of EDMD and BMD may be treatable with antiarrhythmia drugs. A pacemaker may be implanted if these do not provide adequate control. Heart transplants are increasingly common for men with BMD. A complete cardiac evaluation is recommended at least once in all carrier females of DMD and EDMD.

### Respiratory care

People who develop weakness of the diaphragm or other ventilatory muscles may require a mechanical ventilator to continue breathing deeply enough. Air may be administered through a nasal mask or mouthpiece, or through a tracheostomy tube, which is inserted through a surgical incision through the neck and into the windpipe. Most people with muscular dystrophy do not need a tracheostomy, although some may prefer it to continual use of a mask or mouthpiece. Supplemental oxygen is not needed. Good hygiene of the lungs is critical for health and long-term survival of a person with weakened ventilatory muscles. Assisted cough techniques provide the strength needed to clear the airways of secretions; an assisted cough machine is also available and provides excellent results.

### Experimental treatments

Two experimental procedures aiming to cure DMD have attracted a great deal of attention. In myoblast transfer, millions of immature muscle cells are injected into an affected muscle. The goal of the treatment is to promote the growth of the injected cells, replacing the abnormal host cells with healthy new ones. Myoblast transfer is under investigation but remains experimental.

**Gene therapy** introduces unaltered copies of the altered gene into muscle cells. The goal is to allow the existing muscle cells to use the new gene to produce the protein it cannot make with its abnormal gene. Problems with gene therapy research have included immune rejection of the virus used to introduce the gene, loss of gene function after several weeks, and an inability to get the gene to enough cells to make a functional difference in the affected muscle. Researchers are preparing for the first gene therapy trial for LGMD in the United States. The goal will be to replace the missing sarcoglycan gene(s).

### Genetic counseling

Individuals with muscular dystrophy and their families may benefit from **genetic counseling** for information on the condition and recurrence risks for future pregnancies.

## Prognosis

The expected life span for a male with DMD has increased significantly. Most young men will live into their early or mid-twenties. Respiratory infections become an increasing problem as their breathing becomes weaker, and these infections are usually the cause of death.

The course of the other muscular dystrophies is more variable; expected life spans and degrees of disability are hard to predict, but may be related to age of onset and initial symptoms. Prediction is made more difficult because, as new genes are discovered, it is becoming clear that several of the dystrophies are not uniform disorders, but rather symptom groups caused by different genes.

People with dystrophies with significant heart involvement (BMD, EDMD, myotonic dystrophy) may nonetheless have almost normal life spans, provided that cardiac complications are monitored and treated aggressively. The respiratory involvement of BMD and LGMD similarly require careful and prompt treatment.

### Prevention

There is no way to prevent any of the muscular dystrophies in a person who has the genes responsible for these disorders. Accurate genetic tests, including prenatal tests, are available for some of the muscular dystrophies. Results of these tests may be useful for purposes of family planning.

### Resources

**BOOKS**

Emery, Alan. *Muscular Dystrophy: The Facts*. Oxford Medical Publications, 1994.

Swash, Michael, and Martin Schwartz. *Neuromuscular Conditions: A Practical Approach to Diagnosis and Management,* 3rd edition. New York: Springer, 1997.

**ORGANIZATIONS**

Muscular Dystrophy Association. 3300 East Sunrise Dr., Tucson, AZ 85718. (520) 529-2000 or (800) 572-1717. http://www.mda.org.

Online Myotonic & Congenital Dystrophies Support Group International. 185 Unionville Road, Freedom, PA 15042. (724) 775-9448 or (724) 774-0261. http://www. angelfire.com/pa2/MyotonicDystrophy/index.html.

Nada Quercia, Msc, CCGC

# Myasthenia gravis

### Definition

Myasthenia gravis is an autoimmune disease that causes muscle weakness.

### Description

The name myasthenia gravis literally means "grave muscle weakness." Myasthenia gravis (MG) affects the neuromuscular junction, interrupting the communication between nerve and muscle, and thereby causing weakness. A person with MG may have difficulty moving their eyes, walking, speaking clearly, swallowing, and even breathing, depending on the severity and distribution of weakness. Increased weakness with exertion, and improvement with rest, is a characteristic feature of MG.

### Genetic profile

Myasthenia gravis is not inherited directly nor is it contagious. It is usually considered sporadic, meaning that it occurs by chance. One to four percent of cases are familial, which means they occur more than once in a family. Predisposition in a family to develop myasthenia gravis may be due to autoimmunity in general.

### Demographics

About 36,000 people in the United States are affected by MG; roughly 14 people per 100,000. It can occur at any age, but is most common in women under age 40, and in men who are over 60. Occasionally the disease is present in more than one person in a family.

### Signs and symptoms

Myasthenia gravis is an autoimmune disease, meaning it is caused by the body's own immune system. In MG, the immune system attacks a receptor on the surface of muscle cells. This prevents the muscle from receiving the nerve impulses that normally make it respond. MG affects voluntary muscles, which are

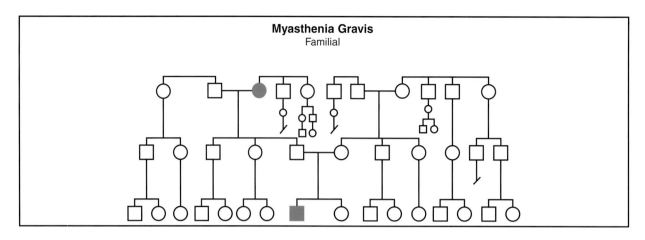

**Familial inheritance of Myasthenia gravis.** *(Gale, a part of Cengage Learning.)*

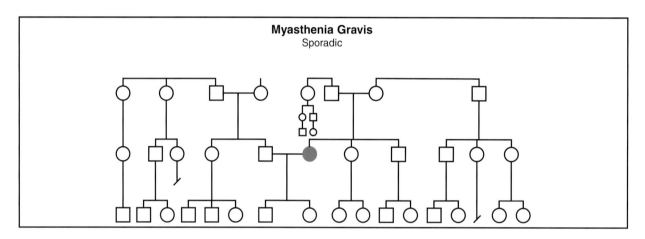

**Sporatic occurrence of Myasthenia gravis in a family.** *(Gale, a part of Cengage Learning.)*

those muscles under conscious control responsible for movement. It does not affect heart muscle or the smooth muscle found in the digestive system and other internal organs.

A muscle is stimulated to contract when the nerve cell controlling it releases acetylcholine molecules onto its surface. The acetylcholine lands on a muscle protein called the acetylcholine receptor. This leads to rapid chemical changes in the muscle, which cause it to contract. Acetylcholine is then broken down by acetylcholinesterase enzyme, to prevent further stimulation.

In MG, immune cells create antibodies against the acetylcholine receptor. Antibodies are proteins normally involved in fighting infection. When these antibodies attach to the receptor, they prevent it from receiving acetylcholine, decreasing the ability of the muscle to respond to stimulation.

Why the immune system creates these self-reactive autoantibodies is unknown, although there are several hypotheses:

- During fetal development, the immune system generates many B cells that can make autoantibodies, but B cells that could harm the body's own tissues are screened out and destroyed before birth. It is possible that the stage is set for MG when some of these cells escape detection.

- Genes controlling other parts of the immune system, called MHC genes, appear to influence how susceptible a person is to developing autoimmune disease.

- Infection may trigger some cases of MG. When activated, the immune system may mistake portions of the acetylcholine receptor for portions of an invading virus, though no candidate virus has yet been identified conclusively.

## KEY TERMS

**Antibody**—A protein produced by the mature B cells of the immune system that attach to invading microorganisms and target them for destruction by other immune system cells.

**Autoantibody**—An antibody that reacts against part of the self.

**Autoimmune disease**—Describes a group of diseases characterized by an inflammatory immune reaction erroneously directed toward 'self' tissues.

**Bulbar muscles**—Muscles that control chewing, swallowing, and speaking.

**Neuromuscular junction**—The site at which nerve impulses are transmitted to muscles.

**Pyridostigmine bromide (Mestinon)**—An anticholinesterase drug used in treating Myasthenia gravis.

**Tensilon test**—A test for diagnosing myasthenia gravis. Tensilon is injected into a vein and, if the person has MG, their muscle strength will improve for about five minutes.

**Thymus gland**—An endocrine gland located in the front of the neck that houses and transports T cells, which help to fight infection.

• About 10% of those with MG also have thymomas, or benign tumors of the thymus gland. The thymus is a principal organ of the immune system, and researchers speculate that thymic irregularities are involved in the progression of MG.

Some or all of these factors (developmental, genetic, infectious, and thymic) may interact to create the autoimmune reaction.

The earliest symptoms of MG often result from weakness of the extraocular muscles, which control eye movements. Symptoms involving the eye (ocular symptoms) include double vision (diplopia), especially when not gazing straight ahead, and difficulty raising the eyelids (ptosis). A person with ptosis may need to tilt their head back to see. Eye-related symptoms remain the only symptoms for about 15% of MG patients. Another common early symptom is difficulty chewing and swallowing, due to weakness in the bulbar muscles, which are in the mouth and throat. Choking becomes more likely, especially with food that requires extensive chewing.

Weakness usually becomes more widespread within several months of the first symptoms, reaching their maximum within a year in two-thirds of patients.

Weakness may involve muscles of the arms, legs, neck, trunk, and face, and affect the ability to lift objects, walk, hold the head up, and speak.

Symptoms of MG become worse upon exertion and better with rest. Heat, including heat from the sun, hot showers, and hot drinks, may increase weakness. Infection and stress may worsen symptoms. Symptoms may vary from day to day and month to month, with intervals of no weakness interspersed with a progressive decline in strength.

Myasthenic crisis is an emergency condition requiring immediate treatment. It may occur when the breathing muscles become too weak to provide adequate respiration. Symptoms include weak and shallow breathing, shortness of breath, pale or bluish skin color, and a racing heart. In patients treated with anticholinesterase agents, myasthenic crisis must be differentiated from cholinergic crisis related to overmedication.

Pregnancy worsens MG in about one third of women, has no effect in one third, and improves symptoms in another third. About 12% of infants born to women with MG have neonatal myasthenia, a temporary but potentially life-threatening condition. It is caused by the transfer of maternal antibodies into the fetal circulation just before birth. Symptoms include weakness, poor muscle tone, feeble cry, and difficulty feeding. The infant may have difficulty breathing, requiring the use of a ventilator. Neonatal myasthenia usually clears up within a month.

### Diagnosis

Myasthenia gravis is often diagnosed accurately by a careful medical history and a neuromuscular exam, but several tests are used to confirm the diagnosis. Other conditions causing worsening of bulbar and skeletal muscles must be considered, including drug-induced myasthenia, thyroid disease, Lambert-Eaton myasthenic syndrome, botulism, and inherited muscular dystrophies.

MG causes characteristic changes in the electrical responses of muscles that may be observed with an electromyogram, which measures muscular response to electrical stimulation. Repetitive nerve stimulation leads to reduction in the height of the measured muscle response, reflecting the muscle's tendency to become fatigued.

Blood tests may confirm the presence of the antibody to the acetylcholine receptor, though up to a quarter of MG patients will not have detectable levels. A chest x ray or chest computed tomography scan (CT scan) may be performed to look for thymoma.

## Treatment and management

While there is no cure for myasthenia gravis, there are a number of treatments that effectively control symptoms in most people.

Edrophonium (Tensilon) blocks the action of acetylcholinesterase, prolonging the effect of acetylcholine and increasing strength. An injection of edrophonium rapidly leads to a marked improvement in most people with MG. An alternate drug, neostigmine, may also be used.

Pyridostigmine (Mestinon) is usually the first drug prescribed. Like edrophonium, pyridostigmine blocks acetylcholinesterase. It is longer-acting, taken by mouth, and well-tolerated. Loss of responsiveness and disease progression combine to eventually make pyridostigmine ineffective in tolerable doses in many patients.

Thymectomy, or removal of the thymus gland, has increasingly become standard treatment for MG. Up to 85% of people with MG improve after thymectomy, with complete remission eventually seen in about 30%. The improvement may take months or even several years to fully develop. Thymectomy is not usually recommended for children with MG, since the thymus continues to play an important immune role throughout childhood.

Immune-suppressing drugs are used to treat MG if response to pyridostigmine and thymectomy are not adequate. Drugs include corticosteroids such as prednisone, and the non-steroids azathioprine (Imuran) and cyclosporine (Sandimmune).

Plasma exchange may be performed to treat myasthenic crisis or to improve very weak patients before thymectomy. In this procedure, blood plasma is removed and replaced with purified plasma free of autoantibodies. It can produce a temporary improvement in symptoms, but is too expensive for long-term treatment. Another blood treatment, intravenous immunoglobulin therapy, is also used for myasthenic crisis. In this procedure, large quantities of purified immune proteins (immunoglobulins) are injected. For unknown reasons, this leads to symptomatic improvement in up to 85% of patients. It is also too expensive for long-term treatment.

People with weakness of the bulbar muscles may need to eat softer foods that are easier to chew and swallow. In more severe cases, it may be necessary to obtain nutrition through a feeding tube placed into the stomach (gastrostomy tube).

Some drugs should be avoided by people with MG because they interfere with normal neuromuscular function. Drugs to be avoided or used with caution include:

- many types of antibiotics, including erythromycin, streptomycin, and ampicillin
- some cardiovascular drugs, including Verapamil, betaxolol, and propranolol
- some drugs used in psychiatric conditions, including chlorpromazine, clozapine, and lithium

Many other drugs may worsen symptoms, so patients should check with the doctor who treats their MG before taking any new medications.

A Medic-Alert card or bracelet provides an important source of information to emergency providers about the special situation of a person with MG. They are available from health care providers.

## Prognosis

Most people with MG can be treated successfully enough to prevent their condition from becoming debilitating. In some cases, however, symptoms may worsen even with vigorous treatment, leading to generalized weakness and disability. MG rarely causes early death except from myasthenic crisis. There is no known way to prevent myasthenia gravis. Thymectomy improves symptoms significantly in many patients, and relieves them entirely in some. Avoiding heat can help minimize symptoms.

## Resources

### BOOKS

Swash, Michael, and Martin Schwarz. *Neuromuscular Diseases: A Practical Approach to Diagnosis and Management. New York:* Springer, 1997.

### PERIODICALS

Drachman, D. B. "Myasthenia Gravis." *New England Journal of Medicine* 330 (1994): 1797-1810.

Robinson, Richard. "The Body At War with Itself." *Quest* 4, no. 3 (1997): 20-24.

### WEBSITES

*Immune Deficiency Foundation.* http://www.primaryimmune.org.

*Myasthenia Gravis Foundation of America.* http://www.myasthenia.org.

*National Institute of Neurological Disorders and Stroke Fact Sheet on Myasthenia Gravis.* http://www.ninds.nih.gov/health_and_medical/pubs/myasthenia_gravis.htm.

### ORGANIZATIONS

Muscular Dystrophy Association. 3300 East Sunrise Dr., Tucson, AZ 85718. (520) 529-2000 or (800) 572-1717. http://www.mda.org.

Myasthenia Gravis Foundation of America. 355 Lexington Ave., 15th Ploor, New York, NY 10017 (212) 297-2156, (800) 541-5454, Fax: (212) 370-9047. http://www.myasthenia.org.

Catherine L. Tesla, MS, CGC

# Myopia

## Definition

Myopia is the medical term for nearsightedness. People with myopia see objects more clearly when they are close to the eye, while distant objects appear blurred or fuzzy. Reading and close–up work may be clear, but distance vision is blurry.

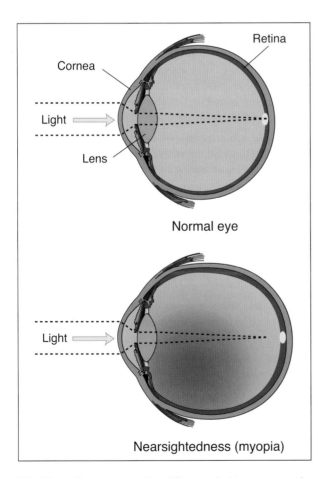

**This illustration compares the difference between a normal eye shape and light refraction versus a myopic eye.** *(Gale, a part of Cengage Learning.)*

## Description

To understand myopia it is necessary to have a basic knowledge of the main parts of the eye's focusing system: the cornea, the lens, and the retina. The cornea is a tough, transparent, dome–shaped tissue that covers the front of the eye (not to be confused with the white, opaque sclera). The cornea lies in front of the iris (the colored part of the eye). The lens is a transparent, dou–ble–convex structure located behind the iris. The retina is a thin membrane that lines the rear of the eyeball. Light–sensitive retinal cells convert incoming light rays into electrical signals that are sent along the optic nerve to the brain, which then interprets the images.

In people with normal vision, parallel light rays enter the eye and are bent by the cornea and lens (a process called refraction) to focus precisely on the retina, providing a crisp, clear image. In the myopic eye, the focusing power of the cornea (the major refracting structure of the eye) and the lens is too great with respect to the length of the eyeball. Light rays are bent too much, and they converge in front of the retina. This inaccuracy is called a refractive error. In other words, an overfocused fuzzy image is sent to the brain.

There are many types of myopia. Some common types include:

- physiologic
- pathologic
- acquired

By far the most common form, physiologic myopia develops in children sometime between the ages of five and 10 years and gradually progresses until the eye is fully grown. Physiologic myopia may include refractive myopia (the cornea and lens–bending properties are too strong) and axial myopia (the eyeball is too long). Patho–logic myopia is a far less common abnormality. This condition begins as physiologic myopia, but rather than stabilizing, the eye continues to enlarge at an abnor–mal rate (progressive myopia). This more advanced type of myopia may lead to degenerative changes in the eye (degenerative myopia). Acquired myopia occurs after infancy. This condition may be seen in association with uncontrolled **diabetes** and certain types of cataracts. Antihypertensive drugs and other medications can also affect the refractive power of the lens.

## Genetic profile

Eye care professionals have debated the role of **genetics** in the development of myopia for many years. Some believe that a tendency toward myopia may be inherited, but that the actual disorder results from a combination of environmental and genetic factors.

## KEY TERMS

**Accommodation**—The ability of the lens to change its focus from distant to near objects. It is achieved through the action of the ciliary muscles that change the shape of the lens.

**Cornea**—The transparent structure of the eye over the lens that is continous with the sclera in forming the outermost, protective, layer of the eye.

**Diopter (D)**—A unit of measure for describing refractive power.

**Epi-LASIK**—A surgical procedure that uses a blunt, plastic oscillating blade called an epithelial separator to cut a flap in the cornea.

**Laser–assisted in–situ keratomileusis (LASIK)**—A surgical procedure that uses a cutting tool and a laser to modify the cornea and correct moderate to high levels of myopia.

**Laser–assisted sub–epithelial keratomileusis (LASEK)**—A surgical procedure in which the epithelium is loosened on the corneal surface. The loosened epithelium is then reflected away from the cornea, and laser ablation performed.

**Lens**—The transparent, elastic, curved structure behind the iris (colored part of the eye) that helps focus light on the retina.

**Ophthalmologist**—A physician specializing in the medical and surgical treatment of eye disorders.

**Optic nerve**—A bundle of nerve fibers that carries visual messages from the retina in the form of electrical signals to the brain.

**Optometrist**—A medical professional who examines and tests the eyes for disease and treats visual disorders by prescribing corrective lenses and/or vision therapy. In many states, optometrists are licensed to use diagnostic and therapeutic drugs to treat certain ocular diseases.

**Orthokeratology**—A method of reshaping the cornea using a contact lens. It is not considered a permanent method to reduce myopia.

**Peripheral vision**—The ability to see objects that are not located directly in front of the eye. Peripheral vision allows people to see objects located on the side or edge of their field of vision.

**Photorefractive keratectomy (PRK)**—A procedure that uses an excimer laser to make modifications to the cornea and permanently correct myopia. As of early 1998, only two lasers have been approved by the FDA for this purpose.

**Radial keratotomy (RK)**—A surgical procedure involving the use of a diamond–tipped blade to make several spoke–like slits in the peripheral (non–viewing) portion of the cornea to improve the focus of the eye and correct myopia by flattening the cornea.

**Refraction**—The bending of light rays as they pass from one medium through another. Used to describe the action of the cornea and lens on light rays as they enter they eye. Also used to describe the determination and measurement of the eye's focusing system by an optometrist or ophthalmologist.

**Refractive eye surgery**—A general term for surgical procedures that can improve or correct refractive errors by permanently changing the shape of the cornea.

**Retina**—The light–sensitive layer of tissue in the back of the eye that receives and transmits visual signals to the brain through the optic nerve.

**Visual acuity**—The ability to distinguish details and shapes of objects.

---

Environmental factors include close work; work with computer monitors or other instruments that emit some light (electron microscopes, photographic equipment, lasers, etc.); emotional stress; and eye strain.

A variety of genetic patterns for inheriting myopia have been suggested, ranging from a recessive pattern with complete penetrance in people who are homozygotic for myopia to an autosomal dominant pattern; an autosomal recessive pattern; and various mixtures of these patterns. One explanation for this lack of agreement is that the genetic profile of high myopia (defined as a refractive error greater than –6 diopters) may differ from that of low myopia. Some researchers believe that high myopia is determined by genetic factors to a greater extent than low myopia.

The lack of clear consensus concerning the role of heredity in myopia may be due to the sensitivity of the human eye to very small changes in its anatomical structure. Since even small deviations from normal structure cause significant refractive errors, it may be difficult to single out any specific genetic or environmental factor as their cause.

### Genetic markers and gene mapping

Since 1992, genetic markers that may be associated with genes for myopia have been located on human chromosomes 1, 2, 12, and 18. There is some genetic information on the short arm of **chromosome** 2 in highly myopic people. Genetic information for low myopia appears to be located on the short arm of chromosome 1, but it is not known whether this information governs the structure of the eye itself or vulnerability to environmental factors.

In 1998, a team of American researchers presented evidence that a **gene** for familial high myopia with an autosomal dominant transmission pattern could be mapped to human chromosome 18 in eight North American families. The same group also found a second locus for this form of myopia on human chromosome 12 in a large German/Italian family. In 1999, a group of French researchers found no linkage between chromosome 18 and 32 French families with familial high myopia. These findings have been taken to indicate that more than one gene is involved in the transmission of the disorder.

As of 2009, the heritability of high–grade myopia had been confirmed. Multiple high–grade myopia genetic loci have been identified, and confirmatory studies identifying high–grade and moderate myopia loci have also occurred. However, myopia susceptibility genes still remain unknown.

### Family studies

It has been known for some years that a family history of myopia is one of the most important risk factors for developing the condition. Only 6–15% of children with myopia come from families in which neither parent is myopic. In families with one myopic parent, 23–40% of the children develop myopia. If both parents are myopic, the rate rises to 33–60% for their children. One American study found that children with two myopic parents are six times as likely to develop myopia themselves as children with only one or no myopic parents. The precise interplay of genetic and environmental factors in these family patterns, however, is not yet known.

One multigenerational study of Chinese patients indicated that third generation family members had a higher risk of developing myopia even if their parents were not myopic. The researchers concluded that, at least in China, the genetic factors in myopia have remained constant over the past three generations while the environmental factors have intensified. The increase in the percentage of people with myopia over the last 50 years in the United States has led American researchers to the same conclusion.

## Demographics

The prevalence of refractive error in the United States has not been evaluated since the early 1970s. According to a 2006 study sponsored by the National Eye Institute (NEI), refractive errors are estimated to affect 42.2 million (35%) of Americans 40 years or older.

Myopia is the most common eye disorder in humans around the world. It affects some 20% of the adult population in the United States. In various reports, incidence frequently varies with age, sex, race, ethnicity, occupation, environment, and other factors. Myopia is more common in central and eastern Europe than in northern Europe, Britain, and the United States. It is also very common in certain populations, such as Chinese, Japanese, Arab, and Jewish persons. Myopia is uncommon in black, Nubian, and Sudanese persons.

Other factors that affect the demographic distribution of myopia are income level and education. The prevalence of myopia is higher among people with above–average incomes and educational attainments. Myopia is also more prevalent among people whose work requires a great deal of close focusing, including work with computers.

## Signs and symptoms

Myopia is said to be caused by an elongation of the eyeball. This means that the oblong (as opposed to normal spherical) shape of the myopic eye causes the cornea and lens to focus at a point in front of the retina. A more precise explanation is that there is an inadequate correlation between the focusing power of the cornea and lens and the length of the eye.

People are generally born with a small amount of hyperopia (farsightedness), but as the eye grows this decreases and myopia does not become evident until later. This change is one reason why some researchers think that myopia is an acquired rather than an inherited trait.

The symptoms of myopia are blurred distance vision, eye discomfort, squinting, and eye strain.

## Diagnosis

The diagnosis of myopia is typically made during the first several years of elementary school when a teacher notices a child having difficulty seeing the chalkboard, reading, or concentrating. The teacher or school nurse often recommends an eye examination by an ophthalmologist or optometrist. An ophthalmologist—M.D. or D.O. (Doctor of Osteopathy)—is a medical doctor trained in the diagnosis and treatment of eye problems. Ophthalmologists also perform eye surgery. An optometrist (O.D.) diagnoses, manages and/or treats eye and visual disorders. In many states, optometrists are licensed to use diagnostic and therapeutic drugs.

A patient's distance vision is tested by reading letters or numbers on a chart posted a set distance away (usually 20 ft, [7 m]). The doctor asks the patient to view images through a variety of lenses to obtain the best correction. The doctor also examines the inside of the eye and the retina. An instrument called a slit lamp is used to examine the cornea and lens. The eyeglass prescription is written in terms of diopters (D), which measure the degree of refractive error. Mild to moderate myopia usually falls between -1.00D and -6.00D. Normal vision is commonly referred to as 20/20 to describe the eye's focusing ability at a distance of 20 ft (7 m) from an object. For example, 20/50 means that a myopic person must stand 20 ft away from an eye chart to see what a normal person can see at 50 ft (7 m). The larger the bottom number, the greater the myopia.

## Treatment and management

People with myopia have three main options for treatment: optical devices, such as eyeglasses and contact lenses, refractive eye surgery, and intraocular surgical procedures.

### Optical devices

**EYEGLASSES.** Eyeglasses are the most common method used to correct myopia. Concave glass or plastic lenses are placed in frames in front of the eyes. The lenses are ground to the thickness and curvature specified in the eyeglass prescription. The lenses cause the light rays to diverge so that they focus further back, directly on the retina, producing clear distance vision.

**CONTACT LENSES.** Contact lenses are a second option for treatment. Contact lenses are extremely thin round discs of plastic that are worn on the eye in front of the cornea. Although there may be some initial discomfort, most people quickly grow accustomed to contact lenses. Hard contact lenses, made from a material called PMMA, are virtually obsolete. Rigid gas permeable lenses (RGP) are made of plastic that holds its shape but allows the passage of some oxygen into the eye. Some believe that RGP lenses may halt or slow the progression of myopia because they maintain a constant, gentle pressure that flattens the cornea. In 2004, results of a NEI–sponsored study called the Contact Lens and Myopia Progression (CLAMP) Study, were published. Researchers found

that RGP contact lenses slowed the progression of myopia in young children. Researchers also found that RGP contact lenses did not slow the growth of the eye, responsible for the majority of myopia in children. Instead of slowing the growth of the eye, RGP lenses kept the cornea from changing shape more than soft contact lenses.

Soft contact lenses are made of flexible plastic and can be up to 80% water. Soft lenses offer increased comfort and the advantage of extended wear; some can be worn continuously for up to one week. While oxygen passes freely through soft lenses, bacterial contamination and other problems can occur, requiring replacement of lenses on a regular basis. It is very important to follow the cleaning and disinfecting regimens prescribed because protein and lipid buildup can occur on the lenses, causing discomfort or increasing the risk of infection. Contact lenses offer several benefits over glasses, including: better vision, less distortion, clear peripheral vision, and cosmetic appeal. In addition, contacts will not fog up from perspiration or changes in temperature.

### Refractive eye surgery

For people who find glasses and contact lenses inconvenient or uncomfortable, and who meet selection criteria regarding age, degree of myopia, general health, etc., refractive eye surgery is a third treatment alternative. Radial keratotomy was the first such procedure developed, but has been replaced since the mid–1990s by photorefractive keratectomy (PRK), laser–assisted in–situ keratomileusis (LASIK), Epi-LASIK, and laser–assisted sub–epithelial keratomileusis (LASEK). Refractive eye surgery improves myopic vision by permanently changing the shape of the cornea so that light rays focus properly on the retina. These procedures are performed on an outpatient basis and generally take 10–30 minutes.

**PHOTOREFRACTIVE KERATECTOMY (PRK).** PRK involves the use of a computer to measure the shape of the cornea. Using these measurements, the surgeon uses a computer–controlled excimer laser to make modifications to the cornea. The PRK procedure flattens the cornea by vaporizing small amounts of tissue from the cornea's surface, thereby improving the cornea's refractive properties in focusing light on the retina. The ultra thin, outer layer of the eye (epithelium) is removed completely by laser energy during the PRK procedure, and eventually grows back. PRK has been approved by the Food and Drug Administration (FDA) for myopia since 1995 and the first excimer lasers used to perform PRK have been improved significantly in terms of size, efficiency, and accuracy. PRK can treat mild to moderate forms of myopia.

**LASER–ASSISTED IN–SITU KERATOMILEUSIS (LASIK).**
LASIK has been approved by the FDA for several different laser platforms. About 5 million procedures have been performed in the United States since the approval of the excimer laser for refractive surgery in late 1995. It is recommended for moderate to severe cases of myopia. LASIK is perhaps best thought of as PRK performed under a flap instead of on the corneal surface. The flap is flipped back to expose the inner layers of the cornea. The cornea is treated with a laser to change the shape and focusing properties,then the flap is replaced. For myopic LASIK ablations, most of the laser energy is directed at the center of the treatment zone with the result that the central cornea is thus flattened.

**LASER–ASSISTED SUB–EPITHELIAL KERATOMILEUSIS (LASEK).** In a LASEK procedure, the epithelium is chemically loosened using dilute alcohol on the corneal surface. The loosened epithelium is then reflected away from the cornea, and laser ablation performed. The procedure preserves the extremely thin epithelial layer by lifting it from the eye's surface before using a laser for reshaping. After the LASEK procedure, the epithelium is replaced on the eye's surface.

**EPI–LASIK.** In Epi–LASIK, the surgeon uses a blunt, plastic oscillating blade called an epithelial separator to cut a flap in the cornea. Instead of the alcohol used in LASEK to loosen the epithelial sheet, the epithelial separator is used to separate the sheet from the eye. This avoids the possibility of an adverse reaction from the alcohol. Because it is more difficult to create the epithelial flap in people with steeper corneas (who have higher amounts of myopia), the procedure is considered more appropriate for people with less steep corneas (who have low myopia).

### Intraocular surgical procedures

These procedures involve extraction of the clear lens with or without lens implantation and the use of intraocular lens (IOL) implants. IOLs have been used since 1999 for correcting large refractive errors in myopia. An IOL is a microscopic lens that can be placed inside the eye to correct certain vision problems. For patients who are extremely nearsighted and may have contraindications to LASIK, an IOL may be implanted in front of the iris to correct their distance vision and provide normal focusing ability and near vision. Although IOLs are intended to be permanent, the procedure is reversible.

### Risks

All of these surgical procedures carry risks, the most serious being corneal scarring, corneal rupture, infection, flap problems, dry eye, cataracts, and loss of vision. The National Eye Institute (NEI) warns that before agreeing to refractive surgery, patients should get a clear picture of what they can expect. Surgeons should explain the risks and possible complications, as well as potential side effects.

Since refractive eye surgery does not guarantee 20/20 vision, it is important to have realistic expectations before choosing this treatment. For example, the American Academy of Ophthalmology (AAO) reports that nine out of 10 patients achieve 20/20 vision, but 20/20 does not always mean perfect vision. Detailed, precise vision may be slightly diminished. Even if the patient gains near-perfect vision, irritating side effects are also possible, such as postoperative pain, poor night vision, variation in visual acuity, light sensitivity and glare, and optical distortion. Finally, refractive eye surgeries are considered elective procedures and are rarely covered by insurance plans.

## Alternative treatments

Some eye care professionals recommend treatments to help improve circulation, reduce eye strain, and relax the eye muscles. It is possible that by combining exercises with changes in behavior, the progression of myopia may be slowed or prevented. Alternative treatments include: visual therapy (also referred to as vision training or eye exercises); discontinuing close work; reducing eye strain (taking a rest break during periods of prolonged near vision tasks); and wearing bifocals to decrease the need to accommodate when doing close–up work.

### Clinical trials

Clinical trials on myopia are currently sponsored by the National Institutes of Health (NIH) and other agencies. As of 2009, NIH reported121 on–going and completed studies.

Examples include:

- The evaluation of neurovision correction (NVC) technology for the treatment of low myopia. (NCT00469612)

- A study of the inheritance of myopia in families of various nationalities and ethnic backgrounds to identify gene changes that cause myopia or similar diseases. (NCT00272376)

- A study to determine whether the MEL 80 Excimer Laser is effective in the treatment of moderate to high myopia, when used as part of the LASIK procedure. (NCT00762541)

Clinical trial information is constantly updated by NIH and the most recent information on myopia trials can be found at: http://clinicaltrials.gov.

## Prognosis

Glasses and contact lenses can (but not always) correct the patient's vision to 20/20. Refractive surgery can make permanent improvements for the right candidates.

While the genetic factors that influence the transmission and severity of myopia cannot be changed, some environmental factors can be modified. They include reducing close work; reading and working in good light; taking frequent breaks when working at a computer or microscope for long periods of time; maintaining good nutrition; and practicing visual therapy (when recommended).

Eye strain can be prevented by using sufficient light for reading and close work, and by wearing corrective lenses as prescribed. Everyone should have regular eye examinations to see if their prescription has changed or if any other problems have developed. This is particularly important for people with high (degenerative) myopia who are at a greater risk of developing retinal detachment, retinal degeneration, **glaucoma**, or other problems.

## Resources

### BOOKS

Caster, Andrew. *Lasik: The Eye Laser Miracle: The Complete Guide to Better Vision*. New York, NY: Ballantine Books, 2008.

De Angelis, David. *The Secret of Perfect Vision: How You Can Prevent and Reverse Nearsightedness*. Berkeley, CA: North Atlantic Books, 2008.

Knobbe, Chris. *Refractive Eye Surgery: A Consumer's Complete Guide*. Charleston, SC: BookSurge Publishing, 2006.

### PERIODICALS

de Benito–Llopis L., et al. "Ten–year Follow–up of Excimer Laser Surface Ablation for Myopia in Thin Corneas." *American Journal of Ophthalmology* 147, no. 5 (2009): 768–773.

Kim, M. J., et al. "Congenital axial high myopia detected by prenatal ultrasound." *American Journal of Pediatric Ophthalmology and Strabismus* 46, no. 1 (January–February 2009): 50–53.

McKone, E., et al. "Blurry means good focus: myopia and visual attention." *Perception* 37, no. 11 (2008): 1765–17.

Schäche, M., et al. "Fine mapping linkage analysis identifies a novel susceptibility locus for myopia on chromosome 2q37 adjacent to but not overlapping MYP12." *Molecular Vision* 15 (2009): 722–730.

Young, T. L. "Molecular genetics of human myopia: an update." *Optometry and Vision Science* 86, no. 1 (January 2009): E8–E22.

### WEBSITES

*Basic Lasik: Tips on Eye Surgery*. Information Page. NEI, October 2008 (April 05, 2009). http://www.ftc.gov/bcp/edu/pubs/consumer/health/hea04.shtm.

*LASIK, Epi–LASIK & LASEK*. Information Page. The Eye Digest, June 17, 2007 (April 05, 2009). http://www.agingeye.net/lasik/lasik.php#.

*Myopia*. Medical Encyclopedia. Medline, August 22, 2008 (April 05, 2009). http://www.nlm.nih.gov/MEDLINEPLUS/ency/article/001023.htm.

*Myopia (Nearsightedness)*. Information Page. AOA. (April 05, 2009). http://www.aoa.org/myopia.xml.

*Nearsightedness*. Information Page. Mayo Clinic, January 17, 2008 (April 05, 2009). http://www.mayoclinic.com/print/nearsightedness/DS00528/DSECTION = all&METHOD = print.

*Nearsightedness*. Fact Sheet. NEI. (April 05, 2009). http://www.nei.nih.gov/healthyeyestoolkit/factsheets/Nearsightedness.pdf.

*Questions and Answers about Refractive Errors*. Information Page. NEI, October 2008 (April 05, 2009). http://www.nei.nih.gov/CanWeSee/qa_refractive.asp.

*Refractive Errors*. Information Page. EyeCare America, May 2007 (April 05, 2009). http://www.nlm.nih.gov/MEDLINEPLUS/ency/article/001023.htm.

### ORGANIZATIONS

American Academy of Ophthalmology (AAO). PO Box 7424, San Francisco, CA 94120-7424. (415) 561-8500. Fax: (415) 561-8533. Email: patientinfo@aao.org. http://www.aao.org.

American Optometric Association (AOA). 243 N. Lindbergh Blvd., St. Louis, MO 63141. (800) 365-2219. http://www.aoa. org.

EyeCare America. P.O. Box 429098, San Francisco, CA 94142-9098. (877) 887-6327. Fax: (415) 561-8567. http://www.eyecareamerica.org/eyecare/.

National Eye Institute (NEI). 2020 Vision Place, Bethesda, MD 20892-3655. (301) 496-5248. http://www.nei.nih.gov.

Rebecca J. Frey, PhD
Risa Palley Flynn

Myotonia atrophica *see* **Myotonic dystrophy**

# Myotonic dystrophy

## Definition

Myotonic dystrophy is a progressive disease in which the muscles are weak and are slow to relax after contraction.

**Relationship between phenotype and CTG repeat length in myotonic dystrophy**

| Phenotype | Clinical signs | CTG repeat size | Age of onset (Years) | Average age of death (Years) |
|---|---|---|---|---|
| Premutation | None | 38 to ~49 | Normal | Normal |
| Mild | Cataracts<br>Mild myotonia | 50 to ~150 | 20–70 | 60—normal |
| Classical | Weakness<br>Myotonia<br>Cataracts<br>Balding<br>Cardiac arrhythmia<br>Others | ~100 to ~1000–1500 | 10–30 | 48–55 |
| Congenital | Infantile hypotonia<br>Respiratory deficits<br>Mental retardation | ~1000 to 2000 | Birth to 10 | 45 |

*(Table by GGS Creative Resources. Reproduced by permission of Gale, a part of Cengage Learning.)*

**Myotonic Dystrophy**

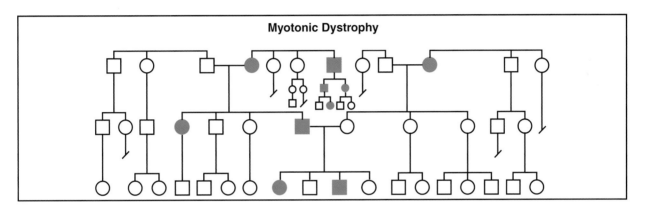

*(Gale, a part of Cengage Learning.)*

## Description

Myotonic dystrophy (DM), also called dystrophia myotonica, myotonia atrophica, or Steinert disease, is a common form of **muscular dystrophy**. DM is an inherited disease, affecting both males and females. About 30,000 people in the United States are affected. Symptoms may appear at any time from infancy to adulthood. DM causes general weakness, usually beginning in the muscles of the hands, feet, neck, or face. It slowly progresses to involve other muscle groups, including the heart. DM affects a wide variety of other organ systems as well.

A severe form of DM, congenital myotonic dystrophy, may appear in newborns of mothers who have DM. Congenital means that the condition is present from birth.

## Genetic profile

The most common type of DM is called DM1 and is caused by a mutation in a **gene** called myotonic

dystrophy protein kinase (DMPK). The DMPK gene is located on **chromosome** 19. When there is a mutation in this gene, a person develops DM1. The specific mutation that causes DM1 is called a trinucleotide repeat expansion.

Some families with symptoms of DM do not have a mutation in the DMPK gene. Scientists found that the DM in many of these families is caused by a mutation in a gene on chromosome 3. However, the specific gene and mutation have not yet been identified. These families are said to have DM2.

### Trinucleotide repeats

In the DMPK gene, there is a section of the genetic code where the three letters CTG are repeated a certain number of times. In people who have DM1, this word is repeated too many times—more than the normal number of 37 times—and thus this section of the gene is too big. This enlarged section of the gene is called a trinucleotide repeat expansion.

## KEY TERMS

**Electrocardiogram (ECG, EKG)**—A test that uses electrodes attached to the chest with an adhesive gel to transmit the electrical impulses of the heart muscle to a recording device.

**Electromyography (EMG)**—A test that uses electrodes to record the electrical activity of muscle. The information gathered is used to diagnose neuromuscular disorders.

**Muscular dystrophy**—A group of inherited diseases characterized by progressive wasting of the muscles.

**Sleep apnea**—Temporary cessation of breathing while sleeping.

**Trinucleotide repeat expansion**—A sequence of three nucleotides that is repeated too many times in a section of a gene.

People who have repeat numbers in the normal range will not develop DM1 and cannot pass it to their children. Having more than 50 repeats causes DM1. People who have 38–49 repeats have a premutation and will not develop DM1, but can pass DM1 onto their children. Having repeats numbers greater than 1,000 causes congenital myotonic dystrophy.

In general, the more repeats in the affected range that someone has, the earlier the age of onset of symptoms and the more severe the symptoms. However, this is a general rule. It is not possible to look at a person's repeat number and predict at what age they will begin to have symptoms or how their condition will progress.

Exactly how the trinucleotide repeat expansion causes myotonia, the inability to relax muscles, is not yet understood. The disease somehow blocks the flow of electrical impulses across the muscle cell membrane. Without proper flow of charged particles, the muscle cannot return to its relaxed state after it has contracted.

### Anticipation

Sometimes when a person who has repeat numbers in the affected or premutation range has children, the expansion grows larger. This is called anticipation. A larger expansion can result in an earlier age of onset in children than in their affected parent. Anticipation happens more often when a mother passes DM1 onto her children then when it is passed from the father. Occasionally repeat sizes stay the same or even get smaller when they are passed to a person's children.

### Inheritance

DM is inherited through autosomal dominant **inheritance**. This means that equal numbers of males and females are affected. It also means that only one gene in the pair needs to have the mutation in order for a person to be affected. Since a person only passes one copy of each gene onto their children, there is a 50% or one in two chance that a person who has DM will pass it onto each of their children. This percentage is not changed by results of other pregnancies. A person with a premutation also has a 50%, or one in two, chance of passing the altered gene on to each of their children. However, whether or not their children will develop DM1 depends on whether the trinucleotide repeat becomes further expanded. A person who has repeat numbers in the normal range cannot pass DM1 onto their children.

### Demographics

DM occurs in about one of 20,000 people and has been described in people from all over the world.

### Signs and symptoms

There is a range in the severity of symptoms in DM and not everyone will have all of the symptoms listed here.

Myotonic dystrophy causes weakness and delayed muscle relaxation called myotonia. Symptoms of DM include facial weakness and a slack jaw, drooping eyelids called ptosis, and muscle wasting in the forearms and calves. A person with DM has difficulty relaxing his or her grasp, especially in the cold. DM affects the heart muscle, causing irregularities in the heartbeat. It also affects the muscles of the digestive system, causing constipation and other digestive problems. DM may cause cataracts, retinal degeneration, low IQ, frontal balding, skin disorders, atrophy of the testicles, and **diabetes**. It can also cause sleep apnea—a condition in which normal breathing is interrupted during sleep. DM increases the need for sleep and decreases motivation. Severe disabilities do not set in until about 20 years after symptoms begin. Most people with myotonic dystrophy maintain the ability to walk, even late in life.

A severe form of DM, congenital myotonic dystrophy, may appear in newborns of mothers who have DM1. Congenital myotonic dystrophy is marked by severe weakness, poor sucking and swallowing responses, respiratory difficulty, delayed motor development, and mental retardation. Death in infancy is common in this type.

Some people who have a trinucleotide repeat expansion in their DMPK gene do not have symptoms or have very mild symptoms that go unnoticed. It is not unusual for a woman to be diagnosed with DM after she has an infant with congenital myotonic dystrophy.

### Predictive testing

It is possible to test someone who is at risk for developing DM1 before they are showing symptoms to see whether they inherited an expanded trinucleotide repeat. This is called predictive testing. Predictive testing cannot determine the age of onset that someone will begin to have symptoms, or the course of the disease.

### Diagnosis

Diagnosis of DM is not difficult once the disease is considered. However, the true problem may be masked because symptoms can begin at any age, can be mild or severe, and can occur with a wide variety of associated complaints. Diagnosis of DM begins with a careful medical history and a thorough physical exam to determine the distribution of symptoms and to rule out other causes. A family history of DM or unexplained weakness helps to establish the diagnosis.

A definitive diagnosis of DM1 is done by **genetic testing**, usually by taking a small amount of blood. The **DNA** in the blood cells is examined and the number of repeats in the DMPK gene is determined. Various other tests may be done to help establish the diagnosis, but only rarely would other testing be needed. An electromyogram (EMG) is a test used to examine the response of the muscles to stimulation. Characteristic changes are seen in DM that helps distinguish it from other muscle diseases. Removing a small piece of muscle tissue for microscopic examination is called a muscle biopsy. DM is marked by characteristic changes in the structure of muscle cells that can be seen on a muscle biopsy. An electrocardiogram could be performed to detect characteristic abnormalities in heart rhythm associated with DM. These symptoms often appear later in the course of the disease.

### Prenatal testing

Testing a pregnancy to determine whether an unborn child is affected is possible if genetic testing in a family has identified a DMPK mutation. This can be done at 10–12 weeks gestation by a procedure called chorionic villus sampling (CVS), which involves removing a tiny piece of the placenta and analyzing DNA from its cells. It can also be done by **amniocentesis** after 16 weeks gestation by removing a small amount of the amniotic fluid surrounding the baby and analyzing the cells in the fluid. Each of these procedures has a small risk of miscarriage associated with it and those who are interested in learning more should check with their doctor or genetic counselor.

Another procedure, called preimplantation diagnosis, allows a couple to have a child that is unaffected with the genetic condition in their family. This procedure is experimental and not widely available. Those interested in learning more about this procedure should check with their doctor or genetic counselor.

## Treatment and management

Myotonic dystrophy cannot be cured, and no treatment can delay its progression. However, many of the symptoms it causes can be treated. Physical therapy can help preserve or increase strength and flexibility in muscles. Ankle and wrist braces can be used to support weakened limbs. Occupational therapy is used to develop tools and techniques to compensate for loss of strength and dexterity. A speech-language pathologist can provide retraining for weakness in the muscles controlling speech and swallowing.

Irregularities in the heartbeat may be treated with medication or a pacemaker. A yearly electrocardiogram is usually recommended to monitor the heartbeat. Diabetes mellitus in DM is treated in the same way that it is in the general population. A high-fiber diet can help prevent constipation. Sleep apnea may be treated with surgical procedures to open the airways or with nighttime ventilation. Treatment of sleep apnea may reduce drowsiness. Lens replacement surgery is available when cataracts develop. Pregnant woman should be followed by an obstetrician familiar with the particular problems of DM because complications can occur during pregnancy, labor and delivery.

Wearing a medical bracelet is advisable. Some emergency medications may have dangerous effects on the heart rhythm in a person with DM. Adverse reactions to general anesthesia may also occur.

## Prognosis

The course of myotonic dystrophy varies. When symptoms appear earlier in life, disability tends to become more severe. Occasionally people with DM may require a wheelchair later in life. Children with congenital DM usually require special educational programs and physical and occupational therapy. For both types of DM, respiratory infections pose a danger when weakness becomes severe.

### Resources

**PERIODICALS**

The International Myotonic Dystrophy Consortium (IDMC). "New nomenclature and DNA testing guidelines for myotonic dystrophy type 1 (DM1)." *Neurology* 54 (2000): 1218–1221.

Meola, Giovanni. "Myotonic Dystrophies." *Current Opinion in Neurology* 13 (2000): 519–525.

**WEBSITES**

*Gene Clinics.* http://www.geneclinics.org.

Myotonic Dystrophy Web site. http://www.umd.necker.fr/myotonic_dystrophy.html.

NCBI Genes and Disease Web Page. http://www.ncbi.nlm.nih.gov/disease/Myotonic.html.

Smith, Corrine O'Sullivan. "Myotonic Dystrophy: Making an Informed Choice About Genetic Testing." *University of Washington.* http://www.depts.washington.edu/neurogen/Myotonic.pdf.

**ORGANIZATIONS**

Muscular Dystrophy Association. 3300 East Sunrise Dr., Tucson, AZ 85718. (520) 529-2000 or (800) 572-1717. http://www.mda.org.

Karen M. Krajewski, MS, CGC

# Myotubular myopathy

## Definition

Myotubular myopathy (MTM) belongs to a rare group of developmental disorders of voluntary muscle called congenital myopathies that present as a "floppy baby" syndrome. This is a genetically inherited disorder with various abnormalities in muscle fiber development, muscle tone, and contraction. MTM refers to the pathological finding of muscle fibers with centrally located nuclei resembling the myotubule stage of muscle development.

## Description

This condition is also called as centronuclear myopathy (CNM), X-linked MTM (MTM1), pericentronuclear myopathy, or type I fiber hypotrophy with central nuclei. It is primarily caused by defective maturation of the muscle. Spiro first described this disorder in 1966. The myotubularin **gene** was identified in 1996.

Muscle fibers normally undergo a complicated series of maturational changes before becoming a fully functional normal adult muscle fiber. The myotubule stage is an intermediate state in the fiber maturational process. It is seen normally only in an 8–20-weeks-old fetus and is characterized by central nuclei. In MTM, the maturation is arrested at this stage and the protein machinery of the muscle fiber needed for contraction is not fully formed. Muscles of patients with MTM thus show an overabundance of immature, poorly functional myotubular fibers.

MTM has different modes of **inheritance**, resulting in a wide variability of symptom onset (birth to early adulthood) and rate of symptom progression. Some researchers classify CNM and MTM as two extreme ends of a spectrum, with CNM being the milder form. Disability arises due to weakness of voluntary muscles and respiratory difficulty, progressing to death.

## Genetic profile

There are three types of MTM, based on the mode of inheritance.

### X-linked MTM (MTM1)

This is the most common form and is inherited usually in an X-linked recessive fashion, although *de novo* (new) mutations can occur rarely. It is due to a mutation in the myotubularin, or MTM1, gene that occurs on the long arm of the X **chromosome** at locus Xq28. Another related gene, called MTMR1, is also found on the X chromosome. About 150 types of myotubularin mutations have been identified, and, depending on the type, the severity of disease expression varies. Mutations that truncate the gene lead to severe or lethal disease expression. Mutations that delete part of the gene or cause misreading of the gene cause less severe disease. The gene encoding for the myotubularin protein is widely expressed, not just in the muscle. The relationship between the gene product and the disease is still being investigated.

**Allele**—One of the different or alternative forms that a gene can exist at a single locus (spot on a chromosome).

**Amniotic fluid**—The liquid that surrounds and cushions the developing fetus inside the mother's womb.

**Autosomal**—A chromosome not involved in sex determination; the human genome consists of a total of 46 chromosomes: 22 pairs of autosomes, and one pair of sex chromosomes (the X and Y chromosomes).

**Carrier**—An individual who possesses an unexpressed abnormal gene of a recessive genetic disorder.

**Contractures**—An abnormal and usually permanent shortening and contraction of a muscle or tendon that causes a deformity or subnormal range of movement.

**Creatine kinase (CK)**—An enzyme that is normally found in the skeletal or voluntary muscle and cardiac muscle; very high levels in the blood usually indicate breakdown of either heart or voluntary muscle.

**Cryptoorchidism**—Failure of descent of the testis from the abdominal cavity into the scrotum.

**De novo**—Latin term for new.

**Dolicocephaly**—Elongated and narrow skull shape due to premature closure of the sagittal suture that runs from the forehead to the back of the skull.

**Electromyography**—A test that assess the activity of the muscles and the nerves that supply the muscles; one part of the test involves passing electrical current through the nerves and studying the response of the muscles to it, while the other part involves studying muscle activity by inserting a thin needle into it.

**G-tube**—A gastrostomy tube, which is inserted surgically into the stomach and used for feeding and for administering medications.

**Hydrocephalus**—A condition caused by abnormal collection of fluid inside the ventricles of the brain, causing an enlarged head.

**Hypotonia**—Low or poor muscle tone, resulting in floppy limbs.

**Linkage analysis**—A gene-hunting technique that traces patterns of heredity in large, high-risk families in an attempt to locate a disease-causing gene mutation by identifying traits that are co-inherited with it.

**Lordosis**—An exaggeration of the normal lumbar curve such that the chest is prominent and the small of the back is hollowed.

**Myopathy**—Any disorder of the muscle, usually associated with weakness.

**Myotubule**—An intermediate stage in muscle fiber development, where the fiber is tubular with a centrally placed nucleus, instead of a peripheral eccentric nucleus.

**Polyhydramnios**—An abnormal condition characterized by excessive build up of amniotic fluid in the mother's womb.

**Ptosis**—Drooping of the upper eyelid.

**Pulmonologist**—A physician who specializes in lung diseases.

**Scoliosis**—An abnormal side-to-side curvature of the spine.

**Spherocytes**—Abnormal spherically shaped red blood cells caused by a disorder in the cell membrane; normally, the red blood cell is biconcave in shape.

**Stent**—A tubular device made of metal or plastic that is inserted into a body duct or tube to prevent collapse, blockage, or overgrowth.

**Skewed inactivation**—Random inactivation of either the paternally or maternally derived X chromosome in the female; also called Lyonization, and occurs early in embryonic development.

**Tendon reflex**—Reflex contraction of the muscle that is observed by tapping on its tendon.

**Tracheostomy**—A surgical opening in the trachea or wind-pipe to help breathing.

---

Each cell has one pair of sex chromosomes. The female has two copies of the X chromosome, one inherited from each parent, while the male has only one X chromosome inherited from the mother and the Y chromosome inherited from the father. A mother that carries one abnormal X chromosome containing

the myotubularin mutation has a 50% chance of passing it to each of her offspring. If the daughter inherits the mutation, she may not exhibit any symptoms as she has an extra normal copy; this makes her a carrier. However, a son who inherits the mutation will express the disease, as he cannot compensate for the mutated gene carried on his single X chromosome. If an affected male child has other affected male siblings, about 90% of the time the abnormal gene has been inherited from the mother in an X-linked fashion. If there are no other affected male siblings, then it is most likely a *de novo* mutation. Father-to-son transmission is not possible in MTM1.

### Carriers of X-linked MTM

Carriers are usually females who have an abnormal gene on one of their X chromosomes. They usually do not express the disease due to compensation from the normal copy. Skewed inactivation of the X chromosome containing the normal gene leads to milder disease expression.

### Autosomal dominant MTM

In this mode of inheritance, one copy of another myotubularin gene (MTMR2, MTMR3) is abnormal on an autosome, chromosome 12. Each cell has two chromosomes 12 carrying the myotubularin gene, and there are two alternate forms (alleles) in which the gene can exist. Therefore, four possible combinations of alleles can exist for this gene. If a person has one normal and one abnormal allele and expresses the normal allele, the individual will have the autosomal dominant form of MTM. Both males and females are equally affected, and the disease is passed on from generation to generation. There will usually be one affected person in each generation, and each child has a 50% chance of inheriting the abnormal gene. Father-to-son transmission is possible.

### Autosomal recessive MTM

This can occur in three ways. The affected person can have two abnormal alleles of the myotubularin gene or can have two different types of abnormal alleles. Finally, the affected person can have one normal and one abnormal allele and expresses the abnormal allele. Males and females are affected equally. Some ethnic predilections occur due to consanguinity where each parent of an affected child is a non-expressing carrier with both a normal and an abnormal allele. Therefore, each of their children has a 25% chance of being affected and a 50% chance of being a non-expressing carrier.

## Demographics

MTM is a rare condition; accurate estimates are unavailable. Approximate estimates for X-linked MTM range from one 50,000–500,000 newborn males. Unlike other congenital myopathies, there is a relatively high incidence in Africans.

## Signs and symptoms

There is a wide spectrum of clinical features seen in MTM depending on the mode of inheritance, but the basic problem arises from poor muscle tone interfering with posture, locomotion, and muscle strength. In general, the earlier the symptoms present, the more severe and progressive is the disorder.

### X-linked MTM

This is the most severe and most studied form, which presents at birth or even prior to birth, typically occurring in males. Mothers who are pregnant with affected boys experience polyhydramnios, which is an excessive amount of amniotic fluid due to decreased fetal swallowing of the fluid. Affected boys also exhibit decreased movements *in utero*. Fetal cardiac rhythm disturbances can also occur. Newborn males with MTM have a weak cry, are floppy at birth, have difficulty suckling and swallowing, exhibit severe generalized muscle weakness, and have serious respiratory difficulty. Life-threatening difficulties are caused by respiratory and swallowing problems. In very severe cases, the infants succumb to the disease quite early in the absence of adequate respiratory support, and death can occur within a few days of birth. Intermediate form of X-linked MTM occurs in adolescents who develop severe muscle weakness and become nonambulatory between early and middle life. Mild forms can present in early adulthood with facial weakness, eye muscle weakness, and mild gait difficulty.

Affected boys have a long slender body with long fingers and toes and appear frail. Length is disproportional to body weight as skeletal growth surpasses muscle growth. This is thought to be a result of endocrine dysfunction leading to rapid skeletal growth. The head can be dolicocephalic (elongated) or enlarged due to **hydrocephalus**. Other facial features, such as high arched palate, dental abnormalities, puffy or droopy eyelids (ptosis) due to eye muscle weakness, and squint, occur. Poor muscle tone leads to decreased blinking during the day and incomplete eye closure during sleep, causing eye irritation. Speech is soft and nasal. The affected children adopt a frog-leg posture due to hypotonia (decreased muscle tone). Skeletal deformities, such as pigeon-chest, **scoliosis**, and joint dislocations, also occur due to hypotonia. Tendon reflexes are absent. Over time, contractures occur in the hip, knee, and ankle joints, making walking difficult. Swallowing difficulty leads to drooling with aspiration of oral secretions into the lungs that can result in pneumonia. Intelligence and cognitive development is usually normal unless there has been a significant birth injury or respiratory distress with prolonged lack of oxygen.

Other associated medical problems include spherically shaped abnormal red blood cells (spherocytes), anemia, enlarged spleen, and gallstones. *Peliosis hepatis* is a disorder in which the liver has large blood-filled cysts that can rupture into the abdominal cavity and cause massive bleeding and death. Some have a vitamin K responsive bleeding disorder. Other genital and urinary problems like undescended testes (cryptoorchidism) and kidney stones also occur. Constipation can be a result of poor gut motility or overall physical immobility. Hearing and vision are unaffected.

### Autosomal dominant MTM

This is the least severe form and tends to affect males twice as often as females. It presents in late childhood or early adulthood and progresses slowly. It is less common than X-linked MTM. The major problem is proximal muscle weakness in the shoulders and hips with leg cramps. Ptosis, joint contractures, and a mild tremor can also be seen.

### Autosomal recessive MTM

This can begin at birth, in late infancy, or in early adulthood, but is much less severe than X-linked MTM. Females are slightly more affected than males. Common features include: weakness of eye muscles and face; thin face with a high, arched palate; hypotonia; mild generalized weakness, including neck, trunk, shoulder, and hip muscles; delayed motor milestones; and respiratory distress. Affected individuals develop a waddling gait due to hip muscle weakness and have lordosis and club-feet. Infants have a slowly progressive paralysis of eye muscles, loss of facial expression, and continuing limb weakness as they grow. Seizures or blackout spells can occur. Intelligence can be normal, or mental deficiency can occur. This condition progresses slowly and eventually leads to loss of ambulation. Many children are never able to run or participate in games with their peers.

### Carriers

These are usually women and they present with mild facial weakness, spinal deformities, such as scoliosis, flat feet, mild muscle weakness, and gait difficulty.

## Diagnosis

There is a considerable overlap in symptom severity among the three forms of MTM in affected males. Thus, in a family with a single affected male child, reliance on clinical features alone to diagnose the pattern of inheritance, to predict its prognosis, and to counsel the family regarding the chance of having another affected child becomes difficult. Detailed and thorough family history should be obtained to detect other family members with possible MTM. There is no absolute biochemical, **DNA**, or pathology test that can tell conclusively the pattern of inheritance in an isolated case. A history of spontaneous abortions or death of male infants in the neonatal period is a clue to X-linked transmission.

Creatine kinase (CK) is an enzyme that indicates muscle breakdown and can be normal or slightly increased. Electromyography (EMG), which involves needle testing of muscle activity, can point to a myopathy without being specific for MTM. Muscle biopsy is diagnostic, whereby a piece of muscle from the thigh or arm is taken and studied under the microscope to highlight the typical central plump nuclei in muscle fibers. The diagnosis depends on demonstrating a large number of muscle fibers with centrally placed nuclei. In X-linked MTM, all muscles are equally affected and about 50–80% of the muscle fibers are abnormal. Muscle biopsy can detect 50–70% of female carriers of X-linked MTM, but the biopsy can also be normal.

**Genetic testing** can be done in specialized laboratories to detect the common types of myotubularin **gene mutations**. If no mutation is found on the X chromosome, this means that either the mutation is transmitted autosomally or that it is a mutation that cannot be detected by currently available methods. The mother of a child with X-linked MTM can be tested genetically to see if she is a carrier, as this helps predict the chances of recurrence in a future pregnancy. Testing for X-linked MTM is available on a commercial basis, but testing for autosomal forms is only available through a research study.

Prenatal diagnosis is possible for detecting X-linked MTM by tracing the family history of the disease by a process of linkage analysis, which works only if there is more than one affected male member in the family. This can be done even if the exact type of genetic mutation is not known. Pre-implantation genetic diagnosis (PGD) is a technique whereby testing is done on the embryo and only unaffected embryos are placed back in the uterus for continuation of pregnancy.

## Treatment and management

There is no proven treatment to cure or stop progression of MTM, but aggressive supportive measures for swallowing and breathing are warranted to preserve good functional ability as these have been shown to prolong life expectancy. A team approach, including a neurologist, pulmonologist, orthopedic surgeon, physiatrist, physical therapist, occupational therapist, and geneticist, ensures the best possible therapy.

Tracheostomy tubes and ventilators help with breathing. In some cases, the muscles become stronger with time, and the tubes can be removed. Stents can be used to widen and support floppy airways. Lung infections can be treated with antibiotics. Chest physiotherapy helps to periodically clear lung secretions and decrease the incidence of pneumonia. Nutrients can be fed via oral feeding tubes and G-tubes. There are no special ingredients to be incorporated in the diet, as no supplement has been consistently proven to improve muscle strength and build muscle bulk. Caloric intake should be tailored to the requirements of each individual child.

Physical therapy plays a very important part in maintaining and improving muscle strength, joint flexibility, range of motion, and gait. Care should be taken not to overexert and fatigue the already weak muscles and a regular exercise program should be devised. Passive stretching, bracing, and surgical-release procedures are done to prevent tendon and joint contractures. Bracing or surgery may be needed to correct spinal deformities. The occupational therapist can help in devising adaptive equipment for walking and for other daily activities.

Speech therapy is important to overcome problems with speaking due to poor phonation and articulation. Passy-Muir speaking valves can be used in patients who have a tracheostomy tube. Orthodontic services are needed to correct dental malocclusion. Some children can learn to communicate using sign language, communication assist devices, or high-tech computerized devices. Intelligence is not affected, and therefore these children may even be able to attend regular schools. Artificial tears should be used to prevent dry eyes. Yearly blood tests and liver function tests should be done to monitor development anemia and liver malfunction. Folic acid is used when the child has anemia and spherical red blood cells. Appropriate precautions should be taken to avoid bleeding during any major surgery.

**Genetic counseling** should be sought after a child has been diagnosed with MTM to discuss the prognosis for the child, to help the couple with future reproductive planning, and to help with prenatal diagnosis. The probability of having another affected child varies with the specific mode of inheritance.

### Prognosis

Only males are severely affected by X-linked MTM and prognosis has been historically poor due to early respiratory failure. The children lack enough strength and endurance in the respiratory muscles to withstand respiratory complications, such as infections and lung collapse. Death used to occur within one to two years of life, with a mean of five months.

Respiratory weakness and frequent pneumonias indicate poor prognosis. Today, with interventions like ventilators and tracheostomy tubes, these complications are delayed and survival is prolonged. Currently, more than two-thirds of children with MTM survive past the first year of life. In X-linked MTM, contrary to prior thinking, the muscle weakness does not appear to be progressive. Children with autosomal recessive MTM usually survive past infancy. Those with autosomal dominant MTM even survive into late adulthood, and the disease is compatible with a normal life expectancy.

### Resources

#### BOOKS

Bradley, Walter G., Robert B. Daroff, Gerald M. Fenichel, and Joseph Jankovic. *Neurology in Clinical Practice*, 4th edition. Philadelphia: Butterworth Heinemann, 2004.

Fenichel, Gerald M. *Clinical Pediatric Neurology*, 4th edition. Philadelphia: W.B. Saunders Company, 2001.

#### PERIODICALS

Das, Soma, and Gale Ellen Herman. "X-linked Myotubular Myopathy." *GeneReviews* (May 2004).

Fan, Hueng-Chuen C,, Chuen-Ming Lee, Horng-Jyh Harn, Shin-Nan Cheng, and Yeong-Seng Yuh. "X-linked Centronuclear Myopathy." *American Journal of Perinatology* 20 (April 2003): 173–179.

Riggs, Jack E., John B. Bodensteiner, and Sydney S. Schochet. "Congenital Myopathies/Dystrophies." *Neurologic Clinics of North America* 21 (2003): 779–794.

#### OTHER

Myotubular Myopathy Resource Group. 2602 Quaker Drive, Texas City, TX 77590. (409) 945 8569. http://www.mtmrg.org.

The University of Chicago. The Division of Biological Sciences. 5841 S. Maryland Avenue, Chicago, IL 60637. (777) 834 0555. http://www.genes.uchicago.edu.

#### ORGANIZATIONS

Gene Clinics. 9725 Third Avenue, NE, Suite 602, Seattle, WA 98115. (206) 221 2943. http://www.geneclinics.org.

Muscular Dystrophy Association. 3300 East Sunrise Drive, Tucson, AZ 85718-3208. (800) 572 1717. http://www.mda.org.

National Institute of Health/National Institute of Neurological Disorders and Stroke Brain Resources and Information Network. PO Box 5801, Bethesda, MD 20824. (301) 496 5751. (800) 352.9484. http://www.ninds.nih.gov.

National Organization for Rare Disorders, Inc. 55 Kenosia Ave, PO Box 1968, Danbury, CT 06813-1968. (800) 999 6673. http://www.rarediseases.org.

Chitra Venkatasubramanian, MBBS, MD

# N

# Nail-patella syndrome

## Definition

Nail-patella syndrome, is a genetic disease of the connective tissue that produces defects in the fingernails, knee caps, and kidneys.

## Description

Nail-patella syndrome is also known as Fong Disease, Hereditary Onycho-Osteodysplasia (H.O.O.D.), Iliac Horn Disease, and Turner-Kieser syndrome. Patients who have nail-patella syndrome may show a variety of physical abnormalities. The hallmark features of this syndrome are poorly developed fingernails, toenails, and patellae (kneecaps). Other common abnormalities include elbow deformities, abnormally shaped pelvis bone (hip bone), and kidney (renal) disease.

Less common medical findings include changes in the upper lip, the roof of the mouth, and unusual skeletal abnormalities. Skeletal abnormalities may include poorly developed scapulae (shoulder blades), sideways bent fingers (clinodactyly), **clubfoot**, **scoliosis**, and unusual neck bones. There are also other effects, such as thickening of the basement membrane in the skin and of the tiny clusters of capillaries (glomeruli) in the kidney. Scientists have recognized an association between nail-patella syndrome and colon **cancer**. Nail-patella syndrome is associated with open-angle **glaucoma**, which, if untreated, may lead to blindness. Patients may also have cataracts, drooping eyelids (ptosis), or corneal problems such as glaucoma.

People with nail-patella syndrome may display only a few or many of the recognized signs of this disease. Symptoms vary widely from person to person. Signs even vary within a single family with multiple affected members.

## Genetic profile

Nail-patella syndrome has been recognized as an inherited disorder for over 100 years. It is caused by mutations in a **gene** known as LIM Homeobox Transcription Factor 1-Beta (LMX1B), located on the long arm of **chromosome** 9.

The LMX1B gene codes for a protein that is important in organizing embryonic limb development. Mutations in this gene have been detected in many unrelated people with nail-patella syndrome. Scientists have also been able to interrupt this gene in mice to produce defects similar to those seen in human nail-patella syndrome.

Nail-patella syndrome is inherited in an autosomal dominant manner. This means that possession of only one copy of the defective gene is enough to cause disease. When a parent has nail-patella syndrome, each of their children has a 50% chance to inherit the disease-causing mutation.

A new mutation causing nail-patella syndrome can occur in a person with no family history. This is called a sporadic occurrence and accounts for approximately 20% of cases of nail-patella syndrome. The children of a person with sporadic nail-patella syndrome are at a 50% risk of developing signs of the disorder.

## Demographics

The incidence of nail-patella syndrome is approximately one in 50,000 births. This disorder affects males and females equally. It is found throughout the world and occurs in all ethnic groups. The strongest risk factor for nail-patella syndrome is a family history of the disease.

## Signs and symptoms

Medical signs of nail-patella syndrome vary widely between patients. Some patients with this

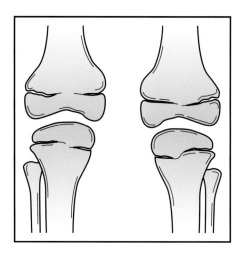

Diagram of two legs affected by nail-patella syndrome. Note the absence of the patella in this image of knees. *(Reproduced by permission of Cengage Learning Gale.)*

disorder do not display symptoms. These patients are discovered to have the nail-patella syndrome only when genetic studies trace their family history. Scientists are now working to learn what causes different people to display such different symptoms of nail-patella syndrome.

The most obvious signs associated with nail-patella syndrome is absent, poorly developed, or unusual fingernails. Fingernail abnormalities are found in over 80% of patients with this disorder. Abnormalities may be found in one or more fingernails. Only rarely are all fingernails affected. This disease most commonly affects the fingernails of the thumbs and index fingers. The pinky fingernail is least likely to be affected. Fingernails may be small and concave with pitting, ridges, splits, and/or discoloration. Toenails are less often affected. The lunulae, or light-colored crescent moons, at the base of the fingernail bed next to the cuticle are sometimes triangularly-shaped in people with nail-patella syndrome.

Kneecap abnormalities are the second most common sign associated with this disorder. Either or both kneecaps may be missing or poorly formed. If present, kneecaps are likely to be dislocated. The knees of people with nail-patella syndrome may have a square appearance. Besides the kneecap, other support structures including bones, ligaments, and tendons may be malformed. These support structures stabilize the knee, therefore patients with some leg malformations may have difficulty in walking.

The hip bones of approximately 80% of patients with nail-patella syndrome have unusual bony projections called posterior iliac horns. These bony projections, or spurs, are internal and not obvious unless they are detected on x ray. This unusual pelvic anatomy is not associated with any other disease.

Kidney disease is present in at least 30% of people with nail-patella syndrome. Biopsy shows lesions that resemble those of inflammation of the clusters of capillaries in the kidneys (glomerulonephritis), but without any infection present. Kidney failure is the most dangerous consequence of nail-patella syndrome. It occurs in about 30% of patients who have kidney involvement. An early sign of kidney involvement is the presence of protein or blood in the urine (chronic, benign proteinuria and hematuria). Kidney involvement is progressive, so early diagnosis and treatment of renal disease is important. Kidney disease has been reported in children with nail-patella syndrome, but renal involvement more commonly develops during adulthood.

Various skeletal symptoms may occur. Patients with nail-patella syndrome may not be able to fully straighten their arms at the elbow. This may create a webbed appearance at the elbow joint. Patients may have sideways bent fingers, poorly developed shoulder blades, clubfoot, hip dislocation, unusual neck bones, or scoliosis.

Eye problems may be present and vary from person to person. Nail-patella syndrome is associated with open angle glaucoma. Open angle glaucoma is caused by fluid blocked into the front chamber of the eye. This blocked fluid builds increasing pressure into the eye. If untreated, this increased pressure may lead to permanent damage of the optic nerve and irreversible blindness. Some patients with nail-patella syndrome have ptosis, or drooping eyelids. Nail-patella syndrome has also been associated with abnormalities of the cornea, cataracts, and astigmatism. Additionally, the irises of the eye may be multicolored, possibly displaying a clover-shaped pattern of color.

### Diagnosis

**Genetic testing** for nail-patella syndrome is available only through research institutions that are working to further characterize this disorder. Genetic testing cannot predict which signs of the disease will develop, nor can genetic testing predict the severity of disease symptoms. Improved genetic testing for nail-patella syndrome is anticipated in the future.

Diagnosis of this disease is most often made on visual medical clues such as the characteristic abnormalities of the fingernails and kneecaps. Diagnosis is confirmed by x ray images of the affected bones and, when indicated, kidney biopsy. The bony pelvic spurs found in 80% of patients with nail-patella syndrome are not associated with any other disease.

Prenatal diagnosis for nail-patella syndrome by third-trimester ultrasound was documented in 1998. Prenatal diagnosis via genetic testing of cells obtained by chorionic villus sampling was reported the same year. Prenatal genetic testing for nail-patella syndrome is not yet widely available. There is controversy surrounding the use of prenatal testing for such a variable disorder. Prenatal testing cannot predict the extent of an individual's disease.

### Treatment and management

Treatment is usually not necessary. Treatment, when required, depends on each patient's specific symptoms. Severe kidney disease is treated with dialysis or a kidney transplant. Patients receiving kidney transplant do not develop nail-patella type renal complications in their new kidney.

A wheelchair may be required if walking becomes painful due to bone, tendon, ligament, or muscle defects. Orthopedic surgery may be necessary for congenital clubfoot deformity. Manipulation or surgery may be required to correct hip dislocation. Cataracts are also surgically treated. Medical treatment at early signs of glaucoma prevents progression of the disease to blindness.

---

## QUESTIONS TO ASK YOUR DOCTOR

- How did nail-patella syndrome get its name?
- On what basis does a physician diagnosis a person with nail-patella syndrome?
- Is nail-patella a life-threatening condition and, if not, what are its most serious medical consequences?
- Should my child be monitored on an ongoing basis for his nail-patella syndrome and, if so, what tests are recommended?

---

**Genetic counseling** is offered to persons who have the disease. Parents with this disease have a 50% chance of passing it to each of their children. Current genetic testing technology cannot predict the severity or scope of an individual's symptoms.

Because many possible manifestations of nail-patella syndrome exist, patients are advised to pursue extra medical care including regular urinalysis and special eye exams. Children with nail-patella syndrome should be screened for scoliosis.

### Prognosis

Survival among patients with nail-patella syndrome is not decreased unless a they exhibit renal complications. It is estimated that 8% of individuals with nail-patella syndrome who come to medical attention eventually die of kidney disease.

### Resources

#### BOOKS

Berkow, R., M. H. Beers, A. J. Fletcher, and R. M. Bogin. *The Merck Manual of Medical Information - Home Edition.* McGraw-Hill, 2000.

#### WEBSITES

*Gene Clinics.* http://www.geneclinics.org.
*OMIM—Online Mendelian Inheritance in Man.* http://www.ncbi.nlm.nih.gov/omim.

John Thomas Lohr
Judy C. Hawkins, MS

Naito-Oyanagi disease *see* **Dentatorubral-pallidoluysian atrophy**

# Nance-Insley syndrome

## Definition

Nance-Insley syndrome is a craniofacial anomaly that is caused by a **gene** mutation interfering with prenatal bone development. The observable results are a short physique, flattened face, and overgrowth at joints. Another name for this condition is otospondylomegaepiphyseal **dysplasia**, derived from the Greek words *oto* (referring to the eyes), *spondylos* (referring to the spine), and *epiphysial* (referring to the formative areas of the bones). The Greek word *dysplasia* refers to abnormal tissue formation. Nance-Insley is related to **Stickler syndrome** but is distinct from it. Nance-Insley is more severe in shared symptoms and involves hearing disabilities instead of the visual disability of Stickler.

## Demographics

This condition is very rare. There is an extremely limited number of reports in the literature. No prevalence data were available as of 2009. The gene responsible for this disorder has been determined to be autosomal, which means that males and females are equally affected. The trait is dominant in some cases and recessive in others. Some cases have been shown to be due to a sporadic mutation.

## Description

This disorder is caused by a mutation on the gene COL11A2 responsible for producing collagen XI, an organic gel that influences the development of bones and cartilage in the skeletal system. People with Nance-Insley are affected mostly in their bone development and structure. The distinct facial features are due to weak bone structures under the face. There is no effect on the intellectual function.

The distinct facial features of an affected person include an abnormally small lower jaw and an underdeveloped mid-face. The underdeveloped mid-face is noted by a small nose and flat nasal bridge. In addition to the facial features, the most notable feature of Nance-Insley is the relatively short stature of those affected. Other observable features include an abnormal skeletal framework and wide-set eyes. Almost all affected individuals have a **cleft palate**.

Some of the expected characteristics include the following:

- Shortened limbs
- Short hands and feet
- Enlarged joints
- Flattened vertebrae
- Early onset of arthritis
- Hearing loss
- Joint pain
- Upturned nose

Some of the common problems throughout the life span include pain in the joints and continually diminishing hearing. Many people with Nance-Insley syndrome suffer from the early onset of **osteoarthritis**.

## Causes and symptoms

Nance-Insley syndrome is caused by a mutation on the gene COL11A2 on **chromosome** 6. This gene is responsible for production of the type XI collagen. This collagen produces an organic gel that contributes to the systematic conversion of cartilage into bone and the orderly growth of bone in the developing fetus. Without type XI collagen, there is an overgrowth at the end of long bones contributing to stiff, inflexible joints. Another effect of the lack of type XI collagen is a decrease in bone growth.

A child born with Nance-Insley syndrome will have abnormal bone growth, which is manifested in the characteristic facial features such as a small nose, flat nasal bridge, and underdeveloped mid-face. Other bone problems include the overgrowth at joints and short limbs. Other symptoms occurring in this syndrome include wide-set eyes, hearing loss, and a cleft palate.

The mutation responsible for Nance-Insley syndrome can be inherited in three manners: as an autosomal dominant trait; as an autosomal passive trait; and as a spontaneous mutation. In some cases, the trait is dominant, but in another it is recessive, which is strange but not extraordinarily unusual. If a child is born with Nance-Insley syndrome there is a chance that later siblings may have it also and that current siblings are carriers. The age of either parent has been determined to be inconsequential in the development of this disorder.

## Diagnosis

Signs of this disorder are observable from birth. However, many of these signs are also symptoms of Stickler syndrome. Identifying this condition as Nance-Insley with its accompanying complications is only possible through a genetic test of a blood sample.

The main test for recognizing chromosomal disorders is the fluorescence in-situ hybridization (FISH). This method of analyzing the structures of

## KEY TERMS

**Cartilage**—The stiff yet flexible connective tissue found in many areas in the bodies, which grows and repairs more slowly than other connective tissue.

**Fluorescence in-situ hybridization (FISH)**—A method of analyzing the structures of human genetics that uses fluorescent probes designed to link to specific genetic particles such as proteins, genes, or chromosomal material.

**Osteoarthritis**—A group of diseases and mechanical abnormalities involving degradation of joints.

**Type XI collagen**—A type of collagen that produces an organic gel that helps cartilage to convert into bone and helps bone growth in the developing fetus.

## QUESTIONS TO ASK YOUR DOCTOR

- What corrective surgery should I expect?
- How do other people with Nance-Insley cope with daily living skills?
- Is genetic counseling important for my situation?
- What are the chances that a child of mine will be born with Nance-Insley?
- How often should I be physically evaluated?
- Will my condition get worse?

human **genetics** relies on fluorescent probes designed to link to specific genetic particles such as proteins, genes, or chromosomal material. If the correlating probe cannot link to the material for which it is designed, then the result is accepted as an absence of the material. In testing for Nance-Insley syndrome, the probes specific to the COL11A2 on the chromosome 6 would be injected into genetic material from the affected person. If examination of the probes does not detect a continuous pattern, then the person definitely has a mutation on this gene.

The condition can also be detected prenatally through **amniocentesis**. If a parent suspects that he or she is a carrier for Nance-Insley syndrome, an amniocentesis is able to detect the presence of the mutations. However, a test for Nance-Insley syndrome is complicated, so it is not usually done in amniocentesis analysis. The distinct characteristics, observable at birth, are not usually observable through the **prenatal ultrasound**. The problem with an ultrasound picture of the developing fetus is that as of 2009 ultrasound was not powerful enough to detect the subtle features that would suggest the child has Nance-Insley syndrome.

### Treatment

There is no cure for the underlying condition of the mutation. The damage that is done prenatally remains for a lifetime. The various treatments for Nance-Insley syndrome are concerned with alleviating associated disabilities and delaying any perceived deterioration.

### Traditional treatment

The usual treatment for children involves continuous evaluations of all related conditions. Orthopedic surgery may be necessary at times. Physical therapy and adaptive devices may help alleviate some of the problems. The cleft palate needs to be repaired in childhood, as well as any condition of the ears. If there is no chance for correcting the problems with the ears, therapy designed to help the patient adapt to a loss of hearing is required.

Some problems are less severe with age. However, joint pain and loss of hearing require assessment and treatment throughout the lifespan. Joint replacement may be required at a relatively young age.

### Alternative treatment

The popularity of human growth hormone therapy may lead someone with Nance-Insley to consider it as an acceptable therapy for this condition. However, the short stature of the Nance-Insley patient is due to bone malformations. Such disorders do not respond well to growth hormone therapy.

### Prognosis

There is no cure for Nance-Insley syndrome. Some of the initial bone structure problems may be alleviated with age. However, the early onset of osteoarthritis is fairly certain, as is lifetime hearing problems. Those affected with this syndrome have intellectual skills in normal range and can learn adaptive skills well. Also, there is nothing inherent in this disorder to suggest less than average life expectancy.

### Prevention

As noted above, the presence of the mutation can be detected through a prenatal test such as amniocentesis.

Detecting the mutation is not usually a goal of typical amniocentesis because the condition is so rare. Prenatal counseling is recommended for a couple when one or both are carriers of the mutated gene. Information on this disorder and others that can arise through spontaneous mutations is recommended for parents during pregnancy.

### Resources

#### BOOKS

Bissonnette, Bruno, Igor Luginbuehl, Bruno Marciniak, and Bernard Dalens. *Syndromes: Rapid Recognition and Perioperative Implications..* New York: McGraw-Hill Professional, 2006.

Shapiro, Frederic. *Pediatric Orthopedic Deformities.* San Diego: Academic Press, 2001.

#### PERIODICALS

Spranger, J. "The type XI Collagenopathies." *Pediatric Radiology.* 1998. 10: 745-750.

#### OTHER

Otospondylomegaepiphyseal Dysplasia. U.S. National Library of Medicine. http://ghr.nlm.nih.gov/ condition = otospondylomegaepiphysealdysplasia.

#### ORGANIZATIONS

Human Growth Foundation, 997 Glen Cove Avenue, Suite 5, Glen Head, NY, 11545, 800-451-6434, http:// www.hgfound.org.

Little People of America, 250 El Camino Real, Suite 201, Tustin, CA, 92780, 714-368-3689, 888-LPA-2001, 714-368-3367, info@lpaonline.org, http:// www.lpaonline.org.

Ray F. Brogan, PHD

## Nanocephalic dwarfism *see* Seckel syndrome

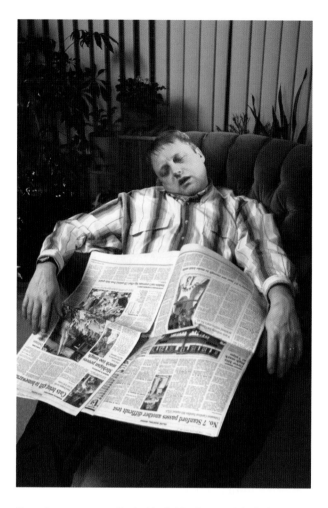

Narcolepsy causes affected individuals to suddenly fall into a deep sleep, even in the middle of an activity. *(Custom Medical Stock Photo, Inc.)*

# Narcolepsy

## Definition

Narcolepsy is a disorder marked by excessive daytime sleepiness, uncontrollable sleep attacks, and cataplexy (a sudden loss of muscle tone, usually lasting up to half an hour).

## Description

Narcolepsy is the second–leading cause of excessive daytime sleepiness (after obstructive sleep apnea). Persistent sleepiness and sleep attacks are the hallmarks of this condition. The sleepiness has been compared to the feeling of trying to stay awake after not sleeping for two or three days.

People with narcolepsy fall asleep suddenly— anywhere, at any time, maybe even in the middle of a conversation. These sleep attacks can last from a few seconds to more than an hour. Depending on where they occur, they may be mildly inconvenient or even dangerous to the individual. Some people continue to function outwardly during the sleep episodes, such as talking or putting things away. But when they wake up, they have no memory of the event.

Narcolepsy is related to the deep, dreaming part of sleep known as rapid eye movement (REM) sleep. Normally when people fall asleep, they experience 90 minutes of non–REM sleep, which is then followed by REM sleep. People with narcolepsy, however, enter REM sleep immediately. In addition, REM sleep occurs inappropriately throughout the day.

## KEY TERMS

**Cataplexy**—A symptom of narcolepsy in which there is a sudden episode of muscle weakness triggered by emotions. The muscle weakness may cause the person's knees to buckle, or the head to drop. In severe cases, the patient may become paralyzed for a few seconds to minutes.

**Hypnagogic hallucinations**—Dream–like auditory or visual hallucinations that occur while falling asleep.

**Hypothalamus**—A part of the forebrain that controls heartbeat, body temperature, thirst, hunger, body temperature and pressure, blood sugar levels, and other functions.

**Sleep paralysis**—An abnormal episode of sleep in which the patient cannot move for a few minutes, usually occurring on falling asleep or waking up. Often found in patients with narcolepsy.

### Genetic profile

In 2005, narcolepsy was reported to have one of the tightest associations with a specific HLA allele. The HLA **gene** family provides instructions for making a group of related proteins known as the human leukocyte antigen (HLA) complex. The HLA complex helps the immune system distinguish the body's own proteins from proteins made by foreign invaders such as viruses and bacteria. From Eighty-eight to ninety-eight percent of patients affected by narcolepsy have been shown to be HLA DQB1*0602 positive. This allele strongly increases the susceptibility for cataplexy although 41% of patients without cataplexy are carriers. DRB1 and DQB1 genes have been sequenced in narcolepsy patients but no mutation has been identified. This suggests that these genes strongly confer susceptibility to narcolepsy without their function being defective. It is accordingly believed that non–HLA genes may also be involved in susceptibility to narcolepsy. In 2004, a study reported significant evidence linking narcolepsy with a locus in a 5 Mb region of **chromosome** 21q.

The disorder sometimes runs in families, but most people with narcolepsy have no relatives with the disorder. Some researchers therefore believe that the **inheritance** of narcolepsy is similar to that of heart disease. In heart disease, several genes play a role in being susceptible to the disorder, but it usually does not develop without an environmental trigger of some sort.

### Demographics

According to the National Institute for Neurological Disorders and Stroke (NINDS), narcolepsy is an underrecognized and underdiagnosed condition in the United States. The exact prevalence is not known, but it is estimated to affect about one in every 2,000 Americans. The disorder occurs worldwide in every racial and ethnic group, affecting males and females equally. However, prevalence varies among populations. For example, narcolepsy is less prevalent in Israel (about one per 500,000) but considerably more prevalent in Japan (about one per 600).

### Signs and symptoms

While the symptoms of narcolepsy usually appear during the teens or 20s, the disease may not be diagnosed for many years. Most often, the first symptom is an overwhelming feeling of fatigue. After several months or years, cataplexy and other symptoms appear.

Cataplexy is the most dramatic symptom of narcolepsy. It affects 75% of people with the disorder. During attacks, the knees buckle and the neck muscles go slack. In extreme cases, the person may become paralyzed and fall to the floor. This loss of muscle tone is temporary, lasting from a few seconds to half an hour, but frightening. The attacks can occur at any time but are often triggered by strong emotions, such as anger, joy, or surprise.

Other symptoms of narcolepsy include:

- Sleep attacks: short, uncontrollable sleep episodes throughout the day
- Sleep paralysis: a frightening inability to move shortly after awakening or dozing off
- Auditory or visual hallucinations: intense, sometimes terrifying experiences at the beginning or end of a sleep period
- Disturbed nighttime sleep: tossing and turning, nightmares, and frequent awakenings during the night

### Diagnosis

If a person experiences both excessive daytime sleepiness and cataplexy, a diagnosis may be made on the patient history alone. Laboratory tests, however, can confirm a diagnosis. These may include an overnight polysomnogram—a test in which sleep is monitored with electrocardiography, video, and respiratory parameters. A Multiple Sleep Latency Test, which measures sleep latency (onset) and how quickly

REM sleep occurs, may be used. People who have narcolepsy usually fall asleep in less than five minutes.

If a diagnosis is in question, a genetic blood test can reveal the existence of certain substances in people who have a tendency to develop narcolepsy. Positive test results suggest, but do not prove, the existence of narcolepsy.

Narcolepsy is a complex disorder, and it is often misdiagnosed. It takes 14 years, on average, for an individual to be correctly diagnosed.

### Treatment and management

There is no cure for narcolepsy. It is not progressive, and it is not fatal, but it is chronic. The symptoms can be managed with medication or lifestyle adjustment. Amphetamine–like stimulant drugs are often prescribed to control drowsiness and sleep attacks. Patients who do not like taking high doses of stimulants may choose to take smaller doses and"manage" their lifestyles, such as by napping every couple of hours, to relieve daytime sleepiness. Antidepressants are often effective in treating symptoms of abnormal REM sleep.

With the recent discovery of the gene that causes narcolepsy, researchers are hopeful that therapies can be designed to relieve the symptoms of the disorder.

### Prognosis

Narcolepsy is not a degenerative disease, and patients do not develop other neurologic symptoms. However, narcolepsy can interfere with a person's ability to work, play, drive, and perform other daily activities. In severe cases, the disorder prevents people from living a normal life, leading to **depression** and a loss of independence.

### Resources

#### BOOKS

Icon Health Publications. *Narcolepsy —A Medical Dictionary, Bibliography, and Annotated Research Guide to Internet References*. San Diego, CA: Icon Health Publications, 2004.

Parker, James N., and Philip M. Parker. *The Official Patient's Sourcebook on Narcolepsy*. San Diego, CA: Icon Health Publications, 2002.

#### PERIODICALS

Billiard, M. "Narcolepsy: current treatment options and future approaches." *Neuropsychiatric Disease and Treatment* 4, no. 3 (June 2008): 557–566.

Dorris, L., et al. "Psychosocial and intellectual functioning in childhood narcolepsy." *Developmental Neurorehabilitation* 11, no. 3 (July–September 2008): 187–194.

Fronczek, R, et al. "Manipulation of skin temperature improves nocturnal sleep in narcolepsy." *Journal of Neurology, Neurosurgery, and Psychiatry* 79, no. 12 (December 2008): 1354–1357.

Nevsimalova, S. "Narcolepsy in childhood." *Sleep Medicine Reviews* 13, no. 2 (April 2009): 169–180.

Todman, D. "Narcolepsy." *European Neurology* 61, no. 4 (2009): 255.

#### WEBSITES

*Narcolepsy Fact Sheet*. Fact Sheet. NINDS, March 4, 2009 (April 25, 2009). http://www.ninds.nih.gov/disorders/narcolepsy/detail_narcolepsy.htm.

*Narcolepsy Information Page*. Information Page. NINDS, March 4, 2009 (April 25, 2009). http://www.ninds.nih.gov/disorders/narcolepsy/narcolepsy.htm.

*Narcolepsy and Sleep*. Information Page. NSF (April 25, 2009). http://www.sleepfoundation.org/site/c.huIXKjM0IxF/b.4814429/k.78A8/Sleep_and_Narcolepsy.htm.

*Sleep Disorders*. Health Topics. Medline, April 20, 2009 (April 25, 2009). http://www.nlm.nih.gov/medlineplus/sleepdisorders.html.

#### ORGANIZATIONS

Narcolepsy Network, Inc. 79A Main St., North Kingstown, RI 02852. (888)292-6522 or (401)667-2523. Fax: (401)633-6567. Email: narnet@narcolepsynetwork.org. http://www.narcolepsynetwork.org.

National Heart, Lung, and Blood Institute (NHLBI). PO Box 30105, Bethesda, MD 20824-0105. (301)592-8573. Email: nhlbiinfo@rover.nhlbi.nih.gov. http://www.nhlbi.nih.gov.

National Institute for Neurological Disorders and Stroke (NINDS). P.O. Box 5801, Bethesda, MD 20824. (800) 352-9424 or (301)496-5751. http://www.ninds.nih.gov.

National Sleep Foundation. 1522 K St. NW, Suite 500, Washington, DC 20005. (202)347-3472. Fax: (202) 347-3472. Email : nsf@sleepfoundation.org. http://www.sleepfoundation.org.

Michelle Lee Brandt

# Nephrogenic diabetes insipidus

### Definition

Nephrogenic **diabetes** insipidus (NDI) is a kidney disorder characterized by the organ's inability to respond to the antidiuretic hormone (ADH), also called arginine vasopressin (AVP), produced in the hypothalamus, a structure of the brain. NDI involves an abnormality in the kidney tubules that prevents the proper amount of water from being reabsorbed from

**Acidosis**—A condition of decreased alkalinity resulting from abnormally high acid levels (low pH) in the blood and tissues. Usually indicated by sickly sweet breath, headaches, nausea, vomiting, and visual impairments.

**Alzheimer disease**—A degenerative disease of the central nervous system characterized by premature senility and other mental deterioration.

**Amyloidosis**—Accumulation of amyloid deposits in various organs and tissues in the body such that normal functioning of an organ is compromised.

**Dehydration**—An extreme loss of water in the body, which, if untreated, can lead to brain damage and death.

**Electrolyte**—A solution or a substance in a solution consisting of various chemicals that can carry electric charges. They exist in the blood as acids, bases, and salts, such as sodium, calcium, potassium, chlorine, and magnesium.

**Fanconi syndrome**—A reabsorbtion disorder in the kidney tubules.

**Kidney tubules**—A portion of the kidneys that causes water to be excreted as urine or reabsorbed into the body.

**Nephrons**—Microscopic-size tubes that filter the water that flows into the kidneys.

**Osmolarity**—The concentration of an osmotic solution, especially when measured in osmols or milliosmols per liter of solution.

**Osmotically**—Referring to the movement of a solvent through a semipermeable membrane (as of a living cell) into a solution of higher solute concentration that tends to equalize the concentrations of solute on the two sides of the membrane.

**Sarcoidosis**—A chronic disease characterized by nodules forming in the lymph nodes, lungs, bones, and skin.

**Sickle cell anemia**—A chronic, inherited blood disorder characterized by sickle-shaped red blood cells. It occurs primarily in people of African descent, and produces symptoms including episodic pain in the joints, fever, leg ulcers, and jaundice.

**Sjögren syndrome**—A chronic inflammatory disease often associated with rheumatoid arthritis.

the kidneys back into the body. Instead, the water is excreted in large amounts as diluted urine.

### Description

There are two categories of nephrogenic diabetes insipidus: inherited and acquired. Within the inherited group, there are three types of NDI: X-linked, autosomal recessive, and autosomal dominant. Unlike the more common diabetic disorder diabetes mellitus, NDI is not related to insulin production or levels of sugar in the blood and urine.

Ninety percent of inherited NDI is X-linked, meaning it is caused by an alteration in a **gene** carried on the X **chromosome**. Since women have two X chromosomes and men have only one, an X-linked recessive condition is expected to effect men since they do not have a second X chromosome with a normal copy of the gene to produce the needed substance. Autosomal recessive NDI is rarer and equally affects males and females. Autosomal dominant NDI is the most rare of the three and affects both males and females.

Inherited NDI is present from birth and symptoms usually manifest within the first several days of

life. If the disorder is not diagnosed and treated early, it will cause the body to lose too much water. This dehydration can lead to brain damage and eventually death. But, with early diagnosis and treatment to avoid severe dehydration, the person can live a normal life span without any mental impairment.

Acquired NDI is the most common type of the disease and can be acquired at any age. It is most frequently acquired through the long-term use of certain prescription medicine, including demeclocycline, methicillin, foscarnet, and some anticancer drugs. In rare instances, it can be caused by an underlying disease or disorder, such as sickle cell anemia, chronic kidney failure, sarcoidosis, amyloidosis, Fanconi syndrome, and Sjögrens syndrome. Other rare causes of acquired NDI are low blood levels of potassium and abnormally high blood calcium levels. Pregnancy can also result in temporary acquired NDI. However, most cases of acquired NDI are caused by long-term use of the prescription drug lithium, used to treat **bipolar disorder** (manic **depression**).

NDI, also called gypsy's curse, is caused by the kidneys inability to respond to the water-saving hormone (ADH), a natural chemical that is manufactured in the brain but works in the kidneys. The body's two kidneys make urine, which is then sent to the bladder, and help to maintain the balance of water, salt, and minerals. A majority of the water is reabsorbed from nephrons in the kidneys into surrounding inner tissue. Each kidney contains hundreds of thousands of nephrons, microscopic-size tubes that filter the water flowing into the kidneys. The water that is not absorbed becomes urine.

The first references to NDI appeared in medical literature in the 1880s, but it wasn't until the 1940s that detailed observations and studies were done. In a landmark 1946 study published in the *American Journal of the Diseases of Children*, authors A. J. Waring, L. Kajdi, and V. Tappan, summarized the main clinical and pathophysiological aspects of the disorder. "The presenting complaints were unexplained fever, failure to gain weight, and constipation. The bouts of dehydration are usually not associated with acidosis. The thirst of one of the patients studied was satisfied only when five to six times the normal requirement of fluid was offered. The levels of (blood) serum sodium and chloride decreased to normal and the infant remained free from fever on this high fluid intake."

### Genetic profile

Genes are the blueprint for the human body that directs the development of cells and tissue. Mutations in some genes can cause **genetic disorders** such as inherited nephrogenic diabetes insipidus. Every cell in the body has 23 pairs of chromosomes, 22 pairs of which are called autosomes and contain two copies of individual genes. The 23rd pair of chromosomes is called the sex chromosome because it determines a person's sex. Men have an X and a Y chromosome while women have two X chromosomes. X-linked nephrogenic diabetes insipidus is caused by a defect in the vasopressin-2 receptor (AVPR2) gene in the X chromosome which renders the kidneys unreceptive to ADH.

Since inherited NDI is usually inherited as an X-linked condition, almost all persons with the disorder are male. Females have two X chromosomes, which means they have two copies of each gene. Males have only one X chromosome and one copy of each gene. If a male has an altered AVPR2 gene, he will have NDI. If a female has one altered gene, she will be a carrier and will be at risk to pass the altered gene on to her children. If her son inherits the altered gene, he will be affected. If her daughter inherits the affected gene, she will be a carrier like her mother. If her son does not inherit the altered gene, he will not be affected and will not pass the altered gene on to his children. If a daughter does not inherit the altered gene, she will not pass it on to her children. If an affected male has children, all of his daughters will be carriers but none of his sons will be affected.

Women who have the abnormal AVPR2 gene may have milder symptoms of NDI than males. This is because early in development, one X-chromosome in each cell of a female is "turned off" at random. If by chance a woman has more than half of the X chromosomes that carry the normal AVPR2 gene turned off, she may have mild symptoms of NDI. Approximately 90% of people with inherited NDI have it as a result of this X-linked gene.

The gene that produces aquaporin-2 (AQP2) can cause autosomal recessive and autosomal dominant NDI when altered. The AQP2 gene produces a protein that helps the kidneys reabsorb water into the body and concentrate urine. Since the AQP2 gene is carried on chromosome 12, a non-sex chromosome, it is carried in both males and females. Also, an abnormal AQP2 gene is recessive, meaning if only one of the person's two AQP2 genes is abnormal, it will not cause NDI. If both genes are abnormal, then that person will have NDI. A child born to a couple who are both carriers of autosomal recessive NDI has a 25% chance to be affected since the child is at risk to receive a copy of the altered gene from its mother and father. In autosomal dominant NDI, either parent may be affected and may pass the altered gene to the child. Also, only one altered gene is necessary to be present for the condition to manifest. Acquired NDI is not hereditary and can not be genetically passed on from parents to their offspring.

### Demographics

In general, the various types of NDI appear to affect people regardless of age, race, or ethnicity. However, in X-linked NDI, the predominance of cases is among males. The exact number of people with NDI is not known. Estimates range from one in every 500,000 to five in every 100,000. In acquired NDI, one of the diseases that can cause it is sickle cell anemia, which occurs primarily in people of African descent.

### Signs and symptoms

The primary symptoms for all types of NDI are generally the same: polyuria (excreting large amounts of dilute urine) and polydipsia, drinking excessive amounts of water, from 3–10 gal (12–38 L) per day. In infants born with NDI, symptoms begin to occur within a few days after birth. But since a child cannot verbally communicate its need for larger than normal amounts of water, parents, physicians, and other caregivers must be alert to other signs of the disorder. Overt signs include fever, irritability, and constipation, all of which may indicate dehydration. The child may also vomit often, be anorexic, and prefer water to milk. Other signs include rapid and severe dehydration if fluids are restricted or withheld, high levels of sodium and chloride in the blood, and urine that does not have a high specific gravity.

Elderly people, usually those with acquired NDI, may need close monitoring for symptoms especially if they are unable to communicate their need for lots of water, such as patients with **Alzheimer disease** or other mental deterioration. Also, elderly persons may be less sensitive to their need for water. Because of this, elderly persons with NDI can be more prone to dehydration, leading to such problems as infection, kidney failure, confusion, lethargy, and constipation.

For acquired NDI, close medical monitoring should be done for people at high risk for the disorder. These include people undergoing long-term treatment with lithium, and people with sickle cell anemia, chronic kidney failure, other kidney problems, very low blood levels of potassium and protein, and high blood levels of calcium.

## Diagnosis

NDI is one of four types of diabetes insipidus (DI). In all four types, the basic symptoms are extreme thirst and excessive urination. Depending on other symptoms and conditions present in the patient, it can often be easy for a physician to suspect NDI. But additional tests are required to confirm it. These include a test of urine concentration to measure the ratio of osmotically active particles (such as sodium) to body water, a blood test to determine plasma concentrations, measuring urine volume, and a test to determine the level of the antidiuretic hormone AVP in blood plasma.

Sometimes physicians will have the patient take a water deprivation test to help determine the type of NDI present. In this test, the patient goes without water or other liquids for up to six hours. The blood plasma concentrations and urine volume are then measured. Even though a patient with NDI will become dehydrated during this test, the doctor monitors the patient's body weight and blood plasma osmolarity levels to insure they remain within safe parameters. At the end of the test, the patient is generally diagnosed with NDI if he or she has high levels of osmotically active particles in the blood and low levels of osmotically active particles in the urine.

The patient is also given desmopressin acetate (DDAVP), a synthetic version of AVP, to determine if the patient has a different form of DI called pituitary diabetes insipidus, also known as central diabetes insipidus. In addition, the physician measures heart rate and diastolic blood pressure to help determine whether the NDI is caused by defective AVPR2 genes or defective AQP2 genes.

## Treatment and management

Although there is no cure for NDI, all forms of the disorder are treatable. Drinking plenty of water is the first and foremost treatment. Regardless of the age of the patient, water must be available at all times. However, it is important for a child to maintain control of their NDI with medication so that they can eat, drink, and grow normally.

Medications used to treat NDI include one or a combination of indomethacin (Indocin), amiloride (Midamor), the thiazide diuretics hydrochlorothiazide (Hydrodiuril) or Chlorothiazide (Diuril), and occasionally desmopressin.

Management of NDI is also accomplished through restricting the intake of sodium and sometimes protein. Thiazide diuretics can reduce a patient's urine output, but they may also cause potassium depletion. Potassium supplements may be required. NDI that occurs during pregnancy usually goes away after delivery of the child. NDI caused by diet abnormalities are usually reversible once the diet becomes balanced. Acquired NDI caused by electrolyte imbalances such as low levels of calcium in the blood plasma or high levels of potassium in the blood plasma can be reversed once the imbalance is corrected.

In patients with lithium-induced NDI, thiazide diuretics are used cautiously since they reduce the kidneys' ability to excrete lithium. In many, but not all cases, people with lithium-induced NDI can improve when the dosage is decreased or stopped. In some cases, the lithium-induced NDI is irreversible.

## Prognosis

Infants and children with inherited NDI can live a normal life span providing they are diagnosed correctly, treated early, and properly manage the disorder. Without early diagnosis and treatment in infancy, NDI can lead to mental retardation and even death. Infants and children with NDI tend to be slightly smaller and weigh less than children without NDI.

As children with NDI mature into adults, they tend to be slightly shorter than their parents, but with a normal weight. With appropriate treatment and management, NDI should not interfere with activities such as school, work, or sports.

### Resources

#### BOOKS

Czernichow, P. *Diabetes Insipidus in Man.* S. Karger Publishing, Basel, Switzerland, 1985.

Narins, Robert G. *Maxwell and Kleeman's Clinical Disorders of Fluid and Electrolyte Metabolism,* Fifth Edition. McGraw-Hill Publishing, Inc., New York, 1994.

Scriver, Charles R., et al. *The Metabolic Basis of Inherited Disease,* Eighth Edition. McGraw-Hill Publishing, Inc., New York, 2000.

#### PERIODICALS

Arthus, M. F., et al. "Report of 33 Novel AVPR2 Mutations and Analysis of 117 Families with X-linked Nephrogenic Diabetes Insipidus." *Journal of the American Society of Nephrology* (June 2000): 1044-1054.

Bichet, D. G. "Nephrogenic Diabetes Insipidus." *American Journal of Medicine* (November 1998): 431-442.

Oksche, A., and W. Rosenthal. "The Molecular Basis of Nephrogenic Diabetes Insipidus." *Journal of Molecular Medicine* (April 1998): 326-337.

Schulz, Pasel K., et al. "Functional Characterization of the Molecular Defects Causing Nephrogenic Diabetes Insipidus in Eight Families." *Journal of Clinical Endocrinology and Metabolism* (April 2000): 1703-1710.

Stone, Dr. Kurt A. "Lithium-induced Nephrogenic Diabetes Insipidus." *Journal of the American Board of Family Practice* (January/February 1999): 43-47.

Van Lieburg, Angenita F., et al. "Clinical Presentation and Follow-up of 30 Patients with Congenital Nephrogenic Diabetes Insipidus." *Journal of the American Society of Nephrology* (October 1999): 1958-1964.

Wildin, R. S., and D. E. Cogdell. "Clinical Utility of Direct Mutation Testing for Congenital Nephrogenic Diabetes Insipidus in Families." *Pediatrics* (March 1999): 632-639.

#### WEBSITES

*Diabetes Insipidus Foundation.* http://diabetesinsipidus.maxinter.net.

#### ORGANIZATIONS

Nephrogenic Diabetes Insipidus Foundation. PO Box 1390, Eastsound, WA 98245. (888) 376-6343. Fax: (888) 376-3842. http://www.ndi.org.

Ken R. Wells

# Neu-Laxova syndrome

### Definition

Neu-Laxova syndrome is a rare disorder characterized by onset of severe growth delay during pregnancy, multiple birth defects, and abnormal physical development of the brain. Affected infants typically die shortly after delivery or are stillborn.

### Description

In 1971, Dr. Neu published the first report of a family that included three children with a unique pattern of multiple birth defects. Each child had an unusually small head (*microcephaly*) and abnormalities of their arms, legs, skin, and external genitalia. The two affected daughters were each stillborn, while the affected son only lived for seven weeks. In 1972, Dr. Laxova described a different family whose children had birth defects similar to those first described by Dr. Neu. The parents in this second family were first cousins to one another. Taken together, these two families were considered evidence of a previously unrecognized genetic syndrome. The disorder was named Neu-Laxova syndrome in honor of these two physicians.

Neu-Laxova syndrome (NLS) has since become known as a rare, lethal inherited condition characterized by a specific pattern of facial, brain, and limb abnormalities. Other associated abnormalities often include dry, scaly skin, generalized swelling of body tissues (edema), and extremely slow growth.

### Genetic profile

Neu-Laxova syndrome is inherited as an autosomal recessive condition. Males and females are equally likely to be affected. It has been reported in a variety of ethnic groups. Proof of autosomal recessive

**Agenesis of the corpus callosum**—Failure of the corpus callosum to form and develop. The corpus callosum is the band of nerve fibers located between the two sides, or hemispheres, of the brain.

**Cataract**—A clouding of the eye lens or its surrounding membrane that obstructs the passage of light resulting in blurry vision. Surgery may be performed to remove the cataract.

**Cerebellum**—A portion of the brain consisting of two cerebellar hemispheres connected by a narrow vermis. The cerebellum is involved in control of skeletal muscles and plays an important role in the coordination of voluntary muscle movement. It interrelates with other areas of the brain to facilitate a variety of movements, including maintaining proper posture and balance, walking, running, and fine motor skills, such as writing, dressing, and eating.

**Cleft lip**—A separation of the upper lip that is present from birth but originates early in fetal development.

A cleft lip may appear on one side (unilateral) or both sides (bilateral) and is occasionally accompanied by a cleft palate. Surgery is needed to completely repair cleft lip.

**Cleft palate**—A congenital malformation in which there is an abnormal opening in the roof of the mouth that allows the nasal passages and the mouth to be improperly connected.

**Dandy-Walker malformation**—A complex structural abnormality of the brain frequently associated with hydrocephalus, or accumulation of excess fluid in the brain. Abnormalities in other areas of the body may also be present. Individuals with Dandy-Walker malformation have varying degrees of mental handicap or none at all.

**Placenta**—The organ responsible for oxygen and nutrition exchange between a pregnant mother and her developing baby.

**Stillbirth**—The birth of a baby who has died sometime during the pregnancy or delivery.

---

**inheritance** includes the birth of more than one affected child to normal parents, and the observed incidence of infants with NLS among the children of two blood relatives. Consanguinity, or the mating of two biologically related individuals, increases the possibility of having a child with a genetic disorder. Since any two relatives will share a portion of their genes in common, they are more likely to each be a carrier of the same autosomal recessive gene.

In order to be affected with NLS, an individual must inherit two copies of the NLS gene, or one copy from each carrier parent. A carrier has one NLS gene and one normal gene; as such, an NLS carrier appears completely normal. However, two carriers face a risk of 25%, or a one in four chance, of having a child with NLS. Conversely, they also have a 75% chance of having an unaffected child. These risks apply to each of their pregnancies together.

Infants with NLS have also been born to non-consanguineous, or unrelated, couples. Anytime a child with NLS is born, the parents must be obligate, or mandatory, carriers of one NLS gene. As such, they face an increased risk in future pregnancies together of having another affected child.

The gene for NLS has not yet been identified. Thus, it is not possible to perform direct **genetic testing** to determine carrier status, confirm a clinical diagnosis, or provide accurate prenatal diagnosis.

### Demographics

Adequate data are not available to provide a specific statistic regarding the frequency of NLS. The condition is very rare. According to a 1995 publication, only 40 cases of Neu-Laxova syndrome had been reported up to that point in the medical literature.

### Signs and symptoms

Stillborn or newborn infants with NLS have a characteristic pattern of internal and external abnormalities. Not all affected infants will have all of the features listed below, and some anomalies are slightly more common than others.

Infants with Neu-Laxova syndrome often have unusual facial features. Their heads are very small, and their foreheads appear to slant backwards. The distance between the eyes is wider than normal (*hypertelorism*), and the eyes are prominent or bulging. Cataracts may be present. The eyelids are typically absent. The bridge of the nose is wide and slightly flattened. The ears are abnormally shaped. The lower jaw appears recessed as compared to the upper jaw (*retrognathia*), and the mouth itself is usually open with abnormally thick lips. **Cleft lip** may be present, with or without **cleft palate**.

The external features of the head and face are a reflection of severe physical abnormalities of the brain. It is not unusual for an infant with NLS to have an underdeveloped cerebellum or even **lissencephaly**, a more serious malformation characterized by a smooth brain surface. Normal development of the brain includes an intricate pattern of grooves, or gyri, on its outer surface. A lack of these grooves leads to profound mental retardation among survivors and an increased frequency of medical complications, such as seizures. Other reported brain malformations include agenesis of the corpus callosum and **Dandy-Walker malformation**.

A variety of limb abnormalities have also been described in NLS. Affected individuals often have shortened arms and legs that are held out from the body in an unusual, fixed position. This positioning is often referred to as flexion contractures. The fingers and toes may appear underdeveloped (hypoplastic) and/or fused together (syndactyly). The heels of the feet are often rounded (rocker-bottom feet), and the neck is short.

Other abnormalities more common to NLS include markedly limited physical growth. This typically begins during pregnancy and, as such, is referred to as intrauterine growth restriction (IUGR). Edema, or an excessive amount of fluid in the tissues of the body, is a hallmark of NLS. The edema may either be generalized and very severe throughout the body or limited only to the face or scalp. The skin is often extremely dry and scaly, a medical condition called **ichthyosis**. The lungs are often hypoplastic (underdeveloped), even when delivery occurs at term. The external genitalia are often abnormal, but this is more obvious in males than in females since males typically have a small, underdeveloped penis.

Finally, in addition to IUGR during pregnancy, an excessive volume of amniotic fluid (polyhydramnios) often develops. This is due to a combination of abnormal fluid production and impaired fetal swallowing from the associated nervous system abnormalities. The placenta is also usually abnormal in appearance and function.

### Diagnosis

Many infants with NLS have been born into families with no previous history of the disorder and/or ones in which the parents are unrelated. Thus, an exact diagnosis of NLS during pregnancy may be very difficult, particularly for a couple with no apparent risk factors. Direct genetic testing for NLS will not be possible until the responsible gene has been identified. Some non-specific prenatal findings should, however, alert the physician that additional prenatal evaluation is warranted. These include IUGR and polyhydramnios. Both findings often lead to an obvious difference in the size of a pregnant woman's uterus and her estimated weeks of pregnancy. A woman whose fetus has severe IUGR and normal amniotic fluid often appears less pregnant than she actually is. In contrast, a woman with polyhydramnios often appears more pregnant, or larger. A detailed **prenatal ultrasound** test may be used to obtain pictures of abnormalities of the fetus as well as possible abnormalities of the placenta whenever there is an apparent discrepancy in a woman's size and her dates.

Two groups have separately reported diagnosis of NLS using ultrasound. However, in both cases, the diagnosis was formally established only after delivery. A number of the physical findings associated with NLS, particularly those involving the face, limbs, and brain, may be apparent following a detailed ultrasound later in pregnancy. In experienced hands and with the knowledge of a previous affected infant, some of these findings may be observed earlier.

In one of the published cases, a diagnosis of NLS was helped by the physical findings of an ultrasound exam at 32 weeks of pregnancy. The fetus was found to have many of the abnormalities associated with NLS. In the second report, ultrasound was used to assess fetal movement patterns at 34 weeks of pregnancy. Abnormal fetal movement is indicative of abnormal brain development. The authors were able to document a lack of normal fetal activity, such as breathing movements, sucking, swallowing, hiccups, and movements of the arms and legs in a fetus diagnosed with NLS after birth.

Accurate diagnosis of this condition is difficult before birth for those couples in which no NLS gene has been identified and no family history of NLS is known. While the combination of abnormal physical development and possibly abnormal fetal activity is highly indicative of a severe genetic condition, both would not be specific enough to pinpoint Neu-Laxova syndrome as the cause in all cases. Other genetic syndromes would be under consideration, pending a clinical examination after delivery.

For this reason, a careful physical evaluation after birth is critical in establishing a diagnosis of NLS. For those infants who are stillborn and for those who die after delivery, an autopsy is also helpful in documenting all of the associated internal abnormalities. A precise diagnosis facilitates accurate **genetic counseling**, including prognosis for an affected child and the risk of recurrence for future pregnancies.

### Treatment and management

For those couples who have had a previous child with Neu-Laxova syndrome, serial prenatal ultrasound evaluations should be offered to monitor fetal growth, screen for physical abnormalities, and, assess fetal well-being later in pregnancy given the increased risk for stillbirth. Ultrasound diagnosis of any of the structural birth defects associated with NLS in these families should be considered evidence of the disorder. Since some of these findings may not become evident until later in pregnancy, termination of the pregnancy may not be an option for some couples. Plans for the remainder of the pregnancy as well as delivery can, however, be discussed. Given the serious prognosis associated with NLS, some parents may find a non-interventionist approach during labor and delivery, such as no fetal monitoring or Cesarean section delivery, acceptable. A clinical examination after birth is recommended.

Most infants with NLS have either been stillborn or died very shortly after delivery. However, there is one reported case of an affected Japanese infant who lived for 134 days. Humane medical care is therefore appropriate in survivors although the prognosis would still be extremely poor.

An autopsy is recommended on all affected infants after death to document and confirm all of the associated physical abnormalities. While this acts as a way to confirm the diagnosis, it is also a useful

way to continue to add to the knowledge about the syndrome and its physical effects.

### Prognosis

The number of infants described with Neu-Laxova syndrome is small. However, with the exception of the reported infant who lived 134 days, all affected children have either died before delivery or shortly thereafter. Neu-Laxova syndrome is a serious genetic condition whose anomalies prevent long-term survival.

### Resources

**BOOKS**

Jones, K. L., ed. "Neu-Laxova syndrome." In *Smith's Recognizable Pattern of Human Malformations*. W. B. Saunders Company, Philadelphia, 1997.

**PERIODICALS**

Kainer, F., et al. "Qualitative analysis of fetal movement patterns in the Neu-Laxova syndrome." *Prenatal Diagnosis* 16, no. 7 (July 1996): 667-669.

Shapiro, I., et al. "Neu-Laxova syndrome: Prenatal ultrasonographic diagnosis, clinical and pathological studies, and new manifestations." *American Journal of Medical Genetics* 43, no. 3 (June 1992): 602-605.

**WEBSITES**

TheFetus.net, http://www.thefetus.net/sections/articles/Syndromes/Neu_Laxova.html.

"OMIM—Online Mendelian Inheritance in Man." http://www.ncbi.nlm.nih.gov/omim.

**ORGANIZATIONS**

Genetic Alliance. 4301 Connecticut Ave. NW, #404, Washington, DC 20008-2304. (800) 336-GENE (Helpline) or (202) 966-5557. Fax: (888) 394-3937 info@geneticalliance. http://www.geneticalliance.org.

Lissencephaly Network, Inc. 716 Autumn Ridge Lane, Fort Wayne, IN 46804-6402. (219) 432-4310. Fax: (219) 432-4310. lissennet@lissencephaly.org. http://www.lissencephaly.org.

Terri A. Knutel, MS, CGC

# Neural tube defects

### Definition

Neural tube defects are a group of severe birth defects in which the brain and spinal cord are malformed and lack the protective skeletal and soft tissue encasement.

## KEY TERMS

**Embryo**—The earliest stage of development of a human infant, usually used to refer to the first eight weeks of pregnancy. The term *fetus* is used from roughly the third month of pregnancy until delivery.

**Hydrocephalus**—The excess accumulation of cerebrospinal fluid around the brain, often causing enlargement of the head.

**Meninges**—The two-layered membrane that covers the brain and spinal cord.

## Description

Incomplete formation and protection of the brain or spinal cord with bony and soft tissue coverings during the fourth week of embryo formation are known collectively as neural tube defects. Lesions may occur anywhere in the midline of the head or spine. These defects are among the most common serious birth defects, but they vary considerably in their severity. In some cases, the brain or spinal cord is completely exposed, in some cases protected by a tough membrane (meninges), and in other cases covered by skin.

**Spina bifida** accounts for about two-thirds of all neural tube defects. The spine defect may appear anywhere from the neck to the buttocks. In its most severe form, termed "spinal rachischisis," the entire spinal canal is open exposing the spinal cord and nerves. More commonly, the defect appears as a localized mass on the back that is covered by skin or by the meninges.

**Anencephaly**, the second most common neural tube defect, accounts for about one-third of cases. Two major subtypes occur. In the most severe form, all of the skull bones are missing and the brain is exposed in its entirety. The second form, in which only a part of the skull is missing and a portion of the brain exposed, is termed "meroacrania."

Encephaloceles are the least common form of neural tube defects, comprising less than 10% of birth defects. With encephaloceles, a portion of the skull bones are missing leaving a bony hole through which the brain and its coverings herniate (protrude). Encephaloceles occur in the midline from the base of the nose, to the junction of the skull and neck. As with spina bifida, the severity varies greatly. In its mildest form, encephaloceles may appear as only a small area of faulty skin development with or without any underlying skull defect. At the severe end of the spectrum, most of the brain may be herniated outside of the skull into a skin-covered sac.

## Genetic profile

Most neural tube defects (80-90%) occur as isolated defects. Neural tube defects of this variety are believed to arise through the combined influence of genetic and environmental forces. This multifactorial causation presumes that one or more predisposing genes collaborate with one or more environmental influences to lead to the birth defect. Poor nutrition is believed to be an environmental risk factor and hereditary defects in the absorption and utilization of folic acid are presumptive genetic predisposing factors. After a couple has one infant with a neural tube defect, the recurrence risk is 3-5%. After the birth of two NTD-affected infants, the risk increases to 8-10%.

When neural tube defects occur concurrently with other malformations there is a greater likelihood of an underlying specific genetic or environmental cause. Genetic causes include **chromosome** aberrations and single **gene mutations**. Environmental causes include maternal **diabetes** mellitus, exposure to prolonged hyperthermia, and seizure medications during the early months of pregnancy.

## Demographics

Neural tube defects occur worldwide. It appears that the highest prevalence (about one in 100 pregnancies) exists in certain northern provinces in China; an intermediate prevalence (about one in 300-500 pregnancies) has been found in Ireland and in Central and South America; and the lowest prevalence (less than one in 2,000 pregnancies) has been found in the Scandinavian countries. In the United States, the highest prevalence has occurred in the Southeast. Worldwide there has been a steady downward trend in prevalence rates over the past 50-70 years.

## Signs and symptoms

Because of the faulty development of the spinal cord and nerves, a number of consequences are commonly seen in spina bifida. As a rule, the nerves below the level of the defect develop in a faulty manner and fail to function, resulting in paralysis and loss of sensation below the level of the spinal lesion. Since most defects occur in the lumbar region, the lower limbs are usually paralyzed and lack normal sensation. Furthermore, the bowel and bladder have inadequate nerve connections, causing inability to control bladder and bowel function. Sexual function is likewise impaired. Hydrocephaly develops in most infants either before or after surgical repair of the spine defect.

In anencephaly, the brain is destroyed by exposure during intrauterine life. Most infants with anencephaly are stillborn, or die within the initial days or weeks after birth.

Infants with encephaloceles have variable neurologic impairments depending on the extent of brain involvement. When only the brain covering is involved, the individual may escape any adverse effect. However, when the brain is involved in the defect, impairments of the special senses such as sight, hearing, and cognitive thinking commonly result.

### Diagnosis

At birth, the diagnosis is usually obvious based on external findings. Prenatal diagnosis may be made with ultrasound examination after 12-14 weeks of pregnancy. Screening of pregnancies can be carried out at 16 weeks by testing the mother's blood for the level of alphafetoprotein. Open neural tube defects leak this fetal chemical into the surrounding amniotic fluid, a small portion of which is absorbed into the mother's blood.

### Treatment and management

No treatment is available for anencephaly. Aggressive surgical and medical management has improved survival and function of infants with spina bifida. Surgery closes the defect, providing protection against injury and infection. A common complication that may occur before or after surgical correction is the accumulation of excessive cerebral spinal fluid (hydrocephaly) in the major cavities (ventricles) within the brain. Hydrocephaly is usually treated with the placement of a mechanical shunt, which allows the cerebral spinal fluid from the ventricles to drain into the circulation or another body cavity. A number of medical and surgical procedures have been used to protect the urinary system as well. Walking may be achieved with orthopedic devices. Encephaloceles are usually repaired by surgery soon after birth. The success of surgery often depends on the amount of brain tissue involved in the **encephalocele**.

It has been found that 400 micrograms of folic acid taken during the periconceptional period (two to three months prior to conception, and two to three months following conceptions) protects against most neural tube defects. While there are a number of foods (green leafy vegetables, legumes, liver, and orange juice) that are good sources of natural folic acid, synthetic folic acid is available in over-the-counter multivitamins and a number of fully fortified breakfast cereals.

Additionally, a population-wide increase in folic acid intake has been achieved through the fortification of enriched cereal grain flours since January 1998, a measure authorized by the United States Food and Drug Administration. The increased blood folic acid levels achieved in recent years has likely resulted from the synergy of dietary, supplementation, and fortification sources of folic acid.

### Prognosis

Infants with anencephaly are usually stillborn or die within the initial days of life. Eighty to ninety percent of infants with spina bifida survive with surgery. Paralysis below the level of the defect, including an inability to control bowel and bladder function, and hydrocephaly are complications experienced by most survivors. Intellectual function is normal in most cases.

The prognosis for infants with encephaloceles varies considerably. Small encephaloceles may cause no disability whether surgical correction is performed or not. Infants with larger encephaloceles may have residual impairment of vision, hearing, nerve function, and intellectual capacity.

### Resources

#### PERIODICALS

Sells, C. J., and J. G. Hall, Guest Editors. "Neural Tube Defects." *Mental Retardation and Developmental Disabilities Research Reviews* 4, no. 4 (1998) Wiley-Liss.

#### ORGANIZATIONS

March of Dimes Birth Defects Foundation. 1275 Mamaroneck Ave., White Plains, NY 10605. (888) 663-4637. resourcecenter@modimes.org. http://www.modimes.org.

National Birth Defects Prevention Network. Atlanta, GA (770) 488-3550. http://www.nbdpn.org.

Shriners Hospitals for Children. International Shrine Headquarters, 2900 Rocky Point Dr., Tampa, FL 33607-1460. (813) 281-0300.

Spina Bifida Association of America. 4590 MacArthur Blvd. NW, Suite 250, Washington, DC 20007-4226. (800) 621-3141 or (202) 944-3285. Fax: (202) 944-3295.

Roger E. Stevenson, MD

# Neuraminidase deficiency

## Definition

Neuraminidase deficiency, or sialidosis, is a rare inherited metabolic disorder with multiple symptoms that can include skeletal abnormalities and progressive neurological degeneration.

## KEY TERMS

**Dysostosis multiplex**—A variety of bone and skeletal malformations.

**Fibroblast**—Cells that form connective tissue fibers like skin.

**Glycoprotein**—A protein with at least one carbohydrate group.

**Heterozygote**—Having two different versions of the same gene.

**Homozygote**—Having two identical copies of a gene or chromosome.

**Lipid**—Large, complex biomolecule, such as a fatty acid, that will not dissolve in water. A major constituent of membranes.

**Lysosome**—Membrane-enclosed compartment in cells, containing many hydrolytic enzymes; where large molecules and cellular components are broken down.

**Myoclonus**—Twitching or spasms of a muscle or an interrelated group of muscles.

**Oligosaccharide**—Several monosaccharide (sugar) groups joined by glycosidic bonds.

**Polysaccharide**—Linear or branched macromolecule composed of numerous monosaccharide (sugar) units linked by glycosidic bonds.

**Recessive**—Genetic trait expressed only when present on both members of a pair of chromosomes, one inherited from each parent.

**Sialic acid**—N-acetylneuraminic acid, a sugar that is often at the end of an oligosaccharide on a glycoprotein.

**Vacuolation**—The formation of multiple vesicles, or vacuoles, within the cytosol of cells.

## Description

### Nomenclature

Neuraminidase deficiency is caused by a mutation, or change, in the NEU1 **gene** that codes for the lysosomal enzyme alpha-N-acetylneuraminidase, or neuraminidase for short. This enzyme sometimes is referred to as sialidase. It is also sometimes called N-acetyl-neuraminic acid hydrolase. The disorder is manifested in one of two forms, known as sialidosis types I and II. Sialidosis type I is the milder form of the disorder, with symptoms typically appearing during adolescence. It is known as the non-dysmorphic or normophormic form of sialidosis. Sialidosis type II is the more severe form of neuraminidase deficiency, with symptoms developing in the fetus, at birth, or during infancy or early childhood. It is known as the dysmorphic form of sialidosis.

Over the years, this disorder has been called by a number of different names, in addition to neuraminidase deficiency, alpha-neuraminidase deficiency, sialidase deficiency, and sialidosis. It sometimes is known as cherry-red spot and myoclonus syndrome, cherry-red spot myoclonus **epilepsy** syndrome, or myoclonus and cherry-red spot syndrome, in reference to characteristic symptoms of the disorder. Other names include glycoprotein neuraminidase deficiency, NEUG deficiency, NEU or NEU1 deficiency, and neuraminidase 1 deficiency. Sialidosis type I sometimes is referred to as juvenile sialidosis and type II as infantile sialidosis, in reference to the age of onset.

### Lysosomal storage diseases

Lysosomes are membrane-bound spherical compartments or vesicles within the cytosol, the semi-fluid areas of cells. Lysosomes contain more than 50 different enzymes that are responsible for digesting, or hydrolyzing, large molecules and cellular components. These include proteins; polysaccharides, which are long, linear or branched chains of sugars; and lipids, which are large insoluble biomolecules that are usually built from fatty acids. The smaller breakdown products from the lysosomes are recycled to the cytosol.

Neuraminidase deficiency is one of at least 41 genetically-distinct lysosomal storage diseases. These disorders result from mutations in the genes encoding the hydrolytic enzymes of the lysosome. In these disorders, some of the macromolecules in the lysosomes cannot be degraded and they, or their partial-breakdown products, accumulate there. The lysosomes swell to the point where cellular function is disrupted.

Neuraminidase deficiency, particularly sialidosis type II, commonly has been classified as the lysosomal storage disease called **mucolipidosis** type I (ML I), formerly lipomucopolysaccharidosis. This is because the symptoms of neuraminidase deficiency are similar to various mucolipidosis disorders. However mucolipidoses are characterized by the accumulation of large and complex lipid-polysaccharides. In contrast, neuraminidase deficiency leads to the accumulation of specific types of short chains of sugar called oligosaccharides and of certain proteins with oligosaccharides attached to them, called glycoproteins. Thus, it may be more appropriate to classify neuraminidase deficiency as an oligosaccharide storage disease, since it leads to the accumulation of excess oligosaccharides in various tissues throughout the body and the excretion of oligosaccharides.

### Neuraminidase

Neuraminidase, or sialidase, is a type of enzyme known as an exoglycosidase because it cleaves terminal sugar units, or residues, off oligosaccharides. Specifically, neuraminidase cleaves, or hydrolyzes, terminal sialic acid residues. Sialic acid, also known as N-acetylneuraminic acid, is a type of sugar molecule that often is at an end of an oligosaccharide. The oligosaccharides with sialic acid residues may be attached to proteins (glycoproteins). Therefore, neuraminidase deficiency prevents the proper breakdown of oligosaccharides and glycoproteins that contain sialic acid and the disorder is characterized by the accumulation and excretion of these substances.

In addition to interfering with the lysosomal breakdown of sialic acid compounds, neuraminidase deficiency can lead to abnormal proteins. Following protein synthesis, some lysosomal enzymes reach the lysosome in an inactive form and require further processing for activation. One such processing step is the neuraminidase-catalyzed removal of sialic acid residues from oligosaccharides on the enzymes. Lysosomal hydrolases that require further processing by neuraminidase include acid phosphatase, alpha-mannosidase, arylsulfatase B, and alpha-glucosidase.

Under conditions of neuraminidase deficiency, sialyloligosaccharides accumulate in various cells, including lymphocytes (white blood cells that produce antibodies), fibroblasts (connective tissue cells), bone marrow cells, Kupffer cells of the liver, and Schwann cells, which form the myelin sheaths of nerve fibers. Furthermore, proteins with sialic acid attachments accumulate and can be detected in fibroblasts and in the urine.

Neuraminidase exists in the lysosome in a high-molecular-weight complex with three other proteins the enzyme beta-galactosidase, the enzyme N-acetylgalactosamine-6-sulfate sulfatase (GALNS), and a multi-functional enzyme called protective protein/cathepsin A (PPCA). Neuraminidase must be associated with PPCA in order for the neuraminidase to reach the lysosome. Once inside the lysosome, PPCA mediates the association of as many as 24 neuraminidase molecules to form active neuraminidase. The active enzyme remains associated with PPCA and beta-galactosidase, which appear to be necessary for protecting and stabilizing the neuraminidase activity. A distinct lysosomal storage disease,

**neuraminidase deficiency with beta-galactosidase deficiency**, or galactosialidosis, results from mutations in the gene encoding PPCA. In this disorder, both neuraminidase and beta-galactosidase are deficient.

## Genetic profile

### Inheritance of neuraminidase deficiency

Neuraminidase deficiency is an autosomal recessive disorder that can be caused by any one of a number of different mutations in the NEU1 gene encoding the lysosomal neuraminidase. The disorder is autosomal because the NEU1 gene is located on **chromosome** 6, rather than on the X or Y sex chromosomes. The disorder is recessive because it only develops when both genes encoding neuraminidase, one inherited from each parent, are defective; however, the two defective NEU1 genes do not need to carry the same mutations. If the two mutations are identical, the individual is a homozygote. If the two mutations are different, the affected individual is called a compound heterozygote. Individuals with one defective gene and one normal gene encoding neuraminidase may have reduced levels of the active enzyme, but they do not have symptoms of neuraminidase deficiency.

All of the offspring of two parents with neuraminidase deficiency will inherit the disorder. All of the offspring of one parent with neuraminidase deficiency and one parent with a single defective NEU1 gene will inherit at least one defective NEU1 gene. They will have a 50% chance of inheriting two defective genes and, therefore, developing neuraminidase deficiency. The offspring of one parent with neuraminidase deficiency and one parent with normal NEU1 genes will inherit a defective gene from the affected parent, but will not develop neuraminidase deficiency. The offspring of parents who both carry one defective NEU1 gene have a 50% chance of inheriting one defective NEU1 gene and a 25% chance of inheriting two genes and developing neuraminidase deficiency. Finally, the children of one parent with a single defective NEU1 gene and one parent with normal NEU1 genes will have a 50% chance of inheriting the defective gene, but will not develop neuraminidase deficiency.

### Mutations in the NEU1 gene

A number of different mutations that can cause neuraminidase deficiency have been identified in the NEU1 gene. The type of neuraminidase deficiency, sialidoses types I or II, as well as the severity of the symptoms, depends on the specific mutation(s) that are present. Some mutations change one amino acid out of the 415 amino acids that compose a single neuraminidase molecule. Other identified mutations result in a shortened enzyme. Many of the identified mutations are clustered in one region on the surface of the protein. These mutations result in a sharp reduction in the activity of the enzyme and lead to the rapid degradation of neuraminidase inside the lysosome.

Some mutations in the NEU1 gene lead to a complete absence of neuraminidase activity, with little or no neuraminidase enzyme present in the lysosomes. These mutations usually result in the severe, infantile-onset, type II sialidosis. Other mutations result in an inactive protein that is present in the lysosome. These mutations generally result in juvenile-onset, type II sialidosis, with symptoms of intermediate severity. Some mutations significantly reduce, but do not obliterate, neuraminidase activity in the lysosome. Individuals with at least one mutated gene of this type are not completely neuraminidase-deficient and have mild, type I sialidosis. Occasionally, individuals have multiple mutations in the NEU1 gene, leading to more severe forms of neuraminidase deficiency.

## Demographics

Neuraminidase deficiency is an extremely rare disorder. Because of its similarities to many other disorders, it has been difficult to determine its frequency. In the United States, it is estimated to occur in one out of every 250,000 live births. In Australia, the estimate is one out of 4.2 million. Since neuraminidase deficiency is an autosomal rather than a sex-linked disorder, it occurs equally in males and females.

As an autosomal recessive disorder, neuraminidase deficiency requires two copies of the defective gene, one inherited from each parent. Thus, neuraminidase deficiency is much more common in the offspring of couples who are related to each other (consanguineous marriages), such as first or second cousins.

Sialidosis type I appears to be more common among Italians. Type 2 sialidosis seems to occur more frequently among Japanese.

## Signs and symptoms

The clinical symptoms of neuraminidase deficiency are similar to the symptoms of the mucolipidoses, including I-cell disease (mucolipidosis II) and pseudoHurler polydystrophy (mucolipidosis III). Furthermore, the clinical distinctions between sialidoses types I and II may not be clearly defined.

### Sialidosis type I

The symptoms of sialidosis type I do not appear until the second decade of life. Infants and children with this form of neuraminidase deficiency may have a normal appearance and grow normally until adolescence. At that time, the appearance of red spots in both eyes, known as cherry-red macules or cherry-red macular spots, may be one of the first symptoms of neuraminidase deficiency. Eventually, color and/or night blindness may develop. Cataracts may occur and vision may deteriorate gradually into blindness.

Other symptoms of sialidosis type I include myoclonus. These are sudden involuntary muscle contractions, which may eventually develop into myoclonic seizures. The myoclonus may become debilitating, even in sialidosis type I. Individuals with this form of neuraminidase deficiency may have increased deep tendon reflexes and may develop tremors and various other neurological conditions. There may be a progressive loss of muscle coordination, called ataxia, and walking and standing may become increasingly difficult. Speech problems, such as slurring, may develop.

The above symptoms also may occur in sialidosis type II. However, in addition to the age of onset, type I can be distinguished from type II by the absence of skeletal and facial abnormalities. Furthermore, individuals with this form of neuraminidase deficiency have normal intelligence.

### Sialidosis type II

Sialidosis type II has three forms: congenital or neonatal, with symptoms present at or before birth; infantile, with symptoms developing at birth or during the first year of life; and juvenile, with symptoms developing between the ages of two and twenty.

Symptoms of sialidosis type II vary from mild to severe, but are always more severe than in type I sialidosis. With neonatal onset, infants may be born with ascites (accumulation of fluid in the abdominal cavity), swollen liver and spleen (hepatosplenomegaly), hernia of the umbilicus or the groin, and other abnormalities. With severe forms of the disorder, children may die in infancy. With milder forms, they may show no symptoms for the first 10 years of life. Thus, ascites, hepatosplenomegaly, and hernias may develop later. Children with neuraminidase deficiency may grow abnormally fast. Cherry-red macules, myoclonus, and other neurological abnormalities, including tremors, may be present. The myoclonus may progress into a form of epilepsy. These children may have mild to severe mental retardation.

Sialidosis type II is characterized by a variety of skeletal malformations (dysostosis multiplex). Obvious symptoms may include distinctive, coarse facial features (called coarse facies), a short trunk with relatively long legs and arms, and a prominent breast bone (pectus carinatum). In addition, there may be a lack of muscle tone and strength (hypotonia) and the progressive wasting of muscular tissue.

The hearing may be affected in sialidosis type II. Individuals may have difficulty breathing (dyspnea). Cardiac problems may develop and severe congenital sialidosis type II apparently can result in severely-dilated coronary arteries. Loose bowel movements are common with this form of neuraminidase deficiency.

## Diagnosis

### Neuraminidase activity

Typically, neuraminidase deficiency is diagnosed by measuring the activity of the enzyme in cultures of fibroblast cells that have been grown from cells obtained via a skin biopsy. Lysosomal neuraminidase also can be measured in leukocytes (white blood cells). However, human cells have two other types of neuraminidase, encoded by different genes. One of these enzymes is present in the cell membrane and the other is in the cytosol of various cells, including leukocytes. These enzymes are not deficient in sialidosis and their activities can interfere with the measurement of lysosomal neuraminidase.

Neuraminidase activity usually is measured by testing the ability of fibroblast cell preparations to hydrolyze, or cleave, a synthetic compound such as 4-methylumbelliferyl-D-N-acetylneuraminic acid. Hydrolysis by neuraminidase liberates 4-methylumbelliferone, which is a compound with a fluorescence that can be measured accurately. Neuraminidase is an unstable enzyme and special precautions are needed to test for its activity. The normal range of neuraminidase activity in fibroblasts is 95-653 picomoles per minute per milligram of protein. In leukocytes, the normal range is 6-60 picomoles per minute per milligram of protein. Levels of active neuraminidase are much lower in sialidosis type II as compared with type I.

### Urine tests

Neuraminidase deficiency may be diagnosed by screening the urine for the presence of sialyloligosaccharides, using chromatography to separate the components of the urine on the basis of size and charge. In unaffected individuals, sialyloligosaccharides are cleaved by neuraminidase and, therefore, are present in the urine in only very low amounts. With neuraminidase deficiency, urine levels of sialyloligosaccharides may be three to five times higher than normal. Sialylglycopeptides, or partially-degraded proteins with sialyloligosaccharides still attached, also can be detected in the urine under conditions of neuraminidase deficiency.

### Histology

Neuraminidase deficiency and other lysosomal storage diseases interfere with the normal lysosomal breakdown of cellular components. As a result, the lysosomes may fill up with large molecules that are only partially digested. In the case of neuraminidase deficiency, the lysosomes fill up with sialyloligosaccharides and sialylglycopeptides. These swollen lysosomes may form inclusion bodies and give cells a vacuolated appearance that is diagnostic of lysosomal storage disease. Neuraminidase deficiency may be diagnosed by histological, or microscopic, examination of a number of different types of cells that may show this cytosolic vacuolation. These cells include the Kupffer cells of the liver, lymphocytes, bone marrow cells, epithelial skin cells, and fibroblasts.

### Sialidosis type II

Infants with sialidosis type II often have visual symptoms of the disorder at birth, including facial and skeletal abnormalities. Skeletal x rays may be used to diagnose the dysostosis multiplex of this type of neuraminidase deficiency. Magnetic resonance imaging (MRI) may be used to determine brain atrophy.

### Prenatal diagnosis

Neuraminidase deficiency may be diagnosed prenatally. In at-risk fetuses, cultured fetal cells from the amniotic fluid, obtained by **amniocentesis**, or cultured chorionic villi cells, obtained by chorionic villi sampling in the early weeks of pregnancy, may be tested for neuraminidase activity. Since carriers of a single mutated NEU1 gene do not have symptoms of neuraminidase deficiency, it may be difficult to recognize an at-risk fetus unless there is a family history of the disorder.

## Treatment and management

At present, there is no treatment for neuraminidase deficiency. Rather, attempts are made to manage individual symptoms. Myoclonic seizures, in particular, are very difficult to control.

## Prognosis

Individuals with sialidosis type I may have a near-normal life expectancy. However, the myoclonus may be progressively debilitating and myoclonic seizures can be fatal. Children with neonatal-onset sialidosis type II usually are stillborn or die at a young age. Those with infantile-onset sialidosis type II rarely survive through adolescence.

## Resources

### BOOKS

Saito, M., and R. K. Yu. "Biochemistry and Function of Sialidases." *Biology of the Sialic Acids*, edited by A. Rosenberg. New York: Plenum Press, 1995, pp. 7-67.

Thomas, G. H., and A. L. Beaudet. "Disorders of Glyco-protein Degradation and Structure: Alpha-mannosi-dosis, Beta-mannosidosis, Fucosidosis, Sialidosis, Aspartylglucosaminuria and Carbohydrate-deficient Glycoprotein Syndrome." *The Metabolic and Molecular Bases of Inherited Disease*, edited by C. R. Scriver, A. L. Beaudet, W. S. Sly, and D. Valle. New York: McGraw Hill, Inc., 1995, pp. 2529-61.

### PERIODICALS

Bonten, E. J., et al. "Novel Mutations in Lysosomal Neu-raminidase Identify Functional Domains and Determine Clinical Severity in Sialidosis." *Human Molecular Genetics* 9, 18 (November 1, 2000): 2715-25.

Lukong, K. E., et al. "Characterization of the Sialidase Molecular Defects in Sialidosis Patients Suggests the Structural Organization of the Lysosomal Multienzyme Complex." *Human Molecular Genetics* 9, 7 (April 12, 2000): 1075-85.

### WEBSITES

Murphy, Paul. "Lysosomal Storage Diseases: A Family Sourcebook." *Human Genetic Disease: A Layman's Approach.* http://mcrcr2.med.nyu.edu/murphp01/lysosome/bill1a.htm.

### ORGANIZATIONS

Canadian Society for Mucopolysaccharide and Related Diseases. PO Box 64714, Unionville, ONT L3R OM9. Canada (905) 479-8701 or (800) 667-1846. http://www.mpssociety.ca.

International Society for Mannosidosis and Related Diseases. 3210 Batavia Ave., Baltimore, MD 21214. (410) 254-4903. info@mannosidosis.org. http://www.mannosidosis.org.

National MPS Society. 102 Aspen Dr., Downingtown, PA 19335. (610) 942-0100. Fax: (610) 942-7188. info@mpssociety.org. http://www.mpssociety.org.

Margaret Alic, PhD

# Neuraminidase deficiency with beta-galactosidase deficiency

## Definition

**Neuraminidase deficiency** with beta-galactosidase deficiency, commonly-known as galactosialidosis, is a rare inherited metabolic disorder with multiple symptoms that can include skeletal abnormalities, mental retardation, and progressive neurological degeneration.

## Description

Neuraminidase deficiency with beta-galactosidase deficiency, or galactosialidosis, is a very rare genetic disorder with progressive signs and symptoms that are almost identical to those of neuraminidase deficiency alone, a disorder that is often called sialidosis. These symptoms can include skeletal and facial abnormalities, seizures, vision and hearing loss, cardiac and kidney problems, and mental retardation. However, as with sialidosis, the severity of the symptoms of galactosialidosis vary greatly.

Galactosialidosis is also known as Goldberg syndrome, after M. F. Goldberg and colleagues who first described the disorder in 1971. The disorder is also sometimes called protective protein/cathepsin A (or PPCA) deficiency, deficiency of lysosomal protective protein, or deficiency of cathepsin A.

Galactosialidosis is caused by a mutation, or change, in the **gene** encoding an enzyme called protective protein/cathepsin A (PPCA). PPCA forms a very large multi-enzyme complex with three other enzymes: beta-galactosidase, N-acetylgalactosamine-6-sulfate sulfatase (GALNS), and alpha-N-acetylneuraminidase. The latter enzyme is commonly referred to as neuraminidase or sialidase. Whereas sialidosis is caused by a mutation in the gene encoding neuraminidase, a mutation in the gene encoding PPCA can affect the activities of all of the enzymes in the complex. However neuraminidase is the enzyme that is most dependent on PPCA. Without functional PPCA, there is little or no neuraminidase activity. Although beta-galactosidase activity is reduced, a significant amount of active enzyme remains. Therefore, the symptoms of neuraminidase deficiency with beta-galactosidase deficiency are more similar to those of sialidosis than to those of beta-galactosidase deficiency. Mutations in the gene encoding beta-galactosidase can result in the disorders known as **GM1-gangliosidosis** (beta-galactosidosis) or Morquio B disease.

Galactosialidosis is subdivided into three types, depending on the age of onset: severe, neonatal or early-infantile; milder, late-infantile; and juvenile/adult. The juvenile/adult form is the most common. There also is an atypical form of galactosialidosis. The type and severity of the disorder depends on the specific mutation(s) present in the genes encoding PPCA.

### Lysosomal storage diseases

Neuraminidase, beta-galactosidase, PPCA, and GALNS are all enzymes that function inside lysosomes. Lysosomes are membrane-bound spherical compartments or vesicles within the cytosol (fluid part) of cells. Lysosomes contain more than 50 different enzymes that are responsible for digesting, or hydrolyzing, large molecules and cellular components. These include proteins, polysaccharides (long, linear or branched chains of sugars), and lipids, which are large, insoluble biomolecules that are usually built from fatty acids. The smaller breakdown products from the lysosome are recycled back to the cytosol.

Galactosialidosis is one of at least 41 genetically distinct lysosomal storage diseases. In these disorders, some of the macromolecules in the lysosome cannot be degraded. Instead, these large molecules, or their partial-breakdown products, accumulate, and the lysosomes swell to the point that cellular function is disrupted.

### Neuraminidase deficiency

Neuraminidase removes sialic acid from the ends of oligosaccharides, which are relatively short chains of sugars. Sialic acid, also known as N-acetylneuraminic acid, is a type of sugar molecule that often is at an end of an oligosaccharide. These oligosaccharides with terminal sialic acid residues may be attached to proteins, called glycoproteins.

Neuraminidase deficiency prevents the breakdown of oligosaccharides and glycoproteins that contain sialic acid and leads to the accumulation and excretion of these substances. It also can lead to the production of abnormal proteins. Following protein synthesis, some lysosomal enzymes reach the lysosome in an inactive form and require further processing for activation. One such processing step is the neuraminidase-catalyzed removal of sialic acid residues from oligosaccharides on enzymes. Thus, under conditions of neuraminidase deficiency, other lysosomal enzymes may not behave properly.

### Protective protein/cathepsin A

PPCA is required for the transport of neuraminidase to the lysosome. Once inside the lysosome, the enzymatic activity of PPCA may be involved in the activation of neuraminidase. Furthermore, PPCA mediates the association of multiple molecules of neuraminidase and beta-galactosidase, as well as GALNS. In the absence of PPCA, all three enzymes are rapidly degraded in the lysosome. Thus, PPCA protects and stabilizes these enzyme activities. In the absence of PPCA, substrates for these enzymes may accumulate to dangerous levels.

Gangliosides are very complex components of cell membranes. They are made up of a long-chain amino alcohol called sphingosine, a long-chain fatty acid, and a very complex oligosaccharide that contains sialic acid. The lysosomal beta-galactosidase is responsible for hydrolyzing gangliosides.

GALNS catalyzes the first step in the lysosomal breakdown of a special type of sugar called keratan sulfate. Both gangliosides and keratan sulfate may accumulate in galactosialidosis.

In addition to its protective functions, PPCA has at least three enzymatic activities of its own, including the ability to cleave (break apart), or hydrolyze, other proteins. Some of the neurological abnormalities that develop with galactosialidosis may be due to the loss of this activity, particularly PPCAs ability to cleave endothelin-1. This peptide is overabundant and abnormally distributed in the neurons and glial cells of the brain and spinal cord of individuals with galactosialidosis.

### Genetic profile

Galactosialidosis is an autosomal recessive disorder that can be caused by any one of a number of different mutations in the gene encoding PPCA. This gene is known as PPGB, for beta-galactosidase protective protein. The disorder is autosomal since the PPGB gene is located on **chromosome** 20, rather than on the X or Y sex chromosomes. The disorder is recessive because it only develops when both genes encoding PPCA, one inherited from each parent, are abnormal. However, the two defective genes do not need to carry the same mutations. If the two mutations are identical, the individual is a homozygote. If the two mutations are different, the affected individual is called a compound heterozygote.

#### PPCA mutations

The type of galactosialidosis and the severity of the symptoms depend on the specific mutations that are present. In general, the higher the level of PPCA activity in the lysosomes, the milder the characteristics of galactosialidosis, and the later the onset of disease.

With some mutations of the PPGB gene, very little of the precursor protein to PPCA is produced and there is no mature PPCA in the lysosome. With other mutations, the precursor protein may not be correctly processed into mature protein. Some individuals with severe early-infantile galactosialidosis carry mutations that prevent precursor PPCA from being targeted to the lysosome. The lysosomes of these individuals have no PPCA.

In contrast, individuals with the late-infantile form of galactosialidosis carry at least one mutant PPGB gene whose product can reach the lysosome. However, there may be only a small amount of PPCA in the lysosome; the PPCA may lack enzymatic activity; the PPCA chains may be unable to combine to form the normal two-chained form; or the PPCA may be degraded rapidly. Nevertheless, with these mutations, the symptoms of galactosialidosis are mild and progress very slowly with no mental retardation.

Other identified mutations prevent the PPCA molecules from folding properly or shorten the PPCA protein so that it cannot form a complex with the other enzymes.

Compound heterozygotes, with different mutations in their PPGB genes, usually have symptoms that are intermediate in severity between those of homozygotes for each of the two mutations. Occasionally, the symptoms of a compound heterozygote may be more mild than those of either homozygote, because the two mutant PPCA proteins can complement, or compensate, for each other's abnormalities.

### Demographics

As an autosomal recessive disorder, neuraminidase deficiency with beta-galactosidase deficiency occurs with equal frequency among males and females. Since it requires two defective copies of the PPGB gene, one inherited from each parent, it is much more common in the offspring of couples who are related to each other (consanguineous marriages), such as first or second cousins.

Galactosialidosis appears to occur with the highest frequency among Japanese. The juvenile/adult form is particularly common among Japanese and specific mutations in the PPGB gene occur with a high frequency in this population.

### Signs and symptoms

Although the features of galactosialidosis vary greatly, they are very similar to those of neuraminidase deficiency (sialidosis). These progressive symptoms include red spots in the eyes, known as cherry-red macules. Eventually, the corneas may be become cloudy and cataracts and blindness may develop. Hearing loss is also common with galactosialidosis.

Myoclonus are sudden involuntary muscle contractions, which may eventually develop into myoclonic seizures. The myoclonus may become debilitating.

Tremors and various other neurological conditions may develop. There may be a progressive loss of muscle coordination, called ataxia, and walking and standing may become increasingly difficult.

Small red skin lesions called angiokeratoma are signs of galactosialidosis. Swollen liver and spleen (hepatosplenomegaly) may develop. Cardiac disease can be one of the major consequences of the disorder.

Symptoms of the more severe forms of galactosialidosis include coarse or malformed facial features and a variety of skeletal malformations (dysostosis multiplex), including short stature. Mental retardation also may be present. Galactosialidosis is one cause of nonimmune **hydrops fetalis**, the excessive accumulation of fluid in the fetus.

## Diagnosis

### Early-infantile onset

Some findings of the disorder, including facial and skeletal abnormalities, may be apparent at birth. Skeletal x rays may be used to diagnose dysostosis multiplex. Magnetic resonance imaging (MRI) or computer tomography (CT) scans may be used to determine brain atrophy. An electroencephalogram (EEG) may indicate epileptic activity.

### Neuraminidase activity

Typically, neuraminidase deficiency is diagnosed by measuring the activity of the enzyme in cultures of fibroblast cells (connective tissue cells) that have been grown from cells obtained by a skin biopsy. Neuraminidase activity usually is measured by testing the ability of fibroblast cell preparations to hydrolyze, or cleave, a synthetic compound such as 4-methylumbelliferyl-D-N-acetylneuraminic acid. Hydrolysis by neuraminidase liberates 4-methylumbelliferone, which is a compound with a fluorescence that can be measured accurately. The normal range of neuraminidase activity in fibroblasts is 95–653 picomoles per min per mg of protein. With galactosialidosis, neuraminidase activity in fibroblasts may be less than 4% of normal.

### Beta-galactosidase activity

Beta-galactosidase activity in blood cells is measured in much the same way as neuraminidase activity in fibroblasts. Using the substrate 4-methylumbelliferyl-alpha-D-galactopyranoside, the fluorescence of 4-methylumbelliferone that is liberated through the action of beta-galactosidase is measured.

In severe forms of galactosialidosis, beta-galactosidase activity is less than 15% of normal and neuraminidase activity is less than 1% of normal. The combination of low beta-galactosidase and low neuraminidase in fibroblasts, with normal levels of other lysosomal enzymes, is diagnostic for galactosialidosis.

### PPCA activity

The enzymatic activity of PPCA also can be measured in fibroblasts. In the early-infantile form of galactosialidosis, PPCA activity may be completely lacking. A small amount of PPCA activity (2–5% of normal) usually is present in the lysosomes of individuals with other forms of galactosialidosis. The highest levels of PPCA activity are associated with the least severe and later-onset forms of the disorder. Carriers with a single mutated PPGB gene may have only half of the normal level of PPCA activity, although they are without symptoms of the disorder.

### Histology

In neuraminidase deficiency with beta-galactosidase deficiency, the lysosomes fill with sialyloligosaccharides and sialylglycopeptides (partially degraded proteins with sialyloligosaccharides still attached). These swollen lysosomes may form inclusion bodies and give cells a vacuolated appearance that is diagnostic of lysosomal storage disease.

Neuraminidase deficiency may be diagnosed by histological, or microscopic, examination of a number of different types of cells that may show this cytosolic vacuolation. These cells include the Kupffer cells of the liver, lymphocytes (white blood cells that produce antibodies), bone marrow cells, epithelial skin cells, fibroblasts, and Schwann cells, which form the myelin sheaths of nerve fibers.

### Urine tests

Neuraminidase deficiency may be diagnosed by screening the urine for the presence of sialyloligosaccharides, using chromatography to separate the components of the urine on the basis of size and charge. In unaffected individuals, sialyloligosaccharides are cleaved by neuraminidase and, therefore, are present in the urine in only very low amounts. With neuraminidase deficiency, urine levels of sialyloligosaccharides may be three to five times higher than normal.

Sialylglycopeptides can be detected in the urine under conditions of neuraminidase deficiency. In neuraminidase deficiency with beta-galactosidase deficiency, keratan sulfate, which accumulates because of the low activity of GALNS, also can be identified in the urine.

*Prenatal diagnosis*

Galactosialidosis may be diagnosed prenatally. In at-risk fetuses, cultured fetal cells from the amniotic fluid (amniocytes), obtained by **amniocentesis**, or cultured chorionic villi cells, obtained by chorionic villi sampling (CVS) in the early weeks of pregnancy, may be tested for neuraminidase and beta-galactosidase activities. Furthermore, the enzymatic activities of PPCA can be measured in amniocytes and chorionic villi. PPCA activity is normally very high in these cells and low activity is an indication of an affected fetus. However, since carriers of a single mutated PPGB gene do not have symptoms of galactosialidosis, it may be difficult to recognize an at-risk fetus unless there is a family history of the disorder.

## Treatment and management

At present, there is no treatment for neuraminidase deficiency with beta-galactosidase deficiency. Rather, attempts are made to manage individual symptoms. Myoclonic seizures, in particular, are very difficult to control. Bone marrow transplantation is being studied as a treatment for severe galactosialidosis.

## Prognosis

The prognosis for individuals with this disorder varies greatly depending on the specific genetic mutation, which determines the age of onset and severity of the disease. Individuals with mild forms of galactosialidosis may have nearly normal life expectancies. However, the early-infantile form of galactosialidosis usually results in death shortly after birth.

## Resources

### BOOKS

Saito, M., and R. K. Yu. "Biochemistry and Function of Sialidases." In *Biology of the Sialic Acids.* Edited by A. Rosenberg, 7–67. New York: Plenum Press, 1995.

Thomas, G. H., and A. L. Beaudet. "Disorders of Glycoprotein Degradation and Structure: Alpha-mannosidosis, Beta-mannosidosis, Fucosidosis, Sialidosis, Aspartylglucosaminuria and Carbohydrate-deficient Glycoprotein Syndrome." In *The Metabolic and Molecular Bases of Inherited Disease.* Edited by C. R. Scriver, A. L. Beaudet, W. S. Sly, and D. Valle, 2529–61. New York: McGraw Hill, Inc., 1995.

### PERIODICALS

Hiraiwa, M. "Cathepsin A/Protective Protein: An Unusual Lysosomal Multifunctional Protein." *Cellular and Molecular Life Sciences* 56 (December 1999): 894–907.

### WEBSITES

Murphy, Paul. "Lysosomal Storage Diseases: A Family Sourcebook." *Human Genetic Disease: A Layman's Approach.* http://mcrcr2.med.nyu.edu/murphp01/lysosome/bill1a.htm.

### ORGANIZATIONS

The International Society for Mannosidosis and Related Diseases. 3210 Batavia Avenue, Baltimore, MD 21214. (410) 254-4903. info@mannosidosis.org. http://www.mannosidosis.org.

United Leukodystrophy Foundation. 2304 Highland Drive, Sycamore, IL 60178. (815) 895-3211. (800) 728-5483. ulf@tbcnet.com. http://www.ulf.org/.

Margaret Alic, PhD

# Neurofibromatosis

## Definition

Neurofibromatoses (NF) are **genetic disorders** of the nervous system that mostly affect the development of nerve cell tissues. These disorders cause soft tumors (neurofibromas) to grow on nerves and produce other abnormalities such as skin changes and bone deformities. The disorders occur as neurofibromatosis type 1 (NF1) or von Recklinghausen disease, and neurofibromatosis type 2 (NF2), with NF1 being the more common form.

## Description

Neural crest cells are primitive cells which exist during fetal development. These cells eventually turn into cells that form nerves throughout the brain, spinal cord, and body. Collectively, this system of nerve cells is called the nervous system, which coordinates movement and sensation. Some nerve cells carry impulses from the brain to muscles or other peripheral

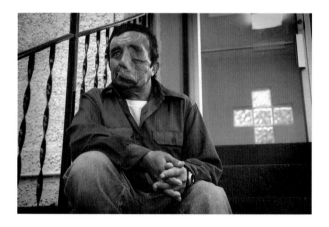

**Neurofibromatosis is a genetic disorder that causes tumors to grow on nerves. It is also characterized by skin changes and bone deformities.** *(AP Images.)*

## KEY TERMS

**Chromosome**—A microscopic thread-like structure found within each cell of the body that consists of a complex of proteins and DNA. Humans have 46 chromosomes arranged into 23 pairs. Changes in either the total number of chromosomes or their shape and size (structure) may lead to physical or mental abnormalities.

**Mutation**—A permanent change in the genetic material that may alter a trait or characteristic of an individual, or manifest as disease, and can be transmitted to offspring.

**Neurofibroma**—A soft tumor usually located on a nerve.

**Tumor**—An abnormal growth of cells. Tumors may be benign (noncancerous) or malignant (cancerous).

structures, hence the name peripheral nervous system. Another group of nerve cells called the central nervous system are capable of transmitting sensation back to the brain for interpretation (such as feeling cold or hot).

In neurofibromatosis, a genetic defect causes these neural crest cells to develop abnormally. This results in numerous tumors and malformations of the nerves, bones, and skin.

### Genetic profile

Both forms of neurofibromatosis are caused by a defective **gene**. NF1 is due to mutations in the NF1 gene located on **chromosome** 17q. This gene provides instructions for making a protein called neurofibromin, produced in many types of cells, including nerve cells and cells that surround nerves, forming myelin sheaths, the fatty layers that protect certain nerve cells. As of 2009, over 1,000 NF1 mutations have been identified. NF2 results from mutations in the NF2 gene on chromosome 22q. The NF2 gene provides instructions for making a protein called merlin (or schwannomin). It is produced in the nervous system, particularly in Schwann cells, which surround and protect nerve cells in the brain and spinal cord. It is believed to act as a tumor suppressor, meaning that it prevents uncontrolled cell growth. A lack of merlin allows Schwann cells to multiply excessively and form the tumors associated with NF2.

Both of these disorders are inherited as a dominant trait. This means that anybody who receives just one defective gene will have the disease. However, a family pattern of NF is only evident for about half of all cases of NF. The other cases of NF occur due to a spontaneous mutation (a spontaneous and permanent change in the structure of a specific gene). Once a spontaneous mutation has been established in an individual it is then possible to be passed on to any offspring. The chance of a person with NF passing on the NF gene to their child is 50%. There are different pathologic alleles (variations of the mutant gene). The frequency of spontaneous (new) mutations is very high and causes for this are still unknown.

### Demographics

According to the National Institute for Neurological Disorders and Stroke (NINDS), an estimated 100,000 Americans have a neurofibromatosis. NF1 occurs in about one of every 3,000 to 4,000 births. It is one of the most common genetic disorders that is dominantly inherited and represents the most common form of NF cases. Recent studies however, now estimate that the incidence of NF2 could be as high as 1 in 25,000 people.

### Signs and symptoms

NF1 has a number of possible signs and can be diagnosed if any two of the following are present:

- The presence of café –au–lait (French for coffee–with–milk) spots. These are patches of tan or light brown skin, usually about 5 to 15 mm in diameter. Nearly all patients with NF1 will display these spots.
- Multiple freckles in the armpit or groin area.
- Most patients with NF1 have tiny tumors called Lisch nodules in the iris (colored area) of the eye.
- Neurofibromas. These soft tumors are the hallmark of NF1. They occur under the skin, often located along nerves or within the gastrointestinal tract. Neurofibromas are small and rubbery, and the skin overlying them may be somewhat purple in color.
- Skeletal deformities, such as a twisted spine (scoliosis), curved spine (humpback), or bowed legs.
- Tumors along the optic nerve (the nerve cells that transmit a visual stimulus to the back part of the brain called the occipital lobe, for intrepretation), which cause vision disturbance occurs in about 20% of patients.
- The presence of NF1 in a patient's parent, child, or sibling.
- Hypertension, or elevated blood pressure.

There are very high rates of speech impairment, learning disabilities, and attention deficit disorder in children with NF1. Other complications include the development of a seizure disorder (an abnormal firing of nerve cells in muscles, causing severe contractions, sometimes involving the whole body), or abnormal accumulation of fluid within the brain (a condition called **hydrocephalus**). A number of cancers are more common in patients with NF1. These include a variety of types of malignant brain tumors, as well as leukemia, and cancerous tumors of certain muscles (rhabdomyosarcoma), the adrenal glands (pheochromocytoma), or the kidneys (Wilms' tumor).

Patients with NF2 do not necessarily have the same characteristic skin symptoms (café–au–lait spots, freckling, and neurofibromas of the skin) that appear in NF1. The characteristic symptoms of NF2 are due to tumors along the acoustic nerve. Interfering with the function of this nerve results in the loss of hearing; and the tumor may spread to neighboring nervous system structures, causing weakness of the muscles of the face, headache, dizziness, poor balance, and uncoordinated walking. Cloudy areas on the lens of the eye (called cataracts) frequently develop at an unusually early age. As in NF1, the chance of brain tumors developing is unusually high.

## Diagnosis

Diagnosis is based on the broad spectrum of clinical signs previously described, which usually can be detected by careful physical examination, ophthalmologic evaluation (visualizing the structures in the eye) and audiogram (test to measure hearing ability). Diagnosis of NF1 requires that at least two of the listed signs are present. Diagnosis of NF2 requires the presence of either a mass on the acoustic nerve or another distinctive nervous system tumor. An important diagnostic clue for either NF1 or NF2 is the presence of the disorder in a patient's parent, child, or sibling. A test to detect a protein (the end–products of a gene) relevant to NF1 mutagenesis has been created, but accuracy for this procedure has not been established.

Monitoring the progression of neurofibromatosis involves careful testing of vision and hearing. X-ray studies of the bones are frequently indicated to detect for the development of deformities. CT scans and MRI scans are performed to track the development/progression of tumors in the brain and along the nerves. Auditory evoked potentials (the electric response evoked in the cerebral cortex by stimulation of the acoustic nerve) may be helpful to determine acoustic nerve involvement, and EEG (electroencephalogram, a record of electrical impulses in the brain) may be required for

patients with suspected seizures. Regular blood pressure monitoring is also advised.

## Treatment and management

There are no available treatments for the disorders which underlie either type of neurofibromatosis. To some extent, the symptoms of NF1 and NF2 can be treated individually. Skin tumors can be surgically removed. Some brain tumors, and tumors along the nerves, can be surgically removed, or treated with drugs (chemotherapy) or x–ray treatments (radiation therapy). Twisting or curving of the spine and bowed legs may require surgical treatment, or the wearing of a special brace.

### Clinical trials

Clinical trials on neurofibromatosis are currently sponsored by the National Institutes of Health (NIH) and other agencies. As of 2009, NIH was reporting 46 on–going and completed studies.

Examples include:

- The evaluation of the safety of Lovastatin in adults with NF1. (NCT00352599)
- The investigation of the outcome of scoliosis and spinal abnormalities in patients with NF1. (NCT00667836)
- A study to identify genes that predict the seriousness of NF1. (NCT00111384)

Clinical trial information is constantly updated by NIH and the most recent information on neurofibromatosis trials can be found at: http://clinicaltrials.gov/search/term = Neurofibromatosis.

## Prognosis

Prognosis varies depending on the tumor type that develops. As tumors grow, they begin to destroy surrounding nerves and structures. Ultimately, this destruction can result in blindness, **deafness**, increasingly poor balance, and increasing difficulty with the coordination necessary for walking. Deformities of the bones and spine can also interfere with walking and movement. When cancers develop, prognosis worsens according to the specific type of **cancer**.

## Prevention

There is no known way to prevent the approximately 50% of all NF cases that occur due to a spontaneous change in the genes (mutation). New cases of inherited NF can be prevented with careful **genetic counseling**. A person with NF can be made to understand that each of his or her offspring has a 50%

chance of also having NF when a parent has NF. Special tests can be performed on the fetus (developing baby) during pregnancy to determine if the fetus will be born with this disorder. **Amniocentesis** (where a needle is passed through the mother's abdomen into the amniotic sac which contains the amniotic fluid and cushions the developing fetus) or chorionic villus sampling (a procedure involving extraction of a tissue sample from the placenta, the structure which connects the fetal blood with the mother, necessary for nutrient and waste exchange) are two techniques that allow small amounts of fetal **DNA (deoxyribonucleic acid,** the chemical that contains specific codes which determine genetic makeup of an individual) removed for analysis. The tissue can then be examined for the presence of the parent's genetic defect. Some families choose to use this information in order to prepare for the arrival of a child with a serious medical condition. Other families may choose not to continue the pregnancy.

## Resources

### BOOKS

Icon Health Publications. *Neurofibromatosis —A Medical Dictionary, Bibliography, and Annotated Research Guide to Internet References.* San Diego, CA: Icon Health Publications, 2004.

Korf, B., and Rubenstein, A. E., editors. *Neurofibromatosis: A Handbook for Patients, Families and Health Care Professionals,* 2nd edition, New York, NY: Thieme New York, 2005.

### PERIODICALS

Ferner, R. E. "Neurofibromatosis 1 and neurofibromatosis 2: a twenty first century perspective." *Lancet Neurology* 6, no. 4 (April 2007): 340–351.

Gerber, P. A., et al. "Neurofibromatosis." *European Journal of Medical Research* 14, no. 3 (March 2009): 102–105.

Huson, S. "Neurofibromatosis: emerging phenotypes, mechanisms and management." *Clinical Medicine* 8, no. 6 (December 2008): 611–617.

Raj, A., et al. "Neurofibromatosis I." *Ophthalmology* 116, no. 3 (March 2009): 598.e1.

Yohav, K. "Neurofibromatosis type 1 and associated malignancies." *Current Neurology and Neuroscience Reports* 9, no. 3 (May 2009): 247–253.

### WEBSITES

*Neurofibromatosis.* Health Topics. Medline Plus, March 13, 2009 (April 25, 2009). http://www.nlm.nih.gov/medline plus/neurofibromatosis.html.

*Neurofibromatosis.* Information Page. JAMA, 2008 (April 25, 2009). http://jama.ama-assn.org/cgi/content/full/300/3/352.

*Neurofibromatosis Fact Sheet.* Fact Sheet. NINDS, March 4, 2009 (April 25, 2009). http://www.ninds.nih.gov/disorders/neurofibromatosis/detail_neurofibromatosis.htm.

*Neurofibromatosis Information Page.* Information Page. NINDS, March 4, 2009 (April 25, 2009). http://www.ninds.nih.gov/disorders/neurofibromatosis/neurofibro matosis.htm.

*What is neurofibromatosis type 1?* Information Page. Genetics Home Reference, March 2007 (April 25, 2009). http://ghr.nlm.nih.gov/condition = neurofibromatosistype1.

*What is neurofibromatosis type 2?* Information Page. Genetics Home Reference, March 2007 (April 25, 2009). http://ghr.nlm.nih.gov/condition = neurofibromatosistype2.

*What is NF?* Information Page. NF (April 25, 2009). http://www.nfinc.org/what.shtml.

### ORGANIZATIONS

Children's Tumor Foundation. 95 Pine St., 16th Floor, New York, NY 10005. (800)323-7938 or (212)344-6633. Fax: (212)747-0004. Email : info@ctf.org. http://www.ctf.org.

National Cancer Institute (NCI). 6116 Executive Blvd., Ste. 3036A, MSC 8322, Bethesda, MD 20892-8322. (800)4-CANCER (422-6237). Email : cancergovstaff@mail. nih.gov. http://cancer.gov.

National Institute for Neurological Disorders and Stroke (NINDS). P.O. Box 5801, Bethesda, MD 20824. (800)352-9424 or (301)496-5751. http://www.ninds. nih.gov.

Neurofibromatosis, Inc. (NF). P.O. Box 66884, Chicago, IL 60666. (630)627-1115 or (800)942-6825. Email: nfinfo@ nfinc.org. http://www.nfinc.org.

Neurofibromatosis Society of Ontario. 2004 Underhill Court, Pickering, ON L1X 2M6, Canada. (905)683-0811 Or (866)843-6376. http://www.nfon.ca.

Laith Farid Gulli, MD

# ▌ Nevoid basal cell carcinoma

## Definition

Nevoid basal cell carcinoma syndrome (NBCCS) is primarily a genetic skin **cancer** condition. The syndrome derives its name from the cancerous skin lesions that typically begin in the third decade of life. However, the name is not completely satisfactory as there are other manifestations of the syndrome.

## Description

A condition that was first described in 1894, nevoid basal cell carcinoma syndrome has been found in mummies dating back to 1000 B.C. However, the condition was brought to medical attention by Dr. Robert Gorlin, and thus also bears the name Gorlin syndrome. Other names include Gorlin-Goltz syndrome and basal cell nevus syndrome.

## KEY TERMS

**Autosomal dominant**—A pattern of inheritance in which only one nonworking gene is needed to display the trait or disease.

**Basal cell carcinoma**—A cancer originating from skin.

**Carcinoma**—Cancer that forms from tissue that covers various surfaces, glands, and organs of the body; an example is skin.

**Cleft lip**—An opening in the upper lip that can extend to the base of one or both nostrils.

**Cleft palate**—A congenital malformation in which there is an abnormal opening in the roof of the mouth, creating a connection between the nasal passages and the mouth.

**Fibroma**—An unusual growth of the tissue that provides stability and support in the body.

**Genes**—The units of inheritance, which contain the instructions to make one or more proteins; genes are located on chromosomes.

**Macrocephaly**—An unusually large head size.

**Medulloblastoma**—A type of brain cancer.

**Mutation**—A change in a gene that causes it to either not function, or malfunction. This will result in manifestation of a disease, or alter a trait.

**Palmar**—Referring to the palms of the hand.

**Plantar**—Referring to the sole of the foot.

**Polydactyly**—The presence of extra fingers or toes.

**Prevalence**—The number of cases of a disease in a population at a specific period of time.

---

While NBCSS often leads to cancer, it can also result in various other physical findings and birth defects. The most common cancer is that of the skin, known as basal cell carcinoma. However, medulloblastoma (brain cancer) and **ovarian cancer** are also possible. Also frequently present are cysts (fluid-filled sacs) of the skin and jaw, palmar and plantar pits (slight depressions on the surface of the skin), a noncancerous growth on the heart known as a fibroma, macrocephaly, and various skeletal problems.

### Genetic profile

NBCCS is caused by mutations in a **gene** known as "patched" (PTCH). PTCH is located on **chromosome** 9. It is believed to be a tumor suppressor gene. The normal role of such genes is to prevent the growth of tumors. They do this by controlling cell growth and division. It is the presence of uncontrolled cell growth that can lead to a tumor.

NBCCS is inherited in an autosomal dominant manner, meaning that only one of the two PTCH genes found in every cell of the body must be mutated in order to have NBCCS. If a person has a mutation in just one of their PTCH genes, the disease will be present. This will include some of the signs and symptoms of the condition.

Fifty percent of the time, a mutation in the PTCH gene may be inherited from a parent with NBCCS. In the other 50% of cases, a mutation can also occur by chance, in an individual without a family history of NBCCS. If the mutated gene is inherited from a parent, the symptoms of the disorder may be very different than those present in the parent. Some individuals will be more severely affected than others, even if they are all from the same family.

Once an individual has a PTCH mutation, there is a 50% chance with each pregnancy that the mutated PTCH gene will be passed on. If inherited, that male or female will have NBCCS.

While an individual with NBCCS will have a mutation in one of their two PTCH genes, it is the development over time of a second PTCH mutation in skin cells that actually leads to the development of the basal cell carcinomas. Such a second mutation is believed to occur by chance, with the exact factors leading to a second mutation not yet fully understood. A second mutation in other cells may also lead to the other types of growths that can occur in NBCCS, including cardiac and ovarian fibromas, as well as medulloblastoma.

### Demographics

NBCCS occurs in an estimated one out of every 57,000 individuals worldwide. However, this may be an underestimate of the true prevalence. While NBCCS is seen in all ethnic groups, individuals of Caucasian descent tend to exhibit more cases of skin cancer than individuals of African descent. Approximately 0.4% of all cases of basal cell carcinoma are caused by the NBCCS.

### Signs and symptoms

The characteristics associated with NBCCS are variable. The most prevalent symptom with this condition is skin cancer. Small growths (1–10 mm [0.04–0.4 in]) in diameter) on the skin can occur during as early as two years of age. However, if not removed, these can develop into basal cell carcinomas by as early an age as puberty. The number of growths may vary from just a few to thousands.

Medulloblastoma, a type of brain cancer, occurs in 3–5% of individuals with NBCSS. It typically presents around two years of life and occurs in males more commonly than females. Seizures have occasionally been seen as part of this condition, but are not felt to be related to the presence of medulloblastoma.

An increased risk for other cancers has been proposed to be associated with this syndrome. However, as of the year 2005 this has not been definitely proven.

Jaw cysts are another common sign of NBCCS. They typically first appear around 15 years of age. Although often large, they rarely cause symptoms other than tooth displacement. The number of cysts can vary greatly and they do have a tendency to recur after surgical removal.

Various birth defects are more common in NBCCS. These can include **polydactyly**, **cleft lip**, **cleft palate**, various eye abnormalities, minor kidney anomalies, rib problems, and spinal anomalies (such as unusually shaped bones of the spinal column). Interestingly, overall height in individuals with NBCCS is slightly higher than average.

There are many possible eye abnormalities, such as cataracts found at birth, unusually small eyeballs, cysts in the eye, failure of the eye to fully develop, shaky or jerky eye movements, and problems with the nerve connecting the eye to the brain.

Rib anomalies are found in 45–60% of individuals with NBCCS. They generally do not cause any problems, although can be a clue to the diagnosis. The different rib problems can include partially missing ribs, ribs that split into two (known as bifid ribs), and ribs that fuse together.

The kidney problems are not as common a symptom, occurring in 14% or less of individuals with NBCCS. The most serious condition is when both kidneys are fused together, known as a horseshoe kidney. Unusual shaped kidneys, cysts, a single missing kidney, and duplication of parts of the kidney can also occur. However, as many of these kidney problems do not tend to cause health issues, they are not always detected unless specifically looked for.

A small percentage of males will have undescended testicles, a lack of smell, unusual breast tissue development, as well as sparse facial and body hair. These can all be signs of hormonal or endocrine disturbance.

Other features often include macrocephaly and growths (fibromas) in the heart and ovaries. Finally, pits or lesions in the palms of the hand or soles of the feet are very common, harmless findings.

## Diagnosis

To make a diagnosis of NBCCS an individual must have at least two major and one minor characteristics that meet the diagnostic criteria. Alternatively, one major and three minor criteria can be present. Since there are many different symptoms that are considered major and minor, no two individuals with NBCCS will be exactly alike in their manifestations.

Examples of major criteria include:

- More than five basal cell carcinomas, or one before the age of 30 years
- Jaw cysts
- Two or more palmar or plantar pits
- Deposits of calcium or other salts on parts of the brain that can be seen on x rays
- A first-degree relative (sibling, parent, or child) known to have NBCCS

Examples of minor criteria include:

- Macrocephaly
- A cleft lip or palate
- Eye abnormalities of various types
- Polydactyly
- Ovarian or cardiac fibromas
- Childhood medulloblastoma
- Rib or spinal anomalies of various types

There is no exact age by which someone can be assured they do not have NBCCS. This is because each possible symptom can develop at a different time. For example, 90% of affected individuals develop jaw cysts by their second decade, but 10% of affected individuals never develop a single basal cell carcinoma. However, enough symptoms are usually present by the time the patient reaches their 20s or 30s that a diagnosis may be possible.

Alternatively, using a blood sample to test the PTCH gene for the presence of a mutation can also make a diagnosis of NBCCS. However, only 65–80% of individuals with NBCCS will actually have a detectable mutation using the technology available as of 2005.

## Treatment and management

Removal of the multiple skin tumors and jaw cysts is recommended. Failure to do so can lead to both the development of basal cell carcinomas and to social difficulties due to the disfiguring nature of these tumors. Removal of jaw cysts should be undertaken by an oral surgeon and the basal cell carcinomas by a plastic surgeon. Radiation therapy should be avoided as these can cause further development of the basal cell carcinomas.

Ovarian fibromas, if present, can be surgically removed. The same is true for cardiac fibromas, although they do not usually cause symptoms.

Since manifestations of NBCCS can vary, any affected individual should be monitored carefully by the appropriate specialist. These include a dermatologist (skin doctor), dentist or orthodontist, ophthalmologist (eye doctor), pediatrician, and geneticist (specialist in **genetics**). Special precautions should be taken to avoid radiation, in the form of both radiation treatment and sun exposure, as this increases the risk to form basal cell carcinomas. Typical methods to reduce sun exposure, such as sun block and hats, should be used.

Phototherapies (treatment of disease by means of light rays) and topical treatments (skin creams based on vitamin A) are currently under investigation as possible means of treatment.

### Prognosis

The life expectancy of individuals with NBCCS is considered to be essentially average. However, the key to this is diagnosis and proper treatment.

Developmental delay can be associated with the enlarged head size, but intelligence is often normal. Therefore, head circumference should be monitored throughout childhood and any rapid changes evaluated by magnetic resonance imaging (MRI) right away.

### Resources

#### WEB SITES

GeneTests, in association with the National Institutes of Health. 9725 Third Avenue NE, Suite 602, Seattle, WA 98115. (206) 221-2943. http://www.genetests.org (March 14, 2005).

#### ORGANIZATIONS

Basal Cell Carcinoma Nevus Syndrome/Gorlin Syndrome Homepage. 3044 Peoria, Steger, IL 60475. (708) 756-3410. http://www.hometown.aol.com/budcaruso/skinindex.html (March 14, 2005).

BCCNS Life Support Network. PO Box 321, Burton, OH 44021. (440) 635-0078. http://www.bccns.org (March 14, 2005).

Sajid Merchant, BSc, MS, CGC

# Niemann-Pick disease

### Definition

Niemann-Pick disease (NPD) is a disorder of fat metabolism that causes abnormalities of the skin, eyes, musculoskeletal system, nervous system, liver, and lymphoid organs. It is named for German pediatricians Albert Niemann (1880-1921) and Ludwig Pick (1898-1935). Six types of the disease have been identified (A, B, C, D, E, and F).

### Description

Niemann-Pick disease is inherited through an autosomal recessive trait. The different types of NPD are characterized by an abnormal accumulation of sphingomyelin. A sphingomyelin is any group of sphingolipids (consists of a lipid and a sphingosine) containing phosphorus. It occurs primarily in the tissue of the nervous system.

Some characteristics of Niemann-Pick disease may be common for all types. Common symptoms include jaundice, hepatosplenomegaly (enlargement of the liver and spleen), physical and mental impairment, and feeding difficulties. Symptoms for most types of NPD (A, B, C, and D) are seen in infancy or early childhood.

Alternate names associated with the NPD disorder are lipid histiocytosis, sphingomyelin lipidosis, and sphingomyelinase deficiency.

### Genetic profile

Niemann-Pick disease is caused by an autosomal recessive genetic trait, therefore the condition will not appear unless a person receives the same defective **gene** for fat metabolism from each parent. This means that if a person is heterozygous for the trait then they will be a carrier and if they are homozygous then they will show the trait. There is a 25% chance for each pregnancy that the disorder will passed onto the child(ren) if both parents are heterozygous for the trait and a 100% chance if both parents are homozygous for the trait.

The gene for Niemann-Pick disease types A and B has been located on the short arm (p) of **chromosome** 11. The gene for types C and D has been located on chromosome 18. NPD types C and D are believed to be allelic disorders. This term means that the two types are due to different mutations (a change in building block sequences) of the same gene. Type E is similar to type C and may be a variant form. It is possible that

## KEY TERMS

**Hepatosplenomegaly**—Enlargement of the liver and spleen.

**Macula**—Abnormal pigmentation in the tissue of the eye.

**Sphingomyelin**—A group of sphingolipids containing phosphorus.

**Sphingomyelinase**—Enzyme required to breakdown sphingomyelin into ceramide.

type F is a mild form of type B but as of the early 2000s there is no supportive research.

### Demographics

Niemann-Pick disease affects males and females equally and has been identified in all races. Type A is the most common form of the disease and is responsible for about 80% of NPD cases.

Types A and B occur mainly in families of eastern European Jewish descent (Ashkenazi). It is estimated that one in 75 may be carriers. Type B is also common in individuals from Tunisia, Morocco, and Algeria. Type C is more common in Spanish-Americans in southern New Mexico and Colorado. As of the early 2000s, it is believed that over 300 people in the United States are affected with type C and an estimated one million worldwide. Type D occurs in French-Canadian descendents from Nova Scotia. Type F has been found to affect people of Spanish descent. As of the early 2000s, it is not clear as to which populations are affected by type E.

### Signs and symptoms

#### Type A

This is the infantile or acute form of Niemann-Pick disease. Abnormal accumulation of sphingomyelin is seen in the developing fetus. Sphingomyelin accumulation could represent 2-5% of the total body weight in individuals with type A. Symptoms may progress rapidly and include the following:

• Hepatosplenomegaly. Enlargement of the liver and spleen is due to the low levels of the enzyme sphingomyelinase. This enzyme is required to breakdown sphingomyelin in the body. The decreased levels of this enzyme cause sphingomyelin content of the liver and spleen to be abnormally high. This occurs between the ages of 6 and 12 months. Accurance of

liver enlargement is seen more commonly than that of the spleen.

• Musculoskeletal abnormalities. Degenerative muscle weakness and floppiness may occur due to a decline in motor and intellectual functioning. This is caused by increased accumulation of sphingomyelin in the nervous system. Seizures and muscular spasms may also occur.

• Macula. Pigmentation in the tissue of the eyes may occur. Formation of cherry-red spots may be seen in approximately 50% of patients diagnosed with NPD type A. This is not visible and can only be detected using special instrumentation.

• Additional abnormalities. These include jaundice, fever, and gastrointestinal (GI) problems such as vomiting, diarrhea, and abdominal distention.

#### Type B

This is the chronic form of Niemann-Pick disease. Symptoms progress slowly and begin during infancy or early childhood. Like type A, type B occurs due to a deficiency of the enzyme sphingomyelinase. Neurological involvement is minimal and usually absent. Symptoms are as follows:

• Hepatosplenomegaly. Abnormal enlargement of the liver and spleen occur due to the accumulation of sphingomyelin.

• Macula. The formation of cherry-red spots on the eyes may be seen in some affected individuals.

• Additional abnormalities. These include a slow growth rate and increased incidence of respiratory infections.

#### Type C

This type of Niemann-Pick disease occurs due to the inability to breakdown cholesterol. This may lead to a secondary deficiency of acid sphingomyelinase. Studies have shown that there may be two types of NPD type C, NPC1 and NPC2. NPC2 is believed to be caused by a deficiency of HE1 (human epididymis-1), which is a cholesterol-binding protein. NPD type C can occur at anytime between infancy and adulthood but is usually seen in children between the ages of 3 and 10. The progression of symptoms in NPD type C is slow and the loss of mental and motor function usually occur in early adulthood. Symptoms are as follows:

• Hepatosplenomegaly. The liver and spleen may be moderately enlarged due to the inability to breakdown cholesterol.

- Musculoskeletal. Psychomotor dysfunction, seizures, tremors, and spasticity of the muscles result due to excessive accumulation of cholesterol in the brain. An individual with NPD type C may also exhibit extreme muscle weakness due to emotional excitement and ataxia. Ataxia is the inability to coordinate voluntary muscle movements.
- Eyes. Type C is characterized by vertical gaze palsy. This results in the difficulty or loss of up and down movement. Some individuals may experience opthalmoplegia (loss of muscle ability to move eyes). This is an impaired function of the muscles of the eyes and may cause the eyes to become stuck or fixed in an upward position.
- Additional abnormalities. These include dysarthria and jaundice. Dysarthria is the inability to form and speak words clearly. Jaundice is a yellow discoloration of the skin, eyes, and possibly the mucous membranes.

### Type D

This is the Nova Scotia variant of Niemann-Pick disease. Like NPD type C, individuals with type D are unable to metabolize cholesterol properly. Individuals with type D do not suffer from a deficiency of acid sphingomyelinase. The symptoms of type D are very similar to type C but vary from case to case.

### Type E

As of the early 2000s, many researchers consider this to be a variant form of type C. NPD type E does not usually begin until adulthood and neurological impairment is rare. Symptoms include the following:

- Hepatosplenomegaly. Enlargement of the liver and spleen may occur due to the accumulation of cholesterol.
- Dementia. This is characterized by confusion, disorientation, deterioration of intellectual capacity and function, and impairment of the memory. Dementia is progressive and irreversible.
- Ataxia. Individuals may have an inability to coordinate voluntary muscle movements.
- Opththalmoplegia. Individuals with type E may have an inability to control the muscle movement of the eyes. This may cause the eyes to become stuck in a certain position.

### Type F

This type of Niemann-Pick disease is characterized by a finding of sea colored blue cells in the blood and/or bone marrow of individuals and therefore may be called sea-blue histocyte disease. It affects people of Spanish descent and may be a mild form of type B. Symptoms may include:

- Hepatosplenomegaly. Abnormal enlargement of the liver and spleen may occur in individuals with NPD type F.
- Cirrhosis. The lobes of the liver may become covered with fibrous tissue (thickened tissue). This fibrous tissue obstructs blood flow through the liver.
- Mild thrombocytopenia. Individuals with NPD type F may suffer from a decrease in the number of platelets found in the blood. Platelets are necessary for coagulation of the blood.
- Macula. Pigmentation in the tissue of the eyes may occur. Individuals may develop a white ring around the maculae of the eyes.
- Hair. Individuals may have an absence of hair in the axillary (armpit) area of the body.

### Diagnosis

As of the early 2000s, there is no objective diagnostic test for Niemann-Pick disease types D, E, and F. Types A and B are diagnosed through **DNA** testing or by a blood test. Blood tests for individuals with types A and B will show low levels of the enzyme sphingomyelinase in white blood cells and elevated sphingomyelin and free cholesterol. Type C can be diagnosed by prenatal testing of fibroclastic cells to determine their ability to process and store cholesterol. This is done by testing the amniotic fluid (liquid which bathes and cushions the fetus). Formation of foam cells occurs in all types of NPD and can be determined through a biopsy of bone marrow tissue. Diagnosis of all types is made possible by taking a detailed family history and a thorough examination of the individual.

Symptoms of Niemann-Pick disease may be similar to those of Refsum syndrome (disorder of fat metabolism associated with abnormal accumulation of phytanic acid in the blood and other body tissues), **Tay-Sachs disease** (disorder found in Eastern European Jewish descendents that results in deterioration of the central nervous system), Sandhoff disease (lipid storage disorder due to a deficiency of the enzyme hexosaminidase), Gaucher's disease (lipid storage disease), and Sialidosis (metabolic disorder due to a deficiency of the enzyme alpha-neuraminidase).

### Treatment and management

As of the early 2000s, there is no specific treatment available for any type of Niemann-Pick disease. Individuals are treated on a symptomatic basis. As of the early 2000s, individuals with NPD types A and B have not benefited from enzyme replacement therapies or

## QUESTIONS TO ASK YOUR DOCTOR

- How do the various types of Niemann-Pick disease differ from each other?
- How is each of these types of the disorder diagnosed?
- In what ways, if at all, is the treatment of Niemann-Pick dependent on the type of the disorder my child has?
- Are there groups interested in Niemann-Pick disease that can provide additional information and counseling about this condition?

organ transplants. Cholesterol lowering drugs and low cholesterol diets are often used for individuals with NPD types C and D, but these have not been effective in slowing the progress of types C and D.

Investigational therapies are being tested for types A, B, C, and D. The possibility of treatment by bone marrow transplantation is being tested for types A and B. Studies have also been completed on the use of stem cell (a cell that produces usable tissues) transplantation as treatment for types A and B. Researchers at the National Institutes of Health are studying combinations of cholesterol lowering drugs for treatment of NPD types C and D.

### Social and lifestyle issues

Individuals diagnosed with Niemann-Pick disease may want to seek counseling or attend support groups that focus on the psychological, physical, and social issues that may result due to the illness.

Parents may want to seek counseling or attend support groups that focus on the lifestyle changes associated with having a child diagnosed with Niemann-Pick disease.

### Prognosis

The prognosis for all types of Niemann-Pick disease varies. In type A, death usually results in early childhood. In individuals with types C and D, death usually results in adolescence or early adulthood. Individuals with type B have a prolonged survival due to the decrease of neurological involvement. As of the early 2000s the prognosis for types E and F has not been adequately researched.

Affected individuals and their families may want to seek **genetic counseling**. Pregnant women can receive prenatal testing for NPD type C. Pregnant women that are carriers and have a partner that is a

carrier should receive genetic counseling regarding the 25% chance of the child having Niemann-Pick disease.

Early diagnosis is important. Due to advances in medicine, an early diagnosis may increase life expectancy.

### Resources

BOOKS

Bowden, Vickey R., Susan B. Dickey, and Cindy Smith Greenberg. *Children and Their Families: The continuum of care*. Philadelphia: W. B. Saunders Company, 1998.
Emery, Alan E. H., MD, and David L. Rimoin, MD, eds. "Sphingomylin Lipidoses (Niemann-Pick disease)." In *Principle and Practice of Medical Genetics*, Volume 2, New York: Churchhill Livingstone, 1983.

Laith F. Gulli, MD
Tanya Bivins, BS

Niikawa-Kuroki syndrome *see* **Kabuki syndrome**

# Nijmegen breakage syndrome

### Definition

Nijmegen breakage syndrome (NBS) is a condition in which chromosomes are susceptible to breakage and symptoms include short stature, small head size, and increased risk for learning disabilities/mental retardation, infections, and **cancer**.

### Description

Nijmegen breakage syndrome gets its name from the fact that the first patient was described in Nijmegen in the Netherlands. A registry of patients is maintained there, and patients with the syndrome are susceptible to having their chromosomes break. These breaks result in rearrangements of chromosomes called translocations, in which two chromosomes exchange pieces, and inversions, in which a section of a **chromosome** breaks off and rejoins the chromosome upside down. Chromosome rearrangements in NBS most commonly involve chromosomes 7 and 14. Genes involved in the immune system, which fights infection, are located on these choromosomes; as a result of disruptions of these genes, most patients with NBS have an increased rate of infections, particularly those involving the respiratory system and the urinary tract. The chromosome breaks also increase susceptibility to cancer. People with NBS are more

## KEY TERMS

**Balanced chromosome translocation**—A rearrangement of the chromosomes in which two chromosomes have broken and exchanged pieces without the loss of genetic material.

**Chromosome inversion**—Rearrangement of a chromosome in which a section of a chromosome breaks off and rejoins the chromosome upside down.

**Microcephaly**—An abnormally small head.

prone to chromosome breaks when exposed to radiation as well. Other defining features of NBS are short stature and small head size.

### Genetic profile

NBS is an autosomal recessive disease, which means that one abnormal **gene** from each parent must be inherited to develop symptoms. A person with only one defective gene copy is called a carrier and will not show signs of NBS but has a 50% chance of passing along the gene to offspring with each pregnancy. Couples in which both parents are carriers of NBS have a 25% chance in each pregnancy of conceiving an affected child. The gene for NBS is on chromosome 8 and is called the NBS1 gene, coding for a protein called nibrin, which is found in all cells throughout the body. Normal nibrin is believed to be important in the repair of **DNA** which has been damaged by breaks in both strands.

Most patients have a specific change in both copies of the nibrin gene in which a string of five DNA bases, ACAAA, is missing from a specific area of the gene, leading to a shortened, or truncated, version of nibrin. A few other mutations have been reported in single patients. All of these mutations also result in a shortened, nonfunctional version of nibrin.

### Demographics

NBS is extremely rare. Approximately 70 patients have been reported. A total of 55 patients from 44 families had been reportedly enrolled in the Nijmegen registry as of the early 2000s. Most patients have been of Slavic or other European descent, with a few patients reported from New Zealand, Mexico, and the United States.

### Signs and symptoms

Virtually all patients with NBS have **microcephaly**, or a small head size (in the lower 3%), with about 75% having this feature present at birth. Young children with NBS show impaired growth. Babies with NBS are either born small or begin to experience growth delay during their first two years. The growth rate is normal after that, but the children always remain small for their ages. According to data available, approximately 40% have normal intelligence, 50% have borderline to mild mental retardation (IQ of 55 to 70), and 10% have moderate mental retardation (IQ of 40 to 54). As of the early 2000s, the 55 patients studied in detail showed no correlation between head circumference at birth and IQ. There is a characteristic facial appearance, which includes a receding forehead, long nose, receding chin, extra folds of skin underneath the eyes, freckles on the nose and cheeks, large ears, and thin hair. Patients frequently have café-au-lait spots (areas of skin that are the color of coffee with milk), and other pigment changes in the skin and eyes.

The incidence of certain birth defects is increased in NBS, with about half of patients having malformed fingers or extra skin between the fingers (called syndactyly). A few patients have been reported to have anal malformations, lack of development of the ovaries and consequent infertility, hip abnormalities, and bone, kidney, and brain abnormalities. Notably lacking is the ataxia, which is progressive loss of coordination, seen in a disorder called ataxia-telangiectasia (A-T), which is otherwise very similar to NBS but is caused by a mutation in a different gene.

People with NBS are at increased risk for infections, most commonly affecting the respiratory tract and urinary tract. Infections of the gastrointestinal tract have also been reported. They are also at increased risk for cancer, mostly B cell lymphoma. Leukemia and other cancers have also been reported.

### Diagnosis

A diagnosis of NBS is suspected in children with small head size, slow growth at birth, characteristic facial features including a receding chin and prominent nose, recurrent infections, cancer (particularly B cell lymphoma), and borderline to moderate mental retardation. Prior to the discovery of the nibrin gene, diagnosis could only be confirmed by studying the levels of immune system proteins called immunoglobulins, looking for particular chromosomal changes involving chromosomes 7 and 14, and assessing radiation sensitivity in cells from patients.

Since the gene for NBS was discovered in 1998, it is now possible to look for a mutation in a patient's nibrin gene. As of the early 2000s, all patients of Slavic origin and approximately 70% of the small number of patients in North America have had two copies of the common five DNA base mutation in the nibrin gene. Other North American patients have had at least one copy of another mutation unique to their family. If a mutation other than the common one is found, it is important to do further investigation to determine whether or not it causes disease, as non-disease causing changes have been reported in the nibrin gene.

Adults who are at risk for having children with NBS, such as siblings of patients, can have carrier testing to determine if they have one altered nibrin gene and are carriers for NBS. During pregnancy, the DNA of a fetus can be tested using cells obtained using the procedures called chorionic villi sampling (CVS), in which cells from the placenta are studied, or **amniocentesis**, in which skin cells from the amniotic fluid surrounding the baby are tested.

### Treatment and management

As of the early 2000s, there is no specific treatment for NBS, although folic acid (a vitamin B derivative) is recommended for prevention of chromosome breaks, since repair of these breaks is compromised in NBS. Similarly, vitamin E is recommended for prevention of further cell damage. For treatment of cancer, high doses of radiation must be avoided, since the damage inflicted on the cells could be fatal.

### Prognosis

Patients with NBS have a decreased life span because of the tendency toward infection and cancer. Of the 55 patients in the NBS registry described in 2000, five had died from infections between infancy and eight years of age. Fourteen had died of cancer between the ages of 2 and 21 years of age. The remaining 36 living patients were between the ages of 4 and 30.

### Resources

#### BOOKS

Wegner, Rolf-Dieter, et al. "Ataxia-Telangiectasia Variants (Nijmegen Breakage Syndrome)." In *Primary Immunodeficiency Diseases: A Molecular and Genetic Approach,* edited by Hans D. Ochs, et al. New York: Oxford University Press, 1999, pp. 324-334.

#### PERIODICALS

The International Nijmegen Breakage Syndrome Study Group. "Nijmegen Breakage Syndrome." *Archives of Disease in Childhood* 82 (2000): 400-406.

#### WEBSITES

Concannon, Patrick J., and Richard A. Gatti. "Nijmegen Breakage Syndrome." *GeneClinics.* University of Washington, Seattle. http://www.geneclinics.org/profiles/nijmegen/index.html. (March 31, 2001).
"Nijmegen Breakage Syndrome." *OMIM—Online Mendelian Inheritance in Man.* http://www.ncbi.nlm.nih.gov/htbin-post/Omim/dispmim?251260. (March 31, 2001).
"Nijmegen Breakage Syndrome." *Virginia Mason Research Center.* http://www.vmresearch.org/nbsinfo.htm. (March 31, 2001).

Toni I. Pollin, MS, CGC

Noack syndrome *see* **Pfeiffer syndrome**

Non-polyposis colon cancer *see* **Muir-Torre syndrome**

# Nonketotic hyperglycemia

## Definition

Nonketotic hyperglycemia, or NKH, results from too much of a molecule called glycine in the body tissues, including the brain. It is a genetic disorder.

## Description

Mutations in one of two genes can cause nonketotic hyperglycemia. Mutations in one of the genes, known as the glycine dehydrogenase (decarboxylating), or GLDC, gene causes more than four-fifths of all cases of this disease. Another 10–15% of cases result from mutations in the other gene, called the aminomethyltransferase or the AMT gene. The remaining 5–10% of cases may be the result of other causes, including mutations of a gene known as the glycine cleavage system protein H (aminomethyl carrier), or GCSH, gene.

GLDC and AMT genes, the two main genes related to nonketotic hyperglycemia, carry the instructions for making enzymes that are an important part of the mechanism involved in breaking down glycine. Glycine is an amino acid (a building block of proteins) that is important in the transmission of nerve impulses.

When one of these genes is defective, glycine does not break down as it should. Instead, it accumulates in organs and tissues, notably the spinal cord and brain, where it can become toxic. When this happens, the person may experience such symptoms as mental retardation and seizures.

Nonketotic hyperglycemia comes in four forms:

- The classical (or neonatal) type, in which symptoms appear soon after birth. This is the most common form of the disease.
- The infantile form, which usually develops when the infant is about six months old
- The late-onset form, which may have severe and rapidly progressing symptoms
- Transient glycine encephalopathy, in which the glycine levels of affected individuals are high at birth, but return to normal or nearly to normal later on. These children often show few if any effects from the temporary spike in glycine levels.

Alternate names associated with nonketotic hyperglycemia are isolated nonketotic hyperglycinemia, glycine encephalopathy, and glycine synthase deficiency.

## Demographics

The overall prevalence of nonketotic hyperglycemia is unknown. Studies in Finland and in British Columbia, Canada, however, have indicated an incidence in newborns of between one in 55,000 and one in 63,000. The British Columbia study also estimated a carrier frequency of about one in 125.

Both males and female children are affected with the disorder with similar frequency, but males with the classical type have milder symptoms and a higher survival rate than females with the classical type. The reason for this disparity is unknown.

## Causes and symptoms

Most cases of NKH result from mutations in the GLDC or AMT genes, both of which lead to an overproduction of glycine. NKH is an autosomal recessive disorder, which means that a child must inherit one copy of the mutated gene from each parent. The parents may not have the condition themselves, but may instead only be carriers. Carriers are individuals who do not develop the disorder, but may pass the gene for the disorder on to their children. If both parents are carriers, each of their children has a 50% chance of being a carrier, and a 25% chance of

acquiring the disorder. If both parents have NKH, all of their children will also acquire the disorder.

### Genetic profile

The GLDC gene is located on **chromosome** 9, and the AMT gene is located on chromosome 3. The GLDC gene carries the instructions for making the enzyme called glycine dehydrogenase, and the AMT gene holds the blueprint for making an enzyme called aminomethyltransferase. These two enzymes are part of an enzyme complex — known as the glycine cleavage system — that works in mitochondria (the powerhouses of the cells) to break down glycine. Normally, the brain has enough glycine to help transmit signals within the central nervous system. When an individual inherits the mutated GLDC or AMT gene from both parents, glycine does not break down properly. As a result, excess glycine builds up to the point that it interferes with the normal transmission of nerve signals.

Not all GLDC or AMT mutations are the same. Scientists know of more than a dozen different mutations in the AMT gene and more than 40 mutations in the GLDC gene that can lead to NKH. Mutations may include:

- substitutions of amino acids
- the insertion of added genetic material into the gene
- the removal of some genetic material from the gene

Depending on the specific mutation, the glycine dehydrogenase or aminomethyltransferase may not function at all, or may function but in a reduced capacity.

GCSH, the gene associated with a much rarer mutation related to this disorder, is located on chromosome 16, and is also part of the glycine cleavage system.

### Symptoms

Symptoms associated with the classical type of NKH may include the following:

- progressive lethargy
- poor muscle tone (hypotonia)
- difficulty breathing, sometimes severe and even life-threatening
- feeding
- jerking of the muscles, sometimes leading to a failure of respiratory muscles and death
- severe mental retardation
- seizures
- coma

Symptoms associated with the infantile form may include the following:

- delayed development beginning at about six months old
- seizures
- mental retardation that develops over time
- behavioral problems

Symptoms associated with the late-onset form may be severe and rapidly worsen. They include:

- spasms and weakness of the legs
- degeneration of the optic nerve, which is the nerve that connects the eye to the brain and helps produce vision
- mild mental retardation
- abnormal movements of the body (choreoathetosis)

Among those individuals with transient glycine encephalopathy, many show no effects from the temporarily high glycine levels, and go on to live normal lives. In some cases, however, patients with this form of the disease may experience seizures and some level of mental disability even after their glycine levels drop to a normal or near-normal amount. Other symptoms that occur in some patients include:

- sporadic episodes of abnormal body movements
- uncontrolled up and down motions of the eye (vertical gaze palsy)

### Diagnosis

#### Examination

A doctor may suspect NKH if the patient has the set of symptoms described here. To form a diagnosis, however, the doctor will order tests.

#### Tests

Common tests for NKH are urine, cerebrospinal, and/or plasma tests, which identify high levels of

glycine, as well as genetic screening, which may check for mutated GLDC, AMT, and/or GCSH genes.

### Treatment and management

No cure exists for NKH. Treatment may be available for some of the symptoms, however.

#### Traditional

Various treatments may be available to ease certain symptoms. For instance, physical therapy may assist with hypotonia.

#### Drugs

Sodium benzoate may help decrease the glycine overload. It may also help reduce convulsions and improve behavioral problems in some individuals. The doctor may prescribe anticonvulsant medications to treat seizures. Studies are continuing on the use of additional drugs, including dextromethorphan, for the treatment of other symptoms, such as decreased brain activity and delayed development.

### Prognosis

People with classical nonketotic hyperglycemia often have severe breathing difficulties, among other symptoms, and frequently die soon after birth. The infants that do survive the initial breathing problems and begin to breathe on their own usually have profound mental retardation as well as repeated seizures that are hard to control even with anti-seizure drugs.

Individuals with the infantile form of NKH have milder, sometimes remittent symptoms, but typically experience at least moderate mental retardation as the years go by. This form, as well as the mild-episodic and the rapidly progressing, late-onset forms of the disorder are so rare that prognosis occurs on a case-by-case basis.

## Prevention

There is no way to prevent NKH. It is an inherited disorder. Adults who are carriers may wish to undergo **genetic counseling** before deciding to have children so that they understand the risks.

## Resources

### PERIODICALS

Alemzadeh, Ramin, Karsten Gammeltoft, and Karla Matteson. " Efficacy of Low-dose Dextromethorphan in the Treatment of Nonketotic Hyperglycinemia." *Pediatrics* 97(1996):924-926.

Hamosh, A., et al. " Dextromethorphan and High-Dose Benzoate Therapy for Nonketotic Hyperglycinemia in an Infant." *The Journal of Pediatrics* 121 (1992): 131–135.

### OTHER

Hamosh, A. " Glycine Encephalopathy." *Gene Reviews.* http://www.ncbi.nlm.nih.gov/bookshelf/br.fcgi?book=gene&part=nkh.

Saudubray, Pr. J.-M. "Hyperglycimemia, isolated nonketotic." *Orphanet.* http://www.orpha.net//consor/cgi-bin/OC_Exp.php?Lng=EN&Expert=407

National Institutes of Health. " Glycine encephalopathy." *Genetics Home Reference.* http://ghr.nlm.nih.gov/condition=glycineencephalopathy.

"What Is Hyperosmolar Hyperglycemic Nonketotic Syndrome (HHNS)?" *American Diabetes Association.* http://www.diabetes.org/type-2-diabetes/treatment-conditions/hhns.jsp.

### ORGANIZATIONS

American Diabetes Association National Call Center, 1701 N. Beauregard St., Alexandria, VA, 22311, (619) 588-2315, AskADA@diabetes.org, http://www.NBIAdisorders.org.

Children Living with Inherited Metabolic Diseases (CLIMB), 176 Nantwich Rd., Crewe, England, CW2 6BG, 0845-241-2173, info.svcs@climb.org.uk, http://www.climb.org.uk/.

Genetic and Rare Diseases Information Center (GARD), P.O. Box 8126, Gaithersburg, MD, 20898-8126, (888) 205-2311, http://rarediseases.info.nih.gov/GARD/.

Inborn Errors of Metabolism Family Support List, http://just4u.com/iem/.

NKH-International Family Network, 1401 Ridgefield Ave., Ocoee, FL, 34761, (407) 656-7456 or (607) 324-3804, wolfieworks@juno.com or catrosenkh@yahoo.com, http://www.nkh-network.org/.

Leslie A. Mertz, PhD

# Noonan syndrome

## Definition

Noonan syndrome is a condition usually involving a heart problem found at birth, short stature, a broad or webbed neck, pectus excavatum and pectus carinatum (chest deformities), as well as a range of developmental delays. Occasionally, café-au-lait spots (a skin finding) and other features of **neurofibromatosis** may be present.

## Description

First described by the pediatrician and heart specialist Jacqueline Noonan in 1963, Noonan syndrome includes numerous specific features. However, no two affected individuals typically have the exact same combination of these characteristics. As of the early 2000s, there still is no defined list of criteria to diagnose the condition, and no molecular **genetic testing** exists to confirm a diagnosis. Therefore, attributing an individual's features to Noonan syndrome is based upon a careful review of medical and family history, a detailed physical examination, and study of other possible diagnoses.

There are three major groups of Noonan syndrome. The classical type is Noonan syndrome, Type 1 (NS1). This is also known as Noonan syndrome, Male **Turner syndrome**, Female pseudo-Turner syndrome, Turner **phenotype** with normal **karyotype**, and Pterygium colli syndrome. NS1 has been called Male Turner syndrome because so many features overlap between NS1 and Turner syndrome. The striking difference between the two conditions is that Turner syndrome is caused by a **chromosome** abnormality, and affects females only. In contrast, men and women are affected with Noonan syndrome equally.

Individuals with NS1 may often have a heart defect, pulmonic stenosis, found at birth. A chest wall abnormality is common, typically with pectus carinatum at the upper portion (near the neck) and pectus excavatum below it, creating a "shield-like" appearance. Developmental delays are sometimes a part of the condition.

Facial features such as a tall forehead, wide-set eyes, low-set ears, and a short neck are common. Young children with NS1 often have very obvious facial features, and may have a "dull" facial expression, similar to conditions caused by muscle weakness. However, facial features may change over time, and adults with Noonan syndrome often have more subtle facial characteristics. This makes the face a less

**Amniocentesis**—A procedure performed at 16-18 weeks of pregnancy in which a needle is inserted through a woman's abdomen into her uterus to draw out a small sample of the amniotic fluid from around the baby. Either the fluid itself or cells from the fluid can be used for a variety of tests to obtain information about genetic disorders and other medical conditions in the fetus.

**Café-au-lait spots**—Birthmarks that may appear anywhere on the skin; named after the French coffee drink because of the light-brown color of the marks.

**Cryptorchidism**—A condition in which one or both testes fail to descend normally.

**Cystic hygroma**—An accumulation of fluid behind the fetal neck, often caused by improper drainage of the lymphatic system *in utero.*

**Karyotype**—A standard arrangement of photographic or computer-generated images of chromosome pairs from a cell in ascending numerical order, from largest to smallest.

**Neurofibromatosis**—Progressive genetic condition often including multiple café-au-lait spots, multiple raised nodules on the skin known as neurofibromas, developmental delays, slightly larger head sizes, and freckling of the armpits, groin area, and iris.

**Nystagmus**—Involuntary, rhythmic movement of the eye.

**Pectus carinatum**—An abnormality of the chest in which the sternum (breastbone) is pushed outward. It is sometimes called "pigeon breast."

**Pectus excavatum**—An abnormality of the chest in which the sternum (breastbone) sinks inward; sometimes called "funnel chest."

**Phenotype**—The physical expression of an individuals genes.

**Pterygium colli**—Webbing or broadening of the neck, usually found at birth, and usually on both sides of the neck.

**Pulmonary stenosis**—Narrowing of the pulmonary valve of the heart, between the right ventricle and the pulmonary artery, limiting the amount of blood going to the lungs.

**Strabismus**—An improper muscle balance of the ocular muscles resulting in crossed or divergent eyes.

**Suture**—"Seam" that joins two surfaces together.

**Turner syndrome**—Chromosome abnormality characterized by short stature and ovarian failure, caused by an absent X chromosome. Occurs only in females.

---

obvious clue of the condition in older individuals. Other associated features in NS1 are smaller genitalia in males, as well as cryptorchidism. Some individuals with the condition develop thrombocytopenia, or a low number of blood platelets, as well as other problems with normal blood coagulation (clotting).

Another type of the condition is Noonan syndrome, Type 2 (NS2). This involves the same characteristic features as Type 1, but the **inheritance** pattern is proposed as recessive, rather than the more commonly seen dominant pattern.

The final type of the syndrome is neurofibromatosis-Noonan syndrome, also known as Noonan-neurofibromatosis syndrome, and neurofibromatosis with Noonan Phenotype. In this, individuals often have some features of both neurofibromatosis and NS1. It has been proposed that this may simply be a chance occurrence of two conditions. This is because these conditions have two distinct **gene** locations, with no apparent overlap.

## Genetic profile

In 1994, Ineke van der Burgt and others discovered that the gene for Noonan syndrome is located on chromosome 12, on the q (large) arm. They found this through careful studies of a large Dutch family, as well as 20 other smaller families, all with people affected by Noonan syndrome. As of the early 2000s, research studies are taking place to further narrow down the gene location. It is proposed to be at 12q24 (band 24 on the q arm of chromosome 12).

Historically, NS1 has been inherited in an autosomal dominant manner, and this is still the most common inheritance pattern for the condition. This means that an affected individual has one copy of the mutated gene, and has a 50% chance to pass it on to each of his or her children, regardless of that child's gender. As of the early 2000s, about half of people with Noonan syndrome have a family history of it. For the other half, the mutated gene presumably occurred as a new event in their conception, so they would likely be the first person in their family to be diagnosed with the condition.

New studies have identified evidence for other inheritance patterns. van der Burgt and Brunner studied four Dutch individuals with Noonan syndrome and their families and proposed an autosomal recessive form of the condition, NS2. In autosomal recessive conditions individuals may be carriers, meaning that they carry a copy of a mutated gene. However, carriers often do not have symptoms of the condition. Someone affected with an autosomal recessive condition has two copies of a mutated gene, having inherited one copy from their mother, and the other from their father. Thus, only two carrier parents can have an affected child. For each pregnancy that two carriers have together, there is a 25% chance for them to have an affected child, regardless of the child's gender. Consanguineous parents (those that are blood-related to each other) are more likely (when compared to unrelated parents) to have similar genes. Therefore, two consanguineous parents may have the same abnormal genes, which together may result in a child with a recessive condition. The hallmark feature of the families in the Dutch study is that the parents of the affected children were consanguineous, making an autosomal recessive form of Noonan syndrome a possibility.

## Demographics

As of the early 2000s, Noonan syndrome is thought to occur between one in 1,000 to one in 2,500 live births. There appears to be no ethnic bias in Noonan syndrome, though many studies have arisen from Holland, Canada, and the United States.

## Signs and symptoms

Occasionally, feeding problems may occur in infants with Noonan syndrome, because of a poor sucking reflex. Short stature by adulthood is common, though birth length is typically normal. Developmental delays may become apparent because individuals are slower to attain milestones, such as sitting and walking. Behavioral problems may be more common, but often are not significant enough for medical attention. Heart defects are common, with pulmonary stenosis being the most common defect. Muscle weakness is sometimes present, as is increased flexibility of the joints. Less common neurologic complications may include schwannomas, or growths (common in neurofibromatosis) of the spinal cord and brain. These schwannomas may also occur in the muscle.

Many facial features are found in Noonan syndrome, often involving the eyes. Eyes may be wide-set, may appear half-closed because of droopy eyelids, and the corners may turn downward. Some other findings, such as nystagmus and strabismus may occur. Interestingly, most people with Noonan syndrome have beautiful pale blue- or green-colored eyes. Often, the ears are low-set (lower than eye-level), and the top portion of cartilage on the ear is folded down more than usual. Hearing loss may occur, most often due to frequent ear infections. A very high and broad forehead is very common. An individual's face may take on an inverted triangular shape. As mentioned earlier, facial features may change over time. An infant may appear more striking than an adult does, as the features may gradually become less obvious. Sometimes, studying childhood photographs of an individual's presumably "unaffected" parents may reveal clues. Parents may have more obvious features of the condition in their childhood photographs.

Chest wall abnormalities such as a shield chest, pectus carinatum, and pectus excavatum occur in the majority of people with NS1. These are thought to occur because of early closure of the sutures underneath these areas. Additionally, widely-spaced nipples are not uncommon. **Scoliosis** (curving of the spine) may occur, along with other spine abnormalities.

Lymphatic abnormalities may be common, often due to abnormal drainage or blockage in the lymph glands. This may cause lymphedema, or swelling, in the limbs. Lymphedema may occur behind the neck (often prenatally) and this is thought to be the cause of the broad/webbed neck in the condition. Prenatal lymphedema is thought to obstruct the proper formation of the ears, eyes, and nipples as well, causing the mentioned abnormalities in all three.

Individuals with Noonan syndrome may have problems with coagulation, shown by abnormal bleeding or mild to severe bruising. **von Willebrand disease** and abnormalities in levels of factors V, VIII, XI, XII, and protein C (all proteins involved in clotting of blood) are common, alone or in combination. These problems may lessen as the person ages, even though the mentioned coagulation proteins may still be present in abnormal amounts. Rarely, some forms of leukemia and other cancers occur.

Kidney problems are often mild, but can occur. The most common finding is a widening of the pelvic (cup-shaped) cavity of the kidney. In males, smaller penis size and cryptorchidism are sometimes seen. Cryptorchidism may lead to improper sperm formation in these men, although sexual function is typically normal. It is not as common to see an affected man have a child with Noonan syndrome, and this is probably due to cryptorchidism. Puberty may be delayed in some women with NS1, but fertility is not usually compromised.

Lastly, follicular keratosis is common on the face and joints. It is a set of dark birthmarks that often show up during the first few months of life, typically along the eyebrows, eyes, cheeks, and scalp. Generally, it progresses until puberty, then stops. Sometimes it may leave scars, which may prevent hair growth in those areas. café-au-lait spots can occur, not unlike those seen in neurofibromatosis.

### Diagnosis

As of the early 2000s, there are no molecular or biochemical tests for Noonan syndrome, which would aid in confirming a diagnosis. Therefore, it is a clinical diagnosis, based on findings and symptoms. The challenge is that there are several conditions that mimic Noonan syndrome. If a female has symptoms, a chromosomal study is crucial to determine whether she has Turner syndrome, as she would have a missing X chromosome. Other chromosomal conditions that are similar include trisomy 8p (three copies of the small arm of chromosome 8) and trisomy 22 mosaicism (mixed cell lines with some having three copies of chromosome 22). A karyotype would help to rule these out.

An extremely similar condition is Cardio-facio-cutaneous syndrome (CFC), which has similar facial features, short stature, lymphedema, and developmental delays, as well as similar heart defects and skin findings. It has been debated as to whether CFC and NS1 are the same condition. The most compelling argument that they are two, distinct condition lies with the fact that all cases of CFC are sporadic (meaning there is no family history), whereas NS1 may often be seen with a family history.

Other similar conditions include Watson and multiple lentigines/LEOPARD syndrome, as they are associated with pulmonary stenosis, wide-set eyes, chest deformities, and mental delays. Careful study would identify Noonan syndrome from these.

Most individuals are diagnosed with NS1 in childhood; however, some signs may present in late stages of a pregnancy. Lymphedema, cystic hygroma, and heart defects can sometimes be seen on a **prenatal ultrasound**. With high-resolution technology, occasionally some facial features may be seen as well. After such findings, an **amniocentesis** would typically be offered (as Turner syndrome would also be suspected) and a normal karyotype would further suspicion of NS1.

## QUESTIONS TO ASK YOUR DOCTOR

- Are there visual signs by which Noonan syndrome can be diagnosed, and are these signs a sufficient basis for diagnosing the condition?
- What are the most serious medical problems associated with this genetic disorder?
- What information or advice can a genetic counselor provide about the possibility of our having a Child with Noonan syndrome?
- Please describe the challenges we would face in the future as the parent of a Child with Noonan syndrome.

### Treatment and management

Treatment is very symptom-specific, as not everyone will have the same needs. For short stature, some individuals have responded to growth hormone therapy. The exact cause of the short stature is not well defined, and therapies are currently being studied. Muscle weakness and early delays often necessitate an early intervention program, which combines physical, speech, and occupational therapies. Heart defects need to be closely followed, and treatment can sometimes include beta-blockers or surgeries, such as opening of the pulmonary valve. For individuals with clotting problems, aspirin and medications containing it should be avoided, as they prevent clotting. Treatments using various blood factors may be necessary to help with proper clotting. Drainage may be necessary for problematic lymphedema, but it is rare. Cryptorchidism may be surgically corrected, and testosterone replacement should be considered in males with abnormal sexual development. Back braces may be needed for scoliosis and other skeletal problems. Unfortunately, medications such as creams for the follicular keratosis are usually not helpful. Developmental delays should be assessed early, and special education classes may help with these. In summary, these various treatment modalities require careful coordination, and many issues are lifelong. A team approach may be beneficial.

### Prognosis

Prognosis for Noonan syndrome is largely dependent on the extent of the various medical problems, particularly the heart defects. Individuals with a severe form of the condition may have a shorter life span than those with a milder presentation. In addition, presence of mental deficiency in 25% of individuals affects the long term prognosis.

### Resources

#### WEBSITES

"Noonan Syndrome." *Ability*. http://www.ability.org.uk/Noonan_Syndrome.html.

"Noonan Syndrome." *Family Village*. http://www.familyvillage.wisc.edu/lib_noon.htm.

"Noonan Syndrome." *Pediatric Database*. http://www.icondata.com/health/pedbase/files/Noonansy.htm.

#### ORGANIZATIONS

The Noonan Syndrome Support Group, Inc. c/o Mrs. Wanda Robinson, PO Box 145, Upperco, MD 21155.(888) 686-2224 or (410) 374-5245. andar@bellatlantic.net. http://www.noonansyndrome.org.

Deepti Babu, MS, CGC

## Norman-Landing disease *see* GM1 gangliosidosis

# Norrie disease

### Definition

Norrie disease (ND) is a severe form of blindness that is evident at birth or within the first few months of life and may involve **deafness**, mental retardation, and behavioral problems.

### Description

ND was first described in the 1920s and 1930s as an inherited form of blindness affecting only males. Recognizable changes in certain parts of the eye were identified that lead to a wasting away or shrinking of the eye over time.

At birth, a grayish yellow, tumor-like mass is observed to cover or replace the retina of the eye, whereas the remainder of the eye is usually of normal shape, size and form. Over time, changes in this mass and progressive deterioration of the lens, iris, and cornea cause the eye to appear milky in color and to become very small and shrunken. ND is always present in both eyes and although some abnormalities in the eye develop later, blindness is often present at birth. Some degree of mental retardation, behavior problems, and deafness may also occur.

ND is inherited in an X-linked recessive manner and so it affects only males. The **gene** for ND was found in the 1990s and **genetic testing** is available.

---

### KEY TERMS

**Cataract**—A clouding of the eye lens or its surrounding membrane that obstructs the passage of light resulting in blurry vision. Surgery may be performed to remove the cataract.

**Cochlea**—A bony structure shaped like a snail shell located in the inner ear. It is responsible for changing sound waves from the environment into electrical messages that the brain can understand, so people can hear.

**Cornea**—The transparent structure of the eye over the lens that is continuous with the sclera in forming the outermost, protective, layer of the eye.

**Iris**—The colored part of the eye, containing pigment and muscle cells that contract and dilate the pupil.

**Lens**—The transparent, elastic, curved structure behind the iris (colored part of the eye) that helps focus light on the retina.

**Retina**—The light-sensitive layer of tissue in the back of the eye that receives and transmits visual signals to the brain through the optic nerve.

---

ND has also been referred to as:

- Norrie-Warburg syndrome
- Atrophia bulborum hereditaria
- Congenital progressive oculo-acoustico-cerebral degeneration
- Episkopi blindness
- Pseudoglioma congenita

### Genetic profile

It has been known for several years by the analysis of many large families, that ND is an inherited condition that affects primarily males. Mothers of affected males do not show any symptoms of the disease. From this observation it was suspected that a gene on the X **chromosome** was responsible for the occurrence of ND. Genetic studies of many families led to the identification of a gene, named NDP (Norrie Disease Protein), located at Xp11. This means the gene is found on the shorter or upper arm of the X chromosome. NDP, a very small gene, was determined to produce a protein named norrin. The function of the norrin protein is not well understood. Preliminary evidence suggests that norrin plays a role in directing how cells interact and grow to become more specialized (differentiation).

Many different kinds of mistakes have been described in the NDP gene that are thought to lead to ND. The majority of these genetic mistakes or mutations alter a single unit of the genetic code and are called point mutations. Most of the identified point mutations are unique to the family studied. Few associations between the type of point mutation and severity of disease have been described. Other occasional errors in the NDP gene are called deletions, which permanently remove a portion of the genetic code from the gene. Individuals with deletions in the NDP gene are thought to have a more severe form of ND that usually includes profound mental retardation, seizures, small head size, and growth delays.

The X chromosome is one of the human sex chromosomes. A human being has 23 pairs of chromosomes in nearly every cell of their body. One of each kind (23) is inherited from the mother and another of each kind (23) is inherited from the father, which makes a total of 46. The 23rd pair is the sex chromosome pair. Females have two X chromosomes and males have an X and a Y chromosome. Females therefore have two copies of all the genes on the X chromosome but males have only one copy. The genes on the Y chromosome are different than those on the X chromosome. Mothers pass on either one of their X chromosomes to all of their children and fathers pass on their X chromosome to their daughters and their Y to their sons.

Males affected with ND have a mutation in their only copy of the NDP gene on their X chromosome and therefore do not make any normal norrin protein. Mothers of such affected males are usually carriers of ND; they have one NDP gene with a mutation and one that is normal. As they have one normal copy of the NDP gene, they usually have a sufficient amount of the norrin protein so that they do not show signs of ND. Women that are carriers for ND have a 50% chance of passing the disease gene onto each of their children. If that child is male, he will be affected with ND. If that child is female, she will be a carrier of ND but not affected. Affected males that have children would pass on their disease gene to all of their daughters who would therefore be carriers of ND. Their sons inherit their Y chromosome and, therefore, would not inherit the gene for ND.

Genetic testing for mutations in the NDP gene is clinically available to help confirm a diagnosis of ND. As of the early 2000s, this testing is able to identify **gene mutations** in about 70% of affected males. If such a mutation were found in an affected individual, accurate carrier testing would be available for females in that family. Additionally, diagnosis of a pregnancy could be offered to women who are at risk for having sons with ND.

### Demographics

ND has been observed to affect males of many ethnic backgrounds and no ethnic group appears to predominate. The incidence is unknown, however.

### Signs and symptoms

The first sign of ND is usually the reflection of a white area from within the eye, which gives the appearance of a white pupil. This is caused by a mass or growth behind the lens of the eye that covers the retina. This mass tends to grow and cause total blindness. It may also develop blood vessels that may burst and further damage the eye. At birth the iris, lens, cornea, and globe of the eye are generally otherwise normal. The problems in the retina evolve over the first few months and until about 10 years of age progressive changes in other parts of the eye develop. Cataracts form and the iris is observed to stick or be attached to the cornea and/or the lens of the eye. The iris will also often decrease in size. Pressure in the fluid within the eye may increase, which can be painful. The retina often becomes detached and may become thickened. Toward the end stages of the disease, the eye globe is seen to shrink considerably in size and appear sunken within the eye socket. The above findings affect both eyes and the changes are usually the same in each eye.

Approximately 50% of affected males have some degree of developmental delay or mental retardation. Some may show behavioral problems or psychosis-like features. Hearing loss may develop in 30–40% of males with ND starting in early childhood. If speech is developed before the onset of deafness, it is usually preserved. Mental impairment and hearing loss do not necessarily occur together. The role that the norrin protein plays in causing mental impairment and hearing loss is unknown.

Much variability in the expression of ND within a family as well as between families has been observed. On rare occasion, carrier females may show some of the retinal problems, such as retinal detachment, and may have some degree of vision loss.

### Diagnosis

The diagnosis of ND is usually made by clinical examination of the eye by an ophthalmologist. Gene testing can be pursued as well, keeping in mind that as many as 30% of affected males cannot be identified using current methods.

The symptoms of ND have considerable overlap with a few other eye diseases and ND must be distinguished from the following conditions:

- Persistent hyperplastic primary vitreous (PHPV)
- Familial exudative vitroeretinopathy (FEVR)
- Retinoblastoma (RB)
- Retinopathy of prematurity (ROP)
- Incontinentia pigmenti type 2 (IP2)

The first two diseases have been shown to also be associated with mutations in the NDP gene and may represent a more mild condition in the broad spectrum of ND.

### Treatment and management

Since the symptoms of ND are often present at birth, little can be done to change them or prevent the disease from progressing. If the retina is still attached to the back of the eye, surgery or laser therapy may be helpful. An ophthalmologist should follow all children with ND to monitor the changes in the disease, including the pressure within the eye. Occasionally, surgery may be necessary. Rarely, the eye is removed because of pain.

The child's hearing should also be monitored regularly so that deafness can be detected early. For individuals with hearing loss, hearing aids are usually quite successful. Cochlear implants may be considered when hearing aids are not helpful in restoring hearing.

Developmental delays or mental retardation as well as lifelong behavioral problems can be a continuous challenge. Educational intervention and therapies may be helpful and can maximize a person's educational potential.

### Prognosis

The life span of an individual with ND may be within the normal range. Risks associated with deafness, blindness, and mental retardation, including

---

injury or illness, might shorten the life span. General health, however, is normal.

### Resources

**WEBSITES**

Sims, Katherine B., MD. "Norrie Disease." [July 19, 1999] *GeneClinics*. University of Washington, Seattle. http://www.geneclinics.org/profiles/norrie/details.html.

**ORGANIZATIONS**

American Council of the Blind. 1155 15th St. NW, Suite 720, Washington, DC 20005. (202) 467-5081 or (800) 424-8666. http://www.acb.org.

American Society for Deaf Children. PO Box 3355, Gettysburg, PA 17325. (800) 942-ASDC or (717) 334-7922 v/tty. http://www.deafchildren.org/asdc2k/home/home.shtml.

National Association of the Deaf. 814 Thayer, Suite 250, Silver Spring, MD 20910-4500. (301) 587-1788. nadinfo@nad.org. http://www.nad.org.

National Federation for the Blind. 1800 Johnson St., Baltimore, MD 21230. (410) 659-9314. epc@roundley.com. http://www.nfb.org.

Norrie Disease Association. Massachusetts General Hospital, E #6217, 149 13th St., Charlestown, MA 02129. (617) 726-5718. sims@helix.mgh.harvard.edu.

Jennifer Elizabeth Neil, MS, CGC

O

Obesity-hypotonia syndrome *see* **Cohen syndrome**

Oculo-auriculo-vertebral spectrum *see* **Goldenhar syndrome**

# Oculo-digito-esophago-duodenal syndrome

## Definition

Oculo-digito-esophago-duodenal syndrome (ODED) is a rare genetic disorder characterized by multiple conditions including various hand and foot abnormalities, small head (**microcephaly**), incompletely formed esophagus and small intestine (esophageal/duodenal atresia), an extra eye fold (short palpebral fissures), and learning disabilities.

## Description

Individuals diagnosed with oculo-digito-esophago-duodenal syndrome usually have a small head (microcephaly), fused toes (syndactyly), shortened fingers (mesobrachyphalangy), permanently outwardly curved fingers (clinodactyly), an extra eyelid fold (palpebral fissures), and learning delays. Other features can include backbone abnormalities (vertebral anomalies), an opening between the esophagus and the windpipe (tracheoesophageal fistula), and/or an incompletely formed esophagus or intestines (esophageal or duodenal atresia). The syndrome was first described by Dr. Murray Feingold in 1975. The underlying cause of the different features of ODED is not fully understood. ODED is also known as Feingold syndrome, microcephaly mesobranchyphalangy tracheoesophageal fistula syndrome (MMT syndrome), and Microcephaly-oculo-digito-esophago-duodenal (MODED) syndrome.

## Genetic profile

The genetic cause of oculo-digito-esophago-duodenal syndrome is not fully understood. One study located an inherited region on the short arm of **chromosome** 2 that appears to cause ODED when mutated. However, it is still not clear if the features of ODED are caused by a single mutation in one gene or the deletion of several side-by-side genes (contiguous genes). Additionally, since this study is the first published molecular genetic study that has determined a specific location for ODED, it is unknown if most cases of ODED are caused by a mutation in this area or if ODED can be caused by genes at other locations as well.

Although the specific location and cause of ODED is not fully determined, it is known that ODED is inherited in families through a specific autosomal dominant pattern. Every individual has approximately 30,000-35,000 genes that tell their bodies how to form and function. Each gene is present in pairs, since one is inherited from their mother and one is inherited from their father. In an autosomal dominant condition, only one non-working copy of the gene for a particular condition is necessary for a person to experience symptoms of the condition. If a parent has an autosomal dominant condition, there is a 50% chance for each child to have the same or similar condition. Thus, individuals inheriting the same non-working gene in the same family can have very different symptoms. For example, approximately 28% of individuals affected by ODED have esophageal or duodenal atresia while hand anomalies are present in almost 100% of affected individuals. The difference in physical findings within the same family is known as variable penetrance or intrafamilial variability.

## Demographics

Oculo-digito-esophago-duodenal syndrome is a rare genetic condition. As of the early 2000s, only 90 patients affected by ODED have been reported in the literature. However, scientists believe that ODED has not been diagnosed in many affected individuals and suggest that ODED is more common than previously thought. The ethnic origin of individuals affected by ODED is varied and is not specific to any one country or group.

### Signs and symptoms

The signs and symptoms of oculo-digito-esophago-duodenal syndrome vary from individual to individual. Most (86-94%) individuals diagnosed with ODED have a small head (microcephaly) and finger anomalies such as shortened fingers (mesobrachyphalangy), permanently curved fingers (clinodactyly), and/or missing fingers. Over half of affected individuals also have fused toes (syndactyly). Between 45% and 85% of individuals affected by ODED have developmental delays and/or mental retardation. Other features can include an extra eyelid fold (palpebral fissures), ear abnormalities/hearing loss, kidney abnormalities, backbone abnormalities (vertebral anomalies), an opening between the esophagus and the windpipe (tracheoesophageal fistula), and/or an incompletely formed esophagus, or intestines (duodenal atresia seen in 20-30%).

### Diagnosis

Diagnosis of oculo-digito-esophago-duodenal syndrome (ODED) is usually made following a physical exam by a medical geneticist using x rays of the hands, feet, and back.

Prenatal diagnosis of ODED can sometimes be made using serial, targeted level II ultrasound imaging, a technique that can provide pictures of the fetal head size, hands, feet, and digestive tract. Ultrasound results indicative of ODED include a "double bubble" sign suggesting incompletely formed intestines (duodenal atresia) and small head size (microcephaly).

Diagnosis by ultrasound before the baby is born is difficult. Prenatal molecular **genetic testing** is not available as of the early 2000s.

### Treatment and management

Since oculo-digito-esophago-duodenal syndrome is a genetic disorder, no specific treatment is available to remove, cure, or fix all conditions associated with the disorder. Treatment for ODED is mainly limited to the treatment of specific symptoms. Individuals with incompletely formed intestinal and esophageal tracts would need immediate surgery to try and extend and open the digestive tract. Individuals with learning difficulties or mental retardation may benefit from special schooling and early intervention programs to help them learn and reach their potential.

### Prognosis

Oculo-digito-esophago-duodenal syndrome results in a variety of different physical and mental signs and symptoms. Accordingly, the prognosis for each affected individual is very different.

Individuals who are affected by physical hand, head, or foot anomalies (with no other physical or mental abnormalities) have an excellent prognosis and most live normal lives.

Babies affected by ODED who have incomplete esophageal or intestinal tracts will have many surgeries and prognosis depends on the severity of the defect and survival of the surgeries.

## Resources

### BOOKS

*Children with Hand Differences: A Guide for Families.* Area Child Amputee Center Publications. Center for Limb Differences in Grand Rapids, MI, phone: 616-454-4988.

### PERIODICALS

Piersall, L. D., et al. "Vertebral anomalies in a new family with ODED syndrome." *Clinical Genetics* 57 (2000): 444-4448.

### WEBSITES

*OMIM—Online Mendelian Inheritance of Man.* http://www3.ncbi.nlm.nih.gov/Omim/.
*Reach.* http://www.reach.org.uk.
*The Family Village.* http://www.familyvillage.wisc.edu.

### ORGANIZATIONS

Cherub Association of Families & Friends of Limb Disorder Children. 8401 Powers Rd., Batavia, NY 14020. (716) 762-9997.
EA/TEF Child and Family Support Connection, Inc. 111 West Jackson Blvd., Suite 1145, Chicago, IL 60604-3502. (312) 987-9085. Fax: (312) 987-9086. eatef2@aol.com. http://www.eatef.org/.

Dawn A. Jacob, MS

## Oculocerebrorenal syndrome of Lowe *see* Lowe syndrome

# Oculodentodigital syndrome

## Definition

Oculodentodigital syndrome (ODDS) is a relatively rare genetic condition with specific medical findings involving the eyes, skeletal system, brain, dentition, and face.

## Description

Most fully described by the German ophthalmologist Dr. Gerard Meyer-Schwickerath and others in 1957, today ODDS is also known as oculodentodigital **dysplasia**, oculodentooseous dysplasia, and Meyer-Schwickerath syndrome.

People with ODDS experience symptoms differently. Overall, the symptoms usually affect the eyes, teeth, hands, feet, face, bones, hair, and brain.

Common signs of ODDS include a slightly indented nasal bone, thin nose with small nasal openings, thin and upturned nostrils, small eyes with iris abnormalities,

---

## KEY TERMS

**Amniocentesis**—A procedure involving removal of a small amniotic fluid sample during pregnancy to obtain fetal chromosome results.

**Cataract**—A change in the eye's lens that causes it to become cloudy in appearance, rather than clear.

**Cleft lip**—Abnormal opening in the upper lip.

**Cleft palate**—Abnormal opening in the upper roof of the mouth.

**Cornea**—Transparent outer layer of the eyeball.

**Glaucoma**—An eye disease that usually involves high pressure in the eye, which can lead to vision problems or blindness if left untreated.

**Iris**—Colored part of the eye, which contains the pupil in the center.

**Magnetic resonance imaging (MRI) scan**—Procedure that shows internal organs and tissues of the body using magnetic fields and signals.

**Mutation**—Small change in the sequence of a gene.

---

small corneas, webbing of the fingers or toes, and weakened enamel on the teeth.

## Genetic profile

ODDS is an inherited disorder caused by mutations in GJA1, also known as the connexin-43 **gene**. This gene is located on **chromosome** 6.

ODDS is most commonly inherited in an autosomal dominant pattern. In this type, family histories are common and the condition may be present in several generations. A person with ODDS has a 50% of having an affected child. The exact signs and symptoms may vary from person to person, even within the same family.

Instances of autosomal dominant **inheritance** with no family history also exist, in which a person develops ODDS from a new mutation that occurred by chance during their conception. There are reports of these chance mutations being possibly associated with an older average age for the father.

Rarely, ODDS has been reported to follow an autosomal recessive pattern of inheritance. In this type, there may be no family history and the condition may only show up in one generation. Two parents would have a 25% chance of having another affected son or daughter once their child is diagnosed with ODDS.

In 1997, Shapiro, et al., reported a unique family history of ODDS. In this family, relatives in successive generations had more severe neurological signs of ODDS than their older relatives, and these signs showed up at an earlier age in each successive generation. Loddenkemper, et al., described a similar family history in 2002, again involving neurological symptoms of ODDS. These patterns suggest the genetic phenomenon called anticipation, which has been described in other genetic conditions. The hallmark of anticipation is people with progressively worse symptoms in successive generations of the same family.

## Demographics

ODDS occurs worldwide, affecting males and females equally. The exact incidence is not known, but it is not a common condition.

## Signs and symptoms

### Ocular and facial findings

Small, sunken eyes that are closer together or wider apart are common features in ODDS. Additionally, one's corneas may be smaller than normal. Other eye findings include **glaucoma**, cataracts, iris abnormalities, poor vision, and an extra fold of skin near the nose at the upper eyelid.

Facial characteristics of people with ODDS can be unique to them and their affected family members. A striking facial feature is the narrow, longer nose seen in the condition. People may also have narrow and upturned nostrils, a prominent jaw, and smaller head size.

### Dental and mouth findings

A common dental finding of ODDS is weaker tooth enamel, making teeth prone to decay and cavities. People with ODDS may also be born with smaller teeth than normal, missing teeth, or have a premature loss of teeth. **Cleft lip** and **cleft palate** have also been seen in ODDS.

### Skeletal and digital findings

People with ODDS can have enlargement of specific bones. These include bones in the hands, feet, ribs, and skull. This can cause the forearm to turn outward in some people. Some with the condition are prone to their hips dislocating.

The hands and feet of people with ODDS can be significantly affected. Some may have severe webbing between their fourth and pinky fingers, so much so that they look like one large, joined finger. The pinky finger may be shortened, curved, or permanently flexed as well. Webbing has also been seen between the third and fourth toes of people with ODDS.

### Neurological findings

Less emphasis has been given to the neurological and other associated symptoms, though they can be very problematic for the person with ODDS. Some people with ODDS have very tight and stiff muscles with increased reflexes. This can result in difficulty with controlled muscle movements such as those needed for walking and speaking. Mental retardation is sometimes seen, and others may have muscle weakness of their limbs that can be similar to paralysis.

Brain changes are seen in people with ODDS. Examples of these are loss in the natural white matter and hardening within some brain structures.

### Other findings

A common finding in ODDS is conductive hearing loss, which is usually related to sound waves not being able to travel through the normal ear pathways.

Thickening of the skin on the palms and soles of people with ODDS is common. It may be yellow-orange in color, but is not usually associated with blisters.

Another occasional finding in ODDS is very fine, dry hair. It may also be sparse and slower to grow than usual.

## Diagnosis

**Genetic testing** from a blood sample is available for those suspected to have a clinical diagnosis. This testing studies the GJA1 gene carefully to look for disease-causing mutations. An abnormal genetic test result is one that finds a mutation in a person's copy of GJA1. Finding this mutation confirms the diagnosis of ODDS. Once a mutation has been found, other at-risk family members can also be tested. Genetic testing can also be offered during the second trimester of a pregnancy via an **amniocentesis** procedure, if a couple desires such information during that time.

Genetic testing should be offered in conjunction with careful **genetic counseling** for the affected individual, the family members, or the expectant couple.

A diagnosis is more often made after the careful identification and study of a person's symptoms and family history. A diagnosis may be suspected by a team of specialists, including an ophthalmologist, dermatologist, dentist, orthopedist, medical geneticist, neurologist, and otolaryngologist.

## Treatment and management

### Ocular and facial findings

The formation or appearance of the eyes cannot be treated and typically do not cause medical complications. Glaucoma, however, can lead to vision loss or blindness if left untreated. It may be treated with prescription eye drops, surgery, or laser treatments. The goal of glaucoma treatments is to reduce the pressure within the eye, thereby reducing the risk of damage to the eye structures and subsequent vision loss.

Some cataracts may be treated with surgery to remove the natural lens of the eye using various procedure options. The ophthalmologist will then replace it with a new, clear artificial lens. Some cataracts, especially those present at birth, may not be treatable and also may not cause serious vision problems for the person.

Facial characteristics seen in ODDS are not treatable and usually cause no medical complications.

### Dental and mouth findings

People with ODDS have teeth that are prone to decay and cavities. Dentists can treat these to prevent further decay; teeth left untreated may need to be removed if the decay is too severe. Common treatment for cavities can include fillings, crowns, or root canal procedures in more complicated cases.

Those with a cleft lip may have it corrected with a surgery in the first few months of life. A cleft palate can be repaired through stages with surgery, often first happening in the first year of life. These surgeries usually require a multidisciplinary team consisting of a plastic surgeon, pediatric dentist, pediatric anesthesiologist, nurses, dietician/feeding specialist, and social worker.

### Skeletal and digital findings

Many of the internal bone changes in people with ODDS cannot be treated. Those with significant webbing between their fingers and toes may find surgery helpful to gain mobility, the use of their digits, or cosmetic improvement. In cases where the bones are not webbed, surgery to separate the fingers or toes may be possible with the help of an orthopedic surgeon and plastic surgeon.

Children with hips that dislocate may require treatment with a harness or splint that keeps the hips in place. If this is not successful, a plaster cast may be

necessary. Sometimes surgery by an orthopedic surgeon is needed to replace a hip in more severe cases.

### Neurological findings

A magnetic resonance imaging (MRI) scan or other imaging study of the brain can document the changes sometimes seen in ODDS. Treatments may help those with increased muscle tone and problems with stiffness. Medications, physical therapy involving motion exercises, active stretching exercises, and occupational therapy can help. A combination of these is important in order for the person with ODDS to gain mobility and independence.

Mental delays and retardation may be assessed by a child development team or early childhood program. Extra assistance is sometimes available through early intervention programs and special education in schools. Social workers are useful to connect families to helpful resources.

### Other findings

Hearing loss is best assessed and treated by an otolaryngologist and audiologist. Once determined as conductive hearing loss, treatments can include the use of antibiotics if an infection is present, ear drops, or hearing aids.

Skin changes are best assessed and treated by a dermatologist. Treatments may include the use of topical ointments or creams. Oral medications or carefully removing the outermost layer of skin to reduce thickness is helpful in some people. Treatments to change the hair texture or thickness is not usually necessary because it causes no medical complications.

A psychologist, genetic counselor, or therapist can be helpful for some with ODDS. Living with visible skin and digit changes can be difficult, and some may find it easier to talk to an objective person or to other families in a support group.

## Prognosis

ODDS can involve a combination of severe medical complications in some cases. Since no two people experience the exact same type of symptoms, it is impossible to predict the ones a child newly diagnosed with the condition will have. No specific lifespan ranges are known, but might be lower in those who have more serious medical concerns. Newer medical treatments continue to offer hope for those with ODDS and their families.

## Resources

### BOOKS

Gorlin, Robert J., M. Michael Cohen, Jr., and Raoul C. M. Hennekam. *Syndromes of the Head and Neck (Oxford Monographs on Medical Genetics, No. 42), Fourth Edition.* Oxford University Press, 2001.

### WEB SITES

*Genetic Alliance.* 2005 (March 15, 2005). http://www.geneticalliance.org.

*Online Mendelian Inheritance in Man.* (March 15, 2005.) http://www.ncbi.nlm.nih.gov/entrez/query.fcgi?db=OMIM.

### ORGANIZATIONS

Oculo-Dento-Digital Dysplasia Support Group. 8810 Orchard Road, Pikesville, MD 21208. Phone: (410) 480-0882. Email: jquasneyjr@comcast.net. http://home.comcast.net/~jquasneyjr.

Deepti Babu, MS, CGC

Okihiro syndrome *see* **Duane retraction syndrome**

Olfactogenitalis of DeMorsier *see* **Kallmann syndrome**

# Oligohydramnios sequence

## Definition

Oligohydramnios sequence occurs as a result of having very little or no fluid (called amniotic fluid) surrounding a developing fetus during a pregnancy. "Oligohydramnios" means that there is less amniotic fluid present around the fetus than normal. A "sequence" is a chain of events that occurs as a result of a single abnormality or problem. Oligohydramnios sequence is therefore used to describe the features that a fetus develops as a result of very low or absent amount of amniotic fluid. In 1946, Dr. Potter first described the physical features seen in oligohydramnios sequence. Because of his description, oligohydramnios sequence has also been known as Potter syndrome or Potter sequence.

## Description

During a pregnancy, the amount of amniotic fluid typically increases through the seventh month and then slightly decreases during the eighth and ninth months. During the first 16 weeks of the pregnancy, the mother's body produces the amniotic fluid. At

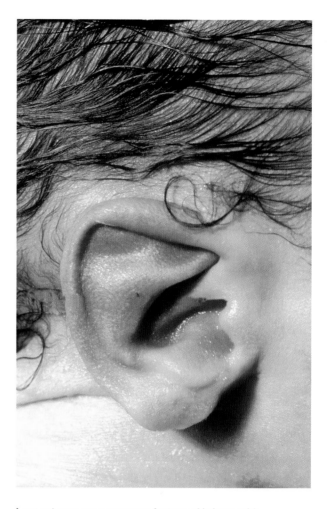

**Low-set ears are a common feature of infants with olioghydramnios sequence.** *(Custom Medical Stock Photo, Inc.)*

approximately 16 weeks, the fetal kidneys begin to function, producing the majority of the amniotic fluid from that point until the end of the pregnancy. The amount of amniotic fluid, as it increases, causes the space around the fetus (amniotic cavity) to expand, allowing enough room for the fetus to grow and develop normally.

Oligohydramnios typically is diagnosed during the second and/or third trimester of a pregnancy. When the oligohydramnios is severe enough and is present for an extended period of time, oligohydramnios sequence tends to develop. There are several problems that can cause oligohydramnios to occur. Severe oligohydramnios can develop when there are abnormalities with the fetal renal system or when there is a constant leakage of amniotic fluid. Sometimes, the cause of the severe oligohydramnios is unknown.

Approximately 50% of the time, fetal renal system abnormalities cause severe oligohydramnios, resulting

## KEY TERMS

**Anomaly**—Different from the normal or expected. Unusual or irregular structure.

**Bilateral**—Relating to or affecting both sides of the body or both of a pair of organs.

**Fetus**—The term used to describe a developing human infant from approximately the third month of pregnancy until delivery. The term embryo is used prior to the third month.

**Hypoplasia**—Incomplete or underdevelopment of a tissue or organ.

**Renal system**—The organs involved with the production and output of urine.

**Syndrome**—A group of signs and symptoms that collectively characterize a disease or disorder.

**Teratogen**—Any drug, chemical, maternal disease, or exposure that can cause physical or functional defects in an exposed embryo or fetus.

**Unilateral**—Refers to one side of the body or only one organ in a pair.

in the fetus developing oligohydramnios sequence. This is because if there is a problem with the fetal renal system, there is the possibility that not enough amniotic fluid is being produced. Renal system abnormalities that have been associated with the development of oligohydramnios sequence include the absence of both kidneys (**renal agenesis**), bilateral cystic kidneys, absence of one kidney with the other kidney being cystic, and obstructions that block the urine from exiting the renal system. In a fetus affected with oligohydramnios sequence, sometimes the renal system abnormality is the only abnormality the fetus has. However, approximately 54% of fetuses with oligohydramnios sequence due to a renal system abnormality will have other birth defects or differences with their growth and development. Sometimes the presence of other abnormalities indicates that the fetus may be affected with a syndrome or condition in which a renal system problem can be a feature. Renal system abnormalities in a fetus can also be associated with certain maternal illnesses, such as insulin dependant **diabetes** mellitus, or the use of certain medications during a pregnancy.

Severe oligohydramnios can also develop even when the fetal renal system appears normal. In this situation, often the oligohydramnios occurs as the result of chronic leakage of amniotic fluid. Chronic leakage of amniotic fluid can result from an infection or prolonged premature rupture of the membranes that surround the fetus (PROM). In chronic leakage of amniotic fluid, the fetus still produces enough amniotic fluid; however, there is an opening in the membrane surrounding the fetus, causing the amniotic fluid to leak out from the amniotic cavity.

### Genetic profile

The chance for oligohydramnios sequence to occur again in a future pregnancy or in a family member's pregnancy is dependant on the underlying problem or syndrome that caused the oligohydramnios sequence to develop. There have been many fetuses affected with oligohydramnios sequence where the underlying cause of the severe oligohydramnios has been a genetic abnormality. However, not all causes of severe oligohydramnios that result in the development of oligohydramnios sequence have a genetic basis. The genetic abnormalities that have caused oligohydramnios developing during a pregnancy include a single gene change, a missing gene, or a **chromosome** anomaly.

Although some fetuses with oligohydramnios sequence have been found to have a chromosome anomaly, the likelihood that a chromosome anomaly is the underlying cause of the renal system anomaly or other problem resulting in the severe oligohydramnios is low. A chromosome anomaly can be a difference in the total number of chromosomes a fetus has (such as having an extra or missing chromosome), a missing piece of a chromosome, an extra piece of a chromosome, or a rearrangement of the chromosomal material. Some of the chromosome anomalies can occur for the first time at the conception of the fetus (sporadic), while other chromosome anomalies can be inherited from a parent. Both sporadic and inherited chromosome anomalies have been seen in fetuses with oligohydramnios sequence. The chance for a chromosome anomaly to occur again in a family is dependent on the specific chromosome anomaly. When the chromosome anomaly is considered to be sporadic, the chance for chromosome anomaly to occur again in a pregnancy is 1% added to the mother's age-related risk to have a baby with a chromosome anomaly. If the chromosome anomaly (typically a rearrangement of chromosomal material) was inherited from a parent, the recurrence risk would be based on the specific chromosome arrangement involved. However, even if a chromosome anomaly were to recur in a future pregnancy, it does not necessarily mean that the fetus would develop oligohydramnios that could cause the development of oligohydramnios sequence.

Many of the genetic conditions that can cause oligohydramnios sequence are inherited in an autosomal recessive manner. An autosomal recessive condition is caused by a difference in a gene. Like chromosomes, the genes also come in pairs. An autosomal recessive condition occurs when both genes in a pair don't function properly. Typically, genes don't function properly because there is a change within the gene causing it not to work or because the gene is missing. An individual has an autosomal recessive condition when they inherit one non-working gene from their mother and the same non-working gene from their father. These parents are called "carriers" for that condition. Carriers of a condition typically do not exhibit any symptoms of that condition. With autosomal recessive **inheritance**, when two carriers for the same condition have a baby, there is a 25% chance for that baby to inherit the condition. There are several autosomal recessive conditions that can cause fetal renal abnormalities potentially resulting in the fetus to develop oligohydramnios sequence.

Oligohydramnios sequence has also been seen in some fetuses with an autosomal dominant conditions. An autosomal dominant condition occurs when only one gene in a pair does not function properly or is missing. This non-working gene can either be inherited from a parent or occur for the first time at conception. There are many autosomal dominant conditions where affected family members have different features and severity of the same condition. If a fetus is felt to have had oligohydramnios sequence that has been associated with an autosomal dominant condition, it would have to be determined if the condition was inherited from a parent or occurred for the first time. If the condition was inherited from a parent, that parent would have a 50% chance of passing the condition on with each future pregnancy.

Sometimes the fetus with oligohydramnios sequence has a condition or syndrome that is known to occur sporadically. Sporadic conditions are conditions that tend to occur once in a family and the pattern of inheritance is unknown. Since there are some families where a sporadic condition has occurred more than one time, a recurrence risk of approximately 1% or less is often given to families where only one pregnancy has been affected with a sporadic condition.

Sometimes examinations of family members of an affected pregnancy can help determine the exact diagnosis and pattern of inheritance. It is estimated that approximately 9% of first-degree relatives (parent, brother, or sister) of a fetus who developed oligohydramnios sequence as a result of a renal abnormality, will also have renal abnormalities that do not cause any problems or symptoms. It is important to remember that if a pregnancy inherits a condition that is associated with oligohydramnios sequence, it does not necessarily mean that the pregnancy will develop oligohydramnios sequence. Therefore, for each subsequent pregnancy, the risk is related to inheriting the condition or syndrome, not necessarily to develop oligohydramnios sequence.

### Demographics

There is no one group of individuals or one particular sex that have a higher risk to develop oligohydramnios sequence. Although, some of the inherited conditions that have been associated with oligohydramnios sequence may be more common in certain regions of the world or in certain ethnic groups.

### Signs and symptoms

With severe oligohydramnios, because of the lack of amniotic fluid, the amniotic cavity remains small, thereby constricting the fetus. As the fetus grows, the amniotic cavity tightens around the fetus, inhibiting normal growth and development. This typically results in the formation of certain facial features, overall small size, wrinkled skin, and prevents the arms and legs from moving.

The facial features seen in oligohydramnios sequence include a flattened face, wide-set eyes, a flattened, beaked nose, ears set lower on the head than expected (low-set ears), and a small, receding chin (micrognathia).

Because the movement of the arms and legs are restricted, a variety of limb deformities can occur, including bilateral **clubfoot** (both feet turned to the side), dislocated hips, broad flat hands, and joint contractures (inability for the joints to fully extend). Contractures tend to be seen more often in fetuses where the oligohydramnios occurred during the second trimester. Broad, flat hands tend to be seen more often in fetuses where the oligohydramnios began during the third trimester.

Fetuses with oligohydramnios sequence also tend to have pulmonary hypoplasia (underdevelopment of the lungs). The pulmonary hypoplasia is felt to occur as a result of the compression of the fetal chest (thorax), although it has been suggested that pulmonary hypoplasia may develop before 16 weeks of pregnancy in some cases. Therefore, regardless of the cause of the severe oligohydramnios, the physical features that develop and are seen in oligohydramnios sequence tend to be the same.

## Diagnosis

An ultrasound examination during the second and/or third trimester of a pregnancy is a good tool to help detect the presence of oligohydramnios. Since oligohydramnios can occur later in a pregnancy, an ultrasound examination performed during the second trimester may not detect the presence of oligohydramnios. In pregnancies affected with oligohydramnios, an ultrasound examination can be difficult to perform because there is less amniotic fluid around the fetus. Therefore, an ultrasound examination may not be able to detect the underlying cause of the oligohydramnios.

In some situations, an amnioinfusion (injection of fluid into the amniotic cavity) is performed. This can sometimes help determine if the cause of the oligohydramnios was leakage of the amniotic fluid. Amnioinfusions may also be used to help visualize the fetus on ultrasound in attempts to detect any fetal abnormalities.

Additionally, maternal serum screening may detect the presence of oligohydramnios in a pregnancy. Maternal serum screening is a blood test offered to pregnant women to help determine the chance that their baby may have **Down syndrome**, **Trisomy 18**, and **spina bifida**. This test is typically performed between the 15th and 20th week of a pregnancy. The test works by measuring amount of certain substances in the maternal circulation.

Alpha-fetoprotein (AFP) is a protein produced mainly by the fetal liver and is one of the substances measured in the mother's blood. The level of AFP in the mother's blood has been used to help find pregnancies at higher risk to have spina bifida. An elevated AFP in the mother's blood, which is greater than 2.5 multiples of the median (MoM), has also been associated with several conditions, including the presence of oligohydramnios in a pregnancy. Since oligohydramnios is just one of several explanations for an elevated AFP level, an ultrasound examination is recommended when there is an elevated AFP level. However, not all pregnancies affected with oligohydramnios will have an elevated AFP level, some pregnancies with oligohydramnios will have the AFP level within the normal range.

Because fetuses with oligohydramnios sequence can have other anomalies, a detailed examination of the fetus should be performed. Knowing all the abnormalities a fetus has is important in making an accurate diagnosis. Knowing the cause of the oligohydramnios and if it is related to a syndrome or genetic condition is essential in predicting the chance for the condition to occur again in a future pregnancy. Sometimes the fetal abnormalities can be detected on a **prenatal ultrasound** examination or on an external examination of the fetus after delivery. However, several studies have shown that an external examination of the fetus can miss some fetal abnormalities and have stressed the importance of performing an autopsy to make an accurate diagnosis.

## Treatment and management

There is currently no treatment or prevention for oligohydramnios sequence. Amnioinfusions, which can assist in determining the cause of the oligohydramnios in a pregnancy, is not recommended as a treatment for oligohydramnios sequence.

## Prognosis

Pregnancies affected with oligohydramnios sequence can miscarry, be stillborn, or die shortly after birth. This condition is almost always fatal because the lungs do not develop completely (pulmonary hypoplasia).

### Resources

#### BOOKS

Larsen, William J. *Human Embryology*. Churchill Livingstone, Inc. 1993.

#### PERIODICALS

Christianson, C., et al. "Limb Deformations in Oligohydramnios Sequence." *American Journal of Medical Genetics* 86 (1999): 430-433.

Curry, C. J. R., et al. "The Potter Sequence: A Clinical Analysis of 80 Cases." *American Journal of Medical Genetics* 19 (1984): 679-702.

Locatelli, Anna, et al. "Role of amnioinfusion in the management of premature rupture of the membranes at less than 26 weeks' gestation." *American Journal of Obstetrics and Gynecology* 183, no. 4 (October 2000): 878-882.

Newbould, M. J., et al. "Oligohydramnios Sequence: The Spectrum of Renal Malformation." *British Journal of Obstetrics and Gynaecology* 101 (1994): 598-604.

Scott, R. J., and S. F. Goodburn. "Potter's Syndrome in the Second Trimester-Prenatal Screening and Pathological Findings in 60 cases of Oligohydramnios Sequence." *Prenatal Diagnosis* 15 (1995): 519-525.

Sharon A. Aufox, MS, CGC

Ollier disease *see* **Chondrosarcoma**

# Omphalocele

## Definition

An omphalocele occurs when the abdominal wall does not close properly during fetal development. The extent to which abdominal contents protrude through the base of the umbilical cord will vary. A membrane usually covers the defect.

## Description

An omphalocele is an abnormal closure of the abdominal wall. Between the sixth and tenth weeks of pregnancy, the intestines normally protrude into the umbilical cord as the baby is developing. During the tenth week, the intestines should return and rotate in such a way that the abdomen is closed around the umbilical cord. An omphalocele occurs when the intestines do not return, and this closure does not occur properly.

## Genetic profile

In one-third of infants, an omphalocele occurs by itself, and is said to be an isolated abnormality. The cause of an isolated omphalocele is suspected to be multifactorial. Multifactorial means that many factors, both genetic and environmental, contribute to the cause. The specific genes involved, as well as the specific environmental factors are largely unknown. The chance for a couple to have another baby with an omphalocele, after they have had one with an isolated omphalocele is approximately one in 100 or 1%.

The remaining two-thirds of babies with an omphalocele have other birth defects, including problems with the heart (heart disease), spine (**spina bifida**), digestive system, urinary system, and the limbs.

Approximately 30% of babies with an omphalocele have a **chromosome** abnormality as the underlying cause of the omphalocele. Babies with chromosome abnormalities usually have multiple birth defects, so many babies will have other medical problems in addition to the omphalocele. Chromosomes are structures in the center of the cell that contain our genes; our genes code for our traits, such as blood type or eye color. The normal number of chromosomes is 46; having extra or missing chromosome material is associated with health problems. Babies with an omphalocele may have an extra chromosome number 13, 18, 21, or others. An omphalocele is sometimes said to occur more often in a mother who is older. This is because the chance for a chromosome abnormality to occur increases with maternal age.

Some infants with an omphalocele have a syndrome (collection of health problems). An example is Beckwith-Wiedemann syndrome, where a baby is born larger than normal (macrosomia), has an omphalocele, and has a large tongue (macroglossia). Finally, in some families, an omphalocele has been reported to be inherited as an autosomal dominant, or autosomal recessive trait. Autosomal means that males and females are equally affected. Dominant means that only one **gene** is necessary to produce the condition, while recessive means that two genes are necessary to have the condition. With autosomal dominant **inheritance**, there is a 50% chance with each pregnancy to have an affected child, while with autosomal recessive inheritance. The recurrence risk is 25%.

## Demographics

Omphalocele is estimated to occur in one in 4,000 to one in 6,000 liveborns. Males are slightly more often affected than females (1.5:1).

## Signs and symptoms

Anytime an infant is born with an omphalocele, a thorough physical examination is performed to determine whether the omphalocele is isolated or associated with other health problems. To determine this, various studies may be performed such as a chromosome study, which is done from a small blood sample. Since the chest cavity may be small in an infant born with an omphalocele, the baby may have underdeveloped lungs requiring breathing assistance with a ventilator (mechanical breathing machine). In 10 to 20% of infants, the sac has torn (ruptured), requiring immediate surgical repair, due to the risk of infection.

## Diagnosis

During pregnancy, two different signs may cause a physician to suspect an omphalocele: increased fluid around the baby (polyhydramnios) on a fetal ultrasound and/or an abnormal maternal serum screening test, showing an elevated amount of alpha-fetoprotein (AFP). Maternal serum screening, measuring analytes present in the mother's bloodstream only during pregnancy, is offered to pregnant women usually over the age of 35. This screening may detect various disorders such as **Down syndrome**, **trisomy 18**, and abnormalities of the spine (such as spina bifida). Other problems can give an abnormal test result, and an omphalocele is an example.

An ultrasound is often performed as the first step when a woman's maternal serum screening is abnormal, if one has not already been performed. Omphalocele is

**Acetylcholinesterase (ACHE)**—An enzyme found in nerve tissue.

**Alpha-fetoprotein (AFP)**—A chemical substance produced by the fetus and found in the fetal circulation. AFP is also found in abnormally high concentrations in most patients with primary liver cancer.

**Amniocentesis**—A procedure performed at 16-18 weeks of pregnancy in which a needle is inserted through a woman's abdomen into her uterus to draw out a small sample of the amniotic fluid from around the baby. Either the fluid itself or cells from the fluid can be used for a variety of tests to obtain information about genetic disorders and other medical conditions in the fetus.

**Amniotic fluid**—The fluid that surrounds a developing baby during pregnancy.

**Analyte**—A chemical substance such as an enzyme, hormone, or protein.

**Autosomal dominant**—A pattern of genetic inheritance where only one abnormal gene is needed to display the trait or disease.

**Autosomal recessive**—A pattern of genetic inheritance where two abnormal genes are needed to display the trait or disease.

**Beckwith-Wiedemann syndrome**—A collection of health problems present at birth including an omphalocele, large tongue, and large body size.

**Chromosome**—A microscopic thread-like structure found within each cell of the body that consists of a complex of proteins and DNA. Humans have 46 chromosomes arranged into 23 pairs. Changes in either the total number of chromosomes or their shape and size (structure) may lead to physical or mental abnormalities.

**Gastroschisis**—A small defect in the abdominal wall normally located to the right of the umbilicus, and not covered by a membrane, where intestines and other organs may protrude.

**Gene**—A building block of inheritance, which contains the instructions for the production of a particular protein, and is made up of a molecular sequence found on a section of DNA. Each gene is found on a precise location on a chromosome.

**Macroglossia**—A large tongue.

**Macrosomia**—Overall large size due to overgrowth.

**Maternal serum screening**—A blood test offered to pregnant women usually under the age of 35, which measures analytes in the mother's blood that are present only during pregnancy, to screen for Down syndrome, trisomy 18, and neural tube defects.

**Multifactorial**—Describes a disease that is the product of the interaction of multiple genetic and environmental factors.

**Omphalocele**—A birth defect where the bowel and sometimes the liver, protrudes through an opening in the baby's abdomen near the umbilical cord.

**Polyhydramnios**—A condition in which there is too much fluid around the fetus in the amniotic sac.

**Thoracic cavity**—The chest.

**Ultrasound**—An imaging technique that uses sound waves to help visualize internal structures in the body.

**Ventilator**—Mechanical breathing machine.

**Ventral wall defect**—An opening in the abdomen (ventral wall). Examples include omphalocele and gastroschisis.

---

usually identifiable on fetal ultrasound. If a woman's fetal ultrasound showed an omphalocele, polyhydramnios, or if she had an abnormal maternal serum screening test, an **amniocentesis** may be offered.

Amniocentesis is a procedure done under ultrasound guidance where a long thin needle is inserted into the mother's abdomen, then into the uterus, to withdraw a couple tablespoons of amniotic fluid (fluid surrounding the developing baby) to study. Measurement of the AFP in the amniotic fluid can then be done to test for problems such as omphalocele. In addition,

a chromosome analysis for the baby can be performed on the cells contained in the amniotic fluid. When the AFP in the amniotic fluid is elevated, an additional test is used to look for the presence or absence of an enzyme found in nerve tissue, called acetylcholinesterase, or ACHE. ACHE is present in the amniotic fluid only when a baby has an opening such as spina bifida or an omphalocele. Not all babies with an omphalocele will cause the maternal serum screening test to be abnormal or to cause extra fluid accumulation, but many will. At birth, an omphalocele is diagnosed by visual/physical examination.

## Treatment and management

Treatment and management of an omphalocele depends upon the size of the abnormality, whether the sac is intact or ruptured, and whether other health problems are present. A small omphalocele is usually repaired by surgery shortly after birth, where an operation is performed to return the organs to the abdomen and close the opening in the abdominal wall. If the omphalocele is large, where most of the intestines, liver, and/or spleen are present outside of the body, the repair is done in stages because the abdomen is small and may not be able to hold all of the organs at once. Initially, sterile protective gauze is placed over the abdominal organs whether the omphalocele is large or small. The exposed organs are then gradually moved back into the abdomen over several days or weeks. The abdominal wall is surgically closed once all of the organs have been returned to the abdomen. Infants are often on a breathing machine (ventilator) until the abdominal cavity increases in size since returning the organs to the abdomen may crowd the lungs in the chest area.

## Prognosis

The prognosis of an infant born with an omphalocele depends upon the size of the defect, whether there was a loss of blood flow to part of the intestines or other organs, and the extent of other abnormalities. The survival rate overall for an infant born with an isolated omphalocele has improved greatly over the past 40 years, from 60% to over 90%.

## Resources

### WEBSITES

Adam.com. "Omphalocele." *Medlineplus*. U.S. National Library of Medicine. http://medlineplus.adam.com/ency/article/000994.htm.

### ORGANIZATIONS

Foundation for Blood Research. PO Box 190, 69 US Route One, Scarborough, ME 04070-0190. (207) 883-4131. Fax: (207) 883-1527. http://www.fbr.org.

Catherine L. Tesla, MS, CGC

# Oncogene

## Definition

In a cell with normal control regulation (non-cancerous), genes produce proteins that provide regulated cell division. **Cancer** is the disease caused by cells that have lost their ability to control their regulation. The abnormal proteins allowing the non-regulated cancerous state are produced by genes known as oncogenes. The normal gene from which the oncogene evolved is called a proto-oncogene.

## Description

### History

The word oncogene comes from the Greek term *oncos*, which means tumor. Oncogenes were originally discovered in certain types of animal viruses that were capable of inducing tumors in the animals they infected. These viral oncogenes, called v-onc, were later found in human tumors, although most human cancers do not appear to be caused by viruses. Since their original discovery, hundreds of oncogenes have been found but only a small number of them are known to affect humans. Although different oncogenes have different functions, they are all somehow involved in the process of transformation (change) of normal cells to cancerous cells.

### The transformation of normal cells into cancerous cells

The process by which normal cells are transformed into cancerous cells is a complex, multi-step process involving a breakdown in the normal cell cycle. Normally, a somatic cell goes through a growth cycle in which it produces new cells. The two main stages of this cycle are interphase (genetic material in the cell duplicates) and mitosis (the cell divides to produce two other identical cells). The process of cell division is necessary for the growth of tissues and organs of the body and for the replacement of damaged cells. Normal cells have a limited life span and only go through the cell cycle a limited number of times.

**Autosomal dominant manner**—An abnormal gene on one of the 22 pairs of non-sex chromosomes that will display the defect when only one copy is inherited.

**Benign**—A non-cancerous tumor that does not spread and is not life-threatening.

**Cell**—The smallest living units of the body which group together to form tissues and help the body perform specific functions.

**Chromosome**—A microscopic thread-like structure found within each cell of the body that consists of a complex of proteins and DNA. Humans have 46 chromosomes arranged into 23 pairs. Changes in either the total number of chromosomes or their shape and size (structure) may lead to physical or mental abnormalities.

**Gene**—A building block of inheritance, which contains the instructions for the production of a particular protein, and is made up of a molecular sequence found on a section of DNA. Each gene is found on a precise location on a chromosome.

**Leukemia**—Cancer of the blood forming organs which results in an overproduction of white blood cells.

**Lymphoma**—A malignant tumor of the lymph nodes.

**Mitosis**—The process by which a somatic cell—a cell not destined to become a sperm or egg—duplicates its chromosomes and divides to produce two new cells.

**Mutation**—A permanent change in the genetic material that may alter a trait or characteristic of an individual, or manifest as disease, and can be transmitted to offspring.

**Nucleus**—The central part of a cell that contains most of its genetic material, including chromosomes and DNA.

**Parathyroid glands**—A pair of glands adjacent to the thyroid gland that primarily regulate blood calcium levels.

**Pheochromocytoma**—A small vascular tumor of the inner region of the adrenal gland. The tumor causes uncontrolled and irregular secretion of certain hormones.

**Proliferation**—The growth or production of cells.

**Protein**—Important building blocks of the body, composed of amino acids, involved in the formation of body structures and controlling the basic functions of the human body.

**Proto-oncogene**—A gene involved in stimulating the normal growth and division of cells in a controlled manner.

**Replicate**—Produce identical copies of itself.

**Somatic cells**—All the cells of the body except for the egg and sperm cells.

**Translocation**—The transfer of one part of a chromosome to another chromosome during cell division. A balanced translocation occurs when pieces from two different chromosomes exchange places without loss or gain of any chromosome material. An unbalanced translocation involves the unequal loss or gain of genetic information between two chromosomes.

**Tumor suppressor gene**—Genes involved in controlling normal cell growth and preventing cancer.

Different cell types are produced by the regulation of which genes in a given cell are allowed to be expressed. One way cancer is caused is by de—regulation of those genes related to control of the cell cycle the development of oncogenes. If the oncogene is present in a skin cell, the patient will have skin cancer; in a breast cell, **breast cancer** will result, and so on.

Cells that lose control of their cell cycle and replicate out of control are called cancer cells. Cancer cells undergo many cell divisions often at a quicker rate than normal cells and do not have a limited life span. This allows them to eventually overwhelm the body with a large number of abnormal cells and eventually affect the functioning of the normal cells.

A cell becomes cancerous only after changes occur in a number of genes that are involved in the regulation of its cell cycle. A change in a regulatory gene can cause it to stop producing a normal regulatory protein or can produce an abnormal protein that does not regulate the cell in a normal manner. When changes occur in one regulatory gene this often causes changes in other regulatory genes. Cancers in different types of cells can be caused by changes in different types of regulatory genes.

Proto-oncogenes and tumor-suppressor genes are the two most common genes involved in regulating the cell cycle. Proto-oncogenes and tumor-suppressor genes have different functions in the cell cycle.

Tumor-suppressor genes produce proteins that are involved in prevention of uncontrolled cell growth and division. Since two of each type of gene are inherited, two of each type of tumor-suppressor gene are also inherited. Both tumor suppressor genes of a pair need to be changed in order for the protein produced to stop functioning as a tumor suppressor. Mutated tumor-suppressor genes therefore act in an autosomal recessive manner.

Proto-oncogenes produce proteins that are largely involved in stimulating the growth and division of cells in a controlled manner. Each proto-oncogene produces a different protein that has a unique role in regulating the cell cycles of particular types of cells. We inherit two of each type of proto-oncogene. A change in only one proto-oncogene of a pair converts it into an oncogene. The oncogene produces an abnormal protein, which is somehow involved in stimulating uncontrolled cell growth. An oncogene acts in an autosomal dominant manner since only one proto-oncogene of a pair needs to be changed in the formation of an oncogene.

### Classes of proto-oncogene

There are five major classes of proto-oncogene/oncogenes: (1) growth factors, (2) growth factor receptors, (3) signal transducers (4) transcription factors, and (5) programmed cell death regulators.

**GROWTH FACTORS.** Some proto-oncogenes produce proteins, called growth factors, which indirectly stimulate growth of the cell by activating receptors on the surface of the cell. Different growth factors activate different receptors, found on different cells of the body. Mutations in growth factor proto-oncogene result in oncogenes that promote uncontrolled growth in cells for which they have a receptor. For example, platelet-derived growth factor (PDGF) is a proto-oncogene that helps to promote wound healing by stimulating the growth of cells around a wound. PDGF can be mutated into an oncogene called v-sis (PDGFB) which is often present in connective-tissue tumors.

**GROWTH FACTOR RECEPTORS.** Growth factor receptors are found on the surface of cells and are activated by growth factors. Growth factors send signals to the center of the cell (nucleus) and stimulate cells that are at rest to enter the cell cycle. Different cells have different growth factors receptors. Mutations in a proto-oncogene that are growth factor receptors can result in oncogenes that produce receptors that do not require growth factors to stimulate cell growth. Overstimulation of cells to enter the cell cycle

can result and promote uncontrolled cell growth. Most proto-oncogene growth factor receptors are called tyrosine kinases and are very involved in controlling cell shape and growth. One example of a tyrosine kinase is called GDFNR. The RET (rearranged during transfection) oncogene is a mutated form of GDFNR and is commonly found in cancerous thyroid cells.

**SIGNAL TRANSDUCERS.** Signal transducers are proteins that relay cell cycle stimulation signals, from growth factor receptors to proteins in the nucleus of the cell. The transfer of signals to the nucleus is a stepwise process that involves a large number of proto-oncogenes and is often called the signal transduction cascade. Mutations in proto-oncogene involved in this cascade can cause unregulated activity, which can result in abnormal cell proliferation. Signal transducer oncogenes are the largest class of oncogenes. The RAS family is a group of 50 related signal transducer oncogenes that are found in approximately 20% of tumors.

**TRANSCRIPTION FACTORS.** Transcription factors are proteins found in the nucleus of the cell that ultimately receive the signals from the growth factor receptors. Transcription factors directly control the expression of genes that are involved in the growth and proliferation of cells. Transcription factors produced by oncogenes typically do not require growth factor receptor stimulation and thus can result in uncontrolled cell proliferation. Transcription factor proto-oncogenes are often changed into oncogenes by chromosomal translocations in leukemias, lymphomas, and solid tumors. C-myc is a common transcription factor oncogene that results from a chromosomal translocation and is often found in leukemias and lymphomas.

**PROGRAMMED CELL DEATH REGULATORS.** Normal cells have a predetermined life span and different genes regulate their growth and death. Cells that have been damaged or have an abnormal cell cycle may develop into cancer cells. Usually these cells are destroyed through a process called programmed cell death (apoptosis). Cells that have developed into cancer cells, however, do not undergo apoptosis. Mutated proto-oncogenes may inhibit the death of abnormal cells, which can lead to the formation and spread of cancer. The bcl-2 oncogene, for example, inhibits cell death in cancerous cells of the immune system.

### Mechanisms of transformation of proto-oncogene into oncogenes

It is not known in most cases what triggers a particular proto-oncogene to change into an oncogene.

There appear to be environmental triggers such as exposure to toxic chemicals. There also appear to be genetic triggers since changes in other genes in a particular cell can trigger changes in proto-oncogenes.

The mechanisms through which proto-oncogenes are changed into oncogenes are, however, better understood. Proto-oncogenes are transformed into oncogenes through: (1) mutation (2) chromosomal translocation, and (3) gene amplification.

A tiny change, called a mutation, in a proto-oncogene can convert it into an oncogene. The mutation results in an oncogene that produces a protein with an abnormal structure. These mutations often make the protein resistant to regulation and cause uncontrolled and continuous activity of the protein. The RAS family of oncogenes, found in approximately 20% of tumors, are examples of oncogenes caused by mutations.

Chromosomal translocations, which result from errors in mitosis, have also been implicated in the transformation of proto-oncogene into oncogenes. Chromosomal translocations result in the transfer of a proto-oncogene from its normal location on a **chromosome** to a different location on another chromosome. Sometimes this translocation results in the transfer of a proto-oncogene next to a gene involved in the immune system. This results in an oncogene that is controlled by the immune system gene and as a result becomes deregulated. One example of this mechanism is the transfer of the c-myc proto-oncogene from its normal location on chromosome 8 to a location near an immune system gene on chromosome 14. This translocation results in the deregulation of c-myc and is involved in the development of Burkitt's lymphoma. The translocated c-myc proto-oncogene is found in the cancer cells of approximately 85% of people with Burkitt's lymphoma.

In other cases, the translocation results in the fusion of a proto-oncogene with another gene. The resulting oncogene produces an unregulated protein that is involved in stimulating uncontrolled cell proliferation. The first discovered fusion oncogene resulted from a Philadelphia chromosome translocation. This type of translocation is found in the leukemia cells of greater than 95% of patients with a chronic form of leukemia. The Philadelphia chromosome translocation results in the fusion of the c-abl proto-oncogene, normally found on chromosome 9 to the bcr gene found on chromosome 22. The fused gene produces an unregulated transcription factor protein that has a different structure than the normal protein. It is not known how this protein contributes to the formation of cancer cells.

Some oncogenes result when multiple copies of a proto-oncogene are created (gene amplification). Gene amplification often results in hundreds of copies of a gene, which results in increased production of proteins and increased cell growth. Multiple copies of proto-oncogenes are found in many tumors. Sometimes amplified genes form separate chromosomes called double minute chromosomes and sometimes they are found within normal chromosomes.

### Inherited oncogenes

In most cases, oncogenes result from changes in proto-oncogenes in select somatic cells and are not passed on to future generations. People with an inherited oncogene, however, do exist. They possess one changed proto-oncogene (oncogene) and one unchanged proto-oncogene in all of their somatic cells. The somatic cells have two of each chromosome and therefore two of each gene since one of each type of chromosome is inherited from the mother in the egg cell and one of each is inherited from the father in the sperm cell. The egg and sperm cells have undergone a number of divisions in their cell cycle and therefore only contain one of each type of chromosome and one of each type of gene. A person with an inherited oncogene has a changed proto-oncogene in approximately 50% of their egg or sperm cells and an unchanged proto-oncogene in the other 50% of their egg or sperm cells, and therefore has a 50% chance of passing this oncogene on to their children.

A person only has to inherit a change in one proto-oncogene of a pair to have an increased risk of cancer. This is called autosomal dominant **inheritance**. Not all people with an inherited oncogene develop cancer, since mutations in other genes that regulate the cell cycle need to occur in a cell for it to be transformed into a cancerous cell. The presence of an oncogene in a cell does, however, make it more likely that changes will occur in other regulatory genes. The degree of cancer risk depends on the type of oncogene inherited as well as other genetic factors and environmental exposures. The type of cancers that are likely to develop depend on the type of oncogene that has been inherited.

Multiple endocrine neoplasia type II (MENII) is one example of a condition caused by an inherited oncogene. People with MENII have usually inherited the RET oncogene. They have approximately a 70% chance of developing thyroid cancer, a 50% chance of developing a tumor of the adrenal glands (pheochromocytoma), and about a 5-10% chance of developing symptomatic parathyroid disease.

*Oncogenes as targets for cancer treatment*

The discovery of oncogenes approximately 20 years ago has played an important role in developing an understanding of cancer. Oncogenes promise to play an even greater role in development of improved cancer therapies since oncogenes may be important targets for drugs that are used for the treatment of cancer. The goal of these therapies is to selectively destroy cancer cells while leaving normal cells intact. Many anti-cancer therapies currently under development are designed to interfere with oncogenic signal transducer proteins, which relay the signals involved in triggering the abnormal growth of tumor cells. Other therapies hope to trigger specific oncogenes to cause programmed cell death in cancer cells. Whatever the mechanism by which they operate, it is hoped that these experimental therapies will offer a great improvement over current cancer treatments.

### Resources

#### BOOKS

Park, Morag. "Oncogenes." In *The Genetic Basis of Human Cancer*, edited by Bert Vogelstein and Kenneth Kinzler. New York: McGraw-Hill, 1998, pp. 205-228.

#### PERIODICALS

Stass, S. A., and J. Mixson. "Oncogenes and tumor suppressor genes: therapeutic implications." *Clinical Cancer Research* 3 (12 Pt 2) (December 1997): 2687-2695.

"What you need to know about Cancer." *Scientific America* (September 1996).

Wong, Todd. "Oncogenes." *Anticancer Research* 6(A) (Nov-Dec 1999): 4729-4726.

#### WEBSITES

Aharchi, Joseph. "Cell division–Overview." *Western Illinois University*. Biology 150. http://www.wiu.edu/users/mfja/cell1.htm. (1998).

"The genetics of cancer–an overview." (February 17, 1999). Robert H. Lurie Comprehensive Cancer Center of Northwestern University. http://www.cancergenetics.org/gncavrvu.htm.

Kimball, John. "Oncogenes." *Kimball's Biology Pages*. (March 22, 2000). http://www.ultranet.com/~jkimball/BiologyPages/O/Oncogenes.html.

Schichman, Stephen, and Carlo Croce. "Oncogenes." (1999) *Cancer Medicine*. http://www.cancernetwork.com/CanMed/Ch005/005-0.htm.

Lisa Maria Andres, MS, CGC

Onychoosteodysplasia *see* **Nail-Patella syndrome**

Opitz-Frias syndrome *see* **Opitz syndrome**

Opitz-Kaveggia syndrome *see* **FG syndrome**

# Opitz syndrome

## Definition

Opitz syndrome is a heterogeneous genetic condition characterized by a range of midline birth defects such as hypertelorism, clefts in the lips and larynx, heart defects, **hypospadias,** and agenesis of the corpus callosum.

## Description

Opitz syndrome or Opitz G/BBB syndrome, as it is sometimes called, includes G syndrome and BBB syndrome, which were originally thought to be two different syndromes. In 1969, Dr. John Opitz described two similar conditions that he called G syndrome and BBB syndrome. G syndrome was named after one family affected with this syndrome whose last name began with the initial G and BBB syndrome was named after the surname of three different families. Subsequent research suggested that these two conditions were one disorder but researchers could not agree on how this disorder was inherited. It wasn't until 1995 that Dr. Nathaniel Robin and his colleagues demonstrated that Opitz syndrome had both X-linked and autosomal dominant forms.

Opitz syndrome is a complex condition that has many symptoms, most of which affect organs along the midline of the body such as clefts in the lip and larynx, heart defects, hypospadias, and agenesis of the corpus callosum. Opitz syndrome has variable expressivity, which means that different people with the disorder can have different symptoms. This condition also has decreased penetrance, which means that not all people who inherit this disorder will have symptoms.

**Frequencies of common conditions associated with Opitz syndrome**

| Condition | % | Condition | % |
|---|---|---|---|
| Hypospadias | 93% | LTE cleft/fistula | 38% |
| Hypertelorism | 91% | Cleft lip and palate | 32% |
| Swallowing problems | 81% | Strabismus | 28% |
| Ear abnormalities | 72% | Heart defects | 27% |
| Developmental delay | 43% | Imperforate anus | 21% |
| Kidney anomalies | 42% | Undescended testes | 20% |

*(Table by GGS Creative Resources. Reproduced by permission of Gale, a part of Cengage Learning.)*

## Genetic profile

Opitz syndrome is a genetically heterogeneous condition. There appear to be at least two to three genes that can cause Opitz syndrome when changed (mutated) or deleted. Opitz syndrome can be caused by changes in genes found on the X **chromosome** (X-linked) and changes in or deletion of a gene found on chromosome 22 (autosomal dominant).

### Chromosomes, genes and proteins

Each cell of the body, except for the egg and sperm cells contain 23 pairs of chromosomes—46 chromosomes in total. The egg and sperm cells contain only one of each type of chromosome and therefore contain 23 chromosomes in total. Males and females have 22 pairs of chromosomes, called the autosomes, numbered 1 to 22 in order of decreasing size. The other pair of chromosomes, called the sex chromosomes, determines the sex of the individual. Women possess two identical chromosomes called the X chromosomes while men possess one X chromosome and one Y chromosome. Since every egg cell contains an X chromosome, women pass on the X chromosome to their daughters and sons. Some sperm cells contain an X chromosome and some sperm cells contain a Y chromosome. Men pass the X chromosome on to their daughters and the Y chromosome on to their sons. Each type of chromosome contains different genes that are found at specific locations along the chromosome. Men and women inherit two of each type of autosomal gene since they inherit two of each type of autosome. Women inherit two of each type of X-linked gene since they possess two X chromosomes. Men inherit only one of each X-linked gene since they posses only one X chromosome.

Each gene contains the instructions for the production of a particular protein. The proteins produced by genes have many functions and work together to create the traits of the human body such as hair and eye color and are involved in controlling the basic functions of the human body. Changes or deletions of genes can cause them to produce abnormal protein, less protein or no protein. This can prevent the protein from functioning normally.

### Autosomal dominant Opitz syndrome

The gene responsible for the autosomal dominant form of Opitz syndrome has not been discovered yet, but it appears to result from a deletion in a segment of chromosome 22 containing the Opitz gene or a change in the gene responsible for Opitz syndrome. In some cases the deletion or gene change is inherited from either the mother or father who have the gene change or deletion in one chromosome 22 in their somatic cells. The other chromosome 22 found in each of their somatic cells is normal. Some of their egg or sperm cells contain the gene change or deletion in chromosome 22 and some contain a normal chromosome 22. In other cases the deletion has occurred spontaneously during conception or is only found in some of the egg or sperm cells of either parent but not found in the other cells of their body.

Parents who have had a child with an autosomal dominant form of Opitz syndrome may or may not be at increased risk for having other affected children. If one of the parents is diagnosed with Opitz syndrome then each of their children has a 50% chance of inheriting the condition. If neither parent has symptoms of Opitz syndrome nor possesses a deletion, then it becomes more difficult to assess their chances of having other affected children.

In many cases they would not be at increased risk since the gene alteration occurred spontaneously in the embryo during conception. It is possible, however, that one of the parents is a carrier, meaning they possess a change in the autosomal dominant Opitz gene but do not have any obvious symptoms. This parent's children would each have a 50% chance of inheriting the Opitz gene.

### X-linked Opitz syndrome

Some people with the X-linked form of Opitz syndrome have a change (mutation) in a gene found on the X chromosome called the MID1 (midline1) gene. Changes in another X-linked gene called the MID2 gene may also cause Opitz syndrome in some cases. It is believed that the MID genes produce proteins involved in the development of midline organs. Changes in the MID gene prevent the production of enough normal protein for normal organ development.

The X-linked form of Opitz syndrome is inherited differently by men and woman. A woman with an X-linked form of Opitz syndrome has typically inherited a changed MID gene from her mother and a changed MID gene from her father. This occurs very infrequently. All of this woman's sons will have Opitz syndrome and all of her daughters will be carriers for Opitz syndrome. Only women can be carriers for Opitz syndrome since carriers possess one changed MID gene and one unchanged MID gene. Most carriers for the X-linked form of Opitz syndrome do not have symptoms since one normal MID gene is usually sufficient to promote normal development. Some carriers do have symptoms but they tend to be very mild.

## KEY TERMS

**Agenesis of the corpus callosum**—Failure of the corpus callosum to form and develop. The corpus callosum is the band of nerve fibers located between the two sides, or hemispheres, of the brain.

**Amniocentesis**—A procedure performed at 16–18 weeks of pregnancy in which a needle is inserted through a woman's abdomen into her uterus to draw out a small sample of the amniotic fluid from around the baby. Either the fluid itself or cells from the fluid can be used for a variety of tests to obtain information about genetic disorders and other medical conditions in the fetus.

**Anomaly**—Different from the normal or expected. Unusual or irregular structure.

**Autosome**—Chromosomes that do not determine the sex of an individual.

**Chromosome**—A microscopic thread-like structure found within each cell of the body that consists of a complex of proteins and DNA. Humans have 46 chromosomes arranged into 23 pairs. Changes in either the total number of chromosomes or their shape and size (structure) may lead to physical or mental abnormalities.

**Cleft**—An elongated opening or slit in an organ.

**Cleft palate**—A congenital malformation in which there is an abnormal opening in the roof of the mouth that allows the nasal passages and the mouth to be improperly connected.

**Congenital**—Refers to a disorder that is present at birth.

**Cryptorchidism**—A condition in which one or both testes fail to descend normally.

**Deletion**—The absence of genetic material that is normally found in a chromosome. Often, the genetic material is missing due to an error in replication of an egg or sperm cell.

**Deoxyribonucleic acid (DNA)**—The genetic material in cells that holds the inherited instructions for growth, development, and cellular functioning.

**DNA testing**—Analysis of DNA (the genetic component of cells) in order to determine changes in genes that may indicate a specific disorder.

**Esophagus**—The part of the digestive tract that connects the mouth and stomach; the foodpipe.

**FISH (fluorescence *in situ* hybridization)**—Technique used to detect small deletions or rearrangements in chromosomes by attempting to attach a

---

Daughters of carriers for Opitz syndrome have a 50% chance of being carriers and sons have a 50% chance of being affected with Opitz syndrome. A man with an X-linked form of Opitz syndrome will have normal sons but all of his daughters will be carriers.

### Demographics

Opitz syndrome is a rare disorder that appears to affect all ethnic groups. The frequency of this disorder is unknown since people with this disorder exhibit a wide range of symptoms, making it difficult to diagnose and many possess mild or non-detectable symptoms.

### Signs and symptoms

People with Opitz syndrome exhibit a wide range of medical problems and in some cases may not exhibit any detectable symptoms. This may be due in part to the genetic heterogeneity of this condition. Even people with Opitz syndrome who are from the same family can have different problems. This may mean there are other genetic and non-genetic factors that influence

the development of symptoms in individuals who have inherited a changed or deleted Opitz gene. Most individuals with Opitz syndrome only have a few symptoms of the disorder such as wide set eyes and a broad prominent forehead. Opitz syndrome can, however, affect many of the organs and structures of the body and primarily affects the development of midline organs. The most common symptoms are: hypertelorism (wide-spaced eyes), broad prominent forehead, heart defects, hypospadias (urinary opening of the penis present on the underside of the penis instead of its normal location at the tip), undescended testicles, an abnormality of the anal opening, agenesis of the corpus callosum (absence of the tissue which connects the two sides of the brain), **cleft lip**, and clefts and abnormalities of the pharynx (throat) and larynx (voice-box), trachea (wind-pipe), and esophagus.

People with Opitz syndrome usually have a distinctive look to the face such as a broad prominent forehead, cleft lip, wide set eyes that may be crossed, wide noses with upturned nostrils, small chins or jaws, malformed ears, crowded, absent or misplaced teeth, fluorescent (glowing) piece of a chromosome to a sample of cells obtained from a patient.

**Gene**—A building block of inheritance, which contains the instructions for the production of a particular protein, and is made up of a molecular sequence found on a section of DNA. Each gene is found on a precise location on a chromosome.

**Geneticist**—A specialist (M.D. or Ph.D.) who has training and certification in diagnosing, managing, and counseling individuals/families with genetic disorders. Genetics counselors hold a master's degree in medical genetics, and provide many of the same services as geneticists.

**Heterogeneous**—A set of symptoms or a disorder caused by several different gene mutations.

**Hypertelorism**—A wider-than-normal space between the eyes.

**Hypospadias**—An abnormality of the penis in which the urethral opening is located on the underside of the penis rather than at its tip.

**Hypotonia**—Reduced or diminished muscle tone.

**Microcephaly**—An abnormally small head.

**Midline defects**—Defects involving organs along the center of the body such as the lips, penis, and corpus callosum.

**Midline organs**—Organs found along the center of the body such as the lips, penis, and corpus callosum.

**Polydactyly**—The presence of extra fingers or toes.

**Prenatal testing**—Testing for a disease such as a genetic condition in an unborn baby.

**Sex chromosomes**—The X and Y chromosomes that determine the sex of the individual.

**Somatic cells**—All the cells of the body except for the egg and sperm cells.

**Strabismus**—An improper muscle balance of the ocular muscles resulting in crossed or divergent eyes.

**Syndactyly**—Webbing or fusion between the fingers or toes.

**Ultrasound**—An imaging technique that uses sound waves to help visualize internal structures in the body.

**Undescended testicles**—Testicles that failed to move from the abdomen to the scrotum during the development of the fetus.

**X–linked gene**—A gene found on the X chromosome.

and hair that may form a "widow's peak". In many cases the head may appear large or small and out of proportion to the rest of the body.

Often people with Opitz syndrome have difficulties swallowing because of abnormalities in the pharynx, larynx, trachea, or esophagus. This can sometimes result in food entering the trachea instead of the esophagus, which can cause damage to the lungs and pneumonia, and can sometimes be fatal in small infants. Abnormalities in the trachea can sometimes make breathing difficult and may result in a hoarse or weak voice and wheezing.

Both males and females may have abnormal genitals and abnormalities in the anal opening. Males can have hypospadias and undescended testicles and girls may have minor malformation of their external genitalia. Heart defects are also often present and abnormalities of the kidney can be present as well. Intelligence is usually normal but mild mental retardation can sometimes be present. Twins appear more common in families affected with Opitz syndrome.

Males and females with the dominant form of Opitz syndrome are equally likely to have symptoms whereas carrier females with the X-linked form of Opitz syndrome are less likely to have symptoms then males with the condition. In general, males with the X-linked form of Opitz syndrome tend to be more severely affected than females and males with the autosomal dominant form of Opitz syndrome. People with X-linked Opitz syndrome and dominant Opitz syndrome generally appear to exhibit the same range of symptoms. The only known exceptions are upturned nostrils and clefts at the back of throat, which appear to only occur in people with X-linked Opitz syndrome.

### Diagnosis

#### Diagnostic testing

The diagnosis and cause of Opitz syndrome is often difficult to establish. In most cases, Opitz syndrome is diagnosed through a clinical evaluation and not through a blood test. This means a genetic specialist (geneticist) has examined the patient and found enough symptoms of Opitz syndrome to make a diagnosis. Since not all patients have obvious symptoms or even any symptoms at all, this can be a difficult task. It can also be difficult to establish whether an individual has an X-linked form or an autosomal dominant form, and whether it has been inherited or occurred spontaneously. In many cases, the geneticist has to rely on physical examinations or pictures of multiple family members and a description of the family's medical history to establish the cause of Opitz syndrome. In some cases the cause cannot be established.

Sometimes a clinical diagnosis is confirmed through fluorescence *in situ* hybridization (FISH). FISH testing can detect whether a person has a deletion of the region of chromosome 22 that is associated with Opitz syndrome. Fluorescent (glowing) pieces of **DNA** containing the region that is deleted in Opitz syndrome are mixed with a sample of cells obtained from a blood sample. If there is a deletion in one of the chromosomes, the DNA will only stick to one chromosome and not the other and only one glowing section of a chromosome will be visible instead of two. Most patients with the autosomal dominant form of Opitz syndrome cannot be diagnosed through FISH testing since they possess a tiny change in the gene that cannot be detected with this procedure. As of 2001, researchers are still trying to discover the specific gene and gene changes that cause autosomal dominant Opitz syndrome.

FISH testing is unable to detect individuals with the X-linked form of Opitz syndrome. As of the early 2000s, DNA testing for the X-linked form of Opitz disease is not available through clinical laboratories. Some research laboratories are looking for changes in the MID1 gene and the MID2 gene as part of their research and may occasionally confirm a clinical diagnosis of X-linked Opitz syndrome.

### Prenatal testing

It is difficult to diagnose Opitz syndrome in a baby prior to its birth. Sometimes doctors and technicians (ultrasonographers) who specialize in performing ultrasound evaluations are able to see physical features of Opitz syndrome in the fetus. Some of the features they may look for in the ultrasound evaluation are heart defects, wide spacing between the eyes, clefts in the lip, hypospadias, and agenesis of the corpus callosum. It is very difficult, however, even for experts to diagnose or rule-out Opitz syndrome through an ultrasound evaluation.

Opitz syndrome can be definitively diagnosed in a baby prior to its birth if a **MID** gene change is detected in the mother or if a deletion in chromosome 22 is detected in the mother or father. Cells from the baby

## QUESTIONS TO ASK YOUR DOCTOR

- What are the characteristic features of Opitz syndrome?
- On what tests or other measures is a differential diagnosis of Opitz syndrome based?
- What kinds of treatments are typically necessary for a child born with Opitz syndrome?
- Can you recommend an organization that provides information about this genetic condition and support for parents who have a child with Opitz syndrome?

are obtained through an **amniocentesis** or chorionic villus sampling. These cells are analyzed for the particular MID gene change or chromosome 22 deletion found in one of the parents.

### Treatment and management

As of the early 2000s there is no cure for Opitz syndrome and no treatment for the underlying condition. Management of the condition involves diagnosing and managing the symptoms. Clefts, heart defects, and genital abnormalities can often be repaired by surgery. Feeding difficulties can sometimes be managed using feeding tubes through the nose, stomach, or small intestine. Early recognition and intervention with special education may help individuals with mental retardation.

### Prognosis

For most patients, the prognosis and quality of life of Opitz syndrome is good, with individuals typically living a normal life span. The prognosis, however, is very dependent on the type of organ abnormality and the quality of medical care. Patients with severe heart defects and major abnormalities in the trachea and esophagus may have a poorer prognosis.

### Resources

**PERIODICALS**

Buchner, G., et al. "MID2, a homologue of the Opitz syndrome gene MID1: Similarities in subcellular localization and differences in expression during development." *Human Molecular Genetics* 8 (August 1998): 1397-407.

Jacobson, Z., et al. "Further delineation of the Opitz G/BBB syndrome: Report of an infant with congenital heart disease and bladder extrophy, and review of the literature." *American Journal of Medical Genetics* (July 7, 1998): 294-299.

Macdonald, M. R., A. H. Olney, and P. Kolodziej. "Opitz syndrome (G/BBB Syndrome)." *Ear Nose & Throat Journal* 77, no. 7 (July 1998): 528-529.

Schweiger, S., et al. "The Opitz syndrome gene product, MID1, associates with microtubules." *Proceedings of the National Academy of Sciences of the United States of America* 96, no. 6 (March 16, 1999): 2794-2799.

**WEBSITES**

McKusick, Victor A. "Hypertelorism with Esophageal Abnormality and Hypospadias." *OMIM—Online Mendelian Inheritance in Man.* http://www3.ncbi.nlm.nih.gov/htbin-post/Omim/dispmim?145410. (March 28, 2000).

McKusick, Victor A. "Opitz syndrome." *OMIM—Online Mendelian Inheritance in Man.* http://www3.ncbi.nlm.nih.gov/htbin-post/Omim/dispmim?300000. (February 6, 2001).

**ORGANIZATIONS**

Canadian Opitz Family Network. Box 892, Errington, BC V0R 1V0. Canada (250) 954-1434. Fax: (250) 954-1465. opitz@apollos.net. http://www.apollos.net/arena/opitz/start.html.

March of Dimes Birth Defects Foundation. 1275 Mamaroneck Ave., White Plains, NY 10605. (888) 663-4637. resourcecenter@modimes.org. http://www.modimes.org.

National Organization for Rare Disorders (NORD). PO Box 8923, New Fairfield, CT 06812-8923. (203) 746-6518 or (800) 999-6673. Fax: (203) 746-6481. http://www.rarediseases.org.

Opitz G/BBB Family Network. PO Box 515, Grand Lake, CO 80447. opitznet@mac.com. http://www.gle.egsd.k12.co.us/opitz/index.html.

Smith-Lemli-Opitz Advocacy and Exchange (RSH/SLO). 2650 Valley Forge Dr., Boothwyn, PA 19061. (610) 485-9663. http://members.aol.com/slo97/index.html.

Lisa Maria Andres, MS, CGC

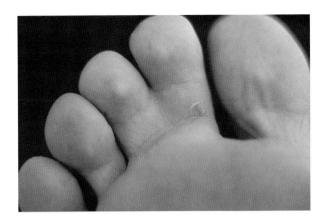

One of the many traits found in individuals with OFD syndrome is webbing of the fingers and toes. *(Custom Medical Stock Photos, Inc.)*

# Oral-facial-digital syndrome

## Definition

Oral-facial-digital (OFD) syndrome is a generic name for a variety of different **genetic disorders** that result in malformations of the mouth, teeth, jaw, facial bones, hands, and feet.

## Description

Oral-facial-digital syndrome includes several different but possibly related genetic disorders. OFD syndromes are also referred to as digito-oro-facial syndromes. As of the early 2000s, there are nine different OFD syndromes, identified as OFD syndrome type I, type II, and so on. OFD syndromes are so named because they all cause changes in the oral structures, including the tongue, teeth, and jaw; the facial structures, including the head, eyes, and nose; and the digits (fingers and toes). OFD syndromes are also frequently associated with developmental delay.

The different OFD syndromes are distinguished from each other based on the specific physical symptoms and the mode of **inheritance**. There are many alternate names for OFD syndromes. A partial list of these is:

- OFD syndrome type I: Gorlin syndrome I, Gorlin-Psaume syndrome, Papillon-Leage syndrome

- OFD syndrome type II: Mohr syndrome, Mohr-Claussen syndrome

- OFD syndrome type III: Sugarman syndrome

- OFD syndrome type IV: Baraitser-Burn syndrome

- OFD syndrome type V: Thurston syndrome

- OFD syndrome type VI: Juberg-Hayward syndrome Varadi syndrome, Varadi-Papp syndrome

- OFD syndrome type VII: Whelan syndrome

## Genetic profile

The mode of inheritance of OFD syndrome depends on the type of the syndrome. Type I is inherited as an X-linked dominant trait and is only found in females because it is fatal in males. X-linked means that the syndrome is carried on the female sex **chromosome**, while dominant means that only one parent has to pass on the **gene** mutation in order for the child to be affected with the syndrome.

**Digit**—A finger or toe. Plural–digits.

OFD syndrome type VII is inherited either as an X-linked or autosomal dominant pattern of inheritance. Autosomal means that the syndrome is not carried on a sex chromosome.

OFD syndrome types II, III, IV, V, and VI are passed on through an autosomal recessive pattern of inheritance. Recessive means that both parents must carry the gene mutation in order for their child to have the disorder.

OFD syndrome types VIII and IX are characterized by either an autosomal or X-linked recessive pattern of inheritance.

The gene location for OFD syndrome type I has been assigned to Xp22.3-22.2, or, on the 22nd band of the p arm of the X chromosome. As of the early 2000s, the specific **gene mutations** responsible for the other types of OFD syndrome have not been identified.

### Demographics

There does not appear to be any clear-cut ethnic pattern to the incidence of OFD syndrome. Most types of OFD syndrome affect males and females with equal probability, although type I, the most common type, affects only females (since it is lethal in males before birth). The overall incidence of OFD syndrome has not been established due to the wide variation between the different types of the syndrome and the difficulty of definitive diagnosis.

### Signs and symptoms

The symptoms observed in people affected by OFD syndrome vary depending on the specific type of the syndrome. In general, the symptoms include the following:

Oral features:

- Cleft lip
- Cleft palate or highly arched palate
- Lobed or split tongue
- Tumors of the tongue
- Missing or extra teeth
- Gum disease
- Misaligned bite
- Smaller than normal jaw

*Facial features:*

- Small or wide set eyes
- Missing structures of the eye
- Broad base or tip of the nose
- One nostril smaller than the other
- Low-set or angled ears

*Digital features:*

- Extra fingers or toes
- Abnormally short fingers
- Webbing between fingers or toes
- Clubfoot
- Permanently flexed fingers

*Mental development and central nervous system:*

- Mental retardation
- Brain abnormalities
- Seizures
- Spasmodic movements or tics
- Delayed motor and speech development

*Other:*

- Growth retardation
- Cardiovascular abnormalities
- Sunken chest
- Susceptibility to respiratory infection

### Diagnosis

Diagnosis is usually made based on the observation of clinical symptoms. There is currently no medical test that can definitively confirm the diagnosis of OFD syndrome, with the exception of genetic screening for OFD syndrome type I.

### Treatment and management

Treatment of OFD syndrome is directed towards the specific symptoms of each case. Surgical correction of the oral and facial malformations associated with OFD syndrome is often required.

### Prognosis

Prognosis depends on the specific type of OFD syndrome and the symptoms present in the individual. OFD syndrome type I is lethal in males before birth. However, other types of OFD syndrome are found in both males and females. Due to the wide variety of symptoms seen in the nine types of the syndrome, overall survival rates are not available.

## Resources

### WEBSITES

"Mohr Syndrome." *OMIM—Online Mendelian Inheritance in Man.* March 20, 2001 [cited April 20, 2001]. http://www.ncbi.nlm.nih.gov/htbin-post/Omim/dispmim?252100.

"Oral-Facial-Digital Syndrome, Type III." *OMIM—Online Mendelian Inheritance in Man.* June 11, 1997 [cited April 20, 2001]. http://www.ncbi.nlm.nih.gov/htbin-post/Omim/dispmim?258850.

"Oral-Facial-Digital Syndrome, Type IV." *OMIM—Online Mendelian Inheritance in Man.* June 11, 1997 [cited April 20, 2001]. http://www.ncbi.nlm.nih.gov/htbin-post/Omim/dispmim?258860.

"Oral-Facial-Digital Syndrome with Retinal Abnormalities." *OMIM—Online Mendelian Inheritance in Man.* April 11, 2002 [cited January 8, 2003]. http://www.ncbi.nlm.nih.gov/htbin-post/Omim/dispmim?258865.

"Orofaciodigital Syndrome I." *OMIM—Online Mendelian Inheritance in Man.* March 16, 2001 [cited April 20, 2001]. http://www.ncbi.nlm.nih.gov/htbin-post/Omim/dispmim?311200.

"Varadi-Papp Syndrome." *OMIM—Online Mendelian Inheritance in Man.* May 9, 1998 [cited April 20, 2001]. http://www.ncbi.nlm.nih.gov/htbin-post/Omim/dispmim?277170.

### ORGANIZATIONS

Children's Craniofacial Association. PO Box 280297, Dallas, TX 75243-4522. (972) 994-9902 or (800) 535-3643. contactcca@ccakids.com. http://www.ccakids.com.

FACES: The National Craniofacial Association. PO Box 11082, Chattanooga, TN 37401. (423) 266-1632 or (800) 332-2373. faces@faces-cranio.org. http://www.faces-cranio.org/.

National Organization for Rare Disorders (NORD). PO Box 8923, New Fairfield, CT 06812-8923. (203) 746-6518 or (800) 999-6673. Fax: (203) 746-6481. http://www.rarediseases.org.

Paul A. Johnson

# Organic acidemias

## Definition

Organic acidemias are a collection of amino and fatty acid oxidation disorders that cause non-amino organic acids to accumulate and be excreted in the urine.

## Description

Organic acidemias are divided into two categories: disorders of amino acid metabolism and disorders involving fatty acid oxidation. There are several dozen different organic acidemia disorders. They are caused by inherited deficiencies in specific enzymes involved in the breakdown of branched-chain amino acids, lysine, and tryptophan, or fatty acids. Some have more than one cause.

Amino acids are chemical compounds from which proteins are made. There are about 40 amino acids in the human body. Proteins in the body are formed through various combinations of roughly half of these amino acids. The other 20 play different roles in metabolism. Organic acidemias involving amino acid metabolism disorders include isovaleric acidemia, 3-methylcrotonylglycemia, combined carboxylase deficiency, hydroxymethylglutaric acidemia, **propionic acidemia**, **methylmalonic acidemia**, beta-ketothiolase deficiency, and glutaric acidemia type I.

Fatty acids, part of a larger group of organic acids, are caused by the breakdown of fats and oils in the body. Organic acidemias caused by fatty acid oxidation disorders include glutaric acidemia type II short-chain acyl-CoA dehydrogenase (SCAD) deficiency, medium-chain acyl-CoA dehydrogenase (MCAD) deficiency, long-chain acyl-CoA dehrdrogenase (LCAD) deficiency, very long-chain acyl-CoA dehydrogenase (VLCAD) deficiency, and long-chain 3-hydroxyacyl-CoA dehydrogenase (LCHAD) deficiency.

Most organic acidemias are considered rare, occurring in less than one in 50,000 persons. However, MCAD occurs in about one in 23,000 births. Most of these disorders produce life-threatening illnesses that can occur in newborns, infants, children, and adults. In nearly all cases, though, the symptoms appear during the first few years of life, usually in children age two or younger. If left undiagnosed and untreated in young children, they can also delay physical development.

## Genetic profile

Genes are the blueprint for the human body, directing the development of cells and tissue. Mutations in

**Acidosis**—A condition of decreased alkalinity resulting from abnormally high acid levels (low pH) in the blood and tissues. Usually indicated by sickly sweet breath, headaches, nausea, vomiting, and visual impairments.

**Alopecia**—Loss of hair or baldness.

**Biotin**—A growth vitamin of the vitamin B complex found naturally in liver, egg yolks, and yeast.

**Branched-chain**—An open chain of atoms having one or more side chains.

**Dystonia**—Painful involuntary muscle cramps or spasms.

**Homocysteine**—An amino acid that is not used to produce proteins in the human body.

**Hyperammonemia**—An excess of ammonia in the blood.

**Hypotonia**—Reduced or diminished muscle tone.

**Ketoacidosis**—A condition that results when organic compounds (such as propionic acid, ketones, and fatty acids) build up in the blood and urine.

**Ketolactic acidosis**—The overproduction of ketones and lactic acid.

**Ketonuria**—The presence of excess ketone bodies (organic carbohydrate-related compounds) in the urine.

**L-carnitine**—A substance made in the body that carries wastes from the body's cells into the urine.

**Lysine**—A crystalline basic amino acid essential to nutrition.

**Metabolic acidosis**—High acidity (low pH) in the body due to abnormal metabolism, excessive acid intake, or retention in the kidneys.

**Neutropenia**—A condition in which the number of leukocytes (a type of white or colorless blood cell) is abnormally low, mainly in neutrophils (a type of blood cell).

**Organic aciduria**—The condition of having organic acid in the urine.

**Pancytopenia**—An abnormal reduction in the number of erythrocytes (red blood cells), leukocytes (a type of white or colorless blood cell), and blood platelets (a type of cell that aids in blood clotting) in the blood.

**Thrombocytopenia**—A persistent decrease in the number of blood platelets usually associated with hemorrhaging.

**Tryptophan**—A crystalline amino acid widely distributed in proteins and essential to human life.

some genes can cause **genetic disorders** such as the organic acidemias. Every cell in the body has 23 pairs of chromosomes, 22 pairs of which contain two copies of individual genes. The 23rd pair of chromosomes is called the sex **chromosome** because it determines a person's gender. Men have an X and a Y chromosome while women have two X chromosomes.

Organic acidemias are generally believed to be autosomal recessive disorders that affect males and females. Autosomal means that the gene does not reside on the sex chromosome. People with only one abnormal gene are carriers but since the gene is recessive, they do not have the disorder. Their children will be carriers of the disorder 50% of the time but not show symptoms of the disease. Both parents must have one of the abnormal genes for a child to have symptoms of an organic acidemia. When both parents have the abnormal gene, there is a 25% chance each child will inherit both abnormal genes and have the disease. There is a 50% chance each child will inherit one abnormal gene and become a carrier of the disorder but not have the disease itself. There is a 25%

chance each child will inherit neither abnormal gene and not have the disease nor be a carrier.

### Demographics

Organic acidemias affect males and females roughly equally. The disorders primarily occur in Caucasian children of northern European ancestry, such as English, Irish, German, French, and Swedish. In a 1994 study by Duke University Medical Center, 120 subjects with MCAD were studied. Of these, 118 were Caucasian, one was African American, and one was Native American; 65 were female and 55 were male; and 112 were from the United States while the other eight were from Great Britain, Canada, Australia, and Ireland.

### Signs and symptoms

Symptoms of organic acidemias vary with type and sometimes even within a specific disorder. Isovaleric acidemia (IA) can present itself in two ways: acute severe or chronic intermittent. Roughly half of IA patients have the acute sever disorder and half the chronic intermittent type. In acute severe cases, patients are healthy at birth but show symptoms between 1 to 14 days later. These symptoms include vomiting, refusal to eat, dehydration, listlessness, and lethargy. Other symptoms can include shaking, twitching, convulsions, low body temperature (under 97.8°F or 36.6°C), and a foul "sweaty feet" odor. If left untreated, the infant can lapse into a coma and die from severe ketoacidosis, hemorrhage, or infections. In the chronic intermittent type, symptoms usually occur within a year after birth and is usually preceded by upper respiratory infections or an increased consumption of protein-rich foods, such as meat and dairy products. Symptoms include vomiting, lethargy, "sweaty feet" odor, acidosis, and ketonuria. Additional symptoms may include diarrhea, thrombocytopenia, neutropenia, or pancytopenia.

There is a wide range of symptoms for 3-methylcrotonglycemia, which can occur in newborns, infants, and young children. These include irritability, drowsiness, unwillingness to eat, vomiting, and rapid breathing. Other symptoms can include hypoglycemia, alopecia, and involuntary body movements.

Approximately 30% of patients with hydroxymethylglutaric acidemia show symptoms within five days after birth and 60% between 3 and 24 months. Symptoms vary and can include vomiting, deficient muscle tone, lethargy, seizures, metabolic acidosis, hypoglycemia, and hyperammonemia.

Symptoms of methylmalonic acidemia (MA) due to methylmalonyl-CoA mutase (MCoAM) deficiency include lethargy, failure to thrive, vomiting, dehydration, trouble breathing, and deficient muscle tone, and they usually present themselves during infancy. In MA due to N-methyltetrahydrofolate, homocysteine methyltransferase deficiency and high homocysteine levels usually occur during the first two months after birth but have been reported in children as old as 14 years. General symptoms are the same as for MA due to MCoAM but can also include fatigue, delirium, **dementia**, spasms, and disorders of the spinal cord or bone marrow.

Symptoms of glutaric acidemia type I usually appear within two years after birth and generally become apparent when a minor infection is followed by deficient muscle tone, seizures, loss of head control, grimacing, and **dystonia** of the face, tongue, neck, back, arms, and hands. Glutaric acidemia type II symptoms fall into three categories:

- Infants with congenital anomalies present symptoms within the first 24 hours after birth, with symptoms of deficient muscle tone, severe hypoglycemia, hepatomegaly (enlarged liver), metabolic acidosis, and

sometimes a "sweaty feet" odor. In some patients, signs include a high forehead, low-set ears, enlarged kidneys, excessive width between the eyes, a mid-face below normal size, and genital anomalies.

- Infants without congenital anomalies have signs of deficient muscle tone, tachypnea (increased breathing rate), metabolic acidosis, hepatomegaly, and a "sweaty feet" odor.
- Mild or later onset symptoms in children that include vomiting, hypoglycemia, hepatomegaly, and myopathy (a disorder of muscle or muscle tissue).

There are two types of propionic acidemia, one caused by propionyl-CoA carboxylase (PCoAC) deficiency and the other caused by multiple carboxylase (MC) deficiency. Symptoms of both disorders are generally the same and include vomiting, refusal to eat, lethargy, hypotonia, dehydration, and seizures. Other symptoms may include skin rash, ketoacidosis, irritability, metabolic acidosis, and a strong smelling urine commonly described as "tom cats'" urine.

There are five types of organic acidemias of fatty acid oxidation that involve deficiencies of acyl-CoA dehydrogenase enzymes: SCAD, MCAD, LCAD, VLCAD, and LCHAD. General symptoms for all five of these disorders include influenza- or cold-like symptoms, hyperammonemia, metabolic acidosis, hyperglycemia, vomiting, a "sweaty feet" odor, and delay in physical development. In young children, other symptoms can include loss of hair, involuntary or uncoordinated muscle movements (ataxia), and a scaly rash (seborrhea rash.) Symptoms generally appear between two months and two years of age, but can appear as early as two days after birth up to six years of age.

There are two combined carboxylase deficiency organic acidemias: holocarboxylase synthetase deficiency and biotindase deficiency. Symptoms of holocarboxylase deficiency include sleep and breathing difficulties, hypotonia, seizures, alopecia, developmental delay, skin rash, metabolic acidosis, ketolactic acidosis, organic aciduria, and hyperammonemia. Symptoms of biotindase deficiency include seizures, involuntary muscular movements, hypotonia, rapid breathing, developmental delay, hearing loss, and visual problems. Skin rash, alopecia, metabolic acidosis, organic acidemia, and hyper ammonemia can also occur.

Symptoms of beta-ketothiolase deficiency vary. In infants, the most common symptoms include severe metabolic acidosis, ketosis, vomiting, diarrhea (often bloody), and upper respiratory or gastrointestinal infections. Adults with the disorder are usually asymptomatic (showing no outward signs of the disease).

## Diagnosis

In all types of organic acidemia, diagnosis cannot be made by simply recognizing the outward appearance of symptoms. Instead, diagnosis is usually made by detecting abnormal levels of organic acid cells in the urine through a urinalysis. The specific test used is called combined gas chromatography-mass spectrometry. In gas chromatography, a sample is vaporized and its components separated and identified. Mass spectrometry electronically weighs molecules. Every molecule has a unique weight (or mass). In newborn screening, mass spectrometry analyzes blood to identify what amino acids and fatty acids are present and the amount present. The results can identify if the person tested has a specific organic acidemia. Many organic acidemias also can be diagnosed in the uterus by using an enzyme assay of cultured cells, or by demonstrating abnormal organic acids in the fluid surrounding the fetus. In some laboratories, analysis is done on blood, skin, liver, or muscle tissue. Molecular **DNA** testing is also available for common mutations of MCAD and LCHAD.

Since most organic acidemias are rare, routine screening of fetuses or newborns is not usually done and are not widely available. In MCAD, a more common organic acidemia, abnormal organic acids are excreted in the urine intermittently so a diagnosis is made by detecting the compound phenylpropionylglycine in the urine.

## Treatment and management

There are few medications available to treat organic acidemias. The primary treatments are dietary restrictions tailored to each disorder, primarily restrictions on the intake of certain amino acids. For example, patients with some acidemias, such as isovaleric and beta-ketothiolase deficiency, must restrict their intake of leucine by cutting back on foods high in protein. Patients with propionic or methylmalonic acidemias must restrict their intake of threonine, valine, methionine, and isoleucine. The intake of the restricted amino acids is based on the percentage of lean body mass rather than body weight. Some patients also benefit from growth hormones. Patients with combined carboxylase deficiency are sometimes treated with large doses of biotin. Some patients with methylmalonic acidemia are treated with large doses of vitamin $B_{12}$.

Glucose infusion (to provide calories and reduce the destructive metabolism of proteins) and bicarbonate infusion (to control acidosis) are often used to treat acute episodes of some acidemias, including isovaleric, 3-methylcrotonylglycemia, and hydroxymethylglutaric.

The primary treatment for MCAD is to not go without food for more than 10 or 12 hours. Children should eat foods high in carbohydrates, such as pasta, rice, cereal, and non-diet drinks, when they are ill. A low fat diet is also recommended. The drug L-carnitine is sometimes used by physicians to prevent low blood sugar when patients have infections or are not eating regularly.

The treatment of LCHAD is similar to that of MCAD, except that L-carnitine is usually not prescribed. Children with LCHAD are often treated with medium chain triglycerides oil.

Holocarboxylase synthetase deficiency is generally treated by administering 10 milligrams (mg) of biotin daily. Eating large amounts of yeast, liver, and egg yolks, which naturally contain biotin, did not improve the condition. **Biotinidase deficiency** is usually treated successfully with pharmacological doses of between 5 and 20 mg of biotin daily. However, hearing and vision problems appear to be less reversible.

## Prognosis

The prognosis of patients with organic acidemias varies with each disorder and usually depends on how quickly and accurately the condition is diagnosed and treated. Some patients with organic acidemias are incorrectly diagnosed with other conditions, such as sudden infant death syndrome (SIDS) or Reye syndrome. Without a quick and accurate diagnosis, the survival rate decreases with each episode of the disorder. Death occurs within the first few years of life, often within the first few months. With a quick diagnosis and aggressive monitoring and treatment, patients can often live relatively normal lives. For example, children with either biotinidase deficiency or holocarboxylase synthetase deficiency, when detected early and treated with biotin, have generally shown resolution of the clinical symptoms and biochemical abnormalities.

## Resources

### BOOKS

Eaton, Simon. *Current Views of Fatty Acid Oxidation and Ketogenesis.* Kluwer Academic Publishers, Dordrecht, the Netherlands, 2000.

Narins, Robert G. *Maxwell and Kleeman's Clinical Disorders of Fluid and Electrolyte Metabolism,* Fifth Edition. McGraw-Hill Publishing, Inc., New York, 1994.

Scriver, Charles R., et al. *The Metabolic Basis of Inherited Disease,* Eighth Edition. McGraw-Hill Publishing, Inc., New York, 2000.

**PERIODICALS**

Brink, Susan. "Little-Used Newborn Test can Prevent Real Heartache." *U.S. News & World Report* (January 17, 2000): 59.

McCarthy, Michael. "Report Calls for Reform of U.S. Newborn Baby Screening Programmes." *The Lancet* (August 12, 2000): 571.

Mitka, Mike. "Neonatal Screening Varies by State of Birth." *JAMA, The Journal of the American Medical Association* (October 25, 2000): 2044.

Thomas, Janet A., et al. "Apparent Decreased Energy Requirements in Children with Organic Acidemias: Preliminary Observations." *Journal of the American Dietetic Association* (September 2000): 1074.

Wang, S. S., et al. "Medium Chain Acyl-CoA-Dehydrogenace Deficiency: Human Genome Epidemiology Review." *Genetic Medicine* (January 1999): 332-339.

**ORGANIZATIONS**

Fatty Oxidation Disorders (FOD) Family Support Group. 805 Montrose Dr., Greensboro, NC 27410. (336) 547-8682. fodgroup@aol.com. http://www.fodsupport.org/welcome.htm.

National Newborn Screening and Genetics Resource Center. 1912 W. Anderson Lane, Suite 210, Austin, TX 78757. Fax: (512) 454-6419. http://www.genes-r-us.uthscsa.edu.

Organic Acidemia Association. 13210 35th Ave. North, Plymouth, MN 55441. (763) 559-1797. Fax: (863) 694-0017. http://www.oaanews.org.

Ken R. Wells

# Ornithine transcarbamylase deficiency

## Definition

Ornithine transcarbamylase deficiency is a disorder in which there is a failure of the body to properly process ammonia, which can lead to coma and death if left untreated.

## Description

Persons with ornithine transcarbamylase deficiency (OTC deficiency) have a problem with nitrogen metabolism. Too much nitrogen in the blood in the form of ammonia can cause brain damage, coma, and death. Ammonia is made up of nitrogen and hydrogen. Ammonia found in humans mostly comes from the breakdown of protein, either protein broken down from muscles, organs, and tissues already in the body, or excess protein that is eaten in the diet. Since excess

---

**KEY TERMS**

**Developmental delay**—When children do not reach certain milestones at appropriate ages. For example, a child should be able to speak by the time he or she is five years old.

**Hyperammonemia**—An excess of ammonia in the blood.

**Urea**—A nitrogen-containing compound that can be excreted through the kidney.

**Urea cycle**—A series of complex biochemical reactions that remove nitrogen from the blood so ammonia does not accumulate.

---

ammonia is harmful, it is immediately excreted in normal humans after passing through the urea cycle and becoming urea. Ornithine transcarbamylase is a **gene** involved in the urea cycle—the process of making ammonia into urea, which occurs in the liver.

It is important to make urea, because unlike ammonia, urea can be excreted by the kidney into the urine. Ammonia on the other hand, cannot be effectively excreted by the kidney. So, if the ornithine transcarbamylase (OTC) function is reduced or impaired, ammonia builds up in the bloodstream. This buildup of ammonia in the bloodstream can lead to consequences as severe as coma and death. The amount of ammonia found in the bloodstream, and the severity of the disorder, depend on how well the OTC gene functions. If it functions reasonably well, the person should have a minor form of the disorder or no disorder. If the gene functions extremely poorly, or not at all, the disorder will be severe.

Synonyms for ornithine transcarbamylase deficiency include Hyperammonemia Type II, Ornithine carbamyl transferase deficiency, OTC deficiency, UCE, Urea cycle disorder, OTC Type, and Hyperammonemia due to ornithine transcarbamylase deficiency.

## Genetic profile

OTC deficiency is an X-linked recessive disorder. This means that it is found on the X **chromosome** (specifically, it is located on the short arm at Xp21.1) Recessive disorders require that only abnormal genes, and no normal genes, be present. For non-sex chromosomes, this means that both copies of a gene (one received from each parent) must be abnormal in order for that person to have the disorder.

In X-linked recessive disorders, however, only one abnormal copy of a gene must be present to cause the disorder in males. Males possess only one X chromosome, from their mother, and one Y chromosome, which they receive from their father. If the mother is a carrier for the disorder (she has one normal gene and one abnormal gene), a male child would have a 50% chance of receiving an abnormal gene from her. If he receives the abnormal gene, he will have the disorder. So male children of a female carrier have a 50% chance of having the disorder.

A female child of a female carrier is much less likely to have the disorder. Unless the father has OTC deficiency, a female child will have one normal and one abnormal gene. Since recessive disorders require that both genes be mutated, the female child cannot have the disorder. Females with only one mutant OTC gene may have a mild form of the disorder because it is not purely recessive. Usually, the normal copy of the gene can sufficiently compensate for the poor functioning of the second, abnormal gene.

Some females do have the full-blown disorder, probably because of a phenomenon called X-inactivation. Although females have two X chromosomes in each cell, only one is active. Therefore, it is possible a female could have the disorder because only the abnormal gene was active in each cell of the liver, which is where OTC function takes place. Not enough is known about X-inactivation to speculate on the likelihood of this occuring. Overall, many more men than women have the disease. This means that OTC disease due to X-inactivation is not very common.

If the father has the gene for the disorder, he cannot pass it on to his male child (he does not give the male child an X chromosome, only a Y). He can give his female child one copy of the gene, which might result in a mild form of the disorder or the full-blown disorder due to X-inactivation.

### Demographics

OTC affects infants at the rate of approximately one birth in every 70,000. As expected with an X-linked disorder, the disorder is more common in males.

### Signs and symptoms

Before birth there are no symptoms of OTC deficiency because the exchange of nutrients and fluids between the mother and fetus allows the excess ammonia to leave the infant's blood and go into the mother's blood. The mother is then able to get rid of the ammonia

as urea because she either lacks the disorder or her ammonia levels are medically well-controlled.

The most severe cases of OTC deficiency usually present in infants before they are a week old, typically in males. It may take several days for symptoms to appear, since it takes that long for protein, and therefore ammonia levels, to build up in the infant. Affected infants generally show periods of inactivity, a failure to feed, and vomiting. Unfortunately, many other disorders may also present with these same general symptoms, and new parents may not recognize these as abnormal in an infant. These symptoms are always accompanied in OTC deficiency by hyperammonemia, or high levels of ammonia in the blood.

Hyperammonemia is the most important symptom for identification and treatment of ornithine transcarbamylase deficiency. It is the cause of all other symptoms seen in OTC deficiency. Additionally, hepatomegaly (an enlarged liver), and seizures may also be present. If the disorder, or at least the hyperammonemia, is not recognized and treated, the symptoms may progress into coma and eventually death. A failure to quickly resolve the hyperammonemia once an infant lapses into a coma may also lead to severe mental retardation or death.

Patients with milder forms of the disorder may show symptoms later in life such as failure to grow at a normal rate or they may experience developmental delay. Developmental delay is an inability to reach recognized milestones like speaking or grasping objects at an appropriate age. These milder symptoms would be accompanied by hyperammonemia, but the levels of ammonia would be much lower than in an episodic attack of hyperammonemia or in the severely ill infant. Other persons with mild forms of the disorder may have no symptoms, or may only experience nausea after a meal with a large protein content.

Persons with a mild form of the disorder and no other symptoms may also learn they have the disorder from an episode of acute hyperammonemia. Acute conditions are brief and immediate, whereas chronic conditions are long-lasting.

An episodic attack of acute hypperammonemia, then, is a an episode where levels of ammonia climb above what may be already high levels of ammonia. A person with an episode of acute hyperammonemia can have symptoms including some, or all, of the following: vomiting, lack of apetite, drowsiness, hepatomegaly, seizures, coma, and death. These episodes can be life-threatening and may require hospitalization depending on their severity and response to medication.

These episodic attacks are probably related to a large increase in the amount of protein being broken down in the body, which results in too much ammonia being produced. This ammonia cannot be immediately excreted, which results in hyperammonemia. The most common reasons for a change in the amount of protein broken down are probably starvation, illness, and surgery. Even persons with no previous symptoms can experience a fatal episode of acute hyperammonemia brought on by an increase in protein breakdown. Since an episodic attack of hyperammonemia can be fatal without any previous symptoms, persons who have at least one family member with OTC deficiency should consider testing to determine whether they have the gene for the disorder. If the disorder is known to be present, an episode of hyperammonemia might be anticipated and its effect lessened.

### Diagnosis

A definitive diagnosis of OTC deficiency is made by laboratory tests, since physical symptoms are very general and common to a large number of disorders. A high level of ammonia in the blood is the hallmark of this disorder and other disorders that affect the urea cycle. In the short term, the levels of two amino acids in the urine, orotate and citrulline, should distinguish between OTC deficiency and other urea cycle deficiencies. In OTC deficiency, citrulline levels are normal or low, and orotate levels are usually high. In the long term, however, the most definitive diagnosis can be made through **DNA** analysis, or through a test of OTC activity in a small piece of liver tissue (a biopsy) taken from the patient.

Prenatal diagnosis of the disorder is difficult and not indicated unless there is an affected family member with the disorder. In that case, if the mutation is known, DNA analysis would reveal the same mutation as in the family member with OTC deficiency. If the mutation is not known, a method called linkage analysis may be used. In linkage analysis, the OTC gene itself is not analyzed, but the DNA near the gene is analyzed. The "near DNA" can then be compared to the "near DNA" of the affected family member. If the DNAs are different, then the fetus should not have the disorder. If they are the same, then the fetus probably has the disorder.

### Treatment and management

#### Long-term management

The severity of the disorder is the most important factor in determining long-term treatment of OTC deficiency. The most severely affected individuals, usually infant males, should have liver transplants. As previously mentioned, the urea cycle and OTCs function occur in the liver. The transplantation immediately corrects OTC deficiency. Episodes of life-threatening ammonemia are prevented, although monitoring of tissue levels of ammonia is suggested. Another important benefit is that the transplant allows the child to develop and grow in a normal manner, without the threat of developmental delay or mental retardation. Transplants are now recommended even for children less than one year of age with a severe form of the disorder.

Two problems with liver transplants exist, however. First, it is difficult to obtain a liver from among the limited supply of donors, especially if the child is not currently hospitalized. The second problem arises from the way in which organs are assigned. Persons who are critically ill receive priority in organ donor lists. This means children whose disease is manageable may not be able to receive a transplant.

Second, children with transplants must have their immune system suppressed. The immune system fights off, and lets one recover from infections like colds, flus, and chicken pox. However, it also fights the introduction of an organ from someone else's body, even a relative—except identical twins. Thus, as long as a person has a transplant, that person must have their immune system suppressed so that the transplanted organ is not killed by the body it is in. The problem with immune suppression is that a person is much more likely to become sick. This disadvantage is far outweighed by the advantages of normal mental development and the prevention of death in patients with severe OTC deficiency.

Patients in rural areas, or areas where there is no immediate access to a hospital equipped to care for a patient with an acute attack of hyperammonemia, should also be strongly considered for a liver transplant if the patient is predisposed to attacks of life-threatening hyperammonemia.

For less severely affected children, or children unable to obtain a liver transplant, long-term therapy consists of a combination of drugs, usually oral; sodium phenylbutyrate; and diet. This bypasses the normal process of the breakdown of protein into urea in the liver, which is the usual way that ammonia leaves the body. Children with OTC deficiency are placed on a low-protein diet so their protein breakdown system does not become overwhelmed and lead to hyperammonemia. Children with OTC deficiency are also given arginine, an amino acid, which, for reasons that are unclear, causes more nitrogen, which is part of ammonia, to be excreted in the urine, and lowers blood ammonia. Dietary regimens vary from patient to patient based on their age, size, and the severity of the disorder. A nutrition expert must be consulted when developing an appropriate diet. The most strict diet consists of vitamin supplements and no protein other than essential amino acids. Essential amino acids are those that cannot be made by the body and must be obtained through food. Since proteins are made up of amino acids, and only amino acids, that means this diet is extremely restrictive. It also means that very little ammonia is left in the bloodstream since most of the otherwise free ammonia is tied up in the synthesis of the non-essential amino acids, amino acids made by the body itself.

Any chronic disease is stressful for a family. Parents and patients should consider support and information groups like the National **Urea Cycle Disorders** Foundation.

### Short-term management

Short-term management of attacks of crisis hyperammonemia (severe acute hyperammonemia) consists of dialysis and drug therapy. Dialysis and large doses of the drugs sodium benzoate and sodium phenylacetate and doses of arginine are used to decrease the levels of ammonia in the blood. These methods are used together due to their synergistic effect.

Dialysis is a process where a toxic substance is removed from the blood. This can best be understood by pouring a small amount of cola into a glass. Now pour a large amount of water into it. In this way, the cola is "watered down" or diluted. Ammonia is diluted in a similar way using dialysis. Blood is removed from a patient and run through a hose. At one point, this hose runs through a tank made up of liquid that contains all the components of blood, but no ammonia (this liquid is like the water in the water and cola example). Thus, ammonia spreads throughout the blood and the liquid surrounding the hose (the same way cola will spread out throughout water added to the glass) and the amount of ammonia in the blood is reduced. By continuously pumping blood through the hose and changing the liquid around the hose, most of the ammonia can be removed from the blood. All of the really large particles, like red blood cells, are also kept in the blood because the hose has holes that are only large enough to let smaller particles like ammonia out while keeping red blood cells in.

### The future

The future treatment of OTC deficiency probably will come from experiments in **gene therapy**. OTC

deficiency is a disorder particularly amenable to gene therapy because only one gene is affected and only one organ, the liver, would need the new gene. However, as of the early 2000s, gene therapy has not been successfully demonstrated in human beings. Many technical problems must still be solved in order to successfully treat OTC deficiency and other disorders like it with gene therapy.

### Prognosis

Only 50% of the most severely affected patients live beyond the time they first attend school. Of those receiving liver transplants, 82% of patients survive five years after receiving the transplant. Children with the severe disorder that receive drug therapy are much more likely to experience mental retardation, developmental delay, and a lack of growth. Also, many infants who experience hyperammonemic comas have severe mental damage.

For individuals not identified at birth or soon after, the prognosis varies widely. The consequences of the disorder are affected by the severity of the disorder and how it is managed, although anyone with the disorder may experience life-threatening attacks of acute hyperammonemia. In terms of long-term survival, puberty appears to be a difficult time for those with OTC deficiency, and persons who survive until after puberty have improved outcomes. The prognosis for this disorder can vary from quite hopeful to very distressing based upon its severity and how well the disorder can be controlled. A severe disorder that is well-controlled may still have a positive outcome.

### Resources

#### PERIODICALS

Maestri, Nancy E., et al. "The Phenotype of Ostensibly Healthy Women Who Are Carriers for Ornithine Transcarbamylase Deficiency." *Medicine* 77, no. 6 (November 1998): 389.

#### WEBSITES

"Ornithine transcarbamylase deficiency." *Aim for Health.* http://www.aim4health.com/family/otc.htm.
"Ornithine transcarbamylase deficiency." *NORD—National Organization for Rare Diseases.* http://www.rarediseases.org.

#### ORGANIZATIONS

National Urea Cycle Disorders Foundation. 4841 Hill Street, La Canada, CA 91011. (800) 38NUCDF. http://www. NUCDF.org/.

Michael V. Zuck, Ph D

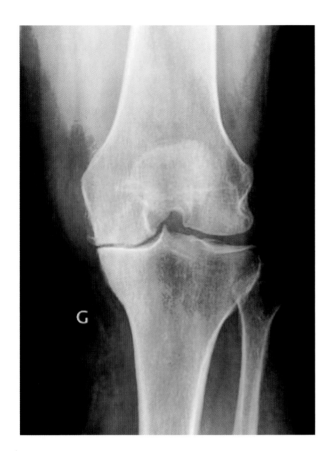

**Colored x ray of the knee showing osteoarthritis.** *(Phanie/ Photo Researchers, Inc.)*

## Description

Osteoarthritis is one of the oldest and most common types of arthritis. With the breakdown of cartilage, the part of the joint that cushions the ends of bones, bones rub against each other, causing pain and loss of movement. Often called "wear-and-tear arthritis" or "old person's arthritis," many factors can cause osteoarthritis.

The biologic causes of the disorder are currently unknown. It does not appear to be caused by aging itself, although osteoarthritis generally accompanies aging. Osteoarthritic cartilage is chemically different from normal aged cartilage.

In many cases, certain conditions seem to trigger osteoarthritis. People with joint injuries from sports, work-related activity, or accidents may be at increased risk, and obesity may lead to osteoarthritis of the knees. Individuals with mismatched surfaces on the joints that could be damaged over time by abnormal stress may be prone to osteoarthritis. One study reported that wearing shoes with 2.5 in (6.3 cm) heels or higher may also be a contributing factor. High heels force women to alter the way they normally maintain balance, putting strain on the areas between the knee-cap and thigh bone and on the inside of the knee joint.

## Demographics

Osteoarthritis is estimated to affect more than 20 million Americans, mostly after age 45. Women are more commonly affected than men.

In the United States about 6% of adults over 30 have osteoarthritis of the knee and about 3% have osteoarthritis of the hip. Prevalence of osteoarthritis in most joints is higher in men than women before age 50, but after this age, more women are affected by osteoarthritis. The occurrence of the disease increases with age. In men, the hip is affected more often while in women, the hands, fingers, and knees are more problematic.

Some forms of osteoarthritis are more prevalent in African American men and women than in Caucasians, possibly because they have a higher bone mineral density. In the case of knee osteoarthritis, it may be related to occupational and physical demands. African American women also have a higher risk of developing bilateral knee osteoarthritis and hip osteoarthritis compared to women of other races. This difference may be because African American women generally have a higher body mass index than the white women, which puts more stress on the joints.

Osteoarthritis is common worldwide, although risk of osteoarthritis varies among ethnic groups. Caucasians have a higher risk than Asians, and the risk of osteoarthritis in the hips is lower in Asia and some Middle East countries than in the United States. Asians appear to have a higher incidence of osteoarthritis in the knee than Caucasians, however, and an equal risk in the spine. Location of affected joints and inherited forms of the disorder can influence age of onset.

## Genetic profile

**Genetics** plays a role in the development of osteoarthritis, particularly in the hands and hips. One study found that heredity may be involved in 30% of people with osteoarthritic hands and 65% of those with osteoarthritic knees. Another study found a higher correlation of osteoarthritis between parents and children and between siblings than between spouses. Other research has shown that a genetic abnormality may promote a breakdown in the protective structure of cartilage.

Abnormal collagen genes have been identified in some families with osteoarthritis. One recent study found that the type IX collagen gene COL9A1 (6q12-q13) may be a susceptibility locus for female hip osteoarthritis. Other research has suggested that mutations in the COL2A1 gene may be associated with osteoarthritis.

Some evidence also suggests that a female-specific susceptibility gene for idiopathic osteoarthritis is located on 11q. There is some evidence of genetic abnormality at the IL1R1 marker on gene 2q12 in individuals with severe osteoarthritis and Heberden nodes (bony lumps on the end joint of fingers).

## Signs and symptoms

Although up to 85% of people over 65 show evidence of osteoarthritis on x ray, only 35-50% experience symptoms. Symptoms range from very mild to very severe, affecting hands and weight-bearing joints such as knees, hips, feet, and the back. The pain of osteoarthritis usually begins gradually and progresses slowly over many years.

Osteoarthritis is commonly identified by aching pain in one or more joints, stiffness, and loss of mobility. The disease can cause significant trouble walking and stair climbing. Inflammation may or may not be present. Extensive use of the joint often exacerbates pain in the joints. Osteoarthritis is often more bothersome at night than in the morning and in humid weather than dry weather. Periods of inactivity, such as sleeping or sitting, may result in stiffness, which can be eased by stretching and exercise. Osteoarthritis pain tends to fade within a year of appearing.

Bony lumps on the end joint of the finger, called Herberden's nodes, and on the middle joint of the finger, called Bouchard's nodes, may also develop.

## Diagnosis

A diagnosis of osteoarthritis is made based on a physical exam and history of symptoms.

X rays are used to confirm diagnosis. In people over 60, the disease can often be observed on x ray. An indication of cartilage loss arises if the normal space between the bones in a joint is narrowed, if there is an abnormal increase in bone density, or if bony projections or erosions are evident. Any cysts that might develop in osteoarthritic joints are also detectable by x ray.

Additional tests can be performed if other conditions are suspected or if the diagnosis is uncertain. Blood tests can rule out **rheumatoid arthritis** or other forms of arthritis.

It is possible to distinguish osteoarthritis from other joint diseases by considering a number of factors together:

- Osteoarthritis usually occurs in older people.
- It is usually located in only one or a few joints.
- The joints are less inflamed than in other arthritic conditions.
- Progression of pain is almost always gradual.

A few of the most common disorders that might be confused with osteoarthritis are rheumatoid arthritis, chondrocalcinosis, and Charcot's joints.

## Treatment and management

There is no known way to prevent osteoarthritis or slow its progression. Some lifestyle changes can reduce or delay symptoms. Treatment often focuses on decreasing pain and improving joint movement. Prevention and treatment measures may include:

- Exercises to maintain joint flexibility and improve muscle strength. By strengthening the supporting muscles, tendons, and ligaments, regular weight-bearing exercise helps protect joints, even possibly stimulating growth of the cartilage.
- Joint protection, which prevents strain and stress on painful joints.
- Heat/cold therapy for temporary pain relief.
- Various pain control medications, including corticosteroids and NSAIDs (nonsteroidal anti-inflammatory drugs such as aspirin, acetaminophen, ibuprofen, and naproxen). For inflamed joints that are not responsive to NSAIDS, injectable glucocorticoids may be used. For mild pain without inflammation, acetaminophen may be used.
- Weight control, which prevents extra stress on weight-bearing joints. One study reported that weight loss seemed to reduce the risk for symptomatic osteoarthritis of the knee in women, and in another,

women who lost 11 pounds or more cut their risk for developing osteoarthritis in half.

- Surgery may be needed to relieve chronic pain in damaged joints. Osteoarthritis is the most common indication for total joint replacement of the hip and knee.

### New treatment findings

Studies have found that estrogen may promote healthy joints in women. Hormone replacement therapy may significantly reduce the risk in postmenopausal women, particularly in the knees.

It has been reported that deficiencies in vitamin D in older people may worsen their condition, so individuals with osteoarthritis should strive to get the recommended 400 IU a day. To protect bones, adults should also consume at least 1,000 mg of calcium daily.

Glucosamine and chondroitin sulfate are popular nutritional supplements that may diminish the symptoms of osteoarthritis. According to some reports, a daily dose of 750–1,500 mg of glucosamine and chondroitin sulfate may result in reduced joint pain, stiffness, and swelling, however these supplements are not approved by the Food and Drug Administration as effective treatment of osteoarthritis. A person with osteoarthritis should consult with a doctor before using dietary supplements to treat symptoms.

### Prognosis

Osteoarthritis is not life threatening, but quality of life can deteriorate significantly due to the pain and loss of mobility that it causes. Advanced osteoarthritis can force the patient to forgo activities, even walking, unless the condition is alleviated by medication or corrected by surgery.

There is no cure for osteoarthritis, and no treatment alters its progression with any certainty. Only

heart disease has a greater impact on work, and 5% of those who leave the work force do so because of osteoarthritis.

### Resources

#### BOOKS

Grelsamer, Ronald P., and Suzanne Loebl, eds. *The Columbia Presbyterian Osteoarthritis Handbook*. New York: Macmillan, 1997.

#### PERIODICALS

Felson, D.T., et al. "Osteoarthritis: New Insights. Part 1: The Disease and Its Risk Factors." *Annals of Internal Medicine* 133, no. 8 (2000): 635+.

Felson, D.T., et al. "Osteoarthritis: New Insights. Part 2: Treatment Approaches." *Annals of Internal Medicine* 133, no. 9 (2000): 726+.

McAlindon, Tim. "Glucosamine for Osteoarthritis: Dawn of a New Era?" *Lancet* 357 (January 27, 2001): 247+.

#### WEBSITES

The Arthritis Research Institute of America. http://www.preventarthritis.org.

National Institute of Arthritis and Musculoskeletal and Skin Diseases. http://www.nih.gov/niams.

#### ORGANIZATIONS

Arthritis Foundation. 1330 West Peachtree St., Atlanta, GA 30309. (800) 283-7800. http://www.arthritis.org.

Jennifer F. Wilson, MS

# Osteogenesis imperfecta

## Definition

Osteogenesis imperfecta (OI) is a group of genetic diseases of collagen in which the bones are formed improperly, making them fragile and prone to breaking.

## Description

Collagen is a fibrous protein material. It serves as the structural foundation of skin, bone, cartilage, and ligaments. In osteogenesis imperfecta, the collagen produced is abnormal and disorganized. This results in a number of abnormalities throughout the body, the most notable being fragile, easily broken bones.

There are four forms of OI, Types I through IV. Of these, Type II is the most severe, and is usually fatal within a short time after birth. Types I, III, and IV have some overlapping and some distinctive symptoms, particularly weak bones.

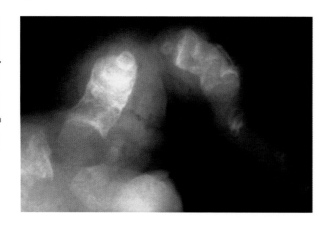

**A radiograph of a patient's left leg affected by osteogenesis imperfecta. This x ray shows light spots and poor bone formation.** *(Photo by Joseph R. Siebert, Ph.D. Custom Medical Stock Photo, Inc.)*

## Genetic profile

Evidence suggests that OI results from mutations in the COL1A1, COL1A2, CRTAP, and LEPRE 1 genes. Mutations in the COL1A1 gene, located on 17q21.3–q22.1, and in COL1A2, located on 7q22.1, are responsible for more than 90% of all cases of OI. These two genes provide instructions for making proteins that are used to assemble type I collagen, the most abundant protein in bone, skin, and other connective tissues. The CRTAP gene, located on 3p22.3, provides instructions for making a protein called "cartilage associated protein," required for normal bone development. The LEPRE1 gene, located on 1p34.1, provides instructions for making an enzyme that works with two other proteins, cartilage associated protein and cyclophilin B, to process certain types of collagen.

OI is usually inherited as an autosomal dominant condition. In autosomal dominant **inheritance**, a single abnormal gene on one of the autosomal chromosomes (one of the first 22 "non–sex" chromosomes) from either parent can cause the disease. One of the parents will have the disease (since it is dominant) and is the carrier. Only one parent needs to be a carrier in order for the child to inherit the disease. A child who has one parent with the disease has a 50% chance of also being a carrier and a 50% chance of not inheriting the dominant gene and thus, not having the disorder.

In OI, the genetic abnormality may direct cells to make an altered collagen protein and the presence of this altered collagen causes OI Type II, III, or IV. Alternately, the dominant altered gene may fail to direct cells to make any collagen protein. Although some collagen is produced by instructions from the normal gene, an overall decrease in the total amount of collagen produced results in OI Type I.

If both parents have OI caused by an autosomal dominant gene change, there is a 75% chance that the child will inherit one or both OI genes. In other words, there is a 25% chance the child will inherit only the mother's OI gene (and the father's unaffected gene), a 25% chance the child will inherit only the father's OI gene (and the mother's unaffected gene), and a 25% chance the child will inherit both parents' OI genes. Because this situation has been uncommon, the outcome of a child inheriting two OI genes is hard to predict. It is likely that the child would have a severe, possibly lethal, form of the disorder.

About 25% of children with OI are born into a family with no history of the disorder. This occurs when the gene spontaneously mutates in either the sperm or the egg before the child's conception. No triggers for this type of mutation are known. This is called a new dominant mutation. The child has a 50% chance of passing the disorder on to his or her children. In most cases, when a family with no history of OI has a child with OI, they are not at greater risk than the general population for having a second child with OI, and unaffected siblings of a person with OI are at no greater risk of having children with OI than the general population.

In studies of families into which infants with OI Type II were born, most of the babies had a new dominant mutation in a collagen gene. In some of these families, however, more than one infant was born with OI. Previously, researchers had seen this recurrence as evidence of recessive inheritance of this form of OI.

More recently, however, researchers have concluded that the rare recurrence of OI to a couple with a child with autosomal dominant OI is more likely due to gonadal mosaicism. Instead of a mutation occurring in an individual sperm or egg, it occurs in a percentage of the cells that give rise to a parent's multiple sperm or eggs. This mutation, present in a percentage of his or her reproductive cells, can result in more than one affected child without affecting the parent with the disorder. An estimated 2–4% of families into which an infant with OI Type II is born are at risk of having another affected child because of gonadal mosaicism.

## Demographics

As of 2009, the prevalence of OI in the United States is unknown. The best estimate suggests a minimum of 20,000 and possibly as many as 50,000 affected individuals.

## Signs and symptoms

### Type I

This is the most common and mildest type. Among the common features of Type I are the following:

- Bones are predisposed to fracture, with most fractures occurring before puberty. People with OI type I typically have about 20–40 fractures before puberty.
- Stature is normal or near–normal.
- Joints are loose and muscle tone is low.
- Usually sclera (whites of the eyes) have blue, purple, or gray tint.
- Face shape is triangular.
- Tendency toward scoliosis (a curvature of the spine).
- Bone deformity is absent or minimal.
- Dentinogenesis imperfecta may occur, causing brittle teeth.
- Hearing loss is a possible symptom, often beginning in the early 20s or 30s.
- Structure of collagen is normal, but the amount is less than normal.

### Type II

Sometimes called the lethal form, Type II is the most severe form of OI. Among the common features of Type II are the following:

- Frequently, OI Type II is lethal at or shortly after birth, often as a result of respiratory problems.
- Fractures are numerous and bone deformity is severe.
- Stature is small with underdeveloped lungs.
- Collagen is formed improperly.

### Type III

Among the common features of Type III are the following:

- Bones fracture easily. Fractures are often present at birth, and x rays may reveal healed fractures that occurred before birth. People with OI Type III may have more than 100 fractures before puberty.
- Stature is significantly shorter than normal.
- Sclera (whites of the eyes) have blue, purple, or gray tint.
- Joints are loose and muscle development is poor in arms and legs.
- Rib cage is barrel–shaped.
- Face shape is triangular.
- Scoliosis (a curvature of the spine) is present.
- Respiratory problems are possible.
- Bones are deformed and deformity is often severe.
- Dentinogenesis imperfecta may occur, causing brittle teeth.
- Hearing loss is possible.
- Collagen is formed improperly.

### Type IV

OI Type IV falls between Type I and Type III in severity. Among the common features of Type IV are the following:

- Bones fracture easily, with most fractures occurring before puberty.
- Stature is shorter than average.
- Sclera (whites of the eyes) are normal in color, appearing white or near–white.
- Bone deformity is mild to moderate.
- Scoliosis (curvature of the spine) is likely.
- Rib cage is barrel–shaped.
- Face is triangular in shape.
- Dentinogenesis imperfecta may occur, causing brittle teeth.
- Hearing loss is possible.
- Collagen is formed improperly.

## Diagnosis

It is often possible to diagnose OI solely on clinical features and x ray findings. Collagen or **DNA** tests may help confirm a diagnosis of OI. These tests generally require several weeks before results are known. Approximately 10–15% of individuals with mild OI who have collagen testing, and approximately 5% of those who have **genetic testing**, test negative for OI despite having the disorder.

Diagnosis is usually suspected when a baby has bone fractures after having suffered no apparent injury. Another indication is small, irregular, isolated bones in the sutures between the bones of the skull (wormian bones). Sometimes the bluish sclera serves as a diagnostic clue. Unfortunately, because of the unusual nature of the fractures occurring in a baby who cannot yet move, some parents have been accused of child abuse before the actual diagnosis of osteogenesis imperfecta was reached.

### Prenatal diagnosis

Testing is available to assist in prenatal diagnosis. Women with OI who become pregnant, or women who conceive a child with a man who has OI, may wish to explore prenatal diagnosis. Because of the relatively small risk (2–4%) of recurrence of OI Type II in a family, families may opt for ultrasound studies to determine if a developing fetus has the disorder.

Ultrasound is the least invasive procedure for prenatal diagnosis, and carries the least risk. Using ultrasound, a doctor can examine the fetus's skeleton for bowing of the leg or arm bones, fractures, shortening, or other bone abnormalities that may indicate OI. Different forms of OI may be detected by ultrasound in the second trimester. The reality is that when it occurs as a new dominant mutation, it is found inadvertently on ultrasound, and it may be difficult to know the diagnosis until after delivery since other genetic conditions can cause bowing and/or fractures prenatally.

Chorionic villus sampling is a procedure to obtain chorionic villi tissue for testing. Examination of fetal collagen proteins in the tissue can reveal information about the quantitative or qualitative collagen changes that lead to OI. When a parent has OI, it is necessary for the affected parent to have the results of his or her own collagen test available. Chorionic villus sampling can be performed at 10–12 weeks of pregnancy.

**Amniocentesis** is a procedure that involves inserting a thin needle into the uterus, into the amniotic sac, and withdrawing a small amount of amniotic fluid. DNA can be extracted from the fetal cells contained in the amniotic fluid and tested for the specific mutation known to cause OI in that family. This technique is useful only when the mutation causing OI in a particular family has been identified through previous genetic testing of affected family members, including previous pregnancies involving a baby with OI. Amniocentesis is performed at 16–18 weeks of pregnancy.

## Treatment and management

There are no treatments available to cure OI, nor to prevent most of its complications. Most treatments are aimed at correcting the fractures and bone abnormalities caused by OI. Splints, casts, braces, and rods are all used. Rodding refers to a surgical procedure in which a metal rod is implanted within a bone (usually the long bones of the thigh and leg). This is done when bowing or repeated fractures of these bones has interfered with a child's ability to begin to walk.

As of 2009, medications are being evaluated for their potential use to treat OI. These include growth hormone treatment, treatment with intravenous and oral drugs called bisphosphonates, an injected drug called teriparatide (for adults only), and gene therapies.

Other treatments include hearing aids and early capping of teeth. Patients may require the use of a walker or wheelchair. Pain may be treated with a variety of medications. Exercise is encouraged as a means to promote muscle and bone strength. Swimming is a form of exercise that puts a minimal amount of strain on muscles, joints, and bones. Walking is encouraged for those who are able.

Smoking, excessive alcohol and caffeine consumption, and steroid medications may deplete bone and increase bone fragility.

Alternative treatment such as acupuncture, naturopathic therapies, hypnosis, relaxation training, visual imagery, and biofeedback have all been used to try to decrease the constant pain of fractures.

### Clinical trials

Clinical trials on osteogenesis imperfecta are currently sponsored by the National Institutes of Health (NIH) and other agencies. As of 2009, NIH was reporting 13 on–going and completed studies.

Examples include:

- The evaluation of bisphosphonate treatment for OI. (NCT00063479)
- The evaluation of the effects of OI. (NCT00001594)
- The evaluation of growth hormone therapy for OI. (NCT00001305)

Clinical trial information is constantly updated by NIH and the most recent information on OI trials can be found at: http://clinicaltrials.gov/.

## Prognosis

Lifespan for people with OI Type I, III, and IV is not generally shortened. The prognosis for people with these types of OI is quite variable, depending on the severity of the disorder and the number and severity of the fractures and bony abnormalities.

Fifty percent of all babies with OI Type II are stillborn. The rest of these babies usually die within a very short time after birth. In recent years, some people with Type II have lived into young adulthood.

## Resources

### BOOKS

Ablon, Joan. *Brittle Bones, Stout Hearts and Minds: Adults with Osteogenesis Imperfecta.* Sudbury, MA: Jones & Bartlett Publishers, 2009.

Minor, Patricia. *What Life Is Like Living with OI: Osteogenesis Imperfecta, Brittle Bones.* Frederick, MD: PublishAmerica, 2006.

Parker, Philip M. *Osteogenesis Imperfecta—A Bibliography and Dictionary for Physicians, Patients, and Genome Researchers.* San Diego, CA: Icon Health Publications, 2007.

### PERIODICALS

Brusin, J. H. "Osteogenesis imperfecta." *Radiologic Technology* 79, no. 16 (July–August 2008): 549–551.

Burnel, G., et al. "Osteogenesis imperfecta: diagnosis and treatment." *Journal of the American Academy of Orthopaedic Surgeons* 16, no. 6 (June 2008): 356–366.

Castillo, H., et al. "Effects of bisphosphonates in children with osteogenesis imperfecta: an AACPDM systematic review." *Developmental Medicine and Child Neurology* 51, no. 1 (January 2009): 17–29.

Hackley. L., and L. Merritt. "Osteogenesis imperfecta in the neonate." *Advances in Neonatal Care* 8, no. 1 (February 2008): 21–39.

Hasegawa, K., et al. "Growth of infants with osteogenesis imperfecta treated with bisphosphonate." *Pediatrics International* 51, no. 1 (February 2009): 54–58.

### WEBSITES

*Fast Facts on Osteogenesis Imperfecta.* Fact Sheet. Osteogenesis Imperfecta Foundation. (April 25, 2009). http://www.oif.org/site/PageServer?pagename = FastFacts.

*Osteogenesis Imperfecta.* Health Topics. Medline Plus, March 18, 2009 (April 25, 2009). http://www.nlm.nih.gov/medlineplus/osteogenesisimperfecta.html.

*Osteogenesis Imperfecta.* Medical Encyclopedia. Medline Plus, April 21, 2009 (April 25, 2009). http://www.nlm.nih.gov/medlineplus/ency/article/001573.htm.

*Osteogenesis Imperfecta Overview.* Information Page. NIAMS (April 25, 2009). http://www.niams.nih.gov/Health_Info/Bone/Osteogenesis_Imperfecta/default.asp.

*What is osteogenesis imperfecta?* Information Page. Genetics Home Reference, November 2007 (April 25, 2009). http://ghr.nlm.nih.gov/condition = osteogenesi simperfecta.

### ORGANIZATIONS

Little People of America. 250 El Camino Real, Suite 201, Tustin, CA 92780. (888)LPA-2001 or (714)368-3689.

Fax: (714)368-3367. Email: info@lpaonline.org. http://www.lpaonline.org.

National Institute of Arthritis and Musculoskeletal and Skin Diseases (NIAMS). 1 AMS Circle, Bethesda, MD 20892-3675. (301)495-4484 or (877)22-NIAMS (226-4267). Fax: (301)718-6366. Email: NIAMSinfo@mail.nih.gov. http://www.niams.nih.gov.

National Organization for Rare Disorders (NORD). 55 Kenosia Avenue, PO Box 1968, Danbury, CT 06813-1968. (203)744-0100 or (800)999-6673. Fax: (203)798-2291. http://www.rarediseases.org.

Osteogenesis Imperfecta Foundation. 804 W. Diamond Ave., Suite 210, Gaithersburg, MD 20878. (301)947-0083 or (800)981-2663. Fax: (301)947-0456. Email: bonelink@oif.org. http://www.oif.org.

Jennifer F. Wilson, MS

# Osteoporosis

## Definition

Osteoporosis is a disease characterized by low bone mass and deterioration of bone tissues, leading to bone fragility and, consequently, an increase in fracture risk.

## Description

The term osteoporosis comes from the Greek word *osteon*, meaning bone, and *porus*, meaning pore or passage. Osteoporosis literally makes bones porous. The amount of calcium stored in bones decreases over time causing the skeleton to weaken.

In the body of early adults, both the mineral portion and the framework of bone is in constant flux. Old tissue is broken down and reabsorbed and new bone is created at approximately the same rate. In later years, this rate of renewal begins to slow behind the rate of removal. This slowing is what leaves the bones thinner and more fragile. The most typical sites of fractures related to osteoporosis are the hip, spine, wrist, and ribs, although the disease can affect any bone in the body.

The average woman acquires 98% of her skeletal mass by approximately age 20. Building strong bones during childhood and adolescence is a key defense against developing osteoporosis later. There are four main steps to preventing osteoporosis: consuming a balanced diet rich in calcium and vitamin D; participating in weight-bearing exercise; following a healthy lifestyle, including no smoking and limited alcohol

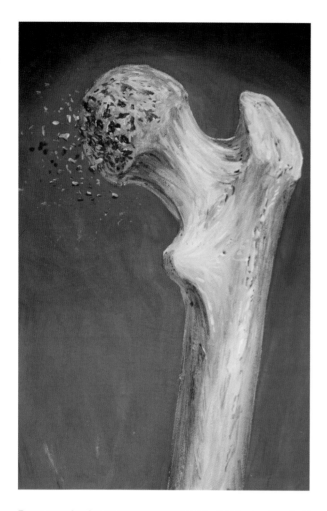

Bone atrophy due to osteoporosis in a human femur. The ball joint has become porous and brittle. *(Custom Medical Stock Photo, Inc.)*

- Lifestyle habits such as smoking, excessive alcohol use, low calcium intake, inadequate physical exercise

Type II, senile osteoporosis, affects both men and women over the age of 70, although women are twice as likely to develop the disorder.

In some cases, osteoporosis is secondary to another cause. It can accompany endocrine disorders such as **acromegaly** and Cushing syndrome. It results from excessive use of drugs such as corticosteroids. In these cases, the treatment is directed at curing the principal ailment or at not using the offending drug. Blood or urine tests will diagnose other causes of bone loss or bone density.

### Genetic profile

Osteoporosis results from a complex interaction between genetic and environmental factors throughout life. Evidence suggests that peak bone mass is inherited, but current genetic markers are only able to explain a small proportion of the variation in individual bone mass or fracture risk. At this time, no specific mode of **inheritance** has been identified. Heritability of bone mass has been estimated to account for 60-90% of its variance. Studies have shown reduced bone mass in daughters of osteoporotic women when compared with controls; in men and women who have first-degree relatives with osteoporosis; and in perimenopausal women who have a family history of hip fracture. Body weight in infancy may be a determinant of adult bone mineral area.

Some scientists think that environmental influences during early life interact with the genome to establish the functional level of a variety of metabolic processes involved in skeletal growth.

intake; and testing bone density and taking medication when appropriate.

Type I, postmenopausal osteoporosis, is the most common. It is usually a consequence of reproductive hormone deficiency, and afflicts mostly women over age 50. The disorder typically appears within the first ten or twenty years after menopause. Men may also develop the disorder, usually around 50-60 years of age, as a result of:

- Prolonged exposure to certain medications such as steroids used to treat asthma or arthritis, anticonvulsants, aluminum-containing antacids, and certain cancer treatments

- Chronic disease that affects the kidneys, lungs, stomach, and intestines and alters hormone levels

- Undiagnosed low levels of the sex hormone testosterone

Many candidate genes exist for osteoporosis, however relatively few have been studied. The first candidate gene to be identified was the vitamin D receptor (VDR) gene, and studies are ongoing as to how much this gene accounts for variance in bone mass. The response of bone mass to dietary supplementation with vitamin D and calcium is known to be dependent, in part, on VDR polymorphisms. Other genes may aid in establishing who would benefit from treatments like hormone replacement therapy, bisphosophonates, or exercise. Associations between bone mass and polymorphisms have also been found in the estrogen receptor gene, the interleukin-6 genes, the transforming growth factor beta, and a binding site of the collagen type I alpha1 (COLIA1) gene.

The risk of osteoporosis is greatly determined by peak bone mass, and any gene linked to fractures in the elderly may possibly be associated with low bone mass in children as well.

Environmental influences such as diet, climate, and physical exercise may have significant impact on gene expression, as well. In particular, malnutrition early in life is likely to have permanent effects resulting in lowered bone mass.

## Demographics

Significant risk has been reported in people of all ethnic backgrounds. Asian and white women are at greatest risk of bone thinning because they generally have the lowest bone density. Although the risk is smaller, African American and Hispanic American women should take precaution, as well. An estimated 10% of African American women over age 50 have osteoporosis and an additional 30% have low bone density that puts them at risk of developing osteoporosis.

Women in general have a four times greater risk than men of developing osteoporosis, and 80% of those affected by osteoporosis are women. In the United States, an estimated eight million American women and two million men have osteoporosis.

An osteoporosis-related fracture will occur in one in two women and one in eight men over the age of 50.

## Signs and symptoms

Often called "the silent disease" because bone loss occurs without symptoms, people may not know that they have osteoporosis until they have a fracture from a minor bump or fall, or a vertebra collapses. Physical signs of osteoporosis include back pain, loss of height over time, stooped posture, and fractures of vertebrae, wrists, or hips. Osteoporosis can be detected by a bone mineral density test or even a regular x ray.

Without preventive treatment, women can lose up to 20% of their bone mass in the first five to seven years following menopause, making them more susceptible to osteoporosis.

Over many years, a sequence of spinal compression fractures may cause kyphosis, the bent-over posture known as dowager's or widow's hump. These fractures rarely require surgery, and they can range from causing minor discomfort to severe painful episodes of backache. In either case, pain generally subsides gradually over one to two months.

## Diagnosis

Since osteoporosis can develop undetected for decades until a fracture occurs, early diagnosis is important.

A bone mineral density test (BMD) is the only way to diagnose osteoporosis and determine risk for future fracture. The painless, noninvasive test measures bone density and helps determine whether medication is needed to help maintain bone mass, prevent further bone loss, and reduce fracture risk.

Several different machines measure bone density. Central machines, such as the dual energy x-ray absorptiometry (DXA or DEXA) and quantitative computed tomography (QCT), measure density in the hip, spine, and total body. Peripheral machines, such as radiographic absorptiometry (RA), peripheral dual energy x-ray absorptiometry (pDXA), and peripheral quantitative computed tomography (pQCT), measure density in the finger, wrist, kneecap, shin bone, and heel.

A physician may be able to observe osteoporotic bone in a routine spinal x ray, however, BMD tests are more accurate and can measure small percentages of lost bone density. In an x ray, osteoporotic bone appears less dense and the image is less distinct, suggesting weaker bone.

There are no official guidelines for osteoporosis screening. Some physicians recommend bone density testing at menopause to begin preventive treatment if necessary. Generally, testing is recommended for postmenopausal women who have suffered a bone fracture after menopause or who have gone through menopause and have at least one risk factor for the disease. The major risk factors are low body weight, low calcium intake, poor health, and a history of osteoporosis in the family. The test is usually recommended for all women over 65.

Testing may also be recommended for elderly men with one of the following risk factors: bone fracture, poor health, or low testosterone levels.

## Treatment and management

There a number of options for preventing and treating bone loss.

### Therapeutic options

Various therapies have been shown to be effective in preventing bone loss and increasing bone mass. These include:

- *Estrogen.* For women with postmenopausal osteoporosis, estrogen replacement therapy helps halt bone loss and exerts a modest bone-building effect. Stopping estrogen therapy restarts bone loss, so long-term treatment is usually recommended. For women entering menopause, some physicians recommend estrogen replacement therapy to replace the decreasing supply of naturally-occurring estrogen in the body and enable the skeleton to slow its rate of absorption and retain calcium. Estrogen is considered the best treatment against osteoporosis. Physicians may recommend combination estrogen and progesterone replacement therapy in women who have an intact uterus in order to reduce endometrial cancer risk. Some studies indicate a relationship between estrogen use and breast cancer while other studies indicate no relationship at all; the issue is still to be determined.
- *Raloxifene.* One of a class of drugs called selective estrogen receptor modulators (SERMs) that appear to prevent bone loss, raloxifene (Evista) produces small increases in bone mass. It is approved for the prevention and treatment of osteoporosis. Like estrogens, SERMs produce changes in blood lipids that may protect against heart disease, although the effects are not as potent as that of estrogen. Unlike estrogens, SERMs do not appear to stimulate uterine or breast tissue.
- *Alendronate.* One of a class of medications called bisphosphonates, alendronate (Fosamax) may prevent bone loss, increase bone mass, and reduce the risk of fractures.
- *Risedronate.* Also from the bisphosphonate family, risedronate (Actonel) has been shown to reduce bone loss, increase bone density, and reduce the risk of fractures.
- *Calcitonin.* A hormone that regulates calcium levels in the blood, calcitonin may prevent bone loss. It is approved for treatment of diagnosed osteoporosis.

### Preventive options

Measures have been identified that improve bone strength over the life span. Physicians recommend that all adult men and women, but particularly men and women over the age of 50, take the following measures to prevent osteoporosis:

- Consume at least 1,000 mg calcium. Foods high in calcium include dairy products, leafy green vegetables, beans, nuts, and whole-grain cereals. Supplements may be taken if adequate intake cannot be achieved through diet.
- Consume 400 IU of vitamin D to enhance calcium absorption.
- Participate in regular weight-bearing exercise, such as walking, jogging, tennis, weight-lifting, and cross-county skiing, to strengthen bones.
- Stop smoking.
- Reduce intake of caffeine to not more than three cups a day.
- Limit alcohol to not more than two drinks per day.
- Avoid excessive amounts of dietary fiber as it binds to calcium and may interfere with absorption.

Making the house a safer place against falls can decrease risk of fracture in people with osteoporosis. Install handrails on the stairs; remove loose throw rugs; keep rooms and hallways well-lit including night lights; install handrails beside the tub, shower and toilet; and place nonskid mats in the bathtub, shower, and on tile bathroom floors.

If fractures occur, treatment may require casts, braces, physical therapy, and surgery to assist bone healing.

## Prognosis

When osteoporosis is untreated, it can cause serious disability. Osteoporosis can be managed with proper medical and self-care.

Osteoporosis is associated with 40,000 deaths annually, mostly from complications of surgery or immobilization after hip fractures.

## Resources

### BOOKS

*Osteoporosis: Diagnosis and management,* edited by Pierre J. Meunier. Mosby, 1998.

*Osteoporosis in Men: The effects of gender on skeletal health,* edited by Eric S. Orwoll. Academic Press, 1999.

### PERIODICALS

Altkorn, Diane, Tamara Vokes, and Alice T. D. Hughes. "Treatment of Postmenopausal Osteoporosis." *JAMA: Journal of the American Medical Association* 11 (2001): 1415+.

NIH Consensus Development Panel on Osteoporosis Prevention, Diagnosis, and Therapy. "Osteoporosis Prevention, Diagnosis, and Therapy." *JAMA: Journal of the American Medical Association* 285 (2001): 785+.

### WEBSITES

National Osteoporosis Foundation. http://www.nof.org.

Osteoporosis and Related Bone Diseases–National Resource Center. National Institutes of Health. http://www.osteo.org.

### ORGANIZATIONS

Foundation for Osteoporosis Research and Education. 300 27th St., Oakland, CA 94612. (888) 266-3015. http://www.fore.org.

Jennifer F. Wilson, MS

---

> ## KEY TERMS
>
> **Alkaline phosphatase (Alk phos)**—A body protein, measurable in the blood, that often appears in high amounts in patients with osteosarcoma. However, many other conditions also elevate the level of alkaline phosphatase.
>
> **Chemotherapy**—A type of treatment for cancer that attempts to kill tumor cells with doses of powerful, often toxic, chemicals.
>
> **Grade**—As a noun: a classification of the cancerous qualities of an individual tumor. A higher grade indicates a more serious disease than does a lower grade. As a verb: to classify the cancerous qualities of an individual tumor.
>
> **Malignant**—Cancerous.
>
> **Metastasize**—To spread to another part of the body.
>
> **Monoclonal antibody**—A protein, produced in large quantities in a laboratory, designed to attack a specific target in the body.
>
> **Osteogenic**—Creating bone.
>
> **Osteogenic sarcoma**—Osteosarcoma.
>
> **Paget's disease**—A non-cancerous disease marked by excessive growth of abnormal bone material.
>
> **Retinoblastoma**—A cancerous tumor of the eye.
>
> **Stage**—As a noun: the extent to which an individual cancer has spread. A higher stage indicates a more serious disease than does a lower stage. As a verb: to determine the extent to which an individual cancer has spread.
>
> **Tumor**—An abnormal growth of cells in the body. Tumors may be benign (non-cancerous) or malignant.

# Osteosarcoma

## Definition

Osteosarcoma, also called osteogenic sarcoma, is a type of **cancer** that develops from bone. Osteosarcoma is destructive at its original area and is likely to spread to other parts of the body.

## Description

Osteosarcoma is a malignant (cancerous) tumor that arises from bone itself, and is thus called a primary bone cancer. Primary bone cancers are relatively rare overall. Approximately 2,400 new cases of osteosarcoma occur in the United States every year.

Osteosarcoma occurs most frequently during childhood or adolescence. About 60% of cases of this disease develop during the second decade of life. The incidence of osteosarcoma rises again among people in their 40s and 50s.

Osteosarcoma may occur in any bone, but develops most commonly in long bones, particularly near the knee or in the upper arm. The cancer starts growing within a bone and forms an expanding, ball-like mass. The tumor eventually breaks through the surface of the bone and begins to invade adjoining structures such as muscles. If untreated, the disease usually appears elsewhere in the same limb and metastasizes to distant parts of the body, such as the lungs.

## Causes and symptoms

There are numerous theories regarding the causes of osteosarcoma. Many cases occur during a time of rapid bone growth, as in teenagers or people with Paget's disease. This suggests that the cancer may develop when the body loses its ability to control the multiplication of certain bone cells. Some cases of osteosarcoma are likely to have a genetic basis, and numerous genetic abnormalities have been found in patients with osteosarcoma. Osteosarcoma is also the most common second cancer to develop in survivors of **retinoblastoma**, a cancer of the eye that often has a genetic cause. Other cases arise in people who have been exposed to radiation, either accidentally or as part of a medical treatment.

The most common early symptoms of osteosarcoma are often vague. There may be pain or swelling at the site of the tumor, but these symptoms initially may not seem serious in a young, active person. Thus, the patient or medical personnel may attribute the symptoms to growing pains, or an injury from sports, for example, and the diagnosis may be delayed. Eventually, it is usually possible to feel a firm lump on the bone, and this lump will be uncomfortable to the touch.

## Diagnosis

The complete diagnosis of osteosarcoma is a complicated process, requiring a variety of tests and the help of several types of medical specialists. Physicians must determine the stage of the cancer (the extent to which it has spread), and the grade of the cancer (the degree of cancerous qualities shown by its cells in a biopsy specimen). A higher grade or stage indicates a more serious disease than does a lower grade or stage.

Initial diagnosis begins with x-ray images of the affected area. These pictures will show a destructive growth within the bone, which is often described as having a "moth-eaten appearance." The patient then requires further imaging tests such as computed tomography (CT, CAT) or magnetic resonance (MR, MRI) scans of the tumor, a chest x-ray series or chest CT, and a nuclear medicine scan of the entire skeleton (bone scan). Blood tests, such as measurements of alkaline phosphatase (alk phos), provide additional information. These tests all help determine the stage of the cancer.

Finally, physicians require a biopsy sample of the diseased bone, obtained with a needle or by a surgical procedure, to be sure that the disease is truly cancer and to identify its grade. There are numerous tests, mostly involving examinations under the microscope, to perform on this biopsy specimen.

## Treatments and prognosis

Before the 1980s, limb amputation was the standard treatment for osteosarcoma. Usually, however, the tumor had already spread elsewhere in the body and the patient eventually died of the disease. Overall results were dismal.

Newer medical developments make it possible to avoid amputation and yet treat many patients with osteosarcoma successfully. Patients almost always receive chemotherapy with more than one drug (multi-drug therapy) before surgery to shrink the original cancer and reduce the likelihood of spread to other areas. Techniques known as limb-sparing surgery often allow removal of the tumor while saving the rest of the extremity. Afterward, patients usually continue to receive chemotherapy, and may require bone grafts or prosthetic devices to replace parts of bones or joints that have been removed.

Future treatments under investigation include monoclonal antibodies that destroy specific cancer cells, techniques to slow cancer growth by controlling certain cellular genes, and bone-seeking substances that directly target areas of active bone growth.

### Alternative and complementary therapies

Current treatments with chemotherapy and surgery offer a substantial improvement over past therapies. Radiation treatment has not been effective. Complementary and alternative medicine techniques may improve a patient's sense of well-being but will not cure this destructive type of cancer.

### Prognosis

Prognosis for an individual patient reflects a complex balance among the extent to which the cancer has already spread at the time of diagnosis, the aggressiveness of the cells within the cancer, and the response to chemotherapy. Early detection is extremely important. The best chance of cure occurs when a tumor shows no sign of metastasis at the time of original surgery, is well-confined within a single bone and is completely removed, and responds well to chemotherapy. The five-year survival rate for osteosarcoma in a long bone of a limb is about 70%. All patients must be followed closely by a physician to watch for cancer recurrence.

## Prevention

Prevention of osteosarcoma is difficult since doctors do not know the cause of most cases. Perhaps research eventually will make prevention possible. Early detection of the disease remains vital. Anyone with persistent pain in a bone or limb should report this to a physician. People with special risk factors including Paget's disease, exposure to significant amounts of radiation, or a family history of certain types of cancer must be especially vigilant.

## Resources

### PERIODICALS

Marina, Neyssa, et al. "Biology and Therapeutic Advances for Pediatric Osteosarcoma." *The Oncologist* 9 (2004): 422-41.

Wittig, James C., et al. "Osteosarcoma: A Multidisciplinary Approach to Diagnosis and Treatment." *American Family Physician* 65 (2002): 1123-32, 1135-6.

Kenneth J. Berniker, M.D.
Abigail V. Berniker, B.A.

# Otopalatodigital syndrome

## Definition

Otopalatodigital (OPD) syndrome, also called digitootopalatal syndrome or palatootodigital syndrome, is a rare X-linked genetic disorder that affects bone and facial structure. OPD is fully expressed in males. Females are only mildly affected.

## Description

There are two forms of OPD syndrome. Type I is inherited through an X-linked trait with intermediate expression in females while type II is inherited through an X-linked recessive trait. OPD syndrome type I is also called Taybi syndrome. OPD syndrome type II is alternately called Andre syndrome, craniooorodigital syndrome, or faciopalatoosseous (FPO) syndrome.

A genetic disorder called frontometaphyseal **dysplasia**, or FMD, has very similar features to type I OPD syndrome.

There are three recognized forms of a genetic disorder called **Larsen syndrome**: an autosomal dominant type, a recessive type, and a lethal type. All three of these syndromes have similar symptoms to those seen in individuals affected with OPD syndrome.

---

**KEY TERMS**

**Brachydactyly**—Abnormal shortness of the fingers and toes.

**Cleft palate**—A congenital malformation in which there is an abnormal opening in the roof of the mouth that allows the nasal passages and the mouth to be improperly connected.

**Clinodactyly**—An abnormal inward curving of the fingers or toes.

**Conductive hearing loss**—Hearing loss that is the result of a dysfunction of the parts of the ear responsible for collecting sound. In this type of hearing loss, the auditory nerve is generally not damaged.

**Hypertelorism**—A wider-than-normal space between the eyes.

**Hypospadias**—An abnormality of the penis in which the urethral opening is located on the underside of the penis rather than at its tip.

**Omphalocele**—A birth defect where the bowel and sometimes the liver protrudes through an opening in the baby's abdomen near the umbilical cord.

**Palpebral fissures**—The opening between the upper and lower eyelids.

**Pectus excavatum**—An abnormality of the chest in which the sternum (breastbone) sinks inward; sometimes called "funnel chest."

---

Recent evidence also suggests that Larsen syndrome, recessive type, may in fact be type II OPD syndrome.

As the various names of OPD syndrome suggest, this disorder is characterized by malformations and/or dysfunctions of the ears (-oto-), palate (-palato-), fingers and toes (-digito-), skull (-cranio-), mouth (-oro-), face (-facio-), and bones (-osseo-). Some of the characteristics common to both types of OPD syndrome include: a **cleft palate**, a prominent forehead, a broad nose, widely spaced eyes (hypertelorism), a downward slanting of the opening between the upper and lower eyelids (palpebral fissures), conductive hearing loss, short fingers and toes (**brachydactyly**), an abnormal inward curving of the fingers (clinodactyly), a caved in chest at birth (pectus excavatum), short stature (dwarfism), and a congenital dislocation of the elbows caused by a misalignment of the head of the large bone in the forearm (radius).

## Genetic profile

Both forms of OPD syndrome are X-linked. The **gene** mutation responsible for the appearance of type I

OPD syndrome has been tentatively assigned to the Xq28 band. It is also believed that type II OPD syndrome is an allelic variant of type I OPD, which is to say that each form of OPD syndrome is caused by different mutations in the same gene or in overlapping genes at the same chromosomal location. Recessive type Larsen syndrome is also believed to be either another allelic variant of OPD syndrome, or identical to type II OPD syndrome. Another extremely rare genetic disorder, Melnick-Needles syndrome, also has an overlapping of symptoms with type II OPD syndrome. It is felt that this syndrome is also possibly an allelic variant of OPD syndrome.

OPD syndrome is transmitted via the X **chromosome**. A female generally possesses two X chromosomes, one from her mother and one from her father. A male generally possesses only a single X chromosome, that from his mother. He gets a Y chromosome from his father. Certain rare exceptions to these **inheritance** patterns are seen, but in general, a female is an XX and a male is an XY. It is for this reason that X-linked disorders are generally seen in greater numbers of males than females. The male does not possess a second X chromosome that can be expressed. A male either has a mutation on his X chromosome, or he does not. A female, on the other hand, can be either homozygous or heterozygous for an X-linked trait. That is, she can either have two identical copies of this trait (homozygous) or only one copy is this trait (heterozygous).

Type I OPD syndrome is transmitted through a dominant trait. A child of a type I OPD syndrome affected parent has a 50% chance of also being affected with type I OPD syndrome.

Type II OPD syndrome is transmitted through an X-linked recessive trait. A child of a type II OPD syndrome affected parent has a 50% chance of also inheriting the gene for the type II OPD syndrome. Subsequently, if that child is male, he will have expression of the disorder. If it is a female child, then she generally will have milder features. Girls who are homozygous for type II OPD syndrome (inheriting the gene from each parent) will exhibit more severe symptoms than girls who are heterozygous for type II OPD syndrome. Males affected with type II OPD syndrome exhibit symptoms similar to those seen in homozygous girls.

### Demographics

As of the early 2000s, the incidence of occurrence of both forms of OPD syndrome has not been determined. The lack of occurrence rate data is partially due to the fact that type I OPD syndrome can often have only very mild clinical and radiological symptoms, such that it is often not diagnosed, or even noticed, until type I OPD syndrome is recognized in a more severely affected member of the family.

Type I OPD syndrome is more common than type II OPD syndrome, and as of the early 2000s, nearly 300 cases had been reported in the medical literature. In 1996, only 25 detailed cases of type II OPD syndrome had been described in the medical literature.

### Signs and symptoms

The severity of symptoms experienced by those people affected with OPD syndrome varies widely from practically asymptomatic to symptoms so severe that they cause infantile or prenatal death. In type II OPD syndrome, males are generally affected with far more severe symptoms than females.

There are six abnormalities of the face and head that characterize OPD syndrome: a cleft palate, downwardly slanting openings between the eyelids, widely spaced eyes (hypertelorism), a prominent forehead, a broad nose, and conductive hearing loss.

Conductive hearing loss results from a blockage of the auditory canal or some other dysfunction of the eardrum or one of the three small bones within the ear (the stapes, the malleus, and the incus) that are responsible for collecting sound. In this type of hearing loss, the auditory nerve is normal. In individuals affected with OPD syndrome, complete **deafness** from birth is often observed. In those individuals with partial hearing, speech disabilities related to this hearing loss are quite common.

In addition to the abnormalities of the head, universal characteristics of OPD syndrome affected individuals also include: abnormally short fingers and toes (brachydactyly); abnormal inward curving of some fingers (clinodactyly); short nails; a congenital dislocation of the elbows, and sometimes the knees; a caved in chest (pectus excavatum) at birth; and growth retardation.

Symptoms that are characteristic of type I OPD syndrome include: curvature of the spine (**scoliosis**); generalized bone malformation, particularly in the bones of the limbs and ribcage; broad distal digits, malformed or missing teeth (hypodontia); and mild mental retardation.

Symptoms that are characteristic of type II OPD syndrome include: low-set ears, flattened vertebrae in the spine, bowing of the bones of the limbs, flexed overlapping digits, a malformation or complete absence of the large bone in the shin (fibula), malformations of the hips, a small opening in the abdominal wall (hernia) at the navel (**omphalocele**), and a malformation of the male genitalia in which the opening of the urethra is located on the underside of the penis, rather than at the tip of the penis (**hypospadias**).

### Diagnosis

A diagnosis of OPD syndrome is suggested when a patient presents the five characteristic abnormalities of the head and face accompanied by conductive hearing loss. This diagnosis is confirmed by the observance of brachdactyly and congenital dislocation of the elbows and/or knees.

Type I OPD syndrome is differentially diagnosed from type II OPD syndrome by the appearance of scoliosis. Type II OPD syndrome is differentially diagnosed from type I OPD by the presence of an omphalocele and greater malformations of the bones of the ribcage.

### Treatment and management

There are currently no treatments aimed specifically at OPD syndrome. Instead, treatment is on a case-by-case and symptom-by-symptom basis.

Malformations of the head and face can generally be corrected, if necessary, by surgeries. In certain instances, the conductive hearing loss experienced by individuals with OPD syndrome may also be corrected through surgery. When it cannot, hearing aids may be required.

Many of the skeletal abnormalities seen in OPD syndrome affected individuals can either be corrected by surgery or can be alleviated through the use of braces until the bones become more fully developed.

Malformations of the male genitalia and the omphalocele observed in type II OPD syndrome affected infants can also be corrected by surgery.

Certain OPD affected individuals may also benefit from treatments with growth hormone.

In cases of mild mental retardation or speech problems, early intervention programs for these types of developmental delays may also be of benefit.

### Prognosis

Most individuals affected with type I OPD syndrome can expect to lead full lives if medical treatments, including corrective surgeries, are sought. Many individuals affected with type II OPD syndrome die either prior to birth or as infants due to respiratory failure associated with the malformation of the bones

## QUESTIONS TO ASK YOUR DOCTOR

- How does the genetic basis of the two types of otopalatodigital syndrome differ from each other?
- What signs and symptoms are characteristic of this disorder?
- What kinds of treatment are available for otopalatodigital syndrome, and at what stage of a child's life should each treatment be used?
- Can you recommend any Web sites that have additional information about this disorder?

of the ribcage. If these individuals survive infancy, they also may expect to live full lives after corrective surgeries and other medical treatments.

### Resources

#### PERIODICALS

Alembik, Y., C. Stoll, and J. Messer. "On the phenotypic overlap between severe oto-palato-digital type II syndrome and Larsen syndrome. Variable manifestations of a single autosomal dominant gene." *Genetic Counseling* (1997): 133-7.

#### WEBSITES

"Entry 304120 Cranioorodigital syndrome." *OMIM— Online Mendelian Inheritance in Man.* http://www.ncbi.nlm.nih.gov/htbin-post/Omim/dispmim?304120.

"Entry 311300: Otopalatodigital syndrome." *OMIM— Online Mendelian Inheritance in Man.* http://www.ncbi.nlm.nih.gov/htbin-post/Omim/dispmim?311300.

"Otopalatodigital (OPD) syndrome I." *Jablonski's Multiple Congenital Anomaly/Mental Retardation (MCA/MR) Syndromes Database.* http://www.nlm.nih.gov/cgi/jablonski/syndrome_cgi?index=517. (February 27, 2001).

"Otopalatodigital (OPD) syndrome II." *Jablonski's Multiple Congenital Anomaly/Mental Retardation (MCA/MR) Syndromes Database.* http://www.nlm.nih.gov/cgi/jablonski/syndrome_cgi?index=518. (February 27, 2001).

"Oto-Palato-Digital Syndrome Type I and II." *NORD— National Organization for Rare Disorders.* http://www.rarediseases.org.

#### ORGANIZATIONS

Children's Craniofacial Association. PO Box 280297, Dallas, TX 75243-4522. (972) 994-9902 or (800) 535-3643. contactcca@ccakids.com. http://www.ccakids.com.

FACES: The National Craniofacial Association. PO Box 11082, Chattanooga, TN 37401. (423) 266-1632 or (800) 332-2373. faces@faces-cranio.org. http://www.faces-cranio.org/.

Let's Face It (USA) PO Box 29972, Bellingham, WA 98228-1972. (360) 676-7325. letsfaceit@faceit.org. http://www.faceit.org/letsfaceit.

National Foundation for Facial Reconstruction. 317 East 34th St. #901, New York, NY 10016. (800) 422-3223. http://www.nffr.org.

Paul A. Johnson

# Ovarian cancer

## Definition

Ovarian **cancer** is a disease in which the cells in the ovaries become abnormal and start to grow uncontrollably, forming tumors. Ninety percent of all ovarian cancers develop in the cells that line the surface of the ovaries and are called "epithelial cell tumors."

## Description

The ovaries are a pair of almond-shaped organs that lie in the pelvis on either side of the uterus. The fallopian tubes connect the ovaries to the uterus. The ovaries produce and release an egg each month during a woman's menstrual cycle. In addition, they also produce the female hormones estrogen and progesterone, which regulate and maintain the proper growth and development of female sexual characteristics.

Ovarian cancer is the fifth most common cancer among women in the United States. It accounts for 4% of all cancers in women. However, ovarian cancer is very difficult to discover in the early stages. This is often because there are no obvious warning signs, and the disease can grow relatively quickly. In addition, the ovaries are situated deep in the abdomen and small tumors may not be detected easily during a routine physical examination. Because of this, the death rate due to ovarian cancer is higher than that of any other cancer among women, since it may only be detected at advanced stages.

Ovarian cancer can develop at any age, but more than half the diagnoses are among women who are 60 years or older. The vast majority of people with ovarian cancer have no family history of the disease. However, for about 5-10% of individuals, there may be a very strong family history of ovarian cancer or other cancers, such as **breast cancer**. In these cases, a specific genetic alteration may be in the family, causing a predisposition to ovarian cancer and other associated cancers.

## Genetic profile

Cells in ovarian tissue normally divide and grow, according to controls and instructions by various genes. If these genes have changes within them, the instructions for cellular growth and division may go awry. Abnormal, uncontrolled cell growth may occur, causing ovarian cancer. Therefore, all ovarian cancers are genetic because they all result from changes within genes. The difference is that most ovarian cancers are caused by sporadic changes within the genes, and only a minority are caused by inherited genetic alterations. Most ovarian cancers occur later in life after years of exposure to various environmental factors (such as the body's own hormones, asbestos exposure, or smoking) that can cause sporadic genetic alterations.

A small proportion of ovarian cancer is caused by inherited genetic alterations. As of 2009, a genetic alteration causing a predisposition solely to ovarian cancer has not yet been identified. However, in 1994 a breast and ovarian cancer susceptibility gene, known as BRCA1 (location 17q21), was identified. The discovery of BRCA2 (location 13q12) followed shortly in 1995. Women with alterations in these genes have an increased risk for breast and ovarian cancer, and men have an increased risk for **prostate cancer**. Men with a BRCA2 alteration have an increased risk for breast cancer. Slightly increased risks for colon and pancreatic cancers (in men and women) are also associated with BRCA2 alterations.

BRCA1 and BRCA2 alterations are inherited in an autosomal dominant manner; an individual who has one copy of a BRCA alteration has a 50% chance to pass it on to each of his or her children, regardless of that child's gender. Nearly all individuals with BRCA alterations have a family history of the alteration, usually a parent with it. In turn, they also may have a very strong family history of breast, ovarian, prostate, colon, and/or pancreatic cancers. Aside from BRCA1 and BRCA2, there likely are other cancer susceptibility genes that are still unknown.

In addition to BRCA1 and BRCA2, ovarian cancer may be present in rare genetic cancer syndromes. In these instances, an individual may have other health problems (unrelated to cancer) and a family history of a wide variety of cancers and symptoms. As an example, Hereditary Non-Polyposis Colorectal Cancer (HNPCC) is a syndrome that often involves cancers of the colon, uterus, ovaries, and stomach. HNPCC is due to changes in several genes including hMLH1, hMSH2, hMSH6, and hPMS2. These genes are unrelated to BRCA1 and BRCA2.

## Demographics

On average, a North American woman faces a lifetime risk of approximately 2% to develop ovarian cancer. The incidence of ovarian cancer is higher among Caucasian women. The American Cancer Society states that in the year 2009 about 21,550 new cases of ovarian cancer will be diagnosed in the United States, and 14,600 women will die from the disease. Specific BRCA alterations are common in certain ethnic groups, which may make hereditary ovarian cancer more common in these populations. As of the 2000s, certain BRCA alterations are more common in the Ashkenazi (Eastern European) Jewish, Icelander, Dutch, French Canadian, and West African populations.

## Signs and symptoms

Ovarian cancer has no specific signs or symptoms in the early stages of the disease. However, one may experience some of the following:

- Pain or swelling in the abdominal area
- Bloating and general feeling of abdominal discomfort
- Constipation, nausea, or vomiting
- Loss of appetite, tiredness
- Unexplained weight gain (generally due to fluid building up from the cancer in the abdomen)
- Vaginal bleeding in women who have already gone through menopause

Only a physician can assess whether or not the symptoms are an indication of early ovarian cancer. This is why it is important for a physician to be informed right away if any of the above symptoms are present.

A family history of ovarian cancer puts a woman at an increased risk for developing the disease. In addition, if a woman has had, or has a family history of, breast cancer she may be at an increased risk for ovarian cancer. Signs of a possible BRCA1 or BRCA2 alteration in a family, signifying hereditary breast or ovarian cancer, include:

- Several relatives with cancer
- A large number of relatives with cancer versus unaffected relatives
- Close genetic relationships between people with cancer, such as parent-child, sibling-sibling
- Earlier ages of cancer onset, such as before ages 45-50
- An individual with both breast and ovarian cancer
- An individual with bilateral or multi-focal breast cancer
- The presence of ovarian, prostate, colon, or pancreatic cancers in the same family
- Case(s) of breast cancer in men

Suspicion of a BRCA alteration may be raised if someone has the above features in their family and they are of a particular ethnic group, such as Ashkenazi Jewish. This is because specific BRCA1 and BRCA2 alterations are known to be more common in this group of individuals.

## Diagnosis

If a woman has symptoms of ovarian cancer, a pelvic examination is usually conducted to feel the ovaries to see if they have enlarged, indicative of a tumor. Blood tests to determine the level of a protein, known as carbohydrate antigen 125 (CA-125), may be done. CA-125 blood levels can be high when a woman has ovarian cancer. Additionally, a pelvic or transvaginal ultrasound (with color Doppler imaging) may be used to get several views of the ovaries, carefully checking their shape and structure. A CT scan may be helpful if the ultrasound is technically unsatisfactory for accurate interpretation.

Biopsy and surgery is necessary in order to determine the type of tumor, as not all tumors are cancerous. If the tumor appears to be small, a procedure known as laparoscopy may be used. A tiny incision is made in the abdomen and a slender, hollow, lighted instrument is inserted through it. This enables the doctor to view the ovary more closely and to obtain a biopsy. If the ovary has suspicious findings on laparoscopy and biopsy, a laparotomy (open surgery performed under general anesthesia) and removal of that ovary is usually performed. Large masses are investigated by open surgery.

Standard imaging techniques such as computed tomography (CT) and magnetic resonance imaging (MRI) may be used to determine if the disease has metastasized (spread) to other parts of the body.

There is DNA-based **genetic testing** to identify a BRCA1 or BRCA2 alteration in an individual. A blood sample is used, and both BRCA genes are studied for alterations. There is also targeted testing for people in high-risk ethnic groups (such as Ashkenazi Jewish), in which only the common BRCA alterations can be tested.

For women without cancer who test positive for a BRCA alteration, this now places them at a significantly increased risk to develop the associated cancers. A woman's risks associated with a BRCA1 alteration are: 40-60% for ovarian cancer by age 70 and 3-85% for breast cancer by age 70. A woman's risks with a BRCA2 alteration are: 16-27% for ovarian cancer by age 70 and 4-86% for breast cancer by age 70.

For women with ovarian cancer who are found to have a BRCA alteration, this now places them at an increased risk to develop breast cancer. For some women, this may be a new risk they were not aware of before the testing, particularly if they have no family history of breast cancer.

For all women with a BRCA2 alteration, there may be a slightly increased risk for colon and pancreatic cancers. Additionally, because the testing process and test results are quite complex (and may have strong emotional consequences) everyone should receive proper **genetic counseling** before pursuing any BRCA1 and BRCA2 testing. Prenatal BRCA testing is available, but is rarely performed unless accompanied by extensive genetic and psychological counseling.

## Treatment and management

As with many other cancers, treatment is determined by the exact size and type of ovarian cancer, so it is often unique to an individual. However, the cornerstone of treatment for ovarian cancer is surgery. This may require a laparotomy procedure in order to remove as much cancerous tissue as possible. Other organs, such as the uterus and fallopian tubes, may also be removed (especially if the cancer has spread there). Chemotherapy, the use of strong chemicals to kill cancer cells, is usually done following surgery. The purpose is to destroy any remaining cancer cells. Radiation therapy (using radioactive waves to kill cancer cells) is not typically used for ovarian cancer because it is not as effective as other treatments.

Screening recommendations for women at high risk to develop ovarian cancer (such as those with a strong family history of the disease) may include:

- Pelvic examination every six months or yearly, starting at age 25-35
- Transvaginal ultrasound with color Doppler imaging every six months or yearly, beginning at age 25-35
- Yearly blood CA-125 testing, starting at age 25-35

For women with a BRCA1 or BRCA2 alteration, they are also at an increased risk for breast cancer. Screening recommendations for them may include:

- Examining their own breasts monthly
- Examination of their breasts by a physician/nurse every six months or yearly, starting at age 25-35
- Mammograms (x rays of the breasts) yearly, starting at age 25-35

Specific screening programs may vary by physician. In addition to cancer screening, women with BRCA1 or BRCA2 alterations should know about their preventive surgery options. They may consider having their healthy ovaries and/or breasts removed, in order to reduce their risks to develop ovarian and/or breast cancer. Women may be more agreeable to having their ovaries removed because ovarian cancer is difficult to detect. However, this ends their ability to have children and automatically begins menopause for them. Both preventive surgeries greatly reduce a woman's cancer risk, but they can never eliminate the risk entirely.

For people with cancer or at high risk for it, there often are support and discussion groups available. These may be invaluable for those who feel alone in their situation, because they can meet others who are dealing with the exact same issues.

---

## QUESTIONS TO ASK YOUR DOCTOR

- Ovarian cancer is common among the women in my family. What tests should I have to monitor my risk for the disease?
- On what information is a diagnosis of ovarian cancer made?
- How does one determine the stage to which my ovarian cancer might have developed?
- What types of treatment are recommended for my ovarian cancer, and what side effects should I expect as a result of these treatments?

### Prognosis

Because ovarian cancer is not usually diagnosed until it is in an advanced stage, it is the most deadly of all the female cancers of the reproductive organs. As of 2009, only 46% of women diagnosed with ovarian cancer will survive past five years. If ovarian cancer is diagnosed before it has spread to other organs, more than 93% of the patients will survive five years or more. Unfortunately, less than 20% of all cancers are found at this early stage.

There appears to be no difference in the survival rates of women with or without a BRCA alteration. Because unaffected people in a family with a BRCA alteration may be in high-risk screening programs, the hope is that they may be able to have any of their cancers detected earlier, giving a better prognosis.

### Resources

**BOOKS**

Dollinger, Malin. *Everyone's Guide to Cancer Therapy*. Somerville House Books Limited, 1994.

Morra, Marion E. *Choices*. Avon Books, 1994.

Murphy, Gerald P. *Informed Decisions: The Complete Book of Cancer Diagnosis, Treatment and Recovery*. American Cancer Society, 1997.

**WEBSITES**

*CancerNet*. http://www.cancernet.nci.nih.gov.

*National Ovarian Cancer Coalition*. http://www.ovarian.org.

"Ovarian Cancer." *CancerNet*. http://www.cancernet.nci.nih.gov/Cancer_Types/Ovarian_Cancer.shtml.

**ORGANIZATIONS**

American Cancer Society. 1599 Clifton Rd. NE, Atlanta, GA 30329. (800) 227-2345. http://www.cancer.org.

Facing Our Risk of Cancer Empowered (FORCE). 934 North University Drive, PMB #213, Coral Springs, FL 33071. (954) 255-8732. info@facingourrisk.org. http://www.facingourrisk.org.

Gilda's Club. 195 West Houston Street, New York, NY 10014. (212) 647-9700. Fax: (212) 647-1151. http://www.gildasclub.org.

Gynecologic Cancer Foundation. 401 North Michigan Avenue, Chicago, IL 60611. (800) 444-4441.

National Cancer Institute. Office of Communications, 31 Center Dr. MSC 2580, Bldg. 1 Room 10A16, Bethesda, MD 20892-2580. (800) 422-6237. http://www.nci.nih.gov.

Deepti Babu, MS

Owren parahemophilia *see* **Factor V leiden thrombophilia**

# Paine syndrome

## Definition

Paine syndrome is a rare genetic condition that is present at birth. Characterized by an undersized head and related abnormalities in the brain, the disease results in severe mental and physical retardation, movement disorders, and vision problems. Most infants with Paine syndrome do not survive their first year of life.

## Description

The cerebellum, which is Latin for "little brain," is the part of the brain that controls involuntary movements, such as maintaining balance and coordinating muscles during physical activity. When shaking hands, for example, the cerebellum plays a primary role in coordinating the dozens of muscles involved in this seemingly simple task. Paine syndrome, which is named after the American pediatrician who first described the condition in 1960, interferes with the proper growth of the cerebellum and other parts of the brain while the fetus is still in the womb. Though this syndrome is considered a single entity, it actually includes several disorders that emerge together. The result is a variety of debilitating effects.

Children born with Paine syndrome have **microcephaly**. This neurological disease, which is also associated with conditions other than Paine syndrome, is characterized by an abnormally small head. The head of an infant with microcephaly is smaller than average when compared to other babies of the same age and gender. This decreased skull size is an indication that the brain did not grow properly during fetal development. The form of microcephaly associated with Paine syndrome causes physical and mental retardation. Aside from a small head, infants with Paine syndrome may have undersized bodies. Motor skills, language abilities, and other aspects of normal development are impaired. Babies with Paine syndrome, for example,

may require a gavage due to feeding difficulties or trouble swallowing. Unlike most infants, they may seem disinterested in the world around them.

Paine syndrome also produces specific problems related to movement. Infants affected by the disease develop spasticity. This nervous system disorder, in which muscles do not relax properly after being stretched, can cause muscle stiffness, pain, or physical deformity. It can also lead to repetitive spasms by a particular muscle or group of muscles (these spasms are known as myoclonic jerks). Aside from spasticity, an infant with Paine syndrome may experience generalized seizures.

Vision can also be affected, resulting in optic atrophy. This eye disorder causes a degeneration of the nerves carrying information from the eyes to the brain. Optic atrophy can lead to blurry vision or other visual disturbances.

The underlying cause of Paine syndrome, which is sometimes referred to as microcephaly-spastic diplegia syndrome, is unknown. The effects of the disease are thought to stem from the limited growth of the cerebellum and other areas of the brain. Autopsies of affected children have revealed underdevelopment of this region, as well as abnormalities in the cerebrum and other brain structures.

Paine syndrome is considered very similar to another genetic, congenital disease known as Seemanova syndrome. Both diseases have a number of symptoms in common, though Seemanova syndrome lacks certain characteristics of the former (such as an underdeveloped cerebellum). Some doctors view both conditions as variations of a more broadly defined disorder called Paine-Seemanova syndrome.

## Genetic profile

The **gene** responsible for Paine syndrome has not been identified, but is believed to lie on the X **chromosome**. For this reason, the disease is referred to as an

X-linked genetic condition. Only males are affected. Females do not usually develop the symptoms of Paine syndrome but they may be carriers of the gene associated with the disease. This is because women have two X chromosomes, while men only possess one. Even if a woman possesses the gene for Paine syndrome on one of her X chromosomes, she still has a second X chromosome that is free of the faulty gene. This second X chromosome is what protects her from developing symptoms of Paine syndrome, though she may be able to transmit the disease to her children.

### Demographics

Paine syndrome is a rare, congenital disease that only affects males. Most children born with it do not survive infancy.

### Signs and symptoms

The most visible symptom of Paine syndrome is often the size of the head, which is smaller than normal. Affected infants may experience feeding difficulties or swallowing problems. They may not appear to be growing properly or may seem disinterested in their environment. The development of motor skills and speech is delayed.

In simple terms, Paine syndrome causes structural abnormalities in the cerebellum, cerebrum, and other parts of the brain. The skull itself is abnormally small, due to the fact that its size is dictated by brain growth. Damage to the optic nerve may also occur. In addition, Paine syndrome produces elevated amino acid levels in the urine and cerebrospinal fluid.

### Diagnosis

The disease is often diagnosed at birth when the size of the head is measured, though a small head circumference may be identified later during a routine exam if it is not detected shortly after delivery. Imaging procedures (such as an x ray, CT scan, or MRI) are used to identify the structural abnormalities of the brain and skull. Analyses of blood and urine are also performed. An electroencephalogram (EEG), a non-invasive test that measures the electrical activity of the brain, may be recommended to help assess developmental problems or detect relevant brain or nervous system abnormalities.

### Treatment and management

There is no cure for Paine syndrome. The changes in brain structure associated with the disease cannot be reversed. When possible, treatment focuses on alleviating symptoms. Anticonvulsants, for example, can be used to help control seizures; dextroamphetamine may also be prescribed to ease symptoms. In addition to drugs, orthopedic surgery is sometimes necessary. Family education and **genetic counseling** for parents is also recommended.

### Prognosis

Due to its debilitating effects on the brain and nervous system, Paine syndrome is usually fatal within one year after birth.

### Resources

**BOOKS**

Victor, Maurice, et al. *Principles of Neurology*. 7th ed. New York: McGraw-Hill, 2001.

**PERIODICALS**

Lubs, H.A., P. Chiurazzi, J.F. Arena, et al. "XLMR genes: Update 1996." *American Journal of Medical Genetics* 64 (1996): 147–57.

Opitz, J.M., et al. "International workshop on the fragile X and X-linked mental retardation." *American Journal of Medical Genetics* 17 (1984): 5–94.

Paine, R.S. "Evaluation of familial biochemically determined mental retardation in children, with special reference to aminoaciduria." *New England Journal of Medicine* 262 (1960): 658–65.

**WEBSITES**

U.S. National Library of Medicine. http://www.nlm.nih.gov.

**ORGANIZATIONS**

U.S. National Library of Medicine. 8600 Rockville Pike, Bethesda, MD 20894.

Greg Annussek

# Pallister–Hall syndrome

## Definition

Pallister–Hall syndrome (PHS) is an extremely rare developmental disorder characterized by a spectrum of features ranging from mild (extra fingers or toes or a non–cancerous malformation in the hypothalamus region of the brain) to severe (laryngotracheal cleft, an opening between the windpipe and voicebox that can cause death in newborns).

## Description

First reported in 1980 by American geneticist Judith G. Hall and American medical doctor Philip D. Pallister, PHS is often diagnosed at birth. Some symptoms are immediately noticeable, including short limbs, extra digits, unusual facial features, or blockage of the anal opening. Some signs, such as mental retardation and abnormalities of the heart, lung, or kidneys, must be diagnosed by a physician.

Newborn infants with PHS must be carefully monitored for signs of hypopituitarism (insufficient production of growth hormones by the pituitary gland), which can cause fatal complications if not promptly treated. Similarly, inadequate activity of the adrenal gland can be lethal in newborns. If not immediately recognized, an imperfectly formed anus can also develop serious complications in a newborn. PHS is sometimes inappropriately considered part of the CAVE (cerebro–acro–visceral early lethality) group of disorders.

## Genetic profile

PHS is believed to have autosomal dominant **inheritance**, meaning that it can occur in either sex, and is passed from generation to generation when an abnormal **gene** is received from one parent and a normal gene is received from the other. Affected patients have a 50% chance of passing the disorder to each offspring. In most such cases, signs and symptoms in affected offspring are similar to those of the parents. However, PHS is more commonly found in isolated cases involving individuals with no family history of the disorder. These cases are thought to result from new, random, genetic mutations with no known cause. Mutations in the GLI3 gene cause PHS (chromosomal locus 7p13). This gene provides instructions for making a protein that controls gene expression, the process that regulates whether genes are turned on or off in particular cells. The GLI3 mutations typically lead to the production of an abnormally short version of the GLI3 protein. Because of the rarity of this disorder and the subtlety of its identifying characteristics, the ratio of these random mutation cases to inherited cases is not known.

## Demographics

Only about 100 cases of this very rare genetic disorder have been diagnosed worldwide. Males seem to be more affected than females. The disorder is not limited to particular ethnic groups. Some researchers have proposed that many patients with Pallister–Hall signs and symptoms have been misdiagnosed as having a related genetic disorder, isolated post–axial **polydactyly** type A (PAP–A).

## Signs and symptoms

This disorder is noted for a wide range of signs and symptoms, including the following:

- Abnormalities of the head, neck, and facial areas including short neck, short midface, flat nasal bridge, small tongue, noticeable underdevelopment of one jaw compared to the other, asymmetric skull, cleft palate and other irregularities of the palate, cleft larynx or epiglottis, cysts on the gums, and ears that are small, low–set, and abnormally rotated toward the back of the head.
- Hypothalamic hamartoblastoma, a non–cancerous tumor in the hypothalamus. It grows at the same rate as nearby brain tissue, up to 4 cm across, taking the place of the hypothalamus. Most hypothalamic hamartomas have no symptoms, but in some cases they can cause neurological problems including gelastic epilepsy, which causes chest and diaphragm movements similar to those that occur during laughter.
- Inhibited flow of cerebrospinal fluid in the brain.
- Limb abnormalities including short limbs, extra fingers or toes (central or postaxial polydactyly), webbing of fingers or toes (syndactyly), abnormally small fingernails or toenails, or absent nails.
- Respiratory abnormalities including underdeveloped or abnormally developed lungs.
- Anus lacking the usual opening.
- Congenital heart defects.
- Kidneys with abnormal development or placement.
- Underdeveloped or abnormally developed adrenal, pituitary, or thyroid glands. This can lead to decreased activity of these glands. Some Pallister–Hall newborns cannot survive due to insufficient activity of the adrenal gland. An underdeveloped pituitary gland can also have lethal consequences. Symptoms of hypopituitarism may include hypoglycemia, jaundice, or unusual drowsiness.
- In males, unusually small penis, underdeveloped testicles, or failure of one or both testes to descend normally.
- Retarded growth in most patients.
- Mild mental retardation.
- Spinal abnormalities.
- Dislocated hips.
- Signs of puberty may appear unusually early.

## Diagnosis

Both clinical examination and family history are used to diagnose PHS.

The hallmark clinical findings are hypothalamic hamartoma (a non–cancerous tumor in the hypothalamus), as well as extra fingers or toes. Another sign useful for diagnostic purposes is bifid epiglottis, a cleft in the thin flap of cartilage behind the base of the tongue. This particular malformation is almost never seen except in cases of PHS. It rarely causes problems.

Prenatal testing may be conducted by ultrasound, however, its effectiveness in detecting PHS is not conclusive.

A molecular genetic test exists to scan the coding regions of the GL13 gene for mutations.

## Treatment and management

Management depends on the specific signs and symptoms present.

Unless there are unusual complications, hamartoblastomas are usually left in place. However, it is sometimes necessary to surgically remove a hamartoblastoma when it causes undue pressure on the brain (**hydrocephalus**). Hamartoblastomas are usually monitored throughout the life of the patient. Typically, magnetic resonance imaging (MRI) is used, because hypothalamic hamartomas are sometimes not visible on computerized tomography (CT) scans or cranial ultrasound examinations.

Because of the dangers posed by adrenal insufficiency, Pallister–Hall patients are often assessed for cortisol deficiency. Cortisol (hydrocortisone) is an important steroid hormone released by the adrenal glands. Patients are also likely to see an endocrinologist to evaluate their growth hormone, luteinizing hormone, follicle–stimulating hormone, and thyroid hormone levels. X rays may be taken of limbs, and the kidneys may be examined by ultrasound. The epiglottis may be examined by laryngoscope, an instrument used to view the larynx through the mouth.

If patients show evidence of aspiration (when breathing forces foreign matter into the lungs) they should be seen immediately by an ear, nose, and throat specialist to determine whether laryngotracheal cleft is present.

Newborns with hypopituitarism should immediately be given hormone replacement therapy and watched closely for life–threatening complications.

A surgical procedure known as a colostomy may be needed to correct an imperforate anus.

Similarly, extra toes or fingers can be surgically corrected on an elective basis.

Seizures, such as those caused by gelastic **epilepsy**, may require symptomatic treatment.

Whenever a new case of PHS is uncovered, it is advisable to also examine the parents and any offspring for the disorder. Evaluation for a parent is likely to include a cranial MRI, x rays of hands and feet, and laryngoscopy.

As of 2009, one clinical trial on PHS was being sponsored by the National Human Genome Research Institute (NHGRI), seeking to evaluate the range of severity, natural history, molecular etiology, and pathophysiology of PHS. Researchers were investigating the relationship between Pallister–Hall and some disorders with similar characteristics, including **Greig cephalopolysyndactyly** syndrome (GCPS), McKusick–Kaufman syndrome (MKS), Bardet–Biedl syndrome (BBS), and oro–facial–digital syndromes (OFDs).

### Prognosis

Because of the broad range and severity of Pallister–Hall signs and symptoms, the prognosis varies widely from case to case.

In families in which multiple cases of PHS exist, the prognosis for any new case is likely to be similar to the existing cases. Mild forms of the syndrome have been identified in a number of large, healthy families believed to have a normal life expectancy.

In cases that occur in isolated individuals, the prognosis is based on the specific malformations present. Reviews of these malformations as reported in scientific literature have limited usefulness because published cases tend to be more severe than those normally encountered. Unless there are life–threatening malformations such as hypopituitarism, the prognosis for these random cases is considered excellent.

There is a 50% chance that any child of a Pallister–Hall patient will be affected.

### Resources

#### BOOKS

Parker, Philip M. *Pallister Hall–Syndrome —A Bibliography and Dictionary for Physicians, Patients, and Genome Researchers*. San Diego, CA: Icon Health Publications, 2007.

#### PERIODICALS

Azzam, A., et al. "Psychiatric and neuropsychological characterization of Pallister–Hall syndrome." *Clinical Genetics* 67, no. 1 (January 2005): 87–92.
Kalff–Suske, M., et al. "Gene symbol: GLI3. Disease: Pallister–Hall syndrome." *Human Genetics* 114, no. 4 (March 2004): 403.

Roscioli, T., et al. "Pallister–Hall syndrome: unreported skeletal features of a GLI3 mutation." *American Journal of Medical Genetics A* 136A, no. 4 (August 2005): 390–394.

#### WEBSITES

*Pallister Hall–Syndrome*. Information Page. NORD, November 26, 2008 (April 25, 2009). http://www.rare diseases.org/search/rdbdetail_abstract.html? disname = Pallister + Hall + Syndrome.
*Pallister–Hall Syndrome*. Information Page. Madisons Foundation, 2009 (April 25, 2009). http://www.madi sonsfoundation.org/index.php/component/option, com_mpower/diseaseID,362/.
*Pallister–Hall Syndrome*. Information Page. NHGRI, June 7, 2005 (April 25, 2009). http://research.nhgri.nih.gov/ phs/.
*Polydactyly*. Medical Encyclopedia. Medline Plus, April 21, 2009 (April 25, 2009). http://www.nlm.nih.gov/medli neplus/ency/article/003176.htm.

#### ORGANIZATIONS

Madisons Foundation. P.O. Box 241956, Los Angeles, CA 90024. (310)264-0826. Fax: (310)264-4766. http:// www.madisonsfoundation.org.
National Organization for Rare Disorders (NORD). 55 Kenosia Avenue, PO Box 1968, Danbury, CT 06813-1968. (203)744-0100 or (800)999-6673. Fax: (203)798-2291. http://www.rarediseases.org.
Pallister–Hall Foundation. RFD Box 3000, Fairground Rd., Bradford, VT 05033. (802)222-9683. Email: messer@sover.net.

David L. Helwig

## Pallister–Killian syndrome

### Definition

Pallister–Killian syndrome (PKS) is a rare **chromosome** abnormality in which a person has four copies of the short arm of chromosome 12 instead of the normal two copies. Affected individuals have unusual facial features, mental retardation, seizures, patchy color differences in the skin, and various other physical abnormalities. Many fetuses with PKS die during pregnancy or soon after birth.

### Description

PKS was first described in 1977. The first two patients reported by Pallister were adults with severe mental retardation, unusual facial features, severe lack of muscle strength, and pale areas on their skin. In

1981, Killian and Teschler–Nicola described a child with mental retardation, unusual facial features, pale skin on the face, and absence of hair at the front of the scalp.

PKS may also be called Killian syndrome, Killian/Teschler–Nicola syndrome, Pallister mosaic syndrome, or Teschler–Nicola/Killian syndrome. This syndrome is also known as tetrasomy 12p mosaicism or isochromosome 12p syndrome based on the characteristic chromosome abnormality detected via laboratory studies. PKS is called mosaic because the characteristic chromosome abnormality that causes the syndrome appears only in a fraction of the total cells examined.

### Genetic profile

PKS is a sporadic disorder, which means that it appears to occur at random. The chromosome problem that causes PKS, tetrasomy 12p, does not appear to run in families. PKS is not specifically associated with any specific chemical or environmental exposures.

Tetrasomy 12p is characterized by the presence of four copies of the short arm of chromosome 12, instead of the normal two copies. This chromosome abnormality is not found throughout an affected person's body. Chromosome analysis performed on the blood of persons with PKS virtually always shows normal results. The characteristic chromosome abnormality can, however, be detected via chromosome analysis on skin cells. Through chromosome analysis, tetrasomy 12p is identified due to the presence of what appears to be an extra chromosome composed of two copies of the short arm of chromosome 12. This chromosome composed of two copies of the short arm of chromosome 12 is called an isochromosome. In tetrasomy 12p, there is a total of four copies of the short arm of chromosome 12: there are the two normal copies, plus the two abnormal copies located on the extra isochromosome.

### Demographics

The incidence of PKS is uncertain and is estimated around one in 25,000. PKS occurs at random; however, an association with advanced maternal age (35 years or greater) has long been documented. Though PKS may occur more frequently in babies born to mothers age 35 or older, the syndrome still may occur in babies born to mothers of any age. PKS occurs strictly due to an abnormality of the chromosomes.

### Signs and symptoms

Many infants with more severe physical defects associated with PKS die in utero or shortly after birth. Other persons with PKS have lived at least into their 20s. All persons with PKS have some level of mental retardation or developmental delay.

The features of PKS may vary significantly between affected persons. The most typical person with PKS will have profound mental retardation, delayed development, lack of muscle tone, light– and/or dark–colored areas of skin, lack of scalp hair above the temples, and unusual facial features. The facial features characteristic for PKS include a large forehead, widely spaced eyes with vertical folds of skin at the inner corners, droopy eyelids, short and upturned nose, full cheeks, lengthened distance between the nose and upper lip, and small chin.

Persons with PKS often have **deafness**, absent or minimal speech, poor vision, and seizures. Individuals with PKS have additionally been reported to have short, wide hands with short fingers, while others have extra fingers or toes. Some affected persons have had **cleft palate** and some have had a bifid uvula (cleft, or split, uvula). The teeth come in later than normal in persons with PKS. Heart defects may be present and the sac normally surrounding the heart, the pericardium, may be missing. Additionally, there may be small patches of exposed tissue where the skin did not develop.

Many individuals with PKS have been reported to have extra nipples, and some have a hernia around the navel. Some persons with PKS have problems with the intestines or anus. Many have birth defects involving the genitals or internal reproductive organs and others have disorganized or cyst–filled kidneys. A small tail–like stub at the bottom of the spine was reported in at least one person affected with PKS.

The features of PKS change over time. The lack of hair above the temples, which is common in younger persons with PKS, mostly resolves by age five. Additionally, an affected individual's initial lack of muscle tone gives way to fixation of the joints later in life.

### Diagnosis

PKS may be suspected from a person's physical features, but a diagnosis requires that a person has the characteristic chromosome abnormality, tetrasomy 12p. PKS is different from many types of chromosomal syndromes in that the causative chromosome abnormality is not found from chromosome studies on the blood. Chromosome testing on skin cells will show the characteristic chromosome abnormality in at least some of the cells. It is believed that the characteristic chromosome abnormality, the isochromosome 12p, does not show up in the blood cells because the abnormal isochromosome is lost in the rapid cell division that creates these blood cells. Diagnosis of PKS has traditionally required a skin biopsy, but recent reports indicate that the diagnosis can be made using cells scraped from the inside the cheek.

Many cases of PKS may be diagnosed prenatally. PKS is detectable by **amniocentesis**, a routine test offered in pregnancies suspected to be at risk for chromosome problems. PKS may be suspected when certain physical abnormalities are detected on an ultrasound during pregnancy. In pregnancies where PKS has been diagnosed in an unborn baby, many ultrasounds have shown an increased amount of fluid around the baby, in addition to other physical abnormalities, including short arms and legs, heart malformations, diaphragmatic hernia, cystic hygroma, and unusually flat profile of the face.

### Treatment and management

There is no treatment or cure for PKS, or for the mental retardation and developmental delays associated with this syndrome. Persons with PKS are treated for the symptoms they display. Individuals with PKS often take medications for seizures; some may have surgeries due to birth defects involving the diaphragm,

intestines, anus, kidneys, genitals, or heart. Physical therapy and occupational therapy may be helpful for development of muscle tone and reduction of joint fixation.

### Prognosis

Many infants with PKS die before they are born (in utero) or soon after birth. Some affected individuals reaching their 20s have been reported. Many have severe to profound mental retardation and very few self–care skills. A few reports have described affected persons with milder intellectual impairment.

### Resources

#### BOOKS

Gorlin, Robert J., Michael M. Cohen, and Raoul C. M. Hennekam. "Pallister–Killian Syndrome." In *Syndromes of the Head and Neck*, 4th edition. New York: Oxford University Press, 2001.

#### PERIODICALS

Baglaj, M., et al. "Pallister–Killian syndrome: a report of 2 cases and review of its surgical aspects." *Journal of Pediatric Surgery* 43, no. 6 (June 2008): 1218–1221.

Theisen, A., et al. "aCGH detects partial tetrasomy of 12p in blood from Pallister–Killian syndrome cases without invasive skin biopsy." *American Journal of Medical Genetics A* 149A, no. 5 (April 2009): 914–918.

#### WEBSITES

*Pallister Killian Mosaic Syndrome.* Information Page. NORD, November 26, 2008 (April 25, 2009). http://www.rarediseases.org/search/rdbdetail_abstract.html?disname=Pallister%20Killian%20Mosaic%20Syndrome.

*Pallister–Killian Syndrome Home Page.* Website. March 2, 2009 (April 25, 2009). http://www.pk-syndrome.org

*What is PKS?* Information Page. PKS Kids, 2009 (April 25, 2009). http://www.pkskids.net/whatispks.htm.

#### ORGANIZATIONS

Chromosome Disorder Outreach, Inc. P.O. Box 724, Boca Raton, FL 33429-0724. (561) 395-4252. Email: info@chromodisorder.org. http://www.chromodisorder.org.

National Organization for Rare Disorders (NORD). 55 Kenosia Avenue, PO Box 1968, Danbury, CT 06813-1968. (203) 744-0100 or (800) 999-6673. Fax: (203) 798-2291. http://www.rarediseases.org.

PKS Kids. 123 Carowinds Dr., Greencastle, PA 17225. Email: onebuddy@comcast.net. http://www.pkskids.net.

Judy C. Hawkins, MS, CGC

# Pancreatic beta cell agenesis

## Definition

Pancreatic beta cell agenesis is a rare disorder in which a child is born with no beta cells—the cells in the pancreas that produce insulin—resulting in **diabetes**.

## Description

Diabetes mellitus is a disease caused by elevated blood sugar and can result in numerous medical problems that can affect the kidney, eyes, cardiovascular system, skin, and joints. There are two common types. Type 1 results from destruction of the insulin-producing cells (beta cells) of the pancreas and usually occurs in children of at least one year of age or young adults. Injected insulin is required to allow glucose (sugar) to enter the body's cells to be used for energy. Type 2 diabetes occurs mostly in older, often obese, adults and results from the body's cells' decreased ability to respond to the insulin the body produces. In contrast to these two types, neonatal diabetes is extremely rare. Neonatal diabetes is usually transient, meaning that it goes away after some time. It appears to be caused by immaturity of the beta cells; babies with this form of the disease usually recover and do not require insulin before about three months of age. Fewer than 40 cases of permanent neonatal diabetes had been reported. Reported causes of neonatal diabetes have included absence of the whole pancreas, absence of the clusters (called islets) that contain the beta cells, and absence of the beta cells themselves. This last form is known as pancreatic beta cell agenesis.

Only one confirmed case of pancreatic beta cell agenesis has been reported (1994). This was an infant girl who had a low birth weight and showed high glucose (sugar) in her blood during a routine test. She was pale, with a low body temperature, rapid breathing and low muscle tone. Her health was further complicated by a diagnosis of an additional metabolic disorder, **methylmalonic acidemia** (MMA). She died at the age of 16 days. An autopsy showed that her pancreas had islets, which are the bundles of cells containing insulin-producing cells as well as cells that produce other hormones. However, the islets did not contain insulin-producing cells.

## Genetic profile

Pancreatic beta cell agenesis may be an autosomal recessive disorder. This means that a child would have to inherit two abnormal copies of a specific gene, one

## KEY TERMS

**Agenesis**—Failure of an organ, tissue, or cell to develop or grow.

**Beta cells**—Specialized cells of the pancreas that make insulin.

**Diabetes mellitus**—The clinical name for common diabetes. It is a chronic disease characterized by inadequate production or use of insulin.

**Insulin**—A hormone produced by the pancreas that is secreted into the bloodstream and regulates blood sugar levels.

**Metabolic disorder**—A disorder that affects the metabolism of the body.

**Metabolism**—The total combination of all the chemical processes that occur within cells and tissues of a living body.

**Pancreas**—An organ located in the abdomen that secretes pancreatic juices for digestion and hormones for maintaining blood sugar levels.

from each parent, in order to have the disorder. The infant described had both pancreatic beta cell agenesis and MMA, also known to be an autosomal recessive disorder. A gene causing MMA is located on **chromosome** 6, and studies of this child's genes and chromosomes showed that she inherited two identical copies of at least part of chromosome 6 from her father, a condition known as paternal uniparental isodisomy, instead of one copy of this region from each parent. The MMA was caused by the **inheritance** of two identical abnormal MMA genes from her father and the beta cell agenesis was then believed to have been caused by the inheritance of two abnormal copies of another gene. On other chromosomes, it has been shown that certain genes only work when they come from the mother and others only from the father. Several cases of transient neonatal diabetes have also had two identical copies of paternal chromosome 6 or other abnormalities of chromosome 6. This suggests that there may be a connection between pancreatic beta cell agenesis and transient neonatal diabetes. It is believed that the relevant region of chromosome 6 contains a gene that delays the production of insulin and only works when inherited from the father. As of 2001, there were no reports in the literature describing the status of the beta cells in infants with transient neonatal diabetes. Presumably, this is because a pancreatic biopsy would be required, and this procedure would be too strenuous for a fragile baby.

## Demographics

The overall incidence of neonatal, or newborn, diabetes mellitus is approximately one in 400,000 to one in 600,000 live births, and many cases are transient, with the infants requiring insulin for an average of three months. These infants do appear to be at an increased risk of developing type 2 diabetes in young adulthood. Fewer than 40 cases of well-documented permanent neonatal diabetes have been reported. Only two infants with neonatal diabetes have demonstrated (by autopsy) a complete lack of insulin-producing cells in the pancreas at birth. The first child had both pancreatic beta cell agenesis and another disorder called methylmalonic acidemia. She also had low birth weight, typical of children with neonatal diabetes because of the inability to metabolize glucose. The second child was of normal birth weight, suggesting that she originally had beta cells that were subsequently destroyed, perhaps by an autoimmune process as in type 1 diabetes. Both of these infants died in the newborn period.

### Signs and symptoms

Symptoms of neonatal diabetes include lethargy, dehydration, and breathing difficulties. In the laboratory, high levels of glucose (sugar) in the blood and urine are demonstrated. Children with neonatal diabetes, including the child with pancreatic beta cell agenesis, are generally of low birth weight.

### Diagnosis

Neonatal diabetes, like other forms of diabetes, is diagnosed by high blood sugar levels. Permanent and transient forms of neonatal diabetes are indistinguishable at initial diagnosis. Determining if the cause of neonatal diabetes is pancreatic beta cell agenesis was done after death in the published cases by studying the pancreas from an autopsy; a pancreatic biopsy would be required to make this diagnosis in a living child.

### Treatment and management

Pancreatic beta cell agenesis, like type 1 and some cases of type 2 diabetes mellitus, is treated by insulin injection.

### Prognosis

Both children reported to have absence of beta cells were diagnosed on autopsy because they died at birth. The second child's prognosis was complicated by the fact that she had the additional MMA disorder. It is not known if any living children have pancreatic beta cell agenesis.

### Resources

#### PERIODICALS

Abramowics, Marc J., et al. "Isodisomy of Chromosome 6 in a Newborn with Methylmalonic Acidemia and Agenesis of Pancreatic Beta Cells Causing Diabetes Mellitus." *Journal of Clinical Investigation* 94 (1994): 418–21.

Blum, D., et al. "Congenital absence of insulin cells in a neonate with diabetes mellitus and mutase-deficient methymalonic acidaemia." *Diabetologia* 36 (1993): 352–7.

#### ORGANIZATIONS

American Diabetes Association. 1701 N. Beauregard St., Alexandria, VA 22311. (703) 549-1500 or (800) 342-2383. http://www.diabetes.org.

Juvenile Diabetes Foundation International (JDF). 120 Wall St., New York, NY 10005. (212) 785-9500 x708 or (800) 533-2873. http://www.jdf.org.

Toni I. Pollin, MS, CGC

# Pancreatic cancer

## Definition

The pancreas is a gland found in the abdomen behind the stomach. The pancreas secretes a fluid that breaks down fats and proteins, and releases hormones, such as insulin, to control blood sugar levels. Pancreatic **cancer** is uncontrolled growth of cells of the pancreas. A higher than average number of pancreatic cancer cases occurring in the same family is known as familial pancreatic cancer.

## Description

Most pancreatic cancer grows from cells from the exocrine pancreas, the secreting portion of the pancreas. The most common appearance of pancreatic cancer cells is gland-like, which is termed adenocarcinoma.

In most cases, it is difficult to determine the cause of pancreatic cancer. Both environmental as well as genetic risk factors have been suggested for pancreatic cancer. A high-fat diet has been linked to increased pancreatic cancer risk, whereas diets high in vegetables and fruits seem to lower the risk. Smoking is known to increase the risk of pancreatic cancer; it is estimated that as many as 30% of pancreatic cancer cases are linked to smoking. Alcohol use and coffee consumption have been linked with increased pancreatic cancer

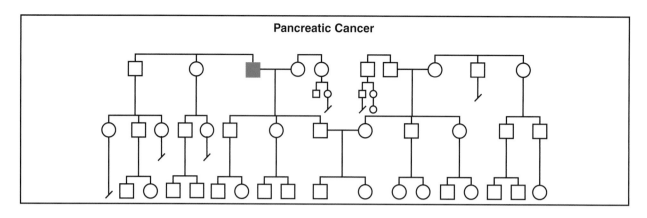

**Pancreatic Cancer**

*(Gale, a part of Cengage Learning.)*

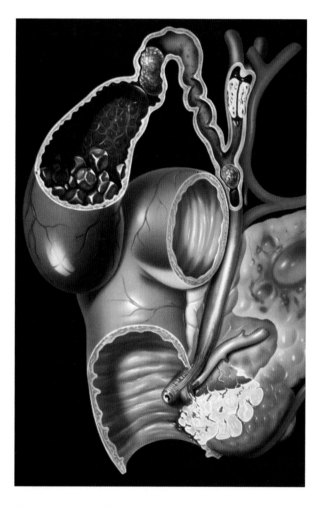

**Illustration of invading cancer of the human pancreas. The gallbladder and gallstones at top right of image are green, and the pink c-shaped tube at left and center are the duodenum.** *(Custom Medical Stock Photo, Inc.)*

risk, in some studies, but this connection has not been proven. Previous stomach surgery also may increase the risk of pancreatic cancer. Aflatoxin, a common fungal contaminant of certain foods, such as rice, corn, and peanuts, is a known cause of liver cancer, and has been postulated to also pose a risk for pancreatic cancer. However, no link has been found.

Certain occupations, such as farming or manufacturing, may increase the risk of pancreatic cancer. Multiple studies have shown that exposure to pesticides increases the risk. The relationship of **diabetes** to pancreatic cancer has been closely studied. It is uncertain whether diabetes is the cause or the symptom of pancreatic cancer. Presence of diabetes, however, may alert health care providers to the presence of pancreatic cancer. Long-term inflammation of the pancreas, chronic pancreatitis, may increase the risk of pancreatic cancer as well. Genetic risk factors have also been reported.

### Genetic profile

Several studies have reported a higher rate of pancreatic cancer in relatives of individuals with the disease. Hereditary causes are estimated to account for about 10% of all pancreatic cancer cases. The most well-known case of familial pancreatic cancer is that of former president Jimmy Carter, whose mother, sister, and brother all died of the disease. Some risk is thought to be due to known hereditary conditions, whereas, in other cases, a known genetic syndrome has not been determined.

There are several known genetic syndromes that increase the risk of pancreatic cancer. Mutations in the BRCA1 and BRCA2 genes have been clearly linked to increases in breast and **ovarian cancer**, as well as a potential increased pancreatic cancer risk. Loss or inactivation of the paternal copy of the DIRAS3 gene (1p31) has also been reported in certain forms of

## KEY TERMS

**Biopsy**—The surgical removal and microscopic examination of living tissue for diagnostic purposes.

**BRCA2**—Gene, when altered, known to cause increased risks of breast, ovarian and, possibly, pancreatic cancer.

**Cationic trypsinogen gene**—Gene known to cause hereditary pancreatitis when significantly altered.

**CDKN2A, or p16**—Gene, when altered, known to cause familial atypical multiple mole melanoma (FAMMM) syndrome and possibly increased pancreatic cancer risk.

**Chemotherapy**—Treatment of cancer with synthetic drugs that destroy the tumor either by inhibiting the growth of the cancerous cells or by killing the cancer cells.

**Computed tomography (CT) scan**—An imaging procedure that produces a three–dimensional picture of organs or structures inside the body, such as the brain.

**Duct**—Tube–like structure that carries secretions from glands.

**Duodenum**—Portion of the small intestine nearest the stomach; the first of three parts of the small intestine.

**Endoscopic retrograde cholangiopancreatography (ERCP)**—A method of viewing the pancreas by inserting a thin tube down the throat into the pancreatic and bile ducts, injection of dye, and performing x rays.

**Exocrine pancreas**—The secreting part of the pancreas.

**Familial adenomatous polyposis (FAP)**—Inherited syndrome causing large numbers of polyps and increased risk of colon cancer and other cancers.

**Hereditary non–polyposis colon cancer (HNPCC)**—A genetic syndrome causing increased cancer risks, most notably colon cancer; also called Lynch syndrome.

**Insulin**—A hormone produced by the pancreas that is secreted into the bloodstream and regulates blood sugar levels.

**Jaundice**—Yellowing of the skin or eyes due to excess of bilirubin in the blood.

**Li–Fraumeni syndrome**—Inherited syndrome known to cause increased risk of different cancers, most notably sarcomas.

**Melanoma**—Tumor, usually of the skin.

**Metastasis**—The spreading of cancer from the original site to other locations in the body.

**Mutation**—A permanent change in the genetic material that may alter a trait or characteristic of an individual, or manifest as disease, and can be transmitted to offspring.

**Palliative**—Treatment done for relief of symptoms rather than a cure.

**Pancreas**—An organ located in the abdomen that secretes pancreatic juices for digestion and hormones for maintaining blood sugar levels.

**Pancreatitis**—Inflammation of the pancreas.

**Peutz–Jeghers syndrome**—Inherited syndrome causing polyps of the digestive tract and spots on the mouth, as well as increased risk of cancer.

**Radiation**—High–energy rays used in cancer treatment to kill or shrink cancer cells.

**Staging**—A method of describing the degree and location of cancer.

**Whipple procedure**—Surgical removal of the pancreas and surrounding areas, including a portion of the small intestine, the duodenum.

---

pancreatic cancer. **Hereditary pancreatitis**, which is due to alterations in the cationic trypsinogen gene on **chromosome** 7 at 7q35, causes long-term, recurrent inflammation of the pancreas. Individuals with hereditary pancreatitis are estimated to have a 40% risk of pancreatic cancer by age 70. Changes, or mutations, in the CDKN2A (p16) gene can increase risks of melanoma, a type of skin cancer and, possibly, pancreatic cancer. Hereditary non-polyposis colon cancer (HNPCC), or Lynch syndrome, increases the risk of

colon cancer and other cancers, including pancreatic cancer, in some families. Peutz-Jeghers (**familial adenomatous polyposis**, FAP) and Li-Fraumeni syndromes cause slightly increased risks of pancreatic cancer, in addition to the other symptoms of the disorders. All of these disorders are inherited in an autosomal dominant pattern. With autosomal dominant **inheritance**, men and women are equally likely to inherit the syndrome, and children of affected individuals are at 50% risk of inheriting the gene alteration.

Other syndromes, some with different inheritance patterns, may be linked to pancreatic cancer as well. **Genetic testing** is available for many of these known syndromes, but due to the complexity of the disorders, **genetic counseling** should be considered before testing.

Some families with increased pancreatic cancer rates do not have a known genetic syndrome as the cause. It is possible that environmental factors or chance could explain some cases of pancreatic cancer in families; however, it is also possible that other as yet unknown genetic causes could explain some cases of familial pancreatic cancer. While genetic testing may not be available in all cases, families may participate in collections, or registries, of familial pancreatic cancer cases for research purposes.

### Demographics

In 2008, the American Cancer Society (ACS) estimated that 37,680 Americans (18,770 men and 18,910 women) would be diagnosed with pancreatic cancer with an estimated 34,290 deaths (17,500 men and 16,790 women), making this type of cancer the fourth leading cause of cancer death overall. Over the past 15 to 25 years, rates of cancer of pancreatic cancer have dropped slightly in men and women. The ACS also estimates that the lifetime risk of developing pancreatic cancer is about 1 in 76 (1.31%).

### Signs and symptoms

Since the symptoms of pancreatic cancer are not specific to the disease, and typically do not develop until the cancer has progressed, it is difficult to diagnosis pancreatic cancer at an early stage.

The symptoms of pancreatic cancer can include:

- weight loss
- loss of appetite
- abdominal or back pain
- jaundice (yellow color to skin and eyes)
- digestive problems, including greasy stool
- sudden diabetes

### Diagnosis

If pancreatic cancer is suspected, regardless of the cause, a physical exam often is done first, and certain body imaging tests may be recommended. One imaging test that may be done is a computed tomography (CT) scan. This exam creates pictures of the interior of the body from computer–analyzed differences in x rays passing through the body. Evidence of substantial tumors or any metastasis (spreading of cancer) can be detected by CT scanning. Once a biopsy is taken, the tissue sample is examined by CT for evidence of cancer and this typically determines the diagnosis.

Ultrasound is another method of viewing internal body structures. In ultrasound, sound waves are passed into the body and a computer develops an image based on the returned sound waves. Ultrasound is generally less expensive and more easily available than CT; however, there are limitations to the use of ultrasound in viewing the pancreas. Ultrasound may be used in addition to CT. Endoscopic retrograde cholangiopancreatography (ERCP) is a method of viewing the pancreas by inserting a thin tube down the throat, injecting of dye into the pancreatic and bile ducts, and taking x rays.

Once the tumor and any metastasis has been identified and the biopsy tissue evaluation has been done, the tumor can be staged. Staging is a ranking system that provides a method of describing the extent and characteristics of a cancer. Staging can be used to help determine the treatment and prognosis for a given cancer.

### Treatment and management

Surgery often provides the best chance of a cure, though it is not often possible due to the spread of cancer. Removal of all or part of the pancreas and other areas, such as the duodenum (the first part of the small intestine), is known as the Whipple procedure. Complications of this surgery include infection and bleeding.

Chemotherapy is cancer–killing medicine that has been found to increase survival in some patients. This drug can be given intravenously or orally. Once in the bloodstream, chemotherapy agents reach other parts of the body. There are different chemotherapy agents and the side effects may be different as well, including nausea, hair loss, low blood counts, and other effects.

Recent improvements in radiation, high–energy rays directed at cancer cells, have made this therapy more effective. Although cures due to radiation therapy are uncommon, relief from pain and increased survival are possible. Side effects of radiation therapy may include skin changes, upset stomach, and other effects.

Sometimes, surgery, radiation, or other therapies are done to relieve symptoms rather than cure the cancer. This is known as palliative treatment.

Involvement in research as part of clinical trials may be offered to certain patients. Although treatments through clinical trials may not be proven, it is an opportunity to potentially benefit from new therapies.

Screening before cancer development may be considered for patients with a higher risk of the disease either due to a known genetic syndrome or to a family history of pancreatic cancer. ERCP and ultrasound have been used for screening purposes; however, the usefulness and cost–effectiveness of these tests for screening needs further evaluation. Surveillance may be considered for persons with two or more close relatives (first–degree family members) with pancreatic cancer, or with one close relative (first–degree) with pancreatic cancer at an early age (before age 50), or with two or more distant relatives (second–degree), one of which was affected before age 50.

Prophylactic pancreatectomy, surgical removal of the pancreas before any cancer development, has been considered in cases with a hereditary risk. The concern with prophylactic pancreatectomy is that there is a risk of serious complications, and consequently the decision must be weighed carefully.

### Clinical trials

Clinical trials on pancreatic cancer are currently sponsored by the National Institutes of Health (NIH) and other agencies. As of 2009, NIH reported 748 on–going and completed studies.

Examples include:

- The evaluation of the response of subjects with pancreatic cancer that have undergone surgical resection and treatment with a vaccine given with chemotherapy and chemoradiation. (NCT00569387)
- The evaluation of the effectiveness of Tarceva (OSI–774) combined with capecitabine in treating patients with metastatic pancreatic cancer. (NCT00125021)
- A study to identify susceptibility genes in high risk familial pancreatic cancer patients. (NCT00526578)
- A study to evaluate patient reported pain and other symptoms for predicting overall survival in advanced pancreatic cancer patients. (NCT00805688)

Clinical trial information is constantly updated by NIH and the most recent information on pancreatic cancer trials can be found at: http://clinicaltrials.gov.

### Prognosis

It is difficult to diagnose pancreatic cancer early and, therefore, the cancer frequently has spread to other locations in the body, such as the liver or lymph nodes (part of the immune system). Survival rates five years after pancreatic cancer, in general, have been reported to be between 3% and 25%. Most long–term survivors originally had smaller tumors and no spreading of the cancer. Of course, every case of pancreatic cancer is different, and it is difficult to predict the course and survival for each individual patient. The prognosis of individuals with hereditary risk factors is dependent on the syndrome, if any, and the aggressiveness of the particular cancer.

### Resources

**BOOKS**

Casil, Amy Sterling. *Pancreatic Cancer: Current and Emerging Trends in Detection and Treatment.* New York, NY: Rosen Publishing Group, 2009.

Lowy, Andrew M., et al., editors. *Pancreatic Cancer.* New York, NY: Springer, 2008.

O'Reilly, Eileen. *100 Q&A About Pancreatic Cancer,* 2nd edition, Sudbury, MA: Jones and Bartlett Publishers, 2009.

Rains, Calvin. *My Journey With Pancreatic Cancer.* Bloomington, IN: AuthorHouse, 2006.

**PERIODICALS**

Bednar, F., and D. M. Simeone. "Pancreatic cancer stem cells and relevance to cancer treatments." *Journal of Cellular Biochemistry* 107, no. 1 (May 2009): 40–45.

Greenhalf, W., et al. "Screening of high–risk families for pancreatic cancer." *Pancreatology* 9, no. 3 (April 2009): 215–222.

Hoimes, C. J., et al. "Therapeutic tools in pancreatic cancer." *Journal of the Pancreas* 10, no. 2 (March 2009): 118–122.

Hruban, R. H., et al. "Emerging molecular biology of pancreatic cancer." *Gastrointestinal Cancer Research* 2, suppl. 4 (July 2008): S10–S159.

Klapman, J., and M. P. Malafa. "Early detection of pancreatic cancer: why, who, and how to screen." *Cancer Control* 15, no. 4 (October 2008): 280–287.

Philip, P. A. "Targeted therapies for pancreatic cancer." *Gastrointestinal Cancer Research* 2, suppl. 4 (July 2008): S16–S19.

Yeh, J. J. "Prognostic signature for pancreatic cancer: are we close?" *Future Oncology* 5, no. 3 (April 2009): 313–321.

**WEBSITES**

*Basics of Pancreatic Cancer.* Information Page. John Hopkins Medicine, 2009 (April 25, 2009). http://pathology.jhu.edu/pancreas/BasicIntro.php?area = ba.

*Detailed Guide: Pancreatic Cancer.* Information Page. ACS, 2009 (April 25, 2009). http://www.cancer.org/docroot/CRI/CRI_2_3x.asp?rnav = cridg&dt = 34.

*General Information About Pancreatic Cancer.* Information Page. NCI, 2009 (April 25, 2009). http://www.cancer.gov/cancertopics/pdq/treatment/pancreatic/patient.

*Pancreatic Cancer.* Information Page. Mayo Clinic, July 1, 2008 (April 25, 2009). http://www.mayoclinic.com/health/pancreatic-cancer/DS00357.

*What is pancreatic cancer?* Information Page. CCS, January 22, 2009 (April 25, 2009). http://www.cancer.ca/ canada-wide/about%20cancer/types%20of%20 cancer/what%20is%20pancreatic%20cancer. aspx?sc_lang=en.

**ORGANIZATIONS**

American Cancer Society (ACS). P.O. Box 22718, Oklahoma City, OK 73123-1718. (800) ACS-2345. http://www. cancer.org.

Canadian Cancer Society (CCS). National Office, Suite 200, 10 Alcorn Ave., Toronto, ON M4V 3B1, Canada. (416) 961-7223. Fax: (416) 961-4189. Email: ccs@ cancer.ca. http://www.cancer.ca.

National Cancer Institute (NCI). 6116 Executive Blvd., Ste. 3036A, MSC 8322, Bethesda, MD 20892-8322. (800) 4-CANCER (422-6237). Email: cancergovstaff@mail. nih.gov. http://cancer.gov.

Pancreatic Cancer UK. 31 Brooklyn Dr., Emmer Green, Reading, Berkshire RG4 8SR, UK. 0118-9472934. Email: enquiries@pancreaticcancer.org.uk. http:// www.pancreaticcancer.org.uk.

Kristin Baker Niendorf, MS, CGC
Edward R. Rosick, DO, MPH, MS

Pancreatic carcinoma *see* **Pancreatic cancer**

# Panic disorder

## Definition

A panic disorder is a psychological state characterized by acute (rapid onset) feelings, which engulf a person with a deep sense of destruction, death and imminent doom. The main feature of panic disorder (PD) is a history of previous panic attacks (PA). The PA symptoms are pronounced and the affected person will gasp for air, have increased breathing (hyperventilate), feel dizzy (light headed), and develop a loss of sensation (parasthesia). Most patients will run outside and symptoms like increased breathing will slow and the PA symptoms will subside. Most PA last three to ten minutes. It is rare for PA to extend in duration over 30 minutes.

## Description

The essential characteristics of panic disorder, consist of specific and common criteria. The affected person usually has recurrent and unexpected panic attacks (the active presentation of panic disorder). The PA is characterized by a discrete, rapid onset feeling of intense fear or discomfort. Affected persons

have several somatic (referring to physical signs) or cognitive (thinking) symptoms. Affected persons usually react in a manner that indicates impending doom. They commonly exhibit signs of a sweating, racing heart beat, chest pain, shortness of breath, and the perception of feeling smothered. The panic attack (PA) is usually followed by one month (or more) of one or more of the following thought processes:

- persistent concern or preoccupation about having future attacks

- worry about the possible consequences, complications, or behavioral changes associated with attacks (e.g. losing control, going crazy, or having a serious medical condition like a heart attack)

## Genetic profile

Panic disorder definitely runs in families and twin studies suggest that about 20% of patients who have the criteria for diagnosis have first–degree relatives with the disorder. In families with no history of affected first–degree relatives the prevalence decreases to 4%. The ratio between monozygotic twins (identical) to dizygotic (non–identical) twins is 5:1 for PD. Recent evidence suggests that there is a genetic mutation in the SLC6A4 **gene**. This gene is related to a brain chemical called serotonin, a chemical in the brain, which is known to effect mood. If the transport of serotonin is imbalanced then certain parts of the brain may not receive the correct stimulus causing alterations in mood. Some studies have demonstrated that there is no positive family history in about 50% of patients diagnosed with PD. Other possible causes of PD include social learning and autonomic responsiveness (the attack will affect the body and hypersensitizes nerve cells in the brain). Another gene possibly associated with panic disorder is the COMT gene that provides instructions for making an enzyme called catechol–O–methyltransferase. Mutations in this gene have been associated with other disorders that affect thought and emotion, with studies suggesting that these conditions may be due to inefficient processing of information in the prefrontal cortex.

## Demographics

PD usually begins during the affected persons late teens or in the twenties, and is uncommon after age 35 and unusual after age 45 years. Global studies suggest that the lifetime prevalence of PD is between 1.5% and 3.5%. In the United States, the National Institute of Mental Health (NIMH) estimates that panic disorder affects about 6 million American adults and is twice as common in women as men.

Agoraphobia (anxiety state about being in situations or places that might make escape embarrassing or difficult) is seen in approximately one–third to one–half of persons who meet the criteria for PD diagnosis. Other reports indicate that about 95% of persons affected with agoraphobia also have a previous history or current diagnosis of PD. In some cultures PA is believed to be associated with magic or witchcraft. Additional causes of PA may include intentional suppression of one's freedoms or public life.

## Signs and symptoms

### Criteria for panic attack:

1. Cardiac palpitations (pounding, racing or accelerated heart rate).
2. Sweating.
3. Shaking (trembling).
4. Breathing difficulties, including shortness of breath or perceptions of being smothered.
5. Feeling of choking.
6. Chest discomfort or pain.
7. Feeling light–headed (faint, dizzy or unsteady).
8. Stomach discomfort or nausea.
9. Affected individuals may lose contact with reality during the attack.
10. A feeling of being detached and out of contact with oneself.
11. Fear of losing control of oneself (going "crazy").
12. Fear of dying.
13. Tingling or numbness sensations.

### Criteria for panic disorder:

1. Recurrent and unexpected PA.
2. Worry about the consequences, implications, or behavioral changes associated with PA (perceptions of going "crazy," losing control of actions, or suffering from a life threatening condition, such as a heart attack).

3. PA is not caused by or associated with a medical condition.
4. PA is not associated with another mental disorder, such as phobia (an exaggerated fear to something like spiders or heights). Exposure to a specific phobia situation or object can promote a PA.

### Criteria for agoraphobia:

1. The essential feature of agoraphobia is anxiety about being in situations or places that make escape embarrassing or difficult. These fears usually involve characteristic clusters of situations that include being on a bridge, being in a crowd, standing in line in a department store, or traveling in a train, bus, or automobile. Elevators are another common cause promoting the occurrence of PA. These situations, which lead to the PA, are often difficult or embarrassing to abruptly flee from.
2. Avoidance of the affected person's fear, which usually limits travel away from home, causing impaired functioning.

### Criteria for PD without agoraphobia:

Recurrent unexpected PA; at least one attack followed by one month or more of one or more of the following symptoms:

- persistent concern about having future attacks
- worry about consequences associated with attacks
- a change in behavioral patterns related to the attacks (e.g., the affected person avoids travel)
- absence of agoraphobia
- PA are not due to a medical condition
- PA not associated with another mental disorder (e.g., phobias)

### Criteria for panic disorder with agoraphobia:

1. Criteria 1, 2, and 5 for PD without agoraphobia must be present.
2. The presence of agoraphobia.

## Diagnosis

There are no specific laboratory findings associated with diagnosing PD. However, evidence suggests that some affected persons may have low levels of carbon dioxide and an important ion in the human body called bicarbonate (helps in regulating blood from becoming to acidic or alkaline). These chemical changes may hypersensitize (making cells excessively sensitive) nerve cells, which can increase the activity of other structures throughout the body, such as sweat glands (sweating) and the heart (racing, accelerated or pounding rate). Additionally, lactic acid (a chemical made in the body from sugar) plays a role in nerve cell hypersensivity. The diagnosis of PD can be made accurately if the specific symptoms and criteria are established.

Neuroimaging studies indicate that the arteries (vessels that deliver oxygen rich blood to cells and tissues) are constricted (smaller diameter) as a result of increased breathing rates during a PA.

The consulting clinician must exclude other possible causes of panic attacks such as intoxication with stimulant drugs (cocaine, caffeine, amphetamines [speed]). Withdrawal from alcohol and barbiturates can also induce panic–like behaviors. Additionally, the consulting therapist should obtain a comprehensive medical history and examination to determine if the PA is caused by a medical condition frequently observed in hormonal diseases (overactive thyroid), tumors that secrete chemicals causing a person to have pronounced "hyper" changes (racing heartbeat, sweating, shaking). Other causes include a possible cardiac (heart) disease such as an irregularly beating heart.

### Treatment and management

Moderate to severe PD is characterized by frequent PA ranging from five to seven times a week or with significant disability associated with anxiety between episodes. In addition to cognitive–behavioral therapy an affected person will usually require medications. There are three classes of medications commonly prescribed for PD patients.

#### Tricyclic antidepressants

Tricyclic antidepressants are a class of medications used to treat **depression** and other closely related mental disorders. Individuals affected with PD are usually given imipramine, which has been shown in some studies to be effective in approximately 70% of cases. Medications in this category usually have a prolonged lag time until a positive response is observed. This is primarily due to adverse side effects, which prevent rapid increases of dosage and also because they act on specific chemical imbalances in the brain, which take time to stabilize.

The first choice of medication treatment for PD is tricyclics (imipramine, desipramine and nortriptyline). These medications require careful dosing and monitoring. The actual blood level (therapeutic level necessary to make improvements) may vary in special populations who have the disorder. Elderly patients may require a smaller dose, due to decrease in metabolism (in this context metabolism refers to the breakdown of large chemicals to smaller ones for usage) and kidney function, which are part of aging. Some patients may develop gastrointestinal (stomach) side effects, which may interfere with absorption from the gut, thereby decreasing beneficial blood levels. Furthermore, patients who receive tricyclics may develop dry mouth and low blood pressure. The heart may be adversely affected (altered rate and rhythm) especially in patients with preexisting diseases, causing direct damage or strain in the heart. Affected persons receiving tricyclics also commonly experience changes in sexual functioning, including loss of desire and ejaculation. Adverse (negative) side effects usually decrease patient compliance (the person stops taking medications to avoid side effects). Recently, a new group of tricyclics was made available. These tricyclics (fluoxetine, sertraline, paroxetine and fluvoxamine) act on specific areas in the brain to correct potential chemical imbalances.

#### Monoamine oxidase inhibitors (MAOIs)

A second line category of medications used to treat PD are the monoamine oxidase (a chemical that assists in storing certain chemicals in nerve cells) inhibitors (MAOI). MAOIs will stop the action of MAO, thereby decreasing the amount of certain chemicals in the brain that may influence PAs. This group of medications is effective in approximately 75–80% of cases, especially for refractory (not active) depression. Affected individuals using MAOIs must avoid specific foods to prevent a hypertensive crisis (when the blood pressure rapidly increases). These foods include cheeses (except cream cheese, cottage cheese, and fresh yogurt); liver of all types; meat and yeast extracts; fermented or aged meats (such as salami and bologna); broad and Chinese bean pods; all types of alcohol–containing products; soy sauce; shrimp and shrimp paste; and sauerkraut. Although MAOIs are effective medications for treatment of PD, they are underutilized due to strict dietary limitations.

#### Benzodiazepines

Benzodiazepines are another class of medications used to treat PD. They include medications such as diazepam (Valium), lorazepam, and clonazepam. They have been reported to be effective in 70–90% of patients with PD. However, the effective dose is approximately two to three times higher for PD than milder forms of simple anxiety (these medications are usually indicated for mild anxiety). This increased dosing in patients with PD is undesirable since there is risk of physical dependence and withdrawal (commonly exhibited when the medication is rapidly tapered down or stopped). However, they are indicated when PD affected patients respond poorly to tricyclics or have a fear of taking MAOIs due to dietary restrictions and problems associated with eating the wrong foods accidentally.

### Long term management

Reassuring the PD patient that anticipated panic attacks are unlikely while taking medication is essential for long–term maintenance. Cognitive–behavioral therapy is also important for long–term treatment. Weaning off medications must be done slowly since patients develop a sense of security that they will not have an attack while actively dosing.

### Clinical trials

Clinical trials on panic disorder are currently sponsored by the National Institutes of Health (NIH) and other agencies. As of 2009, NIH reported 98 on–going and completed studies.

Examples include:

- The evaluation of the effectiveness of psychodynamic psychotherapy in treating adults with panic disorder. (NCT00128388)
- A study to identify genes that increase the risk of developing panic disorder. (NCT00083265)
- A study to examine brain and noradrenaline function in panic disorder. (NCT00103987)
- The evaluation of the relative effectiveness of three psychotherapies in treating people with a panic disorder. (NCT00353470)

Clinical trial information is constantly updated by NIH and the most recent information on panic disorder trials can be found at: http://clinicaltrials.gov.

## Prognosis

The course of PD and agoraphobia varies considerably over time. Some cases may experience spontaneous remissions (the disorder is present but it is not active). The course can be so variable that an affected person may go on for years without a PA, then have several attacks, and then enter a second phase of remission, which may last for years. In some cases a decrease in PA may be closely related to a decrease and avoidance of anxiety–associated situations, which promote agoraphobia. Agoraphobia itself may become chronic (long term or permanent) with or without PA. In general, approximately 50–60% will recover substantially five to 20 years after the initial attack. Approximately 20% will still have long term

> ## QUESTIONS TO ASK YOUR DOCTOR
>
> - Are the symptoms I have described to you typical of panic disorder?
> - If my spouse and I decide to have children, are they likely to inherit this condition from one of us?
> - Are there medications I can take to relieve the symptoms of panic disorder?
> - What side effects, if any, should I expect from these medications?

impairment, which will stay the same or slightly worsen. Generally, the earlier treatment is sought, the better the outcome. The course in children and adolescents is chronic (long term), usually lasting about three years. Generally, PD shows the highest risk of developing new psychological disorders during follow up visits. If PA is treated early, anticipatory anxiety and phobia may be more manageable and responsive to treatment.

## Resources

### BOOKS

Berman, Carol. *100 Q&A About Panic Disorder*. Sudbury, MA: Jones and Bartlett Publishers, 2005.

Burns, David D. *When Panic Attacks: The New, Drug–Free Anxiety Therapy That Can Change Your Life*. New York, NY: Random House, 2007.

Craske, Michelle G., and David H. Barlow. *Mastery of Your Anxiety and Panic: Therapist Guide*. New York, NY: Oxford University Press, 2007.

Peurifoy, Reneau Z. *Anxiety, Phobias, and Panic*. New York, NY: Time Warner Books, 2005.

Wilson, Reid. *Don't Panic Third Edition: Taking Control of Anxiety Attacks*. New York, NY: Harper Collins Publishers, 2009.

### PERIODICALS

Bednar, F., and D. M. Simeone. "Internet–Based Treatment for Panic Disorder: Does Frequency of Therapist Contact Make a Difference?" *Cognitive Behaviour Therapy* (March 18, 2009): 1–14.

Busch, F. N., et al. "A study demonstrating efficacy of a psychoanalytic psychotherapy for panic disorder: implications for psychoanalytic research, theory, and practice." *Journal of the American Psychoanalytic Association* 57, no. 1 (February 2009): 131–148.

Powers, A., and D. Westen. "Personality subtypes in patients with panic disorder." *Comprehensive Psychiatry* 50, no. 2 (March–April 2009): 164–172.

Pull, C. B., and C. Damsa. "Pharmacotherapy of panic disorder." *Neuropsychiatric Disease and Treatment* 4, no. 4 (August 2008): 779–795.

Starcevic, V. "Treatment of panic disorder: recent developments and current status." *Expert Review of Neurotherapeutics* 8, no. 8 (August 2008): 1219–1232.

Teng, E. G., et al. "When anxiety symptoms masquerade as medical symptoms: what medical specialists know about panic disorder and available psychological treatments." *Journal of Clinical Psychology in Medical Settings* 15, no. 4 (December 2008): 314–321.

**WEBSITES**

*Answers to Your Questions About Panic Disorder.* Information Page. APA, 2009 (April 25, 2009). http://www.apa.org/topics/anxietyqanda.html.

*Panic Disorder.* Information Page. NIMH, March 31, 2009 (April 25, 2009). http://www.nimh.nih.gov/health/topics/panic-disorder/index.shtml.

*Panic Disorder.* Health Topic. Medline Plus, April 13, 2009 (April 25, 2009). http://www.nlm.nih.gov/medlineplus/panicdisorder.html.

*Panic Disorder (Panic Attack).* Information Page. Anxiety Disorders Association of America, 2009 (April 25, 2009). http://www.adaa.org/GettingHelp/AnxietyDisorders/Panicattack.asp.

*What is a Panic Attack?* Information Page. American Psychiatric Association, November 2006 (April 25, 2009). http://healthyminds.org/factsheets/LTF-Panic.pdf.

*When Fear Overwhelms: Panic Disorder.* Information Page. NIMH, 2008 (April 25, 2009). http://www.nimh.nih.gov/health/publications/when-fear-overwhelms-panic-disorder/index.shtml.

**ORGANIZATIONS**

American Psychiatric Association. 1000 Wilson Boulevard, Suite 1825, Arlington, VA 22209. (888) 35-77924. Email: apa@psych.org. http://www.psych.org.

American Psychological Association (APA). 750 First St. NE, Washington, DC 20002-4242. (800) 374-2721. Fax: (202) 336-5568. http://www.apa.org.

Mental Health America. 2000 N. Beauregard Street, 6th Floor Alexandria, VA 22311. (703) 684-7722 or (800) 969-6642. Fax: (703) 684-5968 http://www.nmha.org.

National Institute of Mental Health (NIMH). 6001 Executive Boulevard, Bethesda, MD 20892-9663. (866) 615-6464 or (301) 443-4513. Fax: (301) 443-4279. Email: nimhinfor@nih.gov. http://www.nimh.nih.gov.

Laith Farid Gulli, MD
Bilal Nasser, MS

# Pantothenate kinase-associated neurodegeneration (PKAN)

## Definition

Pantothenate kinase-associated neurodegeneration (PKAN) is a genetic disorder of the nervous system. It is characterized by prolonged movement difficulties and an accumulation of iron in the brain.

Alternate names associated with pantothenate kinase-associated neurodegeneration include neurodegeneration with brain iron accumulation 1 (NBIA1), juvenile-onset neuroaxonal dystrophy, Hallervorden-Spatz syndrome or disease, and hypoprebetalipoproteinemia, acanthocytosis, **retinitis pigmentosa**, and pallidal degeneration (HARP). Hallervorden-Spatz disease and HARP were once considered separate disorders and were known by those two names.

## Demographics

PKAN is estimated to affect one to three people per million (an incidence rate of 0.001–0.0003%). Its incidence does not appear to be related to ethnicity, gender, or geographic area. The classic form is more common and accounts for about three-fourths of all cases.

## Description

PKAN is a genetic disorder that usually results when an individual inherits a mutation in a **gene** that makes a protein called pantothenate kinase 2. This mutated gene causes iron to build up in parts of the brain, particularly in the basal ganglia. This region is a collection of three clusters of nerve cells (neurons) that control movement. These three clusters are known as the caudate nucleus, putamen, and globus pallidus, and are located deep in the brain. When iron accumulates in the basal ganglia, involuntary movements can result. These include tremors and jerking movements or rigidity of the limbs.

Two forms of the disease exist. They are:

- Classic form, in which symptoms arise in early childhood. Symptoms are usually severe and worsen rapidly.
- Atypical form, which appears later in childhood or in adolescence. Symptoms are generally less severe and advance more slowly than those in the classic form. The atypical form is less common than the classic form.

## Causes and symptoms

PKAN results from a mutation in the pantothenate kinase 2 gene, which is generally abbreviated PANK2. This disorder is an autosomal recessive one,

## KEY TERMS

**Amino acid**—A building block of proteins.

**Basal ganglia**—A collection of three clusters of neurons in the brain that control movement.

**Dementia**—Significant deterioration of mental ability.

**Dysphagia**—Swallowing problems.

**Dystonia**—Involuntary muscle contractions.

**Mitochondria**—The powerhouses of cells.

**Neuron**—Nerve cell.

so it occurs when an individual inherits a mutated PANK2 gene from each parent. The parents may not have the condition themselves but may instead only be carriers. A carrier is an individual who does not develop the disorder but may pass the gene for the disorder onto a child. If both parents are carriers, each of their children has a 50-percent chance of being a carrier, and a 25-percent chance of acquiring the disorder. If both parents have PKAN, all of their children will also acquire the disorder.

### Genetic profile

Located on the short arm of **chromosome** 20, the PANK2 gene carries the blueprint for making the enzyme pantothenate kinase 2, which is active in the mitochondria (the powerhouses of cells) in nerve cells within the brain. Pantothenate kinase 2 is part of the process that makes the molecule called coenzyme A, which is important in converting carbohydrates and fats into energy.

Individuals who have inherited the mutated PANK2 gene from both parents experience a disruption in the production of coenzyme A, and although scientists were unsure as of late 2009 of the precise mechanism responsible, iron begins to accumulate in the brain, and a range of symptoms develop.

Scientists know of some 100 different mutations in the PANK2 gene that are associated with PKAN. Commonly, the PANK2 mutation results from a substitution in amino acids, the building blocks of proteins. The amino acid glycine is often substituted with the amino acid arginine at a single position in the enzyme. In some patients, usually including those with the classic form of the disease, the mutation completely cuts off production of functional pantothenate kinase 2. In other patients, usually those with the atypical form of the disorder, the enzyme is produced, but it does not function as it should. Either

way, the manufacture of coenzyme A is compromised, and symptoms arise.

### Symptoms

Individuals with PKAN typically begin to experience symptoms as children, and they worsen as they age. Symptoms may include the following:

- Involuntary muscle contractions (dystonia)
- Tremors
- Muscle spasms
- Stiffness or rigidity in the arms and legs
- Difficulty walking
- Weakness
- Abnormal posture
- Repeated words, rapid speech, or slurred speech, particularly in the atypical form
- Swallowing problems (dysphagia)
- Night blindness followed by increasingly impaired vision
- Dementia
- Behavioral problems, particularly in the atypical form
- Personality changes, particularly in the atypical form
- Depression, particularly in the atypical form

## Diagnosis

Patients and/or their parents should inform the doctor of any family history of this (and other inherited neurological or muscular disorders), which will be helpful in making a diagnosis.

### Examination

The doctor will typically conduct or order a neurological examination to check for muscle weakness, rigidity of the limbs, involuntary muscle contractions, and other movement abnormalities.

### Tests

Although not widely available, **genetic testing** can confirm the presence of the mutation associated with PKAN.

### Procedures

A particularly telling diagnostic tool for this disorder is a magnetic resonance imaging (MRI) scan, which can detect a pattern of iron accumulation in the brain that is characteristic to this disorder. This pattern is known as the *eye of the tiger*.

## QUESTIONS TO ASK YOUR DOCTOR

- What is the difference between botulinum toxin and baclofen, and is one safer than the other?
- How long will surgical treatments for dystonia be effective?
- My spouse and I are both carriers and would like to have a child. Is prenatal testing available to determine whether a baby has PKAN? Is there a way, perhaps through preimplantation genetic diagnosis, to ensure that we have a baby that does not have the disorder?
- I have a relative with PKAN. Should I be tested for this disorder? What about my children?
- What is the advantage of early diagnosis for this disorder?

### Treatment and management

No cure for PKAN is available, but treatments exist for a number of the symptoms. Some are as follows:

- Nerve-blocking botulinum toxin, the muscle relaxant baclofen, or other surgical treatments for dystonia
- Evaluations and possible treatments for feeding problems
- Pain medications when necessary

In addition, a medical professional may also recommend physical therapy for movement issues or occupational therapy to assist the day-to-day life of those individuals who have visual, motor, or other impairments.

### Prognosis

Individuals with the classic form of this disease generally experience their first symptoms before they reach 10 years of age, whereas those with the atypical form usually do not have symptoms until they are more than 10 years of age, sometimes not until they reach their 20s. In both cases, the disease worsens over time, but the classic form progresses more quickly. In individuals with the classic form, the ability to walk on their own is lost within 10 to 15 years of the onset of symptoms. Those with the atypical form generally lose the ability to walk unassisted within 15 to 40 years after the onset of symptoms. Many individuals with this disorder live long lives, but some die young due to secondary problems (such as aspiration pneumonia that results from inhaling a inappropriate substance such as saliva or vomit) associated with the illness.

### Prevention

There is no way to prevent PKAN. It is an inherited disorder.

Adults who are carriers may wish to undergo **genetic counseling** before deciding to have children so that they understand the risks. Brothers and sisters of a child with the disorder have a 25-percent chance of having the disorder themselves, and a 50-50 chance of being a carrier for the disorder.

### Resources

#### BOOKS

Jankovic, Joseph. "Movement Disorders.&rdquo *Textbook of Clinical Neurology*, edited by C. G. Goetz. 3rd ed. Philadelphia: Saunders Elsevier, 2007, Chapter 34.

#### PERIODICALS

Dooling, Elizabeth C., et al. "Hallervorden-Spatz Syndrome." *Archives of Neurology*. 1974. 30: 70-83.
Hayflick, Susan J., et al. "Genetic, Clinical, and Radiographic Delineation of Hallervorden-Spatz Syndrome." *New England Journal of Medicine*. 2003. 348: 33-40.
Kotzbauer, Paul T., et al. "Altered Neuronal Mitochondrial Coenzyme A Synthesis in Neurodegeneration with Brain Iron Accumulation Caused by Abnormal Processing, Stability, and Catalytic Activity of Mutant Pantothenate Kinase 2." *Journal of Neuroscience*. 2007. 25: 689-698.

#### OTHER

Gregory, Allison, and Hayflick, Susan J. Pantothenate Kinase-Associated Neurodegeneration. GeneReviews. http://www.ncbi.nlm.nih.gov/bookshelf/br.fcgi?book = gene&part = pkan.
Hallervorden-Spatz Disease. MedHelp. http://www.medhelp.org/medical-information/show/166/Hallervorden-Spatz-disease?page = 1#sec_98.
Hallervorden-Spatz Disease. MedlinePlus. http://www.nlm.nih.gov/medlineplus/ency/article/001225.htm.
National Institutes of Health. Pantothenate Kinase-associated Neurodegeneration. Genetics Home Reference. http://ghr.nlm.nih.gov/condition = pantothenatekinaseassociatedneurodegeneration.

#### ORGANIZATIONS

National Organization for Rare Disorders (NORD), P.O. Box 1968, 55 Kenosia Ave., Danbury, CT, 06813-1968, 203-744-0100, orphan@rarediseases.org, http://www.rarediseases.org.
NBIA Disorders Association, 2082 Monaco Court, El Cajon, CA, 92019-4235, 619-588-2315, info@NBIAdisorders.org, http://www.NBIAdisorders.org.

Leslie A. Mertz, PHD

Parkinson disease-juvenile *see* **Parkinson disease**

# Parkinson disease

## Definition

Parkinson disease (PD) is a progressive movement disorder marked by tremors, rigidity, slow movements (bradykinesia), and posture instability. It occurs when cells in one of the movement-control centers of the brain begin to die for unknown reasons. PD was first noted by British physician James Parkinson in the early 1800s.

## Description

Usually beginning in a person's late fifties or early sixties, Parkinson disease causes a progressive decline in movement control, affecting the ability to control initiation, speed, and smoothness of motion. Symptoms of PD are seen in up to 15% of those ages 65–74, and almost 30% of those ages 75–84.

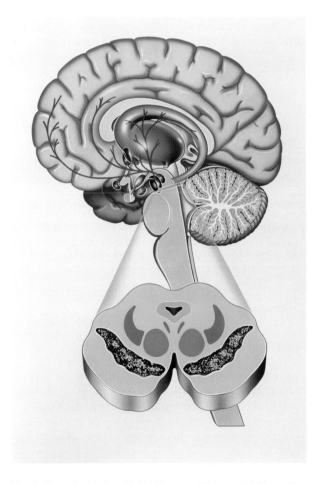

**Illustration of a brain with Parkinson's Disease.** *(J. Bavosi/ Photo Researchers, Inc. Reproduced by permission.)*

### Genetic profile

Most cases of PD are sporadic. This means that there is a spontaneous and permanent change in nucleotide sequences (the building blocks of genes). Sporadic mutations also involve unknown environmental factors in combination with genetic abnormalities. The abnormal gene (mutated gene) will form an altered end-product or protein. This will cause abnormalities in specific areas in the body where the protein is used. Some evidence suggests that the disease is transmitted by autosomal dominant **inheritance**. This implies that an affected parent has a 50% chance of transmitting the disease to any child. This type of inheritance is not commonly observed. The most recent evidence is linking PD with a gene that codes for a protein called alpha-synuclein. Further research is attempting to fully understand the relationship with this protein and nerve cell degeneration.

## Demographics

PD affects approximately 500,000 people in the United States, both men and women, with as many as 50,000 new cases each year.

## Signs and symptoms

The immediate cause of PD is degeneration of brain cells in the area known as the substantia nigra, one of the movement control centers of the brain. Damage to this area leads to the cluster of symptoms known as "parkinsonism." In PD, degenerating brain cells contain Lewy bodies, which help identify the disease. The cell death leading to parkinsonism may be caused by a number of conditions, including infection, trauma, and poisoning. Some drugs given for psychosis, such as haloperidol (Haldol) or chlorpromazine (thorazine), may cause parkinsonism. When no cause for nigral cell degeneration can be found, the disorder is called idiopathic parkinsonism, or Parkinson disease. Parkinsonism may be seen in other degenerative conditions, known as the "parkinsonism plus" syndromes, such as progressive supranuclear palsy.

The substantia nigra, or "black substance," is one of the principal movement control centers in the brain. By releasing the neurotransmitter known as dopamine, it helps to refine movement patterns throughout the body. The dopamine released by nerve cells of substantia nigra stimulates another brain region, the corpus striatum. Without enough dopamine, the corpus striatum cannot control its targets, and so on down the line. Ultimately, the movement patterns of walking, writing, reaching for objects, and other basic actions cannot function properly, resulting in the symptoms of parkinsonism.

There are some known toxins that can cause parkinsonism, most notoriously a chemical called MPTP, found as an impurity in some illegal drugs. Parkinsonian symptoms appear within hours of ingestion, and are permanent. MPTP may exert its effects through generation of toxic molecular fragments called free radicals, and reducing free radicals has been a target of several experimental treatments for PD using antioxidants.

It is possible that early exposure to some as-yet-unidentified environmental toxin or virus leads to undetected nigral cell death, and PD then manifests as normal age-related decline brings the number of functioning nigral cells below the threshold needed for normal movement. It is also possible that, for genetic reasons, some people are simply born with fewer cells in their substantia nigra than others, and they develop PD as a consequence of normal decline.

### Symptoms

The identifying symptoms of PD include:

- Tremors, usually beginning in the hands, often occuring on one side before the other. The classic tremor of PD is called a "pill-rolling tremor," because the movement resembles rolling a pill between the thumb and forefinger. This tremor occurs at a frequency of about three per second.

- Slow movements (bradykinesia) occur, which may involve slowing down or stopping in the middle of familiar tasks such as walking, eating, or shaving. This may include freezing in place during movements (akinesia).

- Muscle rigidity or stiffness, occuring with jerky movements replacing smooth motion.

- Postural instability or balance difficulty occurs. This may lead to a rapid, shuffling gait (festination) to prevent falling.

- In most cases, there is a "masked face," with little facial expression and decreased eye-blinking.

In addition, a wide range of other symptoms may often be seen, some beginning earlier than others:

- depression

- speech changes, including rapid speech without inflection changes

- problems with sleep, including restlessness and nightmares

- emotional changes, including fear, irritability, and insecurity

- incontinence

- constipation

- handwriting changes, with letters becoming smaller across the page (micrographia)

- progressive problems with intellectual function (dementia)

## Diagnosis

The diagnosis of Parkinson disease involves a careful medical history and a neurological exam to look for characteristic symptoms. There are no definitive tests for PD, although a variety of lab tests may be done to rule out other causes of symptoms, especially if only some of the identifying symptoms are present. Tests for other causes of parkinsonism may include brain scans, blood tests, lumbar puncture, and x rays.

## Treatment and management

There is no cure for Parkinson disease. Most drugs treat the symptoms of the disease only, although one drug, selegiline (Eldepryl), may slow degeneration of the substantia nigra.

### Exercise, nutrition, and physical therapy

Regular, moderate exercise has been shown to improve motor function without an increase in medication for a person with PD. Exercise helps maintain range of motion in stiff muscles, improve circulation, and stimulate appetite. An exercise program designed by a physical therapist has the best chance of meeting the specific needs of the person with PD. A physical therapist may also suggest strategies for balance compensation and techniques to stimulate movement during slowdowns or freezes.

Good nutrition is important to maintenance of general health. A person with PD may lose some interest in food, especially if depressed, and may have nausea from the disease or from medications, especially those known as dopamine agonists. Slow movements may make it difficult to eat quickly, and delayed gastric emptying may lead to a feeling of fullness without having eaten much. Increasing fiber in the diet can improve constipation, soft foods can reduce the amount of needed chewing, and a prokinetic drug such as cisapride (Propulsid) can increase the movement of food through the digestive system.

People with PD may need to limit the amount of protein in their diets. The main drug used to treat PD, L-dopa, is an amino acid, and is absorbed by the digestive system by the same transporters that pick up other amino acids broken down from proteins in the diet. Limiting protein, under the direction of the physician or a nutritionist, can improve the absorption of L-dopa.

No evidence indicates that vitamin or mineral supplements can have any effect on the disease other than in the improvement of the patient's general health. No antioxidants used to date have shown promise as a treatment except for selegiline, monoamine oxidase B (MAO-B) inhibitor. A large, carefully controlled study of vitamin E demonstrated that it could not halt disease progression.

### Drugs

The pharmacological treatment of Parkinson disease is complex. While there are a large number of drugs that can be effective, their effectiveness varies with the patient, disease progression, and the length of time the drug has been used. Dose-related side effects may preclude using the most effective dose, or require the introduction of a new drug to counteract them. There are five classes of drugs currently used to treat PD.

**DRUGS THAT REPLACE DOPAMINE.** One drug that helps replace dopamine, levodopa (L-dopa), is the single most effective treatment for the symptoms of PD. L-dopa is a derivative of dopamine, and is converted into dopamine by the brain. It may be started when symptoms begin, or when they become serious enough to interfere with work or daily living.

L-dopa therapy usually remains effective for five years or longer. Following this, many patients develop motor fluctuations, including peak-dose "dyskinesias" (abnormal movements such as tics, twisting, or restlessness), rapid loss of response after dosing (known as the "on-off" phenomenon), and unpredictable drug response. Higher doses are usually tried, but may lead to an increase in dyskinesias. In addition, side effects of L-dopa include nausea and vomiting, and low blood pressure upon standing (orthostatic hypotension), which can cause dizziness. These effects usually lessen after several weeks of therapy.

**ENZYME INHIBITORS.** Dopamine is broken down by several enzyme systems in the brain and elsewhere in the body; blocking these enzymes is a key strategy to prolonging the effect of dopamine. The two most commonly prescribed forms of L-dopa contain a drug to inhibit the amino acid decarboxylase (an AADC inhibitor), one type of enzyme that breaks down dopamine. These combination drugs are Sinemet (L-dopa plus carbidopa) and Madopar (L-dopa plus benzaseride). Controlled-release formulations also aid in prolonging the effective interval of an L-dopa dose.

The enzyme MAO-B inhibitor selegiline may be given as add-on therapy for L-dopa. Research indicates selegiline may have a neuroprotective effect, sparing nigral cells from damage by free radicals. Because of this, and the fact that it has few side effects, it is also frequently prescribed early in the disease before L-dopa is begun. Entacapone and tolcapone, two inhibitors of another enzyme system called catechol-O-methyltransferase (COMT), may reach the market, as early studies suggest that they effectively treat PD symptoms with fewer motor fluctuations and decreased daily L-dopa requirements.

**DOPAMINE AGONISTS.** Dopamine works by stimulating receptors on the surface of corpus striatum cells. Drugs that also stimulate these cells are called dopamine agonists, or DAs. DAs may be used before L-dopa therapy, or added on to avoid requirements for higher L-dopa doses late in the disease. DAs available in the United States as of early 1998, include bromocriptine (Permax, Parlodel), pergolide (Permax), and pramipexole (Mirapex). Two more, cabergoline (Dostinex) and ropinirole (Requip), are expected to be approved soon. Other dopamine agonists in use outside the United States include lisuride (Dopergine) and apomorphine. Side effects of all the DAs are similar to those of dopamine, plus confusion and hallucinations at higher doses.

**ANTICHOLINERGIC DRUGS.** Anticholinergics maintain dopamine balance as levels decrease. However, the side effects of anticholinergics (dry mouth, constipation, confusion, and blurred vision) are usually too severe in older patients or in patients with **dementia**. In addition, anticholinergics rarely work for very long. They are often prescribed for younger patients who have predominant shaking. Trihexyphenidyl (Artane) is the drug most commonly prescribed.

**DRUGS WHOSE MODE OF ACTION IS UNCERTAIN.** Amantadine (Symmetrel) is sometimes used as an early therapy before L-dopa is begun, and as an add-on later in the disease. Its anti-parkinsonian effects are mild and not seen in many patients. Clozapine (Clozaril) is effective especially against psychiatric symptoms of late PD, including psychosis and hallucinations.

### Surgery

Two surgical procedures are used for treatment of PD that cannot be controlled adequately with drug therapy. In PD, a brain structure called the globus pallidus (GPi) receives excess stimulation from the corpus striatum. In a pallidotomy, the GPi is destroyed by heat, delivered by long thin needles inserted under anesthesia. Electrical stimulation of the GPi is another way to reduce its action. In this procedure, fine electrodes are inserted to deliver the stimulation, which may be adjusted or turned off as the response dictates. Other regions of the brain may also be stimulated by electrodes inserted elsewhere. In most patients, these procedures lead to significant improvement for some motor symptoms, including peak-dose dyskinesias. This allows the patient to receive more L-dopa, since these dyskinesias are usually what cause an upper limit on the L-dopa dose.

A third procedure, transplant of fetal nigral cells, is highly experimental. Its benefits to date have been modest, although improvements in technique and patient selection are likely to change that.

### Alternative treatment

Currently, the best treatments for PD involve the use of conventional drugs such as levodopa. Alternative therapies, including acupuncture, massage, and yoga,

---

## QUESTIONS TO ASK YOUR DOCTOR

- What do scientists know about the causes of Parkinson disease?
- How does a physician know that a person has Parkinson disease rather than some other similar medical condition?
- What medications are available for the treatment of Parkinson disease, and how effective are these mediations?
- Are there herbs or other alternative medicines that can be used for the treatment of Parkinson disease?

---

can help relieve some symptoms of the disease and loosen tight muscles. Alternative practitioners have also applied herbal and dietary therapies, including amino acid supplementation, antioxidant (vitamins A, C, E, selenium, and zinc) therapy, B vitamin supplementation, and calcium and magnesium supplementation, to the treatment of PD. Anyone using these therapies in conjunction with conventional drugs should check with their doctor to avoid the possibility of adverse interactions. For example, vitamin B6 (either as a supplement or from foods such as whole grains, bananas, beef, fish, liver, and potatoes) can interfere with the action of L-dopa when the drug is taken without carbidopa.

### Prognosis

Despite medical treatment, the symptoms of Parkinson disease worsen over time, and become less responsive to drug therapy. Late-stage psychiatric symptoms are often the most troubling, including difficulty sleeping, nightmares, intellectual impairment (dementia), hallucinations, and loss of contact with reality (psychosis).

### Prevention

There is no known way to prevent Parkinson disease.

### Resources

**BOOKS**

Biziere, Kathleen, and Matthias Kurth. *Living With Parkinson Disease.* New York: Demos Vermande, 1997.

**PERIODICALS**

"An Algorithm for the Management of Parkinson Disease." *Neurology* 44/supplement 10 (December 1994): 12. http://neuro-chief-e.mgh.harvard.edu/parkinsonsweb/Main/Drugs/ManPark1.html.

**WEBSITES**

AWAKENINGS. http://www.parkinsonsdisease.com.

**ORGANIZATIONS**

National Parkinson Foundation. 1501 NW Ninth Ave., Bob Hope Road, Miami, FL 33136. http://www.parkinson.org.

Parkinson Disease Foundation. 710 West 168th St. New York, NY 10032. (800) 457-6676. http://www.apdaparkinson.com.

Worldwide Education and Awareness for Movement Disorders (WE MOVE). Mt. Sinai Medical Center, 1 Gustave Levy Place, New York, NY 10029. (800) 437-MOV2. http://www.wemove.org.

Laith Farid Gulli, MD

Parkinsonism *see* **Parkinson disease**

# Paroxysmal nocturnal hemoglobinuria

## Definition

Paroxysmal nocturnal hemoglobinuria (PNH) is a rare acquired disease in which the bone marrow produces abnormal blood cells, including red blood cells. Such red blood cells are too easily broken, and the hemoglobin inside them is released. The disease is sometimes characterized by nighttime attacks (nocturnal paroxysms) on red blood cells, when the cells break down and spill hemoglobin into the urine (hemoglobinuria). The result is reddish-brown urine upon rising in the morning.

## Description

Also known as Marchiafava-Micheli syndrome, PNH was first identified in 1882. PNH is caused by a change (mutation) in a **gene** that prevents it from making a fat required by the three types of blood cells: red blood cells, white blood cells, and platelets.

When the fat (glycosylphosphatidylinositol, or GPI) is missing from the outside walls of blood cells, proteins cannot stick to the cells and the cells cannot function normally. In healthy red blood cells, GPI binds proteins that protect the cells from chemical attack. In healthy white blood cells, GPI may attach to proteins that help the cells fight infections. In healthy platelets, GPI helps control the platelets clotting mechanism.

Not only are all types of blood cells abnormal in PNH, but the numbers of blood cells are decreased. The decrease in red blood cells, coupled with their destruction, causes anemia in people affected with PNH.

---

**KEY TERMS**

**Anemia**—A blood condition in which the level of hemoglobin or the number of red blood cells falls below normal values. Common symptoms include paleness, fatigue, and shortness of breath.

**Bone marrow**—A spongy tissue located in the hollow centers of certain bones, such as the skull and hip bones. Bone marrow is the site of blood cell generation.

**Glycosylphosphatidylinositol (GPI)**—A fat that attaches proteins to the outside walls of blood cells.

**Hemoglobin**—Protein-iron compound in the blood that carries oxygen to the cells and carries carbon dioxide away from the cells.

**Platelets**—Small disc-shaped structures that circulate in the bloodstream and participate in blood clotting.

**Red blood cell**—Hemoglobin-containing blood cells that transport oxygen from the lungs to tissues. In the tissues, the red blood cells exchange their oxygen for carbon dioxide, which is brought back to the lungs to be exhaled.

**White blood cell**—A cell in the blood that helps fight infections.

---

The severity of PNH varies greatly from individual to individual. In some affected people, blood in the urine is barely detectable; others lose so much blood that they require repeated transfusions to stay alive. In severe cases, abnormal platelets may cause abnormal clotting, and about one-third of people with PNH die from clots in the veins of the liver, stomach, or brain.

## Genetic profile

Mutations in any of 10 different genes can affect the production of GPI. Only one gene, however, is always altered in PNH. This is the PIG-A gene, located on the X **chromosome**. Females have two X chromosomes (only one is active) and males have one X chromosome.

People are not born with an altered PIG-A gene, probably because such an abnormality would be lethal to an unborn child. Rather, changes occur in the PIG-A gene sometime after birth, resulting in PNH. PNH is thus an acquired genetic disease, not an inherited disease.

## Demographics

PNH is a rare disease. In a million people, only about two to six cases of PNH will be diagnosed. PNH is most common in adults between the ages of 30 and 50, although it has been identified in infants less than one year old and people as old as 82. The disease is slightly more common in females than in males (the ratio is 1.2-to-1). Researchers have not reported that the disease is more common in one population than others, although Asians are much less likely to have clotting problems than are Caucasians.

## Signs and symptoms

Only about one-quarter of people with PNH have the telltale sign, reddish-brown urine, for which the disease is named. Other symptoms vary greatly among affected individuals. All those affected, however, have some degree of red cell breakdown that results in more or less severe anemia.

Contributing to anemia in people with PNH is the decreased production of red blood cells in the center of the bones (bone marrow). When the needed fat, GPI, is missing, the bone marrow fails to produce functioning red blood cells, white blood cells, and platelets, and the numbers of these blood cells drop dangerously low. This condition is called bone marrow failure.

Those affected with PNH may have frequent infections because their white blood cells are decreased in number and the cells that circulate in the blood are abnormal. Individuals with PNH may have stomach pain because abnormal platelets can cause clotting in liver and stomach veins. Headaches may result when clots form in veins that pass through the brain.

## Diagnosis

PNH and other types of blood diseases are usually diagnosed by examining a sample of bone marrow cells or tissue under a microscope for abnormalities. Doctors obtain the sample by performing a bone marrow aspiration or biopsy on the individual. In PNH, the bone marrow usually looks empty because so few blood cells are being produced.

Two tests that are more specific to PNH require the affected person's blood. The Ham test, developed in 1938, has long been the standard laboratory test for confirming PNH. The test determines whether an individual's red blood cells break down when attacked by certain chemicals. The Ham test is very sensitive and identifies minuscule levels of abnormal red blood cells, but it also identifies individuals with another disease of the red blood cells, congenital dyserythropoietic anemia. A second laboratory test, the sugar water test,

works on principles similar to the Ham test. Although the sugar water test is less sensitive to low levels of abnormal red blood cells than the Ham test, it is positive only when the person has PNH.

The most sensitive and specific laboratory test for PNH is flow cytometry. In this test, the individual's blood cells are treated with a chemical that normally binds to proteins on the cell wall. The size of the treated cells is measured to determine if the chemical is attached to the cell. In people with PNH, there are no proteins on the cell wall so the chemical does not bind and the cells appear smaller than normal cells.

## Treatment and management

PNH can be treated with a bone marrow transplant, a procedure in which the diseased bone marrow is destroyed and replaced with healthy bone marrow. The operation can be risky, so bone marrow transplants are most often performed on children. The operation is most successful if the healthy bone marrow is donated by an identical twin of the affected child, but bone marrow from other family members can sometimes be used.

If a suitable bone marrow donor cannot be found or if the affected person is not strong enough to withstand a bone marrow transplant, PNH can be managed by supportive treatment. Those affected may take drugs to prevent clots from forming and to prevent red blood cells from breaking down. If the number of blood cells falls dangerously low, affected individuals may receive multiple transfusions of blood cells or may be given drugs. When a person has lost a lot of red blood cells, doctors may prescribe iron supplements to help build up the blood again.

**Gene therapy** is an experimental treatment for PNH. In gene therapy, the normal PIG-A gene is inserted into the affected person's cells, where it takes the place of the abnormal gene and begins making the missing fat. The effectiveness of gene therapy for PNH has not yet been proven in humans.

## Prognosis

After an affected individual has been diagnosed with PNH, he or she usually lives for another 10 to 20 years. About 25% of people with PNH live more than 25 years after first being diagnosed. In a few people (about 15%), the disease disappears altogether and the person recovers spontaneously.

Most people who die from PNH do so because of abnormal clotting. About 10% of these individuals develop and eventually die from another disease involving red blood cells, aplastic anemia. About 5% of people with PNH develop a disease involving abnormal white blood cells, acute myelogenous leukemia.

### Resources

#### BOOKS

Rosse, Wendell F. "Paroxysmal Nocturnal Hemoglobinuria." In *Hematology: Basic Principles and Practice* 3rd ed. Ed. Ronald Hoffman, et al., 331–342. New York: Churchill Livingstone, 2000.

#### PERIODICALS

Hillmen, Peter, and Stephen J. Richards. "Implications of Recent Insights into the Pathophysiology of Paroxysmal Nocturnal Haemoglobinuria." *British Journal of Haematology* 108 (2000): 470–79.

Nishimura, Jun-ichi, et al. "Paroxysmal Nocturnal Hemoglobinuria: An Acquired Genetic Disease." *American Journal of Hematology* 62 (1999): 175–82.

#### WEBSITES

Paroxysmal Nocturnal Hemoglobinuria (PNH) Support Group. http://www.pnhdisease.org.

#### ORGANIZATIONS

Anemia Institute for Research and Education. 151 Bloor St. West, Suite 600, Toronto, ONT M5S 1S4. Canada (877) 99-ANEMIA. http://www.anemiainstitute.net.

Aplastic Anemia Foundation. 100 Park Ave., Suite 108, Rockville, MD 20850. (800) 747-2820. http://www.aamds.org/aplastic.

National Organization for Rare Disorders (NORD). PO 55 Kenosia Ave., Danbury, CT 06813. (203) 744-0100, or (800) 999-6673. http://www.rarediseases.org.

Linnea E. Wahl, MS

Partial 11q monosomy syndrome *see* **Jacobsen syndrome**

# Patent ductus arteriosus

### Definition

Patent ductus arteriosus (PDA) is a heart abnormality that occurs when the ductus arteriosus (the temporary fetal blood vessel that connects the aorta and the pulmonary artery) does not close at birth.

### Description

The ductus arteriosus is a temporary fetal blood vessel that connects the aorta and the pulmonary artery before birth. The ductus arteriosus should be present and open before birth while the fetus is developing in the uterus. Since oxygen and nutrients are received from the placenta and the umbilical cord instead of the lungs, the ductus arteriosus acts as a "short cut" that allows blood to bypass the deflated lungs and go straight out to the body. After birth, when the lungs are needed to add oxygen to the blood, the ductus arteriosus normally closes. The closure of the ductus arteriosus ensures that blood goes to the lungs to pick up oxygen before going out to the body. Closure of the ductus arteriosus usually occurs at birth as levels of certain chemicals, called prostagladins, change and the lungs fill with air. If the ductus arteriosus closes correctly, the blood pumped from the heart goes to the lungs, back into the heart, and then out to the body through the aorta. The blood returning from the lungs and moving out of the aorta carries oxygen to the cells of the body.

In some infants, the ductus arteriosus remains open (or patent) and the resulting heart defect is known as patent ductus arteriosus (PDA). In most cases, a small PDA does not result in physical symptoms. If the PDA is larger, health complications may occur.

In an average individual's body, the power of blood being pumped by the heart and other forces leads to a certain level of pressure between the heart and lungs. The pressure between the heart and lungs of an individual affected by PDA causes some of the oxygenated blood that should go out to the body (through the aorta) to return back through the PDA into the pulmonary artery. The pulmonary artery takes the blood immediately back to the lungs. The recycling of the already oxygenated blood forces the heart to work harder as it tries to supply enough oxygenated blood to the body. In this case, the left side of the heart usually grows larger as it works harder and must contain all of the extra blood moving back into

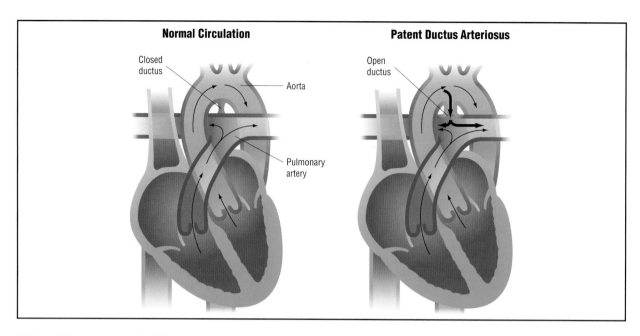

**Normal Circulation**

Closed ductus

Aorta

Pulmonary artery

**Patent Ductus Arteriosus**

Open ductus

**Failure of the temporary fetal blood vessel that connects the aorta and the pulmonary artery (ductus arteriosus) to close after birth results in patent ductus arteriosus. This open duct interferes with proper blood flow through the aorta.**
*(Gale, a part of Cengage Learning.)*

the heart. This is known as a left-to-right or aortic-pulmonary shunt.

The size of the PDA determines how much harder the heart has to work and how much bigger the heart becomes. If the PDA is large, the bottom left side of the heart is forced to pump twice as much blood because it must supply enough blood to recycle back to the lungs and move out to the body. As the heart responds to the increased demands for more oxygenated blood by pumping harder, the pulmonary artery has to change in size and shape in order to adapt to the increased amount and force of the blood. In some cases, the increase in size and shape changes the pressure in the pulmonary artery and lungs. If the pressure in the lungs is higher than that of the heart and body, blood returning to the heart will take the short cut back into the aorta from the pulmonary artery through the PDA instead of going to the lungs. This backward flowing of blood does not carry much oxygen. If blood without much oxygen is being delivered to the body, the legs and toes turn blue or cyanotic. This is called a shunt reversal.

When a PDA results in a large amount of blood being cycled in the wrong order, either through a left-to-right shunt or shunt reversal, the overworked, enlarged heart may stop working (congestive heart failure) and

the lungs can become filled with too much fluid (pulmonary edema). At this time, there is also an increased risk for a bacterial infection that can inflame the lining of the heart (endocarditis). These three complications are very serious.

## Genetic profile

PDA can be a result of an environmental exposure before birth, inheriting a specific changed or mutated **gene** or genes, a symptom of a genetic syndrome, or be caused by a combination of genetic and environmental factors (multifactorial).

Environmental exposures that can increase the chance for a baby to be affected by PDA include fetal exposure to rubella before birth, preterm delivery, and birth at a high altitude location.

PDA can be an inherited condition running in families as isolated PDA or part of a genetic syndrome. In either case, there are specific gene changes or mutations that lead to an abnormality in the elastic tissue forming the walls of the ductus arteriosus. The genes causing isolated PDA have not been identified, but it is known that PDA can be inherited through a family in an autosomal dominant pattern or an autosomal recessive pattern.

## KEY TERMS

**Aorta**—The main artery located above the heart which pumps oxygenated blood out into the body. Many congenital heart defects affect the aorta.

**Catheterization**—The process of inserting a hollow tube into a body cavity or blood vessel.

**Ductus arteriosus**—The temporary channel or blood vessel between the aorta and pulmonary artery in the fetus.

**Echocardiograph**—A record of the internal structures of the heart obtained from beams of ultrasonic waves directed through the wall of the chest.

**Electrocardiogram (ECG, EKG)**—A test used to measure electrical impulses coming from the heart in order to gain information about its structure or function.

**Endocarditis**—A dangerous infection of the heart valves caused by certain bacteria.

**Oxygenated blood**—Blood carrying oxygen through the body.

**Pulmonary artery**—An artery that carries blood from the heart to the lungs.

**Pulmonary edema**—A problem caused when fluid backs up into the veins of the lungs. Increased pressure in these veins forces fluid out of the vein and into the air spaces (alveoli). This interferes with the exchange of oxygen and carbon dioxide in the alveoli.

Every person has approximately 30,000 genes, which tell our bodies how to grow and develop correctly. Each gene is present in pairs since one is inherited from the mother, and one is inherited from the father. In an autosomal dominant condition, only one changed or mutated copy of the gene for PDA is necessary for a person to have PDA. If a parent has an autosomal dominant form of PDA, there is a 50% chance for each child to have the same or similar condition.

PDA can also be inherited in an autosomal recessive manner. A recessive condition occurs when a child receives two changed or mutated copies of the gene for a particular condition, such as PDA (one copy from each parent). Individuals with a single changed or mutated copy of a gene for a recessive condition, are known as carriers, and have no health problems related to the condition. In fact, each individual carries between

five and 10 genes for harmful, recessive conditions. However, when two people who each carry a changed or mutated copy of the same gene for a recessive condition meet, there is a chance, with each pregnancy, for the child to inherit the two changed or mutated copies from each parent. In this case, the child would have PDA. For two known carriers, there is a 25% risk with each child to have a child with PDA, a 50% chance to have a child who is a carrier, and a 25% chance to have a child who is neither affected nor a carrier.

Most cases of PDA occur as the result of **multifactorial inheritance**, which is caused by the combination of genetic factors and environmental factors. The combined factors lead to isolated defects in the elastic tissue forming the walls of the ductus arteriosus. Family studies can provide different recurrence risks depending on the family member affected by multifactorial PDA. If an individual is affected by isolated, multifactorial PDA, they have a 2-4% chance of having a child affected by PDA. If a couple has one child with isolated, multifactorial PDA, there is a 3% chance that another of their children could be affected by PDA. If a couple has two children affected by isolated, multifactorial PDA, there is a 10-25% chance that they could have another child affected by PDA.

Unless a specific pattern of **inheritance**, preterm delivery, or known exposure is found through the examination of a detailed pregnancy and family history, the multifactorial family studies are used to estimated the possible risk of recurrence of PDA in a family.

### Demographics

PDA is a very common heart disorder. Though an exact incidence of PDA is difficult to determine, one review in 1990 found that approximately 8% of live births were found to be affected by PDA. PDA can occur in full-term infants, but is seen most frequently in preterm infants, infants born at a high altitude, and babies whose mothers were affected by German measles (rubella) during pregnancy. PDA is two to three times more common in females than males. PDA occurs in individuals of every ethnic origin and does not occur more frequently in any one country or ethnic population.

### Signs and symptoms

The main sign of PDA is a constant heart murmur that sounds like the hum of a refrigerator or other machinery. This murmur is usually heard by the doctor using a stethoscope. Otherwise, there are no specific symptoms of PDA, unless the ductus arteriosus size is large. Children and adults with a large ductus arteriosus can show difficulty in breathing during moderate physical exercise, an enlarged heart, and failure to gain weight. In some cases, heart failure and pulmonary congestion can indicate a PDA.

### Diagnosis

Diagnosis is most often made by detecting the characteristic "machinery" heart murmur heard by a doctor through a stethoscope. Tests such as a chest x ray, echocardiograph, and ECG are used to support the initial diagnosis. Other indications of PDA include failure to gain weight, frequent chest infections, heavy breathing during mild physical exertion, congestive heart failure, and pulmonary edema. Prenatal ultrasounds are unable to detect PDA because the heart defect does not occur until the time of birth.

### Treatment and management

The treatment and management of PDA depends upon the size of the PDA and symptoms being experienced by the affected individual. In some cases, a PDA can correct itself in the first months of life. In preterm infants experiencing symptoms, the first step in correcting a PDA is treatment through medications such as indomethacin. In preterm infants whose PDA is not closed through medication, full term infants affected by PDA, and adults, surgery is an option for closing the ductus arteriosus. In 2000 and 2001, researchers developed and reviewed alternatives to surgical closure such as interventional cardiac catheterization and video-assisted thorascopic surgical repair. A cardiologist can help individuals determine the best method for treatment based on their physical symptoms and medical history.

### Prognosis

Adults and children can survive with a small opening remaining in the ductus arteriosus. Treatment, including surgery, of a larger PDA is usually successful and frequently occurs without complications. Proper treatment allows children and adults to lead normal lives.

### Resources

#### BOOKS

Alexander, R. W., R. C. Schlant, and V. Fuster, eds. *The Heart*. 9th ed. New York: McGraw-Hill, 1998.

Jaworski, Anna Marie, ed. *The Heart of A Mother*. Temple, Texas: Baby Hearts Press, 1999.

Kleinman, Mary. *What Your Doctor Didn't Tell you About Congenital Heart Disease*. Salt Lake City: Northwest Publishing Inc., 1993.

Neill, Catherine. *The Heart of A Child*. Baltimore: Johns Hopkins University, 1992.

#### WEBSITES

Congenital Heart Defect Resource. http://www.congenital heartdefects.com.

"Congenital Cardiovascular Defects." *American Heart Association* http://www.americanheart.org. 2000.

"Heart Disorders & Defects." *Family Village*. December 23, 2008 (December 11, 2009). http://www.familyvillage. wisc.edu/Lib_heart.html.

#### ORGANIZATIONS

CHASER (Congenital Heart Anomalies Support, Education, and Resources). 2112 North Wilkins Rd., Swanton, OH 43558. (419) 825-5575. http://www.csun.edu/ ~hcmth011/chaser/chaser-news.html.

Kids with Heart. 1578 Careful Dr., Green Bay, WI 54304. (800) 538-5390. http://www.kidswithheart.org.

Dawn A. Jacob, MS

PC deficiency *see* **Pyruvate carboxylase deficiency with lactic acidemia**

# Pedigree analysis

### Definition

A pedigree is a family tree or chart made of symbols and lines that represent a patient's genetic family history. The pedigree is a visual tool for documenting biological relationships in families and the presence of diseases. Pedigree analysis is an assessment made by a medical professional about genetic risk in a family.

## Purpose

Pedigrees are most often constructed by medical geneticists or genetic counselors. People are referred to genetic professionals because of concern about the presence of a genetic condition in a family member. Pedigree analysis can help identify a genetic condition running through a family, aids in making a diagnosis, and aids in determining who in the family is at risk for genetic conditions. During pedigree construction, the family's beliefs about the cause for a genetic disease or emotional issues related to a diagnosis may be revealed. For instance, family members may experience guilt or shame about passing on a genetic trait. Thus, the communication process involved in taking the family history may allow the health care provider to identify areas in which the patient may need reassurance, education, or emotional support.

## Creating a pedigree

### Pedigree symbols

A standard set of symbols has been established for use in creating pedigrees. Some of the most commonly used symbols are shown in this entry. When a person is affected with a birth disorder, mental retardation, or other health problems, the individual is shaded or marked. If more than one condition is present in a family, different identifying marks should be made. A key to decipher these markings should also be included on the pedigree. The meaning of each horizontal and vertical line is also shown.

### Information obtained

A typical pedigree is made of information about three generations of a family. The consultand is the person seeking genetic evaluation, counseling or testing. The proband in a family is the person in a family affected with a genetic disease. Beginning with the consultand, questions should be asked about the health of first, second, and third degree relatives. First-degree relatives are children, parents and siblings. Second-degree relatives are half siblings, nieces, nephews, aunts and uncles, grandparents, and grandchildren. Third-degree relatives are first cousins. Important information to obtain on both sides of the family includes:

- ages or dates of birth
- presence of any birth disorders, learning problems, chronic illnesses, surgeries, or medical treatments
- presence of specific features of a disease if the condition is suspected in the family
- genetic testing results if previously performed in the family

- cause of death for deceased family members
- pregnancy losses, stillbirths or infant deaths and causes
- infertility in the family
- ethnic background of the families
- consanguinity

It is important to establish the accuracy of information given by patients. Therefore, medical records are often requested in order to provide accurate risk assessment.

## Pedigree patterns

### Autosomal dominant inheritance

Pedigree 1 illustrates the occurrence of an autosomal dominant disorder called **neurofibromatosis** (NF). NF is characterized by growths under the skin called neurofibromas, dark spots on the skin called café au lait spots, and an eye finding called Lisch nodules. NF is caused by a single dominant **gene** on **chromosome** 17. Each person who is affected with NF has a 50% chance to pass the gene on to each child. The symptoms of NF are variable so that some family members are affected more seriously than others. The pedigree shows that in autosomal dominant **inheritance**, multiple generations of a family are affected. This is called vertical transmission of a trait through a family. Males and females are equally likely to be affected. In a particular sibship, about half of the siblings are affected.

### Autosomal recessive inheritance

Pedigree 2 illustrates the occurrence of an autosomal recessive disorder called **cystic fibrosis** (CF) in a family. CF is a chronic respiratory disease characterized by digestive problems and a shortened life span. A person with CF has two genes for the condition on chromosome 7. Each parent is an obligate carrier of a gene for the condition. When both parents are carriers, there is a one in four or 25% chance that each child they have together will be affected. In autosomal recessive inheritance, siblings are most often affected rather than people in successive generations. Since siblings are affected, this is called horizontal transmission of a disease in the family. Males and females are equally likely to be affected in this type of inheritance and others in the family have an increased chance to be unaffected carriers of the disease.

### X-linked recessive inheritance

Pedigree 3 illustrates the occurrence of an X-linked disorder called **hemophilia**. Hemophilia is characterized by excessive bleeding and bruising. Depending on the type of hemophilia, a particular blood-clotting factor is deficient. In X-linked recessive inheritance, males are

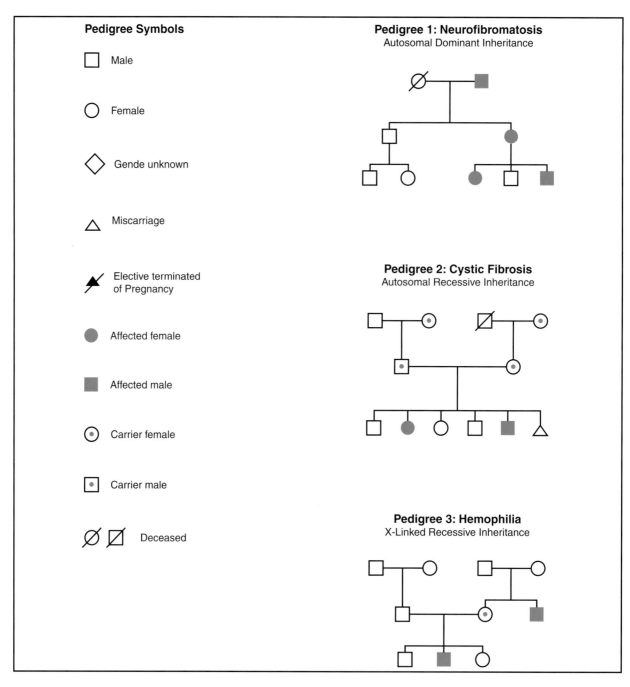

**Pedigree Symbols**

☐ Male

◯ Female

◇ Gende unknown

△ Miscarriage

⚡ Elective terminated of Pregnancy

⬤ Affected female

◼ Affected male

⊙ Carrier female

⊡ Carrier male

∅ ⊘ Deceased

**Pedigree 1: Neurofibromatosis**
Autosomal Dominant Inheritance

**Pedigree 2: Cystic Fibrosis**
Autosomal Recessive Inheritance

**Pedigree 3: Hemophilia**
X-Linked Recessive Inheritance

**The illustration above identifies several common symbols used to represent individuals in a pedigree chart. The three pedigree charts to the side provide examples of different types of inheritance patterns and the transmission of abnormal genes through three generations in a family.** *(Gale, a part of Cengage Learning.)*

affected with the condition while females are unaffected carriers. In X-linked recessive inheritance, vertical transmission of the disease is seen, with skipping of generations. There is no male-to-male transmission of a disease in this type of inheritance. This is because males pass their Y chromosome to each son, instead of the X chromosome with the disease gene. Each daughter of an affected male is an obligate carrier of the disease since they will always inherit his X chromosome. There is a 50% that each son of a carrier woman will be affected. There is a 50% chance that each daughter of a carrier female will be a carrier.

## Resources

### BOOKS

Baker, Diane. *A Guide to Genetic Counseling.* New York: A. Wiley and Sons, Inc. 1998.

Harper, Peter S. *Practical Genetic Counseling.* Oxford: Butterworth Heinmann 1998.

Rose, Peter, and Anneke Lucassen. "Taking a Family History." In *Practical Genetics for Primary Care.* Oxford: Oxford University Press, 1999.

### PERIODICALS

Bennett, Robin et al. "Recommendations for Standardized Human Pedigree Nomenclature." *The Journal of Genetic Counseling* (December 1995): 267–79.

Sonja Rene Eubanks, MS, CGC

# Pelizaeus-Merzbacher disease

## Definition

Pelizaeus-Merzbacher disease (PMD) is a neurological condition that affects myelin, the insulation surrounding the nerves in the brain and spinal cord.

## Description

PMD was named for two German doctors, F. Pelizaeus and L. Merzbacher, who first described the condition in the late 1800s. The severity of characteristics in PMD can range from mild to severe. PMD primarily affects males, but occasionally females have mild or moderate symptoms. PMD is also called a **leukodystrophy**, meaning that it affects the myelin, sometimes called the white matter, in the brain and spinal cord. The brain and the spinal cord together are called the central nervous system.

## Genetic profile

PMD is caused by a mutation or change in the proteolipid protein **gene** (PLP). The PLP gene has the instructions to make proteolipid protein, one of the proteins that make up myelin in the central nervous system. When there is a mutation in the PLP gene, the myelin is not formed properly or is not made at all, resulting in PMD.

Genes are organized on structures called chromosomes. There are hundreds to thousands of genes on each **chromosome**. There are 46 chromosomes in each cell of the body. These are grouped into 23 pairs. The first 22 pairs are the same in both males and females. The 23rd pair is called the sex chromosomes; having

---

one X chromosome and one Y chromosome causes a person to be male; having two X chromosomes causes a person to be female. A fetus acquires one member of each pair from the mother's egg and one member from the father's sperm.

The PLP gene is located on the X chromosome. Since males have only one X chromosome, they have only one copy of the PLP gene. Thus, a male with a mutation in his PLP gene will have PMD. Females have two X chromosomes and, therefore, have two copies of the PLP gene. If they have a mutation in one copy of their PLP genes, they may only have mild symptoms of PMD or no symptoms at all. This is because their normal copy of the PLP gene does make normal myelin. Females who have one copy of the PLP gene with a mutation and one normal copy are called carriers.

### Inheritance

PMD is passed on through families by X-linked recessive **inheritance**. This means that affected males are related through females in the family. A male does not pass PMD on to his sons. Females pass on one of their X chromosomes to their sons or daughters. If the normal X chromosome is passed on, her son or daughter will be unaffected and cannot pass PMD onto their children. However, if the X chromosome with the PLP mutation is passed on, a daughter will be a carrier while the son would have PMD. Therefore, a female PLP mutation carrier has a 50%, or one in two chance of having a normal child (son or daughter), a 25%, or one in four chance of having a carrier daughter, and a 25%, or one in four chance of having an affected son.

Males with PMD usually do not reproduce and therefore do not pass on PMD.

### Mutations

Different types of mutations or changes in the PLP gene cause PMD. Everyone in a family who has the condition or is a carrier has the exact same PLP mutation. The most common type of mutation is a duplication (doubling) of the PLP gene. This means that two copies of the PLP gene are present on one X chromosome. Having this extra copy causes the myelin to be abnormal and leads to PMD. About 50–75% of people with PMD have a PLP duplication. The duplication usually causes a severe form of PMD. Another 15–20% of people with PMD have point mutations within their PLP gene. A point mutation is like a typo in the gene. This typo changes the message of the gene and also causes the myelin to be abnormal. A few patients with PMD have a deletion of the PLP gene as their cause of PMD. This means that they have no copies of the PLP gene if they are male or one copy if they are female. Another 5–20% of patients have characteristics of PMD, but no mutation has been found in their PLP gene. Scientists are working to determine the cause of disease in these people.

## Demographics

PMD has been described in people from all over the world and from many different ethnic backgrounds. The condition is rare and estimated to affect approximately one in 300,000 individuals in the United States.

## Signs and symptoms

There is a range in the severity of symptoms of PMD. Rough categories have been set up based on the age of onset and severity of symptoms. However, many patients do not fall neatly into one of these categories and instead fall somewhere in between. Patients with different severities have been seen in the same family.

In the most severe form of PMD, symptoms are first noticed shortly after birth or in infancy. This is called connatal PMD. One of the first signs usually noticed is nystagmus, a side-to-side jerking of the eyes. This does not usually cause problems with vision. Patients can have significant mental retardation and never learn to walk, talk, or care for themselves. They may have noisy breathing called stridor and difficulty sucking. Seizures may be present in these children. They are often small for their age and have trouble gaining weight. Early on, they have floppy muscles

called hypotonia, but later develop spasticity, which is stiffness or tightness in the muscles and joints.

Those patients who have classical PMD, which is less severe than the connatal type, usually have nystagmus. Nystagmus develops within the first few months of life. Other symptoms typically develop within the first few years. These children also have hypotonia that turns into spasticity. Sometimes these patients will learn to walk. However, they may need a wheelchair as their spasticity increases. Shaking of the head and neck called titubation may occur. Although these children often have moderate mental retardation, they often learn to talk and often understand more than is evident by their speech.

A less severe type of PMD is called the PLP null syndrome. Those affected do not usually have nystagmus and their spasticity may be mild. Symptoms develop in early childhood. This group of patients may also have a peripheral neuropathy, which is a problem with the nerves that run from the spinal cord through the body. This can cause weakness and problems with sensation (telling if something is hot or cold, for example). These patients usually talk and walk. They may have mild to moderate mental retardation.

There are some people who have PLP mutations who are very mildly affected. They have spasticity and sometimes have other problems such as a spastic bladder. Intelligence is normal or mildly impaired. Although these individuals have mutations in the PLP gene, their condition is given a different name, spastic paraplegia 2 (SPG2).

## Diagnosis

When problems are first noticed in an infant or a child, they will usually be referred to a pediatric neurologist who is specially trained in diseases of the nerves and muscles in children. At the initial evaluation, the neurologist will perform a clinical examination to evaluate the child's development and how well the nerves and muscles work. At this time, a thorough family history should be taken to determine if there are others in the family that are affected and if so, how they are related.

One of the initial tests that may be ordered is magnetic resonance imaging (MRI). In this test, pictures of the brain are taken and the amount of white matter in the brain is measured. In people with PMD, the amount of white matter is usually significantly reduced compared to normal. However, a decrease in white matter is seen in other neurological conditions and is not specific to PMD. An MRI can be helpful in making the diagnosis of PMD, but if changes are seen on MRI, it does not confirm the diagnosis of PMD. Changes in the white matter may only be seen after one to two years of age when the brain has matured.

If no one else in the family is known to be affected, testing may be performed to rule out conditions other than PMD. Often PMD may not initially be suspected when no one else is affected in the family. It is not uncommon for people to be misdiagnosed initially. Sometimes the diagnosis of PMD is made only after a second affected child is born into a family.

### Genetic testing

The only way to be absolutely sure that someone has PMD is by **genetic testing**, usually done by a blood test. First, the genetic material is evaluated to see if a PLP gene duplication is present. If this test is negative, additional testing can be done to look for other mutations in the gene. In 80% of people who have clear symptoms of PMD, a mutation can be found in the PLP gene. If a mutation in the PLP gene has been identified in a family member, testing a child suspected of having PMD is possible to look at the mutation known to cause PMD in the family.

## Treatment and management

There is no treatment or cure for PMD. Medical management is aimed at making life as full as possible and keeping people free from illness. Different types of therapy might be suggested. An occupational therapist can suggest adaptive devices to make it easier for an affected person to get around his or her home and perform everyday activities such as eating and using the bathroom. For example, they may suggest installing bars to use in the bathroom or shower or special utensils for eating. Physical therapy can be helpful for reducing spasticity. Some patients with PMD require a feeding tube to help take in more calories. There are also medications that can assist in treating spasticity and seizures.

### Prenatal testing

Testing during pregnancy to determine whether an unborn child is affected is possible if genetic testing in a family has identified a specific PLP mutation. This can be done at 10–12 weeks gestation by a procedure called chorionic villus sampling (CVS), which involves removing a tiny piece of the placenta and examining the cells. It can also be done by **amniocentesis** after 16 weeks gestation by removing a small amount of the amniotic fluid surrounding the baby and analyzing the cells in the fluid. Each of these procedures has a small risk of miscarriage associated with them. Couples interested in these options should have **genetic counseling** to carefully explore all of the benefits and limitations of these procedures.

---

## QUESTIONS TO ASK YOUR DOCTOR

- What are the usual signs and symptoms associated with Pelizaeus-Merzbacher disease?
- What is known about the genetic basis of this disorder?
- At what age can Pelizaeus-Merzbacher disease be diagnosed, and how is that diagnosis made?
- What factors affect the prognosis for a child diagnosed with Pelizaeus-Merzbacher disease?

---

Another procedure, called preimplantation diagnosis, allows a couple to have a child that is unaffected with the genetic condition in their family. This procedure is experimental and not available for all conditions. Those interested in learning more about this procedure should check with their doctor or genetic counselor.

## Prognosis

The prognosis for patients with PMD varies in part due to the severity of the symptoms. The quality of care that patients receive also makes a difference in their quality of life. Boys with connatal PMD may die in infancy or early childhood, although some have survived into their thirties. Those with classic PMD or with the PLP null syndrome usually reach adulthood, and some have survived into their seventies. The symptoms of PMD usually progress very slowly and some people have a plateau of their symptoms over time. Some people may seem to get worse over time but it is likely to be due to factors such as growth spurts, poor nutrition, or frequent illness and not because of progression of the disease. Most patients with PMD die from pulmonary or breathing difficulties.

### Resources

#### PERIODICALS

Cailloux, F., F. Gauthier-Barichard, C. Mimault, V. Isabelle, V. Courtois, G. Giraud, B. Dastugue, O. Boespflug-Tanguy, and the Clinical European Network on Brain Dysmyelinating Disease. "Genotype-phenotype correlation in inherited brain myelination defects due to proteolipid protein gene mutations." *European Journal of Human Genetics* 8, no. 5 (November 2000): 837–45.

Garbern, J., F. Cambi, M. Shy, and J. Kamholz. "The molecular pathogenesis of Pelizaeus-Merzbacher disease." *Archives of Neurology* 56 (October 1999): 1210–14.

Yool, D.A., J.M. Edgar, P. Montague, and S. Malcolm. "The proteolipid protein gene and myelin disorders in man and animal models." *Human Molecular Genetics* 9, no. 6 (2000): 987–992.

**WEBSITES**

"Clinical Programs." *PMD Website at Wayne State University.* http://www.med.wayne.edu/neurology.
GeneClinics. http://www.geneclinics.org.
Online Mendelian Inheritance in Men. http://www.ncbi.nlm.nih.gov/Omim.

**ORGANIZATIONS**

National Organization for Rare Disorders (NORD). 55 Kenosia Ave., PO Box 1948, Danbury, CT 06813. (203) 744-0100. or (800) 999-6673. http://www.rarediseases.org.
PMD Foundation. 1307 White Horse Rd., Suite 603, Voorhees, NJ 08043. (609) 443-9623. http://pmdfoundation.org.
United Leukodystrophy Foundation. 2304 Highland Dr., Sycamore, IL 60178. (815) 895-3211 or (800) 728-5483. Fax: (815) 895-2432. http://www.ulf.org.

Karen M. Krajewski, MS, CGC

# Pendred syndrome

## Definition

Pendred syndrome is an inherited condition that causes hearing loss typically beginning at birth and usually leads to the development of an enlarged thyroid, called a goiter. The thyroid is a gland responsible for normal body growth and metabolism. People with Pendred syndrome often have altered development of certain bones in the inner ear and/or balance problems as well. Vaughan Pendred first described the presence of hearing loss and goiter in two sisters in 1896, and the condition became known as Pendred syndrome. Genetic research has identified a **gene** on **chromosome** 7 that is usually altered in people with Pendred syndrome.

## Description

Pendred syndrome is sometimes called goiter-sensorineural **deafness**, due to the common existence of both goiter and a form of hearing loss called sensorineural hearing loss in affected individuals. In order to understand how goiter occurs, it is helpful to first understand how the thyroid gland normally works. The thyroid is located underneath the larynx (voice box), in the front of the neck. The main role of the thyroid is to trap iodine, an essential nutrient found in various foods as well as salt, and to use it to make two important hormones: T3 and T4. These thyroid hormones allow the body to grow normally and to increase the speed of metabolism (breakdown) of nutrients. The thyroid is able to create these hormones because of a series of chemical reactions. A portion of the brain called the hypothalamus is responsible for controlling many body functions. One of its functions is to make a chemical called thyroid releasing hormone (TRH). This hormone travels to another gland, called the anterior pituitary gland, which is located underneath the brain. The TRH stimulates the anterior pituitary gland, which makes a chemical called thyroid stimulating hormone (TSH). This hormone travels to the thyroid, and activates the release of T3 and T4 into the body.

The word goiter is used to describe an enlargement of the thyroid gland. People with goiter may have hypothyroidism (they make too little T3/T4), hyperthyroidism (they make too much T3/T4), or they may have thyroid glands that work normally. Approximately 44–50% of people with Pendred syndrome have hypothyroidism, while the remaining 50–56% have thyroid glands that create a normal amount of thyroid hormones. However, approximately 75% develop goiter at some point in time, although it is rarely present at birth. Thirty to 40% of individuals develop an enlarged thyroid in late childhood or during their early teen-age years. The remaining 60–70% show symptoms during their early adult years. The enlargement of the thyroid gland happens because the mechanisms that control iodine transfer within the cells of the thyroid do not work well. This transfer is necessary to allow the iodine to bind to (and in doing so, help generate) thyroid hormones stored inside the thyroid. Since the iodine is not moved to the correct area of the thyroid, it becomes "pooled," rather than attaching itself to thyroid hormones. This faulty processing of iodine among people with Pendred syndrome can often be confirmed by the use of a perchlorate discharge test. Perchlorate is a chemical that causes the pooled iodine to be pushed out of the thyroid into the bloodstream where it can be measured. Since people with Pendred syndrome usually have more pooled iodine than normal, they will push out or discharge a larger amount of iodine when they are exposed to perchlorate. However, not all affected individuals show abnormal results, so the test is not perfect.

Pendred syndrome causes a specific type of hearing impairment called sensorineural hearing loss (SNHL). The ear can be divided into three main parts: the outer ear, the middle ear, and the inner ear. The parts of the outer ear include the pinna (the visible portion of the ear), the ear canal and the eardrum. The pinna directs sound waves from the environment through the ear canal, toward the eardrum. The eardrum vibrates, and causes tiny bones (called ossicles), which are located in the middle ear, to move. This movement causes pressure changes in fluids surrounding the parts that make up the inner ear.

**Cochlea**—A bony structure shaped like a snail shell located in the inner ear. It is responsible for changing sound waves from the environment into electrical messages that the brain can understand, so people can hear.

**Cochlear implantation**—A surgical procedure in which a small electronic device is placed under the skin behind the ear and is attached to a wire that stimulates the inner ear, allowing people who have hearing loss to hear useful sounds.

**Enlarged vestibular aqueduct (EVA)**—An enlargement of a structure inside the inner ear called the vestibular aqueduct, which is a narrow canal that allows fluid to move within the inner ear. EVA is seen in approximately 10% of people who have sensorineural hearing loss.

**Goiter**—An enlargement of the thyroid gland, causing tissue swelling that may be seen and/or felt in the front of the neck. May occur in people who have overactive production of thyroid hormones (hyperthyroidism), decreased production of thyroid hormones (hypothyroidism), or among people who have normal production of thyroid hormones.

**Metabolism**—The total combination of all of the chemical processes that occur within cells and tissues of a living body.

**Pendrin**—A protein encoded by the PDS (Pendred syndrome) gene located on chromosome 7q31. Pendrin protein is believed to transport iodide and chloride within the thyroid and the inner ear.

**Perchlorate discharge test**—A test used to check for Pendred syndrome by measuring the amount of iodine stored inside the thyroid gland. Individuals with Pendred syndrome usually have more iodine stored than normal, and thus their thyroid will release a large amount of iodine into the bloodstream when they are exposed to a chemical called perchlorate.

**Sensorineural hearing loss (SNHL)**—Sensorineural hearing loss occurs when parts of the inner ear, such as the cochlea and/or auditory nerve, do not work correctly. It is often defined as mild, moderate, severe, or profound, depending upon how much sound can be heard by the affected individual. SNHL can occur by itself, or as part of a genetic condition such as Pendred syndrome.

**Thyroid gland**—A gland located in the front of the neck that is responsible for normal body growth and metabolism. The thyroid traps a nutrient called iodine and uses it to make thyroid hormones, which allow for the breakdown of nutrients needed for growth, development and body maintenance.

**Vestibular system**—A complex organ located inside the inner ear that sends messages to the brain about movement and body position. Allows people to maintain their balance when moving by sensing changes in their direction and speed.

The main structures of the inner ear are the cochlea and the vestibular system. These structures send information regarding hearing and balance to the brain. The cochlea is shaped like a snail shell, and it contains specialized sensory cells (called hair cells) that change the sound waves into electrical messages. These messages are then sent to the brain through a nerve (called the auditory nerve) that allows the brain to "hear" sounds from the environment. The vestibular system is a specialized organ that helps people maintain their balance. The vestibular system contains three structures called semi-circular canals, which send electrical messages to the brain about movement and body position. This allows people to maintain their balance when moving by sensing changes in their direction and speed.

Sensorineural hearing loss occurs when parts of the inner ear (including the cochlea and/or auditory nerve) do not work correctly. The amount (or degree) of hearing loss can be described by measuring the hearing threshold (the sound level that a person can just barely hear) in decibels (dB). The greater a person's dB hearing level, the louder the sound must be to just barely be heard.

Hearing loss is often defined as mild, moderate, severe, or profound. For people with mild hearing loss (26–45 dB), understanding conversations in a noisy environment, at a distance, or with a soft-spoken person is difficult. Moderate hearing loss (46–65 dB) causes people to have difficulty understanding conversations, even if the environment is quiet. People with severe hearing loss (66–85 dB) have difficulty hearing conversation unless the speaker is standing nearby or is talking loudly. Profound hearing loss (85 dB) may prevent people from hearing sounds from their environment or even loud conversation. People with Pendred syndrome generally have severe to profound SNHL that is congenital (i.e. present at birth) in both ears.

However, some affected individuals develop SNHL during childhood, after they have learned to speak.

People with SNHL often undergo specialized imaging tests, such as computed tomography (CT) and/or magnetic resonance imaging (MRI) scans, which create detailed images of the tissue and bone structures of the inner ear. Approximately 85% of people affected with Pendred syndrome have physical changes in the inner ear that can be seen with these tests. A common finding is a visible change in the snail-shaped cochlea called a Mondini malformation, in which the cochlea is underdeveloped and has too few coils compared to a normal cochlea. Another visible change sometimes seen in the inner ear is called enlarged vestibular aqueduct. The vestibular aqueduct is a narrow canal that allows fluid to move within the inner ear. Enlarged vestibular aqueduct (EVA) is the most common form of inner ear abnormality that is seen with CT or MRI scans. As the name implies, the vestibular aqueduct (canal) is larger than normal in people with EVA. Although EVA is seen in approximately 10–12% of people who are born with SNHL, some people with EVA can have SNHL that fluctuates (comes and goes) or is progressive (gradually worsening) as well as balance problems.

In spite of the fact that Pendred syndrome has typically been diagnosed among people with both SNHL and goiter/thyroid problems, preliminary studies support the finding that some people with EVA and SNHL have a form of Pendred syndrome, even if they do not have goiter or thyroid problems.

Pendred syndrome causes vestibular dysfunction in approximately 66% of affected individuals, which means they have abnormalities in their vestibular (balance) system. This may cause problems such as dizziness because they cannot sense changes in direction or speed when they are moving.

### Genetic profile

Pendred syndrome is inherited in an autosomal recessive manner. Autosomal means that males and females are equally likely to be affected. Recessive refers to a specific type of **inheritance** in which both copies of a person's gene pair (i.e. both alleles) need to be changed or altered in order for the condition to develop. In this situation, an affected individual receives an altered copy of the same gene from each parent. If the parents are not affected, they each have one working copy of the gene and one non-working (altered) copy, and are only carriers for Pendred syndrome. The chance that two carrier parents will have a child affected with Pendred syndrome is 25% for each pregnancy. They also have a 50% chance to have an unaffected child who is simply a carrier, and a 25% chance to have an unaffected child who is not a carrier, with each pregnancy.

The gene for Pendred syndrome is located on chromosome 7q31 and has been named the PDS gene. The gene tells the body how to make a specific protein called pendrin. The pendrin protein is believed to be responsible for transporting negatively charged elements called iodide and chloride (forms of iodine and chlorine) within the thyroid and likely the inner ear as well. Changes within the PDS gene create an altered form of pendrin protein that does not work properly, and thus causes the symptoms of Pendred syndrome. Genetic researchers have identified at least 47 different types of alterations in the PDS gene among different families. However, four of these are more common than the others, and it is estimated that approximately 75% of affected people have these common changes.

Genetic research on the PDS gene has revealed that different types of gene changes can lead to different symptoms. For example, changes that completely inactivate the pendrin protein have been seen among people with Pendred syndrome (i.e. SNHL and goiter), whereas other types of alterations that only decrease the activity of pendrin have been found in people who have an inherited form of deafness called DFNB4. These individuals do have SNHL, but do not develop goiter. The researchers who published this finding in 2000 believed that the small amount of pendrin activity in these individuals likely prevented or delayed the symptoms of goiter. Another study published in 2000 showed that a large portion (greater than 80%) of people with EVA and SNHL were found to have one or more changes in the PDS gene, even though they did not all have thyroid changes such as goiter or abnormal perchlorate discharge test results. Thus, it is believed that changes in the pendrin gene actually cause a number of overlapping conditions. These conditions range from Pendred syndrome (i.e. SNHL and thyroid changes) to SNHL with EVA.

### Demographics

Pendred syndrome has been estimated to occur in approximately 7.5 in 100,000 births in Great Britain, and one in 100,000 births in Scandinavia. It has been diagnosed in many different ethnic groups, including Japanese, East Indian, and other Caucasian groups, as well as among people of African descent. Inherited forms of congenital SNHL occur in approximately one of every 2,000 children. Prior to the discovery of the PDS gene, researchers estimated that up to 10% of all children born with SNHL could actually have Pendred syndrome. However, the percentage may be even higher. This is because changes in the PDS gene have been found in people who have SNHL and EVA, even though they do not have thyroid changes that would have helped make a clear diagnosis of Pendred syndrome in the past. Thus, future genetic studies on large groups of individuals with SNHL will help researchers understand how common Pendred syndrome truly is, as well as the range of symptoms that are caused by changes in the PDS gene.

## Signs and symptoms

Although the symptoms of Pendred syndrome can vary among different individuals, the findings may include:

- sensorineural hearing loss that is usually congenital
- thyroid changes such as goiter, abnormal perchlorate discharge test results, and/or hypothyroidism
- inner ear changes, such as enlarged vestibular aqueduct (EVA) or Mondini malformation
- altered vestibular function that leads to balance problems

## Diagnosis

The diagnosis of Pendred syndrome is typically based upon the results from a variety of tests that measure hearing, thyroid appearance/function, inner ear structure, and balance. Sometimes the diagnosis is not made until a person with SNHL reaches adolescence or adulthood and develops thyroid problems such as goiter or hypothyroidism. These problems are usually detected by physical examination and blood tests, and thus help diagnose Pendred syndrome. Children who are born with SNHL often undergo special imaging tests such as CT or MRI scans. These may show inner ear changes that raise the question of possible changes in the PDS gene, even if the children do not have thyroid problems. In each of these situations, **genetic testing** may provide useful information that can confirm the diagnosis of Pendred syndrome.

Genetic research testing can be done for people with suspected or known Pendred syndrome by studying their **DNA**. The laboratory can check for the four common changes and some unique changes that have been found in the PDS gene. If this testing identifies an affected person's specific genetic changes, other people in the same family who are not affected can have their DNA examined as well. This can determine whether an unaffected person is a carrier for Pendred syndrome or not. In addition, testing could be done during a pregnancy if both of a baby's parents are carriers and have each had specific changes diagnosed in their DNA.

If genetic testing is done for people with known or suspected Pendred syndrome and the laboratory finds only one changed gene or no changes in the PDS gene, the diagnosis of Pendred syndrome cannot be confirmed. However, this does not rule out the possibility of Pendred syndrome. Sometimes this happens simply because the affected person has a very unique change in the PDS gene that the lab cannot clearly identify. Over time, further genetic research could potentially provide useful information about their specific genetic changes as knowledge about the PDS gene grows.

## Treatment and management

There is no known cure for Pendred syndrome. However, there are several ways to treat some of the symptoms.

### Treatment and management of SNHL

Regular visits with an audiologist (a hearing specialist) and an ENT (a physician specializing in the ear, nose, and throat) are important for people with Pendred syndrome. Hearing tests are necessary to check for changes in hearing ability, especially if people have milder forms of hearing loss and have some ability to hear. Among people with milder forms of hearing loss, hearing aids and speech therapy may be useful. However, people with profound SNHL and their families usually benefit from sign language training, which provides a good method of communication. Some people with severe to profound forms of hearing loss may also consider a procedure called cochlear implantation, in which a small electronic device is surgically placed behind the ear (underneath the skin) and is attached to a wire that stimulates the inner ear. This may allow people to hear useful sounds.

### Treatment and management of thyroid problems

Regular examinations by an endocrinologist (a physician specializing in the treatment of hormone problems) who is familiar with Pendred syndrome is important. People who develop goiter and/or hypothyroidism are sometimes treated with a medication called thyroxine, which is basically the hormone called T4. Other people with goiter have most of their thyroid surgically removed. However, this form of treatment is not a cure, and the remaining thyroid tissue can grow and redevelop into goiter again. Among some people, the goiter does not require treatment or it simply disappears on its own.

There are a number of support groups available that provide education, support and advice to help people cope with the symptoms of SNHL and thyroid problems that often occur among individuals with Pendred syndrome.

### Prognosis

Pendred syndrome does not cause a shortened life span for affected individuals. Those who develop hypothyroidism and do not seek treatment may experience a variety of health problems including low energy level, weight gain, constipation, and dry skin. However, hypothyroidism and goiter can usually be well managed with medication or surgery. The degree of hearing loss that occurs is typically severe to profound from an early age and usually changes very little over the years. Among affected people who develop SNHL during childhood (after learning to speak), the degree of hearing loss can worsen over time. Sign language training (and sometimes cochlear implants) allow alternative methods of communication and thus help people reach their full potential. Support groups for people with hearing loss often help individuals with SNHL (whether due to Pendred syndrome or other causes) maintain and/or improve their quality of life as well.

### Resources

#### BOOKS

Gorlin, R. J., H. V. Toriello, and M. M. Cohen. "Goiter and profound congenital sensorineural hearing loss (Pendred syndrome)." In *Hereditary Hearing Loss and Its Syndromes.* Oxford Monographs on Medical Genetics No. 28. New York and Oxford: Oxford University Press, 1995.

#### PERIODICALS

Reardon, William, et al. "Prevalence, age of onset, and natural history of thyroid disease in Pendred syndrome." *Journal of Medical Genetics* 36 (August 1999): 595–98.

Reardon, William, et al. "Enlarged vestibular aqueduct: a radiological marker of Pendred syndrome, and

mutation of the PDS gene." *Quarterly Journal of Medicine* 93, no. 2 (2000): 99–104.

Scott, Daryl A., et al. "Functional differences of the PDS gene product are associated with phenotypic variation in patients with Pendred syndrome and non-syndromic hearing loss (DFNB4)." *Human Molecular Genetics* 9, no. 11 (2000): 1709–15.

Scott, Daryl A., et al. "The Pendred syndrome gene encodes a chloride-iodide transport protein." *Nature Genetics* 21, no. 4 (April 1999): 440–43.

#### WEBSITES

Smith, Richard R. J., MD, and Guy Van Camp, PhD. "Pendred Syndrome DFNB4." *GeneReviews.* April 9, 2008 (December 11, 2009). University of Washington, Seattle. http://www.ncbi.nlm.nih.gov/bookshelf/br.fcgi?book = gene&part = pendred#pendred.

#### ORGANIZATIONS

American Society for Deaf Children. #2047, 800 Florida Ave. NE, Washington, DC 20002-3695. (800) 942-ASDC v/tty. http://www.deafchildren.org.

American Thyroid Association. 6066 Leesburg Pike, Suite 550, Falls Church, VA 22041. (703) 998-8890. http://www.thyroid.org.

Boys Town National Research Hospital. 555 N. 30th St., Omaha, NE 68131. (402) 498-6749. http://www.boystownhospital.org

National Association of the Deaf. 8630 Fenton St., Suite 820, Silver Spring, MD 20910-4500. (301) 587-1788. nadinfo @nad.org. http://www.nad.org.

National Institute on Deafness and Other Communication Disorders. 31 Center Dr., MSC 2320, Bethesda, MD 20814. http://www.nidcd.nih.gov.

Vestibular Disorders Association. PO Box 13305, Portland, OR 97213-0305. (800) 837-8428. http://www.vestibular.org.

Pamela J. Nutting, MS, CGC

Pepper syndrome *see* **Cohen syndrome**

Perinatal sudanophilic leukodystropy *see* **Pelizaeus-Merzbacher disease**

Peroutka sneeze *see* **Achoo syndrome**

# Pervasive developmental disorders

### Definition

The pervasive developmental disorders, or PDDs, are a group of childhood disorders that manifest during the first years of the child's life. They are marked by severe weaknesses in several areas of development: social interaction, communication, or the appearance of stereotyped behavior patterns and interests. The PDDs are also known as autistic spectrum disorders. As the phrase *spectrum disorder* suggests, persons with these disorders fall at different points along a fairly wide continuum of disabilities and associated disorders. As defined by DSM-IV, the pervasive developmental disorders include:

- autistic disorder
- Rett syndrome
- childhood disintegrative disorder (CDD)
- Asperger syndrome
- pervasive developmental disorder not otherwise specified (PDD-NOS)

### Description

The PDDs form a diagnostic category intended to identify children with delays in or deviant forms of social, linguistic, cognitive, and motor (muscular movement) development. The category covers children with a wide variety of developmental delays of differing severity in these four broad areas. The precise cause(s) of the PDDs are still obscure, but are assumed to be abnormalities of the central nervous system.

#### Autistic disorder

Autistic disorder, or **autism**, was first described in 1943. Autistic children are characterized by severe impairment in their interactions with others and delayed or abnormal patterns of communication; about 50% of autistic children do not speak at all. These abnormalities begin in the first weeks of life; it is not unusual for the parents of an autistic child to say that they "knew something was wrong" quite early in the child's development. Another characteristic symptom has been termed "insistence on sameness;" that is, these children may become extremely upset by trivial changes in their environment or daily routine—such as a new picture on the wall or taking a different route to the grocery store. Autistic children often make repetitive or stereotyped gestures or movements with their hands or bodies. Their behavioral symptoms may also include impulsivity, aggressiveness, temper tantrums, and self-biting or other forms of self-injury.

About 75% of children diagnosed with autism are also diagnosed with moderate mental retardation (IQ between 35 and 50). Their cognitive skills frequently develop unevenly, regardless of their general intelligence level. A minority of autistic children have IQs above 70; their condition is sometimes called high-functioning autism, or HFA. In addition to mental retardation, autism is frequently associated with other neurological or medical conditions, including encephalitis, **phenylketonuria**, tuberous sclerosis, **fragile X syndrome**, and underdeveloped reflexes. About 25% of autistic children develop seizure disorders, most often in adolescence.

#### Rett syndrome

Unlike autism, **Rett syndrome** has a very distinctive onset and course. The child develops normally during the first five months of life; after the fifth month, head growth slows down and the child loses whatever purposeful hand movements she had developed during the first five months. After 30 months, the child frequently develops repetitive hand-washing or hand-wringing gestures; over 50% of children with the disorder will develop seizure disorders. Rett syndrome is also associated with severe or profound mental retardation. This disorder is diagnosed only in females.

#### Childhood disintegrative disorder (Heller's syndrome)

Childhood disintegrative disorder, or CDD, was first described by an educator named Theodore Heller in 1908. He referred to it as *dementia infantilis*. Children with CDD have apparently normal development during the first two years of life. Between two and ten years of age, the child loses two or more previously acquired skills, including language skills, social skills, toileting, self-help skills, or motor skills. The child may also lose interest in his or her surroundings, and often comes to "look autistic." CDD has several different patterns of onset and development; it may develop rapidly (within weeks) or more slowly (over a period of months).

CDD is frequently associated with severe mental retardation. In addition, children with CDD have a higher risk of seizures. CDD is occasionally associated with general medical conditions (metachromatic **leukodystrophy** or Schilder's disease) that could account for the developmental losses, but in most cases there is no known medical cause of the child's symptoms.

### Asperger syndrome

**Asperger syndrome** (AS) was first identified in 1944 by a Viennese psychiatrist. It is sometimes called autistic psychopathy. AS is distinguished from autism by later onset of symptoms; these children usually develop normally for the first few years of life and retain relatively strong verbal and self-help skills. They are often physically clumsy or awkward, however, and this symptom may be noticed before the child starts school. AS is diagnosed most frequently when the child is between five and nine years of age. One of the distinctive features of Asperger syndrome is an abnormal degree of fascination or preoccupation with a limited or restricted subject of interest, such as railroad timetables, the weather, astronomical data, French verb forms, etc. In addition, the child's knowledge of the topic reflects rote memorization of facts rather than deep understanding.

Unlike autism, AS does not appear to be associated with a higher risk of seizure disorders or such general conditions as fragile X syndrome.

### Pervasive developmental disorder not otherwise specified

PDD-NOS is regarded as a "sub-threshold" category, which means that it covers cases in which the child has some impairment of social interaction and communication, or has some stereotyped patterns of behavior, but does not meet the full criteria for another PDD. PDD-NOS is sometimes referred to as atypical personality development, atypical autism, or atypical PDD. No diagnostic criteria specific to this category are provided in DSM-IV. Little research has been done on children diagnosed with PDD-NOS because the condition has no clear definition. The available data indicate that children placed in this category are diagnosed at later ages than children with autism, and are less likely to have mental impairment.

## Genetic profile

Of the PDDs, autism has the best-documented genetic component, although more research is required. It is known that the degree of similarity in a pair of twins with respect to autism is significantly higher in identical than in fraternal twins. The likelihood of the biological parents of an autistic child having another child with the disorder is thought to be about 1:20. It is possible that the actual rate is higher, since many parents of one autistic child decide against having more children.

The genetic profile of Asperger syndrome is less well known, although the disorder appears to run in families—most commonly families with histories of **depression** or **bipolar disorder**. Rett syndrome is known only from case studies, so data about its genetic profile is not available. The same lack of information is true also of CDD—partly because the disorder was first reported in 1966 and has only been officially recognized since 1994, and partly because the condition has been frequently misdiagnosed.

## Demographics

Autism is thought to affect between two and five children out of every 10,000. Childhood disintegrative disorder is much less frequent, perhaps only a tenth as common as autism. Rett syndrome is also very rare, and is known only from case series reported in the medical literature. The incidence of Asperger syndrome is not definitely known, but is thought to lie somewhere between 0.024% and 0.36% of the general population.

Some of the PDDs are considerably more common in boys than in girls. The male to female sex ratio in autism is variously given as 4:1 or 5:1. Less is known about the incidence of Asperger syndrome, but one study reported a male/female ratio of 4:1. Initial studies of CDD suggested an equal sex ratio, but more recent data indicate that the disorder is more common among males. Rett syndrome, on the other hand, has been reported only in females.

## Signs and symptoms

The signs and symptoms of each PDD are included in its description.

## Diagnosis

The differential diagnosis of autistic spectrum disorders is complicated by several factors. One is the wide variation in normal rates of children's development. In addition, because some of the symptoms of autism are present in mental retardation, it can be difficult to determine which condition is present in a specific child, or whether both conditions are present. A definitive diagnosis of autism is rarely given to children below the age of three years. Delays or abnormal patterns in cognitive and social development can be more accurately assessed in children age three or four; children with AS or PDD-NOS may not be diagnosed until age five or later. A third factor is the tangled history of differential diagnosis of childhood disorders. Autism was first described by a physician named Leo Kanner in 1943. For several decades after Kanner's initial observations, researchers assumed that there was an association or continuity between autism in children and **schizophrenia** in adults. In fact, the term *autism* was first used to describe the self-focused thinking that characterizes schizophrenia; it was only later that the word was applied to the severe impairment of social behaviors that is a major symptom of autistic disorder. It took years of further research to establish clear diagnostic distinctions between autism and schizophrenia. Furthermore, the early assumption of a connection between autism and schizophrenia led to the hypothesis that autism was caused by painful experiences in early childhood. It is now known that autism and the other PDDs are essentially neurological disturbances.

### Medical or laboratory testing

There are no brain imaging studies or laboratory tests that can be performed to diagnose a pervasive developmental disorder. The examiner may recommend a hearing test to rule out **deafness** as a possible cause of a child's failure to respond to the environment, or a brain scan to rule out other physical conditions.

### Diagnostic interviews

A PDD may be diagnosed by a pediatrician, pediatric neurologist, psychologist, or specialist in child psychiatry. The diagnosis is usually based on a combination of the child's medical and developmental history and clinical interviews or observations of the child. Children who cannot talk can be evaluated for their patterns of nonverbal communication with familiar as well as unfamiliar people. The parents may be asked to describe the child's use of eye contact, gestures, facial expressions, and body language. A clinical psychologist can administer special tests designed to evaluate the child's problem-solving abilities without the use of language.

### Diagnostic questionnaires and other tools

The examiner may use a diagnostic checklist or screener such as the Childhood Autism Rating Scale, or CARS, which was developed in 1993. In addition, the Autism Research Institute (ARI) distributes a Form E-2 questionnaire that can be completed by the parents of a child with a PDD and returned to ARI. Form E-2 is not a diagnostic instrument as such but a checklist that assists ARI in the compilation of a database of symptoms and behaviors associated with autistic spectrum disorders. Parents who complete the form will receive a brief report about their child. Researchers expect that the database will help to improve the accuracy of differential diagnosis as well as contribute to more effective treatments for children with PDDs.

## Treatment and management

The treatment and management of children with PDDs varies considerably according to the severity of the child's impairment and the specific areas of impairment.

### Medications

There are no medications that can cure any of the PDDs, and no single medication that is recommended for the symptoms of all children with PDDs. In addition, there are few comparative medication studies of children with autistic spectrum disorders. The five sites (UCLA, University of Indiana, Ohio State, Yale, and the Kennedy-Krieger Institute) involved in the Research Units in Pediatric Psychopharmacology (RUPP) Program are currently conducting a study of respiridone in PDD children with behavioral problems. The RUPP sites are also testing medications approved for use in adults with self-injuring behaviors, anxiety, aggressive behavior, and obsessive-compulsive disorder on children with PDDs. This research is expected to improve the available treatments for children with these disorders.

### Psychotherapy

The only PDD patients who benefit from individual psychotherapy are persons with AS or with HFA who are intelligent enough to have some insight into their condition. Typically, they become depressed in adolescence or adult life when they recognize the nature and extent of their social disabiliities.

### Educational considerations

Most children with AS and some children with high-functioning autism are educable. Many people with AS, in fact, successfully complete graduate or professional school. Only a small percentage of autistic children, however, complete enough schooling to be able to live independently as adults. Children with CDD must be placed in schools for the severely disabled.

### Employment

Most children with AS can finish school and enter the job market. They do best in occupations that have regular routines or allow them to work in isolation. Only a few high-functioning autistic children are potentially employable.

## Prognosis

The PDDs as a group are lifelong disorders, but the prognoses vary according to the child's degree of impairment. As a general rule, language skills and the child's overall IQ are the most important factors in the prognosis. Children with AS have the most favorable educational prognosis but usually retain some degree of social impairment even as adults. Of autistic children, only about one-third achieve partial or complete independence in adult life. The prognoses for Rett syndrome and CDD are worse than that for autism, as the skill levels of these children often continue to deteriorate. Some, however, make very modest developmental gains in adolescence. Lastly, current information about the prognoses of children with PDDs is derived from treatments given to patients in the 1970s or 1980s. As knowledge of effective treatments for PDDs continues to accumulate, children with these disorders receive treatment earlier than they did two decades ago. It is likely that future prognoses for the PDDs will reflect these improvements.

## Resources

### BOOKS

Psychiatric Association Staff. *Diagnostic and Statistical Manual of Mental Disorders.* 4th ed, revised. Washington, DC: American Psychiatric Association, 2000.

"Psychiatric Conditions in Childhood and Adolescence." In *The Merck Manual of Diagnosis and Therapy.* Edited by Mark H. Beers, MD, and Robert Berkow, MD. Whitehouse Station, NJ: Merck Research Laboratories, 1999.

Thoene, Jess G., ed. *Physicians' Guide to Rare Diseases.* Montvale, NJ: Dowden Publishing Company, 1995.

Waltz, Mitzi. *Pervasive Developmental Disorders: Finding a Diagnosis and Getting Help.* New York: O'Reilly & Associates, Inc., 1999.

### PERIODICALS

Autism Research Institute. *Autism Research Review International.* San Diego, CA: 1987.

---

## QUESTIONS TO ASK YOUR DOCTOR

- What does the phrase "pervasive developmental disorders" mean?
- At what stage of a person's life do pervasive developmental disorders typically manifest?
- Are there medications or other types of treatments that can be used with pervasive developmental disorders?
- Are there organizations that can provide parents with additional information about any one or more of the most common pervasive developmental disorders?

---

### WEBSITES

Center for the Study of Autism Home Page, maintained by Stephen Edelson, PhD. http://www.autism.org.

Yale Child Study Center. http://info.med.Yale.edu/chldstdy/autism.

### ORGANIZATIONS

Autism Research Institute. 4182 Adams Ave., San Diego, 92116. http://autisim.com.

National Organization for Rare Disorders (NORD). 55 Kenosia Ave., PO Box 1968, Danbury, CT 06813. (203) 744-0100 or (800) 999-6673. Fax: (203) 746-6481. http://www.rarediseases.org.

Yale-LDA Social Learning Disabilities Project. Yale Child Study Center, 230 South Frontage Road, New Haven, CT 06520-7900. (203) 785-3420. http://childstudycenter.yale.edu/autisim.

Rebecca J. Frey, PhD

---

# Peutz-Jeghers syndrome

## Definition

Peutz-Jeghers syndrome (PJS) is named after two doctors who first studied and described it in 1921. It is an association of three very specific conditions in any one person. The first condition is the appearance of freckles on parts of the body where freckles are not normally found. The second condition is the presence of multiple gastrointestinal polyps. The third condition is a risk, greater than the risk seen in the general population, of developing certain kinds of cancers.

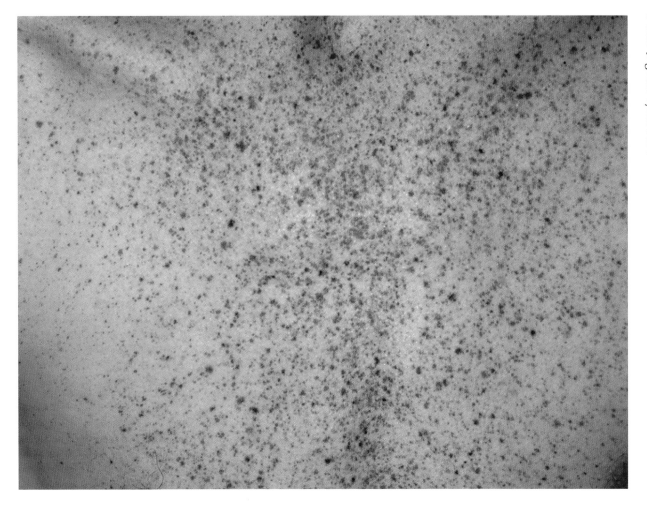

**The chest of a person afflicted with Peutz-Jeghers syndrome.** *(Custom Medical Stock Photo, Inc. Reproduced by permission.)*

## Description

The freckles associated with PJS are dark brown, dark blue, or greenish black. In almost all people with PJS, these freckles are present at birth on the lining of the cheeks inside the mouth. By the time most children reach one or two years old, freckles develop around the lips, nostrils, eyes, anus, and genitals. This is in contrast to ordinary freckles, which are absent at birth and rarely develop in these locations. The freckles seen in PJS are sometimes called macules (discolored spot or patch on the skin of various colors, sizes, and shapes), or areas of hyperpigmentation (increased pigmentation of the skin).

Some people with PJS also have these freckles on the palms of their hands or feet or on their fingertips. Freckles may merge together. The freckles on the skin often fade or disappear by adolescence, but the freckles inside the mouth generally remain throughout the person's life.

Gastrointestinal polyps can develop in children as young as one or two years old. The age at which polyps appear and the number of polyps vary widely from patient to patient. The polyps can occur in infants and cause spasms and pain in the abdomen. On average, polyps appear by the time a child with PJS is 10 years old. There may be anywhere from dozens to hundreds of polyps throughout the gastrointestinal tract. For this reason, PJS is sometimes called polyposis, which means "too many polyps." Most PJS polyps occur in the small intestine, but they can also develop in the esophagus, stomach, and colon. In some people with PJS, polyps have been found in the mouth or nose.

The polyps seen in PJS have a unique structure. They consist of overgrowths of normal tissue that smooth muscle bands of the stomach and instestines run through. This kind of overgrowth is called a hamartoma. Consequently, PJS is sometimes called hamartomatous intestinal polyposis. A hamartoma is a non-cancerous tumor, and hamartomatous polyps are

## KEY TERMS

**Biopsy**—The surgical removal and microscopic examination of living tissue for diagnostic purposes.

**Colon**—The large intestine.

**Colonoscopy**—Procedure for viewing the large intestine (colon) by inserting an illuminated tube into the rectum and guiding it up the large intestine.

**Endoscopy**—A slender, tubular optical instrument used as a viewing system for examining an inner part of the body and, with an attached instrument, for biopsy or surgery.

**Enteroscopy**—A procedure used to examine the small intestine.

**Esophagus**—The part of the digestive tract that connects the mouth and stomach; the food pipe.

**Gastrointestinal**—Concerning the stomach and intestine.

**Hamartoma.**—An overgrowth of normal tissue.

**Hyperpigmentation.**—An abnormal condition characterized by an excess of melanin in localized areas of the skin, which produces areas that are much darker than the surrounding unaffected skin.

**Laparoscopy**—A diagnostic procedure in which a small incision is made in the abdomen and a slender, hollow, lighted instrument is passed through it. The doctor can view the ovaries more closely through the laparoscope, and if necessary, obtain tissue samples for biopsy.

**Macule**—A flat, discolored spot or patch on the skin.

**Mammogram**—A procedure in which both breasts are compressed/flattened and exposed to low doses of x rays, in an attempt to visualize the inner breast tissue.

**Polyp**—A mass of tissue bulging out from the normal surface of a mucous membrane.

**Polypectomy**—Surgical removal of polyps.

**Tumor suppressor gene**—Genes involved in controlling normal cell growth and preventing cancer.

not cancerous. However, they can take up too much space, causing obstruction, pain, and even bleeding. They can also become cancerous, or malignant, if a genetic change results in uncontrolled cell growth.

It is this potential for malignant change that increases **cancer** risk in people with PJS. As might be expected, the gastrointestinal tract is the most common site for cancer in people with PJS. The small intestine, stomach, gallbladder, pancreas, colon, and rectum are all susceptible. However, cancer can also occur outside the gastrointestinal tract. When this happens, the sites most likely to be involved are the breasts, ovaries, uterus, cervix, or testicles.

PJS does not affect intelligence or behavior.

### Genetic profile

Researchers have identified the **gene** responsible for about seven out of ten PJS cases. The gene is named STK11, and it is located at the 19p13 site on **chromosome** 19. In some older studies, the same gene is referred to as LKB1. Researchers have connected more than 50 different STK11 mutations to cases of PJS.

However, some cases do not appear to be connected to STK11. As a result, PJS qualifies as a genetically heterogeneous condition; this means that it has more than one known genetic cause. Research continues in order to locate the genes involved in the three out of ten cases not related to STK11.

When linked to STK11, PJS is an autosomal dominant disorder. This means that the condition occurs even when an individual inherits only one abnormal copy of STK11 from either parent. In some people with PJS, the condition is limited to freckles on the lining of the cheeks inside the mouth. Many of these people also have gastrointestinal polyps. One abnormal copy of STK11 also increases a person's risk of developing the kinds of cancer associated with PJS.

Since only one abnormal copy of STK11 is needed to cause PJS, most people with the condition still have one normal copy of the gene. One normal copy is usually enough to protect against the kinds of cancer associated with PJS. This is because STK11 is a tumor suppressor gene. A properly working tumor suppressor gene makes a product that controls cell growth. Since cancer is the result of uncontrolled cell growth, tumor suppressors prevent cancer. Even one working copy of STK11 protects against cancer.

The reason people with PJS have an increased risk of developing cancer is that one STK11 gene is already abnormal at birth. If damage to the normal STK11 gene occurs later, the ability to control cell growth is lost, leading to the kinds of cancers associated with PJS.

Damage to normal genes can occur in anyone. However, it generally takes less time to damage one gene than two genes. Therefore, people with PJS are likely to develop cancer at earlier ages than are people born with two normal STK11 genes.

About half of all PJS cases occur because a child inherits a changed gene from a parent with PJS. The other half are due to a mutation in the cell from which the child develops. A person born with one abnormal gene can pass that gene on to the next generation. One out of two of this person's children will inherit the gene. In addition, if PJS is inherited, each parent or sibling of the affected person has a one out of two chance of carrying the gene.

## Demographics

PJS occurs in about one out of 25,000 people. It affects males and females of all races and ethnic groups. The particular genetic mutation may differ among groups and even among families within a group.

## Signs and symptoms

The first sign of PJS, freckling inside the mouth or in unusual places, generally appears in infants. Polyps usually begin causing symptoms by age 10. Polyps make themselves known in a variety of ways. They can cause abdominal pain or intestinal bleeding. Sometimes the blood loss leads to anemia (a condition where there is a reduction in circulating red blood cells, the amount of hemoglobin, or the volume of packed red cells). Polyps sometimes protrude outside the rectum or obstruct the gastrointestinal tract. Untreated obstructions can be fatal.

Tumors may appear in childhood. Children as young as six may develop a particular kind of ovarian or testicular tumor that causes early puberty. Affected boys sometimes begin to develop breasts. These tumors can be non-cancerous, but they have the potential to become malignant.

A few patients develop malignant tumors in the first decade of life. Other patients have stomach, breast, or cervical cancer before age 30. The specific form of cervical cancer is extremely rare in the general population.

## Diagnosis

Because the peculiar freckling seen in PJS is present so early, doctors familiar with the condition may suspect PJS even before other symptoms occur. This is ideal, since early diagnosis greatly improves the prognosis.

Many children or young adults come to medical attention due to the pain, bleeding, or anemia caused by polyps. Doctors can confirm the presence of multiple polyps using a variety of methods. Noninvasive methods include ultrasound and x ray techniques. Invasive methods use a tube and an optical system to conduct an internal inspection of the gastrointestinal tract. These methods include endoscopy, enteroscopy, and colonoscopy, all of which involve entry to the gastrointestinal tract through an existing body orifice. Laparoscopy is another invasive method; it involves entering the gastrointestinal tract through an incision in the abdomen. All invasive methods allow for removal of polyps found during the exam. Once the polyps are removed and examined, their unique structure and large number lead to diagnosis of PJS. The average age at PJS diagnosis is 17.

Freckles and polyps occur in more than 95% of people with PJS. Sometimes, though, the freckles fade before symptoms of polyps appear. It is important to take a medical history in order to determine if freckles were present on the skin earlier in life. The doctor should also examine the lining of the cheeks inside the mouth, where freckles are likely to remain throughout life.

The number and intensity of the freckles do not predict the severity of gastrointestinal symptoms or the risk of developing cancer. Any patient diagnosed with PJS needs regular cancer screening.

The presence of the rare cervical cancer, ovarian tumor, or testicular tumor associated with PJS leads to diagnosis in some patients.

A family history of PJS is suspicious but not required for diagnosis, since PJS can occur as a new mutation. Once PJS has occurred in a family, parents, siblings, and children of the affected person should seek medical attention.

**Genetic testing** is available to confirm clinical diagnosis or to determine if a person carries an abnormal STK11 gene. Using a swab, cells are removed from the lining of the cheeks inside the mouth. **DNA** is extracted and analyzed. The test confirms PJS if analysis reveals an STK11 mutation. However, the test cannot rule out PJS if an STK11 mutation is not found, since some cases are due to other genetic causes.

Prenatal diagnosis of PJS is possible only if the family's specific STK11 mutation has previously been identified. Prenatal testing is done by **amniocentesis** or chorionic villus sampling. Amniocentesis involves removal of a small amount of amniotic fluid from the uterus. Chorionic villus sampling involves removal of a small sample of placental tissue. In either case, DNA is extracted from sample cells and analyzed.

Even without genetic testing, diagnosis of PJS is fairly straightforward. Although several other conditions cause multiple intestinal polyps or hyperpigmentation, the distinctive structure of PJS polyps and the unusual location of PJS freckles eliminate other conditions from consideration.

## Treatment and management

For people with a family history of PJS, treatment and management of the condition may begin even before diagnosis. If PJS freckles do not appear at birth and if there are no symptoms of polyps, affected families may desire genetic testing for their children.

For most genetic conditions, testing is delayed until children are old enough to understand the disease, its consequences, and the advantages and disadvantages of genetic screening. However, since PJS can affect children under the age of 10, any delay could be risky. Therefore, it is appropriate for families with PJS to consider genetic testing for their children. Children who do carry an STK11 mutation can begin a preventive care program immediately, and children who do not carry an STK11 mutation can avoid unnecessary intervention.

The decision to seek genetic testing requires careful consideration. A positive test for PJS cannot predict the precise age of onset, symptoms, severity, or progress of the condition. A genetic counselor can assist interested family members as they confront the medical, social, personal, and economic issues involved in genetic testing.

Parents, siblings, and children of people with STK11 mutations may not wish to undergo genetic testing. In this case, they should have a thorough clinical exam to confirm or rule out PJS. The exam includes a careful inspection for freckles. In addition, people age 10 or older require gastrointestinal screening, abdominal ultrasound, and a blood test for anemia. Males over age 10 should have a testicular exam. Females should have a pelvic exam and ultrasound, pap smear, and breast exam annually, by age 20. Women age 35 or older should have a mammogram.

For people with no family history of PJS, treatment and management usually begin when PJS is diagnosed.

In past generations, polyp complications such as intestinal obstruction or hemorrhage were a frequent cause of death in PJS patients. However, treatment of polyps is now widely available. The doctor performs a polypectomy to remove the polyps. Polypectomy may be done at the same time as endoscopy, enteroscopy, colonoscopy, or laparoscopy. Anesthesia is used to make the patient more comfortable.

To manage polyps and screen for early signs of cancer, all people who have PJS and are age 10 or older need preventive screening on a regular basis. Gastrointestinal screening is the first test, and polypectomy is performed at the same time. Also at age 10, the person begins an annual screening program that includes a blood test for anemia and a testicular exam for boys.

After age 10, gastrointestinal screening with polypectomy is performed every two years.

By age 20, annual screening is expanded to include an abdominal ultrasound for both males and females, as well as a pelvic exam and ultrasound, pap smear, and breast exam for females.

By age 35, a woman with PJS should have her first mammogram; mammograms should be repeated every two years until the woman is 50. At that time, a mammogram should be added to the annual screening program.

Polyps found during preventive screening are immediately treated by polypectomy. Preventive screening may also reveal suspicious growths in the gastrointestinal tract or outside of it. These growths require urgent medical attention, since they may be precancerous or cancerous. Diagnosis may require additional tests or biopsy. Treatment is determined on an individual basis, depending on the patient's medical condition and the nature of the growth.

Some people with PJS do not care for the appearance of their freckles. Removal of freckles using laser therapy is an available treatment option.

Many people with PJS find the preventive screening program psychologically exhausting, and young children can find it frightening. These individuals often need the ongoing support and understanding of friends, family, and community. Several organizations composed of people with PJS, their family members, and medical professionals offer additional support and information. There is also an on-line support group dedicated to PJS.

People with PJS may find it helpful to consult a genetic counselor. Genetic counselors can provide up-to-date information about PJS research, therapy, and management.

## Prognosis

Early detection of PJS is the key to its prognosis. Polyps cause less pain and fewer complications when found and removed early. In addition, the patient can begin a preventive screening program at an early age. This increases the likelihood of finding suspicious growths before they become malignant.

Unless they undergo regular screening, people with PJS have a one in two chance of dying from cancer before the age of 60. Moreover, the average age of cancer death in unscreened people with PJS is 39.

Researchers are actively investigating cancer screening, prevention, and treatment methods. In the meantime, regular preventive screening may reduce the illness and premature death associated with PJS.

## Resources

### BOOKS

Rimoin, David L., et al., eds. *Emery and Rimoin's Principles and Practice of Medical Genetics.* Third Edition. New York: Churchill Livingstone, 1996.

Sybert, Virginia P. *Genetic Skin Disorders.* New York: Oxford University Press, 1997.

### PERIODICALS

Boardman, Lisa A., et al. "Genetic Heterogeneity in Peutz-Jeghers syndrome." *Human Mutation* 16, no. 1 (2000): 23-30.

Hemminki, Akseli. "The molecular basis and clinical aspects of Peutz-Jeghers syndrome." *Cellular and Molecular Life Sciences* 55 (2000): 735-750.

Westerman, Anne Marie, et al. "Peutz-Jeghers syndrome: 78-year follow-up of the original family." *The Lancet* 353 (April 1999): 1211-1215.

### WEBSITES

*Association of Cancer Online Resources.* http://www.acor.org.

*National Cancer Institute.* http://www.cancer.gov.

*GeneTests.* http://www.ncbi.nlm.nih.gov/sites/GeneTests/ ?db = GeneTests.

*Network for Peutz-Jeghers and Juvenile Polyposis Syndrome.* http://www.cge.mdanderson.org/npjs.

OMIM: Online Mendelian Inheritance in Man. http://www. ncbi.nlm.nih.gov/omim

### ORGANIZATIONS

Genetic Alliance. 4301 Connecticut Ave. NW, #404, Washington, DC 20008-2304. (800) 336-GENE (Helpline) or (202) 966-5557. Fax: (888) 394-3937 info@geneticalliance. http://www.geneticalliance.org.

IMPACC (Intestinal Multiple Polyposis and Colorectal Cancer). PO Box 11, Conyngham, PA 18219. (570) 788-1818.

International Peutz-Jeghers Support Group. Johns Hopkins Hospital, Blalock 1008, 600 North Wolfe St., Baltimore, MD 21287-4922.

Avis L. Gibons

# Pfeiffer syndrome

## Definition

Pfeiffer syndrome is one of a group of disorders defined by premature closure of the sutures of the skull, resulting in an abnormal skull shape. People affected with these conditions, known as **craniosynostosis** syndromes, may also have differences in facial structure and hand and foot abnormalities. The defining features of Pfeiffer syndrome are abnormalities of the hands, feet, and shape of the skull.

## Description

Pfeiffer syndrome is a complex disorder. Three subtypes of Pfeiffer have been defined based on symptoms. The syndrome is caused by a mutation (alteration) in either of two different genes. As the genes that cause craniosynostosis syndromes were discovered throughout the 1990s, scientists realized that these syndromes have overlapping underlying causes. Crouzon, Apert, Jackson-Weiss, and other syndromes are related to Pfeiffer syndrome by genetic causation as well as associated symptoms. Noack syndrome, once thought to be a separate condition, is now known to be the same as Pfeiffer syndrome. Acrocephalosyndactyly, Type V (ACS5) and Noack syndrome both refer to Pfeiffer syndrome.

## Genetic profile

Pfeiffer syndrome is an autosomal dominant condition. Every person has two copies of every **gene**, one maternally inherited and one paternally inherited. Autosomal dominant conditions occur if a person has a change in one member of a gene pair. The chance for an affected individual to have an affected child is 50% with each pregnancy.

A person who has an autosomal dominant condition may have it because he or she inherited the altered gene from an affected parent or because of a new mutation. A new mutation occurs when the gene is altered for the first time in that individual. A person with an autosomal dominant condition due to a new mutation is the first person in his or her family to be affected.

Nearly all of the individuals with Pfeiffer syndrome types 2 and 3 described in the medical literature have new mutations. When a person has a new mutation, his or her parents are usually not at risk to have another child with the condition. The milder form, Pfeiffer syndrome type 1, is more likely to be inherited. When the mutation is inherited, the child's symptoms are often similar to those of the affected parent. Pfeiffer syndrome is fully penetrant. This means that all of the individuals who have the mutated gene associated with the condition are expected to have symptoms. In other words, the mutant gene is always expressed.

The two genes that cause Pfeiffer syndrome are called FGFR1 and FGFR2. FGFR1 is on **chromosome** 8. FGFR2 is on chromosome 11. These genes are members of a group of genes called the fibroblast growth factor receptors.

Fibroblasts play an important role in the development of connective tissue (e.g. skin and bone). Fibroblast growth factors (FGFs) stimulate certain cells to divide, differentiate (specialize to perform a specific function different than the function of the original cell), and migrate. FGFs are important in limb development, wound healing and repair, and other biological processes. FGFs communicate with targeted cells through the action of the fibroblast growth factor receptors. Fibroblast growth factor receptors (FGFRs) on the targeted cells bind the FGFs and relay their message within the cell.

In 1999, 11 conditions were known to be caused by mutations in three of the four FGFR genes. However, only one condition is present in each affected family. Mutations in FGFR2 may cause Pfeiffer syndrome as well as Apert, Jackson-Weiss, and Crouzon syndromes. Nonetheless, a parent with Pfeiffer syndrome is at risk to have a child with Pfeiffer but is not at risk to have a child with Crouzon, Apert, or Jackson-Weiss syndromes. Because family members in multiple generations all have the same condition, the condition is said to "breed true" within families. A few exceptions—families with more than one FGFR-associated condition—are reported in the medical literature.

A given genetic condition may be associated with mutations in one particular gene, and mutations in a given gene may cause only one genetic condition. Alternatively, mutations in a gene may be associated with more than one genetic condition, and a particular genetic condition may be caused by any mutation in a number of multiple genes. FGFR2 causing both Pfeiffer and Apert syndromes is an example of the former; FGFR1 and FGFR2 causing Pfeiffer syndrome is an example of the latter. Various mutations of a particular gene are called alleles. Sometimes a gene causes different genetic conditions because each allele leads to a specific set of symptoms.

The exact same mutation in the FGFR2 gene may cause Pfeiffer syndrome in one family and cause a different craniosynostosis syndrome in another family. However, each family continues to have the same symptoms (the conditions breed true in each family). Differing effects of genes are sometimes explained by differing environmental influences and by differing interactions with other genes. However, the diverse effects of the FGFR2 gene probably have a more specific explanation/mechanism. The underlying reasons for these phenomena may be explained when fibroblast growth factors and their receptors are better understood. At that time, criteria defining various craniosynostosis syndromes (e.g. Pfeiffer, Crouzon, and Jackson-Weiss) may be re-examined and revised.

### Demographics

The incidence of Pfeiffer syndrome is approximately one in 100,000. The incidence of craniosynostosis is one in 2,000 to one in 2,500, which includes syndromic and non-syndromic cases. In non-syndromic cases, the craniosynostosis is an isolated finding; no other abnormalities are present. Non-syndromic craniosynostosis is much more common than syndromic craniosynostosis. Usually isolated craniosynostosis is sporadic (not familial).

### Signs and symptoms

Individuals with Pfeiffer syndrome have a high forehead, a tower shaped skull, and broad, deviated thumbs and great toes. The symptoms of type 1 are milder than those of types 2 and 3. Undergrowth of the midface leads to down-slanting, low-placed, widely spaced eyes; a small upper jaw bone; and a low nasal bridge. The larynx (voice organ below the base of the tongue) and the pharynx (tube that connects the larynx to the lungs) may be abnormal. Additional symptoms include a projecting chin, divergent visual axes, abnormalities of the passage between the nose and the pharynx, and hearing loss. Fingers and toes may be short and/or partially grown together. The palate may be especially high, and teeth may be crowded. In type 2, the elbow joint is frozen in place.

The skull is composed of many bones that fuse when the brain has finished growing. If the bones of the skull fuse prematurely (craniosynostosis), the skull continues to grow in an abnormal pattern. The places where the bones of the skull fuse are called sutures.

The suture that fuses prematurely in Pfeiffer syndrome is the coronal suture. This suture separates the frontal bone of the skull from the two middle bones (called the parietal bones). When the coronal suture closes prematurely, upward growth of the skull is increased and growth toward the front and back is decreased. Sometimes the sagittal suture will also be fused prematurely in individuals with Pfeiffer syndrome. This suture separates the right and left sides of the middle of the skull. If both the coronal and sagittal sutures fuse prematurely, the skull develops a somewhat cloverleaf shape. Individuals with Pfeiffer type 2 have cloverleaf skulls more often than individuals with types 1 and 3.

The coronal suture is also fused prematurely in Crouzon, Jackson-Weiss, Apert, and Beare-Stevenson syndromes. The thumbs and big toes are normal in Beare-Stevenson and Crouzon syndromes. Additional associated abnormalities distinguish Apert and Jackson-Weiss syndromes.

Serious complications of Pfeiffer syndrome include respiratory problems and **hydrocephalus**. Hydrocephalus is excessive fluid in the brain, which leads to mental impairment if untreated. Breathing problems may be caused by trachea abnormalities or be related to undergrowth of the midface. Some individuals may require an incision in the trachea (tracheostomy). Serious complications are more common in Pfeiffer types 2 and 3. Individuals with types 2 and 3 are severely affected, and often do not survive past infancy. Death may result from severe brain abnormalities, breathing problems, prematurity, and surgical complications. Even without accompanying hydrocephalus, developmental delays and mental retardation are common (in types 2 and 3). Lower displacement of the eyes may be so severe that the infant is unable to close his or her eyelids. Individuals with types 2 and 3 may also have seizures. Intellect is usually normal in Pfeiffer type 1.

## Diagnosis

The diagnosis of Pfeiffer syndrome is based primarily on clinical findings (symptoms). Although **genetic testing** is available, the diagnosis is usually made based on physical examination and radiological testing.

Often the doctor can determine which cranial suture closed prematurely by physical examination. For confirmation, an x ray or computerized tomography (CT) scan of the head may be performed. Determining which suture is involved is crucial in making the correct craniosynostosis diagnosis.

Craniosynostosis may be caused by an underlying genetic abnormality, or it may be due to other, nongenetic factors. In Pfeiffer syndrome, the tissue itself is abnormal and causes the suture to fuse prematurely. The doctor will consider nongenetic causes of craniosynostosis. These secondary causes include external forces such as abnormal head positioning (in the uterus or in infancy) and a small brain.

Genetic testing may be useful for prenatal diagnosis, confirmation of the diagnosis, and to provide information to other family members. Mutations are not detected in all individuals with Pfeiffer syndrome. Approximately one-third of affected individuals with Pfeiffer syndrome do not have an identifiable mutation in the FGFR1 or FGFR2 gene. People with Pfeiffer syndrome due to a mutation in the FGFR1 gene may have less severe abnormalities than people who have Pfeiffer due to mutations in the FGFR2 gene.

Prenatal diagnosis is available by chorionic villus sampling (CVS) or **amniocentesis** if a mutation has been identified in the affected parent. Amniocentesis is performed after the fifteenth week of pregnancy and CVS is usually performed in the tenth and twelfth weeks of pregnancy.

Craniosynostosis may be visible by fetal ultrasound. Conditions caused by mutations in the FGFR genes account for only a small portion of craniosynostosis. Assuming that the fetus does not have a family history of one of these conditions, genetic testing for the FGFR genes is unlikely to provide useful additional information.

## Treatment and management

Children with Pfeiffer syndrome usually see a team of medical specialists at regular intervals. This team typically includes plastic surgeons, neurosurgeons, orthopedists, ear, nose and throat doctors (otolaryngologists), dentists, and other specialists. The affected person may see the specialists all at once in a craniofacial clinic at a hospital. Many physical problems must be addressed.

## QUESTIONS TO ASK YOUR DOCTOR

- Please describe the process that occurs during craniosynostosis.
- Why is Pfeiffer syndrome regarded as a genetic disorder?
- How are the major symptoms of Pfeiffer syndrome treated?
- What organizations are available for support and guidance for families dealing with Pfeiffer syndrome?

Developmental, psychosocial, and financial issues are additional concerns. Treatment is aimed at the symptoms, not the underlying cause. Even if craniosynostosis is discovered prenatally, only the symptoms can be treated.

Multiple surgeries are usually performed to progressively correct the craniosynostosis and to normalize facial appearance. A team of surgeons is often involved, including a neurosurgeon and a specialized plastic surgeon. The timing and order of surgeries vary. Patients with syndromic craniosynostosis often require surgery earlier than patients with nonsyndromic craniosynostosis. The first surgery is usually performed early in the first year of life, even in the first few months.

Additional surgeries may be performed for other physical problems. Limb abnormalities often are not correctable. If the limb malformations do not lead to a loss of function, surgery is usually not required. Fixation of the elbow joints may be partially corrected, or at least altered to enable better functioning.

Hydrocephalus, airway obstruction, hearing loss, incomplete eyelid closure, and spine abnormalities require immediate medical attention.

### Prognosis

The prognosis for an individual is based on the symptoms he or she has. Individuals with Pfeiffer syndrome type 1 have a better prognosis than individuals with types 2 or 3. But the designation of type is based on that person's symptoms.

Although people with Pfeiffer syndrome may not obtain a completely normal appearance, significant improvement is possible. Timing the surgeries correctly is an important factor in whether they are successful and whether repeat surgeries are required.

Although Pfeiffer syndrome is rare, craniosynostosis is relatively common. Multiple agencies and organizations exist to help families face the challenges of having a child with craniosynostosis and facial differences. The identification of the FGFR genes that cause Pfeiffer (and other) craniosynostosis syndromes has promoted research into the underlying process that causes Pfeiffer syndrome. It will be another enormous challenge to go from understanding the process to treating the process. When the process that causes Pfeiffer and related conditions is better understood, a much clearer knowledge of human development in general will also be established.

### Resources

#### BOOKS

Lansdown, Richard. *Children in the Hospital, A Guide for Family and Care Givers.* New York: Oxford University Press, Inc., 1996.

#### PERIODICALS

Marino, Dan. "A New Face for Nicole." *Parents* (July 2000): 77–80.
McIntyre, Floyd L. "Craniosynostosis." *American Family Physician* (March 1997): 1173–77.

#### WEBSITES

*Craniofacial Anomalies.* Fact Sheet. Pediatric Surgery, Columbia University. http://cpmcnet.columbia.edu/dept/nsg/PNS/Craniofacial.html.
*Pfeiffer Syndrome Fact Sheet.* FACES. http://www.faces-cranio.org/.

#### OTHER

*Our child was just diagnosed with Craniosynostosis—What do we do now?* Fact sheet. Craniosynostosis and Parents Support, Inc. http://www.caps2000.org.
*My child looks different: a guide for parents.* Booklet. Changing Faces. http://www.cfaces.demon.co.uk/resources.html.
*Exploring faces through fiction.* Booklet. Changing Faces. http://www.cfaces.demon.co.uk/resources.html.

#### ORGANIZATIONS

AboutFace International. 123 Edwards St., Suite 1003, Toronto, ONT M5G 1E2. Canada (800) 665-FACE. info@aboutfaceinternational.org. http://www.aboutfaceinternational.org.
Children's Craniofacial Association. 13140 CoitRD, Suite517, Dallas, TX 75240. (972) 994-9902 or (800) 535-3643. contactcca@ccakids.com. http://www.ccakids.com.
Cleft Palate Foundation. 1504 E. Franklin St., Suite 102 Chapel Hill, NC 27514. (919) 993-9044. Fax: (919) 933-9604. http://www.cleftline.org.
FACES: The National Craniofacial Association. PO Box 11082, Chattanooga, TN 37401. (423) 266-1632 or (800) 332-2373. faces@faces-cranio.org. http://www.faces-cranio.org/.

Headlines: the Craniofacial Support Group. http://www. headlines.org.uk.

Let's Face It. University of Michigan, School of Dentistry, 1011 N. University, Ann Arbor, MI 48109. http://desica. dent.umich.edu/faceit.

World Craniofacial Foundation. PO Box 515838, 7777 Forest Lane, Ste C-621, Dallas, TX 75251-5838. (972) 566-6669 or (800) 533-3315. worldcf@worldnet.att.net. http://www.worldcf.org.

Michelle Queneau Bosworth, MS, CGC

# Pharmacogenetics

## Definition

Pharmacogenetics is one of the newest subspecialties of **genetics** that deals with the relationship between inherited genes and the ability of the body to metabolize drugs.

## Description

Medicine today relies on the use of therapeutic drugs to treat disease, but one of the longstanding problems has been the documented variation in patient response to drug therapy. The "recommended" dosage is usually established at a level shown to be effective in 50% of a test population, and based on the patient's initial response, the dosage may be increased, decreased, or discontinued. In rare situations, the patient may experience an adverse reaction to the drug and be shown to have a pharmacogenetic disorder. The unique feature of this group of diseases is that the problem does not occur until after the drug is given, so a person may have a pharmacogenetic defect and never know it if the specific drug required to trigger the reaction is never administered.

### Adverse reactions

Consider the case of a 35-year-old male who is scheduled for surgical repair of a hernia. The patient is otherwise in excellent health and has no family history of any serious medical problems. After entering the operating theater, an inhalation anesthetic and/or muscle relaxant is administered to render the patient unconscious. Unexpectedly, there is a significant increase in body temperature, and the patient experiences sustained muscle contraction. If this condition is not reversed promptly, it can lead to death. Anesthesiologists are now very familiar with this type of reaction. It occurs only rarely, but it uniquely identifies the patient as having **malignant hyperthermia**, a rare autosomal dominant disorder that affects the body's ability to respond normally to anesthetics. Once diagnosed with malignant hyperthermia, it is quite easy to avoid future episodes by simply using a different type of anesthetic when surgery is necessary, but it often takes one negative, and potentially life-threatening, experience to know the condition exists.

An incident that occurred in the 1950s further shows the diversity of pharmacogenetic disorders. During the Korean War, service personnel were deployed in a region of the world where they were at increased risk for malaria. To reduce the likelihood of acquiring that disease, the antimalarial drug primaquine was administered prophylactically. Shortly thereafter, approximately 10% of the African-American servicemen were diagnosed with acute anemia and a smaller percentage of soldiers of Mediterranean ancestry showed a more severe hemolytic anemia. Investigation revealed that the affected individuals had a mutation in the glucose 6-phosphate dehydrogenase (G6PD) gene. Functional G6PD is important in the maintenance of a balance between oxidized and reduced molecules in the cells, and, under normal circumstances, a mutation that eliminates the normal enzyme function can be compensated for by other cellular processes. However, mutation carriers are compromised when their cells are stressed, such as when the primaquine is administered. The system becomes overloaded, and the result is oxidative damage of the red blood cells and anemia. Clearly, both the medics who administered the primaquine and the men who took the drug were unaware of the potential consequences. Fortunately, once the drug treatment was discontinued, the individuals recovered.

### Research efforts

Drugs are essential to modern medical practice, but, as in the cases of malignant hyperthermia and G6PD deficiency, it has become clear that not all individuals respond equally to each drug. Reactions can vary from positive improvement in the quality of life to life threatening episodes. Annually, in the United States, there are over two million reported cases of adverse drug reactions and a further 100,000 deaths per year as a result of drug treatments. The **Human Genome Project** and other research endeavors are now providing information that is allowing a better understanding of the underlying causes of pharmacogenetic anomalies with the hope that eventually the number of negative episodes can be reduced.

Research on one enzyme family is beginning to revolutionize the concepts of drug therapy. The cytochrome P450 system is a group of related enzymes that are key components in the metabolic conversion of over 50% of all currently used drugs. Studies involving one member of this family, CYP2D6, have revealed the presence of several polymorphic genetic variations (poor, intermediate, extensive, and ultra) that result in different clinical phenotypes with respect to drug metabolism. For example, a poor metabolizer has difficulty converting the therapeutic drug into a useable form, so the unmodified chemical will accumulate in the body and may cause a toxic overdose. To prevent this from happening, the prescribed dosage of the drug must be reduced.

An ultra metabolizer, on the other hand, shows exceedingly rapid breakdown of the drug to the point that the substance may be destroyed so quickly that therapeutic levels may not be reached, and the patient may never show any benefit from treatment. In these cases, switching to another type of drug that is not associated with CYP2D6 metabolism may prove more beneficial.

The third phenotypic class, the extensive metabolizers, is less extreme than the ultra metabolism category, but nevertheless presents a relatively rapid turnover of drug that may require a higher than normal dosage to maintain a proper level within the cells. The intermediate **phenotype** falls between the poor and extensive categories and gives reasonable metabolism and turnover of the drug. This is the group for whom most "recommended" drug dosages appear to be appropriate.

The elucidation of the four different metabolic classes has clearly shown that the usual "one size fits all" recommended drug dose is not appropriate for all individuals. In the future, it will become increasingly necessary to know the patient's metabolic phenotype with respect to the drug being given to determine the most appropriate regimen of therapy for that individual.

### Future applications

Based on current studies, it is possible to envision many different applications in the future. In addition to providing patient specific drug therapies, pharmacogenetics will aid in the clinician's ability to predict adverse reactions before they occur and identify the potential for drug addiction or overdose. New tests will be developed to monitor the effects of drugs, and new medications will be found that specifically target a particular genetic abnormality. Increased knowledge in this field should provide a better understanding of the metabolic effects of food additives, work related chemicals, and industrial by–products. In time, these advances will improve the practice of medicine and become the standard of care.

Constance K. Stein, PhD

Phenotype *see* **Genotypes and phenotypes**

# Phenylketonuria

### Definition

Phenylketonuria (PKU) can be defined as a rare metabolic disorder caused by a deficiency in the production of the hepatic (liver) enzyme phenylalanine

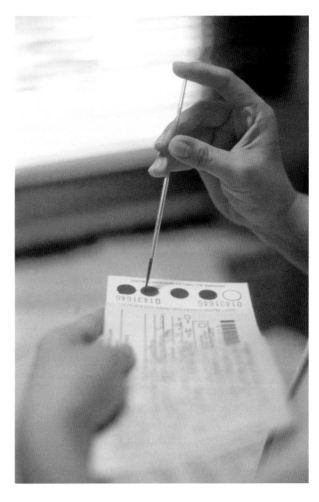

**A technician is performing a test to screen for PKU.** *(Custom Medical Stock Photo, Inc.)*

# KEY TERMS

**Amino acid**—Organic compounds that form the building blocks of protein. There are 20 types of amino acids (eight are "essential amino acids" which the body cannot make and must therefore be obtained from food).

**Axon**—Skinny, wire-like extension of nerve cells.

**Enzyme**—A protein that catalyzes a biochemical reaction or change without changing its own structure or function.

**Gene**—A building block of inheritance, which contains the instructions for the production of a particular protein, and is made up of a molecular sequence found on a section of DNA. Each gene is found on a precise location on a chromosome.

**Genetic disease**—A disease that is (partly or completely) the result of the abnormal function or expression of a gene; a disease caused by the inheritance and expression of a genetic mutation.

**IQ**—Abbreviation for Intelligence Quotient. Compares an individual's mental age to his/her true or chronological age and multiplies that ratio by 100.

**Metabolism**—The total combination of all of the chemical processes that occur within cells and tissues of a living body.

**Mutation**—A permanent change in the genetic material that may alter a trait or characteristic of an individual, or manifest as disease, and can be transmitted to offspring.

**Myelin**—A fatty sheath surrounding nerves in the peripheral nervous system, which help them conduct impulses more quickly.

**Nervous system**—The complete network of nerves, sense organs, and brain in the body.

**Phenylalanine**—An essential amino acid that must be obtained from food since the human body cannot manufacture it.

**Protein**—Important building blocks of the body, composed of amino acids, involved in the formation of body structures and controlling the basic functions of the human body.

**Recessive**—Genetic trait expressed only when present on both members of a pair of chromosomes, one inherited from each parent.

hydroxylase (PAH). PKU is the most serious form of a class of diseases referred to as "hyperphenylalaninemia," all of which involve above normal (elevated) levels of phenylalanine in the blood. The primary symptom of untreated PKU, mental retardation, is the result of consuming foods that contain the amino acid phenylalanine, which is toxic to brain tissue.

PKU is an inherited, autosomal recessive disorder. It is the most common genetic disease involving amino acid metabolism. PKU is incurable, but early, effective treatment can prevent the development of serious mental incapacity.

## Description

PKU is a disease caused by the liver's inability to produce a particular type of PAH enzyme. This enzyme converts (metabolizes) the amino acid called phenylalanine into another amino acid, tyrosine. This is the only role of PAH in the body. A lack of PAH results in the build–up of abnormally high phenylalanine concentrations (or levels) in the blood and brain. Above normal levels of phenylalanine are toxic to the cells that make up the nervous system and causes irreversible abnormalities in brain structure and

function in PKU patients. Phenylalanine is a type of **teratogen**. Teratogens are any substance or organism that can cause birth disorders in a developing fetus.

The liver is the body's chief protein processing center. Proteins are one of the major food nutrients. They are generally very large molecules composed of strings of smaller building blocks or molecules called amino acids. About twenty amino acids exist in nature. The body breaks down proteins from food into individual amino acids and then reassembles them into "human" proteins. Proteins are needed for growth and repair of cells and tissues, and are the key components of enzymes, antibodies, and other essential substances.

### PKU and the human nervous system

The extensive network of nerves in the brain and the rest of the nervous system are made up of nerve cells. Nerve cells have specialized extensions called dendrites and axons. Stimulating a nerve cell triggers nerve impulses, or signals, that speed down the axon. These nerve impulses then stimulate the end of an axon to release chemicals called neurotransmitters that spread out and communicate with the dendrites of neighboring nerve cells.

Many nerve cells have long, wire-like axons that are covered by an insulating layer called the myelin sheath. This covering helps speed nerve impulses along the axon. In untreated PKU patients, abnormally high phenylalanine levels in the blood and brain can produce nerve cells with abnormal axons and dendrites, and cause imperfections in the myelin sheath referred to as hypomyelination and demyelenation. This loss of myelin can "short circuit" nerve impulses (messages) and interrupt cell communication. A number of brain scan studies also indicate a degeneration of the white matter in the brains of older patients who have not maintained adequate dietary control.

PKU can also affect the production of one of the major neurotransmitters in the brain, called dopamine. The brain makes dopamine from the amino acid tyrosine. PKU patients who do not consume enough tyrosine in their diet cannot produce sufficient amounts of dopamine. Low dopamine levels in the brain disrupt normal communication between nerve cells, which results in impaired cognitive (mental) function.

Some preliminary research suggests that nerve cells of PKU patients also have difficulty absorbing tyrosine. This abnormality may explain why many PKU patients who receive sufficient dietary tyrosine still experience some form of learning disability.

### Behavior and academic performance

IQ (intelligence quotient) tests provide a measure of cognitive function. The IQ of PKU patients is generally lower than the IQ of their healthy peers. Students with PKU often find academic tasks difficult and must work harder to succeed than their non-PKU peers. They may require special tutoring and need to repeat some of their courses. Even patients undergoing treatment programs may experience problems with typical academic tasks such as math, reading, and spelling. Visual perception, visual-motor skills, and critical thinking skills can also be affected. Ten years of age seems to be an important milestone for PKU patients. After age 10, variations in a patient's diet seems to have less influence on their IQ development.

People with PKU tend to avoid contact with others, appear anxious, and show signs of **depression**. However, some patients may be much more expressive and tend to have hyperactive, talkative, and impulsive personalities. It is also interesting to note that people with PKU are less likely to display such habits as lying, teasing, and active disobedience. It should be emphasized that current research findings are still quite preliminary and more extensive research is needed to clearly show how abnormal phenylalanine levels in

the blood and brain might affect behavior and academic performance.

### Genetic profile

PKU symptoms are caused by alterations or mutations in the genetic code for the PAH enzyme. Mutations in the PAH gene prevent the liver from producing adequate levels of the PAH enzyme needed to break down phenylalanine. The PAH gene and its PKU mutations are found on **chromosome** 12 in the human genome. In more detail, PKU mutations can involve many different types of changes, such as deletions and insertions, in the **DNA** of the gene that codes for the PAH enzyme.

PKU is described as an inherited, autosomal recessive disorder. The term autosomal means that the gene for PKU is not located on either the X or Y sex chromosome. The normal PAH gene is dominant to recessive PKU mutations. A recessive genetic trait, such as PKU, is one that is expressed—or shows up—only when two copies are inherited (one from each parent).

A person with one normal and one PKU gene is called a carrier. A carrier does not display any symptoms of the disease because their liver produces normal quantities of the PAH enzyme. However, PKU carriers can pass the PKU genetic mutation onto their children. Two carrier parents have a 25% chance of producing a baby with PKU symptoms, and a 50% chance having a baby that is a carrier for the disease. Although PKU conforms to these basic genetic patterns of **inheritance**, the actual expression, or **phenotype**, of the disease is not strictly an "either/or" situation. This is because there are at least 400 different types of PKU mutations. Although some PKU mutations cause rather mild forms of the disease, others can initiate much more severe symptoms in untreated individuals. The more severe the PKU mutation, the greater the effect on cognitive development and performance (mental ability).

Also, it must be remembered that human cells contain two copies of each type of gene. Different combinations of any two PKU mutations tend to produce a wide spectrum of physiological and psychological symptoms. For example, patients who receive two "severe" PKU mutations from their parents can potentially develop more serious symptoms than people who possess a combination of one severe type and one milder form of mutation. To further complicate the genetic picture of PKU, other types of genes have been identified which seem to be responsible for the abnormal processing of phenylalanine in brain tissue. These abnormalities add to the severity of PKU symptoms experienced by patients who inherit these genes. In more detail, the association of multiple types of genes with a single condition, such as PKU, is referred to as molecular heterogeneity.

## Demographics

One in 50 individuals in the United States have inherited a gene for PKU. About five million Americans are PKU carriers. About one in 15,000 babies test positive for PKU in the United States. Studies indicate that the incidence of this disease in Caucasian and Native American populations is higher than in African-American, Hispanic, and Asian populations.

## Signs and symptoms

Untreated PKU patients develop a broad range of symptoms related to severely impaired cognitive function, sometimes referred to as mental retardation. Other symptoms can include extreme patterns of behavior, delayed speech development, seizures, a characteristic body odor, and light body pigmentation. The light pigmentation is due to a lack of melanin, which normally colors the hair, skin and eyes. Melanin is made from the amino acid tyrosine, which is lacking in untreated cases of PKU. Physiologically, PKU patients show high levels of phenylalanine and low levels of tyrosine in the blood. Babies do not show any visible symptoms of the disease for the first few months of life. However, typical PKU symptoms usually do show up by a baby's first birthday.

## Diagnosis

The primary diagnostic test for PKU is the measurement of phenylalanine levels in a drop of blood taken from the heel of a newborn baby's foot. This screening procedure is referred to as the Guthrie test (Guthrie bacterial inhibition assay). In this test, PKU is confirmed by the appearance of bacteria growing around high concentrations of phenylalanine in the blood spot. PKU testing was introduced in the early 1960s and is the largest genetic screening program in the United States. It is required by law in all 50 states. Early diagnosis is critical. It ensures the early treatment PKU babies need to develop normally and avoid the complications of PKU.

The American Academy of Pediatrics recommends that this test be performed on infants between 24 hours and seven days after birth. The preferred time for testing is after the baby's first feeding. If the initial PKU test produces a positive result, then follow-up tests are performed to confirm the diagnosis and to determine if the elevated phenylalanine levels may be caused by some medical condition other than PKU. Treatment for PKU is recommended for babies that show a blood phenylalanine level of 7–10 mg/dL or higher for more than a few consecutive days. Another, more accurate test procedure for PKU measures the ratio (comparison) of the amount of phenylalanine to the amount of tyrosine in the blood.

Newer diagnostic procedures (called mutation analysis and **genotype** determination) can actually identify the specific types of PAH **gene mutations** inherited by PKU infants. Large-scale studies have helped to clarify how various mutations affect the ability of patients to process phenylalanine. This information can help doctors develop more effective customized treatment plans for each of their PKU patients.

## Treatment and management

The severity of the PKU symptoms experienced by people with this disease is determined by both lifestyle and genetic factors. In the early 1950s, researchers first demonstrated that phenylalanine-restricted diets could eliminate most of the typical PKU symptoms—except for mental retardation. Dietary therapy (also called nutrition therapy) is the most common form of treatment for PKU patients. PKU patients who receive early and consistent dietary therapy can develop fairly normal mental capacity to within about five IQ points of their healthy peers. By comparison, untreated PKU patients generally have IQ scores below 50.

Infants with PKU should be put on a specialized diet as soon as they are diagnosed to avoid progressive brain damage and other problems caused by an accumulation of phenylalanine in the body. A PKU diet helps patients maintain very low blood levels of phenylalanine by restricting the intake of natural foods that contain this amino acid. Even breast milk is a problem for PKU babies. Special PKU dietary mixtures or formulas are usually obtained from medical clinics or pharmacies.

Phenylalanine is actually an essential amino acid. This means that it has to be obtained from food because the body cannot produce this substance on its own. Typical diets prescribed for PKU patients provide very small amounts of phenylalanine and higher quantities of other amino acids, including tyrosine. The amount of allowable phenylalanine can be increased slightly as a child becomes older.

In addition, PKU diets include all the nutrients normally required for good health and normal growth, such as carbohydrates, fats, vitamins, and minerals. High protein foods like meat, fish, chicken, eggs, nuts, beans, milk, and other dairy products are banned from PKU diets. Small amounts of moderate protein foods (such as grains and potatoes) and low protein foods (some fruits and vegetables, low protein breads and pastas) are allowed. Sugar-free foods, such as diet soda, which contain the artificial sweetener aspartame, are also prohibited foods for patients with PKU. That is because aspartame contains the amino acid phenylalanine.

Ideally, school-age children with PKU should be taught to assume responsibility for managing their diet, recording food intake, and for performing simple blood tests to monitor their phenylalanine levels. Blood tests should be done in the early morning when phenylalanine levels are highest. Infants and young children require more frequent blood tests than older children and adults. The amount of natural foods allowed in a diet could be adjusted to ensure that the level of phenylalanine in the blood is kept within a safe range—two to 6 mg/dL before 12 years of age and 2–15 mg/dL for PKU patients over 12 years old.

A specialized PKU diet can cause abnormal fluctuations in tyrosine levels throughout the day. Thus, some health professionals recommend adding time released tyrosine that can provide a more constant supply of this amino acid to the body. It should be noted that some PKU patients show signs of learning disabilities even with a special diet containing extra tyrosine. Research studies suggest that these patients may not be able to process tyrosine normally.

For PKU caregivers, providing a diet that is appealing as well as healthy and nutritious is a constant challenge. Many patients with PKU, especially teenagers, find it difficult to stick to the relatively bland PKU diet for extended periods of time. Some older patients decide to go off their diet plan simply because they feel healthy. However, many patients who abandon careful nutritional management develop cognitive problems, such as difficulties remembering, maintaining focus, and paying attention. Many PKU health professionals contend that all patients with PKU should adhere to a strictly controlled diet for life.

One promising line of PKU research involves the synthesis (manufacturing) of a new type of enzyme that can break down phenylalanine in food consumed by the patient. This medication would be taken orally and could prevent the absorption of digested phenylalanine into the patient's bloodstream.

In general, medical researchers express concern about the great variation in treatment programs currently available to PKU patients around the world. They have highlighted the urgent need for new, consistent international standards for proper management of

PKU patients, which should emphasize comprehensive psychological as well as physiological monitoring and assessment.

### PKU and pregnancy

Women with PKU must be especially careful with their diets if they want to have children. They should ensure that phenylalanine blood levels are under control before conception and throughout pregnancy. Mothers with elevated (higher than normal) phenylalanine levels are high risk for having babies with significant birth disorders, such as microencephaly (smaller than normal head size), and **congenital heart disease** (abnormal heart structure and function), stunted growth, mental impairment, and psychomotor (coordination) difficulties. This condition is referred to as maternal PKU and can even affect babies who do not have the PKU disease.

### Prognosis

Early newborn screening, careful monitoring, and a life-long strict dietary management can help PKU patients to live normal, healthy, and long lives.

### Resources

**BOOKS**

Brust, John C. M. *The Practice Of Neural Science: From Synapses To Symptoms.* New York: McGraw-Hill, 2000.

Gilroy, John. *Basic Neurology.* 3rd ed. New York: McGraw-Hill, 2000.

Koch, Jean Holt. *Robert Guthrie—The PKU Story: Crusade Against Mental Retardation.* Pasadena, CA: Hope Publishing House, 1997.

Ratey, John J. *A User's Guide To The Brain: Perception, Attention, And The Four Theaters Of The Brain.* 1st ed. New York: Pantheon Books, 2001.

Schuett, Virginia E. *Low Protein Cookery For Phenylketonuria.* 3rd ed. Madison: University of Wisconsin Press, 1997.

Walker, John M. *Genetics and You.* Totowa, NJ: Humana Press, 1996.

Weiner, William J., Christopher G. Goetz, eds. *Neurology For The Non-Neurologist.* 4th ed. Philadelphia: Lippincott, Williams & Wilkins, 1999.

## PERIODICALS

Burgard, P. "Development of intelligence in early treated phenylketonuria." *European Journal of Pediatrics* 159, Suppl. 2 (October 2000): S74–9.

Chang, Pi-Nian, Robert M. Gray, and Lisa Lehn O'Brien. "Review: Patterns of academic achievement among patients treated early with phenylketonuria." *European Journal of Pediatrics* 159, no.14 (2000): S96–9.

Eastman, J.W., et al. "Use of the phenylalanine: Tyrosine ratio to test newborns for phenylketonuria in a large public health screening programme." *Journal of Medical Screening* 7, no. 3 (2000): 131–5.

MacDonald, A. "Diet and compliance in phenylketonuria." *European Journal of Pediatrics* 159, Suppl. 2 (Oct. 2000): S136–41.

Smith, Isabel, and Julie Knowles. "Behaviour in early treated phenylketonuria: A systematic review." *European Journal of Pediatrics* 159, no. 14 (2000): S89–93.

Stemerdink, B.A., et al. "Behaviour and school achievement in patients with early and continuously treated phenyl-ketonuria." *Journal of Inherited Metabolic Disorders* 23, no. 6 (2000): 548–62.

van Spronsen, F.J.F., et al. "Phenylketonuria: Tyrosine supplementation in phenylalanine-restricted diets." *American Journal of Clinical Nutrition* 73, no. 2 (2001): 153–7.

Wappner, Rebecca, et al. "Management of Phenylketonuria for Optimal Outcome: A Review of Guidelines for Phenylketonuria Management and a Report of Surveys of Parents, Patients, and Clinic Directors." *Pediatrics* 104, no. 6 (December 1999): e68.

## WEBSITES

Consensus Development Conference on Phenylketonuria (PKU): Screening and Management, October 16–18, 2000. http://odp.od.nih.gov/consensus/news/upcoming/pku/pku_info.htm#overview.

Genetics and Public Health in the 21st Century. Using Genetic Information to Improve Health and Prevent Disease. http://www.cdc.gov/genetics/_archive/publications/Table.

## ORGANIZATIONS

Allergy and Asthma Network. Mothers of Asthmatics, Inc. 2751 Prosperity Ave., Suite 150, Fairfax, VA 22031. (800) 878-4403. Fax: (703)573-7794.

American Academy of Allergy, Asthma & Immunology. 611 E. Wells St, Milwaukee, WI 53202. (414) 272-6071. Fax: (414) 272-6070. http://www.aaaai.org/default.stm.

Centers for Disease Control. GDP Office, 4770 Buford Highway NE, Atlanta, GA 30341-3724. (770) 488-3235. http://www.cdc.gov/genetics.

Children's PKU Network. 1520 State St., Suite 111, San Diego, CA 92101-2930. (619) 233-3202. Fax: (619) 233 0838. pkunetwork@aol.com.

March of Dimes Birth Defects Foundation. 1275 Mamaro-neck Ave., White Plains, NY 10605. (888) 663-4637. resourcecenter@modimes.org. http://www.modimes.org.

National PKU News. Virginia Schuett, editor/dietician. 6869 Woodlawn Avenue NE #116, Seattle, WA 98115-5469. (206) 525-8140. Fax: (206) 525-5023. http://www.pkunews.org.

University of Washington PKU Clinic. CHDD, Box 357920, University of Washington, Seattle, WA. (206) 685-3015. Within Washington State: (877) 685-3015. Clinic Coordinator: vam@u.washington.edu. http://depts.washington.edu/pku/contact.html..

Marshall G. Letcher, MA

Phocomelia *see* **Roberts SC phocomelia**

Phytanic acid oxidase deficiency *see* **Refsum disease**

Phytanic acid storage disease *see* **Infantile refsum disease**

Pierre-Robin syndrome *see* **Pierre-Robin sequence**

Pierre-Robin syndrome with fetal chrondro-dysplasia *see* **Weissenbacher-Zweymuller syndrome**

# Pierre-Robin sequence

## Definition

Pierre-Robin sequence consists of the micrognathia, (small lower jaw), or retrognathia (lower jaw displaced to the back), glossoptosis (displacement of the tongue into the throat) and obstruction of the airway. It is usually accompanied by a **cleft palate** (an opening in the roof of the mouth). The term sequence is used to describe the pattern of multiple anomalies derived from a single known prior anomaly or mechanical factor.

## Description

Children born with Pierre-Robin sequence are found to have small mandibles (lower jaws), or mandibles that are displaced back, tongues that are pushed back into the throat, and difficulty breathing of varying degrees. They also have difficulty feeding. Pierre-Robin sequence is usually accompanied by a cleft palate. It is also known as Pierre-Robin syndrome.

### Genetic profile

Pierre-Robin sequence can occur in association with other syndromes; isolated (not associated with other malformations); or in associations with other developmental disorders that do not represent a specific syndrome. Heredity has not been proven to be a factor in the cause of isolated Pierre-Robin sequence. Pierre-Robin sequence found in association with numerous syndromes may have a mode of **inheritance** that is related to the syndrome itself. The mode of inheritance includes single **gene** as well as **chromosomal abnormalities**.

The cause of the abnormal lower jaw in Pierre-Robin syndrome may be mechanical, genetic, teratogenic, or multi-factorial. Mechanical factors such as fibroids inside the uterus may constrict the lower jaw preventing it from growing. Single gene or chromosomal abnormalities produce syndromes that have Pierre-Robin sequence. Teratogenic (anything that affects development of the embryo) causes include maternal use of alcohol. Multifactorial inheritance means that the cause is a combination of environmental and hereditary factors.

### Demographics

The incidence of Pierre-Robin sequence is reported to be one out of 8,500 live births. Other reports show that the range is one out of 2,000 to one out of 50,000 live births. This wide range is due to different diagnostic criteria and the presence or absence of associated syndromes. Fewer than 20% of newborns born with Pierre-Robin sequence have the isolated type.

### Signs and symptoms

In Pierre-Robin sequence, the lower jaw of the fetus displaces the tongue backwards into the throat. The tongue located in this abnormal position blocks the embryonic structures from joining in the midline in order to form the palate, the roof of the mouth. The result is a cleft palate—an opening in the roof of the mouth. The size of the cleft palate varies as well as its position. It is not present in all patients.

Babies born with Pierre-Robin have difficulty feeding and breathing because the tongue—pushed backwards by the lower jaw—obstructs the throat. Feeding and breathing difficulties may be very mild or very severe.

Affected persons may also develop hearing problems due to fluid collecting in the ears.

### Diagnosis

Prenatal ultrasonic examination may show findings to indicate the possibility of Pierre-Robin sequence alerting the physician to be prepared at birth for the possibility of the baby having breathing and feeding problems.

### Treatment and management

The type of treatment varies according to the severity of the symptoms and their duration. Babies may not require any therapy if they have no symptoms of breathing difficulties and no feeding difficulties

If breathing difficulties are mild, the easiest management is keeping the baby in the prone position. This position causes the tongue to fall forward, relieving the obstruction. A thorough evaluation of these patients must be conducted, which includes endoscopy of the airways and upper digestive tract. Close monitoring must be maintained because the prone position may obscure breathing difficulties.

If positioning the patient prone fails, a nasopharyngeal airway may be used but only for a short time. The airway is a tube passed through the nose into the upper airway, which the baby can breath through.

If the above methods fail or are required for a prolonged length of time, then some type of surgical intervention will be required. Surgical procedures include glossopexy, in which the tongue is sutured to the lower lip in order to prevent it from moving back into the throat causing obstruction. Subperiosteal release of the floor of the mouth muscles on the lower jaw is an operation in which the tongue can no longer move back into the throat because muscles are released from their insertions. Tracheotomy is performed by surgically cutting an opening in the trachea (windpipe). This opening bypasses the obstruction. The choice of surgical intervention varies according to the duration and severity of respiratory obstruction; other causes of respiratory obstruction that may be present; and the experience of the surgeon. Glossopexy and tracheotomy are temporary and reversed when the baby can breath adequately on its own.

The treatment of feeding difficulty varies according to the degree of difficulty. It has been found that the severity of feeding difficulty is proportional to the severity of airway obstruction. Feeding is usually accomplished with specialized cleft palate nipples and bottles or nasogastric tubes (a feeding tube passed through the nose and into the stomach). Sometimes a gastrotomy tube is needed for feeding. This is a tube passed through a surgical opening made in the abdominal wall and stomach.

Children with Pierre-Robin sequence are prone to hearing loss due to fluid collecting behind the tympanic membrane (ear drum), and may require drainage tubes placed into the ear.

If the child has a cleft palate, it is usually surgically repaired between the ages of nine and 18 months.

## Prognosis

The prognosis for individuals with Pierre-Robin sequence varies with the severity of symptoms and if it is associated with other congenital abnormalities. The more severe the symptoms and associated congenital abnormalities, the greater the risk of complications.

The rate at which the lower jaw starts to catch up in growth depends on the cause of Pierre-Robin sequence. The majority of children with the isolated type will achieve near normal jaw size within a few years of birth. If Pierre-Robin sequence is part of a syndrome that has a small jaw, the jaw may remain small throughout life.

## Resources

### PERIODICALS

Bath, A. P. "Management of the upper airway obstruction in Pierre-Robin Sequence." *Journal of Laryngology and Otology* 111, no. 12 (December 1997): 1155–7.

Cohen, N. M. Jr. "Pierre-Robin Sequences and complexes: causal heterogeneity and pathogenetic/phenotypic variability." (Editorial). *American Journal of Medical Genetics* 84, no. 4 (June 4, 1999): 311–5.

Cruz, M. "Pierre-Robin Sequences: secondary respiratory difficulties and intrinsic feeding abnormalities." *Layrngoscope* 109, no. 10 (October 1999): 1632–6.

Hsieh, Y. Y. "The Prenatal Diagnosis of Pierre-Robin Sequence" *Prenatal Diagnosis* 19, no. 6 (June 1999): 567–9.

Marques, I. L. "Etiopathogenesis of isolated Robin Sequence." *Cleft Palate-Craniofacial Journal* 35, no. 6 (November 1998): 517–25.

Myer, C. M. "Airway management in Pierre-Robin Sequence." *Otolaryngology–Head and Neck Surgery* 118, no. 5 (May 1998): 630–5.

Prows, C. A. "Beyond Pierre-Robin Syndrome." *Neonatal Network* 18, no. 5 (August 1999): 13–9.

Van Der Haven. "The Jaw Index: New guide defining Micrognatia in newborns." *Cleft Palate-Craniofacial Journal* 34, no. 3 (May 1997): 240–1.

Vester, F. "Pierre-Robin Syndrome: Mandibular growth during the first year of life." *Annals of Plastic Surgery* 42, no. 2 (February 1999): 154–7.

### ORGANIZATION

Let's Face It. University of Michigan, School of Dentistry, 1011 N. University, Ann Arbor, MI 48109. http://desic-a.dent.umich.edu/faceit.

### WEBSITES

About Face International. http://aboutfaceinternational.org/.
Pierre-Robin Network. http://www.pierrerobin.org.

Farris F. Gulli, MD

# Pituitary dwarfism

## Definition

Dwarfism is a condition in which the growth of the individual is very slow or delayed. There are many forms of dwarfism. The word pituitary is in reference to the pituitary gland in the body. This gland regulates certain chemicals (hormones) in the body. Therefore, pituitary dwarfism is decreased bodily growth due to hormonal problems. The end result is a proportionate little person, because the height as well as the growth of all other structures of the individual are decreased.

## Description

Pituitary dwarfism is caused by problems arising in the pituitary gland. The pituitary gland is also called the hypophysis. The pituitary gland is divided into two halves: the anterior (front) and posterior (back) halves. The anterior half produces six hormones: growth hormone, adrenocorticotropin (corticotropin), thyroid stimulating homone (thyrotropin), prolactin, follicle stimulating hormone, and lutenizing hormone. The posterior pituitary gland only produces two hormones. It produces antidiuretic hormone (vasopressin) and oxytocin.

Most forms of dwarfism are a result of decreased production of hormones from the anterior half of the

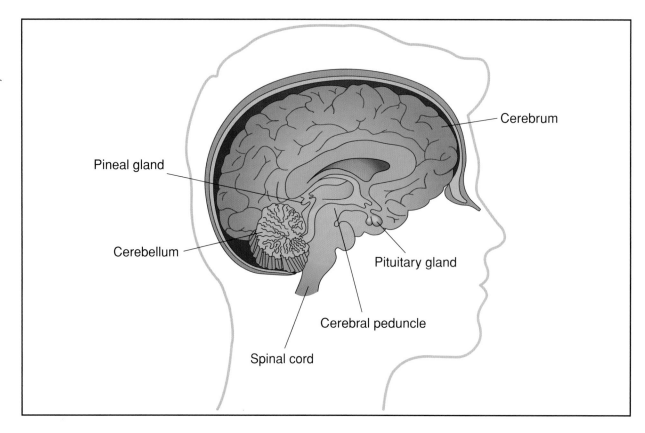

*(Gale, a part of Cengage Learning.)*

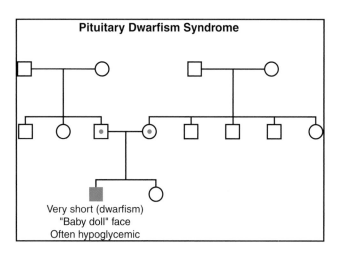

*(Gale, a part of Cengage Learning.)*

pituitary gland. The most common form is due to decreases of growth hormone. These decreases during childhood cause the individual's arms, legs, and other structures to develop normal proportions for their bodies, but at a decreased rate.

When all of the hormones of the anterior pituitary gland are not produced, this is called panhypopituitarism. Another type of dwarfism occurs when only the growth hormone is decreased. Dwarfism can also result from a lack of somatomedin C (also called insulin like growth factor, IGF-1) production. Somatomedin C is a hormone produced in the liver that increases bone growth when growth hormone is present. The African pygmy and the Levi-Lorain dwarfs lack the ability to produce somatomedin C in response to growth hormone. All causes of dwarfism lead to a proportionate little person.

Growth is the body's response to different hormones. The forebrain contains a small organ called the hypothalamus, which is responsible for releasing hormones in response to the body's needs for purposes of regulation. Growth hormone is produced in the anterior pituitary gland when growth hormone-releasing hormone (GHRH) is released by the hypothalamus. Growth hormone is then released and stimulates the liver to produce IGF-1. In return, IGF-1 stimulates the long bones to grow in length. Thus, growth can be slowed down or stopped if there is a problem making any of these hormones or if there is a problem with the cells receiving these hormones.

## KEY TERMS

**Adrenocorticotropin (corticotrophin)**—A hormone that acts on cells of the adrenal cortex, causing them to produce male sex hormones and hormones that control water and mineral balance in the body.

**Antidiuretic hormone (vasopressin)**—A hormone that acts on the kidneys to regulate water balance.

**Craniopharyngioma**—A tumor near the pituitary gland in the craniopharyngeal canal that often results in intracranial pressure.

**Deprivational dwarfism**—A condition where emotional disturbances are associated with growth failure and abnormalities of pituitary function.

**Follicle-stimulating hormone (FSH)**—A hormone that in females stimulates estrogen and in males stimulates sperm production.

**Growth hormone**—A hormone that eventually stimulates growth. Also called somatotropin.

**Hormone**—A chemical messenger produced by the body that is involved in regulating specific bodily functions such as growth, development, and reproduction.

**Lutenizing hormone**—A hormone secreted by the pituitary gland that regulates the menstrual cycle and triggers ovulation in females. In males it stimulates the testes to produce testosterone.

**Oxytocin**—A hormone that stimulates the uterus to contract during child birth and the breasts to release milk.

**Panhypopituitarism**—Generalized decrease of all of the anterior pituitary hormones.

**Prolactin**—A hormone that helps the breast prepare for milk production during pregnancy.

**Puberty**—Point in development when the gonads begin to function and secondary sexual characteristics begin to appear.

**Thyroid stimulating hormone (thyrotropin)**—A hormone that stimulates the thyroid gland to produce hormones that regulate metabolism.

### Genetic profile

Pituitary dwarfism has been shown to run in families. New investigations are underway to determine the specific cause and location of the **gene** responsible for dwarfism. The human cell contains 46 chromosomes arranged in 23 pairs. Most of the genes in the two chromosomes of each pair are identical or almost identical with each other. However, with dwarfism, there appears to be disruption on different areas of **chromosome** 3 and 7. Some studies have isolated defects for the production of pituitary hormones to the short arm (the "p" end) of chromosome 3 at a specific location of 3p11. Other studies have found changes on the short arm of chromosome 7.

### Demographics

Some estimates show that there are between 10,000 and 15,000 children in the United States who have growth problems due to a deficiency of growth hormone.

### Signs and symptoms

A child with a growth hormone deficiency is often small with an immature face and chubby body build. The child's growth will slow down and not follow the normal growth curve patterns. In cases of tumor, most commonly craniopharyngioma (a tumor near the pituitary gland), children and adolescents may present with neurological symptoms such as headaches, vomiting, and problems with vision. The patient may also have symptoms of double vision. Symptoms such as truly bizarre and excessive drinking behaviors (polydipsia) and sleep disturbances may be common.

### Diagnosis

The primary symptom of pituitary dwarfism is lack of height. Therefore, a change in the individual's growth habits will help lead to a diagnosis. Another diagnostic technique uses an x ray of the child's hand to determine the child's bone age by comparing this to the child's actual chronological age. The bone age in affected children is usually two years or more behind the chronological age. This means that if a child is ten years old, his or her bones will look like they are those of an eight-year-old child. The levels of growth hormone and somatomedin C must also be measured with blood tests.

Hypopituitarism may be gained or acquired following birth for several reasons. It could be due to trauma to the pituitary gland such as a fall or following surgery to the brain for removal of a tumor. It may also be due to the child's environment (deprivational dwarfism).

On examination by the doctor there may be optic nerve atrophy, if the dwarfism is due to a type of tumor. X rays of the area where the pituitary gland is located (sella turcica) or more advanced imaging such as magnetic resonance imaging (MRI) or computed tomography (CT) may show changes of the pituitary gland itself. Computed tomography is an advanced form of x ray that will help determine the integrity of the bone and how much calcification the tumor is producing. Magnetic resonance imaging will also help in the diagnosis. MRI is a type of imaging device that can visualize soft tissues such as muscle and fat.

If the dwarfism is due to environmental and emotional problems, the individual may be hospitalized to monitor hormone levels. Following a few days of hospitalization, hormone levels may become normal due to avoidance of the original environment.

### Treatment and management

The main course of therapy is growth hormone replacement therapy when there is lack of growth hormone in the body. A pediatric endocrinologist, a doctor specializing in the hormones of children, usually administers this type of therapy before a child's growth plates have fused or joined together. Once the growth plates have fused, GH replacement therapy is rarely effective.

Growth hormone used to be collected from recently deceased humans. However, frequent disease complications resulting from human growth hormone collected from deceased bodies led to the banning of this method. In the mid-1980s, techniques were discovered that could produce growth hormones in the lab. Now, the only growth hormone used for treatment is that made in a laboratory.

A careful balancing of all of the hormones produced by the pituitary gland is necessary for patients with panhypopituitarism. This form of dwarfism is very difficult to manage.

### Prognosis

The prognosis for each type of dwarfism varies. A panhypopituitarism dwarf does not pass through the initial onset of adult sexual development (puberty) and never produces enough gonadotropic hormones to develop adult sexual function. These individuals also have a great deal of other medical conditions. Dwarfism due to only growth hormone deficiency has a different prognosis. These individuals do pass through puberty and mature sexually, however, they remain proportionately small in stature.

If the individual is lacking only growth hormone then growth hormone replacement therapy can be administered. The success of treatment with growth hormone varies. An increase in height of 4–6 in (10–15 cm) can occur in the first year of treatment. Following this first year, the response to the hormone is not as

## QUESTIONS TO ASK YOUR DOCTOR

- How does pituitary dwarfism differ from other forms of dwarfism?
- What information does current research provide about the genetic cause of pituitary dwarfism?
- Please explain the process involved in growth hormone replacement therapy.
- What is the prognosis for a child born with pituitary dwarfism?

successful. Therefore, the amount of growth hormone administered must be tripled to maintain this rate. Long-term use is considered successful if the individual grows at least 0.75 in (2 cm) per year more than they would without the hormone. However, if the growth hormone treatment is not administered before the long bones—such as the legs and arms—fuse, then the individual will never grow. This fusion is completed by adult age.

Improvement for individuals with dwarfism due to other causes such as a tumor, varies greatly. If the dwarfism is due to deprevational causes, then removing that child from that environment should help to alleviate the problem.

### Resources

#### BOOKS

Guyton, Arthur C., and John E. Hall. "The Pituitary Hormones and Their Control by the Hypothalamus." *Textbook of Medical Physiology,* 9th ed. Philadelphia: W.B. Saunders Company, 1996.

"Pituitary Dwarfism." In *Merck Manual.* Ed. Mark H. Beers, Robert Berkow, and Mark Burs, 2378–80. Rahway, NJ: Merck & Co., Inc., 1999.

Rogol, Alan D. "Hypothalamic and Pituitary Disorders in Infancy and Childhood." In *Principles and Practice of Endocrinology and Metabolism,* 2nd ed. Edited by Kenneth L. Becker et. al., 180–88. Philadelphia: J.B. Lippencott Company, 1995.

#### PERIODICALS

Maheshwari, H. G., et. al. "Phenotype and Genetic Analysis of a Syndrome Caused by an Inactivating Mutation in the Growth Hormone-Releasing Hormone Receptor: Dwarfism of Sindh." *Journal of Clinical Endocrinology and Metabolism* 83, no. 11 (1998): 4065–81.

Nagel, B. H. P. "Magnetic resonance images of 91 children with different causes of short stature: Pituitary size reflects growth hormone secretion." *European Journal of Pediatrics* 156 (1997): 758–63.

Raskin, S., et. al. "Genetic mapping of the human pituitary-specific transcriptional factor gene and its analysis in familial panhypopituitary dwarfism." *Human Genetics* 98 (1996): 703–5.

### WEBSITES

"Clinical Growth Charts by the National Center for Health Statistics." *Center for Disease Control.* http://www.cdc.gov/nchs/about/major/nhanes/growthcharts/clinical_charts.htm.

"Entry 312000: Panhypopituitarism; PHP." *OMIM—Online Mendelian Inheritance in Men.* National Institutes of Health. http://www.ncbi.nlm.nih.gov/htbin-post/Omim/dispmim?312000.

Hill, Mark. "Development of the Endocrine System—Pituitary." *The University of New South Wales, Sydney, Australia—Department of Embryology* http://anatomy.med.unsw.edu.au/CBL/Embryo/OMIMfind/endocrine/pitlist.htm.

### ORGANIZATIONS

Human Growth Foundation. 997 Glen Cove Ave., Glen Head, NY 11545. (800) 451-6434. Fax: (516) 671-4055. http://www.hgfl@hgfound.org.

Little People of America, Inc. National Headquarters, PO Box 745, Lubbock, TX 79408. (806) 737-8186 or (888) LPA-2001. lpadatabase@juno.com. http://www.lpaonline.org.

MAGIC Foundation for Children's Growth. 1327 N. Harlem Ave., Oak Park, IL 60302. (708) 383-0808 or (800) 362-4423. Fax: (708) 383-0899. mary@magicfoundation.org. http://www.magicfoundation.org/ghd.html.

Jason S. Schliesser, DC

# PK deficiency *see* Pyruvate kinase deficiency
# PKD *see* Polycystic kidney disease
# PKU *see* Phenylketonuria

# Poland anomaly

## Definition

Poland anomaly is a rare pattern of malformations present at birth that includes unilateral changes in the chest and shoulder girdle muscles, forearm bones, and fingers. Although there are other associated features, the most recognized characteristics are abnormalities of the major chest muscles (pectoralis) and the presence of syndactyly or webbing that joins the fingers of the hand. Treatment of this anomaly is mainly through reconstructive surgery.

### KEY TERMS

**Autosomal dominant**—A pattern of genetic inheritance where only one abnormal gene is needed to display the trait or disease.

**Dextrocardia**—Defect in which the position of the heart is the mirror image of its normal position.

**Pectoralis muscles**—Major muscles of the chest wall.

**Renal agenesis**—Absence or failure of one or both kidneys to develop normally.

**Sporadic**—Isolated or appearing occasionally with no apparent pattern.

**Syndactyly**—Webbing or fusion between the fingers or toes.

## Description

Poland anomaly (also known as Poland syndactyly, Poland syndrome, Poland sequence, or Pectoral dysplasia-dysdactyly) was first described in 1841 by Alfred Poland, who was a medical student at Guy's Hospital in London when he noted malformations in the body of a deceased convict named George Elt. The diagnosis of Poland anomaly may encompass various combinations of the following abnormalities:

- absence of major chest muscles: pectoralis major, pectoralis minor
- hand anomalies: syndactyly (webbed or fused fingers), shortened fingers
- underdeveloped forearm bones: ulna, radius
- underdeveloped or absence of the nipple and, in females, the breast
- absence of groups of rib cartilage
- absence of shoulder girdle muscles: latissimus dorsi, serratus anterior
- underdeveloped skin and underlying tissue of the chest
- abnormal curvature of the spine
- patchy hair growth under the arm
- rare associations with abnormalities in the heart, kidney or development of certain cancers

In most cases, physical abnormalities are confined to one side of the body and tend to favor the right side by almost two to one. The manifestations of Poland anomaly are extremely variable and rarely are all the features recognized in one individual. Involvement of the pectoralis muscle and fingers is the most consistent feature.

The exact cause of Poland anomaly is not known, but may result from the interruption of fetal growth at about the forty-sixth day of pregnancy, when the fetal fingers and pectoralis muscle are developing. Several researchers have suggested that there may be too little blood flow through the fetal subclavian artery that goes to the chest and arm; the more severe the blood flow disruption, the more numerous and severe the resulting malformations. However, the final proof for this idea has not been found.

## Genetic profile

Most occurrences of Poland anomaly appear to be sporadic (i.e., random, and not associated with a inherited disorder) and are not passed on from parent to child. However, there have been rare reports of Poland anomaly that appear in multiple members of the same family. In at least one case, this familial occurrence of Poland anomaly appears to be inherited in an autosomal dominant pattern. The fact that other organs systems (kidney, heart) and increased risks of certain cancers are associated with this condition supports the hypothesis that there may be some genetic abnormality. However, if there is some sort of genetic or inherited cause in some patients with Poland anomaly, it has not been identified. For purposes of **genetic counseling**, the Poland anomaly can be regarded as a sporadic condition with an extremely low risk of being transmitted from parent to child.

## Demographics

Poland anomaly is not common. It affects one child in about 20,000 to 30,000. Geographically, estimates of the frequency range from one in 17,213 in Japanese school children, to an average of one in 32,000 live births in British Columbia, with a low incidence, one in 52,530, in Hungary. For reasons that are unclear, Poland anomaly is three times more frequent in boys than girls.

## Signs and symptoms

The manifestations of Poland anomaly are most often limited to the physical manifestations described above. The degree to which this condition is disabling depends on which manifestations are present and their individual severity, but most often relate to disabilities in the affected arm and hand. Upon rare occasions, the Poland anomaly is associated with dextrocardia (the position of the heart is the mirror image of its normal position), **renal agenesis** (maldevelopment of the kidney) or the association with cancers such as leukemia, leiomyosarcoma and non-Hodgkin lymphoma. Intelligence is not impaired by Poland anomaly.

## Diagnosis

The diagnosis of Poland anomaly relies on physical exam and radiographic evaluation, such as the use of x rays or other imaging techniques to define abnormal or missing structures that are consistent with the criteria for Poland anomaly. There is no laboratory blood or genetic test that can be used to identify people with Poland anomaly.

## Treatment and management

During early development and progressing through until young adulthood, children with Poland anomaly should be educated and trained in behavioral and mechanical methods to adapt to their disabilities. This program is usually initiated and overseen by a team of health care professionals including a pediatrician, physical therapist, and occupational therapist. A counselor specially trained to deal with issues of disabilities in children is often helpful in assessing problem areas and encouraging healthy development of self-esteem. Support groups and community organizations for people with Poland anomaly or other disabilities often prove useful as well.

After growth development is advanced enough (usually late adolescence or early adulthood), reconstructive plastic surgery may be offered, primarily to correct cosmetic appearance. The goal of reconstruction is to restore the natural contour of the chest wall while stabilizing the chest wall defect. Chest wall reconstruction must be tailored to the requirements of each patient, but often involves moving and grafting ribs and muscles from other parts of the body to reconstruct the chest wall and breast. In addition, bioengineered cartilage or breast implants can be used to help give the chest a more normal appearance. Hand abnormalities are treated according to the severity, and requires individual consultation with a reconstructive plastic surgeon.

## Prognosis

The prognosis for people with Poland anomaly is excellent. Reconstructive surgery is safe and cosmetic corrections achieved can be significant. Associated symptoms of heart and kidney defects as well as **cancer** association are rare, but indicate that patients with

Poland anomaly should be followed closely by a physician familiar with the condition.

### Resources

**BOOKS**

Canale, S.T. *Campbell's Operative Orthopaedics*. St. Louis: Mosby, 1998.

Sabiston, D.C. *Textbook of Surgery*. Philadelphia: W.B. Saunders, 1997.

**PERIODICALS**

Urschel, H.C. "Poland's syndrome." *Chest Surgery Clinics of North America* 10 (May 2000): 393–403.

**WEBSITES**

"Poland anomaly." In *Online Mendelian Inheritance in Man*. http://www.ncbi.nlm.nih.gov/entrez/dispomim.cgi?id=173800.

**ORGANIZATIONS**

National Organization for Rare Disorders (NORD). 55 Kenosia Ave., Suite 1968, Danbury, CT 06813. (203) 744-0100 or (800) 999-6673.http://www.rarediseases.org.

Oren Traub, MD, PhD

Poland syndactyly *see* **Poland anomaly**

Poland syndrome *see* **Poland anomaly**

# Polycystic kidney disease

## Definition

Polycystic kidney disease (PKD) is one of the most common of all life-threatening human **genetic disorders**. It is an incurable genetic disorder characterized by the formation of fluid-filled cysts in the kidneys of affected individuals. These cysts multiply over time. It was originally believed that the cysts eventually caused kidney failure by crowding out the healthy kidney tissue. It is now thought that the kidney damage seen in PKD is actually the result of the body's immune system. The immune system, in its attempts to rid the kidney of the cysts, instead progressively destroys the formerly healthy kidney tissue.

## Description

A healthy kidney is about the same size as a human fist. PKD cysts, which can be as small as the head of a pin or as large as a grapefruit, can expand the kidneys until each one is bigger than a football and weighs as much as 38 lbs (17 kg).

There are two types of PKD: infantile PKD, which generally shows symptoms prior to birth; and adult onset PKD. Individuals affected with infantile PKD are often stillborn. Among the liveborn individuals affected with infantile PKD, very few of these children survive to the age of two. The adult onset form of PKD is much more common. The time and degree of symptom onset in the adult form of PKD can vary widely, even within a single family with two or more affected individuals. Symptoms of this form of PKD usually start to appear between the ages of 20 and 50. Organ deterioration progresses more slowly in adult onset PKD than it does in the infantile form; but, if left untreated, adult onset PKD also eventually leads to kidney failure.

## Genetic profile

Polycystic kidney disease is expressed as both a recessive and a dominant trait. A recessive genetic trait will not cause disease in a child unless it it inheritied from both parents. A dominant genetic trait can be inherited from just one parent. Those people affected with autosomal dominant PKD (ADPKD) have the much more common adult onset form. Those with autosomal recessive PKD (ARPKD) have the infantile form.

There are mutations on at least three genes that cause adult onset PKD. Approximately 85% of these cases are known to arise from mutations in the PKD1 gene that has been mapped to a region on the short arm of **chromosome** 16 (16p13.3-p13.12). Another 10–15% of cases of adult onset PKD are thought to be caused by mutations in the PKD2 gene that has been mapped to a region on the long arm of chromosome 4 (4q21-q23). It is thought that the remainder of the cases of PKD are caused by mutations in the

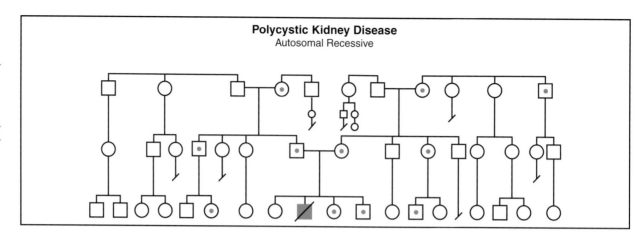

**Polycystic Kidney Disease**
Autosomal Recessive

*(Gale, a part of Cengage Learning.)*

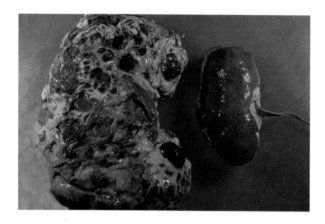

**The cyst covered kidney on the left is substantially larger than the normal kidney on the right.** *(Photo Researchers, Inc.)*

PKD3 gene, which has not yet been mapped. This unidentified "PKD3 gene" may, in fact, be more than one gene.

Adult onset PKD is transmitted from parents to their offspring as a non-sex linked (autosomal) dominant trait. This means that if either parent carries this genetic mutation, there is a 50% chance that their child will inherit this disease. In the case of two affected parents, there is a 75% probability that their children will be affected with adult onset PKD.

Infantile PKD is caused by a non-sex linked (autosomal) recessive genetic mutation that has been mapped to a region on the short arm of chromosome 6 (6p21). Both parents must be carriers of this mutation for their children to be affected with infantile PKD. In the case of two carrier parents, the probability is 25% that their child will be affected by infantile PKD.

## Demographics

One of the most common of all life-threatening genetic diseases, PKD affects more than 60,000 Americans. Over 12.5 million people worldwide are affected with PKD. Approximately one in every 400 to 1,000 people is affected with ADPKD. Another one in 10,000 are affected with ARPKD. PKD is observed in both males and females. PKD is also observed with equal probability among ethnic groups.

## Signs and symptoms

A baby born with infantile PKD has floppy, low-set ears, a pointed nose, a small chin, and folds of skin surrounding the eyes (epicanthal folds). Large, rigid masses can be felt on the back of both thighs (flanks), and the baby usually has trouble breathing.

In the early stages of adult onset PKD, many people show no symptoms. Generally, the first symptoms to develop are: high blood pressure (hypertension); general fatigue; pain in the lower back or the backs of the thighs; headaches; and/or urinary tract infections accompanied by frequent urination.

As PKD becomes more advanced, the kidneys' inability to function properly becomes more pronounced. The cysts on the kidney may begin to rupture and the kidneys tend to be much larger than normal. Individuals affected with PKD have a much higher rate of kidney stones than the rest of the population at this, and later stages, of the disease. Approximately 60% of those individuals affected with PKD develop cysts in the liver, while 10% develop cysts in the pancreas.

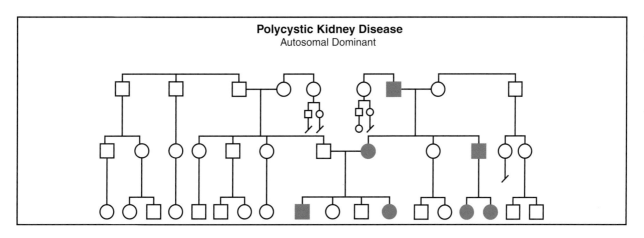

**Polycystic Kidney Disease**
Autosomal Dominant

*(Gale, a part of Cengage Learning.)*

Because the kidneys are primarily responsible for cleaning the blood, individuals affected with PKD often have problems involving the circulatory system. These include: an underproduction of red blood cells which results in an insufficient supply of oxygen to the tissues and organs (anemia); an enlarged heart (cardiac hypertrophy) probably caused by long term hypertension; and a leakage of the valve between the left chambers (auricle and ventricle) of the heart (mitral valve prolapse). Less common (affecting approximately 5% of PKD patients) are brain aneurysms. An aneurysm is an abnormal and localized bulging of the wall of a blood vessel. If an aneurysm within the brain leaks or bursts, it may cause a stroke or even death.

Other health problems associated with adult onset PKD include: chronic leg or back pain; frequent infections; and, herniations of the groin and abdomen, including herniation of the colon (diverticular disease). A herniation, or hernia, is caused when a tissue, designed to hold the shape of an underlying tissue, becomes weakened at a particular spot. The underlying tissue pushes against this weakened area until the area is no longer able to hold back the underlying tissue and the area forms an abnormal bulge through which the underlying tissue projects. Diverticular disease is caused by a weakening of the muscles that hold the shape of the organs of the digestive tract. These muscles weaken allowing these organs, particularly one section of the colon, to form sac-like projections that can trap feces and become infected, or rupture.

In the final stages of PKD, the major symptom is kidney (renal) failure. Renal failure is indicated by an increase of nitrogen (in the form of urea) in the blood (uremia, or uremic poisoning). Uremia is a rapidly fatal condition without treatment.

### Diagnosis

Many patients who have PKD do not have any symptoms. Their condition may not be discovered unless tests that detect it are performed for other reasons.

When symptoms of PKD are present, the diagnostic procedure begins with a family medical history and physical examination of the patient. If several family members have PKD, there is a strong likelihood that the patient has it too. If the disease is advanced, the doctor will be able to feel the patient's enlarged kidneys. Heart murmur, high blood pressure, and other signs of cardiac impairment can also be detected.

Urinalysis and a blood test called creatine clearance can indicate how effectively the kidneys are functioning. Scanning procedures using intravenous dye reveal kidney enlargement or deformity and scarring caused by cysts. Ultrasound and computed tomography (CT) scans can reveal kidney enlargement and the cysts that caused it. CT scans can highlight cyst-damaged areas of the kidneys. A sampling of the kidney cells (biopsy) may be performed to verify the diagnosis.

### Treatment and management

There is no way to prevent cysts from forming or becoming enlarged, or to prevent PKD from progressing to kidney failure. Treatment goals include preserving healthy kidney tissue; controlling symptoms; and preventing infection and other complications.

If adult PKD is diagnosed before symptoms become evident, urinalysis and other diagnostic tests are performed at six-week intervals to monitor the patient's health status. If results indicate the presence of infection or another PKD-related health problem, aggressive antibiotic therapy is initiated to prevent inflammation that can accelerate disease progression; iron supplements or infusion of red blood cells are used to treat anemia; and surgery may be needed to drain cysts that bleed, cause pain, have become infected, or interfere with normal kidney function.

Lowering high blood pressure can slow loss of kidney function. Blood-pressure control, which is the cornerstone of PKD treatment, is difficult to achieve. Therapy may include anti-hypertensive medications, diuretic medications, and/or a low-salt diet. As kidney function declines, some patients need dialysis and/or a kidney transplant.

There is no known way to prevent PKD, but certain lifestyle modifications can help control symptoms. People who have PKD should not drink heavily or smoke. They should not use aspirin, non-steroidal anti-inflammatory drugs (NSAIDs), or other prescription or over-the-counter medications that can impair kidney function. Individuals affected with PKD should eat a balanced diet, exercise regularly, and maintain a weight appropriate for their height, age, and body type. Regular medical monitoring is also recommended.

### Prognosis

There is no known cure for PKD. Those affected with infantile PKD generally die before the age of two. In adults, untreated disease can be rapidly fatal or continue to progress slowly, even after symptoms of kidney failure appear. About half of all adults with PKD also develop kidney failure. Unless the patient undergoes dialysis or has a kidney transplant, they usually do not survive more than four years after diagnosis.

Although medical treatment can temporarily alleviate symptoms of PKD, the expanding cysts continue to increase pressure on the kidneys. Kidney failure and uremic poisoning (accumulation of waste products the body is unable to eliminate) generally cause death about 10 years after symptoms first appear.

Medications used to fight **cancer** and reduce elevated cholesterol levels have slowed the advance of PKD in laboratory animals. They may soon be used to treat adults and children who have the disease. Researchers are also evaluating the potential benefits of anti-inflammatory drugs, which may prevent the scarring that destroys kidney function.

## Resources

### BOOKS

Shaw, Michael, ed. *Everything You Need to Know About Diseases.* Springhouse, PA: Springhouse Corporation, 1996.

### PERIODICALS

Koptides, M., and C. Deltas. "Autosomal dominant polycystic kidney disease: Molecular genetics and molecular pathogenesis." *Human Genetics* (August 2000): 115–26.

Pei, Y., et al.,"Bilineal disease and trans-heterozygotes in autosmal dominant polycystic kidney disease." *American Journal of Human Genetics* (February 2001): 355–63.

### WEBSITES

Brochert, Adam, MD. "Polycystic Kidney Disease." (September 4, 2000). *HealthAnswers.* http://www.health answers.com/library/library_fset.asp.

Cooper, Joel R. "Treating Polycystic Kidney Disease. What Does the Future Hold?" *Coolware, Inc.* http://www.coolware.com/health/medical_reporter/kidney1.html.

Online Mendelian Inheritance in Man (OMIM). http://www.ncbi.nlm.nih.gov.

*Polycystic Kidney Disease Access Center.* http://www.nhpress.com/pkd/.

### ORGANIZATIONS

Polycystic Kidney Disease Foundation. 4901 Main Street, Kansas City, MO 64112-2634. (800) PKD-CURE. http://www.pkdcure.org/home.htm.

Paul A. Johnson

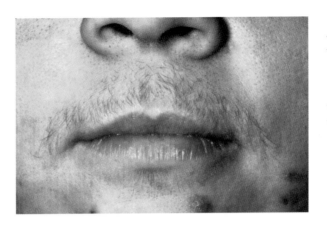

**Females affected with Polycystic ovary syndrome often have excessive facial hair, known as hirsutism.** *(Photo Researchers, Inc.)*

# Polycystic ovary syndrome

## Definition

Polycystic ovary syndrome (PCOS), formerly Stein-Leventhal syndrome, is a disorder in which women do not experience normal release of eggs from the ovaries, they have an abnormal production of male hormones, and their body is resistant to the effects of the hormone insulin. The disorder results in infertility, abnormal masculinization, and increased risk of developing heart disease and certain cancers.

## Description

The normal function of the female reproductive system is complex, requiring the interplay of different organ systems. One set of important organs are the ovaries. The ovaries are two small structures contained in the lower abdomen, on either side of the uterus, that contain small immature eggs, called ova. Ova are stored within the ovaries in individual structures called follicles.

In a monthly cycle, a part of the brain called the pituitary gland secretes two substances into the blood stream—lutenizing hormone (LH) and follicle-stimulating hormone (FSH). As certain levels of LH and FSH build in the blood stream, the follicles of the eggs begin to swell and grow, creating cysts. Eventually, the changing levels of LH and FSH cause one of the ovarian cysts to burst open, releasing a mature egg. This process by which an egg is released from the ovary is called ovulation.

Once a mature egg is released from the ovary, it passes into the fallopian tubes, tube-like structures that are passageways to the uterus. If sperm cells from the male are present within the fallopian tubes, they will join with the egg in a process called fertilization. The fertilized egg can then pass into the uterus and implant into the thickened wall of the uterus where it can develop into a fetus. If no sperm cells are present, the mature egg goes unfertilized and is lost, along with the thickened later of the uterus, in a monthly process called menstruation.

Polycystic ovary syndrome (PCOS), first described by I. F. Stein and M. L. Leventhal in 1935, is a disorder in which normal ovulation does not occur. The term "polycystic" derives from the fact that the egg-containing cysts in the ovaries do not burst open, resulting in enlarged ovaries containing many swelled cysts. The reason for this problem in ovulation is unclear, however several abnormalities have been characterized in women with PCOS. First, there is a disturbance in the production of LH and FSH by the pituitary, leading to altered levels of the substances in the blood stream. There is also evidence that the ovaries do not respond appropriately to the FH and LSH that is present. Second, there is an abnormal over-production of male hormones, called

## KEY TERMS

**Acanthosis nigricans**—A skin condition characterized by darkly pigmented areas of velvety wart-like growths. Acanthosis nigricans usually affects the skin of the armpits, neck, and groin.

**Androgens**—A group of steroid hormones that stimulate the development of male sex organs and male secondary sexual characteristics.

**Diabetes**—An inability to control the levels of sugar in the blood due to an abnormality in the production of, or response to, the hormone insulin.

**Fallopian tube**—Either of a pair of tubes that conduct ova from the ovaries to the uterus.

**Follicle**—A pouch-like depression.

**Follicle-stimulating hormone (FSH)**—A hormone that stimulates estrogen in females and sperm production in males.

**Hirsuitism**—The presence of coarse hair on the face, chest, upper back, or abdomen in a female as a result of excessive androgen production.

**Hormone**—A chemical messenger produced by the body that is involved in regulating specific bodily functions such as growth, development, and reproduction.

**Infertility**—Inability in a woman to become pregnant.

**Insulin**—A hormone produced by the pancreas that is secreted into the bloodstream and regulates blood sugar levels.

**Lutenizing hormone (LH)**—A hormone secreted by the pituitary gland that regulates the menstrual cycle

and triggers ovulation in females. In males it stimulates the testes to produce testosterone.

**Masculinization**—Development of excess body and facial hair, deepening of the voice, and increase in muscle bulk in a female due to a hormone disorder.

**Menstruation**—Discharge of blood and fragments of the uterine wall from the vagina in a monthly cycle in the absence of pregnancy.

**Mutation**—A permanent change in the genetic material that may alter a trait or characteristic of an individual, or manifest as disease, and can be transmitted to offspring.

**Ova**—Another name for the egg cells that are located in the ovaries.

**Ovary**—The female reproductive organ that produces the reproductive cell (ovum) and female hormones.

**Ovulation**—The monthly process by which an ovarian follicle or cyst ruptures, releasing a mature egg cell.

**Pituitary gland**—A small gland at the base of the brain responsible for releasing many hormones, including luteinizing hormone (LH) and follicle-stimulating hormone (FSH).

**Uterus**—A muscular, hollow organ of the female reproductive tract. The uterus contains and nourishes the embryo and fetus from the time the fertilized egg is implanted until birth.

androgens, by the ovaries and the adrenal gland. Finally, women with PCOS are resistant to the effects of the hormone, insulin. Insulin is a hormone made in the pancreas that is responsible for transport of sugar from the blood into the cells. While these abnormalities have been well characterized, it is unclear whether they cause PCOS, or whether they are a result the disease.

### Genetic profile

Women diagnosed with PCOS frequently have relatives with symptoms similar to that seen in the disorder. As a result of these observations, many scientists have proposed that genetic factors play a role in the disease. Over the past few decades, researchers have identified families in which PCOS appears to be inherited with an autosomal dominant or an X-linked pattern. However, these cases are rare and do not hold true for the majority of people with PCOS.

Current theories suggest that different genetic changes may result in PCOS or that multiple genetic factors are needed for the full manifestation of the disease. Abnormalities in several genes have been associated with PCOS, including mutations in the genes for follistatin (locus 5p14), 17-beta-hydroxysteroid dehydrogenase (locus 9p22), and a cytochrome P450 enzyme (locus 15q23-q24). Each of these genes plays a different role in the response to LH and FSH, or in the conversion of male hormones to female hormones, although their relationship to PCOS is unclear. Ongoing research is likely to identify further genetic mutations that are associated with PCOS.

### Demographics

Estimates of the prevalence of PCOS in the general population have ranged from 2-20% with recent studies suggesting that 3-6% of women of reproductive age are affected by the disorder. This makes PCOS one of the most common hormone disorders in women of reproductive age.

It is unclear whether this disease is distributed uniformly among different geographical areas and ethnic groups, however, studies performed in 1999 show the prevalence of this disorder in the United States is just over 3% in African-American females and almost 5% in Caucasian females. The prevalence of PCOS in Greek women was shown to be higher, nearly 7%.

### Signs and symptoms

The first signs of PCOS tend to manifest at puberty. As a result of the failure to ovulate normally, young women with PCOS may fail to menstruate or menstruate only erratically. A small percentage of women may have normal menstrual cycles. Women affected with PCOS often experience infertility, an inability to become pregnant. Additionally, women with PCOS tend to gain weight, and 70% eventually become obese.

The overproduction of androgens leads to changes in the body that are more typical of male development. For example, approximately 70% of women with PCOS will show hair growth on the face, chest, stomach, and thighs (hirsuitism). Simultaneously, they show thinning of the hair more typical of male-pattern baldness. Other male characteristics, such as deep voice, acne, and increased sex drive may also be present, and affected women often have decreased breast size.

Women with PCOS do not respond appropriately to the hormone, insulin. As a result, 15% of women with PCOS may develop high levels of sugar in the blood later in life, a condition known as **diabetes**. Resistance to insulin is also associated with dark, warty skin growths in the groin and armpits, known as acanthosis nigricans.

Untreated PCOS is a risk factor for the development of several dangerous conditions. The hormone abnormalities in PCOS place women at considerable risk for endometrial **cancer** and possibly **breast cancer**. The risk of endometrial cancer is three times higher in women with PCOS than in normal women, and small studies suggest that the risk of breast cancer may by three to four times higher. PCOS also results in increased risk of high blood pressure, diabetes, and high cholesterol, all of which contribute to heart disease and stroke.

### Diagnosis

A diagnostic search for PCOS is usually initiated when women experience an absence of menstrual periods for at least six months, an inability to become pregnant, and/or abnormal hair growth or acne. A comprehensive physical exam performed at that time may reveal excessive body hair, low voice, acanthosis nigricans, or obesity. Enlarged ovaries are also identifiable on pelvic examination in about 50% of patients.

Blood tests can be performed that may yield results consistent with PCOS, including abnormal levels of LH and FSH (typically in a ratio of 3:1), abnormally high levels of androgens (testosterone, DHEA, DHEAS), abnormally high levels of insulin, and abnormally low levels of a substance called sex hormone-binding globulin. In addition, a physician may perform a diagnostic test called a progesterone challenge. In this test, a physician administers a hormone called progesterone to the patient to determine if it will provoke menstruation. If menstruation does occur in response to the progesterone, it is likely that a patient has PCOS.

Finally, an ultrasound examination of the ovaries may be performed to determine if large cystic follicles can be documented. With this approach, the diagnosis of PCOS is based on the finding of more than eight enlarged follicles in the ovary.

### Treatment and management

There is no cure for PCOS, thus treatment focuses on several goals, including the restoration of the menstrual cycle, blocking the effect of androgens, reducing insulin resistance, lowering the risk of cancer and heart disease, and possibly restoring ovulation and fertility.

In patients who do not desire pregnancy, hormones can be administered in the form of birth control pills, which may result in normal menstrual cycles, decreased hair growth and acne, and a lower risk of developing endometrial cancer. Although women will note a decrease in hair growth after approximately six months of treatment with birth control pills, additional cosmetic hair removal therapy is often necessary. In women who do not respond appropriately to birth control pills, another medication known as luprolide (Lupron) can be used, but with more long term side effects (e.g., hot flushes, bone demineralization, atrophic vaginitis).

Other types of medication can be used to block the effects of androgens. When these medications are taken with birth control pills, 75% of women report decreased body hair growth. The most commonly used medications to block androgen effects are spironolactone (Aldactone), flutamide (Eulexin), and cyproterone (Cyprostat).

Treatment with medications that restore the body's normal response to insulin has been shown to decrease LH and androgen levels. Recent studies have demonstrated that such agents restore the menstrual cycle in 68-95% of patients treated for as short a time as four to six months. One of the most commonly used medications to improve the effects of insulin is metformin (Glucophage).

In patients who are trying to become pregnant, a physician can administer medications that will cause ovulation. The main medication used to induce ovulation is clomiphene citrate (Clomid). Ovulation is successful in approximately 75% of women treated with clomiphene, but only 30-40% of women will successfully become pregnant. Another medication, follitropin alpha (Gonal- F), has achieved pregnancy rates of 58-82%, but may cause more side effects and frequently results in more than one baby per pregnancy.

Some women who do not respond to medications may undergo surgery to remove portions of the ovary. For reasons that are not completely understood, removal of a portion of the ovary may result in some degree of normal menstrual cycles.

While medications and surgery may provide a degree of symptomatic relief for some women, other simultaneous strategies can increase their benefits. Behavior modifications, including weight reduction, diet and exercise, are recommended for all women with PCOS. As little as a 7% reduction in body weight can lead to a significant decrease in androgen levels and to the resumption of ovulation in obese women with PCOS. Cosmetic techniques, including electrolysis (destruction of the hair follicle using electricity) and laser therapy, may be used to decrease hair growth. Finally, women should be seen regularly for full physical examinations including pelvic exams to aid in the early detection of ovarian, breast, and uterine cancer and should be managed by an interdisciplinary health care team including a primary care physician, obstetrician/gynecologist and reproductive endocrinologist.

### Prognosis

While PCOS is one of the most common hormone disorders in young women, proper diagnosis and treatment has greatly increased the quality of life in these individuals. Roughly half of women with PCOS will be able to achieve pregnancy, and about three-fourths will see reduction in masculine traits such as hair growth with proper medical treatment. Initiation of vigorous exercise and a restricted diet may result in even better outcomes. Patients with PCOS are at higher risk of developing diabetes, heart disease, and certain cancers and should be seen regularly by a physician. Barring these developments, life span in

## QUESTIONS TO ASK YOUR DOCTOR

- How common is polycystic ovary syndrome in the general public?
- What medical conditions are associated with this disorder?
- How is polycystic ovary syndrome treated, and how effective are those treatments?
- Can you recommend an Internet site or two that will provide additional information on this condition?

patients with PCOS is approximately the same as the general population.

### Resources

#### BOOKS

"Disorders of Ovarian Function" In *Williams Textbook of Endocrinology,* edited by J. D. Wilson. Philadelphia: W.B. Saunders, 1998, pp 781-801.

"Hypofunction of the Ovaries." In *Nelson Textbook of Pediatrics,* edited by R.E. Behrman. Philadelphia: W.B. Saunders, 2000, pp 1752-1758.

*Kistner's Gynecology and Women's Health,* edited by K. J. Ryan. St. Louis: Mosby, 1999.

#### PERIODICALS

Hunter, M.H. "Polycystic Ovary Syndrome: It's Not Just Infertility." *American Family Physician* 62 (September 2000): 1079-1088.

#### WEBSITES

"Polycystic Ovary Syndrome 1." *OMIM—Online Mendelian Inheritance in Man.*http://www.ncbi.nlm.nih.gov/entrez/dispomim.cgi?id=184700.

#### ORGANIZATIONS

Polycystic Ovarian Syndrome Association. PO Box 80517, Portland, OR 97280. (877) 775-PCOS. http://www.pcosupport.org.

Oren Traub, MD, PhD

# Polydactyly

### Definition

Polydactyly is the presence of extra fingers and toes (digits) at birth. Rather than having five fingers per hand or five toes per foot, an infant with polydactyly will have

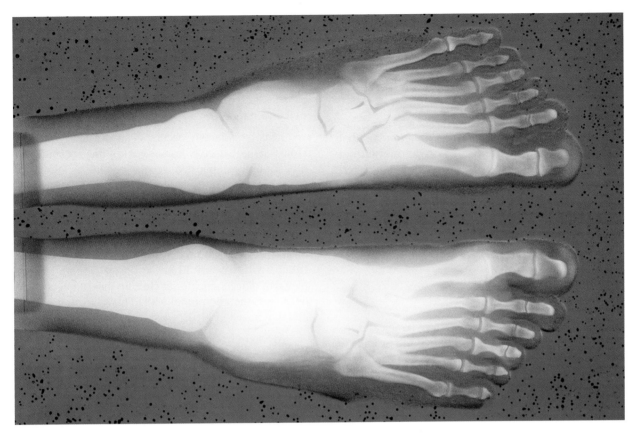

**An enhanced x ray showing feet with six toes each.** *(Chris Bjornberg / Photo Researchers, Inc.)*

six or more digits on either the hands or feet that may or may not be fully formed.

### Description

Polydactyly, also called supernumerary digits or extra digits, can occur on either the hands or feet and the extent of the digit development is variable. Individuals with polydactyly can have one small extra rudimentary finger or toe on one of their hands or feet or they can have fully formed extra digits on both their hands and feet. Extra digits can be fully formed or rudimentary and may contain no bones at all. Rudimentary digits may only be attached by a thin stalk of skin. Individual are described as having isolated polydactyly if they only have extra digits and have no other obvious malformations. Most of the time, polydactyly occurs as an isolated condition, but it can occur as a symptom of different genetic syndromes. There are more than 100 different genetic syndromes that have polydactyly as one of their findings.

Different experts have different systems for describing polydactyly. The two most common systems describe the location and extent of the polydactyly. Preaxial, central, and postaxial are the terms used to describe the location of the extra digit. If the extra digit is located on the side of the hand by the thumb or on the side of the foot by the big toe, then a person is diagnosed with preaxial polydactyly. Postaxial polydactyly occurs when the extra digit is located on the side of the hand or foot by the fifth digit (the pinky or small toe), and central polydactyly occurs when the extra digit is located in between the thumb and pinky or between the big and little toes.

Type A and type B are used to describe the variable size of the digits in polydactyly. Extra digits can be fully formed with the right number of joints and bones, or they can be poorly formed with the wrong number of joints and no bones (rudimentary digits). Fully formed digits are type A polydactyly and poorly formed or rudimentary digits are type B polydactyly. Thus, a person with a small rudimentary digit on the outside of the pinky is diagnosed with isolated postaxial polydactyly type B.

### Genetic profile

Polydactyly is caused by errors that occur during the process of fetal development. There are a number of genes that determine the pattern of hands and feet. Genes are the basic unit of **inheritance** and provide the instructions for how a body is to form. A difference or error in one of these genes can lead to one of the different types of polydactyly. The exact genes responsible for polydactyly have not been found.

The three different types of polydactyly, postaxial, central, and preaxial, appear to have different patterns of inheritance. Postaxial polydactyly is inherited as an autosomal dominant that shows variable expressivity. The inheritance patterns for postaxial and central polydactyly are not well understood.

Genes are made of **deoxyribonucleic acid (DNA)** and located on chromosomes. DNA is composed of four units (called bases) that are designated A, T, G, and C. The sequence of the bases contains the instructions for making each of the body's structures. A change in one of the DNA letters making up a gene is a mutation. In some cases, mutations can alter the instructions and lead to malformations.

All individuals pass their chromosomes on to their children, and therefore pass down their DNA instructions (genes). Genes always come in pairs: one pair each from the mother and one from the father. In an autosomal dominant disorder, only one gene needs to be altered for an individual to have the disorder or malformation. If an individual has the gene change (mutation) that causes postaxial polydactyly, there is a 50% chance that the disorder will be passed onto an offspring.

While the gene for polydactyly is passed unchanged from generation to generation, it often manifests itself very differently in different individuals. For example, a father may have the gene for polydactyly and have had a very small nubbin of soft skin on the outer edge of his hand. However, his child with the same gene may have extra fully formed digits on both hands and feet. This difference in how the gene manifests is called variable expression. The causes of variable expression are not well understood.

Most polydactyly occurs as an isolated condition. However, polydactyly can occur as one symptom of other more complicated genetic conditions. Some of the syndromes that polydactyly is a feature of are **trisomy 13** syndrome, **Meckel-Gruber syndrome**, **Bardet-Biedl syndrome**, and **Ellis-van Creveld syndrome**.

Trisomy 13 is a rare, usually lethal, genetic syndrome cause by an extra number 13 **chromosome**. Infants with trisomy 13 have poor growth and multiple birth defects, including **cleft lip**, heart defects, and defects of the abdominal wall. This syndrome is usually diagnosed at birth.

Meckel-Gruber syndrome is an autosomal recessive syndrome characterized by poor growth, **encephalocele** (opening on the spine), postaxial polydactyly, and cystic kidneys. This syndrome is usually diagnosed at birth.

Bardet-Biedl is a rare autosomal recessive genetic syndrome characterized by obesity, postaxial polydactyly, retina (eye) abnormalities, and mental retardation. Often, individuals with this syndrome are not diagnosed until childhood.

Ellis-van Creveld syndrome is a rare autosomal recessive genetic syndrome common in the Amish population. Infants with this syndrome have skeletal abnormalities, short arms and legs, and polydactyly. About half of these infants also have a heart defect. Most infants with this syndrome are diagnosed shortly after birth or in infancy.

### Demographics

Polydactyly is a relatively common birth defect that occurs in all ethnic groups. Postaxial polydactyly is the most common form of polydactyly and accounts for about 80% of cases. It occurs in about one in 2,000 Caucasian births, and is about 10 times more common in individuals with African ancestry. In about 30% of cases of polydactyly, there is a positive family history and about 50% of polydactyly is bilateral (affects both sides of the body). Preaxial polydactyly is the most common form of polydactyly in individuals of Asian ancestry.

### Signs and symptoms

The presence of polydactyly is most often noted at birth. While it can be shocking for some parents, the presence of isolated polydactyly poses no immediate health risks for the infant. It is a very common malformation that is easily treated (surgically removed).

Individuals with polydactyly can have one small extra rudimentary finger or toe on one of their hands or feet or they can have fully formed extra digits on both their hands and feet. Extra digits can be fully formed or rudimentary and may contain no bones at all. Rudimentary digits may only be attached by a thin stalk of skin.

## Diagnosis

The diagnosis of polydactyly is usually made shortly after birth by physical examination. It can also be diagnosed prenatally or before a baby is born. Polydactyly can sometimes be seen on a **prenatal ultrasound** (sonogram) as early as 18 weeks gestation. If polydactyly is noticed on a sonogram, other medical tests may be suggested to make sure that the fetus does not have any of the problems associated with other genetic syndromes. A detailed sonogram should be done to measure the limbs and growth of the baby, while an **amniocentesis** may be offered to do a chromosomal analysis of the fetus. A fetal echocardiograph (heart ultrasound) may be performed to rule out heart abnormalities. In addition, other tests may be done to rule out other syndromes.

## Treatment and management

When polydactyly is noted in an infant, a number of the following tests may be done, including:

- A very thorough medical examination to make sure that there are no other birth defects or abnormalities.
- A medical family history to determine if anyone else in the family has had polydactyly or any other syndromes associated with polydactyly.
- X rays to determine the extent of the polydactyly (i.e., whether the digit contains bone or is just skin).
- Laboratory tests, such as chromosome analysis, enzyme assays, and further x rays, may be ordered to determine is a suspected disorder is present.

While the initial diagnosis may shocking to most parents, isolated polydactyly has no health consequences and is usually surgically corrected before the infant leaves the hospital.

Polydactyly is rarely a functional concern and the removal of the extra digit is often for cosmetic purposes or to aid in the wearing of shoes. The age at which surgery is performed depends on the extent and degree of the polydactlyly. A type B, or partially formed, digit that contains no bone may be removed before the infant leaves the hospital. A type A polydactyly is often corrected when the patient is one year of age.

Complex polydactlyly (central polydactyly) may require multiple surgeries to improve function and cosmetic appearance.

## Prognosis

The prognosis for isolated polydactyly is excellent. When polydactyly is associated with another genetic syndrome, the prognosis is dependent on the presence of other features of that syndrome. Many of the genetic syndromes that have polydactyly as one of their symptoms are quite serious, and early death and significant disability are possibilities.

## Resources

### WEB SITES

National Library of Medicine, Medline Plus. (April 11, 2005.) http://www.nlm.nih.gov/medlineplus/ency/article/003176.htm.

Kathleen A. Fergus, MS, CGC

Polyps and spots syndrome *see* **Peutz-Jeghers syndrome**

Polysplenia syndrome *see* **Asplenia**

# Pompe disease

## Definition

Pompe disease, also called acid maltase deficiency, is a non-sex linked recessive genetic disorder that is the most serious of the **glycogen storage diseases** affecting muscle tissue. It is one of several known congenital (present at birth) muscular diseases (myopathies), as distinct from a **muscular dystrophy**, which is a family of muscle disorders arising from faulty nutrition. The Dutch pathologist J. C. Pompe first described this genetic disorder in 1932.

## Description

Pompe disease is also known as glycogen storage disease type II (GSD II) because it is characterized by a buildup of glycogen in the muscle cells. Glycogen is the chemical substance muscles use to store sugars and starches for later use. Some of the sugars and starches from the diet that are not immediately put to use are converted into glycogen and then stored in the muscle cells. These stores of glycogen are then broken down

## KEY TERMS

**Acid maltase**—The enzyme that regulates the amount of glycogen stored in muscle cells. When too much glycogen is present, acid maltase is released to break it down into waste products.

**Acidosis**—A condition of decreased alkalinity resulting from abnormally high acid levels (low pH) in the blood and tissues. Usually indicated by sickly sweet breath, headaches, nausea, vomiting, and visual impairments.

**Catalyze**—Facilitate. A catalyst lowers the amount of energy required for a specific chemical reaction to occur. Catalysts are not used up in the chemical reactions they facilitate.

**Enzyme**—A protein that catalyzes a biochemical reaction or change without changing its own structure or function.

**Exon**—The expressed portion of a gene. The exons of genes are those portions that actually chemically code for the protein or polypeptide that the gene is responsible for producing.

**Fibroblast**—Cells that form connective tissue fibers like skin.

**Glycogen**—The chemical substance used by muscles to store sugars and starches for later use. It is composed of repeating units of glucose.

**Hypoglycemia**—An abnormally low glucose (blood sugar) concentration in the blood.

**Intron**—That portion of the DNA sequence of a gene that is not directly involved in the formation of the chemical that the gene codes for.

**Myopathy**—Any abnormal condition or disease of the muscle.

**Serum CK test**—A blood test that determines the amount of the enzyme creatine kinase (CK) in the blood serum. An elevated level of CK in the blood indicates that muscular degeneration has occurred and/or is occurring.

into sugars, as the muscles require them. Acid maltase is the chemical substance that regulates the amount of glycogen stored in muscle cells. When too much glycogen begins to accumulate in a muscle cell, acid maltase is released to break down this excess glycogen into products that will be either reabsorbed for later use in other cells or passed out of the body via the digestive system. Individuals affected with Pompe disease have either a complete inability or a severely limited ability

to produce acid maltase. Since these individuals cannot produce the amounts of acid maltase required to process excess glycogen in the muscle cells, the muscle cells become overrun with glycogen. This excess glycogen in the muscle cells causes a progressive degeneration of the muscle tissues.

Acid maltase is an enzyme. An enzyme is a chemical that facilitates (catalyzes) the chemical reaction of another chemical or of other chemicals; it is neither a reactant nor a product in the chemical reaction that it catalyzes. As a result, enzymes are not used up in chemical reactions, but rather recycled. One molecule of an enzyme may be used to catalyze the same chemical reaction over and over again several hundreds of thousands of times. All the enzymes necessary for catalyzing the various reactions of human life are produced within the body by genes. Genetic enzyme deficiency disorders, such as Pompe disease, result from only one cause: the affected individual cannot produce enough of the necessary enzyme because the **gene** designed to make the enzyme is faulty. Enzymes are not used up in chemical reactions, but they do eventually wear out, or accidentally get expelled. Also, as an individual grows, they may require greater quantities of an enzyme. Therefore, most enzyme deficiency disorders will have a time component to them. Individuals with no ability to produce a particular enzyme may show effects of this deficiency at birth or shortly thereafter. Individuals with only a partial ability to produce a particular enzyme may not show the effects of this deficiency until their need for the enzyme, because of growth or maturation, has outpaced their ability to produce it.

The level of ability of individuals with Pompe disease to produce acid maltase, or thier ability to sustain existing levels of acid maltase, are the sole determinants of the severity of the observed symptoms in individuals and the age of onset of these symptoms.

Pompe disease is categorized into three separate types based on the age of onset of symptoms in the affected individual. Type a, or infantile, Pompe disease usually begins to produce observable symptoms in affected individuals between the ages of two and five months. Type b, or childhood, Pompe disease usually begins to produce observable symptoms in affected individuals in early childhood. This type generally progresses much more slowly than infantile Pompe disease. Type c, or adult, Pompe disease generally begins to produce observable symptoms in affected individuals in the third or fourth decades of life. This type progresses even more slowly than childhood Pompe disease.

## Genetic profile

The locus of the gene responsible for Pompe disease has been localized to 17q23. The severity of the associated symptoms and the age of onset in affected individuals have been closely tied to the particular mutation at this locus. Three specific mutations and one additional mutation type have been demonstrated to occur along the gene responsible for Pompe disease. Each of these is associated with varying symptoms.

A gene is a particular segment of a particular **chromosome**. However, within the segment containing a particular gene there are two types of areas: introns and exons. Introns are sections of the segment that do not actively participate in the functioning of the gene. Exons are those sections that do actively participate in gene function. A typical gene consists of several areas that are exons divided by several areas of introns.

One mutation on the gene responsible for the production of acid maltase is a deletion of exon 18. A second mutation on the gene responsible for the production of acid maltase is the deletion of a single base pair of exon 2. Both these mutations are associated with a complete inability of the affected individual to produce acid maltase. Individuals with these mutations will invariably be affected with infantile (type a) Pompe disease.

The third mutation on the gene responsible for the production of acid maltase is a complicated mutation within intron 1 that causes the cutting out of exon 2. This mutation is generally not complete in every copy of the gene within a given individual so it is associated with a partial ability of the affected individual to produce acid maltase. Individuals with this mutation will be affected with either childhood (type b), or, more commonly, adult (type c) Pompe disease. In fact, greater than 70% of all individuals affected with adult Pompe disease possess this particular mutation.

The final mutation class known to occur on the gene responsible for the production of acid maltase is missense at various locations along the various exons. Missense is the alteration of a single coding sequence (codon) that codes for a single amino acid that will be used to build the protein that is the precursor to the acid maltase molecule. These missense mutations generally prevent the production of acid maltase and lead to infantile (type a) Pompe disease.

The exact mutations responsible for the other 30% of the adult (type c) and the remainder of the childhood (type b) Pompe disease cases have not yet been determined.

## Demographics

Pompe disease is observed in approximately one in every 100,000 live births. In 2000, it was estimated that between 5,000 and 10,000 people were living somewhere in the developed world with a diagnosed case of Pompe disease. It is observed in equal numbers of males and females and across all ethnic subpopulations.

Since Pompe disease is a recessive disorder, both parents must be carriers of the disorder for it to be passed to their children. In the case of carrier parents with one child affected by Pompe disease, there is a 25% likelihood that their next child will also be affected with the disorder. However, because type c (adult) Pompe disease generally does not show symptoms in the affected individual until that individual is past 30, it is possible for an affected individual to parent children. In this case, the probability of a second child being affected with Pompe disease is 50%. Should two affected individuals bear offspring; the probability of their child being affected with Pompe disease is 100%.

In families with more than one affected child, the symptoms of the siblings will closely correspond. That is, if one child develops infantile Pompe disease, a second child, if affected with the disorder, will also develop the infantile form.

## Signs and symptoms

The symptoms of Pompe disease vary depending on the severity of the deficiency of acid maltase in the affected individual. The most acid maltase deficient individuals will develop infantile Pompe disease and will exhibit the most severe symptoms. Likewise, the least acid maltase deficient individuals will develop adult Pompe disease and have less severe symptoms.

Infantile (type a) Pompe disease is characterized by the so-called "floppy baby" syndrome. This condition is caused by extreme weakness and lack of tone of the skeletal muscles. This observed weakness in the skeletal muscles is accompanied by the much more serious problems of overall weakness of the heart muscle (cardiomyopathy) and the muscles of the respiratory system, primarily the diaphragm. Enlargement of the heart (cardiomegaly), tongue and liver are also observed. Glycogen accumulation is observed in most tissues of the body.

Childhood (type b) Pompe disease is characterized by weakness of the muscles of the trunk and large muscle mass with little muscle tone. This is due to a buildup of glycogen in the muscle cells. The heart and liver of those affected with childhood maltase deficiency are generally normal. However, there is a progressive weakening of the skeletal and respiratory muscles. The observed muscle weakness in childhood Pompe disease affected individuals gradually progresses from the muscles of the trunk to the muscles of the arms and the legs. Glycogen accumulation is observed primarily in the muscle tissues.

Adult (type c) Pompe disease is characterized by fatigue in younger affected individuals and by weakness of the muscles of the trunk in older affected individuals. The observed muscle weakness in adult Pompe disease affected individuals gradually progresses from the muscles of the trunk to the muscles of the arms and the legs. High blood pressure in the artery that delivers blood to the lungs (pulmonary hypertension) is also generally observed in affected adults. Glycogen accumulation is observed primarily in the muscle tissues.

### Diagnosis

Infantile Pompe disease is generally diagnosed between the ages of two and five months when symptoms begin to appear. The first indicator of infantile Pompe disease is general weakness and lack of tone (hypotonia) of the skeletal muscles, particularly those of the trunk.

A blood test called a serum CK test is the most commonly used test to determine whether muscular degeneration is causing an observed muscular weakness. It is used to rule out other possible causes of muscle weakness, such as nerve problems. To determine the CK serum level, blood is drawn and separated into the part containing the cells and the liquid remaining (the serum). The serum is then tested for the amount of creatine kinase (CK) present. Creatine kinase is an enzyme found almost exclusively in the muscle cells and not typically in high amounts in the bloodstream. Higher than normal amounts of CK in the blood serum indicate that muscular degeneration is occurring: that the muscle cells are breaking open and spilling their contents, including the enzyme creatine kinase into the bloodstream. Individuals affected with Pompe disease have extremely high serum CK levels. Those affected with infantile Pompe disease have much higher serum CK levels than those affected with the childhood or adult forms. The actual serum CK level, once observed to be higher than normal, can also be used to differentiate between various types of muscular degeneration.

Serum CK levels cannot be used to distinguish Pompe disease from other glycogen storage diseases. Pompe disease (type II glycogen storage disease) is differentially diagnosed from type I glycogen storage disease by blood tests for abnormally low levels of glucose (hypoglycemia) and a low pH, or high acidity, (acidosis). Hypoglycemia and acidosis are both characteristic of type I glycogen storage disease, but neither is characteristic of Pompe disease.

It is sometimes possible to determine the abnormally low levels of the acid maltase enzyme in the white blood cells (leukocytes) removed during the above blood serum tests. If these levels can be determined and they are abnormally low, a definitive diagnosis of Pompe disease can be made. When the results of this leukocyte test are not clear, Pompe disease types a and b may be positively diagnosed by testing muscles cells removed from the affected individual (muscle biopsy) for the actual absence or lack of sufficient acid maltase. This test is 100% accurate for type a and type b Pompe disease, but it may give improper results for type c Pompe disease. In these hard-to-identify cases of type c Pompe disease, an identical test to that performed on the leukocytes may be performed on cultured fibroblasts grown from a sample from the affected individual. This test is 100% accurate for type c Pompe disease.

### Treatment and management

The only potential treatment for this deficiency is enzyme replacement therapy. This approach was initially undertaken in the 1970s for Pompe disease with no success. A new enzyme replacement therapy is, however, currently in human clinical trials that began in 1999.

### Prognosis

Pompe disease of all three types is 100% fatal. Individuals affected with infantile Pompe disease generally die from heart or respiratory failure prior to age one. Individuals affected with childhood Pompe disease generally die from respiratory failure between the ages of three and 24. Individuals affected with adult Pompe disease generally die from respiratory failure within 10 to 20 years of the onset of symptoms.

Human clinical trials involving enzyme replacement therapy, in which a synthetic form of acid maltase is administered to affected individuals, were begun in 1999 at Duke University Medical Center in North Carolina and Erasmus University Rotterdam in the Netherlands. Genzyme Corporation and Pharming Group N. V. announced the first results of these trials in a joint press release on October 5, 2000. These two companies currently own the worldwide patent rights to the synthetic enzyme being studied. As of early 2001, these clinical trials were in phase I/II of the three-stage testing process for use in humans.

## Resources

### PERIODICALS

Chen, Y., and A. Amalfitano. "Towards a molecular therapy for glycogen storage disease type II (Pompe disease)." *Molecular Medicine Today* (June 2000): 245-51.

Poenaru, L. "Approach to gene therapy of glycogenosis type II (Pompe disease)." *Molecular Genetics and Metabolism* (July 2000): 162-9.

### WEBSITES

*Neuromuscular Disease Center* http://www.neuro.wustl.edu/neuromuscular/msys/glycogen.html.

"Glycogen Storage Disease". *OMIM—Online Mendelian Inheritance in Man.* November 29, 2009 (December 11, 2009). http://www. ncbi.nlm.nih.gov/entrez/dispomim. cgi?id = 232300.

*The Pompe's Disease Page.* http://www.cix.co.uk/~embra/pompe/Welcome.html (February 12, 2001).

### OTHER

"Genzyme General and Pharming Group Reports Results From First Two Clinical Trials for Pompe Disease." *Genzyme Corporation Press Release* (October 5, 2000).

"Pompe disease therapy to be tested." *Duke University Medical Center Press Release* (May 24, 1999).

### ORGANIZATIONS

Acid Maltase Deficiency Association (AMDA). PO Box 700248, San Antonio, TX 78270-0248. (210) 494-6144 or (210) 490-7161. Fax: (210) 490-7161 or 210-497-3810. http://www.amda-pompe.org.

Association for Glycogen Storage Disease (United Kingdom). 0131 554 2791. Fax: 0131 244 8926. http://www.agsd.org.uk.

Paul A. Johnson

# Porphyrias

## Definition

The porphyrias are a group of disorders in which the body produces too much porphyrin and insufficient heme, the iron–containing molecule found for example in hemoglobin, the oxygen–carrier protein. Porphyrins are precursor molecules for heme and certain enzymes. Excess porphyrins are excreted as waste in the urine and stool. Overproduction and overexcretion of porphyrins causes low, unhealthy levels of heme and certain important enzymes creating various physical symptoms.

## Description

Biosynthesis of heme is a multistep process that begins with simple molecules and ends with a large, complex heme molecule. Each step of the chemical pathway is directed by its own task–specific protein, called an enzyme. As a heme precursor molecule moves through each step, an enzyme modifies the precursor for the next step. If a precursor molecule is not modified, it cannot proceed further in the pathway, causing a build–up of that specific precursor.

The precursors prevented from proceeding further along the pathway accumulate at the stage of the enzyme defect, causing an array of physical symptoms in an affected person. Specific symptoms depend on the point at which heme biosynthesis is blocked and which precursors accumulate. In general, the porphyrias primarily affect the skin and the nervous system. Symptoms can be debilitating or life–threatening in some cases. Porphyria is most commonly an inherited condition. It can also, however, be acquired after exposure to poisonous substances.

### Heme

Heme is produced in several tissues in the body, but its primary biosynthesis sites are the liver and bone marrow. Heme synthesis for immature red blood cells, namely the erythroblasts and the reticulocytes, occurs in the bone marrow.

Although production is concentrated in the liver and bone marrow, heme is utilized in various capacities in virtually every tissue in the body. In most cells, heme is a key building block in the construction of factors that oversee metabolism and transport of oxygen and energy. In the liver, heme is a component of several vital enzymes, particularly cytochrome P450. Cytochrome P450 is involved in the metabolism of chemicals, vitamins, fatty acids, and hormones; it is very important in transforming toxic substances into easily excretable materials. In immature red blood cells, heme is the crucial component of hemoglobin, the biomolecule that carries oxygen in red blood cells.

### Heme biosynthesis

The heme molecule consists of a cyclic porphyrin molecule containing a central iron atom. The heme biosynthesis pathway is a series of steps building the complete heme molecule, and the last step involves incorporation of the iron atom.

The production of heme may be compared to a factory assembly line. At the start of the line, raw materials are fed into the process. At specific points

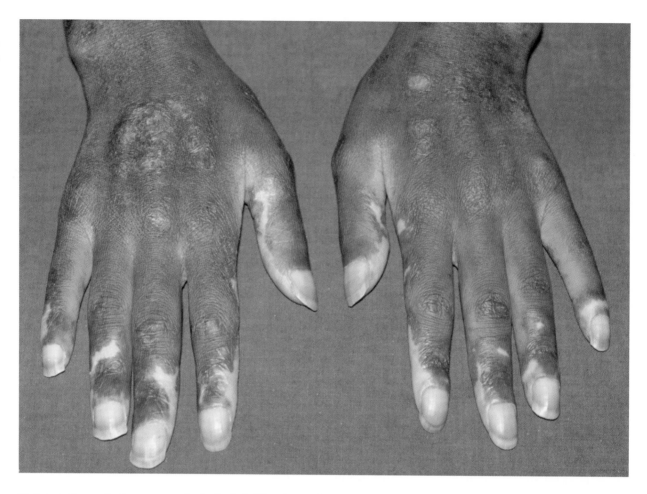

**Early symptoms of cutaneous porphyrias include blistering on the hands, face, and arms following minor injuries or exposure to sunlight.** *(Custom Medical Stock Photo, Inc.)*

along the line, an addition or adjustment is made to further development. Once additions and adjustments are complete, the final product rolls off the end of the line.

Heme biosynthesis is an eight–step process, requiring eight different and properly functioning enzymes:

- delta–aminolevulinic acid synthase
- delta–aminolevulinic acid dehydratase
- porphobilinogen deaminase
- uroporphyrinogen III cosynthase
- uroporphyrinogen decarboxylase
- coproporphyrinogen oxidase
- protoporphyrinogen oxidase
- ferrochelatase

The control of heme biosynthesis is complex. Various chemical signals can trigger increased or decreased production. These signals can affect the enzymes themselves or the production of these enzymes, starting at the genetic level. For example, one point at which heme biosynthesis may be controlled is at the first step. When heme levels are low, greater quantities of delta–aminolevulinic acid (ALA) synthase are produced. As a result, larger quantities of heme precursors are fed into the biosynthesis pathway to step up heme production.

### Types of Porphyrias

Under normal circumstances, when heme concentrations are at an appropriate level, precursor production decreases. However, a defective enzyme can prevent heme biosynthesis from reaching completion. Because heme levels remain low, the synthesis pathway continues to churn out precursor molecules in an attempt to correct the heme deficit.

The net effect of this continued production is an abnormal accumulation of precursor molecules and development of some type of porphyria. Each type of porphyria corresponds to a specific enzyme defect and an accumulation of the associated precursor.

## KEY TERMS

**Autosomal dominant**—A pattern of genetic inheritance where only one abnormal gene is needed to display the trait or disease.

**Autosomal recessive**—A pattern of genetic inheritance where two abnormal genes are needed to display the trait or disease.

**Biosynthesis**—The manufacture of materials in a biological system.

**Bone marrow**—A spongy tissue located in the hollow centers of certain bones, such as the skull and hip bones. Bone marrow is the site of blood cell generation.

**Enzyme**—A protein that catalyzes a biochemical reaction or change without changing its own structure or function.

**Erythropoiesis**—The process through which new red blood cells are created; it begins in the bone marrow.

**Erythropoietic**—Referring to the creation of new red blood cells.

**Gene**—A building block of inheritance, which contains the instructions for the production of a particular protein, and is made up of a molecular sequence found on a section of DNA. Each gene is found on a precise location on a chromosome.

**Hematin**—A drug administered intravenously to halt an acute porphyria attack. It causes heme biosynthesis to decrease, preventing the further accumulation of heme precursors.

**Heme**—The iron–containing molecule in hemoglobin that serves as the site for oxygen binding.

**Hemoglobin**—Protein–iron compound in the blood that carries oxygen to the cells and carries carbon dioxide away from the cells.

**Hepatic**—Referring to the liver.

**Neuropathy**—A condition caused by nerve damage. Major symptoms include weakness, numbness, paralysis, or pain in the affected area.

**Porphyrin**—A large cyclic molecule shaped like a four–leaf clover. Combined with an iron atom, it forms a heme molecule.

**Protoporphyrin**—A precursor molecule to the porphyrin molecule.

Although there are eight steps in heme biosynthesis, there are only seven types of porphyrias; a change in ALA synthase activity does not have a corresponding porphyria.

Enzymes involved in heme biosynthesis display subtle, tissue–specific variations; therefore, heme biosynthesis may be impaired in the liver, but normal in the immature red blood cells, or vice–versa. Incidence of porphyria varies widely between types and occasionally by geographic location. Although certain porphyrias are more common than others, their greater frequency is only relative to other types. All porphyrias are considered to be rare disorders.

In the past, the porphyrias were divided into two general categories based on the location of the porphyrin production. Porphyrias affecting heme biosynthesis in the liver were referred to as hepatic porphyrias. Porphyrias affecting heme biosynthesis in immature red blood cells were referred to as erythropoietic porphyrias (erythropoiesis is the process through which red blood cells are produced). Porphyrias are usually grouped into acute and non–acute types. Acute porphyrias produce severe attacks of pain and neurological effects. Non–acute porphyrias present as chronic diseases.

The acute porphyrias, and the heme biosynthesis steps at which enzyme problems occur, are:

- ALA dehydratase deficiency porphyria (step 2): the enzyme aminolaevulinic acid dehydratase is deficient.

- Acute intermittent porphyria, also known as Swedish porphyria, pyrroloporphyria, and intermittent acute porphyria (step 3): the enzyme porphobilinogen deaminase id deficient.

- Hereditary coproporphyria (step 6): the enzyme coproporphyrinogen oxidase is deficient.

- Variegate porphyria (VP), also known as porphyria variegata, protocoproporphyria, South African genetic porphyria, and Royal malady (supposedly King George III of England and Mary, Queen of Scots, had VP) (step 7): the enzyme protoporphyrinogen oxidase is deficient.

The non–acute porphyrias, and the steps of heme biosynthesis at which they occur, are:

- Congenital erythropoietic porphyria (CEP), also called Gunther's disease, erythropoietic porphyria, congenital porphyria, congenital hematoporphyria, or erythropoietic uroporphyria, is a rare disease (step 4): the enzyme uroporphyrinogen III synthase is deficient.

- Porphyria cutanea tarda (PCT), also called symptomatic porphyria, porphyria cutanea symptomatica, or idiosyncratic porphyria (step 5): the enzyme uroporphyrinogen decarboxylase is deficient. PCT may be acquired, typically as a result of disease (especially hepatitis C), or inherited. Most people remain latent—that is, symptoms never develop.

- Hepatoerythopoietic porphyria (HEP) (also step 5). HEP affects heme biosynthesis in both the liver and the bone marrow. HEP also results from a defect in uroporphyrinogen decarboxylase activity. Disease symptoms, however, strongly resemble congenital erythropoietic porphyria.

- Erythropoietic protoporphyria (EPP), also known as protoporphyria and erythrohepatic protoporphyria (step 8): ferrochelatase is the defiecient enzyme.

### Genetic profile

The underlying cause of all porphyrias is a deficiency of one of the enzymes involved in the heme biosynthesis pathway. Porphyrias are inherited conditions, and in virtually all types, an inherited factor causes the enzyme deficiency. An environmental factor—such as diet, drugs, or sun exposure—may trigger symptoms, but in many cases, symptoms never develop.

Each of the seven porphyrias has a specific **inheritance** pattern and a **gene** mutation responsible for its occurrence:

- ALA dehydratase porphyria: autosomal recessive inheritance, due to a mutation of the ALAD gene in chromosome 9q34. This porphyria type is very rare. In autosomal recessively inherited disorders, a person must inherit two defective genes, one from each parent. A parent with only one gene for an autosomal recessive disorder does not display symptoms of the disease.

- Acute intermittent porphyria: autosomal dominant inheritance, due to a mutation of the PBGD gene in chromosome 11q23.3. An autosomal dominant pattern, which means that only one copy of the abnormal gene needs to be present for the disorder to occur. Simply inheriting this gene, however, does not necessarily mean that a person will develop the disease. Approximately five to 10 per 100,000 persons in the United States carry a gene for AIP, but only 10% of these people ever develop symptoms of the disease.

- Congenital erythropoietic porphyria: autosomal recessive inheritance, due to a mutation of the UROS gene in chromosome 10q25.2–q26.3.

- Porphyria cutanea tarda: autosomal dominant or sporadic inheritance, due to a mutation of the UROD gene in chromosome 1p34.

- Hereditary coproporphyria: autosomal dominant inheritance, due to a mutation of the CPOX gene in chromosome 3q12.

- Variegate porphyria: autosomal dominant inheritance, due to a mutation of the PPOX gene in chromosome 1q22.

- Erythropoietic protoporphyria: autosomal dominant inheritance, due to a mutation of the FECH gene in chromosome 18q21.3.

### Demographics

Porphyrias are rare conditions and are often misdiagnosed because their symptoms are easily confused with other diseases. The most common form of porphyria worldwide is porphyria cutanea tarda. As of 2009, the prevalence of PCT in the United States is estimated at 1 case in 25,000–50,000 population and 1 in 25,000 in the UK. The most common form of acute porphyria is acute intermittent porphyria. **Erythropoietic porphyria** has been reported in diverse populations, but it is very rare: the total number of cases reported worldwide is less than 200. Variegate porphyria has been mostly reported in South Africans of Dutch descent. Among that population, the incidence is approximately three in 1,000 persons. It is estimated that there are 10,000 cases in South Africa. It would appear that the affected South Africans are descendants of two affected Dutch settlers who came to South Africa in 1680. Among other populations, the incidence is estimated to be one to two cases per 100,000 persons

### Signs and symptoms

#### General characteristics

All of the hepatic porphyrias—except porphyria cutanea tarda—follow a pattern of acute attacks separated by periods in which no symptoms are present. For this reason, this group is often referred to as the acute porphyrias. The erythropoietic porphyrias and porphyria cutanea tarda do not follow this pattern and are considered to be chronic conditions.

The specific symptoms of each porphyria vary based on which enzyme is affected and whether that enzyme occurs in the liver or in the bone marrow. The severity of symptoms can vary widely, even within the same type of porphyria. If the porphyria becomes symptomatic, the common factor between all types is an abnormal accumulation of protoporphyrins or porphyrin.

### ALA dehydratase porphyria (ADP)

ADP is characterized by a deficiency of ALA dehydratase. Of the few cases on record, the prominent symptoms were vomiting, pain in the abdomen, arms, and legs, and neuropathy. (Neuropathy refers to nerve damage that can cause pain, numbness, or paralysis.) The nerve damage associated with ADP could cause breathing impairment or lead to weakness or paralysis of the arms and legs.

### Acute intermittent porphyria (AIP)

Symptoms of AIP usually do not occur unless a person with the deficiency encounters a trigger substance. Trigger substances can include hormones (for example oral contraceptives, menstruation, pregnancy), drugs, and dietary factors. Most people with this deficiency never develop symptoms.

Attacks occur after puberty and commonly feature severe abdominal pain, nausea, vomiting, and constipation. Muscle weakness and pain in the back, arms, and legs are also typical symptoms. During an attack, the urine is a deep reddish color. The central nervous system may also be involved. Possible psychological symptoms include hallucinations, confusion, seizures, and mood changes.

### Congenital erythropoietic porphyria (CEP)

Symptoms of CEP are often apparent in infancy and include reddish urine and possibly an enlarged spleen. The skin is unusually sensitive to light and blisters easily if exposed to sunlight. (Sunlight induces protoporphyrin changes in the plasma and skin. These altered protoporphyrin molecules can cause skin damage.) Increased hair growth is common. Damage from recurrent blistering and associated skin infections can be severe. In some cases facial features and fingers may be lost to recurrent damage and infection. Deposits of protoporphyrins can sometimes lead to red staining of the teeth and bones.

### Porphyria cutanea tarda (PCT)

PCT may occur as an acquired or an inherited condition. The acquired form usually does not appear until adulthood. The inherited form may appear in childhood, but often demonstrates no symptoms. Early symptoms include blistering on the hands, face, and arms following minor injuries or exposure to

sunlight. Lightening or darkening of the skin may occur along with increased hair growth or loss of hair. Liver function is abnormal but the signs are mild.

### Hepatoerythopoietic porphyria (HEP)

The symptoms of HEP are similar to those of CEP.

### Hereditary coproporphyria (HCP)

HCP is similar to AIP, but the symptoms are typically milder. The greatest difference between HCP and AIP is that people with HCP may have some skin sensitivity to sunlight. However, extensive damage to the skin is rarely seen.

### Variegate porphyria (VP)

Like AIP, symptoms of VP occur only during attacks. Major symptoms of this type of porphyria include neurological problems and sensitivity to light. Areas of the skin that are exposed to sunlight are susceptible to burning, blistering, and scarring.

### Erythropoietic protoporphyria (EPP)

Owing to deficient ferrochelatase, the last step in the heme biosynthesis pathway—the insertion of an iron atom into a porphyrin molecule—cannot be completed. The major symptoms of this disorder are related to sensitivity to light—including both artificial and natural light sources. Following exposure to light, a person with EPP experiences burning, itching, swelling, and reddening of the skin. Blistering and scarring may occur but are neither common nor severe. EPP is associated with increased risks for gallstones and liver complications. Symptoms can appear in childhood and tend to be more severe during the summer when exposure to sunlight is more likely.

## Diagnosis

Depending on the array of symptoms an individual may exhibit, the possibility of porphyria may not immediately come to a physician's mind. In the absence of a family history of porphyria, non–specific symptoms, such as abdominal pain and vomiting, may be attributed to other disorders. Neurological symptoms, including confusion and hallucinations, can lead to an initial suspicion of psychiatric disease. Diagnosis is more easily accomplished in cases in which non–specific symptoms appear in combination with symptoms more specific to porphyria, like neuropathy, sensitivity to sunlight, or certain other manifestations. Certain symptoms, such as urine the color of port wine, are hallmark signs very specific to porphyria. **DNA** analysis is not yet of routine diagnostic value.

A common initial test measures protoporphyrins in the urine. However, if skin sensitivity to light is a symptom, a blood plasma test is indicated. If these tests reveal abnormal levels of protoporphyrins, further tests are done to measure heme precursor levels in red blood cells and the stool. The presence and estimated quantity of porphyrin and protoporphyrins in biological samples are easily detected using spectrofluorometric testing. Spectrofluorometric testing uses a spectrofluorometer that directs light of a specific strength at a fluid sample. The porphyrins and protoporphyrins in the sample absorb the light energy and fluoresce, or glow. The spectrofluorometer detects and measures fluorescence, which indicates the amount of porphyrins and protoporphyrins in the sample.

Whether heme precursors occur in the blood, urine, or stool gives some indication of the type of porphyria, but more detailed biochemical testing is required to determine their exact identity. Making this determination yields a strong indicator of which enzyme in the heme biosynthesis pathway is defective; which, in turn, allows a diagnosis of the particular type of porphyria.

Biochemical tests rely on the color, chemical properties, and other unique features of each heme precursor. For example, a screening test for acute intermittent porphyria (AIP) is the Watson–Schwartz test. In this test, a special dye is added to a urine sample. If one of two heme precursors—porphobilinogen or urobilinogen—is present, the sample turns pink or red. Further testing is necessary to determine whether the precursor present is porphobilinogen or urobilinogen—only porphobilinogen is indicative of AIP.

Other biochemical tests rely on the fact that heme precursors become less soluble in water (able to be dissolved in water) as they progress further through the heme biosynthesis pathway. For example, to determine whether the Watson–Schwartz urine test is positive for porphobilinogen or urobilinogen, chloroform is added to the test tube. Chloroform is a water–insoluble substance. Even after vigorous mixing, the water and chloroform separate into two distinct layers. Urobilinogen is slightly insoluble in water, while porphobilinogen tends to be water–soluble. The porphobilinogen mixes more readily in water than chloroform, so if the water layer is pink (from the dye added to the urine sample), that indicates the presence of porphobilinogen, and a diagnosis of AIP is probable.

As a final test, measuring specific enzymes and their activities may be done for some types of porphyrias; however, such tests are not done as a screening method. Certain enzymes, such as porphobilinogen deaminase (the abnormal enzyme in AIP), can be easily extracted from red blood cells; other enzymes, however, are less readily collected or tested. Basically, an enzyme test involves adding a certain amount of the enzyme to a test tube that contains the precursor it is supposed to modify. Both the production of modified precursor and the rate at which it appears can be measured using laboratory equipment. If a modified precursor is produced, the test indicates that the enzyme is doing its job. The rate at which the modified precursor is produced can be compared to a standard to measure the efficiency of the enzyme.

### Treatment and management

Treatment for porphyria revolves around avoiding acute attacks, limiting potential effects, and treating symptoms. Treatment options vary depending on the specific type of porphyria diagnosed. **Gene therapy** has been successful for both CEP and EPP. In the future, scientists expect development of gene therapy for the remaining porphyrias. Given the rarity of ALA dehydratase porphyria, definitive treatment guidelines for this rare type have not been developed.

#### *Acute intermittent porphyria, hereditary coproporphyria, and variegate porphyria*

Treatment for acute intermittent porphyria, **hereditary coproporphyria**, and variegate porphyria follows the same basic regime. A person who has been diagnosed with one of these porphyrias can prevent most attacks by avoiding precipitating factors, such as certain drugs that have been identified as triggers for acute porphyria attacks. Individuals must maintain adequate nutrition, particularly in respect to carbohydrates. In some cases, an attack can be stopped by increasing carbohydrate consumption or by receiving carbohydrates intravenously.

When attacks occur, prompt medical attention is necessary. Pain is usually severe, and narcotic analgesics are the best option for relief. Phenothiazines can be used to counter nausea, vomiting, and anxiety, and chloral hydrate or diazepam is useful for sedation or to induce sleep. Hematin, a drug administered intravenously, may be used to halt an attack. Hematin seems to work by signaling the pathway of heme biosynthesis to slow production of precursors. Women, who tend to develop symptoms more frequently than men owing to hormonal fluctuations, may find ovulation–inhibiting hormone therapy to be helpful.

Gene therapy is a possible future treatment for these porphyrias. An experimental animal model of AIP has been developed and research is in progress.

### Congenital erythropoietic porphyria

The key points of congenital erythropoietic porphyria treatment are avoiding exposure to sunlight and prevention of skin trauma or skin infection. Liberal use of sunscreens and consumption of beta–carotene supplements can provide some protection from sun–induced damage. Medical treatments such as removing the spleen or administering transfusions of red blood cells can create short–term benefits, but these treatments do not offer a cure. Remission can sometimes be achieved after treatment with oral doses of activated charcoal. Severely affected patients may be offered bone marrow transplantation, which appears to confer long–term benefits.

### Porphyria cutanea tarda

As with other porphyrias, the first line of defense is avoidance of factors, especially alcohol, that could bring about symptoms. Regular blood withdrawal is a proven therapy for pushing symptoms into remission. If an individual is anemic or cannot have blood drawn for other reasons, chloroquine therapy may be used.

### Erythropoietic protoporphyria

Avoiding sunlight, using sunscreens, and taking beta–carotene supplements are typical treatment options for erythropoietic protoporphyria. The drug, cholestyramine, may reduce the skin's sensitivity to sunlight as well as the accumulated heme precursors in the liver. Liver transplantation has been used in cases of liver failure, but it has not provided a long–term cure of the porphyria.

## Alternative treatment

Acute porphyria attacks can be life–threatening events, so attempts at self–treatment can be dangerous. Alternative treatments can be useful adjuncts to conventional therapy. For example, some people may find relief for the pain associated with acute intermittent porphyria, hereditary coproporphyria, or variegate porphyria through acupuncture or hypnosis. Relaxation techniques, such as yoga or meditation, may also prove helpful in pain management.

### Clinical trials

Clinical trials on porphyrias are currently sponsored by the National Institutes of Health (NIH) and other agencies. As of 2009, NIH was reporting 16 on–going and completed studies.

Examples include:

- The evaluation of the efficacy of heme arginate, singly or in combination with tin mesoporphyrin, in lowering porphyrin precursors in patients with asymptomatic acute intermittent porphyria. (NCT00004396)
- The evaluation of the efficacy and tolerability of deferasirox in the treatment of porphyria cutanea tarda. (NCT00599326)
- A study of nutritional factors in porphyria. (NCT00004788)
- The evaluation of enzyme defects in patients with known or suspected porphyria and their family members. (NCT00004331)

Clinical trial information is constantly updated by NIH and the most recent information on porphyria trials can be found at: http://clinicaltrials.gov.

## Prognosis

Even when porphyria is inherited, symptom development depends on a variety of factors. In the majority of cases, a person remains asymptomatic throughout life. About one percent of acute attacks can be fatal. Other symptoms may be associated with temporarily debilitating or permanently disfiguring consequences. Measures to avoid these consequences are not always successful, regardless of how diligently they are pursued. Although pregnancy has been known to trigger porphyria attacks, dangers associated with pregnancy as not as great as was once thought.

## Prevention

For the most part, the porphyrias are attributed to inherited genes; such inheritance cannot be prevented. However, symptoms can be limited or prevented by avoiding factors that trigger symptom development.

People with a family history of an acute porphyria should be screened for the disease. Even if symptoms are absent, it is useful to know about the presence of the gene to assess the risks of developing the associated porphyria. This knowledge also reveals whether a person's offspring may be at risk. Prenatal testing for certain porphyrias is possible. Prenatal diagnosis of congenital erythropoietic porphyria has been successfully accomplished. Any prenatal tests, however, would not indicate whether a child would develop porphyria symptoms; only that they might have the potential to do so.

## Resources

### BOOKS

Icon Health Publications. *Porphyria —A Medical Dictionary, Bibliography, and Annotated Research Guide to Internet References.* San Diego, CA: Icon Health Publications, 2004.

Lyon Howe, Desiree. *100Porphyria: A Lyon's Share of Trouble.* Los Angeles, CA: Digital Data Werks Inc., 2004.

Parker, Philip M. *Porphyria —A Bibliography and Dictionary for Physicians, Patients, and Genome Researchers.* San Diego, CA: Icon Health Publications, 2007.

### PERIODICALS

Aarsand, A. K., et al. "Familial and sporadic porphyria cutanea tarda: characterization and diagnostic strategies." *Clinical Chemistry* 55, no. 4 (April 2009): 795–803.

Jackson, R., et al. "A confusing case of confusion. Acute porphyrias." *Journal of the Oklahoma State Medical Association* 101, no. 4 (April 2008): 779–795.

Kauppinen, R. "Porphyrias." *Lancet* 365, no. 9455 (January 2005): 2411–252.

Sarkany, R. P. "Making sense of the porphyrias." *Photodermatology, Photoimmunology & Photomedicine* 24, no. 2 (April 2008): 102–108.

Solinas, C., and F. J. Vajda. "Neurological complications of porphyria." *Journal of Clinical Neuroscience* 15, no. 3 (March 2008): 263–268.

Song, G., et al. "Structural insight into acute intermittent porphyria." *FASEB Journal* 23, no. 2 (February 2008): 85–86.

### WEBSITES

*A Guide To Porphyria.* Information Page. Canadian Association for Porphyria, (April 26, 2009). http://www.cpf-inc.ca/guide.htm.

*Acute Intermittent Porphyria.* Information Page. Merck Manuals, August 2008 (April 26, 2009). http://www.merck.com/mmhe/sec12/ch160/ch160c.html.

*Porphyria.* Medical Encyclopedia. Medline Plus, March 2, 2009 (April 26, 2009). http://www.nlm.nih.gov/medlineplus/ency/article/001208.htm.

*Porphyria, Acute Intermittent.* Information Page. NORD, November 26, 2008 (April 26, 2009). http://rarediseases.org/search/rdbdetail_abstract.html?disname=Porphyria%2C%20Acute%20Intermittent.

*Porphyrias.* Information Page. Patient UK, January 24, 2008 (April 26, 2009). http://www.patient.co.uk/showdoc/40001141/.

*Types of Porphyria.* Information Page. APF, 2009 (April 26, 2009). http://www.porphyriafoundation.com/about-porphyria/types-of-porphyria.

### ORGANIZATIONS

American Porphyria Foundation (APF). 4900 Woodway, Suite 780, Houston, TX 77056. (866)APF-3635 or (713)266-9617. E-mail: porphyrus@aol.com. http://www.porphyriafoundation.com.

Canadian Association for Porphyria. P.O. Box 1206, Neepawa, Manitoba ROJ 1HO, Canada. (866)476-2801. E-mail: porphyria@cpf-inc.ca. http://www.cpf-inc.ca.

National Organization for Rare Disorders (NORD). 55 Kenosia Avenue, PO Box 1968, Danbury, CT 06813-1968. (203)744-0100 or (800)999-6673. Fax: (203)798-2291. http://www.rarediseases.org.

Julia Barrett
Judy Hawkins, MS

**Portosystemic venous shunt-congenital** *see* **Patent ductus arteriosus**

**Potter sequence** *see* **Oligohydramnios sequence**

# Prader-Willi syndrome

## Definition

Prader-Willi syndrome (PWS) is a genetic condition caused by the absence of chromosomal material from **chromosome** 15. The genetic basis of PWS is complex. Characteristics of the syndrome include developmental delay, poor muscle tone, short stature, small hands and feet, incomplete sexual development, and unique facial features. Insatiable appetite is a classic feature of PWS. This uncontrollable appetite can lead to health problems and behavior disturbances.

**Amniocentesis**—A procedure performed at 16-18 weeks of pregnancy in which a needle is inserted through a woman's abdomen into her uterus to draw out a small sample of the amniotic fluid from around the baby. Either the fluid itself or cells from the fluid can be used for a variety of tests to obtain information about genetic disorders and other medical conditions in the fetus.

**Centromere**—The centromere is the constricted region of a chromosome. It performs certain functions during cell division.

**Deletion**—The absence of genetic material that is normally found in a chromosome. Often, the genetic material is missing due to an error in replication of an egg or sperm cell.

**Deoxyribonucleic acid (DNA)**—The genetic material in cells that holds the inherited instructions for growth, development, and cellular functioning.

**FISH (fluorescence *in situ* hybridization)**—Technique used to detect small deletions or rearrangements in chromosomes by attempting to attach a fluorescent (glowing) piece of a chromosome to a sample of cells obtained from a patient.

**Gene**—A building block of inheritance, which contains the instructions for the production of a particular protein, and is made up of a molecular sequence found on a section of DNA. Each gene is found on a precise location on a chromosome.

**Hyperphagia**—Over-eating.

**Hypotonia**—Reduced or diminished muscle tone.

**Imprinting**—Process that silences a gene or group of genes. The genes are silenced depending on if they are inherited through the egg or the sperm.

**Maternal**—Relating to the mother.

**Maternal uniparental disomy**—Chromosome abnormality in which both chromosomes in a pair are inherited from one's mother.

**Methylation testing**—DNA testing that detects if a gene is active, or if it is imprinted.

**Mutation**—A permanent change in the genetic material that may alter a trait or characteristic of an individual, or manifest as disease, and can be transmitted to offspring.

**Paternal**—Relating to one's father.

**Translocation**—The transfer of one part of a chromosome to another chromosome during cell division. A balanced translocation occurs when pieces from two different chromosomes exchange places without loss or gain of any chromosome material. An unbalanced translocation involves the unequal loss or gain of genetic information between two chromosomes.

**Uniparental disomy**—Chromosome abnormality in which both chromosomes in a pair are inherited from the same parent.

## Description

The first patients with features of PWS were described by Drs. Prader, Willi, and Lambert in 1956. Since that time, the complex genetic basis of PWS has begun to be understood. Initially, scientists found that individuals with PWS have a portion of genetic material deleted (erased) from chromosome 15. In order to have PWS, the genetic material must be deleted from the chromosome 15 received from one's father. If the deletion is on the chromosome 15 inherited from one's mother, a different syndrome develops. This was an important discovery. It demonstrated for the first time that the genes inherited from one's mother can be expressed differently than the genes inherited from one's father.

Over time, scientists realized that some individuals with PWS do not have a deletion of genetic material from chromosome 15. Further studies found that these patients inherit both copies of chromosome 15 from their mother. This is not typical. Normally, an individual should receive one chromosome 15 from one's father and one chromosome 15 from one's mother. When a person receives both chromosomes from the same parent it is called uniparental disomy. When a person receives both chromosomes from one's mother it is called maternal uniparental disomy.

Scientists are still discovering other causes of PWS. A small number of patients with PWS have a change (mutation) in the genetic material on the chromosome 15 inherited from their father. This mutation prevents certain genes on chromosome 15 from working properly. PWS develops when these genes do not work normally.

Newborns with PWS generally have poor muscle tone (hypotonia) and do not feed well. This can lead to poor weight gain and failure to thrive. Genitalia can be smaller than normal. Hands and feet are also typically smaller than normal. Some patients with PWS have unique facial characteristics. These unique facial features are typically subtle and only detectable by physicians.

As children with PWS age, development is typically slower than normal. Developmental milestones, such as crawling, walking, and talking occur later than usual. Developmental delay continues into adulthood for approximately 50% of individuals with PWS. At about one to two years of age, children with PWS develop an uncontrollable, insatiable appetite. Left to their own devices, individuals with PWS will eat until they have life-threatening obesity. The desire to eat can lead to significant behavior problems.

The symptoms and features of PWS require lifelong support and care. If food intake is strictly monitored and various therapies provided, individuals with PWS have a normal life expectancy.

### Genetic profile

In order to comprehend the various causes of PWS, the nature of chromosomes and genes must be well-understood. Human beings have 46 chromosomes in the cells of their body. Chromosomes contain genes. Genes regulate the function and development of the body. An individual's chromosomes are inherited from their parents. A child should receive 23 chromosomes from the mother and 23 chromosomes from the father.

The 46 chromosomes in the human body are divided into pairs. Each pair is assigned a number or a letter. Chromosomes are divided into pairs based on their physical characteristics. Chromosomes can only be seen when viewed under a microscope. Chromosomes within the same pair appear identical because they contain the same genes.

Most chromosomes have a constriction near the center called the centromere. The centromere separates the chromosome into long and short arms. The short arm of a chromosome is called the "p arm." The long arm of a chromosome is called the "q arm."

Chromosomes in the same pair contain the same genes. However, some genes work differently depending on if they were inherited from the egg or the sperm. Sometimes, genes are silenced when inherited from the mother. Other times, genes are silenced when inherited from the father. When genes in a certain region on a chromosome are silenced, they are said to be "imprinted." **Imprinting** is a normal process. Imprinting does not typically cause disease. If normal imprinting is disrupted a genetic disease can develop.

Individuals should have two complete copies of chromosome 15. One chromosome 15 should be inherited from the mother, or be "maternal" in origin. The other chromosome 15 should be inherited from the father, or be "paternal" in origin.

Several genes found on the q arm of chromosome 15 are imprinted. A gene called SNPRN is an example of one of these genes. It is normally imprinted, or silenced, if inherited from the mother. The imprinting of this group of maternal genes does not typically cause disease. The genes in this region should not be imprinted if paternal in origin. Normal development depends on these paternal genes being present and active. If these genes are deleted, not inherited, or incorrectly imprinted, PWS develops.

Seventy percent of the cases of PWS are caused when a piece of material is deleted, or erased, from the paternal chromosome 15. This deletion happens in a specific region on the q arm of chromosome 15. The piece of chromosomal material that is deleted contains genes that must be present for normal development. These paternal genes must be working normally, because the same genes on the chromosome 15 inherited from the mother are imprinted. When these paternal genes are missing, the brain and other parts of the body do not develop as expected. This is what causes the symptoms associated with PWS.

In 99% of the cases of PWS the deletion is sporadic. This means that it happens randomly and there is not an apparent cause. It does not run in the family. If a child has PWS due to a sporadic deletion in the paternal chromosome 15, the chance the parents could have another child with PWS is less than 1%. In less than 1% of the cases of PWS there is a chromosomal rearrangement in the family which causes the deletion. This chromosomal rearrangement is called a translocation. If a parent has a translocation the risk of having a child with PWS is higher than 1%.

PWS can also develop if a child receives both chromosome 15s from his or her mother. This is seen in approximately 25% of the cases of PWS. Maternal uniparental disomy for chromosome 15 leads to PWS because the genes on the chromosome 15 that should have been inherited from the father are missing. These paternal genes must be present, since the same genes on both the chromosome 15s inherited from the mother are imprinted.

PWS caused by maternal uniparental disomy is sporadic. This means that it happens randomly and there is no apparent cause. If a child has PWS due to maternal uniparental disomy the chance the parents could have another child with PWS is less than 1%.

Approximately 3–4% of patients with PWS have a change (mutation) in a gene located on the q arm of chromosome 15. This mutation leads to incorrect imprinting and causes genes inherited from the father to be imprinted or silenced. These genes should not normally be imprinted. If a child has PWS due to a mutation that changes imprinting, the chance the parents could have another child with PWS is approximately 5%.

It should be noted that if an individual has a deletion of the same material from the q arm of the maternal chromosome 15 a different syndrome develops. This syndrome is called **Angelman syndrome**. Angelman syndrome can also happen if an individual receives both chromosome 15s from the father.

### Demographics

PWS affects approximately one in 10,000 to 25,000 live births. It is the most common genetic cause of life-threatening obesity. It affects both males and females. PWS can be seen in all races and ethnic groups.

### Signs and symptoms

Infants with PWS have weak muscle tone (hypotonia). This hypotonia causes problems with sucking and eating. Infants with PWS may have problems gaining weight. Some infants with PWS are diagnosed with failure to thrive due to slow growth and development. During infancy, babies with PWS may also sleep more than normal and have problems controlling their temperature.

Some of the unique physical features associated with PWS can be seen during infancy. Genitalia that is smaller than normal is common. This may be more evident in males with PWS. Hands and feet may also be smaller than average. The unique facial features seen in some patients with PWS may be difficult to detect in infancy. These facial features are very mild and do not cause physical problems.

As early as six months, but more commonly between one and two years of age, a compulsive desire to eat develops. This uncontrollable appetite is a classic feature of PWS. Individuals with PWS lack the ability to feel full or satiated. This uncontrollable desire to eat is thought to be related to a difference in the brain, which controls hunger. Over-eating (hyperpahgia), a lack of a desire to exercise, and a slow metabolism places individuals with PWS at high risk for severe obesity. Some individuals with PWS may also have a reduced ability to vomit.

Behavior problems are a common feature of PWS. Some behavior problems develop from the desire to eat. Other reported problems include obsessive/compulsive behaviors, **depression**, and temper tantrums. Individuals with PWS may also pick their own skin (skin picking). This unusual behavior may be due to a reduced pain threshold.

Developmental delay, learning disabilities, and mental retardation are associated with PWS. Approximately 50% of individuals with PWS have developmental delay. The remaining 50% are described as having mild mental retardation. The mental retardation can occasionally be more severe. Infants and children with PWS are often delayed in development.

Puberty may occur early or late, but it is usually incomplete. In addition to the effects on sexual development and fertility, individuals do not undergo the normal adolescent growth spurt and may be short as adults. Muscles often remain underdeveloped and body fat increased.

### Diagnosis

During infancy, the diagnosis of PWS may be suspected if poor muscle tone, feeding problems, small genitalia, or the unique facial features are present. If an infant has these features, testing for PWS should be performed. This testing should also be offered to children and adults who display features commonly seen in PWS (developmental delay, uncontrollable appetite, small genitalia, etc.). There are several different genetic tests that can detect PWS. All of these tests can be performed from a blood sample.

Methylation testing detects 99% of the cases of PWS. Methylation testing can detect the absence of the paternal genes that should be normally active on chromosome 15. Although methylation testing can accurately diagnose PWS, it can not determine if the PWS is caused by a deletion, maternal uniparental disomy, or a mutation that disrupts imprinting. This information is important for **genetic counseling**. Therefore, additional testing should be performed.

Chromosome analysis can determine if the PWS is the result of a deletion in the q arm of chromosome 15. Chromosome analysis, also called karyotyping, involves staining the chromosomes and examining them under a microscope. In some cases the deletion of material from chromosome 15 can be easily seen. In other cases, further testing must be performed. FISH (fluorescence in-situ hybridization) is a special technique that detects small deletions that cause PWS.

More specialized **DNA** testing is required to detect maternal uniparental disomy or a mutation that disrupts imprinting. This DNA testing identifies unique DNA patterns in the mother and father. The unique DNA patterns are then compared with the DNA from the child with PWS.

PWS can be detected before birth if the mother undergoes **amniocentesis** testing or chorionic villus sampling (CVS). This testing would only be recommended if the mother or father is known to have a chromosome rearrangement or if they already have a child with PWS syndrome.

### Treatment and management

There is currently no cure for PWS. Treatment during infancy includes therapies to improve muscle tone. Some infants with PWS also require special nipples and feeding techniques to improve weight gain.

Treatment and management during childhood, adolescence, and adulthood is typically focused on weight control. Strict control of food intake is vital to prevent severe obesity. In many cases, food must be made inaccessible. This may involve unconventional measures such as locking the refrigerator or kitchen cabinets. A lifelong restricted-calorie diet and regular exercise program are also suggested. Unfortunately, diet medications have not been shown to significantly prevent obesity in PWS. However, growth hormone therapy has been shown to improve the poor muscle tone and reduced height typically associated with PWS.

Special education may be helpful in treating developmental delays and behavior problems.

Individuals with PWS typically excel in highly structured environments.

### Prognosis

Life expectancy is normal and the prognosis good if weight gain is well controlled.

### Resources

**BOOKS**

Couch, Cheryl. *My Rag Doll*. Couch Publishing, 2000.

Jones, Kenneth Lyons. "Prader-Willi Syndrome." In *Smith's Recognizable Patterns of Human Malformation*. 5th ed. Philadelphia: W.B. Saunders, 1997.

**PERIODICALS**

Butler, Merlin G., and Travis Thompson. "Prader-Willi Syndrome: Clinical and Genetic Findings." *The Endocrinologist* 10 (2000): 3S–16S.

State, Matthew W., and Elisabeth Dykens. "Genetics of Childhood Disorders: XV. Prader-Willi Syndrome: Genes, Brain and Behavior." *Journal of the American Academy of Child and Adolescent Psychiatry* 39, no. 6 (June 2000): 797–800.

**WEBSITES**

Cassidy, Suzanne B., and Stuart Schwartz. "Prader-Willi Syndrome." *GeneReviews*. September 3, 2009 (December 11, 2009). http://ncbi.nlm.nih.gov/bookshelf/br.fcgi?book = gene&part = pws.

"Prader-Willi Syndrome; PWS." *OMIM—Online Mendelian Inheritance in Man*. January 20, 2009. (December 11, 2009). http://www.ncbi.nlm.nih.gov/entrez/dispomim.cgi?id = 176270.

**ORGANIZATIONS**

Alliance of Genetic Support Groups. 4301 Connecticut Ave. NW, Suite 404, Washington, DC 20008. (202) 966-5557. Fax: (202) 966-8553. http://www.geneticalliance.org.

International Prader-Willi Syndrome Organization. Bizio 1, 36023 Costozza, Vicenza, Italy + 39 0444 555557. Fax: + 39 0444 555557. http://www.ipwso.org.

National Organization for Rare Disorders (NORD). 55 Kenosia Ave., PO Box 1968, Danbury, CT 06813. (203) 744-0100 or (800) 999-6673. http://www.rarediseases.org.

Prader-Willi Foundation. 223 Main St., Port Washington, NY 11050. (800) 253-7993. http://www.prader-willi.org.

Prader-Willi Syndrome Association. 5700 Midnight Pass Rd., Suite 6, Sarasota, FL 34242-3000. (941) 312-0400 or (800) 926-4797. Fax: (941) 312-0142. http://www.pwsausa.org PWSAUSA@aol.com.

Holly Ann Ishmael, MS, CGC

# Prenatal ultrasound

## Definition

Prenatal ultrasound is a procedure performed during pregnancy to obtain images of the fetus.

## Description

A prenatal ultrasound, also known as a sonogram, is a procedure in which a tool called a transducer is placed on a woman's abdomen so that images of the fetus in the women's uterus can be viewed on a monitor. The most commonly used ultrasound produces a two-dimensional image of the fetus, although the technology exists to create a three-dimensional image as well. Electrical energy coming in to the transducer is converted to high-frequency sound waves. The sound waves reflect off of any structures they contact and return to the transducer and are converted back to electrical energy. Generally, more dense structures, like fetal bones, are seen as bright white images on the screen. Less dense tissue, like organs and fluid, shows darker on the screen. Gel placed on the woman's abdomen acts as a medium and allows for more rapid transmission of the sound waves and a better image.

There are many reasons an obstetrician may recommend an ultrasound for a pregnant woman. Some of these reasons include getting an accurate gestational age (dating) of the pregnancy, determining viability of a fetus (i.e., heartbeat), determining if any structural changes are present in the fetus, and determining if there are problems in the fetal environment. A prenatal ultrasound is performed by a health care professional, including an obstetrician, a radiologist, and a maternal-fetal medicine specialist. The American Institute of Ultrasound Medicine recommends that physicians performing ultrasound complete an approved residency program, a fellowship, or postgraduate training that includes three months and 500 supervised ultrasound procedures. An ultrasound technician often performs the initial measurements and, if needed, the physician reviews the procedure and obtains additional images. Ultrasounds are sometimes referred to as either basic (level 1) or comprehensive (level 2 or 3), depending on the quality of the equipment used, the amount and detail of the fetal anatomy studied, and the training of the person performing the procedure.

Most pregnant women in the United States have one prenatal ultrasound. There is some debate about when this ultrasound should take place. Early ultrasounds, in the first trimester of pregnancy, are the

KEY TERMS

**Aneuploidy**—A change in the number of chromosomes present, so that there are additional or missing chromosomes.

**Cystic hygroma**—An accumulation of fluid around the head and neck caused by the blockage of drainage of lymphatic fluid.

**Diaphragmatic hernia**—A defect that occurs when the diaphragm does not close properly, and the intestines are able to be herniated through the diaphragm into the chest cavity.

**Gestational age**—An estimation of the age of the pregnancy. The beginning of gestation or pregnancy is counted from the first day of the woman's last menstrual period, although conception usually takes place about two weeks later.

**Holoprosencephaly**—A malformation of the brain in which the two hemispheres or lobes of the brain do not separate properly.

**Hydrocephalus**—The presence of extra cerebrospinal fluid in the ventricles of the brain.

**Neural tube defect**—A defect in closure of the bones of the spine or skull; defects of the brain and skull are called anencephaly, while defects of the spine are called spina bifida.

most accurate way to determine how far advanced a pregnancy is and to set an accurate due date. However, these early ultrasounds do not allow for a detailed study of the fetal anatomy for any changes in development. An anatomical study of the fetus is best performed at about 18–20 weeks gestation. Women who are at increased risk for birth defects, genetic conditions, or pregnancy complications may have multiple ultrasounds. Studies have shown, and the American Institute of Ultrasound Medicine Bioeffects Committee has concluded, that there is no association between prenatal ultrasounds using sound waves and an increased chance for birth defects or other pregnancy complications. Studies have also shown that there is significant psychological benefit to parents from having ultrasounds performed. Prenatal ultrasounds provide parents with reassurance that the fetus is developing normally, or identify problems that can be investigated further.

### First-trimester ultrasounds

The first trimester of pregnancy is considered to be the first 12 weeks of pregnancy, or the first three months. Prenatal ultrasounds in the first trimester may be performed either on the abdomen or vaginally; however, to get the clearest images in the first trimester, a vaginal ultrasound is performed. In this type of ultrasound, a smaller transducer is placed into the vagina, up to the cervix. By having the transducer closer to the uterus, the fetus, which is very small in the first trimester, can be more clearly viewed.

First-trimester ultrasounds are often performed for women, unsure of the dating of their last menstrual period, who want to determine the correct gestational age. Early ultrasounds are best for dating because, early in a pregnancy, all fetuses grow at about the same rate. Therefore, measurements correspond well to gestational age. However, later in pregnancy, fetuses show more characteristics of their own growth pattern, and correlation to gestational age is not as clear. In general, first-trimester ultrasound measurements of gestational age are accurate to within about five days. Second-trimester ultrasound measurements of growth are accurate to about 8–12 days. Pinpointing a correct gestational age aids in determining an accurate due date and, consequently, in scheduling the proper tests at the proper times. One test that is offered to all pregnant women is called a maternal serum multiple marker screening test. This test screens a pregnancy to determine if there is an increased chance for **Down syndrome**, open spine defects, and another chromosomal condition called **trisomy 18**. This test can be performed between 15 and 20 weeks of pregnancy, and may result in a false/negative or false/positive result if the due date of the pregnancy is not accurate.

First-trimester ultrasounds can also be used to detect multiple pregnancies, ectopic pregnancies (pregnancies located outside of the uterus), and the location of the placenta. The placenta is the organ between the mother and fetus that allows for the crossing of nutrients and oxygenated blood. Sometimes the placenta is located over the cervix, blocking the path the fetus would normally take to exit the uterus. Complications of this condition, called placenta previa, can be avoided by performing a cesarean section rather than a vaginal delivery. Another common reason for a first-trimester ultrasound is vaginal bleeding. First-trimester ultrasounds may be able to detect a pregnancy loss or a pregnancy that is not progressing normally. In general, the fetus is too small in the first trimester to view the anatomy in detail. However, a few serious structural changes to the fetus can be identified in the first trimester. These include conditions like **anencephaly** (a condition in which the fetal brain and skull does not

develop), cystic hygromas (large fluid-filled sacs around the fetal neck), and **conjoined twins**.

### Nuchal translucency

First-trimester ultrasounds can also be used to screen a pregnancy for chromosomal conditions, including Down syndrome. People with Down syndrome have mild to moderate mental retardation, a characteristic facial appearance, an increased chance for heart defects and other structural changes, and short stature. By measuring the translucent, or fluid-filled, area at the back of the fetal neck, it can be determined if there is an increased chance for a chromosomal change. An increased nuchal translucency indicates an increased chance for a chromosomal change. This measurement, in combination with an analysis of two proteins in the mother's blood called beta-hCG (human chorionic gonadotropin) and pregnancy-associated plasma protein A (PAPPA) in the first trimester of pregnancy, is referred to as first-trimester screening for aneuploidy (changes in **chromosome** number).

By performing a first-trimester screening between 10 and 14 weeks of pregnancy, about 80% of fetuses with Down syndrome can be detected. Most fetuses with two other chromosomal conditions, **trisomy 13** and 18, can also be detected by first-trimester screenings. Therefore, first-trimester screening for aneuploidy is considered as effective as the more traditional screening for aneuploidy performed in the second trimester. However, The American College of Obstetricians and Gynecologist recommended that individuals who perform prenatal ultrasounds and take measurements of the nuchal translucency complete additional training to ensure that they are taking this measurement correctly. The recommendation also stated that there should be ongoing monitoring of the accuracy of this measurement, that appropriate counseling about screening and testing options for aneuploidy should be provided to women wishing to have first-trimester screening, and that the screening should only be performed when further diagnostic testing indicates an increased risk for aneuploidy. The diagnostic test for chromosomal changes available in the first trimester of pregnancy is called a chorionic villus sampling (CVS). This test can be performed between 10 and 12 weeks of gestation. However, CVS is not as commonly available as **amniocentesis**, the second-trimester test for chromosomal changes.

Screening for aneuploidy in the first trimester is a more recent event and allows women to have diagnostic testing earlier and to make decisions about continuing or discontinuing a pregnancy earlier. Ending a pregnancy in the first trimester or early second trimester is safer for the mother than later pregnancy terminations. In fetuses with an increased nuchal translucency and normal chromosomes, follow-up ultrasounds are recommended as heart defects, other structural changes in development, and other genetic syndromes can still be present.

### Second-trimester ultrasound

Ultrasounds in the second trimester of pregnancy are most often performed using the transducer on the maternal abdomen. Vaginal ultrasound may be used in situations where there is a problem with good visualization of the fetus, such as in obese women. In the second trimester, the fetus is larger and it is possible to see more detail of the development of the fetal anatomy. Anatomy scans of the fetus are most often performed at 18–20 weeks of gestation and can also include images of the placenta, amniotic fluid, umbilical cord, and the sac containing the fetus.

It is also important to look for fetal movement. The absence of movement can indicate the presence of a condition affecting the muscles, bones, or central nervous system. There are many other fetal anomalies that can be detected as well. The finding of a structural anomaly often increases the chance for aneuploidy. Patients may be offered additional tests for more information. When one fetal anomaly is noted on ultrasound, it is important to study the fetus carefully for the presence of other anomalies, since anomalies often occur simultaneously. The prognosis for a fetus when an anomaly is found depends on the severity of the anomaly, the presence of other anomalies, and the presence of a chromosomal condition. Fetuses with mild isolated anomalies have the best prognosis.

### Fetal anomalies

A detailed second-trimester ultrasound allows for the identification of structural changes in development which, in themselves, may be a significant concern, or may be a sign that additional problems like chromosomal changes are present. About 2–3% of all live born infants have a birth defect.

A detailed ultrasound studies many structures in the fetal head and brain. There is a measurement of the amount of fluid in the ventricles, or areas, of cerebrospinal fluid in the brain. Too much fluid in the ventricles of the brain is a condition called **hydrocephalus**. Depending on the degree of hydrocephalus, there can be underdevelopment of the brain and severe mental retardation. The presence of the two main lobes of the brain and the skull are noted to rule out a type of open spine defect called anencephaly. The lobes of the brain are studied to detect midline defects of the brain such as **holoprosencephaly**, in which the lobes of the brain

have not divided properly. The cerebellum, an organ at the back of the brain, is studied because changes in the shape of the cerebellum or the bones in the front of the skull are indicative of an open spine defect, or **spina bifida**. The size of the head is measured, because a small head size, called **microcephaly**, can result in mental retardation. The face is studied for the presence of a **cleft lip**, a small jaw, or either widely or narrowly spaced eyes.

A study of the fetal chest and abdomen will determine if the organs are located on the normal side, or if they are reversed. Ultrasound can detect the presence of diaphragmatic hernia, in which there is a hole in the diaphragm and the intestines are herniated through it into the chest. Abdominal wall defects, in which there is an opening in the abdomen and the intestines are located outside the body, can be detected. Changes to the kidneys, such as cystic, or missing, kidneys and cystic malformations of the lungs, can be detected. The heart is a particularly complex organ and can be difficult to study with ultrasound. The more severe heart defects can be identified with ultrasound, but many smaller structural changes to the heart are missed with ultrasound. When a heart defect is suspected, a more specialized ultrasound of the fetal heart, called an echocardiogram, can be performed. Ultrasound evaluation should also include views of the fetal bladder and stomach. The sex of the fetus can often be seen after 18 weeks of gestation.

A careful study of the fetal spine can detect the presence of spina bifida. Changes in the bones of the arms and legs can also be noted. In particular, an inward curving of the feet or club feet can be seen as well as missing limbs. Shortened or curved long bones are a sign of a **skeletal dysplasia**. There are many types of skeletal dysplasias with varying degrees of severity. Some skeletal dysplasias also include broken bones, short ribs, or changes to the bones in the spine.

Not all changes in development can be detected by ultrasound. The detection rate for individual anomalies with ultrasound varies, and centers that perform ultrasound should collect their own data before providing statistical detection rates to patients. In addition, there can be instances when a condition is diagnosed by ultrasound, but not truly present, or when a condition is misdiagnosed. Patients should be informed of the limitations of ultrasound before the procedure is performed.

### Ultrasound markers

With the advancement of ultrasound technology, additional findings on ultrasound have been identified. These findings are not anomalies, or structural changes, that in themselves cause any problem in development. However, these findings have been associated with an increased chance for chromosomal changes in a fetus. Therefore, these findings have been referred to as markers, or soft signs, of aneuploidy. For instance, fluid-filled cysts called choroids plexus cysts have been seen in fetuses with aneuploidy. The finding of a marker alone in a woman with no other increased risk for aneuploidy is not likely to be significant. Finding multiple markers does increase the chance for aneuploidy. When a marker is seen in the fetus of a woman at increased risk for aneuploidy based on advanced maternal age, maternal serum multiple marker screening, or family history, the patient should receive additional **genetic counseling** to discuss the finding and how it affects the risk for aneuploidy and the additional testing options. When not associated with aneuploidy, these markers are most often of no significance to the health of the fetus.

Fetuses with several chromosomal conditions can survive to full term. Those conditions include trisomy 21 (Down syndrome), trisomy 18, trisomy 13, and **Turner syndrome** (45,X).

About half of children with Down syndrome have a heart defect, some of which can be detected by ultrasound. In addition, fetuses with Down syndrome may have various gastrointestinal changes or a cystic hygroma (fluid-filled cyst around the neck) that may be detected by ultrasound. Ultrasound markers for Down syndrome include inward curving of the fifth finger, an increase of fluid in the kidney, short long bones in the upper arm or leg, extra skin at the back of the neck, a bright spot in either the heart or bowel, absence of the nasal bone, and fluid-filled cysts in the brain. When any of these findings is seen in a woman with an increased chance for Down syndrome, her risks may be increased. If an ultrasound is performed in a woman with an increased risk for Down syndrome, and none of these findings is seen, her risks may be lower than previously estimated. Risk reduction based on ultrasound is controversial and should not be done unless an ultrasound center has collected their own data on detection of Down syndrome with ultrasound.

Trisomy 18 is a rare, severe condition caused by the presence of an extra chromosome 18. Babies with trisomy 18 have severe neurological problems and mental retardation and usually do not survive more than a few months. The most common ultrasound findings in fetuses with trisomy 18 include heart defects and skeletal changes. Fetuses with trisomy 18 have a characteristic hand position that can be noted, clubbed feet, an unusual shape to the feet called rocker-bottom feet, and an unusual shape to the skull called a strawberry-shaped skull. Many other anomalies of other organs have also been noted in fetuses with trisomy 18, including diaphragmatic hernia, open spine defects, and significant growth delay. Markers for trisomy 18 include a thickened nuchal fold, extra fluid in the kidneys, choroids plexus cysts, and a single umbilical artery. Most, but not all, fetuses with trisomy 18 will have some feature of the condition identified on ultrasound.

Trisomy 13 is also a rare, severe condition caused by the presence of an extra chromosome 13 and associated with multiple birth defects, mental retardation, and a shortened lifespan. Ultrasound findings in fetuses with trisomy 13 include heart defects, brain malformations like holoprosencephaly, small head size, cleft lip, kidney malformations, extra fingers or toes, and growth delay. Markers for trisomy 13 include an increased nuchal fold and a bright spot in the heart. Most, but not all, fetuses with Trisomy 13 will have a feature of the condition noted on ultrasound.

Turner syndrome is a condition in which a female is missing the second X chromosome. Females born with Turner syndrome have an increased chance for heart defects and kidney problems. Girls with Turner syndrome have short stature, and will experience infertility as adults. Many pregnancies of fetuses with Turner syndrome miscarry. Ultrasound appearance of these pregnancies often includes a large cystic hygroma, and generalized fluid accumulation throughout the fetal body, called hydrops or edema. Fetuses with Turner syndrome that survive to delivery will sometimes show heart defects, kidney problems, or a cystic hygroma on an ultrasound.

Another way to study the fetal well-being is to study the fetal environment and associated pregnancy structures. If a fetus has oligohydramnios (a low amount of amniotic fluid) in the sac surrounding it, the lungs may not develop and the fetus may not survive. Oligohydramnios may occur because of absence of the kidneys, other structural defects, or due to a rupturing of the membranes or sac surrounding the fetus. Polyhydramnios (an excess of amniotic fluid) may also be a sign of structural changes, especially blockages in the urinary tract system, and can lead to premature delivery of a fetus. There can also be problems when the inner membrane of the sac that holds the fetus tears. The torn strands of amnion can wrap around the fetus and cut off blood flow to those areas. The presence of amniotic bands can disrupt the formation of limbs or any structure they wrap around and cause deformations that range from mild to lethal. There can be problems with the umbilical cord if the cord is too long or too short, has knots in it, is entangled around the fetus, has cysts in it, or is not inserted into the center of the placenta. The placenta may also cause or be associated with problems if it is too small, too large, split, located over the cervical opening, detaches from the uterus, or has tumors in it. Molar pregnancies occur when the placenta is swollen and cystic and no fetus is present. In a partial molar pregnancy, a small, malformed fetus with a chromosomal abnormality called **triploidy** is often present. In triploidy, a fetus has a whole extra set of chromosomes, so that the total number is 69 instead of the usual 46.

### Third-trimester ultrasound

Ultrasounds in the third trimester, or last three months, of the pregnancy are often done to monitor fetal growth. If a fetus is macrosomic (large), as is often the case in maternal **diabetes**, then the fetus is monitored for timing of delivery. Some fetal anomalies that are present earlier do not show features until the third trimester, and some fetal anomalies, like hydrocephalus, may not develop until the third trimester. Ultrasound may be used in the third trimester for fetuses with known anomalies to monitor progression and consider delivery techniques and timing.

Another important use of ultrasound is to guide prenatal procedures such as chorionic villus sampling (CVS) and amniocentesis. In CVS, a physician inserts a catheter into the vagina, through the cervix, and into the placental tissue using ultrasound guidance. By suctioning a small sample of the placental tissue, a sample can be obtained for chromosomal studies. CVS is performed at 10–12 weeks gestation. Amniocentesis is a test performed at 15–20 weeks gestation to obtain a sample of amniotic fluid from the sac of fluid around the fetus. This fluid contains fetal cells that can be used for chromosomal analysis of the fetus. During amniocentesis, a pocket of amniotic fluid located away from the fetus is targeted. Ultrasound is used to identify a pocket of fluid and used to guide the insertion of the needle into the targeted area.

Ultrasound is useful tool in the care of pregnant women. There are many uses for prenatal ultrasound and no identified risk with the procedure.

### Resources

#### BOOKS

Chervenak, F., and S. Gabbe. "Obstetric Ultrasound: Assessment of Fetal Growth and Anatomy." In *Obstetrics: Normal and Problem Pregnancies, Fourth Edition*, edited by Gabbe, S., J. Niebyl, J. L. Simpson. Philadelphia: Churchill Livingston, 2002.

Ville, Y., K. Nicolaides, and S. Campbell. "Prenatal Diagnosis of Fetal Malformations by Ultrasound." In *Genetic Disorders and the Fetus: Diagnosis, Prevention and Treatment, Fifth Edition*, edited by Aubrey Milunski. Baltimore, MD: The Johns Hopkins University Press, 2004.

#### PERIODICALS

American College of Obstetrics and Gynecology, Committee on Obstetric Practice and Committee on Genetics, Committee Opinion No. 296. "First-trimester Screening for Fetal Aneuploidy." *Obstet Gynecol* 104 (2004): 215–217.

Brigatti, K. W., and F. D. Malone. "First-trimester Screening for Aneuploidy." *Obstet Gynecol Clin N Am* 31 (2004): 1–20.

Goldberg, James. "Routine Screening for Fetal Anomalies: Expectations." *Obstet Gynecol Clin N Am* 31 (2004): 35–50.

Lazarus, Elizabeth. "What's New in First-trimester Ultrasound." *Radiol Clin N Am* 41 (2003): 663–679.

Marino, Teresa. "Ultrasound Abnormalities of the Amniotic Fluid, Membranes, Umbilical Cord, and Placenta." *Obstet Gynecol Clin N Am* 31 (2004): 177–200.

Nicolaides, Kypros. "Nuchal Translucency and Other First-trimester Sonographic Markers of Chromosomal Abnormalities." *American Journal of Obstetrics and Gynecology* 191 (2004): 45–67.

Stewart, Teresa. "Screening for Aneuploidy: The Genetic Sonogram." *Obstet Gynecol Clin N Am* 31 (2004): 21–33.

Sonja R. Eubanks, MS, CGC

# Prion diseases

## Definition

Prion diseases are a class of degenerative central nervous system disorders. They are unique in that while a genetic component of the syndrome exists, prion diseases may also be transmitted, and the infectious agent of the disease is a protein. Dr. Stanley Prusiner coined the term "prion," meaning "proteinaceous infectious particle," in 1982. Dr. Prusiner's controversial, but finally accepted, research in the area of prion diseases led to his winning the Nobel Prize in Medicine in 1997.

## Description

There are five forms of prion disease known to occur in humans: kuru, Creutzfeldt-Jakob disease (CJD), Gertsmann-Straussler-Scheinker disease (GSS), fatal familial insomnia (FFI), and new variant Creutzfeld-Jakob disease, popularly known as "mad cow disease." The prion diseases are also called transmissible

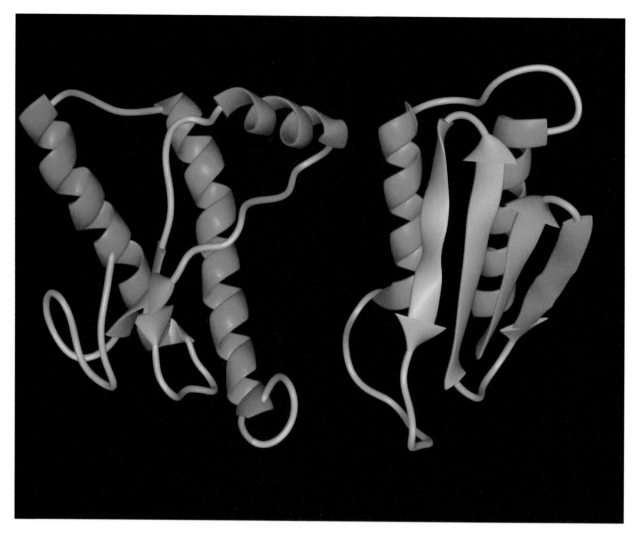

**Computer-generated illustration of human prion protein in its normal shape at molecular level (I) and of disease-causing prion protein in its abnormal shape.** *(AP Images.)*

spongiform encephalopathies because they can be transmitted between unrelated individuals and they sometimes cause a sponge-like encephalopathy, or degeneration of the brain tissue, in which holes and other abnormal structures are formed in the brain. Prion diseases have also been identified in animals and include scrapie in sheep and goats, bovine spongiform encephalopathy (BSE) in cows, feline spongiform encephalopathy in cats, and chronic wasting disease in mule, deer and elk.

Prion diseases have all been associated with the function of a specific cellular protein named the prion protein (PrP). Like all cellular proteins, PrP is a long-chain molecule consisting of linked amino acids. A protein can assume many shapes: twisted into a spiral helix as in **DNA**, extended into linear strands, or folded into sheets of aligned strands. Different shapes of the

same molecular sequence are called isomers. It is theorized that the normal form of cellular PrP is a compact shape consisting mainly of four helix regions, whereas in the abnormal isomer (the prion), the protein is refolded into a sheet-helix combination. Furthermore, this prion, through an unknown mechanism, triggers the conversion of normal PrP to the abnormal shape. The abnormal isomer acts as a template to change more and more normal PrP to the abnormal structure. Therefore, once the protein exists in the abnormal form, it is an infectious agent that can be transmitted from one person to another.

Normal proteins are processed by proteases, which are enzymes present in the body that act to break down excess proteins. However, the abnormal isomer of the prion protein is protease resistant and cannot be broken down by the body's protease

## KEY TERMS

**Ataxia**—A deficiency of muscular coordination, especially when voluntary movements are attempted, such as grasping or walking.

**Iatrogenic**—Caused by (-genic) doctor (iatro-). An iatrogenic condition is a condition that is caused by the diagnosis or treatment administered by medical professionals. Iatrogenic conditions may be caused by any number of things, including: unsterile medical instruments or devices, contaminated blood or implantations, or contaminated air within the medical facility.

**Isomers**—Two chemicals identical in chemical composition (contain the same atoms in the same amounts) that have differing structures. The normal prion protein and the infectious prion protein are conformational isomers of one another. They have the same chemical structures, but for some reason, assume different shapes.

**Myoclonus**—Twitching or spasms of a muscle or an interrelated group of muscles.

**Prion**—A term coined to mean "proteinaceous infectious particle." Prior to the 1982 discovery of prions, it was not believed that proteins could serve as infectious agents.

**Protease**—An enzyme that acts as a catalyst in the breakdown of peptide bonds.

**Spongiform encephalopathy**—A form of brain disease characterized by a "sponge-like" appearance of the brain either on autopsy or via magnetic resonance imaging (MRI).

enzymes. Therefore, the abnormal prion protein continues to be produced without being processed. This leads to an accumulation of the abnormal protein in the body. In several forms of prion disease, the abnormal prion protein aggregates in deposits, or plaques, in the brain tissue. It is believed that once the abnormal prion protein accumulates to a certain level in the body, the physical symptoms of impaired mental and physical functioning begin to show themselves. However, the exact mechanisms by which the abnormal isomer causes disease are not known. The onset of symptoms often does not occur until the patient is elderly, suggesting that either the rate of accumulation of the abnormal protein is initially slow, or that some triggering event late in life causes the initial formation of the abnormal isomer, after which the disease can spread.

The normal function of the prion protein is not completely understood, but it is known to be involved with the functions of the synapses (nerve connections) in the brain. PrP is found in the highest concentrations in the brain. PrP is also found in the eyes, lungs, heart, kidney, pancreas, testes, blood, and in the neuromuscular junction. The conversion of normal PrP to the infectious, abnormal isomer form may disrupt the normal functions of the prion protein, and this may be another cause of the degenerative symptoms of the disease.

Body tissues containing the abnormal isomer are a source of transmission of the disease between people and even across species. Prion diseases are also found in animals, and in animal studies it has been shown that the disease can be spread through the ingestion of infected brain tissue. The transmission can also cross the species barrier; it has been found that cows became affected by prion disease after eating feed contaminated with infected sheep brain tissue. It is widely speculated that the outbreak of "mad cow" disease, the most publicized prion disease, was caused by infection from affected cows in the United Kingdom, although the mode of transmission has still not been determined. Transmission through oral ingestion was also shown to be the cause of kuru in the Fore tribe of New Guinea. After the Fore abandoned their practice of ritual cannibalism in which they consumed the brain tissue of ancestors, the incidence of kuru all but disappeared. Other cases of human infection have been shown to be iatrogenic; in other words, transmitted inadvertently during medical treatment. Most of these iatrogenic cases involve direct contact with brain and nervous system tissue. For example, CJD has been reported to result from the use of contaminated surgical instruments, corneal implants, implantation of dura matter or electrodes in the brain, and from the injection of human growth hormones derived from cadaverous pituitary glands.

Other modes of transmission have been shown to be less efficient in animal studies. The recent outbreak of new variant CJD caused increased concern about possible transmission through blood transfusions and plasma-derived products, but no case of new variant CJD has been proven to result from blood transfusion. Laboratory and epidemiological evidence supporting a strong risk of the spread of prion disease through blood transfusion is not present, even though this area has been intensively studied.

### Genetic profile

The **gene** that encodes the prion protein has been mapped to **chromosome** 20p12. This gene has been named the PRNP gene. Mutations in the PRNP gene can cause alterations in the chemical sequence of amino acids in the prion protein, and this change is believed to make the protein more susceptible to assuming the abnormal conformation. Over 20 different mutations of the gene have been identified, encompassing point mutations (one base pair substituted for another in the gene sequence), insertions (additions to the gene sequence), and deletions (missing parts of the gene sequence). Depending on the specific mutation, different types of prion disease can appear in the patient.

It is estimated that 10-15% of prion disease cases are caused by inherited mutations of the PRNP gene. Because of the delayed onset of the disease and the wide variation in symptoms, more exact statistics are difficult to determine. The **inheritance** pattern is autosomal dominant, meaning that if either parent passes the mutated gene to their offspring, the child will be affected by the disease. A parent with prion disease has a 50% probability of passing on the mutated gene to his or her child.

Another genetic factor important in prion disease is the genetic sequence of the PRNP gene. Like all genes, the PRNP gene is made up of two strands of DNA. Each DNA strand consists of a sequence of chemical structures called bases, and the two strands together form a sequence of base pairs. Three base pairs together form a unit called a codon, and each codon codes for a specific amino acid. At codon 129 of the PRNP gene, either the amino acid methionine (Met) or valine (Val) can be encoded. Since one gene is inherited from each parent, an individual may either be homozygous, having two of the same amino acids (Met-Met or Val-Val) at this position; or, heterozygous, having different amino acids (Met-Val). Individuals who are homozygous appear to be more susceptible to infection of prion diseases, because it has been shown that a greater percentage of those infected are homozygous than in the general population. Also, the clinical symptoms, or **phenotype**, of the prion disease can differ based on whether the individual is Met-Met or Val-Val homozygous, and whether the individual has Met or Val on the same gene as another mutation. For example, a specific point mutation at codon 178 has been found to cause familial CJD if the individual has Val at codon 129 on the mutated gene, while the same mutation causes FFI when the individual has Met at codon 129.

## Demographics

Prion diseases occur worldwide with a rate of one to two cases per one million. CJD is the most common of the prion diseases, while GSS and FFI are extremely rare, and kuru is now virtually nonexistant due to the abandonment of the practice of cannibalism. There is no gender link to the disease. Several forms of prion disease usually do not cause identifiable symptoms until the individual is more than 60 years old, although other forms have an earlier onset and are seen in teenagers and young adults.

Since prion disease can be either inherited or transmitted through infection, the demographics of the disease have both familial and environmental patterns. Inherited CJD is found with high frequency in Libyan Jews and also in other descendants of Sephardic Jews in Greece, Tunisia, Israel, Italy, Spain, and perhaps South America. Other genetic clusters have been identified in Slovakia, Poland, France, and Germany. Fatal familial insomnia has been linked to family pedigrees in Italy, Australia, and the United States, among others. Families with GSS syndrome have been found in several countries in North America and Europe.

The environmental clusters of the disease include the Fore, a remote tribe of New Guinea in which kuru was transmitted through the practice of ritual cannibalism; a group of over 80 cases in Japan resulting from dura mater (brain membrane) grafts from a single surgical supply company; over 100 cases resulting from cadaveric human growth hormone injections in Europe and the United States; and, most famously, the 40-plus cases of new variant CJD or "mad cow" disease in the United Kingdom.

## Signs and symptoms

Prion disease primarily affects the brain and central nervous system, so the symptoms associated with the disease are all related to neurological function. These may include loss of muscular coordination and uncontrollable body movements (ataxia), visual problems, hallucinations, behavioral changes, difficulty in thinking clearly or remembering, sleep disturbances, speech impairment, and insanity. General complaints such as headache, diminished appetitie, and fatigue may occur prior to the onset of the more serious symptoms. The exact combination and severity of these symptoms varies widely between cases and types of prion disease.

CJD, the most common of the human prion diseases, is characterized by a rapid deterioration in mental function from confusion and memory loss into severe **dementia**, accompanied by loss of muscular control (ataxia) and twitching or spasmodic motion (myoclonus). Other symptoms include vision and speech impairment. A scan of electrical activity in the brain, called an electroencephalogram (EEG), will often show an abnormal periodic spike pattern. The onset of symptoms usually occurs when the patient is over age 50 and death follows within one to five years. Microsopic holes, or vacuoles, in the brain tissue, which give it a "spongiform" appearance, are characteristic of CJD.

Gertsmann-Straussler-Scheinker syndrome (GSS) encompasses a variety of disorders. One form of the disease (the ataxic form) is first characterized by an unsteady walk sometimes accompanied by leg pains. These motor problems get worse over several years and are finally accompanied by mental and behavioral breakdown. By contrast, dementia is the main characteristic of the telencephalic form of GSS, accompanied by rigidity, the inability to make facial expressions, tremors, and stuttering or stammering. In another form of the disease, GSS with neurofibrillary tangles, the main features are loss of muscle coordination (ataxia), tremors, and progressive insanity. As in CJD, the affected individuals are usually in their fifties or older, and the progression of the disease may take from two to six years.

The most noticeable sign of fatal familial insomnia (FFI) is the untreatable and progressively worse difficulty in sleeping. The affected individual then begins to experience complex hallucinations which are often enacted dreams. Excessive sweating, irregular heartbeat, high blood pressure, and hyperventilation are other symptoms. Motor impairment may be present. Shortened attention span and memory loss has been observed. In the terminal stages, stupor and coma precede death. The average age at onset of symptoms is the mid-forties, and the disease progresses rapidly with death resulting after about one year. Autopsy reveals the formation of dense tangles of neural fibers and astrocytes in the thalamus region of the brain.

Kuru was called the "shivering" disease by the Fore tribe members because its primary symptom was twitching and shaking of the body. This twitching began slowly and was not present when the person was completely still, but then progressively worsened until any attempt at motion led to drastic and uncontrollable body movements, and the individual could no longer stand or walk. Mental insanity usually did not appear until the terminal stages of the disease. The onset of symptoms usually occurred in middle-aged individuals and the course of the disease was short: three to 12 months.

The early signs of new variant CJD are most often psychiatric disturbances. Abnormal sensations of prickling or itching (paresthesia) or pain even from light touches (dysesthesia) are often present. So far,

individuals affected with new variant CJD are much younger in age, typically teenagers and young adults. The duration of the disease is one to two years. As in CJD, vacuoles are present in the brain, but they are associated with dense deposits, or plaques, of the abnormal PrP isomer.

### Diagnosis

Because of the many different forms of the disease and the overlap in symptoms with other common syndromes such as **Alzheimer disease**, prion diseases are often difficult to diagnosis. A diagnosis of prion disease should be considered in any adult patient with signs of neurological impairment such as uncontrollable body movements, confusion, loss of memory, and cognitive degeneration, or psychiatric abnormality. Periodic discharges of brain waves, as observed on an electroencephalogram (EEG), are present in many, but not all, cases of prion disease. A magnetic resonance imaging (MRI) scan of the brain can rule out other causes of brain disease and potentially identify some abnormalities associated with prion disease. A biopsy, or sampling, of brain tissue can reveal the presence of abnormal PrP, although this procedure is generally not used in elderly patients. **Genetic testing** can reveal those cases of prion disease that are caused by mutations. Bismuth, mercury, or lithium poisoning result in symptoms quite similar to prion disease. These poisonings can be differentially diagnosed by blood tests.

The diagnosis of prion disease can be definitively confirmed by the transmission of the disease to an animal host such as a genetically engineered mouse. However, the transmission period may be quite long, as much as six to seven months. After death, prion disease can also be validated by autopsy of the brain tissue.

Patients eventually identified with prion disease have been initially diagnosed with many other diseases including Alzheimer disease, **Huntington disease**, **Parkinson disease**, **schizophrenia**, **multiple sclerosis**, and myoclonic **epilepsy**. This illustrates the difficulty in identifying the disease and the importance of careful diagnosis to avoid unnecessary treatments.

### Treatment and management

At present, there is no known treatment that can prevent or reverse the transformation of the prion protein into its aberrant form. All treatments for prion disease are directed towards management of the symptoms. These treatments may include psychoactive drugs, electroconvulsive therapy (ECT), and professional care to ensure that the loss of physical

- What is a prion?
- How does a person "catch" a prion? Is the process similar to a viral or bacterial infection?
- How are prion infections treated?
- What is the direction of current research on prion diseases?

and mental functions do not lead to accidental injury or death. Research into more advanced treatments is focusing on the application of gene therapies to block the formation of infectious PrP and drugs, which could act to stabilize the normal PrP structure. As with any inherited disease, **genetic counseling** is important in the management of the familial forms of prion disease.

## Prognosis

Since the forms of prion diseases vary widely, the age at onset and rate of worsening of symptoms are also quite variable, but all prion diseases are incurable and fatal with a duration anywhere from a few months to several years after onset.

## Resources

### PERIODICALS

Mastrianni, J., R. Roos "The prion diseases." *Seminars in Neurology* (October 2000): 337-352.

Prusiner, Stanley. "The prion diseases." *Scientific American* (January 1995): 48-57.

### WEBSITES

*CJD Voice.* (December 11, 2009) http://cjdvoice.org.

*Johns Hopkins Department of Neurology Resource on Prion Disease.* http://www.jhu-prion.org.

*The Official Mad Cow Disease Home Page.* http://www. mad-cow.org (February 23, 2001).

### ORGANIZATIONS

Creutzfeldt-Jakob Disease Foundation, Inc. PO Box 611625, Miami, FL 33261-1625. Fax: (954) 436-7591. http://www.cjdfoundation.org.

Human BSE Foundation (United Kingdom). 0191 389 4157. http://humanbse.foundation@virgin.net.

Paul A. Johnson

# Progeria syndrome

## Definition

Progeria syndrome is an extremely rare genetic disorder of unknown origin that manifests as premature aging in children. Progeria affects many parts of the body including the skin, bones, and arteries.

## Description

Dr. Jonathan Hutchinson in 1886 and Dr. Hastings Gilford in 1904 first described this syndrome. The word progeria is coined from the Greek word *geras*, which means old age. Progeria syndrome is also known as Hutchinson-Gilford progeria syndrome, HGPS or Gilford syndrome.

Most patients appear normal at birth. Signs and symptoms usually begin to develop within the first one to two years of life. Changes in skin and failure to thrive (failure to gain weight) are usually evident first, the exception being four reported cases of possible neonatal progeria. All four infants died before twenty months of age. Death in these cases appears to be related to intrauterine growth retardation and presentation of progeria signs and symptoms at birth. The neonatal cases did not exhibit the development of arteriosclerosis (hardening of the arteries). Arteriosclerosis is the most serious complication of progeria. Complications secondary to arteriosclerosis in childhood, adolescence, or adulthood are the leading cause of death.

Patients with progeria syndrome develop many other signs and symptoms which present a classical appearance. The majority of patients with progeria resemble each other. Common external findings include aging at an accelerated rate, alopecia (hair loss),

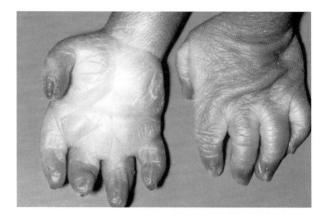

**Signs of premature aging in the hands of a patient diagnosed with progeria.** *(Custom Medical Stock Photo, Inc.)*

## KEY TERMS

**Arteriosclerosis**—Hardening of the arteries that often results in decreased ability of blood to flow smoothly.

**Failure to thrive**—Significantly reduced or delayed physical growth.

**Progeria**—Genetic abnormality that presents initially as premature aging and failure to thrive in children.

**Scleroderma**—A relatively rare autoimmune disease affecting blood vessels and connective tissue that makes skin appear thickened.

prominent scalp veins, absence of fat under the skin (subcutaneous fat), **scleroderma** (thickening of the skin), a pinched nose, small face and jaw (micrognathia) relative to head size (bird face), delayed tooth formation, high pitched voice, and impaired or absence of sexual development. Patients are also known to experience stiffening of various joints, bone structure abnormalities, and the development of arteriosclerosis. Patients with progeria syndrome experience average intelligence and their cognitive abilities are usually not affected.

### Genetic profile

Evidence suggests that the **gene** for progeria may be located on **chromosome** 1. Progeria is believed to be passed on in an autosomal dominant new mutation fashion. The disorder is transmitted to children by autosomal dominant **inheritance**. This means that either affected parent (father or mother) has a 50% chance of having a child (regardless of gender) with the disorder. New mutation refers to the chance change in the structure of a gene resulting in alterations in its function. This new mutation is believed to happen at conception sporadically and permanently (since neither parent is affected). New mutations occur as a result of both genetic and environmental factors. New mutations can be either **chromosomal abnormalities** or point mutations (specific alterations in the building blocks of genes called nucleotides). Research is ongoing to identify a more specific genetic mutation that causes progeria syndrome.

### Demographics

Occurrence of progeria is sporadic and rare, though studies suggest frequency may be related to increased parental age and increased average difference in age of parents. Approximately 100 cases have

been reported to date in the world with the reported incidence (number of absolute occurrence) being one in eight million.

### Signs and symptoms

Progeria syndrome is progressive. Signs develop over time.

- General—Patients are short and weigh less than is appropriate for height. Patients usually do not grow taller than 3.7 ft (1.15 m) or weigh over 40 lb (15 kg). Patients with progeria do not usually exhibit mental impairment.
- Skin—Skin is usually thin, dry and wrinkled. The skin in the hands and feet is pushed inwards. The skin also exhibits color (pigmentation) changes, which presents clinically as yellow-brownish spots. Patients also have a decrease in fat below the skin (subcutaneous) except in the area below the navel. The nails of patients with progeria are small, thin, and poorly developed. Patients experience alopecia (hair loss) of the scalp, eyelashes, and eyebrows. Scalp veins become visible and prominent as hair loss progresses.
- Bones—There are several abnormalities in the skeletal structure.
- Eyes—Patients often appear to have prominent eyes. This is in part secondary to the alterations in bone structure of the face. Patients also may experience farsightedness (hyperopia) and astigmatism. Astigmatism refers to changes in the structure of the lens and cornea (parts of the internal structure of the eyes), which alter the eyes' ability to focus incoming visual images.

### Diagnosis

Diagnosis is based upon physical appearance. Diagnosis is usually made within the first two years of life when patients develop skin changes and fail to grow.

Patients with progeria eventually develop skeletal system (bone and joint) changes. Patients show characteristic radiographic (x ray) findings. In general the skeleton is hypoplastic (underdeveloped). Patients have persistent anterior fontanelles (soft spots of skull in newborn children). Patients with progeria may also develop deterioration of the collarbone and end of the fingers. Hip joints are affected because of alteration in the bone structure of the femur (the bone which extends from the knee upwards to the pelvis). This causes the femur to sit in more of a straight-line relationship to the hip joint. This is abnormal and causes a wide-based gait (walking) and the appearance of a horse-riding stance. It is described as *coxa valga*. Some patients also show an increase in the amount of hyaluronic acid secreted in the urine. Hyaluronic acid is a substance in the body that is found in tissues such as cartilage. Cartilage is a flexible connective tissue that works as a joint stabilizer.

## Treatment and management

There is no cure for progeria. Treatment is symptomatic and aimed at providing psychological support. Palliative measures such as wearing a wig may be beneficial. Relief from chest pain due to changes in arteries can be accomplished by nitroglycerin. Nitroglycerin is a medication that relaxes muscle fibers in blood vessels causing them to expand or dilate. This permits proper blood flow to affected areas, which enables cells and tissues to receive adequate amounts of the oxygen necessary for cell maintenance.

### Experimental research management

Recent evidence suggested the benefit of giving nutritional therapy and growth hormone supplementation. The combination treatment of nutritional therapy and growth hormone supplementation demonstrated an increase in growth of Progeria patients, an increase in growth factors (chemicals which promote formation) within the blood, and a decrease in the patient's basal metabolic rate. Basal metabolic rate is the minimum amount of energy (calories) that an individual needs to ingest on a daily basis in order to execute normal activities and tasks.

Arteriosclerosis is most prominent in coronary (heart) arteries and the aorta (the largest artery in the body, which has many branches supplying oxygen filled blood to cells and tissues). Research indicates successful outcome from aggressive treatment of arteriosclerosis utilizing techniques such as coronary artery bypass (reconstruction of the heart arteries) or coronary artery balloon dilation (stretching the heart arteries in an attempt to allow increased blood flow).

## Prognosis

Age of death ranges from seven to 27 years. One documented case reports an individual living to be 45 years of age. Death is usually secondary to arteriosclerosis complications such as heart failure, myocardial infarction (heart attack), or coronary thrombosis (when a clot from the heart moves to another location cutting the flow of blood to the new location).

## Resources

### BOOKS

Nora, J.J., and F.C. Fraser. *Medical Genetics: Principles and Practice*. Philadelphia: Lea & Febiger, 1989.

Wiedemann, H.R., J. Kunze, and F.R. Grosse. "Progeria." In *Clinical Syndromes*. 3rd ed. Edited by Gina Almond, 306–7. St. Louis: Mosby, Inc., 1997.

### PERIODICALS

Sivaraman, D.M. Thappa., M. D'Souza, and C. Ratnakar. "Progeria (Hutchinson-Gilford): A Case Report." *Journal of Dermatology* 26, no. 5 (May 1999): 324–28.

### WEBSITES

The Council of Regional Networks for Genetic Services. http://www.cc.emory.edu/PEDIATRICS/corn/corn.htm.

The National Society of Genetic Counselors. http://www.nsgc.org/Resource.

### ORGANIZATIONS

Children Living with Inherited Metabolic Diseases. The Quadrangle, Crewe Hall, Weston Rd., Crewe, Cheshire, CW1-6UR. UK 127 025 0221. Fax: 0870-7700-327. http://www.climb.org.uk.

International Progeria Registry. IBR Dept. of Human Genetics, 1050 Forest Hill Rd., Staten Island, NY 10314. (718) 494-5333. wtbibr@aol.com.

Laith Farid Gulli, MD
Nicole Mallory, MS

Progressive tapetochoroidal dystrophy *see* **Choroideremia**

# Propionic acidemia

## Definition

Propionic acidemia is an inborn error of metabolism: a rare inherited disorder in which the body is unable to break down and use certain proteins properly. As a result, massive amounts of organic compounds (such as propionic acid, ketones, and fatty acids) build up in the blood and urine, interfering with normal body functions and development.

## Description

Propionic acidemia, first described in 1961, usually shows up in the first few weeks after birth and, if untreated, results in mental and physical impairment. The disorder can have a broad range of clinical outcomes, ranging from the severe form that is fatal to newborns to the mild, late-onset form associated with periodic attacks of ketoacidosis, when organic compounds build up in the blood and urine. Other names for the disorder include ketotic hyperglycinemia, hyperglycinemia with ketoacidosis and lactic acidosis (propionic type), and propionyl CoA carboxylase (PCC) deficiency, types I and II.

Propionic acidemia can occur in isolation, or it can be a feature of multiple carboxylase deficiency, a condition involving abnormal production of many enzymes—all of which need biotin (a form of vitamin B)—as the result of an abnormality in biotin metabolism. Propionic acidemia is characterized by deficiency of an enzyme, propionyl CoA carboxylase, which the body requires to break down the amino acids isoleucine, valine, threonine, and methionine (chemical building blocks of proteins). The deficiency can be caused by abnormal genes for making propionyl CoA carboxylase (isolated propionic acidemia) or by abnormal genes for metabolizing biotin (propionic acidemia resulting from multiple carboxylase deficiency).

## Genetic profile

Propionic acidemia is an autosomal recessive disorder; that is, if a man and woman each carry one abnormal **gene**, then 25% of their children are expected to be born with the disorder. Two genes, PCCA and PCCA, code for the two parts (alpha and beta subunits) of the propionyl CoA carboxylase molecule.

The PCCA gene controls the production of alpha subunit and is on **chromosome** 13. Alterations in the PCCA gene result in Type I propionic acidemia.

Researchers have identified 19 disease-causing mutations in the PCCA gene. Eight of these mutations result in an incomplete alpha subunit. Six mutations prevent the alpha subunit from binding biotin, which is required for propionyl CoA carboxylase to work properly, and results in multiple carboxylase deficiency. People who inherit two abnormal PCCA genes (homozygotes) produce only 1–5% of the normal amount of propionyl CoA carboxylase. People who inherit one normal and one abnormal PCCA gene (heterozygotes) produce 50% of the normal amount of enzyme.

The PCCA gene, which controls the production of beta subunit, is on chromosome 3. Mutations in this gene are responsible for Type II propionic acidemia.

Twenty-eight disease-causing mutations have been found in the PCCA gene. In people of Caucasian, Spanish, and Latin American heritage, researchers have found the most frequent mutation in about 32% of those with propionic acidemia. In people of Japanese heritage, two other mutations are most prevalent, occurring in 25% and 31% of Japanese patients. Homozygotes for the PCCA gene produce propionyl CoA carboxylase in amounts similar to homozygotes for the PCCA gene, but heterozygotes for the PCCA gene produce nearly normal amounts of propionyl CoA carboxylase. This is probably because many more beta subunits (four to five times more) are produced than alpha subunits, so even with decreased

PCCA gene activity, enough beta subunits are available to combine with alpha subunits to make a complete molecule of propionyl CoA carboxylase.

## Demographics

The frequency with which propionic acidemia occurs throughout the world is unknown because it is a rare disorder. Its occurrence does not appear to be specific to any particular population group. Considered to be prevalent among Inuits in Greenland, propionic acidemia has also been identified in other populations, including Austrian, Spanish, Latin American, Saudi Arabian, Amish, and Japanese people. Males and females are equally likely to be affected.

## Signs and symptoms

Newborns with propionic acidemia are typically small and pale with poorly developed muscles. Symptoms that usually appear in the first weeks of life include poor feeding, vomiting, listlessness (lethargy), and ketoacidosis. Less often, infants with the disorder experience loss of body fluids (dehydration), seizures, and enlarged livers.

In some patients, the disorder appears later in life. Signs include facial abnormalities, such as puffy cheeks and an exaggerated "Cupid's bow" upper lip. Patients with late-onset propionic acidemia may have acute inflammation of the brain (encephalopathy) or be developmentally delayed. These patients may have periodic attacks of ketoacidosis, usually brought on by eating too much protein, becoming constipated, or having frequent infections.

Patients with propionic acidemia as the result of having multiple carboxylase deficiency often have ketoacidosis and their urine may have a distinct "tom cat's urine" odor. These patients may also have skin rash and loss of hair (alopecia).

## Diagnosis

Physicians have only a few tests available that allow them to differentiate propionic acidemia from other inborn errors of metabolism. Tests that are absolutely specific for the disorder involve the measurement of propionyl CoA carboxylase and chemicals related to the reactions it affects. These tests are fairly uncommon and do not have published normal values.

Prenatal diagnosis of propionic acidemia is possible using cells obtained by **amniocentesis**. The cells can be tested for decreased activity of propionyl CoA carboxylase, for their ability to bind propionic acid, or for their methylcitrate levels.

In a newborn child, propionyl CoA carboxylase activity can be measured in white blood cells (leukocytes) from cord blood (blood from the umbilical cord). The infant's blood and urine can be tested for increased levels of propionic acid. These levels are tested as well in older children and adults who are suspected of having the disorder.

Physicians can use genetic tests to analyze **DNA** and identify the specific gene, PCCA or PCCA, that is abnormal.

## Treatment and management

The accepted treatment for propionic acidosis is a low-protein diet. Daily protein intake must be limited to 0.5–1.5 g/kg. Patients should eat frequent meals and avoid fasting, because fasting increases the body's need for propionyl CoA carboxylate.

A low-protein diet keeps the number of ketoacidosis attacks to a minimum; however, such a diet does not prevent attacks. Physicians treat attacks of ketoacidosis by removing all protein from the patient's diet and giving the patient sodium bicarbonate and glucose. If the attack is severe, proteins may be removed from the patient's stomach by peritoneal dialysis.

Some patients may respond to a single oral dose (100 mg/kg) of L-carnitine, an organic compound. Others may be helped by antibiotics, which reduce the number of bacteria that produce propionic acid in the stomach. These are experimental treatments and have not been tested for long-term effects.

Patients with multiple carboxylase deficiency may receive biotin supplements (10 mg daily), which provide immediate, long-lasting improvement. Biotin supplements are not effective, however, for patients with other types of propionic acidemia.

## Prognosis

The future of patients with propionic acidemia depends on the severity of the disorder. Left untreated, propionic acidemia in infants results in coma and death. With early diagnosis and treatment, some children are intellectually normal, while others' lives may be complicated by mental retardation and abnormal physical development. Some with popionic acidemia may be identified only during family studies. For patients with late-onset propionic acidemia, the disease can be controlled

Propionyl CoA carboxylase (PCC) deficiency
*see* **Propionic acidemia**

# Prostate cancer

### Definition

The prostate, a gland found only in men, is part of the reproductive system. Prostate **cancer** is a disease in which the cells of the prostate become abnormal and start to grow uncontrollably, forming tumors. Tumors that can spread to other parts of the body are called malignant tumors or cancers. Tumors that are not capable of spreading are said to be benign.

### Description

The prostate is a gland that produces the semen, the fluid that contains sperm. The prostate is about the size of a walnut and lies just beneath the urinary bladder. Usually prostate cancer is slow growing, but it can grow faster in some instances. As the prostate cancer grows, some of the cells break off and spread to other parts of the body through the lymphatic or the blood systems. This is known as metastasis. The most common sites of spreading are the lymph nodes and various bones in the spine and pelvic region.

The cause of prostate cancer is not clear; however, several risk factors are known. The average age at diagnosis of prostate cancer is around 72. In fact, 80% of prostate cancer cases occur in men over the age of 65. As men grow older, the likelihood of getting prostate cancer increases. Hence, age appears to be a

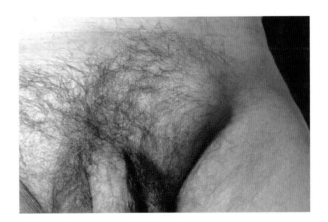

**The enlarged lymph node in the groin area of this male patient is a sign of prostate cancer.** *(Photo Researchers, Inc.)*

to some extent by diet, but many of these patients will also be mentally and physically delayed.

### Resources

#### BOOKS

Fenton, Wayne A., Roy A. Gravel, and David S. Rosenblatt. "Disorders of Propionate and Methylmalonate Metabolism." In *The Metabolic and Molecular Bases of Inherited Disease.* 8th ed. Vol. 2. Ed. Charles R. Scriver, et al. New York: McGraw-Hill, 2001.

#### PERIODICALS

Campeau, Eric, et al. "Detection of a Normally Rare Transcript in Propionic Acidemia Patients with mRNA Destabilizing Mutations in the PCCA Gene." *Human Molecular Genetics* 8, no. 1 (1999): 107–13.

Muro, Silvia, et al. "Identification of Novel Mutations in the PCCA Gene in European Propionic Acidemia Patients." *Human Mutation: Mutation in Brief* no. 253 (1999).

Ravn, Kirstine, et al. "High Incidence of Propionic Acidemia in Greenland is Due to a Prevalent Mutation, 1540insCCC, in the Gene for the Beta-Subunit of Propionyl CoA Carboxylase." *American Journal of Human Genetics* 67 (2000): 203–6.

#### WEBSITES

Propionyl CoA Carboxylase Website. http://www.uchsc.edu/sm/cbs/pcc/pccmain.htm.

#### ORGANIZATIONS

Children Living with Inherited Metabolic Diseases. The Quadrangle, Crewe Hall, Weston Rd., Crewe, Cheshire, CW1-6UR. UK 127 025 0221. Fax: 0870-7700-327. http://www.climb.org.uk.

Organic Acidemia Association. 13210 35th Ave. North, Plymouth, MN 55441. (763) 559-1797. Fax: (863) 694-0017. http://www.oaanews.org.

Organic Acidemias UK. 5 Saxon Rd., Ashford, Middlesex, TW15 1QL. UK (178)424-5989.

Linnea E. Wahl, MS

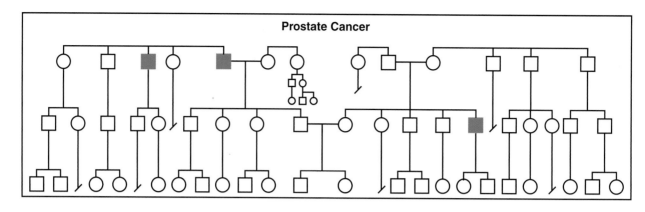

**Prostate Cancer**

*(Gale, a part of Cengage Learning.)*

risk factor for prostate cancer. Race may be another contributing factor. African-Americans have the highest rate of prostate cancer in the world, while the rate in Asians is one of the lowest. However, although the rate of prostate cancer in native Japanese is low, the rate in Japanese-Americans is closer to that of white American men. This suggests that environmental factors also play a role in prostate cancer.

There is some evidence to suggest that a diet high in fat increases the risk of prostate cancer. Studies also suggest that nutrients such as soy isoflavones, vitamin E, selenium, vitamin D and carotenoids (including lycopene, the red color agent in tomatoes and beets) may decrease prostate cancer risk. Vasectomy may be linked to increased prostate cancer rates as well. Workers in industries, such as welding, with exposure to the metal cadmium appear to have a higher than average risk of prostate cancer. Male sex hormone levels also may be linked to the rate of prostate cancer. In addition, some studies have linked increased prostate cancer risk to smoking.

### Genetic profile

An estimated 5–10% of prostate cancer is due to a hereditary cause. Among men with early prostate cancer, a hereditary cause is likely in up to a third of cases before age 60, and almost half of men diagnosed at age 55 or less. Studies have found around a two- to three-fold increased rate of prostate cancer in close relatives of men with the disease. Hereditary prostate cancer is likely in a family if there are three cases of prostate cancer in close relatives or three affected generations (either mother's or father's side), or two relatives with prostate cancer before age 55.

Studies suggest that hereditary prostate cancer is likely to be caused by several different genes instead of a single **gene**. A gene, HPC1 (hereditary prostate cancer gene 1), located on the first **chromosome** pair at 1q24-25, was the first gene suggested to cause hereditary prostate cancer. At least four other genes have been reported, including one thought to increase the risk of both prostate and brain tumors. Other genes known to increase the risk of other cancers, such as **breast cancer**, may be linked to increased prostate cancer risk. Common variations in certain genes also may increase susceptibility to prostate cancer including one gene linked to male sex hormones. Since no clear cause has been identified for the majority of hereditary prostate cancer, **genetic testing**, is typically done through research studies.

### Demographics

Prostate cancer is the most common cancer among men in the United States, and is the second leading cause of cancer deaths. One in six men in the United States will be diagnosed with prostate cancer. Prostate cancer affects African-American men about twice as often as it does caucasian men, and the mortality rate among African-Americans is also higher. African-Americans have the highest rate of prostate cancer in the world. The prostate cancer rate varies considerably around the world. The highest rates are in North America and Western Europe, whereas the rates are moderate in Africa and lowest in Asia. It is unclear what roles **genetics**, diet, economics, and health care access play in these rates.

### Signs and symptoms

Frequently, prostate cancer has no symptoms, and the disease is diagnosed when the patient goes for a routine screening examination. However, occasionally,

## KEY TERMS

**Anti-androgen drugs**—Drugs that block the activity of the male hormone.

**Benign**—A non-cancerous tumor that does not spread and is not life-threatening.

**Benign prostatic hyperplasia (BPH)**—A noncancerous condition of the prostate that causes growth of the prostate tissue, thus enlarging the prostate and blocking urination.

**Biopsy**—The surgical removal and microscopic examination of living tissue for diagnostic purposes.

**Chemotherapy**—Treatment of cancer with synthetic drugs that destroy the tumor either by inhibiting the growth of the cancerous cells or by killing the cancer cells.

**Estrogen**—A female sex hormone.

**Hormone therapy**—Treatment of cancer by changing the hormonal environment, such as testosterone and estrogen.

**Lymph node**—A bean-sized mass of tissue that is part of the immune system and is found in different areas of the body.

**Malignant**—A tumor growth that spreads to another part of the body, usually cancerous.

**Metastasis**—The spreading of cancer from the original site to other locations in the body.

**Prostatectomy**—The surgical removal of the prostate gland.

**Radiation therapy**—Treatment using high-energy radiation from x ray machines, cobalt, radium, or other sources.

**Rectum**—The end portion of the intestine that leads to the anus.

**Semen**—A whitish, opaque fluid released at ejaculation that contains sperm.

**Seminal vesicles**—The pouches above the prostate that store semen.

**Testicles**—Two egg-shaped glands that produce sperm and sex hormones.

**Testosterone**—Hormone produced in the testicles that is involved in male secondary sex characteristics.

**Trans-rectal ultrasound**—A procedure where a probe is placed in the rectum. High-frequency sound waves that cannot be heard by humans are sent out from the probe and reflected by the prostate. These sound waves produce a pattern of echoes that are then used by the computer to create sonograms or pictures of areas inside the body.

---

when the tumor is larger or the cancer has spread to the nearby tissues, the following symptoms may occur:

- weak or interrupted flow of the urine
- frequent urination (especially at night)
- difficulty starting urination
- inability to urinate
- pain or burning sensation when urinating
- blood in the urine
- persistent pain in lower back, hips, or thighs (bone pain)
- difficulty having or keeping an erection (impotence)

### Diagnosis

Although prostate cancer may be very slow-growing, it can be quite aggressive, especially in younger men. When the disease is slow-growing, it may go undetected. Because it may take many years for the cancer to develop, many men with the disease are likely to die of other causes rather than from the cancer.

Prostate cancer is frequently curable when detected early. However, because the early stages of prostate cancer may not have any symptoms, it often remains undetected until the patient goes for a routine physical examination. Diagnosis of the disease is made using some or all of the following tests.

#### Digital rectal examination (DRE)

In order to perform this test, the doctor puts a gloved, lubricated finger (digit) into the rectum to feel for any lumps in the prostate. The rectum lies just behind the prostate gland, and a majority of prostate tumors begin in the posterior region of the prostate. If the doctor does detect an abnormality, he or she may order more tests in order to confirm these findings.

#### Blood tests

Blood tests are used to measure the amounts of certain protein markers, such as prostate-specific antigen (PSA), found circulating in the blood. The cells lining the prostate generally make this protein and a small amount can be detected in the bloodstream.

Prostate cancers typically produce a lot of this protein, and it can be easily detected in the blood. Hence, when PSA is found in the blood in higher than normal amounts (for the patient's age group), cancer may be present. Occasionally, other blood tests also are used to help with the diagnosis.

### Transrectal ultrasound

A small probe is placed in the rectum and sound waves are released from the probe. These sound waves bounce off the prostate tissue and an image is created. Since normal prostate tissue and prostate tumors reflect the sound waves differently, the test can be used to detect tumors. Though the insertion of the probe into the rectum may be slightly uncomfortable, the procedure is generally painless and takes only about 20 minutes.

### Prostate biopsy

If cancer is suspected from the results of any of the above tests, the doctor will remove a small piece of prostate tissue with a hollow needle. This sample is then checked under the microscope for the presence of cancerous cells. Prostate biopsy is the most definitive diagnostic tool for prostate cancer.

If cancer is detected during the microscopic examination of the prostate tissue, the pathologist will "grade" the tumor. This means that the tumor will be scored on a scale of 2-10 to indicate how aggressive the tumor is. Tumors with a lower score are less likely to grow and spread than are tumors with higher scores. This method of grading tumors is called the Gleason system. This is different from "staging" of the cancer. When a doctor stages a cancer, the doctor gives it a number that indicates whether it has spread and the extent of spread of the disease. In Stage I, the cancer is localized in the prostate in one area, while in the last stage, Stage IV, the cancer cells have spread to other parts of the body.

### X rays and imaging techniques

X-ray studies may be ordered to determine whether the cancer has spread to other areas. Imaging techniques (such as computed tomography scans and magnetic resonance imaging), where a computer is used to generate a detailed picture of the prostate and areas nearby, may be done to get a clearer view of the internal organs. A bone scan may be used to check whether the cancer has spread to the bone.

The American Cancer Society and other organizations recommend that PSA blood testing and DRE be offered to men with at least a 10-year life expectancy beginning at age 50. Men at higher risk for prostate cancer, such as those with a family history of the disease or African American men, may wish to consider screening at an earlier age such as 45. A low-fat diet may slow the progression of prostate cancer. Hence, the American Cancer Society recommends a diet rich in fruits, vegetables and dietary fiber, and low in red meat and saturated fats, in order to reduce the risk of prostate cancer.

## Treatment and management

The doctor and the patient will decide on the treatment after considering many factors. For example, the patient's age, the stage of the tumor, his general health, and the presence of any co-existing illnesses have to be considered. In addition, the patient's personal preferences and the risks and benefits of each treatment method are also taken into account before any decision is made.

### Surgery

For early stage prostate cancer, surgery is frequently considered. Radical prostatectomy involves complete removal of the prostate. During the surgery, a sample of the lymph nodes near the prostate is removed to determine whether the cancer has spread beyond the prostate gland. Because the seminal vesicles (the gland where the sperm is made) are removed along with the prostate, infertility is a side effect of this type of surgery. In order to minimize the risk of impotence (inability to have an erection) and incontinence (inability to control urine flow), a procedure known as "nerve-sparing" prostatectomy is used.

In a different surgical method, known as the transurethral resection procedure or TURP, only the cancerous portion of the prostate is removed, by using a small wire loop that is introduced into the prostate through the urethra. This technique is most often used in men who cannot have a radical prostatectomy due to age or other illness, and it is rarely recommended.

### Radiation therapy

Radiation therapy involves the use of high-energy x rays to kill cancer cells or to shrink tumors. It can be used instead of surgery for early stage cancer. The radiation can either be administered from a machine outside the body (external beam radiation), or small radioactive pellets can be implanted in the prostate gland in the area surrounding the tumor.

### Hormone therapy

Hormone therapy is commonly used when the cancer is in an advanced stage and has spread to other parts of the body. Prostate cells need the male

## QUESTIONS TO ASK YOUR DOCTOR

- Why is prostate cancer designated as a genetic disorder?
- Are genetic tests available to determine whether or not a person is at risk for prostate cancer?
- What kind of tests should a man have to determine if he has early stage prostate cancer, and at what age should he have those tests?
- What is the prognosis for a man diagnosed with prostate cancer, and what factors affect this prognosis?

hormone testosterone to grow. Decreasing the levels of this hormone, or inhibiting its activity, may cause the cancer to shrink or stop growing. Hormone levels can be decreased in several ways. Orchiectomy is a surgical procedure that involves complete removal of the testicles, leading to a decrease in the levels of testosterone. Alternatively, drugs (such as LHRH agonists or anti-androgens) that bind to the male hormone testosterone and block its activity can be given. Another method tricks the body by administering the female hormone estrogen. When this is given, the body senses the presence of a sex hormone and stops making the male hormone testosterone. However, there are some side effects to hormone therapy. Men may have hot flashes, enlargement and tenderness of the breasts, or impotence and loss of sexual desire, as well as blood clots, heart attacks, and strokes, depending on the dose of estrogen.

### Chemotherapy

Chemotherapy is the use of drugs to kill cancer cells. The drugs can either be taken as a pill or injected into the body through a needle that is inserted into a blood vessel. This type of treatment is called systemic treatment because the drug enters the blood stream, travels through the whole body, and kills the cancer cells that are outside the prostate. Chemotherapy is sometimes used to treat prostate cancer that has recurred after other treatment. Research is ongoing to find more drugs that are effective for the treatment of prostate cancer.

### Watchful waiting

Watchful waiting means no immediate treatment is recommended, but doctors keep the patient under careful observation. This option is generally used in older patients when the tumor is not very aggressive

and the patients have other, more life-threatening illnesses. Prostate cancer in older men tends to be slow-growing. Therefore, the risk of the patient dying from prostate cancer, rather than from other causes, is relatively small.

### Prognosis

According to the American Cancer Society, the survival rate for all stages of prostate cancer combined has increased from 50% to 87% over the last 30 years. Due to early detection and better screening methods, nearly 60% of the tumors are diagnosed while they are still confined to the prostate gland. The five-year survival rate for early stage cancers is almost 99%. Sixty-three percent of the patients survive 10 years, and 51% survive 15 years after initial diagnosis. Studies on the prognosis of hereditary prostate cancer are ongoing.

### Resources

#### BOOKS

Bostwick, David, et al. *Prostate Cancer: What Every Man—And His Family—Needs to Know.* New York: Villard Books, 1999.

Naros, Steven, et al. "Cancers of the Prostate and Testes." In *Inherited Susceptibility to Cancer: Clinical, Predictive and Ethical Perspectives.* Ed. William D. Foulkes and Shirley V. Hodgson, 246–54. Cambridge: Cambridge University Press, 1998.

#### WEBSITES

National Prostate Cancer Coalition. http://www.4npcc.org.
US TOO! International, Inc. http://www.ustoo.com.

#### ORGANIZATIONS

American Cancer Society. 1599 Clifton Rd. NE, Atlanta, GA 30329. (800) 227-2345. http://www.cancer.org.
American Foundation for Urologic Disease, Inc. 1128 North Charles St., Baltimore, MD 21201-5559. (410)468-1808. http://www.afud.org.
National Cancer Institute. Office of Communications, 31 Center Dr. MSC 2580, Bldg. 1 Room 10A16, Bethesda, MD 20892-2580. (800) 422-6237. http://www.cancer.gov.

Kristin Baker Niendorf, MS, CGC

# Protein C deficiency

## Definition

Protein C deficiency is a lack of sufficient functioning protein C in the blood. Protein C is a substance that helps to prevent blood clots. Persons with this disorder may have no symptoms, mild symptoms, or severe and even life-threatening symptoms.

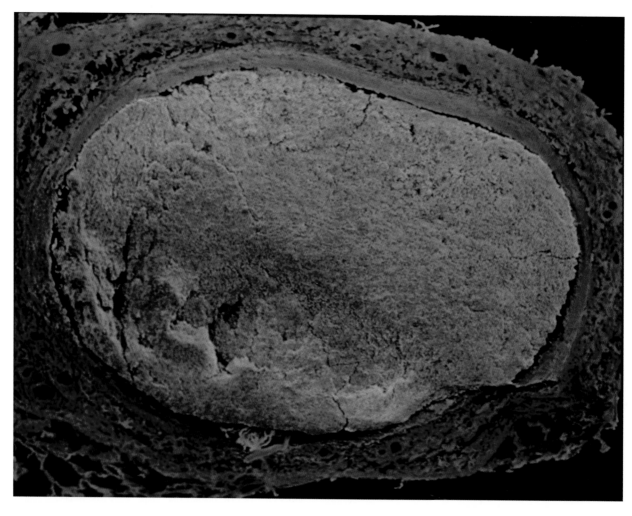

One possible symptom of protein C deficiency is recurring venous thromboembolism, which may result in a pulmonary embolism, or blood clot in the lungs. *(Moredun Animal Health LTD/National Audubon Society Collection/Photo Researchers, Inc. Reproduced by permission.)*

## Demographics

Many people have some level of protein C deficiency, although they have no symptoms. It is estimated that one in 200 to 500 individuals has such a deficiency. Significant protein C deficiency is much rarer, occurring in just one person of every 20,000. The most severe form the disorder, homozygous protein C deficiency, occurs when an individual inherits an abnormal protein C **gene** from each parent. Homozygous protein C deficiency is exceptionally rare. Estimates for the incidence of homozygous protein C deficiency range from one in 500,000 to less than one per million.

## Description

Protein C deficiency was discovered in 1981, just six years after protein C was first isolated. In a 1981 paper published in the *Journal of Clinical Investigations*, researchers described a connection between low concentrations of protein C in the blood plasma (the liquid portion of the blood) and blood clotting. It is now known that protein C plays a crucial role in the series of steps involved in blood clotting. One of protein C's roles in this pathway is to regulate the blood-coagulation protein thrombin. With too little properly functioning protein C to control thrombin's activity, multiple clots can form.

Low levels of protein C may have explicit effects, and in some individuals, these include dark, reddish-purple blotches, which sometimes extend over considerable areas of the body. Such blotching is known as purpura fulminans. Newborns with severe protein deficiency may display considerable blotching, as well as painful black sores, particularly on the back of the head and the buttocks. This is a life-threatening condition.

While in the past many young patients died from the effects of severe protein C deficiency, medical advancements coupled with a better understanding of protein C have led to intensive treatment and monitoring options that allow many patients to survive and thrive.

## Causes and symptoms

Protein C deficiency comes in two types:

- Type I protein C deficiency occurs when an individual has perfectly functioning protein C but has too little of it. Kidney disease or a number of other diseases can prompt an individual's body to produce too little protein C. Type I may also result when individuals have inherited one abnormal protein C gene from one of their parents. Regardless of its cause, people who have too low a level of protein C cannot control thrombin, and this situation causes blood clots to form.
- Type II protein C deficiency occurs when individuals are able to make sufficient protein C, but the protein C that is made does not function correctly and cannot play its proper role in the coagulation cascade. Genetic mutations can cause the production of non-functioning protein C.

Scientists have found that protein C not only interacts with thrombin, but also with other molecules involved in blood clotting, and as of 2008, they have identified more than 160 mutations that can occur in the protein C gene.

### Genetic profile

Protein C deficiency often results from an abnormal protein C gene, which is located on **chromosome 2**. Hereditary protein C deficiency is inherited in an autosomal dominant manner, which means that an individual need only inherit the abnormal gene from one parent. This circumstance often occurs when one parent is heterozygous for the trait or has one normal copy of the gene and one abnormal copy of the gene. When such is the case, that parent's children have a 50-percent chance of inheriting the abnormal gene. If both parents are heterozygous for the trait, a child's chance of inheriting the abnormal gene jumps to 75%, but the child also has a 25% chance of inheriting two copies of the abnormal gene—one from each parent. A child with two copies of the abnormal gene is said to have homozygous protein C deficiency.

### Symptoms

The symptoms of homozygous protein C deficiency and severe heterozygous protein C deficiency are typically evident very soon after birth. They include:

- Appearance and rapid progression of purpura fulminans, which often begin as large red to purple lesions, often at the back of the head or on the buttocks. Purpura fulminans result from clots in small blood vessels that would otherwise feed that tissue. They typically develop quickly into black scabs of dead tissue known as eschars, which are extremely painful.
- Blindness due to blood clots in the veins of the retina.
- Blood clots in large blood vessels, including those of the kidneys.

As patients with severe protein C deficiency age, they typically have recurring problems with purpura fulminans, particularly following injuries, infections, or changes in anti-clotting therapeutic regimens.

Individuals with moderately severe protein C deficiency may not have their first symptoms until they reach their teens or older. These symptoms may include:

- Recurring venous thromboembolism, which is a blood clot that breaks free of its location in a vein and moves elsewhere in the body, sometimes into the lungs (a pulmonary embolism).
- Deep vein thrombosis, or a blood clot in a deep vein, usually in the legs.
- Clots in organ tissues (parenchyma).
- Blood-clotting proteins that become overly active and disseminated (intravascular coagulation).

In the mild form of protein C deficiency, the patient's body makes functional protein C but makes it in insufficient amounts. Some people who have this condition may experience no problems at all. Others may have one or more of the following symptoms:

- recurring blood clots that may affect blood flow and may lead to a pulmonary embolism
- deep vein thrombosis
- arterial ischemic stroke, due to a blood clot in an artery that feeds the brain
- clots in the mesentery, a double-layered fold in the peritoneum of the abdomen
- blood clots that occur during pregnancy

## Diagnosis

### Examination

Doctors will suspect protein C deficiency in infants born with obvious purpura fulminans, particularly those who quickly develop eschars. They may also suspect this disorder in older patients who develop the reddish-purple patches or who experience recurring blood clots.

**Deep vein thrombosis**—A blood clot in a deep vein, usually in the legs.

**Eschars**—Painful patches of dead, blackened tissue.

**Mesentery**—Double-layered fold in the peritoneum.

**Parenchyma** —Functional (rather than structural) tissues of an organ.

**Pulmonary embolism**—A blood clot in the lungs.

**Purpura fulminans**—Dark, reddish-purple patches of dying tissue that result from clots in small blood vessels that would otherwise feed that tissue.

**Venous thromboembolism**—A blood clot that breaks free of its location in a vein and moves elsewhere in the body.

QUESTIONS TO ASK YOUR DOCTOR

- I have mild protein C deficiency and would like to have a baby. Am I at risk for developing venous thrombosis, and if so, what precautions can I take? Are there other risks I should know about?
- My child has just been diagnosed with protein C deficiency, but my other children seem fine. At what age should they be tested for this disorder?
- I understand that several tests are available to test for protein C deficiency. Which do you recommend and why?
- I have protein C deficiency and am going to undergo surgery that will keep me off my feet for more than a week. What special care should I expect at the hospital, and what precautions can I follow once I return home to avoid blood clots while I am recovering?

*Tests*

Doctors will order blood tests to measure the amount of functional protein C and/or to measure the total amount of protein C—functional or not—in the bloodstream. The doctor may repeat the test to make sure that the measured rate is not fluctuating. Another test that a doctor may order involves making tiny nicks in the arm to measure how long the patient continues to bleed and to learn about the clotting activity in the patient.

## Treatment and management

The treatment for patients with protein C deficiency varies based on the severity of the disorder and the individual's symptoms.

*Traditional*

The doctor may order the administration of protein C, usually as fresh frozen plasma or as protein C concentrate. This is a typical treatment for patients with infantile protein C deficiency.

*Drugs*

Some patients may receive anticoagulants, such as a form of heparin or warfarin, to counter current clots and, in some cases, to help prevent future clots.

## Prognosis

Individuals who have homozygous protein C deficiency often experience fatal thrombosis unless they receive replacement protein C through fresh frozen plasma or through protein C concentrate. Patients who have milder forms of the disorder and have associated symptoms typically have a good outcome with treatment, although they may experience symptoms now and again. Many people who have protein C deficiency never have any symptoms and lead normal lives.

## Prevention

Individuals who have protein C deficiency can take various measures to reduce the occurrence of blood clots. These include making typical healthy-lifestyle choices such as eating a balanced diet, remaining physically active, maintaining a healthy weight, and refraining from tobacco use. Avoiding prolonged immobility, such as sitting still on long car rides or plane trips, can also be helpful. Persons who are (or expect to be) bedridden due to surgery or illness should discuss with their doctor options for reducing their risk of blood clots.

**Resources**

**PERIODICALS**

Goldenberg, N. A., and M. J. Manco-Johnson. "Protein C Deficiency." *Haemophilia*, 14 (November 2008): 1214-1221.

Griffin J. H., et al. "Deficiency of Protein C in Congenital Thrombotic Disease." *Journal of Clinical Investigations*, 68 (1981): 1370-1373.

Schafer, A. I. "Thrombotic Disorders: Hypercoagulable States." *Cecil Medicine*, Chapter 182, 23rd ed. Philadelphia: Saunders Elsevier, 2007.

**OTHER**

"Congenital Protein C or S Deficiency." Medline Plus. http://www.nlm.nih.gov/medlineplus/ency/article/000559.htm

"Protein C Deficiency." Lifeblood: The Thrombosis Charity. http://www.thrombosis-charity.org.uk/old/aboutthrom_thrombophilia_congenital_proteinc.htm

University of Illinois, Urbana/Champaign Carle Cancer Center. "Protein C Deficiency." *Hematology Resource Page.* http://www.med.illinois.edu/hematology/PtProtC.htm

UW Health. "Protein C Deficiency." *Health Facts for You.* http://www.uwhealth.org/healthfacts/B_EXTRANET_HEALTH_INFORMATION-FlexMember-Show_Public_HFFY_1126651807773.html

**ORGANIZATIONS**

Lifeblood: The Thrombosis Charity c/o The Thrombosis & Haemostasis Centre, Level 1, North Wing, St. Thomas' Hospital, London, UK, SE1 7EH, 0207 633 9937, lifeblood.charity@googlemail.com, http://www.thrombosis-charity.org.uk.

Leslie A. Mertz, PHD

# Protein S deficiency

## Definition

Protein S deficiency is a disorder caused by an insufficient amount of functioning protein S in the blood. Protein S is a substance that helps to prevent blood clots. Normally, the body has a balance between components that promote clotting and those that prevent it, so that clots form only under certain conditions. In individuals with protein S deficiency, too many clots occur. Some people are born with this deficiency, whereas others develop it because of liver disease or due to a lack of vitamin K. Some people with protein S deficiency never have symptoms, but others experience blood clots, embolisms, miscarriages, and, in a few cases, death.

## Demographics

Protein S deficiency occurs in about one of every 700 individuals. Some individuals may have no symptoms and, therefore, be unaware they have the condition. In others, first symptoms may not appear until adulthood, but they usually materialize before middle age. A much rarer form of the protein S deficiency is the hereditary form of the disorder, known as homozygous protein S deficiency. Homozygous protein S deficiency generally makes its presence known in newborns or infants as purpura fulminans, which is the formation of sometimes-quite-large, purplish patches of dying tissue on the body. These patches are caused by blood clots in small blood vessels that would otherwise feed that tissue.

## Description

Protein S is a relatively new discovery. Researchers first identified it in the late 1970s. This protein is vitamin K-dependent, which means that vitamin K is necessary for its production. Protein S plays an important role in the steps necessary to control coagulation in the human body, and without it, blood clotting becomes abnormal. In particular, protein S is involved in the action of various blood-clotting substances (such as protein C, factor V, and factor VIII). When the levels of protein S are too low, blood clots can occur. People can obtain vitamin K by eating certain foods, such as leafy greens, but they mainly get their vitamin K from bacteria in the large intestine. These bacteria actually make vitamin K, and they usually make plenty to provide all the vitamin K that a person needs.

The main health problem associated with protein S deficiency is blood clotting, or thrombosis. Protein S is important in the blood-clotting pathway because it is one of a number of anti-coagulation proteins that keep the blood from clotting abnormally. In particular, protein S joins with another anticoagulant, protein C, to shut down the clotting action of the enzyme thrombin. Without enough functioning protein S, protein C alone cannot stop thrombin's clotting activity, and it is left to produce clots when it should not. These clots can lodge in blood vessels, where they can limit or stop blood flow. This hindrance of blood flow can be dangerous, and even lethal. Fortunately, various treatments exist to treat abnormal blood clotting.

## Causes and symptoms

Protein S deficiency can result from liver disease or insufficient vitamin K, but it is often a congenital condition resulting from at least one mutated protein S **gene** that is inherited from a parent.

### Genetic profile

Hereditary protein D deficiency results from mutations in the protein S gene PROS1. PROS1 is located on **chromosome** 3. Two of the known mutations of this gene—and several others probably exist—include deletions of parts of the gene such that the mutated gene's instructions for making the protein are no longer complete. A short, improperly functioning protein results.

Hereditary protein S deficiency is inherited in an autosomal dominant manner, which means that an individual need only inherit the abnormal gene from one parent. This situation often occurs when one parent is heterozygous for the trait or has one normal copy of the gene and one abnormal copy of the gene. When such is the case, that parent's children have a 50% chance of inheriting the abnormal gene. If both parents are heterozygous for the trait, the child's chance of inheriting the abnormal gene not only jumps to 75%, but the child also has a 25% chance of inheriting two copies of the abnormal gene—one from each parent. A child with two copies of the abnormal gene is said to have homozygous protein D deficiency.

### Symptoms

Many individuals with protein S deficiency never experience any symptoms, and some only become aware that they have it when they undergo testing because a close relative develops the disorder. Among those who do experience problems associated with the disorder, symptoms can range from mild to severe. Symptoms may include the following:

- purpura fulminans, mainly in individuals with homozygous protein S deficiency
- recurring blood clots that may affect blood flow and may move into the lungs (pulmonary embolism)
- blood clot in a deep vein, usually in the legs (deep vein thrombosis)
- inflammation of veins due to blood clots (thrombophlebitis)
- miscarriage
- swelling and pain in the legs due to venous thrombosis

## Diagnosis

### Examination

Doctors may want to test a patient for protein S deficiency when they learn of a family history of the disorder, particularly when it is combined with the presence of one or more of the following symptoms:

- deep vein thrombosis
- thrombophlebitis
- purpura fulminans
- swelling and pain in the legs, possibly accompanied by redness
- recurring blood clots, particularly in individuals of middle age or younger
- cord-like, hard veins, which are indicative of clotting

## KEY TERMS

**Deep vein thrombosis**—A blood clot in a deep vein, usually in the legs.

**Pulmonary embolism**—A blood clot in the lungs.

**Purpura fulminans**—Dark, reddish-purple patches of dying tissue that result from clots in small blood vessels that would otherwise feed that tissue.

**Thrombophlebitis**—Inflammation of veins due to blood clots.

**Vitamin K**—A vital substance that is obtained by eating certain foods, such as leafy greens, but mainly through bacterial manufacture in the large intestine.

### Tests

Doctors will order blood tests to measure the amount of functional protein S and/or to measure the total amount of protein S—functional or not—in the bloodstream. Doctors may repeat the test to make sure that the measured rate is not fluctuating. Another test that may order involves making small nicks in the arm to measure how long the patient continues to bleed and, therefore, to provide information about the patient's clotting activity.

## Treatment and management

The treatment for protein S deficiency varies based on the patient's symptoms. Symptoms are wide-ranging because numerous protein S mutations can occur, and these can have different effects.

### Traditional

For patients diagnosed with protein S deficiency, doctors typically recommend that the person follow a healthy lifestyle in terms of diet and exercise to lower the risk of blood clots. To treat an already existing clot, a doctor may recommend that the patient receive fresh frozen human plasma, which contains protein S.

### Drugs

Some patients may receive anticoagulants, such as a form of heparin or warfarin, to counter current clots and, in some cases, to help prevent future clots. The use of such drugs is particularly common for women who are pregnant, because even in a person without this disorder, the level of protein S dips during pregnancy. In addition, women who take some forms of birth control pills or certain types of hormone-replacement therapies may experience additional drops in protein S.

### Prognosis

Some individuals with mild forms of this disorder never experience any symptoms and have no problems associated with the condition. Others may have symptoms ranging from mild to severe. Many people with protein S deficiency have a good outcome, particularly when they follow the advice of a physician. Even with the use of anticoagulants, however, life-threatening blood clots do occur occasionally, and some patients die from them.

### Prevention

Individuals who have protein S deficiency can take various measures to reduce the occurrence of blood clots. These include making typical healthy-lifestyle choices such as eating a balanced diet, remaining physically active, maintaining a healthy weight, and refraining from tobacco use. Avoiding prolonged immobility, such as sitting still on long car rides or plane trips, can also be helpful. Persons who are (or who expect to be) bedridden due to surgery or illness should discuss with a doctor options for reducing the risk of blood clots. Women who are considering a pregnancy or beginning birth-control or hormone-replacement therapies should consult a doctor first.

### Resources

**BOOKS**

Schafer, A. I. "Thrombotic disorders: Hypercoagulable States." *Cecil Medicine*, 23rd ed. Chapter 182. Philadelphia: Saunders Elsevier, 2007.

**OTHER**

"Congenital Protein C or S Deficiency." Medline Plus. http://www.nlm.nih.gov/medlineplus/ency/article/000559.htm.
Lifeblood: The Thrombosis Charity. "Protein S Deficiency." Lifeblood: The Thrombosis Charity. http://www.thrombosis-charity.org.uk/old/aboutthrom_thrombophilia_congenital_proteinS.htm.
University of Illinois, Urbana/Champaign Carle Cancer Center. "Protein S Deficiency." Hematology Resource Page. http://www.med.illinois.edu/hematology/PtProtS.htm.

**ORGANIZATIONS**

Lifeblood: The Thrombosis Charity c/o The Thrombosis & Haemostasis Centre, Level 1, North Wing, St. Thomas' Hospital, London, UK, SE1 7EH, 0207 633 9937, lifeblood.charity@googlemail.com, http://www.thrombosis-charity.org.uk.

Leslie A. Mertz, PHD

# Proteus syndrome

### Definition

Proteus syndrome is characterized by excessive growth of cells. This can result in asymmetrical growth, benign (noncancerous) tumors, and pigmented skin lesions.

### Description

Proteus syndrome is a rare condition. It was first described in 1979 by Michael Cohen. Hans-Rudolf Wiedemann named the condition after the Greek god Proteus, who could assume many forms. The disorder gained wide recognition when it became publicized that Joseph (John) Merrick, the person depicted in the movie *The Elephant Man*, probably had Proteus syndrome.

The excess growth of tissue that characterizes Proteus syndrome is progressive. It also tends to affect some tissues and not others. This can result in asymmetrical growth in the body, such as the skull, bones, spine, hands, feet, fingers, and toes. Proteus syndrome often results in overgrowth of one side of the body and not the other. Benign tumors on the surface of the skin or inside the body may also occur. Raised brown patches on the skin and an overgrowth of tissues on the soles of the feet or the palms of the hands are

## KEY TERMS

**Autosomal dominant**—A pattern of genetic inheritance where only one abnormal gene is needed to display the trait or disease.

**Benign tumor**—An abnormal proliferation of cells that does not spread to other sites.

**Chromosome**—A microscopic thread-like structure found within each cell of the body and consists of a complex of proteins and DNA. Humans have 46 chromosomes arranged into 23 pairs. Changes in either the total number of chromosomes or their shape and size (structure) may lead to physical or mental abnormalities.

**Connective tissue**—A group of tissues responsible for support throughout the body; includes cartilage, bone, fat, tissue underlying skin, and tissues that support organs, blood vessels, and nerves throughout the body.

**Cyst**—An abnormal sac or closed cavity filled with liquid or semisolid matter.

**Deoxyribonucleic acid (DNA)**—The genetic material in cells that holds the inherited instructions for growth, development, and cellular functioning.

**Gene**—A building block of inheritance, which contains the instructions for the production of a particular protein, and is made up of a molecular sequence found on a section of DNA. Each gene is found on a precise location on a chromosome.

**Mosaicism**—A genetic condition resulting from a mutation, crossing over, or nondisjunction of chromosomes during cell division, causing a variation in the number of chromosomes in the cells.

**Nevi**—Plural of nevus.

**Nevus**—Any anomaly of the skin present at birth, including moles and various types of birthmarks.

**Protein**—Important building blocks of the body, composed of amino acids, involved in the formation of body structures and controlling the basic functions of the human body.

**Spleen**—Organ located in the upper abdominal cavity that filters out old red blood cells and helps fight bacterial infections. Responsible for breaking down spherocytes at a rapid rate.

**Spontaneous**—Occurring by chance.

**Thymus gland**—An endocrine gland located in the front of the neck that houses and transports T cells, which help to fight infection.

**Tissue**—Group of similar cells that work together to perform a particular function. The four basic types of tissue include muscle, nerve, epithelial, and connective tissues.

**Vascular malformation**—Abnormality of the blood vessels that often appears as a red or pink patch on the surface of the skin.

**Vertebra**—One of the 23 bones which comprise the spine. *Vertebrae* is the plural form.

---

common. The types of tissues and organs that are affected and the severity of the effects vary from person to person and within the course of a lifetime. Proteus syndrome is sometimes associated with mental delay.

### Genetic profile

The specific cause of Proteus syndrome is unclear. Proteus syndrome appears to occur randomly, suggesting that it is not inherited. Research suggests that Proteus syndrome results from an unknown **gene** that is changed (mutated) in some cells, but normal in other cells of the body. This is called mosaicism.

The tissues and organs that are affected in Proteus syndrome and the severity of effects probably depend on how many cells contain the mutated gene, and what type of cells contain it. Someone with many cells containing the changed Proteus gene are more likely to have more severe effects then someone with only a few cells changed. Someone with many cells changed in a particular part of the body, such as the hand, are more likely to have excessive growth in that area. The changed Proteus gene will affect cell growth even after the baby is fully developed, since cell division continues to take place and is necessary for the growth of tissues and organs and for the replacement of damaged cells. The changed Proteus gene mainly results in excessive growth of cells and tissues from infancy to adolescence.

### Demographics

Only 100 to 200 cases of Proteus syndrome have been reported around the world. Both males and females are equally likely to be affected with Proteus syndrome.

## Signs and symptoms

Individuals with Proteus syndrome can have a wide range of manifestations. The effects can also range from mild to severe. The most common manifestations of Proteus syndrome include:

- overgrowth of hands, feet, fingers, or toes (gigantism)
- overgrowth of one side of the limbs, face, or body (hemihypertrophy)
- overgrowth of the connective tissue on the soles of the feet or palms of the hand or, less commonly, in the abdomen or nose (connective tissue nevi)
- darkened, discolored, and often rough and raised patches of skin (skin surface nevi)
- benign tumors on the skin surface and under the skin
- benign tumors of the fat cells (lipoma) or areas of significantly decreased or increased body fat
- abnormalities of the skull resulting in a large or asymmetrical head
- benign bony growths projecting outward from the end of the bones (exostosis)

People with Proteus syndrome can have curvature of the spine. They may also have an enlarged spleen or thymus. Approximately 12–13% of people with the disorder have cystic abnormalities of the lungs, which can interfere with the normal functioning of the lungs. Abnormalities in the blood vessels called vascular malformations, which appear as pink or red patches on the surface of the skin, are common. About one-third of people with Proteus syndrome are mentally impaired; skull abnormalities are often seen in those with impairment. People with Proteus syndrome can have a distinctive facial appearance, with a long and narrow face, down-slanting eyes, wide and forward-tipping nostrils, a low nose bridge, and a mouth that remains open when at rest. Many effects can result from the presence of tumors and bony growths that affect other organs and tissues.

Sometimes mild or moderate effects of Proteus syndrome, such as benign tumors, are present at birth. As a person grows and develops, the tissue overgrowth progresses and changes. This progression is often irregular; it is characterized by periods of major overgrowth and other periods of absent overgrowth. The effects therefore change over the course of a lifetime. However, most changes occur before adolescence, since tissue overgrowth tends to plateau at that time.

## Diagnosis

There is no blood test available to diagnose Proteus syndrome. A diagnosis can be made only by

---

careful observation of the individual, perhaps over a period of time, and through imaging studies. These may include x ray evaluations of the skull and skeletal system; magnetic resonance imaging (MRI) of the limbs, nervous system, and abdomen; and computed tomography (CT) scans of the chest.

The great variability of Proteus syndrome from person to person makes it hard to diagnose. There are no definitive and universal diagnostic guidelines. Some tentative guidelines were established, at the First National Conference on Proteus Syndrome Diagnostic Criteria.

## Treatment and management

There is no cure for Proteus syndrome. Treatment largely involves the management of effects of the disorder, such as the removal of tumors or bony overgrowths. Removal of tumors is not recommended, though, unless they are causing major problems, since these tumors usually grow back. Surgery to remove an overgrown portion of the bone should be performed only if the bony overgrowth is affecting normal functioning. Bony overgrowths in the ear, for example, may need to be removed if they are interfering with hearing. This type of surgery, however, can sometimes increase the growth of the remaining bone. Psychological counseling to help children with Proteus syndrome deal with the disorder should be considered. In order for counseling to be effective, it is preferable that it begins at a young age.

## Prognosis

The long-term prognosis of Proteus syndrome is not known. The life expectancy is likely to vary greatly from person to person. Those with tumors and bony overgrowths affecting critical organs are likely to have a poorer prognosis.

## Resources

### PERIODICALS

Barona-Mazuera, Maria, et al. "Proteus Syndrome: New Findings in Seven Patients." *Pediatric Dermatology* 14, no. 1 (1997): 1–5.

Biesecker, Leslie, et al. "Proteus Syndrome: Diagnostic Criteria, Differential Diagnosis, and Patient Evaluation." *American Journal of Medical Genetics* 84, no. 5 (1999): 389–95.

Cavero, Juan, Evelyn Castro, and Luz Junco. "Proteus Syndrome." *International Journal of Dermatology* 39 (2000): 698–709.

De Becker, Inge. "Ocular Manifestations in Proteus Syndrome." *American Journal of Medical Genetics* 92 (2000): 350–52.

Gilbert-Barness, Enid, Michael Cohen, and John Opitz. "Multiple Meningiomas, Craniofacial Hyperostosis and Retinal Abnormalities in Proteus Syndrome." *American Journal of Medical Genetics* 93 (2000): 234–40.

### WEBSITES

McKusick, Victor A. "Proteus Syndrome." Online Mendelian Inheritance in Man. October 20, 2008 (December 12, 2009). http://www.ncbi.nlm.nih.gov/entrez/dispomim.cgi?id = 176920.

Proteus Syndrome Foundation. http://www.proteus-syndrome.org.

### ORGANIZATIONS

Proteus Syndrome Foundation. 6235 Whetstone Dr., Colorado Springs, CO 80918. (719)264-8445. abscit@aol.com. http://www.Proteus-syndrome.org.

Lisa Maria Andres, MS, CGC

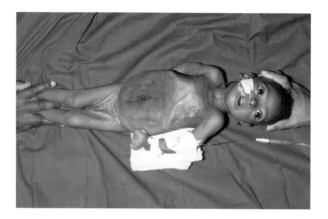

**The distinctive "prune-like" appearance of the abdominal area is evident in this infant.** *(Custom Medical Stock Photo, Inc.)*

# Prune-belly syndrome

## Definition

Prune-belly syndrome is characterized by the following three findings: lack of abdominal muscles, undescended testes, and abnormal development of the urinary tract. Also known as Eagle-Barrett syndrome, this rare disorder was first described in 1839.

## Description

Prune-belly syndrome displays a wide range of severity. Affected individuals will have little to no muscle in their abdominal wall. The abdomen will appear wrinkled, like a prune. In male infants, the testicles, although present, are usually not seen. They remain inside the infant's abdomen. They fail to move to the normal position during development of the fetus. Undescended testes are a risk factor for infertility and testicular **cancer** later in the infant's life.

There are a variety of urinary tract abnormalities that occur in this syndrome. The kidneys may not form fully, and the level of development of the kidneys varies. The ureters, the tubes that connect the kidneys to the bladder, may be very large. In the portions that are very large, the urine may not be able to flow as well as normal. The bladder, the organ that holds the urine, may also be very large. A connection between the umbilicus and bladder may be present as well. The urethra may have areas that are very dilated and others that are very narrow. The narrowing may not allow the urine to flow out well. This blockage causes the bladder to become very large. The drainage of the fetus' bladder is what makes up the amniotic fluid during pregnancy. If the bladder cannot be drained, then not enough amniotic fluid will be present. The lack of amniotic fluid, or oligohydramnios, can cause poor formation of the fetus' lungs. The bladder in these patients may become so large that a mass can be seen and felt on the baby.

Ten percent of cases may have various abnormalities of the heart or large blood vessels. A percentage of cases have abnormalities of the musculoskeletal system such as: dislocation of the hips, abnormal indentation of their chest, malformed feet or fingers, and a spine that is not aligned properly.

## Genetic profile

A specific genetic defect is unknown. Multiple cases in families are rare but have been reported. The risk of recurrence in future pregnancies is unknown but is thought to be low.

### Demographics

Despite the lack of a specific genetic defect or pattern of **inheritance**, over 95% of affected individuals are male. The incidence of this syndrome is estimated at one in 40,000 births.

### Signs and symptoms

There are many symptoms that infants may experience in the newborn period. Most of these depend on the extent of damage that exists in the lungs and urinary tract. Infants who have poorly developed lungs, may be unable to breathe on their own at birth. They may also develop a collapsed lung or pneumothorax. If the infant does not have a normal rib cage then their ability to move air into and out of their lungs is impaired. This can lead to infections in the lung.

Since infants may not be able to eliminate of all their urine, they are at risk of having repeated urinary tract infections.

### Diagnosis

At birth, the syndrome is easily diagnosed based on the three findings that have been described. There is no specific prenatal or genetic test that can diagnose prune-belly syndrome. The diagnosis of prune-belly syndrome can be made in the prenatal period by ultrasound. Ultrasound can show some of the findings in this syndrome such as: distended bladder and ureters, oligohydramnios, and cryptorchidism. An enlarged bladder can be seen in other syndromes besides prune-belly, however, these findings on ultrasound should alert a physician to prune-belly as a possible cause.

### Treatment and management

The potential treatments for prune-belly syndrome depend upon whether the diagnosis is made at birth or in utero. It also varies depending upon how severe the abnormalities are. Over the past two decades, different surgical procedures have been performed on fetuses in an attempt to correct the urinary tract obstructions that occur. One of these procedures is the vesicoamniotic shunt. This procedure relieves bladder obstructions by placing a tube in the fetal bladder allowing amniotic fluid to be produced as usual. The production of amniotic fluid allows for normal development of the lungs. There is not much information regarding the long-term outcomes for persons who receive these shunts. In infants who survive but have renal failure, kidney transplantation has been attempted with some success.

### Prognosis

Approximately 20% of patients with this syndrome are stillborn. Thirty percent of infants do not survive past two years due to renal failure or infection. The remaining 50% of the infants will have a variety of urinary tract problems. A recent study looked at what factors may predict which children with prune-belly syndrome will develop renal failure. In this study, 35 patients with prune-belly syndrome between 1960 and 1997 were examined. Developing pyelonephritis (infection and inflammation of the kidney) at some point in time, having an elevated baseline creatinine, and having both kidneys look abnormal on an ultrasound were predictive for developing renal failure.

### Resources

**BOOKS**

Behrman, Richard, et al. "Prune-Belly Syndrome." In *Nelson Textbook of Pediatrics*. Philadelphia: W.B. Saunders Company, 2000.

**PERIODICALS**

Freedman, A.L., et al. "Long-term outcome in children after antenatal intervention for obstructive uropathies." *The Lancet* 354 (July 1999): 374–7.

Leeners, B., et al. "Prune-Belly Syndrome: Therapeutic Options Including In Utero Placement of a Vesicoamniotic Shunt." *Journal of Clinical Ultrasound* 28, no. 9 (November/December 2000): 500–7.

WEBSITES

Online Mendelian Inheritance in Man (OMIM). http://www.ncbi.nlm.nih.gov/omim/dispmim.

ORGANIZATIONS

National Organization for Rare Disorders (NORD). 55 Kenosia Ave., PO Box 1968, Danbury, CT 06813. (203) 744-0100 or (800) 999-6673. http://www.rarediseases.org.

David Elihu Greenberg, MD

# Pseudo-Gaucher disease

## Definition

Pseudo-Gaucher disease is a rare genetic disorder with characteristics very different from those of **Gaucher disease** but caused by the same genetic mutation as that responsible for Gaucher disease. The condition is transmitted as an autosomal recessive trait. The disorder is also known as Gaucher-like disease.

## Demographics

No prevalence estimates are available for pseudo-Gaucher disease. Approximately 20 cases worldwide have been reported since 1984.

## Description

Gaucher disease is a well-studied genetic disorder transmitted as an autosomal recessive trait. It has a wide variety of manifestations, involving a number of different body systems. It has traditionally been divided into three major types, based on significant differences in those manifestations. Since the mid-1980s, a handful of cases have been reported in patients with some Gaucher-like symptoms, but other symptoms—especially cardiovascular calcification—that appear to justify its classification as a distinct form of genetic disorder, now called Gaucher disease Type IIIC.

## Causes and symptoms

Pseudo-Gaucher disease is caused by one or more mutations on the GBA (glucosidase, beta; acid [includes glucosylceramidase]) **gene**, the same gene that is responsible for other forms of Gaucher disease. The GBA gene is responsible for production of the

enzyme beta-glucocerebrosidase, which catalyzes the breakdown of a large lipid molecule, glucocerebroside, into glucose and ceramide, a simpler lipid molecule. More than 200 mutations in the GBA gene have been implicated in the development of various forms of Gaucher disease. A specific mutation in the same gene has also been found to be associated with the development of pseudo-Gaucher disease. That mutation occurs at position 409 with the substitution of a histidine amino acid for aspartic acid. Although the genotypes of the four forms of Gaucher disease, types I, II, III, and IIIC (pseudo-Gaucher) are similar, the phenotypes produced are very different for the first three categories and pseudo-Gaucher.

The distinguishing characteristic of pseudo-Gaucher disease is cardiovascular calcification, primarily of the aortic and mitral valves. Neurological dysfunction of the eyes, resulting in corneal opacity, has been characteristic of many cases also. Enlargement of the spleen has also been observed in a small number of cases.

## Diagnosis

The presence of cardiovascular insufficiency and ocular opacity are initial indications of the possibility of Gaucher-like disease. Further standard cardiac tests, such as diastolic murmur, cardiac enlargement, and arrhythmia may suggest the presence of cardiovascular disease. Confirmatory test for the disorder consists of a genetic test for the presence of a mutation at position 409 in the GBA gene.

### Treatment and management

No treatments are available for the cure of pseudo-Gaucher disease. Heart valve replacement has been attempted for the most severe cases of valve calcification, but generally without success. Three Spanish sisters who received this surgery all died, at the ages of 13, 15, and 16.

### Prognosis

Prognosis is generally poor for pseudo-Gaucher disease since no successful treatment for manifestations of the disorder have been developed. A number of individuals with the disorder have died during childhood or adolescence.

### Prevention

No steps can be taken to prevent the occurrence of pseudo-Gaucher disease among individuals who carry the characteristic **genotype**. Early detection of the disease may make possible early intervention that may prolong the life of an affected individual.

### Resources

#### PERIODICALS

Abrahamov, Aya. "Gaucher's Disease Variant Characterised by Progressive Calcification of Heart Valves and Unique Genotype." *Lancet.* 346, no. 8981 (1995): 1000-1003.

Beutler, Ernest. "Gaucher Disease Phenotypes Outflanked?" *Genome Research.* 7, no. 10 (1997): 950-951.

Chabás, Amparo, et al. "Unusual Expression of Gaucher's Disease: Cardiovascular Calcifications in Three Sibs Homozygous for the D409H Mutation." *Journal of Medical Genetics.* 32, no. 9 (1995): 740-742.

Uyama, E., et al. "Hydrocephalus, Corneal Opacities, Deafness, Valvular Heart Disease, Deformed Toes and Leptomeningeal Fibrous Thickening in Adult Siblings: A New Syndrome Associated with Beta-Glucocerebrosidase Deficiency and a Mosaic Population of Storage Cells." *Acta Neurologica Scandinavica.* 86, no. 4 (1992): 407-420.

#### OTHER

Gaucher Disease. Genetics Home Reference. http://ghr.nlm.nih.gov/condition = gaucherdisease.

Gaucher-like Disease. Medic8. http://www.medic8.com/genetics/gaucher-like-disease.htm.

Online Mendelian Inheritance in Man. http://www.ncbi.nlm.nih.gov/omim/.

#### ORGANIZATIONS

European Organization for Rare Diseases, 102, rue Didot, Paris, France, 75014, + 33 1 56.53.52.10, + 33 1 56.53.52.15, eurordiseurordis.org, http://www.eurordis.org.

National Gaucher Foundation, 2227 Idlewood Road, Suite 12, Tucker, GA, 30084, 800-504-3189, 770-934-2911, ngf@gaucherdisease.org, http://www.gaucherdisease.org.

David E. Newton, Ed.D.

## Pseudo-Hurler disease *see* GM1 gangliosidosis

## Pseudoachondroplasia

### Definition

Pseudoachondroplasia is moderately severe **skeletal dysplasia** characterized by disproportionate short stature, hypermobile joints, normal head size, and normal length and appearance at birth. Individuals with this condition are usually not diagnosed until early childhood. Complications of this disorder include early-onset arthritis of the weight-bearing joints and other orthopedic complications. This genetic disorder has autosomal dominant **inheritance**.

### Description

Pseudoachondroplasia is a rare genetic skeletal **dysplasia** first described by Drs. Maroteaux and Lamy in 1959. It is sometimes also referred to as pseudoachondroplastic dysplasia and pseudoachondroplastic **spondyloepiphyseal dysplasia** and is one of more than 200 rare skeletal dysplasias. Skeletal dysplasias are a group of disorders that result from problems in bone growth and formation. The term dwarfism is losing favor to the more technical term of skeletal dysplasia. There are many causes of growth problems, including hormone imbalances, metabolic problems, and problems with bone growth.

Pseudoachondroplasia is one of the most common skeletal dysplasias. Individuals with pseudoachondroplasia have normal growth parameters (height and weight) at birth, and it usually is not until the second year of life that growth retardation becomes evident. During this phase, their body proportions resemble those of individuals with achondroplasia—the most common form of skeletal dysplasia. Because of this resemblance, this type is skeletal dysplasia was termed "pseudo" **achondroplasia**.

As the name implies, pseudoachondroplasia was once thought to be closely related to achondroplasia. However, geneticists have since learned otherwise. In appearance, individuals with pseudoachondroplasia share the same height as those with achondroplasia, but their head size is the same as that of average-size people, and they lack the distinct facial features characteristic of achondroplasia. Children with pseudoachondroplasia are usually not diagnosed until they are two or three years old when their growth parameters become abnormal. The most serious complications of pseudoachondroplasia are short stature, orthopedic problems, and early-onset **osteoarthritis** of the weight-bearing joints. Many individuals with pseudoachondroplasia experience significant joint pain, and undergo multiple orthopedic surgeries and joint replacements.

Pseudoachondroplasia is easily recognizable. Individuals with pseudoachondroplasia have disproportionate short stature, normal size head, normal facial features, joint laxity, and disproportionate shortening of their limbs. Most individuals with pseudoachondroplasia have a normal IQ. The early motor development of infants with pseudoachondroplasia is normal until the advent of walking when a waddling gait is often noted. Individuals with pseudoachondroplasia can have medical complications that range from mild to severe. Because of the differences in their bone structure and their joints, they are at increased risk to develop osteoarthritis at an early age (sometimes in their teens and usually by their twenties). They also have a small risk for neurologic problems caused by spinal cord compression due to abnormal vertebra and joint laxity.

The short stature of pseudoachondroplasia can be socially isolating and physically challenging. Most public places are not adapted to individuals of short stature, and this can limit their activities. Children and adults with pseudoachondroplasia can be socially ostracized due to their physical appearance. Many individuals erroneously assume that people with pseudoachondroplasia have limited abilities.

### Genetic profile

Pseudoachondroplasia is caused by a mutation, or change, in the cartilage oligomeric matrix protein 3 **gene** (COMP) that is located on the short arm of **chromosome** 19 (19p13.1).

Genes contain the instructions that tell a body how to form. They are composed of four different chemical bases: adenine (A), thymine (T), cytosine (C), and guanine (G). When these bases are arranged in a specific order, they provide the instructions that a cell needs to form a protein. Every three bases codes for one amino acid. Amino acids are the building blocks of proteins.

The COMP (cartilage oligomeric matrix protein) gene provides the instruction for the formation of a particular protein that is made by cartilage cells and is then transported into the cellular matrix surrounding these cells. Cartilage plays a very important role in bone formation. Because of abnormalities in the formation of this protein, the protein cannot be transported out of the cell. This results in a deficiency of the protein in the cartilage matrix and a buildup of the protein within the cartilage cells. This leads to the development of pseudoachondroplasia. Because cartilage plays a role in the normal growth and development of bones, any problems with cartilage will lead to problems with bone growth.

Pseudoachondroplasia is caused by mutations in the COMP gene. One specific mutation accounts for approximately 30% of the cases of pseudoachondroplasia. The COMP gene is comprised of 757 amino acids. In a normal (non-mutated) gene, amino acid 372 codes for aspartic acid. In most individuals with pseudoachondroplasia, this amino acid has been deleted. Other mutations have been detected in the COMP gene, most of which are small substitutions or deletions of base pairs.

Mutations in the COMP gene are inherited in an autosomal dominant manner. Every individual has two COMP genes: one from their father and one from their mother. In an autosomal dominant disorder, only one gene has to have a mutation for the person to have the disorder. Most individuals with pseudoachondroplasia are born to parents with average stature. Their pseudoachondroplasia is the result of a *de novo*, or new, mutation. No one knows the cause of *de novo* mutations or why they occur so frequently in pseudoachondroplasia. However, once a couple has had a child with pseudoachondroplasia, there is a 4% recurrence risk to have a second similarly affected child. This increased recurrence risk is due to germline mosaicism, or the chance that the *de novo* mutation is present in others of their sperm and egg cells.

An individual with pseudoachondroplasia has a 50% chance of passing on their mutated gene to their children. Often individuals with short stature will marry other individuals with short stature. If the partner of a person with pseudoachondroplasia also has an autosomal dominant inherited skeletal dysplasia, then there is a 25% chance that they will have a child with average stature, a 25% chance that they will have a child with one pseudoachondroplasia gene (a heterozygote), a 25% chance that their child will have the other autosomal dominant skeletal dysplasia (a heterozygote), and a 25% chance that a child will get a double dose of the gene for pseudoachondroplasia and the gene for the other skeletal dysplasia (a double heterozygote). Babies with two skeletal dysplasias (double dose) can be much more severely affected than babies with a single pseudoachondroplasia gene. Couples with skeletal dysplasias should seek **genetic counseling** to understand their exact risks before undertaking a pregnancy.

### Demographics

The exact prevalence of pseudoachondroplasia is unknown, but it is estimated to occur in about one in 30,000 individuals. Pseudoachondroplasia affects males and females in equal numbers. Most individuals with pseudoachondroplasia are born to parents with average stature. This is due to a new mutation that occurs on the COMP gene of the child with pseudoachondroplasia.

### Signs and symptoms

Individuals with pseudoachondroplasia have disproportionate short stature, normal-sized heads, limb differences, and rhizomelic shortening of their limbs; rhizomelic means "root limb." Rhizomelic shortening

of the limbs means that those segments of a limb closest to the body (the root of the limb) are more severely affected. In individuals with pseudoachondroplasia, the upper arms are shorter than the forearms, and the upper leg (thigh) is shorter than the lower leg.

In addition to shortened limbs, individuals with pseudoachondroplasia have other characteristic limb differences. They have a limited ability to rotate and extend their elbows. They also have joint laxity, particularly of the hands, ankles, and knees. Because of this joint laxity, they can be bow-legged or knock-kneed and may have in-turned toes. Their hands and feet are short and broad, as are their fingers and toes. Their fingers and other joints are hyperextensible, or very flexible.

In addition to limb differences, individuals with pseudoachondroplasia have other characteristic skeletal differences. Because of malformed vertebra and lax ligaments, individuals with pseudoachondroplasia can have spinal problems, including kyphosis (hunchback), lordosis (swayback), and **scoliosis**.

Individuals with pseudoachondroplasia have normal facial features and a normal-sized head. This is one of the major features that differentiate pseudoachondroplasia from achondroplasia. Individuals with pseudoachondroplasia have shortening of their long bones. The average adult height of individuals with pseudoachondroplasia ranges from 32–52 in (80–130 cm).

### Diagnosis

Pseudoachondroplasia is diagnosed by a combination of physical exam, x rays, and molecular testing. The characteristic findings of short stature and rhizomelic shortening of the limbs become apparent around two years of age and become more pronounced over time. In addition to being diagnosed by physical examination, individuals with pseudoachondroplasia have some specific bone changes that can be seen on an x ray. A **DNA** blood test to look for mutations in the COMP gene may also help clarify the diagnosis.

Unlike other skeletal dysplasias, pseudoachondroplasia cannot be diagnosed by a **prenatal ultrasound** or sonogram because the characteristic changes in the bones and the growth delays do not appear until the child is two years of age.

The diagnosis of pseudoachondroplasia can be made prenatally by DNA testing if the mutation for that family has been characterized. A sample of tissue from a fetus is obtained by either chorionic villi sampling (CVS) or by **amniocentesis**. Chorionic villi sampling is generally done between 10 and 12 weeks of pregnancy, and amniocentesis is done between 14 and 18 weeks of pregnancy. Chorionic villi sampling involves removing a small amount of tissue from the developing placenta. The tissue in the placenta contains the same DNA as the fetus. Amniocentesis involves removing a small amount of fluid from around the fetus. This fluid contains some fetal skin cells from which DNA can be isolated. The fetal DNA is then tested to determine if it contains the mutation that is responsible for pseudoachondroplasia in that family.

Prenatal DNA testing for pseudoachondroplasia is not routinely performed in low-risk pregnancies. This type of testing is generally limited to high-risk pregnancies, such as those in which both parents have pseudoachondroplasia or one in which one parent has pseudoachondroplasia and the other parent has another autosomal dominant form of skeletal dysplasia. It is particularly helpful in determining if a fetus has received two dominant skeletal mutations. Infants who have inherited two autosomal dominant skeletal dysplasias may have very severe complications that may result in death.

DNA testing can also be performed on blood samples from children or adults. This is usually done as part of a genetic work-up to establish the exact form of skeletal dysplasia. Many skeletal dysplasias can be hard to differentiate from one another, and DNA testing can often clarify the diagnosis.

### Treatment and management

There is no cure for pseudoachondroplasia. All children with pseudoachondroplasia should have their height, weight, and head circumference measured and plotted on growth curves specifically developed for children with pseudoachondroplasia. The most common medical complication is early-onset osteoarthritis and other orthopedic problems. Some patients experience significant pain that can be controlled by analgesics, although the effectiveness of various forms of analgesics has not been thoroughly studied in pseudoachondroplasia. Early-onset osteoarthritis is caused by malformations of the weight-bearing joints and deficient cartilage production. Approximately 50% of patients with pseudoachondroplasia will require hip replacements. By being aware of the potential medical complications and by taking some preventative measures, it may be possible to avoid or delay the onset of some of the long-term consequences of these complications.

Weight management is extremely important for an individual with pseudoachondroplasia. Excess weight can exacerbate many of the potential orthopedic problems, such as bowed legs, curvature of the spine, and joint and lower back pain. Excess weight can also contribute to sleep apnea problems. Development of good eating habits and appropriate exercise programs should be encouraged in individuals with pseudoachondroplasia. However, because of the potential for spinal cord compression, care should be used in choosing appropriate forms of exercise.

The social adaptation of children with pseudoachondroplasia and their families should be closely monitored. Children with visible physical differences can have difficulties in school and socially. Support groups such as Little People of America can be a source of guidance on how to deal with these issues. It is important that children with pseudoachondroplasia not be limited in activities that pose no danger. In addition to monitoring their social adaptation, every effort should be made to physically adapt their surroundings for convenience and to improve independence. Physical adaptations can include step stools to increase accessibility and lowering of light switches and counters.

The two treatments that have been used to try to increase the final adult height of individuals with pseudoachondroplasia are limb-lengthening and growth hormone therapy.

Limb-lengthening involves surgically attaching external rods to the long bones in the arms and legs. These rods run parallel to the bone on the outside of the body. Over a period of 18–24 months, the tension on these rods is increased, which results in the lengthening of the underlying bone. This procedure is long, costly, and has potential complications, including pain, infections, and nerve problems. Limb-lengthening can increase overall height by 12–14 in (30.5–35.6 cm) in some skeletal dysplasias. It does not change the other physical manifestations of pseudoachondroplasia, such as the appearance of the hands and feet. This is an elective surgery, and individuals must decide for themselves if it would be of benefit to them. The optimal age to perform this surgery is not known.

Growth hormone therapy has been used to treat some children with pseudoachondroplasia. Originally, there was doubt about the effectiveness of this treatment because children with pseudoachondroplasia are not growth-hormone deficient. This doubt has proven to be justified. While this treatment seems to have some success for individuals with other forms of skeletal dysplasia, at least one study has found that it actually decreases the height of children with pseudoachondroplasia. Growth hormone therapy is not recommended for pseudoachondroplasia.

## Prognosis

The prognosis for most people with pseudoachondroplasia is very good. In general, they have minimal medical problems, normal IQ, and most achieve success and have a long life, regardless of their stature. The most serious medical barriers to an excellent prognosis are the orthopedic complications and early-onset arthritis that can limit the activities of an individual and cause significant pain. Most individuals with pseudoachondroplasia will have multiple orthopedic surgeries over their lifetime.

Successful social adaptation plays an important role in the ultimate success and happiness of an individual with pseudoachondroplasia. It is very important that the career and life choices of an individual with pseudoachondroplasia not be limited by preconceived ideas about their abilities.

## Resources

### BOOKS

Ablon, Joan. *Living with Difference: Families with Dwarf Children*. Westport, CT: Praeger Publishing, 1988.

### PERIODICALS

American Academy of Pediatrics Committee on Genetics. "Health Supervision for Children with Pseudoachondroplasia." *Pediatrics* 95, no 3 (March 1995): 443–451.

### WEB SITES

The Human Growth Foundation. http://www.hgfound.org/
.

Little People of America: An Organization for People of Short Stature. http://www.lpaonline. org/lpa.html.

### ORGANIZATIONS

Little People of America National Headquarters. Box 745, Lubbock, TX 79408. (888) LPA-2001. E-mail: LPADataBase@juno.com.

Kathleen A. Fergus, MS, CGC

## Pseudothalidomide syndrome *see* **Roberts SC phocomelia**

# Pseudoxanthoma elasticum

## Definition

Pseudoxanthoma elascticum (PXE) is an inherited connective tissue disorder in which the elastic fibers present in the skin, eyes, and cardiovascular system gradually become calcified and inelastic.

## Description

PXE was first reported in 1881 by Rigal, but the problem with elastic fibers was described in 1986 by Darier who gave the condition its name. PXE is also known as Grönblad-Strandberg-Touraine syndrome and systemic elastorrhexis.

The course of PXE varies greatly between individuals. Typically, it is first noticed during adolescence as yellow-orange bumps on the side of the neck. Similar bumps may appear at other places where the skin bends a lot, like the backs of the knees and the insides of the elbows. The skin in these areas tends to get thick, leathery, inelastic, and acquire extra folds. These skin problems have no serious consequences, and for some people, the disease progresses no further.

Bruch's membrane, a layer of elastic fibers in front of the retina, becomes calcified in some people with PXE. Calcification causes cracks in Bruch's membrane, which can be seen through an ophthalmoscope as red, brown, or gray streaks called angioid streaks. The cracks can eventually (e.g., in 10–20 years) cause bleeding, and the usual resultant scarring leads to central vision deterioration. However, peripheral vision is unaffected.

Arterial walls and heart valves contain elastic fibers that can become calcified. This leads to a greater susceptibility to the conditions that are associated with hardening of the arteries in the normal aging population—high blood pressure, heart attack, stroke, and arterial obstruction—and, similarly, mitral valve prolapse. Heart disease and hypertension associated with PXE have been reported in children as young as four to 13 years of age. Although often appearing at a younger age, the overall incidence of these conditions is only slightly higher for people with PXE than it is in the general population.

Arterial inelasticity can lead to bleeding from the gastrointestinal tract and, rarely, acute vomiting of blood.

## Genetic profile

PXE is caused by changes in the genetic material, called mutations, that are inherited in either a dominant or recessive mode. A person with the recessive form of the disease (which is most common) must possess two copies of the PXE gene to be affected, and, therefore, must have received one from each parent. In the dominant form, one copy of the abnormal gene is sufficient to cause the disease. In some cases, a person with the dominant form inherits the abnormal gene from a parent with PXE. More commonly, the mutation arises as a spontaneous change in

## KEY TERMS

**Angioid streaks**—Gray, orange, or red wavy branching lines in Bruch's membrane.

**Bruch's membrane**—A membrane in the eye between the choroid membrane and the retina.

**Carrier**—A person who possesses a gene for an abnormal trait without showing signs of the disorder. The person may pass the abnormal gene on to offspring.

**Claudication**—Pain in the lower legs after exercise caused by insufficient blood supply.

**Connective tissue**—A group of tissues responsible for support throughout the body; includes cartilage, bone, fat, tissue underlying skin, and tissues that support organs, blood vessels, and nerves throughout the body.

**Deletion**—The absence of genetic material that is normally found in a chromosome. Often, the genetic material is missing due to an error in replication of an egg or sperm cell.

**Dominant trait**—A genetic trait where one copy of the gene is sufficient to yield an outward display of the trait; dominant genes mask the presence of recessive genes; dominant traits can be inherited from a single parent.

**Elastic fiber**—Fibrous, stretchable connective tissue made primarily from proteins, elastin, collagen, and fibrillin.

**Gene**—A building block of inheritance, which contains the instructions for the production of a particular protein, and is made up of a molecular sequence found on a section of DNA. Each gene is found on a precise location on a chromosome.

**Mitral valve**—The heart valve that prevents blood from flowing backwards from the left ventricle into the left atrium. Also known as bicuspid valve.

**Mutation**—A permanent change in the genetic material that may alter a trait or characteristic of an individual, or manifest as disease, and can be transmitted to offspring.

**Recessive trait**—An inherited trait or characteristic that is outwardly obvious only when two copies of the gene for that trait are present.

the genetic material of the affected person. These cases are called "sporadic" and do not affect parents or siblings, although each child of a person with sporadic PXE has a 50% risk to inherit the condition.

Both males and females can develop PXE, although the skin findings seem to be somewhat more common in females.

The actual genetic causes of this condition were not discovered until 2000. The recessive, dominant, and sporadic forms of PXE all appear to be caused by different mutations or deletions in a single gene called ABCC6 (also known as MRP6), located on **chromosome** 16. Although the responsible gene has been identified, how it causes PXE is still unknown.

Genetic researchers have since identified mutations in a number of persons with PXE, most of whom have been found to have the recessive type. Affected individuals in these families had mutations in both copies of the gene and parents, who are obligate carriers, had a mutation in only one copy. Contrary to the usual lack of symptoms in carriers of recessive genes, some carriers of recessive PXE have been found to have cardiovascular symptoms typical of PXE.

Although the recessive type is the most common, there are also familial and sporadic cases that have been found to be caused by dominant mutations in the ABCC6 gene.

### Demographics

PXE is rare and occurs in about one in every 160,000 people in the general population. It is likely, though, that PXE is under-diagnosed because of the presence of mild symptoms in some affected persons and the lack of awareness of the condition among primary care physicians.

### Signs and symptoms

A wide range in the type and severity of symptoms exists between people with PXE. The age of onset also varies, although most people notice initial symptoms during adolescence or early adulthood. Often, the first symptoms to appear are thickened skin with yellow bumps in localized areas such as the folds of the groin, arms, knees, and armpits. These changes can also occur in the mucous membranes, most often in the inner portion of the lower lip. The appearance of the skin in PXE has been likened to a plucked chicken or Moroccan leather.

Angioid streaks in front of the retina are present in most people with PXE and an ophthalmologic examination can be used as an initial screen for the condition. Persons with PXE often complain of sensitivity to light. Because of the progressive breakdown of Bruch's membrane, affected persons are at increased risk for bleeding and scarring of the retina, which can lead to decreased central vision but does not usually cause complete blindness.

Calcium deposits in the artery walls contribute to early-onset atherosclerosis, and another condition called claudication, inadequate blood flow that results in pain in the legs after exertion. Abnormal bleeding, caused by calcification of the inner layer of the arteries, can occur in the brain, retina, uterus, bladder, and joints but is most common in the gastrointestinal tract.

### Diagnosis

The presence of calcium in elastic fibers, as revealed by microscopic examination of biopsied skin, unequivocally establishes the diagnosis of PXE.

### Treatment and management

PXE cannot be cured, but plastic surgery can treat PXE skin lesions, and laser surgery is used to prevent or slow the progression of vision loss. Excessive blood loss due to bleeding into the gastrointestinal tract or other organ systems may be treated by transfusion. Mitral valve prolapse (protrusion of one or both cusps of the mitral heart valve back into the atrium during heart beating) can be corrected by surgery, if necessary.

Measures should be taken to prevent or lessen cardiovascular complications. People with PXE should control their cholesterol and blood pressure, and maintain normal weight. They should exercise for cardiovascular health and to prevent or reduce claudication later in life. They should also avoid the use of tobacco, thiazide antihypertensive drugs, blood thinners like coumadin, and non-steroidal anti-inflammatory drugs like aspirin and ibuprofen. In addition, they should avoid strain, heavy lifting, and contact sports, since these activities could trigger retinal and gastrointestinal bleeding.

People with PXE should have regular eye examinations by an ophthalmologist and report any eye problems immediately. Regular check-ups with a physician are also recommended, including periodic blood pressure readings.

### QUESTIONS TO ASK YOUR DOCTOR

- Please explain the meaning of the name "pseudoxanthoma elasticum."
- What is the probability that this genetic disorder will be transmitted from parents to children?
- On what basis is pseudoxanthoma elasticum syndrome diagnosed?
- What ongoing medical attention is needed to monitor the progress of this disease?

Some people have advocated a calcium-restricted diet, but it is not yet known whether this aids the problems brought about by PXE. It is known, however, that calcium-restriction can lead to bone disorders.

### Prognosis

The prognosis is for a normal life span with an increased chance of cardiovascular and circulatory problems, hypertension, gastrointestinal bleeding, and impaired vision. Now that the gene for PXE has been identified, the groundwork for research to provide effective treatment has been laid. Studying the role of the ABCC6 protein in elastic fibers may lead to drugs that will improve or prevent the problems caused by PXE.

Genetic tests are now available that can provide knowledge needed to both diagnose PXE in symptomatic persons and predict it prior to the onset of symptoms in persons at risk. Prenatal diagnosis of PXE, by testing fetal cells for mutations in the ABCC6 gene, can be done in early pregnancy by procedures such as **amniocentesis** or chorionic villus sampling. For most people, PXE is compatible with a reasonably normal life, and prenatal diagnosis is not likely to be highly desired.

**Genetic testing** to predict whether an at-risk child will develop PXE may be helpful for medical management. A child who is found to carry a mutation can be monitored more closely for eye problems and bleeding, and can begin the appropriate lifestyle changes to prevent cardiovascular problems.

### Resources

**BOOKS**

Pope, F. Michael. "Pseudoxanthoma Elasticum, Cutis Laxa, and Other Disorders of Elastic Tissue." In *Emery and Rimoin's Principles and Practice of Medical Genetics.* 3rd ed. Ed. David L. Rimoin, J. Michael Connor, and Reed E. Pyeritz. New York: Churchill Livingstone, 1997.

**PERIODICALS**

Ringpfeil, F., et al. "Pseudoxanthoma Elasticum: Mutations in the MRP6 Gene Encoding a Transmembrane AFP-binding Cassette (ABC) Transporter." *Proceedings of the National Academy of Sciences* 97 (May 2000): 6001–6.

Sherer, D.W., et al. "Pseudoxanthoma Elasticum: An Update." *Dermatology* 199 (1999): 3–7.

**ORGANIZATIONS**

National Association for Pseudoxanthoma Elasticum. 3500 East 12th Avenue, Denver, CO 80206. (303) 355-3866. Fax: (303) 355-3859. Pxenape@estreet.com. http://www.napxe.org.

PXE International, Inc. 23 Mountain Street, Sharon, MA 02067. (781) 784-3817. Fax: (781) 784-6672. PXEInter @aol.com. http://www.pxe.org/.

Barbara J. Pettersen, MS, CGC

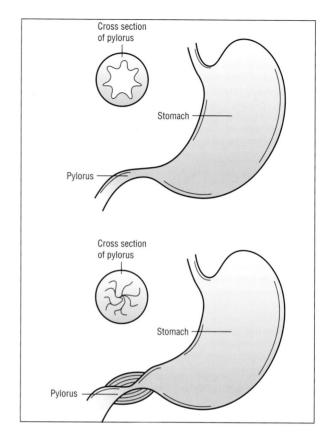

These diagrams show the cross section of a normal pylorus in relation to a stomach with pyloric stenosis where the pylorus has become extremely narrowed. Constriction of the pylorus results from enlargement of the muscle surrounding it. *(Gale, a part of Cengage Learning.)*

# Pyloric stenosis

## Definition

Pyloric stenosis is a disorder that occurs when the pyloric sphincter muscle, which is found at the outlet of the stomach, thickens and becomes enlarged causing the cavity (lumen) of the pylorus to narrow and lengthen. This blocks the passage of food from the stomach to the small intestine (the portion of bowel that continues digestion after food leaves the stomach).

## Description

Pyloric stenosis occurs due to enlargement of the walls of the pyloric sphincter. The pyloric sphincter is a circular smooth muscle at the outlet of the stomach that controls the flow of food from the stomach to the small intestine. The muscle cells become enlarged (hypertrophied) causing a narrowing (stenosis) of the pyloric lumen. This causes food to be pushed back into the stomach. Symptoms of pyloric stenosis typically appear two to six weeks after birth. In rare cases it occurs in older adults, not of genetic cause but due to an ulcer (inflammatory lesion of the mucous-like tissue in the stomach) or hardening of the tissue (fibrosis) at the outlet of the stomach. Alternate names associated with the disorder are hypertrophic pyloric stenosis and infantile hypertrophic pyloric stenosis.

## Genetic profile

The exact cause of pyloric stenosis is unknown. It generally occurs in one in 300 births. The incidence of pyloric stenosis may be higher if a parent or sibling had the condition. It is also more common in the first-born child. Family correlation studies have shown that there is higher expression (concordance) of pyloric stenosis in identical twins (monozygotic) than in fraternal twins (dizygotic). The risk for first-degree relatives (brothers, sisters) of females is higher than those of males. This is also true of second-degree relatives (cousins).

It has been suggested that motilin receptors, which are responsible for motility, might have an involvement in pyloric stenosis. The development of functional motilin receptors occurs around the age of onset for most cases of pyloric stenosis. Studies have found that the use of an antibiotic, called erythromycin for pertussis (a contagious respiratory disease also known as whooping cough) prophylaxis may increase the risk for pyloric stenosis. Erythromycin is a motilin agonist (acts on something to produce a predictable response) and high doses can cause an increase in non-propagated contractions and motility. The lack of neuronal nitric oxide synthase in pyloric tissue may cause a spasm (a twitching or involuntary contraction) in the pyloric muscle in individuals with pyloric stenosis. Neuronal nitric oxide synthase is needed for the synthesis of nitric oxide, which opposes the contraction force in active muscle.

### Demographics

Pyloric stenosis affects males three to four times more than females and appears to have an increased incidence in caucasians.

### Signs and symptoms

Symptoms include:

- Regurgitation and non-bilious vomiting. Infants may bring food back up during or after feeding. Vomiting may become projectile (expelled with force) and vomit may have a "coffee ground" color. Vomit should not contain stomach bile, which is acidic and a brownish-green color. This would be contraindicative of pyloric stenosis.
- Olive-sized abdominal mass. A mass about the size of an olive may be felt in the upper abdomen. The mass should be hard, mobile, and non-tender.
- Pylorospasm. A spasm of the pyloric muscle may occur due to increased motility.
- Additional abnormalities. These include hunger, irritability, lethargy (prolonged sleepiness or sluggishness), weight loss, decreased urine output, constipation, and gastric (stomach) peristalsis (rhythmic contraction of smooth muscle) from the left to right.

### Diagnosis

An individual's medical history and physical assessment by a doctor are necessary for a diagnosis of pyloric stenosis. A palpable mass, the size of an olive, in the upper abdominal area usually confirms a diagnosis of pyloric stenosis. When physical findings are inconclusive, an abdominal ultrasound or barium study may be performed to confirm diagnosis. An ultrasound, the preferred method of confirmation, is a non-invasive study that uses high frequency sound waves to distinguish the image of internal structures of the body. A barium study involves the ingestion of a radiographic dye. The movement of the dye through the gastrointestinal (GI) tract can be followed by fluoroscopy or x ray studies. It has been suggested that the Lipper GI series may be an effective step in confirming pyloric stenosis. This test consists of aspirating (withdrawal of fluid) and measuring gastric contents. The amount of aspirated contents is indicative of pyloric stenosis and studies have demonstrated this method to be a reliable diagnostic tool.

In adults with symptoms of pyloric stenosis, a barium swallow study is used to diagnose the disorder. X rays are taken of the abdominal structures after the ingestion of the barium radioisotope (a radioactive form of a chemical element).

### Treatment and management

The only treatment for pyloric stenosis is surgical pyloromyotomy. Making an incision into the pyloric muscle and spreading the walls of the muscle apart completes the surgery. This allows gastric mucosa to push up through the incision and relieve the blockage.

Blood analysis should be performed before surgery and intravenous (going into the vein) fluids should be given to correct electrolyte (sodium, potassium, calcium etc.) imbalances and rehydrate infants. Following surgery the infant should start on an oral electrolyte (elements necessary for cell functioning) solution (Pedialyte). Feedings will be gradually increased until the infant is tolerating 2-3 oz (60ml) of breast-milk or formula without complications. The stomach needs time to heal; therefore vomiting due to increased feedings is common. Infants are usually discharged 24–48 hours following surgery. It has been suggested that rapid advancement of the strength and volume of feedings is effective and may allow for quicker discharge from the hospital.

Adults being treated for pyloric stenosis usually have a stomach tube inserted into the muscle that remains in place after sugery.

Recurrence of pyloric stenosis after surgery is rare. There has been no occurrence of conditions later in life related to the occurrence of pyloric stenosis during infancy.

### Prognosis

The prognosis of pyloric stenosis is very good for those that are diagnosed early and treated with surgery. Life expectancy of infants diagnosed with pyloric stenosis is the same as that of the average individual. Parents should contact a doctor if pyloric stenosis is suspected.

### Resources

#### BOOKS

Bowden, V. R., S. B. Dickey, and C. Smith-Greenberg. *Children and their families: The continuum of care.* Philadelphia: W.B. Saunders Company, 1991.

Connor, J.M., and M. A. Fergusen-Smith. *Essential Medical Genetics.* 4th ed. Oxford: Blackwell Scientific Publications, 1993.

"Congenital Pyloric Stenosis." In *Principles and Practice of Medical Genetics.* Vol. 2. Ed. Alan E.H. Emery and David L. Rimoin. New York: Churchill Livingstone, 1983.

#### PERIODICALS

Gollin, G., et al. "Rapid advancement of feedings after pyloromyotomy for Pyloric Stenosis." *Clinical Pediatrics* 39 (2000): 187–90.

Honein, M.A., et al. "Infantile hypertrophic pyloric stenosis after pertussis prophylxis with erythromycin: a case review and cohort study." *The Lancet* 354 (1999): 2101–5.

Huffman, G.B. "Evaluating infants with possible pyloric stenosis." *American Family Physician* 60 (1999): 2108–9.

Patterson, L., et al. "Hypertrophy pyloric stenosis in infants following pertussis prophylaxis with erythromycin—Knoxville, Tennessee, 1999." *Morbidity and Mortality Weekly Report* 48 (1999): 1117–20.

#### WEBSITES

Healthgate. http://www.healthgate.com.

McKusick, V.A., ed. Pyloric Stenosis, Infantile." April 14, 2008 (December 12, 2009). *Online Mendelian Inheritance in Man (OMIM).* http://www.ncbi.nlm.nih.gov/entrez/dispomim.cgi?id = 179010.

McKusick, V.A., ed. "Nitric Oxide Synthase 1; NOS1."-January 9, 2009 (December 12, 2009). *Online Mendelian Inheritance in Man (OMIM).* http://www.ncbi.nlm.nih.gov/entrez/dispomim.cgi?id = 163731.

Yale University Department of Surgery. http://www.yalesurgery.med.yale.edu.

Laith Farid Gulli, MD
Tanya Bivins, BS

# Pyruvate carboxylase deficiency

### Definition

Pyruvate carboxylase deficiency (PCD) is a rare non-sex linked (autosomal) disorder that results from an insufficient amount of the enzyme pyruvate carboxylase. This disorder is inherited as a recessive trait and it is known to be caused by more than one different mutation in the same **gene** (allelic variants).

### Description

There are two recognized types of pyruvate carboxylase deficiency, neonatal PCD (type B) and infantile onset PCD (type A). Neonatal PCD is associated with a complete, or near complete, inability to produce pyruvate carboxylase. Infantile onset PCD is associated with a chemical change in the pyruvate carboxylase enzyme that prevents this slightly different chemical from functioning as efficiently as the normal pyruvate carboxylase enzyme.

In order for the cells of the body to function properly, they must have energy. This energy comes in the form of the chemical ATP. ATP is primarily produced by breaking down carbohydrates and blood sugar (glucose) molecules. To begin the process of converting glucose and carbohydrates into usable energy, these molecules are first converted into pyruvate molecules. Once pyruvate molecules have been formed, one of two things will happen: if more energy is required by the cell, the molecules will be further broken down into ATP; or, if no additional energy is needed by the cell, the pyruvate molecules will be put back together to reform a glucose molecule.

These transformations of pyruvate are accomplished primarily by two enzymes: pyruvate dehydrogenase (PDH), an enzyme that begins the breakdown of the pyruvate into ATP, and pyruvate carboxylase, an enzyme that begins the chemical process to reform

## KEY TERMS

**Allelic variants**—A disease is said to have allelic variants when different mutations in the same allele result in identical, or nearly identical, symptoms. An allele is the combined locations of a gene on the two paired chromosomes that contain this gene.

**Autosomal**—Relating to any chromosome besides the X and Y sex chromosomes. Human cells contain 22 pairs of autosomes and one pair of sex chromosomes.

**Biotin**—A growth vitamin of the vitamin B complex found naturally in liver, egg yolks, and yeast.

**Enzyme efficiency**—The rate at which an enzyme can perform the chemical transformation that it is expected to accomplish. This is also called turnover rate. Individuals affected with type A PCD produce an enzyme that is much slower than the normal pyruvate carboxylase enzyme.

**Necrotizing encephalomyelopathy**—A progressive degeneration of the brain and central nervous system. This condition is fatal in nearly all individuals affected with type A pyruvate carboxylase deficiency.

**Pyruvate carboxylase**—The enzyme that is responsible for the first step in the conversion of pyruvate molecules into glucose molecules. Individuals with Type A PCD produce an highly inefficient form of pyruvate carboxylase. Individuals with Type B PCD either completely lack the ability to produce this enzyme, or they cannot produce it in sufficient quantities to sustain life.

glucose molecules. The reformation of glucose from pyruvate is a vital step in cellular metabolism. It allows carbohydrate molecules to be converted into a more readily usable form (glucose). Glucose is not only easier to breakdown into the energy required by the cells, but it is also more able to be transported through the bloodstream than most other fuel sources. This is particularly important because certain cells (primarily those of the brain and nervous system) cannot breakdown larger molecules; they must get their energy directly from glucose.

Pyruvate carboxylase is, in effect, part of the "off switch" for the production of ATP from pyruvate. After a cell has received the amount of ATP it requires, it is the job of pyruvate carboxylase to re-convert the excess pyruvate molecules in that cell back into glucose molecules for storage or transport to another part of the body where they may be needed. Any molecules that are not

put back together will degrade into lactic acid. This lactic acid will either be released into the bloodstream or it will buildup in the tissues. The buildup of lactic acid in the muscle tissues and red blood cells is normal during strenuous exercise. However, the accumulation of lactic acid in other tissues without exercise or without oxygen deprivation is symptomatic of an underlying problem in the normal metabolism of the cells.

People with PCD have either a complete inability or a severely limited ability to produce pyruvate carboxylase. Since these individuals cannot produce the amounts of this enzyme required to form glucose from pyruvate, this pyruvate is converted instead into lactic acid, which builds up in the cells. Additionally, since glucose cannot be adequately formed within the body of a pyruvate carboxylase deficient individual, all the glucose required by the body must be ingested. This causes a glucose shortage that leads to low blood sugar (hypoglycemia) and a progressive degeneration of the tissues, with the most profound effects observed in the brain and central nervous system, since these tissues are the most reliant on the use of glucose for energy.

Pyruvate carboxylase is also important in the process that removes excess nitrogen from the body (the urea cycle). Since pyruvate carboxylase deficient individuals do not have sufficient quantities of pyruvate carboxylase, they develop a build-up of nitrogen, in the form of ammonia, in the bloodstream and the tissues.

### Genetic profile

The gene that is responsible for the production of pyruvate carboxylase has been localized to a small region of **chromosome** 11. There are at least three mutations in this gene that lead to type B PCD. There is only one known mutation that leads to type A PCD.

Both types of PCD are transmitted via a recessive trait which means that both parents must be carriers of the mutation in order for it to occur in their children. In the case of parents with one child affected with PCD, the likelihood that a second child will be affected with PCD is 25%.

### Demographics

PCD is estimated to occur in approximately one in every 250,000 live births, although only 39 cases had been described in the literature prior to 2001.

Type A PCD is also called North American PCD because it occurs almost exclusively in Algonquin language-speaking Native North Americans. In the

Micmac, Cree, and Ojibwa tribes of Canada, it is estimated that as high as one in 10 individuals are carriers of the mutation that causes type A PCD. This suggests a founder effect in these populations. A founder effect is a genetic term that means a single individual brought a mutation into a subpopulation at a time when the subpopulation was quite small. As a result, a large majority of the members of the subpopulation carry the mutation derived through direct ancestry to this one individual.

Type B PCD is also called French PCD because it has a much higher incidence among the French than among any other subpopulation.

### Signs and symptoms

Type A, or infantile onset, PCD may be fatal prior to birth, or it may not present any symptoms until approximately three months of age. These individuals will show severe physical and mental delay. Additionally, children affected with type A PCD have a progressive degeneration of the entire brain and nervous system (necrotizing encephalomyelopathy) that eventually leads to death.

Type B, or neonatal, PCD is generally fatal prior to birth. In the rare instances of a liveborn child affected with type B PCD, severe growth delay (extremely low birth weight) and severe mental impairment are to be expected. Children born with type B PCD fail to thrive and generally do not survive past the first three months of life.

### Diagnosis

PCD is diagnosed primarily through blood tests to determine the blood concentrations of lactate and pyruvate. Extremely high levels of both of these chemicals in the blood indicate that a congenital problem in cellular metabolism is most likely present. PCD is often differentiated from other cellular metabolic disorders by the extreme speed with which glucose levels in the blood drop during fasting (fasting hypoglycemia) and the abnormally low levels of the chemical aspartic acid in the blood.

PCD can be tested prenatally by measuring the activity of pyruvate carboxylase in chorionic villi samples.

### Treatment and management

Administration of aspartic acid has been successful in decreasing the pyruvate and lactate concentrations in the blood of some PCD affected individuals. But, this treatment does not repair the damage to the

## QUESTIONS TO ASK YOUR DOCTOR

- What does the term "pyruvate carboxylase" mean?
- How do type A and type B forms of this disorder differ from each other?
- What treatments are available for this disorder, and do the treatments differ from each type of the condition?
- What information can a genetic counselor provide about pyruvate carboxylase deficiency disorder?

pyruvate carboxylase enzyme, so progressive degeneration of the nervous system is slowed only slightly and the outcome is still death.

Biotin (a B-complex vitamin) is a coenzyme to pyruvate carboxylase. It has been shown that type B PCD is responsive to treatment with biotin while type A is not. Therefore, in the rare instance of a liveborn child with type B PCD, life may be extended through the administration of biotin.

### Prognosis

Without prenatal administration of enzyme replacement therapy (which is currently not available), in which the developing fetus is given an artificial form of pyruvate carboxylase, individuals affected with either type A or type B PCD will die either prior to birth or, generally, within the first six months of life. Without prenatal enzyme replacement therapy, most children affected with PCD are born with such brain and nervous system dysfunction that a decision has to be made about treatment to sustain life.

### Resources

**BOOKS**

Al-Essa, M. A., and P. T. Ozand. *Manual of Metabolic Disease*. Riyadh, Saudi Arabia: King Faisal Specialist Hospital and Research Centre, 1998.

**PERIODICALS**

Brun, N., et al. "Pyruvate carboxylase deficiency: prenatal onset of ischemia-like brain lesions in two sibs with the acute neonatal form." *American Journal of Medical Genetics* (May 1999): 94–101.

Van Costner, R. N., S. Janssens, and J. P. Mission. "Prenatal diagnosis of pyruvate carboxylase deficiency by direct measurement of catalytic activity on chorionic villi samples." *Prenatal Diagnosis* (October 1998): 1041–4.

**WEBSITES**

Frye, Richard E., et al. "Pyruvate carboxylase deficiency." *eMedicine* November 6, 2001 [cited February 27, 2001]. http://www.emedicine.com/ped/topic1967.htm.

Kuang, Wanli, Patricia Sun, Katrina Traber, and Hilary Weiss. "Pyruvate Carboxylase Deficiency." American Medical Association at New York University School of Medicine. 1999 [cited February 27, 2001]. http://endeavor. med. nyu.edu/student-org/ama/docs/mgb1999-2000/ab12.htm.

"Pyruvate Carboxylase Deficiency." Online Mendelian Inheritance in Man (OMIM). September 10, 2002 [cited February 27, 2001]. http://www.ncbi.nlm.nih.gov/entrez/dispomim.cgi?id = 266150.

**ORGANIZATIONS**

Children Living with Inherited Metabolic Diseases. The Quadrangle, Crewe Hall, Weston Rd., Crewe, Cheshire, CW1-6UR. UK 127 025 0221. Fax: 0870-7700-327. http://www.climb.org.uk.

United Mitochondrial Disease Foundation. PO Box 1151, Monroeville, PA 15146-1151. (412) 793-8077. Fax: (412) 793-6477. http://www.umdf.org.

Paul A. Johnson

## KEY TERMS

**ATP**—Adenosine triphosphate. The chemical used by the cells of the body for energy.

**Enzyme**—A protein that catalyzes a biochemical reaction or change without changing its own structure or function.

**Highly aerobic tissues**—Tissue that requires the greatest amount of oxygen to thrive.

**Hypotonia**—Reduced or diminished muscle tone.

**Lactic acid**—The major by-product of anaerobic (without oxygen) metabolism.

**Mitochondria**—Organelles within the cell responsible for energy production.

**Pyruvate dehydrogenase complex**—A series of enzymes and co-factors that allow pyruvate to be converted into a chemical that can enter the TCA cycle.

**TCA cycle**—Formerly know as the Kreb's cycle, this is the process by which glucose and other chemicals are broken down into forms that are directly useable as energy in the cells.

# Pyruvate dehydrogenase complex deficiency

## Definition

Pyruvate dehydrogenase complex deficiency (PDHA) is a genetic disorder that results in a malfunctioning of the Krebs, or tricarboxylic acid (TCA), cycle. It is sex-linked and appears to be a dominant trait.

## Description

PDHA is one of the most common of the **genetic disorders** that cause abnormalities of mitochondrial metabolism. The mitochondria are the organelles inside cells that are responsible for energy production and respiration at the cellular level. One of the most important processes in the mitochondria is the TCA cycle (also known as the Krebs cycle). The TCA cycle produces the majority of the ATP (chemical energy) necessary for maintenance (homeostasis) of the cell. The production of this ATP is accomplished by chemically converting molecules of the chemical pyruvate into carbon dioxide, water, and ATP. After a blood sugar (glucose) molecule has been broken down into two pyruvate molecules, one of two things will occur: if energy is required by the cell, the molecules will be further broken down into ATP, carbon dioxide, and water; or, if energy is not needed by the cell, the pyruvate molecules will be put back together to reform a glucose molecule. These transformations of pyruvate are accomplished primarily by two enzymes: pyruvate carboxylase, an enzyme that converts pyruvate molecules into oxaloacetate molecules in preparation to reform glucose molecules; and pyruvate dehydrogenase (PDH), an enzyme that begins the breakdown of the pyruvate into the eventual products of carbon dioxide, water, and ATP. To break down the pyruvate, PDH gets some help from two other enzymes: dihydrolipoyl transacetylase and dihydrolipoyl dehydrogenase. These three enzymes and the five coenzymes (CoA, NAD +, FAD +, lipoic adic, and TPP) that assist these enzymes are collectively known as the pyruvate dehydrogenase complex (PDH complex).

Individuals affected with PDHA have deficiencies in one or more of the three enzymes within the PDH complex. Most have a deficiency of the PDH enzyme itself. Tissues that require the greatest amounts of oxygen (highly aerobic tissues), such as those of the brain and the rest of the central nervous system, are most sensitive to deficiencies in the PDH complex.

People with PDHA have either a complete inability or a severely limited ability to produce PDH. Since these individuals cannot produce the amounts of PDH required to break down pyruvate, the cells cannot produce enough energy, in the form of ATP, to maintain themselves. This causes a progressive degeneration of the tissues, with the most profound effects observed in the brain and central nervous system.

PDH is an enzyme. An enzyme is a chemical that facilitates (catalyzes) the chemical reaction of another chemical or of other chemicals; it is neither a reactant nor a product in the chemical reaction that it facilitates (catalyzes). As a result, enzymes are not used up in chemical reactions; they are recycled. One molecule of an enzyme may be used to facilitate (catalyze) the same chemical reaction over and over again several hundreds of thousands of times. All the enzymes necessary for catalyzing the various reactions of human life are produced within the body by genes. Genetic enzyme deficiency disorders, such as PDHA, result from only one cause: the affected individual cannot produce enough of the necessary enzyme because the gene designed to make the enzyme is faulty. Enzymes are not used up in chemical reactions, but they do eventually wear out, or accidentally get expelled. Also, as an individual grows, they may require greater quantities of an enzyme. Therefore, most enzyme deficiency disorders will have a time component to them. Individuals with no ability to produce a particular enzyme may show effects of this deficiency at birth or shortly thereafter. Individuals with only a partial ability to produce a particular enzyme may not show the effects of this deficiency until their need for the enzyme, because of growth or maturation, has outpaced their ability to produce it.

The level of ability of the pyruvate dehydrogenase complex deficiency affected individual to produce PDH, or his or her ability to sustain existing levels of PDH, are the sole determinants of the severity of the observed symptoms in that individual and the age of onset of these symptoms.

PDHA is the most common cause of non-exercise-related build-up of lactic acid in the tissues (primary lactic acidosis). When a tissue requires more energy than it can gain from aerobic processing (TCA cycle), it begins to break down carbohydrates, via an anaerobic process, in order to gain the necessary energy. Lactic acid is the by-product of carbohydrate metabolism. The build-up of lactic acid in the muscle tissues and red blood cells is normal during strenuous exercise. However, the accumulation of lactic acid in other tissues without exercise or without oxygen deprivation is symptomatic of an underlying problem in the normal aerobic process (TCA cycle).

## Genetic profile

The gene responsible for PDHA has been mapped to Xp22.2-p22.1. This gene is now termed the PDHA1 gene. At least 50 different mutations of this gene resulting in varying symptoms of PDHA have been identified. Because the gene for PDHA is on the X **chromosome**, it is called a sex-linked disease. PDHA shows a dominant **inheritance** pattern: therefore, females with only one affected X chromosome also exhibit symptoms of the disease.

## Demographics

Almost equal numbers of males and females have been identified as being affected with PDHA. Even though PDHA is known to be transmitted as a sex-linked dominant trait on the X chromosome, it is not necessarily lethal in affected males (who possess only a single X chromosome), because the symptoms of PHDA are quite different depending on the precise mutation responsible for the symptoms in each individual. The genetic mutations are linked to the sex of the affected individual. Affected liveborn males tend to have minor (missense/nonsense type) mutations, while affected females tend to have more major (insertion/deletion type) mutations. The almost unobserved insertion/deletion mutations in males with PDHA suggests that these mutations are fatal to males with only a single X chromosome (homozygous males). Females with two X chromosomes, only one of which contains an insertion/deletion type mutation (heterozygous females) and males with an extra X chromosome (XXY males) with this type of mutation on only one chromosome (heterozygous males) are affected with non-lethal forms of PDHA.

A fixed sequence difference between African and non-African samples of the PDHA1 gene has been identified. That is, those of African descent carry a different version of the PDHA1 gene than those of non-African descent. It has been established that these differences in the subpopulations arose more than 200,000 years ago, which predates the earliest known modern human fossils. This genetic evidence is interesting in that it suggests that the modern human emerged from already genetically divided subpopulations.

## Signs and symptoms

PDHA affects primarily the brain and central nervous system. In individuals with extreme deficiencies of PDH, the brain may fail to reach normal size during fetal development leading to a small brain and skull (**microcephaly**). Abnormal development of the cerebrum, cerebellum, and brainstem are the most common brain dysfunctions associated with PDHA. The normal hollow cavities (ventricles) within the brain are usually much larger than normal (dilated) in individuals affected with PDHA. The connection between the left and right hemispheres of the brain (corpus callosum) is generally underdeveloped or completely absent as well.

A condition in which the normal insulating layer (myelin) that surrounds the neurons is either absent or insufficent (**leukodystrophy**) is observed in many individuals affected with PDHA. Some PDHA affected individuals also have periods of brain malfunctioning in which the neurons within the cerebellum temporarily lose the ability to act in a coordinated fashion (cerebellar ataxia). These attacks of cerebellar ataxia generally last from a few days to a few weeks and reoccur every three to six months thoughout life with decreasing severity after puberty. Lactic acid accumulation in the brain may also lead to breathing (respiratory) and kidney (renal) problems.

Some individuals affected with PDHA experience increased muscle tone in both legs (spastic diplegia) or in all four limbs (spastic tetraplegia) similar to that seen in the classic case of **cerebral palsy**. Seizures occur in almost all individuals affected with PDHA. A seizure is the result of sudden abnormal electrical activity in the brain. This electrical activity can result in a wide variety of clinical symptoms including muscle twitches; tongue biting; fixed, staring eyes; a loss of bladder control resulting in involuntary urination; total body shaking (convulsions); and/or loss of consciousness.

Unusual, or dysmorphic, facial features are sometimes associated with PDHA. These include a broad or upturned nose; low-set ears; downward-slanted eyes, drooping eyelids; and a staring or squinting appearance. Other physical symptoms of PDHA include short fingers and arms, urogenital malformations, low muscle tone (hypotonia), and feeding difficulties. Mental impairment is present in some cases. Delayed physical and motor development can also occur.

### Diagnosis

Improper brain development in individuals with PDHA is observable in the womb via ultrasound or via MRI after birth, although brain malformations may result from any number of other factors. Babies born with PDHA may exhibit low birth weight, a weak suck, failure to thrive, lack of muscle tone, and unusual appearance of the head, face, and limbs. Convulsions, developmental delay, and eye problems may develop a few months after birth. A diagnosis of PDHA is generally confirmed with a blood test for severe lactic acidosis,

an observance of deficient PDH activity in sampled or cultured fibroblasts, or by an observance of elevated amounts of lactate and pyruvate in the cerebrospinal fluid drawn in a spinal tap.

### Treatment and management

Treatment of PDHA is on a case-by-case basis depending on the observed symptoms. These treatments may include early and continuing intervention programs for developmental delays and mental retardation, anticonvulsants to control seizures, muscle relaxants to control spasticity, and/or surgery to release the permanent muscle, tendon, and ligament tightening (contracture) at the joints that is characteristic of longer term spasticity.

A high fat diet including beer as an alternative source of the chemical acetyl-CoA that is not produced in high enough supply because of the deficiency of PDH enzyme is often recommended for those individuals affected with PDHA. Dietary supplements of thiamine, liproic acid and L-carnitine have also proven beneficial in some cases.

### Prognosis

The prognosis for PDHA affected individuals varies widely with the severity of the symptoms. Until gene or enzyme replacement therapy becomes available, the most seriously affected individuals are not likely to receive relief from their symptoms and many will die at early ages. For those less seriously affected, several treatments are available to improve quality of life. Many less severely affected individuals live normal lifespans with their abilities and quality of life only limited by the degree of mental impairment and muscle spasticity that is present.

**Resources**

**PERIODICALS**

Harris, E. and J. Hey "X chromosome evidence for ancient human histories." *Proceedings of the National Academy of Sciences of the United States of America* (March 1999): 3320-4.

Hesterlee, S. "Mitochondrial disease in prespecitve: Symptoms, diagnosis and hope for the future." *Quest* (October 1999).

Lissens, W. et al. "Mutations in the X-linked pyruvate dehydrogenase (E1) alpha subunit gene (PDHA1) in patients with a pyruvate dehydrogenase complex deficiency." *Human Mutations* (2000): 209-19.

**WEBSITES**

*International Mitochondrial Disease Network.* http://www.imdn.org/index.html (February 15, 2001).

*Jablonski's Multiple Congenital Anomaly/Mental Retardation (MCA/MR) Syndromes Database* http://www.nlm.nih.gov/cgi/jablonski/syndrome_cgi?index=548. (February 15, 2001).

Kniffin, Cassandra. "Pyruvate decarboxylase deficency." *OMIM - Online Mendelian Inheritance in Man.* July 14, 2004 (December 12, 2009). http://www.ncbi.nlm.nih.gov/entrez/dispomim.cgi?id=312170.

*Neuromuscular Center of the Presbyterian Hospital of Dallas.* http://www.texashealth.org/nmc/pyruvate_dehydrogenase.htm (February 15, 2001).

**ORGANIZATIONS**

Children's Mitochondrial Disease Network. Mayfield House, 30 Heber Walk, Chester Way, Northwich, CW9 5JB. UK 01606 44733. http://www.emdn-mitonet.co.uk.

United Mitochondrial Disease Foundation. PO Box 1151, Monroeville, PA 15146-1151. (412) 793-8077. Fax: (412) 793-6477. http://www.umdf.org.

Paul A. Johnson

---

**KEY TERMS**

**Anemia**—A blood condition in which the level of hemoglobin or the number of red blood cells falls below normal values. Common symptoms include paleness, fatigue, and shortness of breath.

**Catalyst**—A substance that changes the rate of a chemical reaction, but is not physically changed by the process.

**Compound heterozygotes**—Having two different mutated versions of a gene.

**Enzyme**—A protein that catalyzes a biochemical reaction or change without changing its own structure or function.

**Glycolysis**—The pathway in which a cell breaks down glucose into energy.

**Hemolytic anemia**—Anemia that results from premature destruction and decreased numbers of red blood cells.

**Heterozygote**—Having two different versions of the same gene.

**Homozygote**—Having two identical copies of a gene or chromosome.

**Isozyme/Isoenzyme**—A group of enzymes that perform the same function, but are different from one another in their structure or how they move.

**Mutation**—A permanent change in the genetic material that may alter a trait or characteristic of an individual, or manifest as disease, and can be transmitted to offspring.

**Nonspherocytic**—Literally means not sphere–shaped. Refers to the shape of red blood cells in nonspherocytic hemolytic anemia.

# Pyruvate kinase deficiency

## Definition

Pyruvate kinase deficiency (PKD) is part of a group of disorders called hereditary nonspherocytic hemolytic anemias. Hereditary nonspherocytic anemias are rare genetic conditions that affect the red blood cells. PKD is caused by a deficiency in the enzyme, pyruvate kinase.

## Description

In PKD, there is a functional abnormality with the enzyme pyruvate kinase. Usually, pyruvate kinase acts as a catalyst in the glycolysis pathway, and is considered an essential component in this pathway.

Glycolysis is the method by which cells produce their own energy. A problem with any of the key components in glycolysis can alter the amount of energy produced. In the red blood cells, glycolysis is the only method available to produce energy. Without the proper amount of energy, the red blood cells do not function normally. Since pyruvate kinase is one of the key components in glycolysis, when there is a problem with this enzyme in the red blood cells, there is a problem with the production of energy, causing the red blood cells to not function properly.

There are four different forms of the pyruvate kinase enzyme in the human body. These forms, called isozymes, all perform the same function but each isozyme of pyruvate kinase is structurally different and works in different tissues and organs. The four isozymes of pyruvate kinase are labeled M1, M2, L, and R. The isozyme M1 is found in the skeletal muscle and brain, isozyme M2 can be found in most fetal and adult tissues, isozyme L works in the liver, and isozyme R works in the red blood cells. In PKD, only the pyruvate kinase isozyme found in red blood cells, called PKR, is abnormal. Therefore, PKD only affects the red blood cells and does not directly affect the energy production in the other organs and tissues of the body.

## Genetic profile

There are two PK genes and each **gene** produces two of the four isozymes of pyruvate kinase. The M1 and M2 isozymes are produced by the pyruvate kinase gene called PKM2 and pyruvate kinase isozymes, L and R, are products of the pyruvate kinase gene, PKLR. The PKLR gene is located on **chromosome** 1, on the q arm (the top half of the chromosome), in region 21 (written as 1q21). There have been over 125 different mutations described in the PKLR gene that have been detected in individuals with PKD.

PKD is mainly inherited in an autosomal recessive manner. There have been a few families where it appeared that PKD was inherited in either an autosomal dominant manner or where the carriers of PKD exhibited mild problems with their red blood cells. As with all autosomal recessive conditions, affected individuals have a mutation in both pair of genes. Most individuals with PKD are compound heterozygotes, meaning that each PKLR gene in a pair contains a different mutation. There are individuals who have the same mutation on each PKLR gene, but these individuals tend to be children of parents who are related to each other.

There are three mutations in the PKLR gene called, 1529A, 1456T, and 1468T, that are seen more frequently in individuals with PKD than the other mutations. The mutation 1529A is most frequently seen in Caucasians of northern and central European descent and is the most common mutation seen in PKD. The mutation 1456T is more common in individuals of southern European descent and the mutation 1468T is more common in individuals of Asian descent.

For most of the mutations seen in the PKLR gene, no correlation between the specific mutation and the severity of the disorder has been observed. However, for two of the mutations, there has been speculation on their affect on the severity of PKD. When the mutation 1456T has been seen in the homozygous state (when both PKLR genes contain the same mutation), those rare individuals experienced very mild symptoms of PKD. Also, there have been individuals who were homozygous for the 1529A mutation. These individuals had a very severe form of PKD. Therefore, it is thought that the 1456T mutation is associated with a milder form of the disease and the 1529A mutation is associated with a more severe form of the disease. It is not known how these mutations affect the severity of PKD when paired with different mutations.

## Demographics

Although PKD is the second most common of the hereditary nonspherocytic anemias, it is still rare, with the incidence estimated to be 51 cases per million. It occurs worldwide but most cases have been reported in northern Europe, Japan and the United States. In general, PKD not does appear to affect one gender more than another or be more common in certain regions. However, there are studies of an Amish group in Pennsylvania where a severe form of PKD is more common. The three mutations found in the PKLR gene have been linked to individuals of specific descents. Caucasians of northern and central European descent are more likely to have the 1529A mutations, individuals of southern European descent usually have the 1456T mutation, and individuals of Asian descent are more likely to have the 1468T mutation.

## Signs and symptoms

In general, the more severe the PKD, the earlier in life symptoms tend to be detected. Individuals with the more severe form of PKD often show symptoms soon after birth, but most individuals with PKD begin to exhibit symptoms during infancy or childhood. In individuals with the more mild form of PKD, the condition is sometimes not diagnosed until late adulthood, after an acute illness, or during a pregnancy evaluation.

Symptoms of PKD are similar to those symptoms seen in individuals who have long–term hemolytic anemia. The more common symptoms include variable degrees of jaundice (a yellowish pigment of the skin), slightly to moderately enlarged spleen (splenomegaly), and increased incidence of gallstones. Other physical effects of PKD can include smaller head size and the forehead appearing prominent and rounded (called frontal bossing). If a child with PKD has their spleen removed, their growth tends to improve. Even within the same family, individuals can have different symptoms and severity of PKD.

In individuals with PKD, the red blood cells are taken out of their circulation earlier than normal (shorter life span). Because of this, individuals with PKD have hemolytic anemia. Additionally, the anemia or other symptoms of PKD may worsen during a sudden illness or pregnancy.

## Diagnosis

A diagnosis of PKD can be made by measuring the amount of pyruvate kinase in red blood cells. Individuals with PKD tend to have 5–25% of the normal amount of pyruvate kinase. Carriers of PKD also can have less pyruvate kinase in their red blood cells, approximately 40–60% of the normal value. However, there is an overlap between the normal range of pyruvate kinase and the ranges seen with carriers of PKD. Therefore, measuring the amount of pyruvate kinase in the red blood cells is not a good method of detecting carriers of PKD. If the mutations causing PKD in a family are known, it may be possible to perform mutation analysis to determine carrier status of an individual and to help diagnose individuals with PKD.

## Treatment and management

In the severest cases, individuals with PKD will require multiple blood transfusions. In some of those cases, the spleen may be removed (splenectomy). Red blood cells are normally removed from circulation by the spleen. By removing an individual's spleen (usually a child), the red blood cells are allowed to stay in circulation longer than normal; thereby reducing the severity of the anemia. After a splenectomy, or once an individual with PKD is older, the number of transfusions tends to decrease.

## Prognosis

The prognosis of PKD is extremely variable. Early intervention and treatment of symptoms frequently improve the individual's health. Without treatment, individuals may experience severe complications that could become fatal. Individuals with a mild form of PKD may appear to have no symptoms at all.

## Resources

### BOOKS

Bridges, Kenneth, and Howard A. Pearson. *Anemias and Other Red Cell Disorders*. New York, NY: McGraw-Hill, 2008.

Segel, G. B. "Enzymatic Defects" in *Kliegman: Nelson Textbook of Pediatrics,* 18th edition, Philadelphia, PA: Saunders Elsevier, 2007.

### PERIODICALS

Durand, P. M., and T. L. Coetzer. "Pyruvate kinase deficiency protects against malaria in humans." *Haematologica* 93, no. 6 (June 2008): 939–940.

Raphaël, M. F., et al. "Pyruvate kinase deficiency associated with severe liver dysfunction in the newborn." *American Journal of Hematology* 82, no. 11 (November 2007): 1025–1028.

Wax, J. R., et al. "Pyruvate kinase deficiency complicating pregnancy." *Obstetrics and Gynecology* 109, no. 2 (February 2007): 553–555.

Zanella, A., et al. "Pyruvate kinase deficiency." *Haematologica* 92, no. 16 (June 2007): 721–723.

### WEBSITES

*Hemolytic Anemia*. Medical Encyclopedia. Medline Plus, April 21, 2009 (April 26, 2009). http://www.nlm.nih.gov/medlineplus/ency/article/000571.htm.

*Pyruvate Kinase Deficiency*. Medical Encyclopedia. Medline Plus, May 15, 2008 (April 26, 2009). http://www.nlm.nih.gov/medlineplus/ency/article/001197.htm.

*Pyruvate Kinase Deficiency*. Information Page. Genetic and Rare Diseases information Center (April 26, 2009). http://rarediseases.info.nih.gov/GARD/Disease.aspx?PageID=4&diseaseID=7514.

*Pyruvate Kinase Deficiency*. Information Page. Patient UK, February 20, 2009 (April 26, 2009). http://www.patient.co.uk/showdoc/40001770/.

*Pyruvate Kinase Deficiency —Overview*. Information Page. University of Maryland Medical Center, May 15, 2008 (April 26, 2009). http://www.umm.edu/ency/article/001197.htm.

### ORGANIZATIONS

National Organization for Rare Disorders (NORD). 55 Kenosia Avenue, PO Box 1968, Danbury, CT 06813-1968. (203)744-0100 or (800)999-6673. Fax: (203)798-2291. http://www.rarediseases.org.

Office of Rare Diseases Research (ORDR). 6100 Executive Blvd., Room 3B01, MSC 7518, Bethesda, MD 20892-7518. (301)402-4336. Fax: (301)480-9655. Email: ordr@od.nih.gov. http://rarediseases.info.nih.gov.

Sharon A. Aufox, MS, CGC

Rapp-Hodgkin syndrome *see* **Ectodermal dysplasia**

# Raynaud disease

## Definition

Raynaud disease refers to a disorder in which the fingers or toes (digits) suddenly experience decreased blood circulation. It is characterized by repeated episodes of color changes of the skin of digits during cold exposure or emotional stress.

## Description

Raynaud disease can be classified as one of two types: primary (or idiopathic) and secondary (also called Raynaud phenomenon). Primary Raynaud disease has no predisposing factor, is more mild, and causes fewer complications. About half of all cases of Raynaud disease are of this type. Women are five times more likely than men to develop primary Raynaud disease. The average age of diagnosis is between 20 and 40 years. Approximately three out of ten people with primary Raynaud disease eventually progress to secondary Raynaud disease after diagnosis. About 15% of individuals improve.

Secondary Raynaud disease is the same as primary Raynaud disease, but occurs in individuals with a predisposing factor, usually a form of collagen vascular disease. What is typically identified as primary Raynaud may be later identified as secondary once a predisposing disease is diagnosed. This occurs in approximately 30% of patients. As a result of the predisposing disease, the secondary type is often more complicated and severe, and is more likely to worsen.

Several related conditions that predispose persons to secondary Raynaud disease include **scleroderma**, lupus erythematosus, **rheumatoid arthritis** and polymyositis.

Pulmonary hypertension and some nervous system disorders such as herniated discs and tumors within the spinal column, strokes, and polio can progress to Raynaud disease. Finally, injuries due to mechanical trauma caused by vibration (such as that associated with chain saws and jackhammers), repetitive motion (carpal tunnel syndrome), electrical shock, and exposure to extreme cold can led to the development of Raynaud disease. Some drugs used to control high blood pressure or migraine headaches have been known to cause Raynaud disease.

## Genetic profile

There is significant familial aggregation of primary Raynaud disease. However, as of 2009, no causative **gene** has been identified.

Risk factors for Raynaud disease differ between males and females. Age and smoking seem to be associated with Raynaud disease only in men, while the associations of marital status and alcohol use with Raynaud disease are usually only observed in women. These findings suggest that different mechanisms influence the expression of Raynaud disease in men and women.

## Demographics

The prevalence of Raynaud phenomena in the general population varies from 4–15%. Females are seven times more likely to develop Raynaud diseases than are men. The problem has not been correlated with coffee consumption, dietary habits, occupational history (excepting exposure to vibration), or exposure to most drugs. An association between Raynaud disease and migraine headaches has been reported. Secondary Raynaud disease is common among individuals with systemic lupus erythematosus in tropical countries.

## Signs and symptoms

Both primary and secondary Raynaud disease signs and symptoms are thought to be due to arterioles overreacting to stimuli. Cold normally causes the tiny

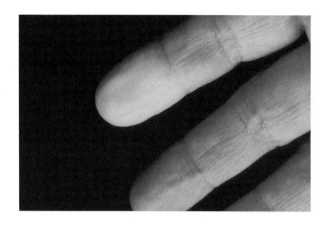

A phenomenon of Raynaud disease occurs when blood flow is temporarily interrupted, causing extremities to become pale due to poor blood circulation. (Custom Medical Stock Photo, Inc.)

muscles in the walls of arteries to contract, thus reducing the amount of blood that can flow through them. In people with Raynaud disease, the extent of constriction is extreme, thus severely restricting blood flow. Attacks or their effects may be brought on or worsened by anxiety or emotional distress.

There are three distinct phases to an episode of Raynaud disease. When first exposed to cold, small arteries respond with intense contractions (vasoconstriction). The affected fingers or toes (in rare instances, the tip of the nose or tongue) become pale and white because they are deprived of blood and, thus, oxygen. In response, capillaries and veins expand

(dilate). Because these vessels are carrying deoxygenated blood, the affected area then becomes blue in color. The area often feels cold and tingly or numb. After the area begins to warm up, the arteries dilate. Blood flow is significantly increased. This changes the color of the area to a bright red. During this phase, persons often describe the affected area as feeling warm and throbbing painfully.

Raynaud disease may initially affect only the tips of fingers or toes. As the disease progresses, it may eventually involve all of one or two digits. Ultimately, all the fingers or toes may be affected. About one person in ten will experience a complication called sclerodactyly. In sclerodactyly, the skin over the involved digits becomes tight, white, thick, smooth and shiny. In approximately 1% of cases of Raynaud disease, deep sores (ulcers) may develop in the skin. In rare cases of frequent, repetitive bouts of severe ischemia (decreased supply of oxygenated blood to tissues or organs), tissue loss, or gangrene, may result and amputation may be required.

### Diagnosis

Primary Raynaud disease is diagnosed following the Allen Brown criteria. There are four components. The certainty of the diagnosis and severity of the disease increase as more criteria are met. The first is that at least two of the three color changes must occur during attacks provoked by cold and/or stress. The second is that episodes must occur periodically for at

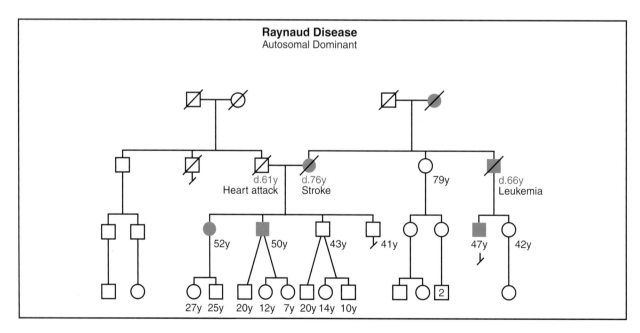

(Gale, a part of Cengage Learning.)

## KEY TERMS

**Arteriole**—The smallest type of artery.

**Artery**—A blood vessel that carries blood away from the heart to peripheral tissues.

**Gangrene**—Death of a tissue, usually caused by insufficient blood supply and followed by bacterial infection of the tissue.

**Idiopathic**—Of unknown origin.

**Lupus erythematosus**—A chronic inflammatory disease that affects many tissues and parts of the body including the skin.

**Polymyositis**—An inflammation of many muscles.

**Pulmonary hypertension**—A severe form of high blood pressure caused by diseased arteries in the lung.

**Rheumatoid arthritis**—Chronic, autoimmune disease marked by inflammation of the membranes surrounding joints.

**Scleroderma**—A relatively rare autoimmune disease affecting blood vessels and connective tissue that makes skin appear thickened.

least two years. The third is that attacks must occur in both the hands and the feet in the absence of vascular occlusive disease. The last is that there is no other identifiable cause for the Raynaud episodes.

A cold stimulation test may also be performed to help to confirm a diagnosis of Raynaud disease. The temperature of affected fingers or toes is taken. The hand or foot is then placed completely into a container of ice water for 20 seconds. After removal from the water, the temperature of the affected digits is immediately recorded. The temperature is taken every five minutes until it returns to the pre-immersion level. Most individuals recover normal temperature within 15 minutes. People with Raynaud disease may require 20 minutes or more to reach their pre-immersion temperature.

Laboratory testing is performed frequently. However, these results are often inconclusive for several reasons. Provocative testing such as the ice immersion just described, is difficult to interpret because there is considerable overlap between normal and abnormal results. The antinuclear antibody test of blood is usually negative in Raynaud disease. Capillary beds under fingernails usually appear normal. Erythrocyte sedimentation rates are often abnormal in people with connective tissue diseases. Unfortunately, this finding is not consistent in people with Raynaud disease.

### Treatment and management

There is no known way to prevent the development of Raynaud disease. Further, there is no known cure for this condition. Therefore, avoidance of the trigger is the best supportive management available. Most cases of primary Raynaud disease can be controlled with proper medical care and avoidance.

Many people are able to find relief by simply adjusting their lifestyles. Affected individuals need to stay warm and keep their hands and feet well covered in cold weather. Layered clothing, scarves, heavy coats, heavy socks, and mittens over gloves are suggested because gloves alone allow heat to escape. It is also recommended that patients cover or close the space between their sleeves and mittens. Indoors, they should wear socks and comfortable shoes. Excessive emotional stress should be avoided. Smokers should quit as nicotine worsens the problem. The use of vibrating tools should be avoided as well.

Biofeedback has been used with some success in treating primary Raynaud. This involves teaching people to "think" their fingers and toes to be warm by willing blood to flow through affected arterioles. Biofeedback has had only limited success. Occasionally, medications such as calcium-channel blockers, reserpine or nitroglycerin may be prescribed to relax artery walls and improve blood flow.

Because episodes of Raynaud disease have also been associated with stress and emotional upset, the condition may be improved by learning to manage stress. Regular exercise is known to decrease stress and lower anxiety. Hypnosis, relaxation techniques, and visualization are also useful methods to help control emotions.

Biofeedback training is a technique during which a patient is given continuous information on the temperature of his or her digits, and then taught to voluntarily control this temperature. Some alternative practitioners believe that certain dietary supplements and herbs may be helpful in decreasing the vessel spasm of Raynaud disease. Suggested supplements include vitamin E (found in fruits, vegetables, seeds, and nuts), magnesium (found in seeds, nuts, fish, beans, and dark green vegetables), and fish oils. The circulatory herbs cayenne, ginger and prickly ash may help enhance circulation to affected areas.

### Prognosis

The prognosis for most people with Raynaud disease is very good. In general, primary Raynaud disease has the best prognosis, with a relatively small chance (1%) of serious complications. Approximately half of all affected individuals do well by taking simple precautions, and never require medication. The prognosis for people with secondary Raynaud disease (or phenomenon) is less predictable. This prognosis depends greatly on the severity of other associated conditions such as scleroderma, lupus, or Sjögren syndrome.

### Resources

#### BOOKS

Coffman, Jay D. *Raynaud Phenomenon.* New York: Oxford University Press, 1989.

Fauci, Anthony S. "The Vasculitis Syndromes." In *Harrison's Principles of Internal Medicine,* edited by Anthony Fauci et al., 14th ed. New York: McGraw Hill, 1998, 1910-1922.

Rosenwasser, Lanny J. "The Vasaculitic Syndromes." In *Cecil Textbook of Medicine,* edited by Lee Goldman, et al. 21st ed. Philadelphia: Saunders, 2000, pp. 1524-1527.

#### PERIODICALS

Brand, F. N., M. G. Larson, W. B. Kannel, and J. M. McGuirk. "The occurrence of Raynaud phenomenon in a general population: the Framingham Study." *Vascular Medicine* 2, no. 4 (November 1997): 296-301.

Fraenkel, L., et al. "Different factors influencing the expression of Raynaud phenomenon in men and women." *Arthritis and Rheumatology* 42, no. 2 (February 1999): 306-310.

Voulgari, P. V., et al. "Prevalence of Raynaud phenomenon in a healthy Greek population." *Annals of Rheumatic Disease* 59, no. 3 (March 2000): 206-210.

#### WEBSITES

*Arthritis Foundation.* Dublin, Ireland. http//www.arthritis-foundation.com/.&gt;

*British Sjögren's Syndrome Association.* http://ourworld.copmpuserve.com/homepages/BSSAssociation.

*Raynaud & Scleroderma Association.* United Kingdom. http://www.Raunaud's.demon.co,uk/.

Rodriguez, J., and S. Wasson. "Raynaud Disease." *Wayne State University School of Medicine.* http://www.med.wayne.edu/raynauds/.

#### ORGANIZATIONS

American Heart Association. 7272 Greenville Ave., Dallas, TX 75231-4596. (214) 373-6300 or (800) 242-8721. inquire@heart.org. http://www.americanheart.org.

Irish Raynaud and Scleroderma Society. PO Box 2958 Foxrock, Dublin 18, Ireland. (01) 235 0900. irss@indigo.ie.

National Heart, Lung, and Blood Institute. PO Box 30105, Bethesda, MD 20824-0105. (301) 592-8573. nhlbiinfo @rover.nhlbi.nih.gov. http://www.nhlbi.nih.gov.

National Organization for Rare Disorders (NORD). PO Box 8923, New Fairfield, CT 06812-8923. (203) 746-6518 or (800) 999-6673. Fax: (203) 746-6481. http://www.rarediseases.org.

Raynaud & Scleroderma Association (UK). 112 Crewe Road, Alsager, Cheshire, ST7 2JA, UK. (44) (0) 1270 872776. webmaster@raynauds.demon.co.uk. http://www.raynauds.demon.co.uk.

L. Fleming Fallon, Jr., MD, PhD, DrPH

Recurrent polyserositis *see* **Familial mediterranean fever**

# Refsum disease

### Definition

Refsum disease is an inherited disorder in which the enzyme responsible for processing phytanic acid is defective. Accumulation of phytanic acid in the tissues and the blood leads to damage of the brain, nerves, eyes, skin, and bones.

### Description

Refsum disease was first characterized by the Norwegian physician, Sigvald Refsum, in the 1940s and is known by other names, such as classical Refsum disease, adult Refsum disease, phytanic acid alpha-hydroxylase deficiency, phytanic acid storage disease, hypertrophic neuropathy of Refsum, heredopathia atactica polyneuritiformis, and hereditary motor and sensory neuropathy IV. Refsum disease should not be confused with

## KEY TERMS

**Autosomal recessive**—A pattern of genetic inheritance where two abnormal genes are needed to display the trait or disease.

**Carrier**—A person who possesses a gene for an abnormal trait without showing signs of the disorder. The person may pass the abnormal gene on to offspring.

**Cerebellar ataxia**—Unsteadiness and lack of coordination caused by a progressive degeneration of the part of the brain known as the cerebellum.

**Enzyme**—A protein that catalyzes a biochemical reaction or change without changing its own structure or function.

**Ichthyosis**—Rough, dry, scaly skin that forms as a result of a defect in skin formation.

**Mutant**—A change in the genetic material that may alter a trait or characteristic of an individual or manifest as disease.

**Organelle**—Small, sub-cellular structures that carry out different functions necessary for cellular survival and proper cellular functioning.

**Peripheral neuropathy**—Any disease of the nerves outside of the spinal cord, usually resulting in weakness and/or numbness.

**Peroxisome**—A cellular organelle containing different enzymes responsible for the breakdown of waste or other products.

**Phytanic acid**—A substance found in various foods that, if allowed to accumulate, is toxic to various tissues. It is metabolized in the peroxisome by phytanic acid hydroxylase.

**Phytanic acid hydroxylase**—A peroxisomal enzyme responsible for processing phytanic acid. It is defective in Refsum disease.

**Plasmapheresis**—A procedure in which the fluid component of blood is removed from the bloodstream and sometimes replaced with other fluids or plasma.

**Retinitis pigmentosa**—Progressive deterioration of the retina, often leading to vision loss and blindness.

infantile **Refsum disease**, which was once thought to be a variant of the disorder but is now known to be a genetically and biochemically distinct entity. Sometimes infantile Refsum disease is simply referred to as "Refsum disease," furthering the confusion.

Living bodies are made up of millions of individual cells that are specifically adapted to carry out particular functions. Within cells are even smaller structures, called organelles, that perform jobs and enable the cell to serve its ultimate purpose. One type of organelle is the peroxisome, whose main function is to break down waste materials or to process materials that, if allowed to accumulate, would prove toxic to the cells.

Phytanic acid is a substance found in foods, such as dairy products, beef, lamb, and some fish. Normally, phytanic acid is processed by a set of enzymes within the cell to convert it to another form. In the past, scientists were unsure where in the cell this process took place, hypothesizing that it may occur in the peroxisome or another organelle, called the mitochondrion. However, recent research has definitively determined that the enzymes responsible for processing phytanic acid are located in the peroxisome.

Refsum disease is an inherited disorder in which one of the peroxisomal enzymes, phytanic acid hydroxylase (also called phytanic acid oxidase, or phytanyl CoA hydroxylase), is defective, resulting in unprocessed phytanic acid. Consequently, high levels of phytanic acid build up in the tissues of the body and the bloodstream, causing damage to different organ systems.

### Genetic profile

Refsum disease is a genetic condition and can be inherited or passed on in a family. The genetic defect for the disorder is inherited as an autosomal recessive trait, meaning that two abnormal genes are needed to display the disease. A person who carries one abnormal gene does not display the disease and is called a carrier. A carrier has a 50% chance of transmitting the gene to his or her children. A child must inherit the same abnormal gene from each parent to display the disease.

Refsum disease is caused by a deficiency in an enzyme, phytanic acid hydroxylase. The gene encoding for this enzyme, called PAHX or PHYH, was identified in 1997 and mapped to human **chromosome** 10 (locus: 10pter-p11.2). Several common mutations have been identified in the gene that result in Refsum disease.

### Demographics

Refsum disease is rare, but the exact incidence and prevalence of the disorder in the general population is not known. Refsum disease may not be distributed equally among geographical areas or different ethnic groups, as most of the diagnosed cases have been found in children and young adults of Scandinavian heritage.

## Signs and symptoms

Patients with Refsum disease generally do not show obvious defects at birth, and growth and development initially appears normal. The onset of clinical symptoms varies from early childhood to age 50, but symptoms usually appear before 20 years of age. The manifestations of Refsum disease primarily involve the nervous system, the eye, the skin, the bones, and, in rare cases, the heart and kidneys.

Phytanic acid deposits in the fatty sheaths surrounding nerves, causing damage and resulting in peripheral neuropathy in 90% of patients with Refsum disease. Peripheral neuropathy is the term for dysfunction of the nerves outside of the spinal cord, causing loss of sensation, muscle weakness, pain, and loss of reflexes. Nerves leading to the nose and ears can also be affected, resulting in anosmia (loss of the sense of smell) in 35% of patients and hearing loss or **deafness** in 50% of patients. Finally, Refsum disease results in cerebellar ataxia in 75% of patients. Cerebellar ataxia is a defect in a specific part of the brain (the cerebellum), resulting in loss of coordination and unsteadiness. In contrast to infantile Refsum disease, people with Refsum disease do not show mental retardation and generally have normal intelligence.

Accumulation of phytanic acid also results in disorders of the eye. The most common finding is **retinitis pigmentosa**, a degeneration of the retina resulting in poor nighttime vision and sometimes blindness. Disorders of pupil movement and nystagmus (uncontrollable movements of the eye) may also be present due to related nervous system damage. Other eye manifestations of Refsum disease may include **glaucoma** (abnormally high pressure in the eye, leading to vision loss) and cataracts (clouding of the lens of the eye).

People with Refsum disease often develop dry, rough, scaly skin. These skin changes, called **ichthyosis**, can occur over the entire body, but sometimes will appear only on the palms and soles of the feet. In addition to these skin abnormalities, 60% of affected people may experience abnormal bone growth, manifesting as shortened limbs or fingers, or abnormal curvatures of the spine.

Patients with Refsum disease usually first present to a physician complaining of weakness in the arms and legs, physical unsteadiness and/or nightblindness or failing vision. The symptoms associated with Refsum disease are progressive and, if untreated, will become more numerous and severe as the patient ages. For reasons that are not completely understood, clinical deterioration can be sometimes be interrupted by periods of good health without symptoms.

## Diagnosis

Refsum disease is diagnosed though a combination of consistent medical history, physical exam findings, and laboratory and **genetic testing**. When patients with Refsum disease present to their physicians complaining of visual problems or muscle weakness, physical signs of retinitis pigmentosa, peripheral neuropathy, cerebellar ataxia, or skin and bone changes (as discussed above) are often noted. These findings raise suspicion for a genetic syndrome or metabolic disorder, and further tests are conducted.

Laboratory tests reveal several abnormalities. Normally, phytanic acid levels are essentially undetectable in the plasma. Thus, the presence of high levels of phytanic acid in the bloodstream is highly indicative of Refsum disease. If necessary, a small portion of the patient's connective tissue can be sampled and grown in a laboratory and tested to demonstrate a failure to process phytanic acid appropriately. Other associated laboratory abnormalities include the presence of high amounts of protein in the fluid that bathes the spinal cord, or abnormal electrical responses recorded from the brain, muscles, heart, ears, retina, and various nerves as a result of nervous system damage.

Genetic testing can also be performed. When a diagnosis of Refsum disease is made in a child, genetic testing of the PAHX/PHYH gene can be offered to determine if a specific gene change can be identified. If a specific change is identified, carrier testing can be offered to relatives. In families where the parents have been identified to be carriers of the abnormal gene, diagnosis of Refsum disease before birth is possible. Prenatal diagnosis is performed on cells obtained by **amniocentesis** (withdrawal of the fluid surrounding a fetus in the womb using a needle) at about 16–18 weeks of pregnancy or from the chorionic villi (a part of the placenta) at 10–12 weeks of pregnancy.

## Treatment and management

There is no cure for Refsum disease, thus treatment focuses on reducing levels of phytanic acid in the bloodstream to prevent the progression of tissue damage. Phytanic acid is not made in the human body and comes exclusively from the diet. Restriction of phytanic acid-containing foods can slow progress of the disease or reverse some of the symptoms. Patients are advised to maintain consumption of phytanic acid below 10 mg/day (the normal intake is approximately 100 mg/day). Sources of high levels of phytanic acid to be avoided include meats (beef, lamb, goat), dairy products (cream, milk, butter, cheese), and some fish (tuna, cod, haddock). Plasma levels of phytanic acid can be monitored periodically by a physician to investigate the effectiveness of the restricted diet and determine if changes are required. As a result of dietary restriction, nutritional deficiencies may result. Consultation with a nutritionist is recommended to assure proper amounts of calories, protein, and vitamins are obtained through the diet, and nutritional supplements may be required.

Because phytanic acid is stored in fat deposits within the body, it is important for patients with Refsum disease to have regular eating patterns; with even brief periods of fasting, fat stores are converted to energy, resulting in the release of stored phytanic acid into the blood stream. Thus, unless a patient assumes a regular eating pattern, repeated and periodic liberation of phytanic acid stores results in greater tissue damage and symptom development. For these same reasons, intentional weight loss though calorie-restricted diets or vigorous exercise is discouraged.

Another useful adjunct to dietary treatment is plasmapheresis. Plasmapheresis is a procedure by which determined amounts of plasma (the fluid component of blood that contains phytanic acid) is removed from the blood and replaced with fluids or plasma that do not contain phytanic acid. Regular utilization of this technique allows people who fail to follow a restricted diet to maintain lower phytanic acid levels and experience less tissue damage and symptoms.

Patients with Refsum disease should be seen regularly by a multidisciplinary team of health care providers, including a pediatrician, neurologist, ophthal mologist, cardiologist, medical geneticist specializing in metabolic disease, nutritionist, and physical/occupational therapist. People with Refsum disease, or those who are carriers of the abnormal gene or who have an relative with the disorder, can be referred for **genetic counseling** to assist in making reproductive decisions.

### Prognosis

The prognosis of Refsum disease varies dramatically. The disorder is slowly progressive and, if left untreated, severe symptoms will develop with considerably shortened life expectancy. However, if diagnosed early, strict adherence to a phytanic acid-free dietary regimen can prevent progression of the disease and reverse skin disease and some of the symptoms of peripheral neuropathy. Unfortunately, treatment cannot undo existing damage to vision and hearing.

## QUESTIONS TO ASK YOUR DOCTOR

- What is the role of phytanic acid in Refsum disease?
- What treatments are available to control the progress of Refsum disease?
- How does a physician determine the prognosis for a child with Refsum disease?
- Can you recommend a Web site that will provide additional information on Refsum disease?

### Resources

#### BOOKS

"Peroxisomal Disorders." In *Nelson Textbook of Pediatrics.* Edited by R. E. Behrman. Philadelphia: W.B. Saunders, 2000, pp 318-384.

#### PERIODICALS

Weinstein, R. "Phytanic acid storage disease (Refsum's disease): Clinical characteristics, pathophysiology and the role of therapeutic apheresis in its management." *Journal of Clinical Apheresis* 14 (1999): 181-184.

#### WEBSITES

"Entry 266500: Refsum Disease." *OMIM—Online Mendelian Inheritance in Man.* http://www.ncbi.nlm.nih.gov/htbin-post/Omim/dispmim?266500.

Oren Traub, MD, PhD

Refsum disease, infantile form *see* **Infantile refsum disease**

Reis-Pucklers corneal dystrophy *see* **Corneal dystrophy**

# Renal agenesis

### Definition

Renal agenesis is the failure of kidney formation during fetal development. Renal agenesis can be unilateral, with one kidney present, or bilateral, with no kidneys or very little kidney present. The two types of renal agenesis have very different clinical courses, with unilateral agenesis being more favorable.

**Amniotic sample**—Sample of amniotic fluid, the protective fluid surrounding a fetus in the womb.

**Anemia**—Condition in which there are low levels of red blood cells.

**Asymptomatic**—Without symptoms.

**Creatinine**—A normal component of blood kept in low levels in urine by functioning kidneys.

**Dialysis**—Filtering of blood to remove waste products that the kidneys would normally remove if they were present and functioning.

**DNA**—Deoxyribonucleic acid, inheritable material that constitutes the building blocks of life.

**Gastrointestinal tract**—The food intake and waste export system that runs from the mouth, through the esophagus, stomach, and intestines, to the rectum and anus.

**Growth factors**—Cellular-signaling components that stimulate cell division or other cell processes.

**Neonate**—A newborn infant up to six weeks of age.

**Oligohydramnios**—An abnormally small amount of amniotic fluid.

**Pulmonary hypoplasia**—Underdevelopment of the lungs.

**RNA**—Ribonucleic acid, the intermediate step between DNA and its final expression product. DNA is transcribed into RNA and RNA is translated into protein.

**Transcription**—The process by which DNA is changed into RNA.

**Transcription factors**—Cellular-signaling components that cause the transcription of a gene.

## Description

Kidneys perform many important bodily functions. Having at least one kidney is necessary for life. Kidneys filter waste and extra fluid from the blood, keep a healthy blood level of electrolytes and minerals, such as sodium, phosphorus, calcium, and potassium, help to maintain healthy blood pressure, and release hormones that are important for bodily functions. Normally, there are two fist-sized kidneys present, one on each side of the spinal column at the back just below the ribcage. Each kidney contains microscopic filter lobules called nephrons that transfer bodily waste products from the bloodstream to the urinary system. Functional nephrons are critical for maintaining bodily functions and for eliminating the buildup of waste products that can be life-threatening.

### Unilateral renal agenesis

Unilateral renal agenesis results from defects in fetal development that cause only one kidney to form. Having a solitary kidney instead of two is not necessarily life-threatening. The solitary kidney usually enlarges, and is able to perform most bodily functions to a degree sufficient for life. When a solitary kidney does negatively affect health, it is through very subtle and gradual changes that may not be noticed initially. Over long periods of time, changes, such as an increase in blood pressure, may require specific preventative measures or treatments. Having a solitary kidney also means that if injury or disease leads to renal failure, there is no back-up kidney to take over. In this circumstance, the consequences of a diseased unilateral kidney can be life-threatening.

### Bilateral renal agenesis

Bilateral renal agenesis is a genetic disorder involving the failure of both kidneys to form during fetal development. Fetal kidney development begins between five and seven weeks of gestation. During development, the fetus is cushioned, protected, and maintained at constant temperature in a substance known as amniotic fluid. Fetal urine production begins in early gestation and is responsible for the majority of the amniotic fluid present in the second and third trimesters of pregnancy. The fetus continuously swallows amniotic fluid, which is reabsorbed in the fetal gastrointestinal tract and excreted back into the amniotic cavity by the kidneys. Because amniotic fluid is maintained by fetal urine, a fetus with no kidneys has little amniotic fluid to surround and protect it in the amniotic sac. This condition is known as oligohydramnios, and results in physical compression of the fetus in the womb. Bilateral renal agenesis causes a set of physical complications known as Potter's syndrome. While bilateral renal agenesis is not the only cause of Potter's syndrome, the lack of both kidneys naturally results in Potter's syndrome symptoms. Only 20% of all Potter syndrome cases are caused by bilateral renal agenesis. The amniotic membrane sticking to the fetus, and the compression, cause further physical malformations, including the squashed facial features characteristic of Potter syndrome.

Compression and lack of amniotic fluid also lead to a serious defect in lung development. The fetal urine is critical for proper lung development. Fetal urine helps to expand the airways and supplies the amino acid proline, a critical amino acid for lung development. Upon leaving the womb, an infant must rely on the lungs and on breathing air to receive oxygen for life. Alveoli are the many small sacs deep in the lungs that are responsible for exchanging oxygen with the blood. If the alveoli are underdeveloped (pulmonary hypoplasia) at birth, the infant cannot breathe properly and will go into respiratory distress. In most cases, the condition is fatal within the first few months of postnatal life. The cause of death is pulmonary hypoplasia, with consequent respiratory insufficiency. There are rare cases in which a portion of one kidney has formed and some lung development occurs. These cases are also often fatal. If sufficient lung development is present, an infant with bilateral renal agenesis may be rescued through dialysis and eventual kidney transplant.

## Genetic profile

Bilateral renal agenesis (BRA) is a rare condition thought to occur in sporadic and autosomal recessive forms. Sporadic forms of BRA have an unknown cause that may or may not be genetic. It is thought that BRA can be inherited in an autosomal recessive form, caused by the **inheritance** of two defective copies of a gene. Each parent contributes one copy of a gene. In autosomal recessive inheritance, if both copies are defective, the result is disease. If only one defective copy is present, the disease does not occur, but the defective gene can still be passed on to subsequent generations. If both parents are carrying a defective gene, each offspring has a one in four (25%) chance of inheriting the disease. Populations with a high frequency of healthy individuals carrying defective genes will also have higher prevalence of offspring with the disease.

BRA is also more common when a parent has a distinct kidney malformation, especially unilateral renal agenesis. Research has demonstrated that unilateral renal agenesis and bilateral renal agenesis are genetically related. For this reason, when bilateral renal agenesis is detected in an infant, an ultrasound is performed on the kidneys of parents and siblings. Approximately 9% of first-degree relatives of infants with bilateral renal agenesis have some type of asymptomatic renal malformation.

As of 2009, the exact genetic causes of both unilateral and bilateral renal agenesis are unknown. It is speculated that both conditions are caused by mutations in the genes involved in fetal kidney development. Normal fetal kidney development involves an essential interaction between the forming kidney buds (ureteric bud) and a tissue known as the metanephric mesenchyme. The interaction of the ureteric bud with the metanephric mesenchyme is necessary for kidney formation. The interaction is controlled by a combination of genes, cellular-signaling molecules that control gene expression (transcription factors), and cellular-signaling molecules that control cell growth (growth factors). Animal studies have identified several of the factors that can be mutated to cause renal agenesis. Research is ongoing to determine the cause in humans.

As of 2009, the cutting edge of renal agenesis research is at the Potter syndrome tissue bank where scientists are running experiments on tissue donations from parents of children born with bilateral renal agenesis. Researchers are collecting tissue samples from the neonates and blood samples from family members in an effort to discover the **gene mutations** responsible for the condition. The Potter syndrome tissue bank is the only one of its kind in the world.

## Demographics

Unilateral kidney agenesis is fairly common, occurring in approximately one per 1,000 live births in the United States. Bilateral renal agenesis occurs in one per 3,000 live births. There is no association of renal agenesis with race. Males have a higher rate of developing Potter syndrome than females. Individuals with bilateral renal agenesis present with the condition as neonates, whereas individuals with unilateral renal agenesis may not be aware of their condition even as adults. Unilateral renal agenesis is usually discovered in an adult undergoing tests for some other condition.

## Signs and symptoms

### Unilateral renal agenesis

Most people born with a solitary kidney do not experience any noticeable signs or symptoms that would indicate they have unilateral renal agenesis. A solitary kidney is usually discovered when the individual is having ultrasound imaging or surgery for some other problem. However, having unilateral renal agenesis can cause gradual changes in bodily functions that lead to unhealthy clinical conditions. A potential complication of a solitary kidney is high blood pressure.

Kidneys normally contribute to maintaining a healthy blood pressure in two ways. Kidneys regulate how much fluid flows through the bloodstream and how much fluid is excreted from the body. The more fluid that flows through the bloodstream, the more the blood pressure increases. Kidneys also release a hormone called renin that works as part of a team of hormones to expand or contract blood vessels. The more contraction of blood vessels there is, the higher the blood pressure. Many individuals who are born with a solitary kidney eventually develop slightly higher blood pressure.

In addition, one kidney doing the work of two kidneys can cause more wear and tear than normally would occur. A solitary kidney may eventually be slightly damaged, causing excessive protein to be excreted from the body through the urine. This condition is known as proteinuria, and is a sign of kidney damage. Another potential complication of having a solitary kidney is reduced efficiency at removing waste from the bloodstream. The portion of the kidney that acts as a filter is the glomerulus. A reduced ability to filter the blood is known as a reduced glomerular filtration rate (GFR), a potential complication of unilateral renal agenesis. As long as these complications are controlled, individuals with a solitary kidney often experience no actual symptoms.

### Bilateral renal agenesis

There are many signs of bilateral renal agenesis during neonatal (first six weeks of life) care. Potter facies are facial features associated with Potter syndrome from bilateral renal agenesis. The facies include a squashed facial appearance, flattened nose, recessed chin, prominent epicanthal folds (fold of skin from root of nose to eyebrow), and low-set abnormal ears. A poor or absent urine output during the first 48 hours of life, respiratory distress, and poorly developed lungs are all indicative signs. The degree of lung development corresponds with the extent and duration of the oligohydramnios. Respiratory distress is often the cause of death.

## Diagnosis

### Unilateral renal agenesis

A diagnosis of unilateral renal agenesis can be made using various imaging techniques such as an ultrasound, or directly through surgery. Diagnosis of unilateral renal agenesis is usually made in asymptomatic adults, while they are investigating some other condition. Complications of unilateral renal agenesis may include proteinuria and reduced GFR. A diagnosis of proteinuria is made through urinalysis. High levels of protein in the urine indicate kidney damage. Highly sensitive urinalysis tests are also performed to diagnose proteinuria. These tests calculate the protein-to-creatinine ratio. A high protein-to-creatinine ratio in urine indicates that the kidney is leaking protein that should be kept in the blood, and indicates kidney damage. The GFR can be measured by injecting a contrast medium into the bloodstream. The injection is followed by a 24-hour period of urine collection to determine how much of the medium was filtered through the kidney. A more recent method of determining GFR is by measuring blood creatinine levels and performing calculations that involve weight, age, and values assigned for sex and race. If GFR remains consistently below 60, a diagnosis of chronic kidney disease is made.

### Bilateral renal agenesis

Bilateral renal agenesis is investigated if there is a history of oligohydramnios, prenatal sonograms depicting renal agenesis, or unilateral renal agenesis in the family. If an infant has bilateral renal agenesis, blood tests will show altered levels of electrolytes and minerals that the kidney typically filters and normalizes. Renal function and GFR can be assessed through measuring blood levels of creatinine. Urinalysis, if any urine is present, is used to detect proteinuria. Ultrasound imaging can reveal renal agenesis both before and after birth, but the prenatal condition is not as easily visualized. Chest x rays, although undesirable in an infant, can be used to assess lung development. In neonates who die from this condition, an autopsy is recommended to confirm the diagnosis.

## Treatment and management

### Unilateral renal agenesis

No treatment is necessary for unilateral renal agenesis other than controlling complications if they arise. Kidney function is monitored by regular physical examinations that check blood pressure and blood and urine tests. These tests are usually done once a year, and are designed to assess whether the unilateral kidney is functioning properly. Regular monitoring is critical because if the solitary kidney becomes diseased or damaged, there is no back-up kidney available to maintain life.

Normal blood pressure is defined as a measurement of 120/80 or lower. High blood pressure is defined as a measurement of 140/90 or higher. Individuals with unilateral renal agenesis are advised to maintain blood pressure levels below 130/80 to prevent kidney damage. If medication is required to control blood pressure, individuals with unilateral renal agenesis may need blood pressure medications that also protect kidney functions. Angiotensin-converting enzyme (ACE) inhibitors and angiotensin receptor blockers are two classes of blood pressure medication that can also protect kidney function and reduce proteinuria. Diuretics may also be used to help lower blood pressure by removing excess fluid from the body.

Individuals with unilateral renal agenesis do not need to follow a special diet, but should limit daily sodium intake to avoid developing high blood pressure. While a special diet is not required, some methods of dieting are contraindicated. High-protein diets are not advised for individuals with unilateral renal agenesis.

Because protein breakdown products add stress to the kidneys as they remove waste from the bloodstream, excessive protein intake puts an extra burden on the solitary kidney. Normal, moderate amounts of protein intake are recommended in unilateral renal agenesis. Alcohol and caffeine intake should also be limited. Individuals with unilateral renal agenesis are often advised to avoid contact sports unless protective gear is worn. Damage to the single functional kidney could quickly become life-threatening.

### Bilateral renal agenesis

Neonates born with bilateral renal agenesis are immediately placed in the neonatal intensive care unit. The level of renal and respiratory function is immediately assessed. Evaluation is also made of any other malformations in bodily systems. Once the long-term prognosis of survival is determined, a treatment plan can be addressed. If a neonate with bilateral renal agenesis has severe respiratory distress from severe pulmonary hypoplasia, no further treatment may be the decided course of action. If lung development is sufficient to respond to treatment, mechanical ventilation can supply respiratory support. Management of renal failure involves a complex course of action taken to address all the consequent complications. Adequate nutrition with restricted sodium and fluid intake may be achieved through a nasogastric feeding tube. Medications and vitamin supplementation can be used to address electrolyte imbalances from lack of kidney function. Because the kidney is responsible for vitamin D formation, vitamin D therapy is important. Calcium carbonate is also supplemented because the kidneys are not present to regulate calcium levels in the blood.

Children with chronic renal failure often have poor growth and require supplemental human growth hormone (Genotropin, Humatrope, Nutropin). Human growth hormone stimulates the growth of bone, skeletal muscle, and organs. Human growth hormone acts in conjunction with another medication, erythropoietin, to increase the number of red blood cells and address the additional complication of anemia. Anemia occurs because the kidneys are not present to produce erythropoietin, which is responsible for the stimulation of red blood cell production in the bone marrow. Epoetin alfa (Epogen, Procrit) is a synthetic form of erythropoietin used in the treatment of bilateral renal agenesis. Anemia is also treated with iron supplements, which can be given orally or administered through an injection.

Renal failure causes hypertension; infants with bilateral renal agenesis may require hypertension medications in addition to restricted sodium and fluids. In renal failure, hypertension is caused by fluid overload.

To treat the hypertension associated with bilateral renal agenesis, diuretic agents (Lasix) are used. Diuretic agents promote the excretion of water and electrolytes from the body. They decrease blood pressure by decreasing the amount of fluid present in the blood vessels. Other hypertensive medications may also be used, as is appropriate for the patient's age. Dialysis is required to function as a blood filter replacement for the kidney. Frequent dialysis treatments remain necessary until the infant is old enough to receive a kidney transplant.

## Prognosis

In the absence of kidney injury or disease, the prognosis for unilateral renal agenesis is excellent. Individuals with unilateral renal agenesis usually lead normal, healthy lives. Avoidance of injury and basic health practices are important to maintain this quality of life.

Bilateral renal agenesis has a very poor prognosis. It is usually fatal in the first few days of life. The usual cause of death is respiratory failure and acute renal failure during the neonatal period. If survival progresses to early childhood, patients may have chronic lung disease or chronic renal failure. If the lungs have sufficient development, a kidney transplant is necessary for survival. After a kidney transplant, the prognosis is improved.

### Resources

#### BOOKS

Moore, Keith L., and T. V. N. Persaud. *The Developing Human, Clinically Oriented Embryology, Seventh Edition*. St. Louis, MO: Elsevier Science, 2003.

#### WEB SITES

Parent Permission for Participation in the Potter Syndrome Tissue Bank. (April 14, 2005.) http://potterssyndrome.org/bendonconsent.html.

Sairam, Vellore K., Luther Travis. "Potter Syndrome." E-medicine. April 1, 2003 (April 14, 2005). http://www.emedicine.com/ped/topic1878.htm.

"Solitary Kidney." National Kidney and Urologic Diseases Information Clearinghouse. May 2004 (April 14, 2005). http://kidney.niddk.nih.gov/kudiseases/pubs/solitarykidney/.

#### ORGANIZATIONS

National Kidney and Urologic Diseases Information Clearinghouse. 3 Information Way, Bethesda, MD 20892-3580. (800) 891-5390. E-mail: nkudic@info.niddk.nih.gov. (April 22, 2005.) http://kidney.niddk.nih.gov/about/index.htm.

Potter's Syndrome Support Group Main Forum. (April 22, 2005.) http://forums.delphiforums.com/n/main.asp?webtag=potterssyndrome&nav=start&prettyurl=%2Fpotters syndrome%2Fstart.

Maria Basile, PhD

# Renal failure due to hypertension

## Definition

Renal failure (kidney failure) is caused primarily by chronic high blood pressure (hypertension) over many years. Hypertension is the second major cause, after **diabetes**, of end stage renal disease (ESRD) and is responsible for 25–30% of all reported cases. In addition, many people with diabetes also have hypertension, thus high blood pressure plays an even larger role in kidney failure.

## Description

About 398,000 people were diagnosed with end-stage renal disease in 1998. Of these, about 83,000 had hypertension and about 133,000 had diabetes. That same year, approximately 63,000 people with ESRD passed away. Most people with ESRD have had symptoms for a long time and may have had kidney disease (nephropathy) for as many as 20 years or more prior to experiencing kidney failure.

## Genetic profile

It is believed that most cases of hypertension leading to kidney failure have a genetic element. Finding a genetic link is complicated by the fact that nearly half of all people with renal failure have three or more serious disorders, such as diabetes. Animal studies have been done to find genetic linkages to hypertension and kidney failure, but genetic studies on humans are in their infancy. A recent breakthrough came in a study of African American subjects with hypertensive end-stage renal disease. Researchers found a significant association between severe hypertension and mutations on the HSD11B2 gene. This is a gene that plays a role in sodium retention and related factors. Their data suggested that the 16q22.1 **chromosome** region was the location of the mutation.

In another study, researchers studied an Israeli family of Iraqi-Jewish origin whose members suffered

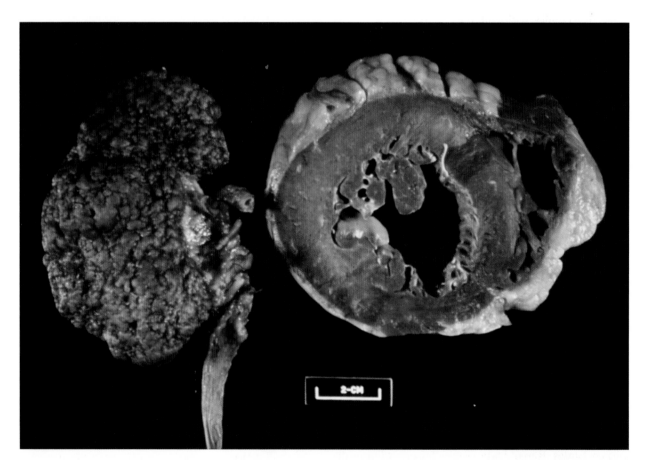

**The effects of hypertension on the kidney (l) and the heart.** ((c) Dr. E. Walker/SPL/Photo Researchers, Inc. Reproduced by permission.)

## KEY TERMS

**Dialysis**—Process by which special equipment purifies the blood of a patient whose kidneys have failed.

**Nephropathy**—Kidney disease.

**Proteinuria**—Excess protein in the urine.

**Serum creatinine**—A chemical in the urine of kidney patients used to determine kidney disease and failure. Elevated levels of serum creatinine are an early marker for severe kidney disease or failure.

**Transplantation**—The implanting of an organ from either a deceased person (cadaver) or from a live donor to a person whose organ has failed.

from hypertension and renal failure. The researchers found a genetic locus at 1q21 that was autosomal dominant. They also hypothesized that the gene encoding atrial natriutetic peptide receptor-1 (NPR1) was the disease gene that led to the hypertension/renal failure.

Other families with high rates of hypertension have also been studied. For example, researchers observed a family of Old Order Amish in Lancaster, Pennsylvania and found a genetic link for hypertension to chromosome 2q31-34. The subjects were not experiencing kidney failure, thus, further study would be needed to determine if the identified genetic locus also coded for ESRD.

### Demographics

People of all ages, races, and both sexes may develop kidney failure due to hypertension. However, some groups are at much greater risk than others. African Americans are at particularly high risk for both hypertension and renal failure and have four times the number of ESRD cases as Caucasians. They also experience kidney failure at a younger age, with an onset at about age 56 compared to an onset at age 62 for Caucasians. African Americans also have a higher rate of diabetes than non-African Americans, another reason for their increased risk for kidney failures. Native Americans and Alaskan Natives are also at high risk for ESRD. There are about the same number of males and females with newly diagnosed ESRD.

In general, according to the National Institutes of Health, the risk for ESRD increases with age, and those who are over age 65 are at greatest risk for ESRD. The United States Renal Data Service (USRDS) of the National Institutes of Health tracks kidney failure statistics in the United States. According to the USRDS,

in 1998, the rate of new cases for those under age 20 was just 13 per million, and the rate increased to 109 for those ages 20–44. A sharp upturn of five times that rate occurred in the 45–64 age group, when the rate is 545 per million people. The rate for those over 65 is about double, at 1,296 per million people. The mean age for individuals with ESRD was 62 years in 1998.

### Signs and symptoms

Universal symptoms of ESRD are severe fatigue, fluid retention (edema) and elevated blood pressure readings. Other symptoms include a failure to eat (anorexia) and skin color changes such as a change to a yellow-brown skin color. Urea from perspiration may appear on the skin as whitish crystals, similar to frost. Pruritis (severe itching of the skin) is common. Patients may have muscle cramps and convulsions. Many have malnutrition from anorexia and vomiting. Gastric ulcers are common, as are cardiac symptoms stemming from the retention of sodium and water. Anemia (low levels of iron in the blood) is also common.

### Diagnosis

Diagnosis is based on the results of a physical examination and laboratory blood and urine tests. A patient who has end stage renal disease looks very ill and has obvious fluid retention and clear indicators of severe disease. Anemia is common. Blood pressure is elevated, and even patients who did not have hypertension prior to the onset of ESRD will develop hypertension. Patients also usually have massive amounts of protein in the urine and high levels of serum creatinine. Urea levels are also raised.

### Treatment and management

Once physicians diagnose end stage renal disease, they must make a plan for dialysis. In addition, patients may be placed on restricted fluids. Anemia is treated and transfusions are given if anemia is severe. ACE inhibitor drugs may be prescribed at low doses to treat cardiac symptoms. Diuretics may be prescribed to reduce fluid retention. Multivitamins may be recommended because of food restrictions.

All patients with kidney failure, despite the cause of the failure, must receive kidney dialysis or kidney transplantation. Eventually, those on dialysis will require transplantation of a kidney, either from a recently deceased person or a live donor. (Each person has two kidneys and can live normally with only one kidney.) About 13,000 kidney transplants are performed in the United States each year and about 47,000 people wait for a donated kidney per year.

There are two types of dialysis. The most common type of treatment is "hemodialysis," a procedure that uses a machine called a dialyzer to clean and filter the blood, since the kidneys can no longer perform that function. A connection from the machine is made to the patient's bloodstream and the blood travels through the dialyzer where it is cleaned for 2–4 hours. This procedure is generally performed three times a week. Patients must also change their diets to carefully limit the amount of salt, potassium, and fluids that are consumed, among other dietary restrictions that are given.

Peritoneal dialysis is another option for patients with kidney failure. In this procedure, the patient's own abdominal lining (the peritoneal membrane) is used to help clean the blood. Rather than the patients own blood traveling to a machine, as with a dialyzer, a cleansing solution is transferred through a special tube (catheter) directly into the body. The catheter remains in the body. The number of treatments and time to perform the cleansing procedures vary.

### Prognosis

Most patients will eventually need a transplanted kidney to continue to live. The survival rate for those on kidney dialysis after one year is about 80% and after two years, about 66%. However, the five year survival rate with dialysis is 29% and the 10 year survival rate is only 8%.

In contrast, the survival rate for those who receive a transplanted kidney from a deceased person is 94% after one year, 92% after two years and 80% after five years. The 10 year survival rate with a cadaver transplantation is 57%. The survival rates are higher when the kidney is from a live donor; for example, the survival rate after 5 years with a live donor kidney is 89% and about 77% after 10 years.

### Resources

#### BOOKS

Beers, Mark H. MD, and Robert Berkow, MD, eds. *The Merck Manual of Diagnosis and Therapy.* 1999. Available at http://www.merck.com/pubs/manual/.

National Institutes of Health. "Chronic Kidney Disease." In *Healthy People 2010.* National Institutes of Health, 2000.

"Patient characteristics at the beginning of ESRD." *2000 Atlas of ESRD in the United States.* U.S. Renal Data System, 2000

#### PERIODICALS

Cohn, Daniel H., et al. "A locus for an autosomal dominant form of progressive renal failure and hypertension at Chromosome 1q21." *American Journal of Human Genetics* 67 (2000): 647-651.

Hsueh, Wen-Chi, PhD, et al. "QTL influencing blood pressure maps to the region of PPH1 On Chromosome 2q31-34 in Old Order Amish." *Circulation* 101 (2000): 2810.

Watson Jr., Bracie, et al. "Genetic association of 11B-hydroxysteroid dehydrogenase type 2 (HSD11B2) flanking microsatellites with essential hypertension in blacks." *Hypertension* 28 (1996): 478-482.

#### WEBSITES

"Entry 161900: Renal Failure, Progressive, with Hypertension." *OMIM—Online Mendelian Inheritance in Man.* http://www.ncbi.nlm.nih.gov/htbin-post/Omim/dispmim?161900.

#### ORGANIZATIONS

American Association of Kidney Patients. 100 S. Ashley Dr., Suite 280, Tampa, FL 33602. (800) 749-2257. www.aakp.org.

American Kidney Fund. Suite 1010, 6110 Executive Blvd., Rockville, MD 20852. (899) 638-8299.

National Kidney and Urologic Diseases Information Clearinghouse. 3 Information Way, Bethesda, MD 20892-3560.

National Kidney Foundation. 30 East 33rd St., New York, NY 10016. (800) 622-9010. http://www.kidney.org.

Christine Adamec

# Renpenning syndrome

## Definition

Renpenning syndrome is an inherited X-linked disorder that manifests itself in males. It is characterized by mental retardation, short stature, a smaller

## KEY TERMS

**Microcephaly**—An abnormally small head.

**Renpenning syndrome**—X-linked mental retardation with short stature and microcephaly not associated with the fragile X chromosome and occurring more frequently in males, although some females may also be affected.

**Short stature**—Shorter than normal height, can include dwarfism.

**Small testes**—Refers to the size of the male reproductive glands, located in the cavity of the scrotum.

**X-linked mental retardation**—Subaverage general intellectual functioning that originates during the developmental period and is associated with impairment in adaptive behavior. Pertains to genes on the X chromosome.

than normal head circumference (**microcephaly**), and small testes. The syndrome was first described by Hans Renpenning, in 1962, in a large Mennonite family living in Manitoba, Canada. The term "Renpenning syndrome" came to be used as a general designation for **X-linked mental retardation**. However, as the syndrome has been mapped to Xp11.2-p11.4, the term "Renpenning syndrome" should be limited to the condition that maps to this region and is characterized by severe mental retardation, microcephaly, short stature, and small testes. The prevalence is unknown.

### Description

Renpenning syndrome is among the group of **genetic disorders** known as X-linked mental retardation (XLMR) syndromes. Developmental delay is present early with males learning to walk at age 2–3 years and able to say simple words at age 3–4 years. Although an affected male may appear physically normal, his head circumference and height will be at the lower limits of normal. After puberty, testes will be smaller than normal. Diagnosis is very difficult especially if there is only one male with mental retardation in a family. The diagnosis is exclusively based on evidence of **inheritance** of the above clinical findings in an X-linked manner and localization to the short arm (Xp11.1-p11.4) of the X **chromosome**.

### Genetic profile

Renpenning syndrome is caused by an alteration in an unknown **gene** located on the short arm (Xp11.2-p11.4) of the X chromosome. The altered gene in affected males is inherited, in most cases, from a carrier mother. Since males have only one X chromosome, a gene mutation on the X is fully expressed in males. Carrier females, with one normal X chromosome and one affected X chromosome, do not have any of the **phenotype** associated with Renpenning syndrome.

Female carriers have a 50/50 chance of transmitting the altered gene to a daughter or a son. A son inheriting the altered gene will have Renpenning syndrome. The affected son will likely not reproduce.

### Demographics

Only males are affected with Renpenning syndrome. Carrier females do not express any of the signs or symptoms. Although Renpenning syndrome has been reported in a single Canadian family, it is believed to be present in all racial/ethnic groups.

### Signs and symptoms

Manifestations of Renpenning syndrome may be present at birth. One male was reported to have global developmental delay at birth. All affected males had delay in reaching developmental milestones—by walking at age 18–24 months and having little or no speech by age three.

Affected males have a small head circumference (microcephaly), are of short stature, and have small testes. Facial features may include central balding, an upslant to the eye openings, and a short distance between the nose and the upper lip. Other clinical findings present in some of the affected males are blindness, seizures and **diabetes** mellitus.

Mental impairment is severe with IQ ranging from 15 to 40.

### Diagnosis

The diagnosis of Renpenning can tentatively be made on the basis of the clinical findings, including an analysis of the family history for evidence of X-linked inheritance. Linkage or segregation analysis using **DNA** markers in Xp11.4-p11.2 would be warrented to possibly rule out other X-linked mental retardation syndromes. Unfortunately, there are no laboratory or radiographic changes that are specific for Renpenning syndrome.

**Sutherland-Haan syndrome**, another X-linked mental retardation syndrome, also has microcephaly, short stature, small testes, and upslanting of the eye openings. Furthermore, this syndrome is localized from Xp11.3 to Xq12, which overlaps with the localization of Renpenning syndrome. However, males with Sutherland-Haan also have spasticity, brachycephaly(disproportionate shortness of the head), and a thin appearance. It is possible these two syndromes have different mutations in the same gene.

The Chudley-Lowry syndrome, which also has microcephaly, short stature, and small testes, has yet to be localized. However, males have distinct facial features, similar to those observed in XLMR-hypotonic facies, and obesity. As this syndrome has not been mapped, it is possible that Chudley-Lowry syndrome results from a mutation in the same unknown gene responsible for Renpenning syndrome.

Three other X-linked mental retardation syndromes (Borjeson-Forssman-Lehman, X-linked hereditary bullous dystrophy, and XLMR-hypotonic facies) have microcephaly, short stature, and small testes. However, these conditions are located in different regions on the X chromosome and can be ruled out if DNA marker analysis is done in the family.

### Treatment and management

As of 2009, there is neither treatment nor cure for Renpenning syndrome. Early educational intervention may prove to be of some benefit for affected males. As some males have had seizures or diabetes mellitus, medication to control these conditions may be required at some point. Also some males may become blind. Some affected males may eventually have to live in facilities outside the home.

### Prognosis

Life threatening or other health concerns have not been associated with Renpenning syndrome. However, the presence of severe mental impairment likely will result in some affected males living in a more controlled environment outside the home.

### Resources

**PERIODICALS**

Fox, P., D. Fox, and J. W. Gerrard. "X-linked mental retardation: Renpenning revisited." *American Journal of Medical Genetics* 7 (1980): 491-495

Renpenning, H., et al. "Familial sex-linked mental retardation." *Canadian Medical Association Journal* 87 (1962): 954-956

Stevenson, R. E., et al. "Renpenning syndrome maps to Xq11." *American Journal of Human Genetics* 62 (1998): 1092-1101

Charles E. Schwartz, PhD

# Retinitis pigmentosa

## Definition

Retinitis pigmentosa (RP) refers to a group of inherited disorders that slowly leads to blindness due to abnormalities of the photoreceptors (primarily the rods) in the retina.

## Description

The retina lines the interior surface of the back of the eye. The retina is made up of several layers. One layer contains two types of photoreceptor cells referred to as the rods and cones. The cones are responsible for sharp central vision, distinguishing and recognizing colors, and seeing fine details. The cones are primarily located in a small area of the retina called the fovea.

The area surrounding the fovea and on the perimeter of the retina contains the rods, which are necessary for vision on the sides, as well as vision in dark and dimly lit conditions. The number of rods increases in the periphery.

The rod and cone photoreceptors normally convert light that enters the eye into electrical impulses; these impulses are sent to the brain along the optic nerve at the back of the eye and an image is recognized by the brain. Another layer of the retina is called the retinal pigmented epithelium (RPE).

In RP, the photoreceptors begin to break down and lose their ability to function. The rods are primarily affected, and as a result it becomes difficult to see in dim light and in the peripheral areas. The ability to see color is also lost in some cases. In the late stages of the disease, only a small area of central vision remains and this can also be lost.

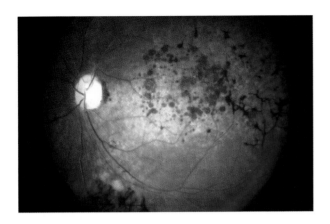

A retinal photo showing retinitis pigmentosa. *(Custom Medical Stock Photo, Inc.)*

There are many forms of retinitis pigmentosa and all of them are genetic. Sometimes the disorder is classified by the age of onset or by the **inheritance** pattern. RP can also be part of a medical syndrome, in which other medical problems are present. This entry focuses on non-syndromic RP, the type that is not associated with other medical complications.

## Genetic profile

RP is an inherited disease associated with different inheritance patterns. It is felt that as many as 100 genes can cause the various types of the condition. The RP may be a familial condition, in which multiple family members are affected. It may also be isolated (or simplex), in which there is only one person with RP in the family. People with isolated RP represent 10–40% of all cases. Some of these may be the result of new gene changes (or mutations). Other isolated cases are those in which the person has a relative with a gene mutation, but that relative has no obvious signs of RP.

RP is most commonly inherited as an autosomal dominant, autosomal recessive, or sex-linked condition in a family. Autosomal dominant RP (ADRP) occurs in about 15–25% of affected individuals. At least 14 different genes have been identified as causing ADRP, with significant ones called the RHO, RP1, RDS, and ROM1 genes. People with ADRP often have an affected parent and other relatives in multiple generations. Someone with ADRP has a 50% chance to have a son or daughter with the same type of RP.

Autosomal recessive RP (ARRP) occurs in about 5–20% of affected individuals. At least 22 genes have been identified that cause this type of RP, including significant ones called RPE65, PDE6A, and PDE6B. In ARRP, each parent of the affected person is a carrier of a gene mutation that causes ARRP. Neither of these

parents has symptoms of ARRP, and they have a 25% chance to have an affected son or daughter in every pregnancy together. All of the children of someone with ARRP would be a carrier for the condition.

Five to 15% of people with RP have the sex-linked form of recessive RP, which is most often X-linked recessive RP (XLRP). At least five genes have been identified with XLRP, with the most significant called RP2 and RP3. Males are usually more affected than females with XLRP and females carry an XLRP mutation on their X **chromosome**. Carrier females may not have signs of XLRP or they may have mild symptoms. In some cases, carriers have serious vision loss associated with XLRP. A female carrier's sons have a 50% chance of being affected, and her daughters have a 50% chance to be carriers. For a male with XLRP, his daughters would all be carriers, but none of his sons would be affected. RP is rarely inherited in an X-linked dominant manner. The risks to family members are very similar to XLRP, but females typically have some symptoms of RP instead. The family history pattern can be very similar to ADRP, and the difference may only be the gene mutation causing the RP in the family.

Rarely, RP is inherited by **gene mutations** in the MTTS2 gene. This gene is located in the cell's mitochondria, as opposed to the cell's nucleus like all of the other genes. When the MTTS2 gene is involved, only a female's sons and daughters would be at risk for RP. If a male has RP caused by the MTTS2 gene, his children would not be at risk for RP.

Also very rarely, RP is caused by the involvement of both the RDS gene and the ROM1 gene in the same family. An individual with RP may have a mutation in each of these genes. The risks to family members would be similar to those found in ADRP.

### Demographics

RP is the most common form of blindness in people between the ages of 20 and 60 years old. It is thought to affect about 1.5 million men and women worldwide and approximately one out of every 4,000 people in the United States and Europe. Haim, et al., reported the lifetime risk for RP in Denmark to be one in 2,500 people. For other parts of the world, there are no published data on exact prevalence, but RP is seen in all ethnic groups.

### Signs and symptoms

The first symptoms are typically difficulties seeing in dimly lit conditions or night blindness. People may notice that they are uncomfortable with an oncoming car's bright headlights when driving at night, or they may have a hard time finding their seat in a darkened movie theatre. People may begin to notice this as young as in childhood, adolescence, or later on in adulthood. In general, the earlier one notices this the more severe their RP may be over time. XLRP is usually associated with a more severe progression of symptoms than other forms of RP.

Eventually, people with RP experience a loss of peripheral vision and this may first start in childhood or early adolescence. This peripheral visual field loss typically progresses to tunnel vision, akin to seeing the world through two narrow straws. Prior to complete constriction of their visual fields, people with undiagnosed RP may be considered clumsy by those who know them, because they may not see the things that are in the normal visual field.

People with RP usually maintain crisp central vision for a very long time, because the cones are not usually involved until the later stages of the condition. Once the cones become involved, people may have their central vision affected, with difficulty distinguishing colors. Occasionally, the loss of the ability to see color occurs before the loss of peripheral vision. Additionally, RP sometimes significantly affects one's visual acuity; men with XLRP may have a visual acuity less than or equal to that of legal blindness.

Specific changes in the eye are consistent with RP. In the early stages of RP, visual testing indicates abnormal rod functioning, but there may be no physical changes in the retina. People may see occasional flickering or small lights flashing in their eyes. Over time this can progress. There may be narrowing to the blood vessels in the retina, fine dust-like coloring within the retina, and floating in the eye's natural liquid. There is often loss of pigment from the layer of tissue underneath the retina. As the rods break down, clumps of dark-colored melanin cause a bone spicule formation along the retina's periphery. These are very characteristic of RP. Eventually, the optic nerve and retinal blood vessels can become pale in color. Others may have white dots deep in the retina, and other abnormalities of the optic nerve.

Those with RP often develop a specific type of cataracts, known as a posterior subcapsular cataract (PSC). These are different than the cataracts found in the general population. PSCs have a yellowish crystal-like appearance in the eye's lens, and this looks different than typical cataracts seen in those without RP. These cataracts may be removed by an ophthalmologist, but this does not help tunnel vision or night blindness.

People with RP usually have these changes in both of their eyes. However, some only have them in one section or one half of an eye. This is called sector RP. People with this usually have no problems with night blindness, though visual testing can identify abnormal rod and cone functioning. Sector RP usually is inherited in a dominant manner, but is also seen in some female carriers of XLRP.

### Diagnosis

A diagnosis of RP is usually made based on analysis of a person's symptoms, visual test results, and family history. **Genetic testing** is available for some types of RP.

When a person complains of problems with night vision, an ophthalmologist or optometrist usually performs a careful eye examination, including pupil dilation, to determine if there are physical changes to the retina and back of the eye that are suggestive of RP. Other retinal problems can cause night blindness and must be ruled out. However, these may not have the retinal changes that are typical of RP. A careful eye examination can also determine one's visual acuity and color vision.

An electroretinogram (ERG) tests how well the photoreceptors in the retina are functioning.

Specifically for RP, this test is very good at identifying how well the rod cells are working. It can also show how well the cone cells are working. A dark adaptation curve (DAC) test can document the exact amount of time one's eyes take to adjust to darkness.

Testing of the visual fields can determine how much is being seen from left to right, and up and down. The full field of vision is studied to identify any blind spots or clarify whether the central vision is affected.

Fluorescein angiography (FA) can be helpful to determine whether blood flow is normal throughout the back of the eye. These detailed photographs of the eye's blood vessels can help identify any circulatory problems at the back of the eye, as well as changes in the retina's structure.

Fundus photographs can be taken to document changes in the eye structure, shape, and color.

A consensus conference documented by Marmor, et al., in 1983 established criteria to establish the diagnosis of RP. They are:

- Rod dysfunction as measured by DAC or ERG
- Progressive loss in photoreceptor function
- Loss of peripheral vision
- Involvement of both eyes

Other eye conditions can mimic RP, but do not have the specific eye changes and visual test results of RP. Gyrate atrophy of the choroid and retina, a recessive disorder, may seem like RP in its symptoms. However, it may be associated with round patches affecting the choroids and retina, which occur in the middle of the retina. **Choroideremia**, an X-linked recessive disorder, causes progressive blindness. However, it usually causes fine dark lines and patches on the choroids, which progress into pale yellow areas.

**Leber congenital amaurosis** is a group of recessive retinal abnormalities that cause serious vision problems or blindness that appear at or shortly after birth. Children affected with this condition usually have roving eye movements. **Cone-rod dystrophy** is a retinal problem in which the rods function well, but the cones progressively worsen. The symptoms may be similar to RP, but occur in the reverse order.

There are a few syndromes that involve RP. These include **Usher syndrome** and **Bardet-Biedl syndrome**. Usher syndrome is a group of recessive conditions that combine RP with **deafness** of varying degrees. Bardet-Biedl syndrome is a group of recessive conditions that combine RP with extra fingers and toes, mental delays, obesity, genital abnormalities, kidney abnormalities, and other medical complications. Genetic blood testing is available for some forms of Usher and Bardet-Biedl syndromes.

Genetic testing from a blood sample is available for some types of non-syndromic RP on a clinical basis. In these cases, an abnormal result would identify a mutation (or mutations) in the gene causing RP for that individual. Other at-risk family members can sometimes be offered genetic testing once a mutation is identified in a family. In some cases, prenatal testing is available through an **amniocentesis** procedure. All genetic testing should be accompanied by careful **genetic counseling**.

### Treatment and management

There is no cure for RP, or known way to stop the disease progression altogether. However, some things can help maintain good retinal function and health.

It is felt that a diet rich in leafy green vegetables and fish may be good for the retina. In addition, certain fish contain omega-3 fatty acids, such as docosahexanoic acid (DHA) that is naturally found in the retina in very high concentrations. Eating a diet of fish like salmon, tuna, mackerel, or whitefish twice a week should naturally provide good DHA levels. Otherwise, good fish oil capsules containing DHA and other omega fatty acids can be obtained with a prescription or purchased at specialty health stores.

Multivitamins containing vitamins A, E, and C may be useful. These have antioxidant properties, which may be protective for the eyes. However, large doses of certain vitamins may be toxic, and affected individuals should speak to their doctors before taking supplements.

Protecting the eyes from harmful ultraviolet rays is essential to cone cell health. People with RP should wear good sunglasses outdoors and especially when over water or near snow on a bright, sunny day.

Smoking has been associated with deteriorating retinal health. Even quitting smoking late in life can make a positive impact on eye health.

PSCs do not usually severely impact the vision of those with RP. However, in some cases an ophthalmologist can remove the eye's lens and replace it with an artificial one to remove the cataract.

Low vision aids can be helpful for those in school or at work. Binocular lens and magnifying screens, large-print reading materials, closed-circuit television, special eyeglass lenses, and other tools can be helpful and are often available from organizations supporting those with vision loss.

Living with a chronic vision problem makes a significant impact on a person's life and family. It is often helpful for families to have a social worker connect them to helpful resources. Others may find genetic counseling, psychotherapy, or meeting other individuals with RP through support groups helpful.

### Prognosis

Life expectancy is normal in RP. It eventually leads to serious visual impairment or blindness. The more severe forms will lead to blindness sooner than the milder forms, but each person's experience with the condition is unique and impossible to predict. Research and future treatments continue to offer hope for those with RP.

### Resources

#### BOOKS

Newell, Frank W. *Ophthalmology: Principles and Concepts,* 7th ed. St. Louis, MO: Mosby Year Book, 1992.

#### ORGANIZATIONS

American Academy of Ophthalmology. P.O. Box 7424, San Francisco, CA 94120-7424. Phone: (415) 561-8500. http://www.eyenet.org.

American Association of the Deaf-Blind. 814 Thayer Ave., Suite 302, Silver Spring, MD 20910. Phone: (301) 495-4403. TTY Phone: (301) 495-4402. Fax: (301) 495-4404. Email: info@aadb.org. http://www.aadb.org/.

The Foundation Fighting Blindness. 11435 Cronhill Drive, Owings Mills, MD 21117-2220. Local phone: (410) 568-0150. Local TDD: (410) 363-7139. Toll-free phone: (888) 394-3937. Toll-free TDD: (800) 683-5555. Email: info@blindness.org. http://www.blindness.org/.

The Foundation Fighting Blindness–Canada. 60 St. Clair Ave., East Suite 703, Toronto, ON, Canada M4T 1N5. Phone: (416) 360-4200. Toll-free phone: (800) 461-3331. Fax: (416) 360-0060. Email: info@ffb.ca. http://www. ffb.ca/.

Retinitis Pigmentosa International. P.O. Box 900, Woodland Hills, CA 91365. Phone: (818) 992-0500. Fax: (818) 992-3265. Email: info@rpinternational.org. http://www. rpinternational.org.

#### WEB SITES

*Genetic Alliance*. 2005 (March 15, 2005). http://www. geneticalliance.org.

*OMIM–Online Mendelian Inheritance in Man*. National Center for Biotechnology Information. (March 15, 2005.) http://www.ncbi.nlm.nih.gov/Omim/ searchomim.html.

*RetNet–Retinal Information Network*. 2005 (March 15, 2005). http://www.sph.uth.tmc.edu/Retnet/.

Deepti Babu, MS, CGC
Amy Vance, MS
Dorothy Elinor Stonely

# Retinoblastoma

## Definition

Retinoblastoma is a rare **cancer** affecting one or both eyes. It occurs mainly in children under the age of five. Its name is derived from the area of the eye that is affected, the retina. The retina is the part of the eye that captures the images of the outside world and transfers these images to the brain. If the eye is thought of as a camera, the retina can be thought of as the film in the camera.

## Description

Retinoblastoma accounts for about 4% of all cancers in children younger than 15 years. In most cases, retinoblastoma only affects one eye; when this occurs, it is referred to as unilateral retinoblastoma. In one out of three cases, it affects both eyes, and is referred to as bilateral retinoblastoma. Retinoblastoma cancer cells can, in rare cases, spread to other areas of the body, including the bone marrow.

Many of the early symptoms of retinoblastoma, such as intermittent pain of the eye, inflammation of the eye, and poor vision, are often overlooked. It is often a parent who notices the most visible sign of retinoblastoma, that being a whitish appearing pupil, known as leukocoria. If retinoblastoma is detected early enough, treatment such as surgery or radiation can result in a 95% cure and survival rate.

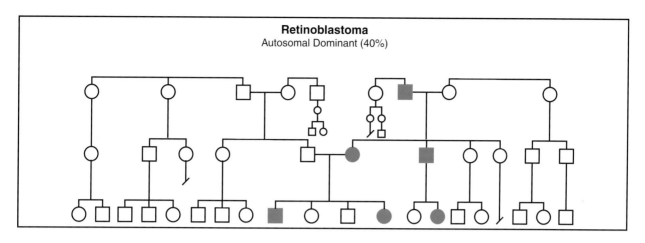

(Gale, a part of Cengage Learning.)

## Genetic profile

Mutations in the "retinoblastoma 1" (RB1) **gene** are responsible for most cases of retinoblastoma. This gene provides instructions for making a protein that acts as a tumor suppressor because it regulates cell growth, preventing cells from dividing too fast or abnormally. Hundreds of RB1 mutations have been identified in people with retinoblastoma. As a result, certain cells in the retina can divide uncontrollably to form cancerous tumors. When the RB1 mutations occur in all of the body's cells, they can be passed to the next generation and the retinoblastoma is called germinal, which is the case for 40% of all retinoblastomas. The other 60% are non–germinal, meaning that RB1 mutations occur only in the eye and cannot be passed to the next generation.

it is estimated that a small percentage of retinoblastoma cases result from deletions in the region of **chromosome** 13 that contains the RB1 gene. Because these chromosomal changes involve other genes besides RB1, affected children usually display other symptoms such as intellectual disability, slow growth, and distinctive abnormal facial features.

In germinal retinoblastoma, the RB1 **gene mutations** are inherited in an autosomal dominant pattern. This means that one copy of the mutated gene in each cell is sufficient to increase cancer risk. The mutated copy of the gene may be inherited from one parent, or the altered gene may be the result of a new mutation that occurs in an egg or sperm cell. For retinoblastoma to develop, a mutation involving the other copy of the RB1 gene must occur in retinal cells during the person's lifetime. It is believed that this second mutation usually occurs in childhood, with the result that retinoblastoma develops in both eyes. In non–germinal retinoblastoma, only one eye is usually affected and there is no family history of the disease. Affected individuals are born with two normal copies of the

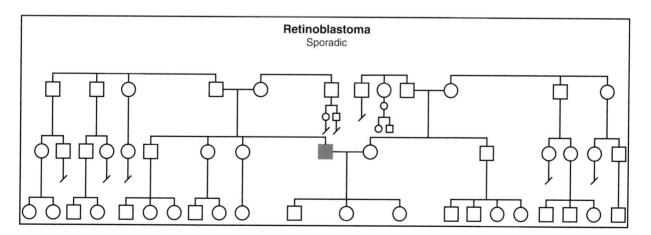

**Pedigree analysis showing sporadic occurrence of retinoblastoma within a family.** *(Gale, a part of Cengage Learning.)*

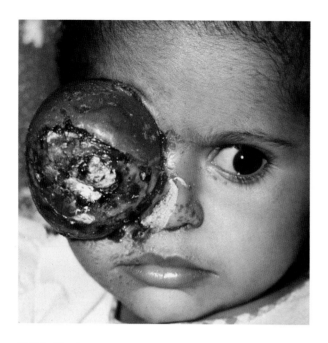

**Child with a large tumor protruding from the right eye socket.**
*(Custom Medical Stock Photo, Inc.)*

RB1 gene. The RB1 gene copies in retinal cells then mutate in early childhood. People with non–germinal retinoblastoma are not at risk of passing these RB1 mutations to their children. However, **genetic testing** is required to ascertain whether a person with retino-blastoma in one eye has the germinal or the non–germinal form of the disease.

### Demographics

Retinoblastoma is the most common type of eye cancer in children. It occurs worldwide in approxi-mately one in 15,000–20,000 births. According to the National Cancer Institute, approximately 300 children and adolescents younger than 20 years of age are diag-nosed with retinoblastomas each year in the United States. Most retinoblastoma cases occur among young children, with almost 63% of all retinoblastomas occur-ring before the age of two and 95% occurring before the age of five. Over the 1975–1995 period, rates of retino-blastoma were essentially equal among males (3.7 per million) and females (3.8 per million) and among whites (3.7 per million) and blacks (4.0 per million).

### Signs and symptoms

Since the successful management of retinoblas-toma depends on detecting it early, the recognition of the signs and symptoms of the condition is critical. This is especially true for primary care physicians, who are often the first medical personnel to see infants or children with retinoblastoma.

There are many ways that retinoblastoma can present itself in infants and children. More than half of all patients with the condition will have a white pupil reflex, called leukocoria. In healthy infants and children, their pupils will appear black, or, when photographed, red. However, patients with retino-blastoma will often have a pupil that appears gray or white.

The second most common presenting sign of ret-inoblastoma, occurring about 25% of the time, is a crossed eye, a medical condition referred to as strabis-mus. The child's eye may appear to be looking out towards the ear, called *exotropia*, or inward towards the nose, called *esotropia*. It should be noted that three to four percent of all American children present with some form of strabismus, but not all of these children have retinoblastoma. However, since 25% of children with retinoblastoma have strabismus, any child with this condition should have a detailed eye exam to rule out retinoblastoma.

While leukocoria and strabismus are the two most common presenting signs of retinoblastoma, there are other ways the condition may present itself. Other symp-toms may include a red, painful eye, poor vision, orbital cellultis (inflammation of the skin and tissue around the eye), and amblyopia, or "lazy eye.". Heterochromia, a diiference in coloration of the irises (the colored part in the center of the eye surrounding the pupil), may also be the first signs of retinoblastoma.

## Diagnosis

The diagnosis of retinoblastoma is frequently made by the parents of an infant or child with the condition. Often, the parents will tell the physician that they have noticed that their child's eye looks "white," or that the child's eye or eyes seem to drift to one side or the other.

When a child is born into a family that has a history of retinoblastoma, diagnosis of the condition can often be made before the baby leaves the hospital by an eye specialist, or ophthalmologist. If there is no family history, and the initial diagnosis is made by the parents or family physician, then the child can be sent to an ophthalmologist for a more thorough eye exam.

To examine a child for retinoblastoma, dilating drops are placed in both eyes to dilate (enlarge) the pupils and allow the ophthalmologist to view the retina. If a tumor is seen or suspected, an ultrasound examination, which uses sound waves to penetrate and outline structures in the eye, is used to confirm the presence of a tumor. Computed tomography (CT) scans use computers to take very detailed pictures of the inside of the body and can be used to see if there are tumors in other parts of the body.

Since the gene responsible for retinoblastoma has been identified, genetic testing is also available to detect the condition.

## Treatment and management

Treatment options for retinoblastoma have significantly increased over the past twenty years. The earliest form of treatment for retinoblastoma was *enucleation*, the removal of the major portion of the affected eye. This led to total loss of vision in that eye. While enucleation is still used, especially when the tumor is very large, newer, more sophisticated treatments have emerged that offer the chance to save at least some vision in the affected eye.

Lasers can be used in a treatment known as photocoagulation. This treatment is best used when the tumor is small and confined to the retina. The laser is actually used to burn and destroy blood vessels that feed the tumor, rather then directly on the tumor itself. The treatment can be repeated one or two times, and in some studies complete remission of the retinoblastoma was achieved in 70% of patients.

Another modality that works well with tumors that are confined to the retina is cryotherapy. It may be used as either the primary mode of treatment or in conjunction with other treatment modalities. Like photocogulation, cryotherapy has its highest success rates with smaller tumors. Unlike photocoagulation, cryotherapy uses extreme cold to destroy the tumor itself.

Thermotherapy uses heat generated from ultrasound or microwaves to destroy the retinoblastoma tumor. While thermotherapy works well on its own with small tumors, it is even more effective when used with chemotherapy or radiation therapy, which are thought to make the tumor more susceptible to the heat generated by thermotherapy.

The use of conventional external beam radiation is still used for retinoblastoma, especially for tumors that are larger and have spread outside the retina. While radiation is applied directly to the tumor, with careful application the eye itself can be saved from destruction in about 75% of patients. In 35% of patients who receive external beam radiation, there is an increased risk for a retinoblastoma tumor to develop in the other eye within a 30–year time frame. Therefore, external beam radiation is generally only used when other conservative measures, such as cryotherapy or photocoagulation fail or cannot be used due to large tumor size.

Probably the most significant advancement in the treatment and management of retinoblastoma has come about in the use of chemotherapy. While in the past chemotherapy was only used to treat patients whose tumors had spread outside the eye, newer chemotherapy agents such as carboplatin and etoposide, along with older agents such as vincristine, are being used to treat tumors that are confined to the eye with significant success. Using these chemotherapeautic agents, it has been shown that tumors typically decrease in size 30–45%. This then allows more conservative and eye–sparing therapy such as cryotherapy and photocoagulation to be used much more effectively.

### Clinical trials

Clinical trials on retinoblastoma are currently sponsored by the National Institutes of Health (NIH) and other agencies. As of 2009, NIH was reporting 43 on–going and completed studies.

Examples include:

- The evaluation of proton beam radiation therapy in children with retinoblastoma as a means of local tumor control and ocular retention. (NCT00432445)
- A study to investigate genetic mutations and environmental exposure in young patients with retinoblastoma and in their parents and young healthy unrelated volunteers. (NCT00690469)
- The evaluation of the effectiveness of combination chemotherapy in treating patients with retinoblastoma. (NCT00002675)

Clinical trial information is constantly updated by NIH and the most recent information on retinoblastoma trials can be found at: http://clinicaltrials.gov/search/condition = %22retinoblastoma%22

### Prognosis

The prognosis for the vast majority of patients with retinoblastoma is excellent. In the United States, over 95% of children with retinoblastoma survive and lead healthy, productive lives.

Children who have unilateral retinoblastoma have at least one normal eye and can lead normal childhood lives, and even drive cars as they get older. The majority of children with bilateral retinoblastoma retain some vision in one eye, and sometimes both eyes. However, all children affected with bilateral retinoblastoma and 15% of children with familial unilateral retinoblastoma have a higher risk of developing other cancers throughout their lives. Therefore, children in these categories need to have regular medical checkups throughout their lives to watch for any signs of secondary cancers in areas such as bone, muscle, skin, and brain.

### Resources

#### BOOKS

Parker, Philip M. *Retinoblastoma —A Bibliography and Dictionary for Physicians, Patients, and Genome Researchers.* San Diego, CA: Icon Health Publications, 2007.
Shields, Jerry A., and Carol L. Shields. *Intraocular Tumors: An Atlas and Text,* 2nd edition, Philadelphia, PA: Lippincott Williams & Wilkins, 2007.

#### PERIODICALS

Leiderman, Y. I., et al. "Molecular genetics of RB1—the retinoblastoma gene." *Seminars in Ophthalmology* 22, no. 4 (October–December 2007): 247–254.
Madhavan, J., et al. "Retinoblastoma: from disease to discovery." *Ophthalmic Research* 40, no. 5 (2008): 221–226.
Mastrangelo, D., et al. "The retinoblastoma paradigm revisited." *Medical Science Monitor* 14, no. 12 (December 2008): RA231–RA240.
Poulaki, V., and S. Mukai. "Retinoblastoma: genetics and pathology." *International Ophthalmology Clinics* 49, no. 1 (2009): 155–164.
Schefler, A. C., and D. H. Abramson. "Retinoblastoma: what is new in 2007–2008." *Current Opinion in Ophthalmology* 19, no. 6 (November 2008): 526–534.

#### ORGANIZATIONS

American Cancer Society (ACS). P.O. Box 22718, Oklahoma City, OK 73123-1718. (800)ACS-2345. http://www.cancer.org..
Canadian Cancer Society (CCS). National Office, Suite 200, 10 Alcorn Ave., Toronto, ON M4V 3B1, Canada. (416)961-7223. Fax: (416)961-4189. Email: ccs@cancer.ca. http://www.cancer.ca..
EyeCare America. 655 Beach St., San Francisco, CA 94109-1336. (877)887-6327 or (800)222-3937. http://www.eyecareamerica.org.
National Cancer Institute (NCI). 6116 Executive Blvd., Ste. 3036A, MSC 8322, Bethesda, MD 20892-8322. (800)4-CANCER (422-6237). Email: cancergovstaff@mail.nih.gov. http://cancer.gov..
National Eye Institute (NEI). 2020 Vision Place, Bethesda, MD 20892-3655. (301)496-5248. http://www.nei.nih.gov.
Retinoblastoma International. 4650 Sunset Blvd., MS #88, Los Angeles, CA 90027. (323)669-2299. http://www.retinoblastoma.net.

#### WEBSITES

*Eye Cancer.* Health Topic, Medline Plus, March 24, 2009 (April 30, 2009). http://www.nlm.nih.gov/medlineplus/eyecancer.html
*Information About Retinoblastoma.* Information Page. NEI, November 2008 (April 30, 2009). http://www.nei.nih.gov/health/blastoma/
*Retinoblastoma.* Medical Encyclopedia, Medline Plus, April 28, 2009 (April 30, 2009). http://www.nlm.nih.gov/medlineplus/ency/article/001030.htm
*Retinoblastoma.* Information Page. NCI, 2009 (April 25, 2009). http://www.cancer.gov/CancerInformation/CancerType/retinoblastoma
*Retinoblastoma.* Information Page. Madisons Foundation, February 4, 2004 (April 30, 2009). http://www.madisonsfoundation.org/index.php/component/option,com_mpower/diseaseID,302/
*Retinoblastoma.* Information Page. Children's Hospital Boston, 2009 (April 30, 2009). http://www.childrenshospital.org/az/Site1523/mainpageS1523P0.html

Edward R. Rosick, DO, MPH, MS

Retinoic acid embryopathy *see* **Accutane embryopathy**

# Rett syndrome

## Definition

Rett syndrome is a progressive neurological disorder seen almost exclusively in females. The most common symptoms include decreased speech, mental retardation, severe lack of coordination, small head size, and unusual hand movements.

## Description

Dr. Andreas Rett first reported females with the symptoms of Rett syndrome in 1966. Females with this X-linked dominant genetic condition are healthy and of average size at birth. During infancy, head growth is abnormally slow and **microcephaly** (small head size) develops. Babies with Rett syndrome initially have normal development. At approximately one year of age, development slows and eventually stops. Patients with Rett syndrome develop autistic features. Involuntary hand movements are a classic feature of Rett syndrome.

Females with Rett syndrome may also develop seizures, curvature of the spine (**scoliosis**), irregular breathing patterns, swallowing problems, constipation, and difficulties walking. Some females with Rett syndrome are unable to walk. There is currently no cure for Rett syndrome. Most girls with Rett syndrome live until adulthood. The **gene** responsible for Rett syndrome has been identified and **genetic testing** is available.

## Genetic profile

Rett syndrome is an X-linked condition. This means that the mutation (genetic change) responsible for Rett syndrome affects a gene located on the X **chromosome**. The affected gene is the methyl CpG-binding protein 2 (MECP2) gene. This gene makes a protein that regulates other genes. When there is a mutation in MECP2, the protein it makes does not work properly. This is thought to prevent normal neuron (nerve cell) development.

Rett syndrome is considered to be X-linked dominant in nature. Males have one X chromosome and one Y chromosome. Females have two X chromosomes. Males with a mutation in their MECP2 gene typically die as infants or are miscarried before birth. Rett syndrome is usually considered fatal in males because the Y chromosome cannot compensate for the MECP2 mutation on the X chromosome. Females with a mutation in the MECP2 gene develop Rett syndrome, but the presence of the second X

chromosome in females carrying a normal MECP2 gene enables them to survive.

The severity of the syndrome in females is related to the type of mutation in the MECP2 gene and the activity of the X chromosomes. Normally, both X chromosomes have the same activity. However, the activity can be unequal. If the X chromosome with the mutation in the MECP2 gene is more active than the X chromosome without the mutation, the female is more severely affected. The reverse is also true. If the X chromosome without the mutation is more active than the X chromosome with the mutation, the female is less severely affected.

If a woman has a mutation in her MECP2 gene, she has a 50% risk with any pregnancy to pass on her X chromosome with the mutation. However, it is uncommon for women with Rett syndrome to have children due to the severity of the disorder.

## Demographics

The incidence of Rett syndrome is thought to be between 1 in 10,000 and 1 in 20,000 live births. It is seen almost exclusively in females. The vast majority of cases of Rett syndrome are sporadic in nature.

Therefore, the risk of a family having more than one affected daughter is typically very low.

### Signs and symptoms

Infants with Rett syndrome typically have normal size at birth. They develop normally until approximately 6–18 months of age. Development then slows, eventually stops, and soon regresses. Affected individuals are unable to do things they were once able to do. Girls with Rett syndrome lose the ability to speak, become uninterested in interacting with others, and stop voluntarily using their hands. The loss of language and eye contact causes girls with Rett syndrome to appear to be autistic. Between one and three years of age, girls with Rett syndrome develop the unusual hand movements that are associated with the disease. Patients wring their hands, clap their hands, and put their hands in their mouth involuntarily. Some patients with Rett syndrome also lose the ability to walk. If the ability to walk is maintained, the gait is very ataxic (uncoordinated, clumsy).

By preschool age the developmental deterioration of girls with Rett syndrome stops, but they continue to have lack of speech, inability to understand language, poor eye contact, mental retardation, ataxia, and apraxia (inability to make purposeful movements). Other common symptoms associated with Rett syndrome include seizures, constipation, irregular breathing, scoliosis, swallowing problems, teeth grinding, sleep disturbances, and poor circulation. As patients with Rett syndrome get older, their ability to move decreases and spasticity (rigidity of muscles) increases.

### Diagnosis

The diagnosis of Rett syndrome is made when the majority of the symptoms associated with the disease are present. If a physician suspects an individual has Rett syndrome, **DNA** testing is recommended. Approximately 75% of patients with Rett syndrome have a mutation in the MECP2 gene. DNA testing can be performed on a blood sample, or other types of tissue from the body. If a mutation is found in the MECP2 gene, the diagnosis of Rett syndrome is confirmed.

### Treatment and management

As of 2001, there is not a cure for Rett syndrome. Treatment of patients with Rett syndrome focuses on the symptoms present. Treatment may include medications that inhibit seizures, reduce spasticity, and prevent sleep disturbances. Nutrition is monitored in

## QUESTIONS TO ASK YOUR DOCTOR

- What are the typical signs and symptoms of Rett syndrome?
- Why does this disorder occur almost exclusively among females?
- Given that we already have one daughter with Rett syndrome, what is the probability of having a second child with the same genetic disorder?
- What is the prognosis for our daughter with Rett syndrome, and on what information do you base that prognosis?

females with Rett syndrome due to their small stature and the constipation associated with the disorder.

### Prognosis

In the absence of severe medical problems, most patients with Rett syndrome live into adulthood.

### Resources

#### BOOKS

Zoghbi, Huda, and Uta Francke. "Rett Syndrome." In *The Metabolic and Molecular Bases of Inherited Disease.* New York: McGraw-Hill, 2001.

#### PERIODICALS

Percy, Alan. "Genetics of Rett Syndrome: Properties of the Newly Discovered Gene and Pathophysiology of the Disorder." *Current Opinion in Pediatrics* 12 (2000): 589-595.

#### WEBSITES

"Rett Syndrome." *Online Mendelian Inheritance in Man.*http://www.ncbi.nlm.nih.gov/entrez/dispomim. cgi?id = 312750 (May 24, 2000).

#### ORGANIZATIONS

Alliance of Genetic Support Groups. 4301 Connecticut Ave. NW, Suite 404, Washington, DC 20008. (202) 966-5557. Fax: (202) 966-8553. http://www.geneticalliance.org.

International Rett Syndrome Association. 9121 Piscataway Rd., Clinton, MD 20735. (800) 818-RETT. http://www.rettsyndrome.org.

National Organization for Rare Disorders (NORD). PO Box 8923, New Fairfield, CT 06812-8923. (203) 746-6518 or (800) 999-6673. Fax: (203) 746-6481. http://www.rarediseases.org.

Rett Syndrome Research Foundation. 4600 Devitt Dr., Cincinnati, OH 45246. http://www.rsfr.org.

Holly A. Ishmael, MS, CGC

## RFH1 *see* **Renal failure due to hypertension**

# Rheumatoid arthritis

## Definition

Rheumatoid arthritis (RA) is a chronic inflammatory disease affecting the joints, most often in the hands and feet. It results in swelling, stiffness, pain, and sometimes joint, bone, and cartilage destruction.

## Description

Although the exact cause of RA is unknown, the disease belongs to a group of diseases called autoimmune disorders. In these disorders, the immune system, the function of which is to protect the body, produces antibodies that attack the soft tissues lining the joints and may also attack connective tissue in many other parts of the body, including the blood vessels and lungs. Eventually, the cartilage, bone, and ligaments of the joint deteriorate, causing deformity, instability, and scarring within the joint. The rate at which the joints deteriorate varies with the individual. A number of risk factors, including genetic predisposition, gender, and unspecified environmental factors, may put a person at risk for developing the disease as well as influence the pattern of the disease.

As with other forms of arthritis, RA involves inflammation of the joints. A membrane called the synovium lines each of the body's movable joints. In RA, white blood cells, which usually attack foreign invaders such as bacteria and viruses, move from the bloodstream into the synovium. There, these blood cells appear to play an important role in causing inflammation to the synovial membrane, a condition called synovitis. This inflammation results in the release of proteins that, over months or years, causes thickening

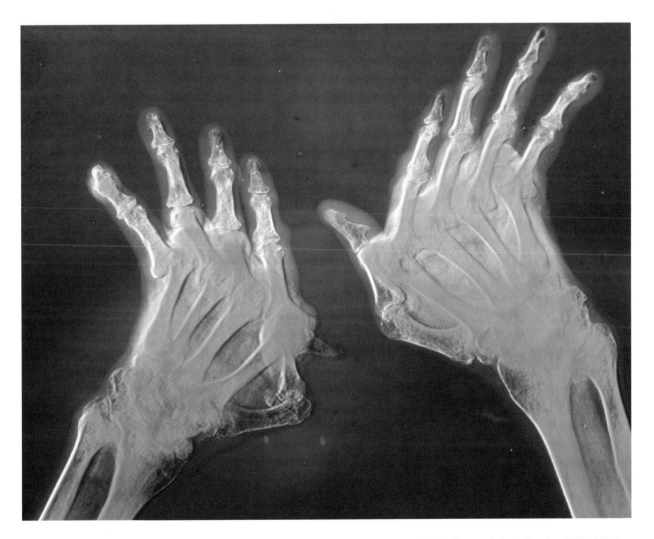

**False-color x ray of hands with extreme rheumatoid arthritis affecting the joints of all the fingers in both hands.** *(CNRI / Photo Researchers, Inc.)*

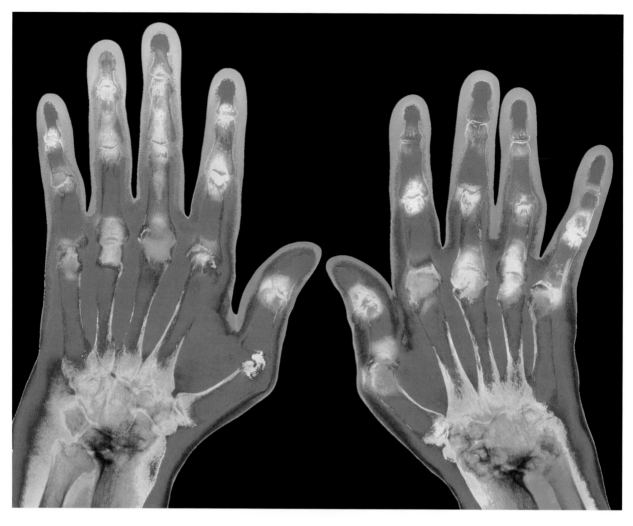

Colored x ray of hands with severe rheumatoid arthritis (RA). Yellow indicates swelling and bone deformation. Most of the joints are ragged because of bone erosion. *(SPL / Photo Researchers, Inc.)*

of the synovium. These proteins can also damage cartilage, bone, tendons, and ligaments. Gradually, the joint loses its shape and alignment, and eventually may be destroyed.

## Genetic profile

Rheumatoid arthritis is a genetically complex disease. Studies in monozygotic (identical) and dizygotic (fraternal) twins indicate that genetic factors are involved in acquiring the susceptibility or tendency to RA rather than the disease itself. People with certain human leukocyte antigen (HLA) genes—specifically, the genetic marker called HLA-DR4 (the DR4 refers to the specific antigen)—are more likely to develop the disease than those without the genes. However, people without this antigen can develop the disease as well.

The HLA-DR4 marker is found in white blood cells and plays a role in helping the body distinguish between its own cells and foreign invaders. In addition, these genes also help predict the severity of the disease and how effectively the disease responds to treatment. The mechanism by which HLA alleles (HLA genetic variations) affect disease risk is still under investigation.

In one study, French scientists found 63 genes that appeared to be linked to the development of rheumatoid arthritis. The group studied and compared the expression of 5,200 genes in the synovial (joint) fluid of a group of patients with RA and another group with **osteoarthritis**. The researchers found 48 known and 15 unknown genes that were either overexpressed or underexpressed in RA patients compared with osteoarthritis patients. Two of the novel genes were located

## KEY TERMS

**Antibodies**—Protein molecules the body produces to fight infection.

**Autoimmune disorder**—Disorder occurring when the body's tissues are attacked by its own immune system, as in RA.

**Cyclooxygenase-2 (COX-2) inhibitors**—Anti-inflammatory drugs that work by blocking the COX-2 enzyme, which plays a role in the inflammatory process, but do not block the COX-1 enzyme, which helps protect the digestive tract.

**Inflammation**—Localized protective response elicited by injury or destruction of tissues and characterized by pain, heat, redness, swelling, or loss of function.

**Tumor necrosis factor**—A protein that plays an early and major role in the rheumatic disease process.

on **chromosome** 6, at the p21 region, which is an area already linked to inflammatory disease. Four other genes were located on the X chromosome. The French scientists hope their findings will lead to the identification of new pathways related to RA, as well as to new diagnostic and treatment options.

However, not all the genes associated with RA have been discovered, and more research is needed.

### Demographics

Rheumatoid arthritis affects approximately 1% of the United States population. Although some people have a mild form of RA, 70% eventually develop chronic problems, and 15% have a severe crippling form of the disease.

The disease occurs in all races and countries. Although RA affects women two to three times more often than men, men tend to be affected more severely by it. The onset of RA most commonly occurs between the ages of 25 and 50, but children and adolescents as well as the elderly may be affected as well. When the disease occurs in children, it is referred to as juvenile RA.

### Signs and symptoms

The course of RA varies with each individual. Some people may have mild symptoms, occasional flare-ups, and long periods without disease (remission), or disease that progresses steadily, either slowly or rapidly. The disease may begin suddenly, with many joints becoming inflamed simultaneously. Most often,

however, RA begins subtly, gradually affecting different joints. Usually the inflammation is symmetric, with joints on both sides of the body affected. Typically, the small joints in the fingers, toes, hands, feet, wrists, elbows, and ankles become inflamed first. The inflamed joints are usually painful and often stiff, especially just after awakening (such stiffness generally lasts for at least 30 minutes and often much longer) or after prolonged inactivity. Some people feel tired and weak, especially in the early afternoon. In addition, RA may produce a low-grade fever.

Affected joints enlarge because of swelling of the soft tissue and can quickly become deformed. Joints may freeze in one position so that they cannot bend or open fully. The fingers may tend to dislocate from their normal position toward the little finger on each hand, causing tendons in the fingers to slip out of place.

Swollen wrists can pinch a nerve and result in numbness or tingling due to carpal tunnel syndrome. Cysts, which may develop behind affected knees, can rupture and cause pain and swelling in the lower legs. Up to 30% of people with RA have hard bumps (called rheumatoid nodules) just under the skin, usually near sites of pressure (such as the back of the forearm near the elbow).

In rare cases, RA causes an inflammation of blood vessels called vasculitis; this condition reduces the blood supply to tissues and may cause nerve damage or leg sores (ulcers) that may become infected. Inflammation of the membranes covering the lungs (pleura) or of the sac surrounding the heart (pericardium), or inflammation and scarring of the lungs can lead to chest pain and shortness of breath. Some people develop swollen lymph nodes, dry eyes or mouth, or red, painful eyes as a result of inflammation.

### Diagnosis

In addition to the important characteristic pattern of symptoms, many tests may be used to support the diagnosis.

Laboratory tests may include rheumatoid factor, white blood cell count, a blood test for anemia, erythrocyte sedimentation rate (ESR, or sed rate), and C-reactive protein, which detects inflammation.

Many people with RA have certain characteristic antibodies in their blood, such as rheumatoid factor, which is present in 70% of people with RA. In addition to RA, rheumatoid factor occurs in several other diseases, such as hepatitis and other infections. Some people even have rheumatoid factor in their blood without any evidence of disease. A higher level of rheumatoid factor in the blood usually results in a more severe RA and a poorer prognosis. The rheumatoid factor level may decrease when joints are less inflamed.

Most people have mild anemia (an insufficient number of red blood cells). Rarely, the white blood cell count becomes abnormally low. When a person with RA has a low white blood cell count and an enlarged spleen, the disorder is called Felty's syndrome.

Nine out of 10 people with RA have an elevated sed rate, a test that measures the rate at which blood cells settle to the bottom of a test tube containing blood; an elevated sed rate suggests that active inflammation is present. The rate depends on certain proteins in the blood. However, this test alone cannot identify the cause of the inflammation. Doctors may monitor the sed rate when symptoms are mild to help determine whether the disease is still active.

A needle biopsy may be recommended. A needle biopsy is an examination of a joint fluid sample or of a tissue sample from rheumatoid nodules, both obtained by a needle.

Characteristic changes in the joints may be seen on x rays.

### Treatment and management

Treatments for RA have improved in recent years. Although most treatments involve medications, in some cases, surgical procedures may be necessary.

Medications for rheumatoid arthritis can relieve its symptoms and slow or halt its progression. Nonsteroidal anti-inflammatory drugs (NSAIDs) help to alleviate both pain and inflammation, if taken on a regular basis. These drugs, which are available without a prescription, include aspirin, ibuprofen (Motrin, Advil), and naproxen (Aleve). These medications are available at higher dosages by prescription. Other NSAIDs available in prescription strength include ketoprofen (Oruvail), tolmetin (Tolectin), diclofenac (Arthrotec, Voltaren), nabumetone (Relafen), and indomethacin (Indocin).

Taking NSAIDs on a regular basis, however, can lead to adverse side effects, such as indigestion and stomach bleeding. Other potential harmful side effects may include damage to the liver and kidneys, ringing in the ears (tinnitus), fluid retention, and hypertension (high blood pressure).

Initially, it was thought that COX-2 inhibitors, another class of NSAIDS, was less damaging to the stomach than the traditional NSAIDS. Like other NSAIDs, COX-2 inhibitors, such as celecoxib (Celebrex), which is one of the few COX-2 inhibitors still on the market in the United States, suppress an enzyme called cyclooxygenase (COX) that is active in joint inflammation. It was believed that NSAIDs work against two versions of the COX enzyme present in the body: COX-1 and COX-2. However, there is increasing evidence to suggest that by suppressing COX-1, the enzyme responsible for protecting the stomach lining, NSAIDs may cause stomach and other problems. Unlike other NSAIDs, COX-2 inhibitors suppress only COX-2, the enzyme involved in inflammation.

Side effects of COX-2 inhibitors may include fluid retention and causing or exacerbating high blood pressure. Furthermore, this class of drugs has been linked to an increased risk of heart attack and stroke. These are reasons why Merck Pharmaceuticals chose to remove its COX-2 inhibitor rofecoxib (Vioxx) from the worldwide market in September 2004. About 1.3 million people in the United States and about 700,000 abroad were using the drug. In April 2005, the COX-2 inhibitor valdecoxib (Bextra) was voluntarily removed from the market by its manufacturer, Pfizer, at the request of the FDA, which stated that the potential risks of heart attack, stroke, and potentially life-threatening skin reactions were greater than its benefits. The FDA also announced new label requirements for both prescription and nonprescription NSAIDS. Prescription labels for COX-2 inhibitors like celecoxib were required to carry a "black box warning" stressing the life-threatening effects associated with the drug.

In December 2004, the FDA issued a Public Health Advisory recommending limited use of COX-2 inhibitors. The guidelines warn patients at high risk of gastrointestinal bleeding, those with a history of intolerance to certain NSAIDS. Individual patient risk for cardiovascular problems and other risks commonly associated with NSAIDS should be taken into account for each patient. Consumers are advised that all nonprescription pain relievers, including NSAIDS, should be used exactly as specified on the label. If NSAIDS are needed for more than 10 days, the FDA suggests that a doctor be consulted.

The FDA's actions differ from the recommendations of an FDA expert advisory panel, which, in February 2005, voted in favor of allowing COX-2 inhibitors celecoxib and valdecoxib to remain available. The panel also voted to allow rofecoxib back on the market, under strict conditions.

Corticosteroids, such as prednisone (Deltasone) and methylprednisolone (Medrol), reduce inflammation and pain and slow the progression of joint damage and destruction associated with RA. In the short term, corticosteroids alleviate pain significantly. When used for many months or years, however, these drugs tend to lose their efficacy and cause serious side effects that may include bruising, thinning of bones, cataracts, weight gain, and **diabetes**. Doctors often prescribe corticosteroids to alleviate acute symptoms, with the goal of gradually tapering off the medication when the patient's pain decreases.

Physicians prescribe disease-modifying antirheumatic drugs (DMARDs) to limit the amount of joint damage that occurs in RA. Taking these drugs during the early stages in the development of RA is especially important in an attempt to slow disease progression and save the joints and other tissues from permanent damage. Because many of these drugs act slowly, it may take weeks to months to detect any benefit. Typically, DMARDs are used in combination with an NSAID or a corticosteroid. Although the NSAID or corticosteroid alleviates any immediate symptoms and limits inflammation, the DMARD acts directly on the disease. Commonly used DMARDs include hydroxychloroquine (Plaquenil), the gold compound auranofin (Ridaura), sulfasalazine (Azulfidine), and minocycline (Dynacin, Minocin). Additional forms of DMARDs include immunosuppressants and tumor necrosis factor (TNF) blockers.

Immunosuppressants act to quiet the immune system, which is overactive in RA. In addition, some of these drugs attack and destroy cells associated with the disease. Some of the commonly used immunosuppressants include methotrexate (Rheumatrex), leflunomide (Arava), azathioprine (Imuran), cyclosporine (Neoral, Sandimmune), and cyclophosphamide (Cytoxan). These medications may have potentially serious adverse side effects, such as increased susceptibility to infection.

The TNFs are a class of DMARDs known as biologic response modifiers. Tumor necrosis factor is a cell protein, or cytokine, that acts as an inflammatory agent in RA. Anti-TNF medications, or TNF blockers, target or block this cytokine and can help reduce pain, morning stiffness, and tender or swollen joints, typically within one or two weeks after initiating treatment. There is evidence that TNF blockers may halt the progression of disease. Often these medications are taken in combination with the immunosuppressant methotrexate. The TNF blockers approved for treatment of RA include etanercept (Enbrel), infliximab (Remicade), and adalimumab (Humira). These medications should not be taken if active infection is present.

Interleukin-1 receptor antagonist (IL-1Ra) is another type of biologic response modifier and is an artificially created (recombinant) form of the naturally occurring interleukin-1 receptor antagonist. Interleukin-1 (IL-1) is a cell protein that promotes inflammation and occurs in excessive amounts in people with RA or other types of inflammatory arthritis. If IL-1 is prevented from binding to its receptor, the inflammatory response is decreased.

The first IL-1Ra approved by the FDA for use in individuals with moderate to severe RA who have not responded adequately to conventional DMARD therapy is anakinra (Kineret). This drug may be used alone or in combination with methotrexate. Anakinra is administered as a daily self-injection. Some potential side effects include injection-site reactions, decreased white blood cell counts, headache, and increased upper respiratory tract infections, especially in people with **asthma** or chronic obstructive pulmonary disease. If active infection is present, anakinra should not be used.

Some people with RA also experience symptoms of **depression**. The most common antidepressants used for RA pain and for sleep that is not restful are amitriptyline (Elavil), nortriptyline (Aventyl, Pamelor), and trazodone (Desyrel).

Although a combination of medication and self-care is the first course of action for RA, other methods are available in severe cases of the disease. The Prosorba column is a blood-filtering technique used to remove certain antibodies that contribute to pain and inflammation in the joints and muscles and is usually performed once a week for 12 weeks on an outpatient basis. Some of the side effects of this procedure include fatigue and a temporary increase in joint pain and swelling for the first few days after the treatment. The Prosorba column treatment is not recommended in combination with angiotensin-converting enzyme (ACE) inhibitors or if heart problems, high blood pressure, or blood-clotting problems are present.

Joint replacement surgery is an option chosen by many people with RA when less invasive methods or medications are not able to alleviate pain and deter joint destruction. When joints are severely damaged, joint replacement surgery can often help restore joint function, reduce pain, or correct a deformity. In some cases, the entire joint may need to be replaced with a metal, ceramic, or plastic prosthesis. Surgery may also involve tightening or loosening tendons, fusing bones to reduce pain, or removing a portion of a diseased bone to improve mobility. The inflamed joint lining may also require removal (synovectomy).

### Prognosis

In rare cases, RA resolves spontaneously. However, at least one out of 10 people with RA eventually becomes severely disabled.

## Resources

### BOOKS

Schlotzhauer, Tammi L., and James L. McGuire. *Living with Rheumatoid Arthritis.* Baltimore, MD: Johns Hopkins University Press, 2003.

Zashin, Scott J., and Laurette Hesser. *Arthritis without Pain: The Miracle of TNF Blockers.* Bangor, ME: Sarah Allison Publishing, 2004–2005.

### PERIODICALS

Drazen, J. M. "Cox-2 Inhibitors: A Lesson in Unexpected Problems." *New England Journal of Medicine* 352 (March 17, 2005): 1131–32.

Silman, A. J., and Jacqueline E. Pearson. "Epidemiology and Genetics of Rheumatoid Arthritis." *Arthritis Research & Therapy* 4 (Supplement 3) (May 9, 2002): S265–S272. Available online: http://arthritis-research.com/content/4/S3/S265.

Smolen, J. S. "The Science of Rheumatoid Arthritis: A Prelude." *Arthritis Research & Therapy* 7 (Supplement 2) (March 16, 2005): S1–S3.

### WEB SITES

Arthritis Research & Therapy. (April 22, 2005.) http://arthritis-research.com/.

### ORGANIZATIONS

American Academy of Orthopaedic Surgeons. P.O. Box 2058, Des Plaines, IL 60017. (800) 824-2263. (April 22, 2005.) http://www.aaos.org.

American College of Rheumatology. 1800 Century Place, Suite 250, Atlanta, GA 30345. (404) 633-3777. (April 22, 2005.) http://www.rheumatology.org/index.asp?.

Arthritis Foundation. 1330 West Peachtree Street, Atlanta, GA 30309. (800) 283-7800. (April 22, 2005.) http://www.arthritis.org.

National Institute of Arthritis and Musculoskeletal and Skin Diseases. National Institutes of Health. 1 AMS Circle, Bethesda, MD 20892-3675 (877) 226-4267. (April 22, 2005.) http://www.niams.nih.gov.

Genevieve T. Slomski, PhD

# Rhizomelic chondrodysplasia punctata

## Definition

Rhizomelic **chondrodysplasia punctata** is a rare, severe, inherited disease. The main features are limb shortening, bone and cartilage abnormalities visible on x ray, abnormal facial appearance, severe mental retardation, profound psychomotor retardation, and cataracts. Skeletal abnormalities can be seen

---

prenatally. Most affected persons die in infancy. No treatments are available.

## Description

Rhizomelic chondrodysplasia punctata (RCDP) is caused by an abnormal protein in a part of the cell called the peroxisome. The inside of the cell contains compartments (called "organelles") that perform specific functions. The peroxisome functions in many metabolic processes, especially those involving lipids (fats) and hydrogen peroxide. Multiple peroxisomes are in almost every human cell. RCDP is one of many peroxisomal disorders, as well as a metabolic disorder.

Three other conditions are also called "chondrodysplasia punctata." These conditions are different from RCDP. They have almost the same name because it describes a feature that is present in all four conditions. However, the causes, features, and patterns of **inheritance** of the other chondrodysplasia punctata conditions are different from those of RCDP.

## Genetic profile

Rhizomelic chondrodysplasia punctata is an autosomal recessive condition. This means that it occurs in both males and females, and often affects people who have no family history of the condition. Humans have two copies of every **gene**, one maternally and one paternally inherited. Autosomal recessive conditions occur when a person has two abnormal copies of the same gene. People who have one abnormal copy and one normal copy of a particular gene are unaffected; they are called "carriers." An affected person has inherited two abnormal RCDP genes, one from each carrier parent. The risk for the carrier parents to have another affected child is then 25% with each pregnancy.

In 1997, the gene that causes RCDP was identified. The gene is called PEX7 and it is on **chromosome** 6. Fifteen genes involved in the synthesis of peroxisomes have been identified in humans. These genes are called PEX genes, and the proteins they code for are called peroxins. Disorders caused by abnormalities of peroxin proteins are often called "peroxisomal biogenesis" disorders.

The PEX7 gene codes for a peroxisomal component that helps transport other important proteins into the peroxisome. The proteins to be transported contain a signal, called "PTS2" (peroxisome targeting sequence 2) that is recognized by the receptor on the peroxisome. When PEX7 is abnormal, the receptor that usually recognizes and helps transport the PTS2 proteins is abnormal. Thus, the abnormality of this one receptor has a cascade effect on many other proteins.

## Demographics

Rhizomelic chondrodysplasia punctata is quite rare. It occurs in fewer than 1/100,000 births. The incidence of peroxisomal biogenesis disorders is approximately 1/50,000 births; RCDP accounts for fewer than one fifth of these.

## Signs and symptoms

"Rhizomelic" refers to shortening of the bones near the center of the body (the bones of the thighs and upper arms more so than the bones of the forearms and lower legs). "Chondro" refers to cartilage and "dysplasia" to abnormal development. "Punctata" refers to specific abnormalities seen on radiological studies such as x ray. The ends of the bones near joints appear to be spotted. The spots represent dense, abnormal cartilage. The spots are also called "punctate calcifications." Other abnormalities include frozen joints (called contractures), abnormal facial features,

cataracts, hearing loss, severe mental retardation, and profound psychomotor retardation. People with RCDP may also have other bone abnormalities, small heads, coarse and sparse hair, and dry, red skin.

The proximal shortening of the bones causes short stature, which is apparent before birth. Growth after birth is retarded as well. The rhizomelic shortening is severe, and occurs to the same degree on both sides of the body. The stippling (spotting) of the bones mainly involves the ends of the bones near the hip, knee, elbow, and shoulder. "Severe" mental retardation describes cognitive deficits worse than those of typical **Down syndrome**. Some researchers have described degeneration of brain tissue after birth. Researchers are not sure of the reason for this; it may be due to toxic effects of excess phytanic acid. Cataracts are symmetrical and occur in both eyes. The abnormal facial features have been called "koala bear facies." Facial features include a broad forehead and a saddle nose.

A subset of people with RCDP do not have some of the typical symptoms, such as shortening of proximal bones and/or severe mental retardation. The diagnosis in these individuals was confirmed to be RCDP. Therefore, the spectrum of features in RCDP is variable; some people are much more mildly affected than is typical. These differences in severity appear to be associated with different mutations in the PEX7 gene.

## Diagnosis

Although suspicion of RCDP is raised by the physical and radiographic features, the diagnosis is made by laboratory testing. People with RCDP have very specific biochemical abnormalities, i.e. abnormal levels of particular substances in bodily fluids. These abnormalities are due to the underlying defect in the peroxisome. The specific abnormalities are: 1) deficient plasmalogen synthesis with very low plasmalogen levels in red blood cells, 2) inability to process (oxidize) phytanic acid leading to elevated levels of phytanic acid in the blood, and 3) an unprocessed form of peroxisomal thiolase. Phytanic acid levels are normal at birth and increase to at least ten times normal by one year of age. Some experts recommend that confimatory studies be performed on cells obtained by skin biopsy.

The biochemical studies diagnostic of RCDP can be performed prenatally on cells obtained by chorionic villus sampling (CVS) or **amniocentesis**. CVS is usually performed from 10–12 weeks of pregnancy and amniocentesis is usually performed after 15 weeks of pregnancy. RCPD may be suspected in a fetus based on ultrasound findings.

Each feature of RCDP is seen in many other conditions, for example rhizomelic limb shortening is seen in other conditions that cause dwarfism. Chondrodysplasia punctata is seen in many inherited conditions but can also be caused by prenatal exposure to the anticoagulant drug, Warfarin. Doctors who specialize in diagnosing rare genetic conditions use subtle differences between the symptoms of these conditions to narrow their search for the suspected diagnosis. Many peroxisomal disorders have abnormal very long chain fatty acids (VLCFAs); VLCFA levels are normal in RCDP.

Two rare conditions cannot be distinguished from RCDP by physical symptoms. These conditions involve specific abnormalities of plasmalogen synthesis. RCDP is caused by abnormal peroxisome synthesis, which leads to multiple biochemical abnormalities including deficient plasmalogen synthesis. In contrast, these two conditions each affect only one protein. The proteins affected are dihydroxyacetone phosphate acyltransferase (DHAPAT) and alkyl dihydroxyacetone phosphate synthase. People with deficiencies in these two proteins have normal thiolase and normal phytanic acid levels.

RCDP is the only condition known to be caused by abnormal PEX7 gene. **Genetic testing** is another method to confirm the diagnosis. A doctor who specializes in medical **genetics** can determine whether this testing is available clinically.

## Treatment and management

The only treatments for RCDP are supportive therapies to treat symptoms. People with RCDP, especially those who are less severely affected, benefit from symptomatic support of various specialties such as ophthalmology and physical therapy. Dietary restrictions or supplements have shown promise in the treatment of some peroxisomal disorders. The enormous obstacle in the severe conditions is that many of the abnormalities develop before birth and are irreversible. The multiple biochemical abnormalities of RCDP also complicate treatment efforts. Some researchers have tried to improve the function of the deficient metabolic process. This treatment, if it works, will probably benefit mildly affected patients more than the typically severely affected person with RCDP.

The underlying cause of the severe mental retardation is not well understood. Some abnormalities of nerve tissue have been described. In many peroxisomal disorders similar to RCDP the nerve tissue migrates abnormally before birth. This abnormal migration is not present in RCDP. It appears that in RCDP the nerve tissue does not differentiate properly once it has migrated to the correct location in the body.

---

## QUESTIONS TO ASK YOUR DOCTOR

- Please explain the meaning of the term "rhizomelic chondrodysplasia punctata."
- What causes this disorder?
- Is there any cure for this disease or any treatment to slow its progress?
- How long does a child with rhizomelic chondrodysplasia punctata typically survive?

---

### Prognosis

The prognosis for the typical individual with RCDP, who is severely affected, is death in infancy. Most affected infants die in the first two years of life. However, exceptions have reported in the medical literature. Individuals who lived past the age of 10 years have been reported. For atypical, mildly affected patients, prognosis is variable.

Scientists' understanding of peroxisomal disorders, and of the peroxisome itself, increased enormously in the last five years. Developing effective treatments of RCDP is a great challenge. But having a better understanding of the underlying cause is the first step. This has also increased awareness of RCDP, probably leading to more accurate diagnoses and higher clinical suspicion. A correct diagnosis is critical in providing accurate recurrence, prognosis, and prenatal diagnosis information.

### Resources

#### PERIODICALS

Bennett, Ruth. "Workshop Looks Into the Challenges, Causes of Dwarfism." *The Oregonian* (July 7, 1999).

Hedley, Lisa Abelow. "A Child of Difference." *New York Times Magazine* 147 (October 1997): 98-99.

#### WEBSITES

"Genetics Tutorial and diagnosis information." Greenberg Center for Skeletal Dysplasias. *Johns Hopkins University*. http://www.med.jhu.edu/Greenberg.Center/Greenbrg.htm.

Gould, Stephen J. "The Peroxisome Website." *John Hopkins University School of Medicine*.http://www.peroxisome.org.

#### ORGANIZATIONS

Footsteps Institute for Rare Diseases. 624 Martin Luther King Way, Tacoma, WA 98405. (253) 383-0985 or (888) 640-4673. rwrfsi@aol.com.

International Patient Advocacy Association. 800 Bellevue Way NE, Suite 400, Bellvue, WA 98004. (425) 462-4037 or (310) 229-5750 or (800) 944-7823 x4037. lvp.ipaa @att.net. http://www.vanpelt-ipaa.com.

National Organization for Rare Disorders (NORD). PO Box 8923, New Fairfield, CT 06812-8923. (203) 746-6518 or (800) 999-6673. Fax: (203) 746-6481. http://www.rarediseases.org.

Rhizomelic Chondrodysplasia Punctata (RCP) Family Support Group. 137 25th Ave., Monroe, WI 53566.

Michelle Queneau Bosworth, MS, CGC

# Rhodopsin

## Definition

Rhodopsin is the visual pigment that "senses" light in the rod cells of the retina.

## Where is rhodopsin?

Rhodopsin is found at the back of the eye, in the retina. The retina is the area of the eye that senses light, interprets that information, and transmits it to the brain for further interpretation. Two types of light-sensing cells are found in the retina: rods and cones. In a simplified explanation, rod cells are responsible for black and white vision, whereas cone cells are responsible for color vision. This is true as far as it goes, but there are many more differences between rods and cones.

In rod cells, rhodopsin is responsible for phototransduction, the process of turning light into chemical and electrical energy. Rhodopsin is responsible for phototransduction in rod cells, but not in cone cells. Three different proteins, similar to rhodopsin, govern phototransduction in the cone cells. Each of these three phototransducers responds to a different color of light, which allows persons with normal color vision to see the entire color spectrum.

In order to understand more of the structure, function, and location of rhodopsin, a discussion of cells and cell membranes is necessary. Every human cell has a cell membrane that separates the environment inside the cell (intracellular environment) from the extracellular (outside the cell) environment. Cell membranes are made up of lipids, which are hydrophobic substances. Hydrophobic literally means fear of water. Oil is an example of a hydrophobic substance. If oil is added to water, the oil will separate itself from the water. Basically, the lipids in the cell membrane form a similar water-excluding ball, but the inside of the ball will contain water (and other intracellular fluids. Each rhodopsin molecule crosses the cell membrane seven times, and each area of the protein in the cell membrane is called a transmembrane domain. These transmembrane domains (which are hydrophobic) dictate an interesting structure for rhodopsin. Imagine folding a hose seven times to hold it in your hand. The structure for rhodopsin is at least that complex. One reason to mention that rhodopsin has seven transmembrane domains is because that structure is common to G proteins, and rhodopsin is a G protein. G proteins are generally involved in a biological cascade. A biological cascade is a system where a small initial input (like a brief flash of light) can result in a rather large output.

## How does rhodopsin turn light into a chemical signal?

Rhodopsin is a combination of two different molecules, retinal and opsin. Retinal is a derivative of vitamin A and opsin is a protein. When rhodopsin is not activated, retinal is in the 11-cis configuration. When light hits 11-cis retinal, it changes its shape to become all-trans retinal. This is the only light-sensitive step in vision (in the rod cells). What the configurations are called, and what those names mean is not as important as the fact that this light-dependent change in conformation results in light being converted into chemical energy.

Once retinal reaches the all-trans conformation, opsin also changes its shape. The new opsin-retinal complex is called metarhodopsin II. Metarhodopsin II is a semistable complex that is the active form of rhodopsin. Metarhodopsin II, unlike the inactive rhodopsin, is able to bind a protein called transducin. Each metarhodopsin II can bind to many transducins (literally hundreds). These transducins then cause a decrease in cGMP concentration, and one transducin molecule can cause the breakdown of more than 1,000 cGMP per second. One can clearly see why the G protein cascades are excellent systems for amplifying a signal.

## Mutations in rhodopsin

Mutations in rhodopsin can result in two different disorders— **retinitis pigmentosa** and congenital stationary night blindness. Retinitis pigmentosa (RP) affects about one in 3,000 persons living in the United States, and about 1.5 million persons worldwide. Many mutations, not just mutations of the rhodopsin **gene**, lead to RP. The disorder may be inherited in an X-linked recessive fashion in 8% of all cases, an autosomal dominant fashion in 19% of cases, or as an autosomal recessive disorder in 19% of all cases. In the rest of the cases (54%), the mutations do not follow classical genetic patterns of **inheritance**. Mutations in rhodopsin have been found to cause approximately 20% of the autosomal dominant form of RP. The rhodopsin gene is located at the 3q locus of the **chromosome**.

Patients with retinitis pigmentosa exhibit symptoms that include night blindness, abnormal pigment accumulation in the retina, and a progressive decrease in the visual fields. The patient's vision decreases from the outermost edges in. The age of onset of the disorder may be as young as six months, but most patients experience the first symptoms between ages 10 and 30. In RP, the patient's rod cells usually degenerate first, followed by a loss of cone cells.

Symptoms may often present after a motor vehicle accident. Not only is the age of onset variable, but the severity of the disease is as well. Patients with the same mutation, even within the same family, exhibit differing severities of the disorder. Mutations in rhodopsin may also cause autosomal recessive cases of RP.

Congenital stationary night blindness (CSNB) is another disorder that can be caused by mutations in the rhodopsin gene. Patients with CSNB, as may be deduced from the name, experience night blindness. However, unlike RP, patients with CSNB do not experience degeneration (death) of cells of the retina (rod and cone cells). Patients with CSNB are thought to have an overactive transducin molecule, which prevents their rods from functioning normally. A mutation in transducin which also causes CSNB supports this theory, since this transducin is also thought to be overly active.

### Treatment and management

As of 2009, no effective treatment for RP exists. However, new treatments are being explored for RP. Experiments in rats have shown that rod cells can be affected by **gene therapy**. Although gene therapy has not been successfully demonstrated as of this printing, at least the hope now exists that eventually gene therapy may be applied to the problem of RP. Previously, addition of a new gene into a non-dividing cell line had been thought to be technically insurmountable. Another experiment in rodents offers hope for those who have autosomal recessive RP. In rats with autosomal recessive RP, retinal pigment transplantation has successfully treated them according to Columbia University's Retinal Transplant newsletter. This technique might prove promising in humans.

### Prognosis

The prognosis for persons with RP is extremely variable. Persons with CSNB will experience night blindness throughout their lives.

### Resources

#### WEBSITES

"A guide to retinitis pigmentosa." *The British Retinitis Pigmentosa Society.* http://www.brps.demon.co.uk/Graphics/G_Guide.html#SYMPTOMS.

Robbins, Alexandra. "Congenital stationary night blindness." http://130.132.19.190/thom/reviews/cnsb.html.

Michael V. Zuck, PhD

# Rieger syndrome

### Definition

Rieger syndrome is a rare disorder characterized by absence and/or malformation of certain teeth, mild craniofacial (relating to the head and the face) abnormalities, and various eye abnormalities. The eye abnormalities, referred to as Rieger eye malformations, may be present separately or as a part of Rieger syndrome.

### Description

First characterized by Herwigh Rieger, an Austrian ophthalmologist in 1935, Rieger syndrome is a dominantly inherited disease. Disease expression is highly variable, including craniofacial, ocular, and dental malformations. Symptoms may also include **myotonic dystrophy** (a condition characterized by delay in the ability to relax muscles), umbilical abnormalities (abnormalities relating to where the umbilical cord attaches to a baby), and other defects. Psychomotor

## KEY TERMS

**Cornea**—The transparent structure of the eye over the lens that is continuous with the sclera in forming the outermost, protective, layer of the eye.

**Craniofacial**—Relating to or involving both the head and the face.

**Hypoplasia**—Incomplete or underdevelopment of a tissue or organ.

**Iris**—The colored part of the eye, containing pigment and muscle cells that contract and dilate the pupil.

**Microcornea**—Abnormal smallness of the cornea.

**Microdontia**—Small teeth.

**Myotonia**—The inability to normally relax a muscle after contracting or tightening it.

**Myotonic dystrophy**—A form of muscular dystrophy, also known as Steinert's condition, characterized by delay in the ability to relax muscles after forceful contraction, wasting of muscles, as well as other abnormalities.

**Ocular**—A broad term that refers to structure and function of the eye.

**Oligodonita**—The absence of one or more teeth.

**Psychomotor**—Movement produced by action of the mind or will.

**Stenosis**—The constricting or narrowing of an opening or passageway.

retardation, a slowing of the motor action directly proceeding from mental activity, occurs in some cases.

Rieger syndrome is also sometimes referred to as goniodysgenesis hypodontia, iridogoniodysgenesis with somatic anomalies, or RGS. It is a multiple congenital anomaly syndrome, a syndrome marked by multiple abnormalities at birth. Currently, there are two genetic types of Rieger syndrome identified. Type I results from a mutation on **chromosome** 4 and Type II on chromosome 13.

### Genetic profile

Rieger syndrome is inherited as an autosomal dominant disease. In autosomal dominant **inheritance**, a single abnormal **gene** on one of the autosomal chromosomes (one of the first 22 non-sex chromosomes) from either parent can cause the disease. One of the parents will have the disease (since it is dominant) and is the carrier. Only one parent needs to be a carrier in order for the child to inherit the disease. A child who

has one parent with the disease has a 50% chance of also having the disease.

There is evidence that there is more than one genetic form of Rieger syndrome. The disease gene responsible for Rieger syndrome Type I is caused by mutations in the RIEG1 gene, which is located on the long arm (q) of chromosome 4 (4q25-Q26).

Linkage studies have indicated that a second type of Rieger syndrome, Type II, maps to the long arm of chromosome 13, at 13q14 (gene RIEG2).

### Demographics

Rieger syndrome is very rare. Little is known in regard to the number of affected individuals or whether certain areas or ethnic groups are at a greater risk. Since the disease appears to be inherited in an autosomal dominant manner, meaning that it is transmitted on one of the non-sex chromosomes, males and females have an equal chance of acquiring the abnormal gene from their parents.

### Signs and symptoms

The symptoms of Rieger syndrome are expressed variably. The main symptoms of Rieger syndrome are:

- Ocular malformations, called Rieger eye malformations, include underdeveloped iris, a small cornea (microcornea), an opaque ring around the outer edge of the cornea, adhesions (abnormal union of surfaces normally separate) in the front of the eye, and/or displacement of the pupil of the eye so that it is not centered.

- Dental abnormalities include a congenital condition causing a fewer number of teeth than normal (hypodontia); a condition in which a single tooth, pairs of teeth, or all the teeth are smaller than normal (microdontia), and/or cone-shaped.

- Craniofacial abnormalities include a protruding lower lip, a broad, flat bridge of the nose, and/or underdeveloped bones of the upper jaw (hypoplasia) causing the face to have a flat appearance.

Other conditions that have been found in some patients with Rieger syndrome are:

- Anal stenosis (a small anal opening).

- Failure of the skin around the navel to decrease in size after birth.

- Protrusion of intestine through a weakness in the abdominal wall around the navel (umbilical hernia).

- Glaucoma (increased pressure within the eyeball) may result from the ocular malformations associated with Rieger syndrome, including defects in the angle of the eye that is created by the iris and cornea (trabeculum), the vein at the corner of the eye that drains the water in the eye into the bloodstream (schlemm), and the associated adhesions. Glaucoma can result in damage to the optic disk and gradual loss of vision, causing blindness in approximately 50% of affected individuals.

Additional conditions have sometimes occurred in conjunction with Rieger syndrome. Whether they are separate entities in which the Rieger eye malformations are present or part of Rieger syndrome is not determined. These conditions are:

- Myotonia (a condition in which the muscles do not relax after contracting).
- Myotonic dystrophy (a chronic progressive disease causing muscles to atrophy, slurred speech, failing vision, droopy eyelids, and general muscle weakness).
- Conductive deafness (hearing loss in which sound does not travel well to the inner ear).
- Less than average intellectual function associated with problems in learning and social behavior.

## Diagnosis

This disorder can be detected soon after birth if the eye defects are visible. When the eye defects are not visible during the first month of life, Rieger syndrome is usually detected in early childhood when the eye and dental defects become apparent.

Molecular **genetic testing** for the RIEG1 and RIEG2 genes is not generally available. But since the molecular structure of the genes has been identified, the possibility now exists for DNA-based testing for diagnosis and **genetic counseling**.

### Genetic counseling

Genetic counseling may be beneficial for patients and their families. Only one parent needs to be a carrier in order for the child to inherit the disease. A child has a 50% chance of having the disease if one parent is diagnosed with the disease and a 75% chance of having the disease if both parents have Rieger syndrome.

### Prenatal testing

For couples known to be at risk for having a baby with Rieger syndrome, testing may be available to assist in prenatal diagnosis. Prior testing of family members is usually necessary for prenatal testing.

Either chorionic villus sampling (CVS) or **amniocentesis** may be performed for prenatal testing. CVS is a procedure to obtain a small sample of placental tissue, called chorionic villi tissue, for testing. Examination of fetal tissue can reveal information about the defects that leads Rieger syndrome. Chorionic villus sampling can be performed at 10–12 weeks gestation.

Amniocentesis is a procedure that involves inserting a thin needle into the uterus and the amniotic sac, and withdrawing a small amount of amniotic fluid. **DNA** can be extracted from the fetal cells contained in the amniotic fluid and tested. Amniocentesis is performed at 16–18 weeks gestation.

Tissue showing the gene mutation for Rieger syndrome Type I or II obtained from CVS or in amniotic fluid is diagnostic.

### Related disorders

A number of disorders are similar to Rieger syndrome. Comparisons may be useful for a differential diagnosis. These related disorders include:

- Cat-eye syndrome, a rare disorder marked by a cleft along the eyeball affecting the iris, the membrane that covers the white of the eyeball (choroid), and/or the retina and causing a vertical pupil; abnormalities such as small polyps or pits near the front of the outer ear; and absence of the opening, duct, or canal of the anus. Other symptoms may include mild mental deficiency and heart defects.
- Ectodermal dysplasias, a group of hereditary syndromes affecting the skin, its derivatives, and some other organs. Symptoms include predisposition to respiratory infection, eczema, poorly functioning sweat glands, abnormal hair and nails, and difficulties with the nasal passages and ear canals.
- Eye, anterior segment dysgenesis, a rare congenital disorder resulting in abnormal tissue development of the outer eye segment. In less severe cases, the back of the outer surface of the cornea is nontransparent (embryotoxin). Symptoms include ocular abnormalities and malformations of the teeth, abdominal wall, skeleton, and heart.

It is generally thought that Axenfeld anomaly, marked by defects limited to the outer part of the field of vision of the eye, should not be considered a separate entity of Rieger syndrome.

## Treatment and management

A physician familiar with the range of problems seen in individuals with Rieger syndrome is important for appropriate health supervision. Treatment should include assistance finding support resources for the family and the individual with Rieger syndrome.

Treatment of Rieger syndrome is focused on treating the symptoms expressed. Depending on what they are, these treatments may include:

- How do the two types of Rieger syndrome differ from each other?
- Are prenatal tests for Rieger syndrome recommended? Why or why not?
- What are the most serious medical complications associated with Rieger syndrome?
- How should the medical progress of a child with Rieger syndrome be monitored throughout his or her life?

- Drug therapy for glaucoma, usually a topical beta blocker in the form of eye drops. Laser surgery may be performed on those patients in whom the pressure in the eye is not relieved by medications.
- Prostheses (false teeth) or other orthodontic interventions for dental malformations.
- Other surgical management of congenital anomalies includes repair of an umbilical hernia that does not close by itself and plastic surgery for craniofacial abnormalities.

### Prognosis

Prognosis depends upon the severity of the disease. Eye defects may lead to severly impaired vision or blindness. Rieger syndrome does not generally lead to a shortened life span.

### Resources

#### BOOKS

Jorde, Lynn B., et al., eds. *Medical Genetics*. 2nd ed. St. Louis: Mosby, 1999.

#### PERIODICALS

Alward, W. L. "Axenfeld-Rieger syndrome in the age of molecular genetics." *American Journal of Ophthalmology* 130 (2000): 107–15.

Amendt, B. A., E. V. Semina, and W. L. Alward. "Rieger syndrome: a clinical, molecular, and biochemical analysis." *Cellular and Molecular Life Sciences* 11 (2000): 1652–66.

Craig, J. E., and D. A. Mackey. "Glaucoma genetics: Where are we? Where will we go?" *Current Opinions in Ophthalmology* 10 (1999): 126–34.

#### OTHER

*OMIM—Online Mendelian Inheritance in Man.*http:// www.ncbi.nlm.nih.gov:80/entrez/query.fcgi?db= OMIM

*Rarelinks*: A site for parents and caregivers dealing with Rieger syndrome. http://rarelinks4parents.homestead. com/index.html

#### ORGANIZATIONS

Blind Children's Fund. 4740 Okemos Rd., Okemos, MI 48864-1637. (517) 347-1357. http:// www.blindchildrensfund.org.

National Association for Parents of the Visually Impaired. PO Box 317, Watertown, MA 02472. (617) 972-7441 or (800) 562-6265. http://www.spedex.com/napvi.

National Association for Visually Handicapped. 22 West 21st Street, New York, NY 10010. (212) 889-3141. http://www.navh.org.

National Eye Institute. Bldg. 31 Rm 6A32, 31 Center Dr., MSC 2510, Bethesda, MD 20892-2510. (301) 496-5248. 2020@nei.nih.gov. http://www.nei.nih.gov.

National Foundation for Ectodermal Dysplasias. PO Box 114, 410 East Main St., Mascoutah, IL 62258-0114. (618) 566-2020. Fax: (618) 566-4718. http://www.nfed. org.

National Organization for Rare Disorders (NORD). PO Box 8923, New Fairfield, CT 06812-8923. (203) 746-6518 or (800) 999-6673. Fax: (203) 746-6481. http:// www.rarediseases.org.

Vision Community Services. 23 A Elm St., Watertown, MA 02472. (617) 926-4232 or (800) 852-3029. http://www. mablind.org.

Jennifer F. Wilson, MS

Riley-Day syndrome *see* **Familial dysautonomia**

# RNA (Ribonucleic acid)

Ribonucleic acid (RNA) conveys genetic information and catalyzes important biochemical reactions. Similar, but not identical, to a single strand of **deoxyribonucleic acid (DNA)**, in some lower organisms, RNA replaces DNA as the genetic material. As with DNA, RNA follows specific base pairing rules, except that in RNA the base uracil replaces the base thymine (i.e., instead of an adenine-thymine or A-T pairing, there is an adenine-uracil or A-U pairing). Accordingly, when RNA acts as a carrier of genetic information, uracil replaces thymine in the genetic code.

In humans, messenger RNA (mRNA) is the product of transcription and acts to convey genetic information from the nucleus to the protein assembly complex at the ribosome. The ribosome is composed of ribosomal RNA (rRNA) and other proteins. Transfer RNAs (tRNA) act to catalyze the translation process by acting

**The molecular structure of RNA.** *(Gale, a part of Cengage Learning.)*

as carriers of specific amino acids. Because tRNAs bind to specific sites on the strand of mRNA, the sequence of amino acids subsequently inserted into the synthesized protein is both specific and genetically determined by the nucleotide sequence in DNA from which the mRNA strand was originally transcribed.

Other forms of RNA perform important roles in other biochemical reactions. Regardless of function, RNA is a biopolymer made up of ribonucleotide units and is present in all living cells and some viruses. The chemical units of RNA are ribonucleotide monomers consisting of a ribose sugar ($C_5H_{10}O_5$) phosphorylated at the third carbon ($C3$) and linked to one of four bases through a type of chemical linkage formed between a sugar and a base by a condensation reaction (glycosidic bond). The four bases found in RNA are adenine (A), guanine (G), cytosine (C), and uracil (U). Other bases may also be found, although they are generally modified versions of these four (e.g., methylated bases are found in parts of tRNA).

The single nucleotides (monomers) of RNA form a linear chain by linking their phosphate groups and sugars in phosphodiester bonds. RNA does not form a double stranded alpha-helix as does DNA. In some parts of the RNA molecule, there is folding into alpha-helical-like regions. Corresponding to their unique functions, messenger RNA (mRNA), ribosomal RNA (rRNA), and transfer RNA (tRNA) all have different three-dimensional structures. In higher eukaryotic organisms, different RNAs are found distributed throughout the cell—in the nucleus, cytoplasm, and also in cytoplasmic organelles such as mitochondria and, in plants, chloroplasts.

The nucleus is the chief site of RNA synthesis and the source of all cytoplasmic RNA, while mitochondria and chloroplasts synthesize their RNA from their own DNA. rRNA is synthesized by the nucleoli within the nucleus, while the high molecular weight precursor to cytoplasmic mRNA, sometimes termed heterogeneous nuclear or hnRNA, is transcribed on the DNA chromatin. Low molecular weight RNA also occurs in the nucleus and consists partly of tRNA and partly of RNA, which has a regulatory function in gene activation. The cytoplasm contains tRNA and rRNA in the ribosomes and mRNA in polysomes, or polyribosomes. The latter are the structural units of protein biosynthesis, consisting of several ribosomes attached to a strand of mRNA.

The function of mRNA is to transcribe the information held in DNA. In the cells of eukaryotic organisms, the first transcriptional product is the long, heterogenous nuclear RNA, or hnRNA. This contains both the nucleotide sequences eventually transcribed into polypeptides and large tracts of sequences not translated. Non-translated sequences are termed introns (or intervening sequences). Removal of introns, and other untranslated portions of the molecule, edits hnRNA into mRNA molecules. After editing removes as much as 90% of hnRNA, the resulting mRNA molecules are transported into the cytoplasm.

rRNA is located within ribosomes, the sites of protein biosynthesis. Ribosomes are large ellipsoid cytoplasmic organelles consisting of RNA and protein.

tRNA, the smallest known functional RNA, is essential for protein biosynthesis. Its purpose is to transfer a specific amino acid from the cytoplasm and incorporate it into the growing polypeptide chain on the polysome. Different tRNAs contain between 70 and 85 nucleotides. The most characteristic feature of tRNA is that it contains the anticodon, a sequence of three nucleotides specific for the mRNA codon sequence. There is at least one tRNA per cell bearing the anticodon for each of the 20 amino acids. The aminoacyl-tRNA (the tRNA carrying the amino acid) binds to the large subunit of a ribosome, where antiparallel base-pairing occurs between the anticodon of the tRNA and the complementary codon of the associated mRNA. The specificity of this base pairing ensures that the amino acid inserts into the correct position in the growing protein polypeptide chain. During translation, the deacylated tRNA (i.e., with its amino acid removed) is released from the ribosome and becomes available once again for recharging with its amino acid.

DNA-dependent RNA synthesis is the process of RNA sythesis on a template of DNA. According to the rules of base pairing, the base sequence of DNA determines the synthesis of a complementary base sequence in RNA. Assisted (catalyzed) by the enzyme RNA polymerase, the growing RNA chain releases from the template so that the process can start again, even before the previous molecule is complete. Termination codons and a termination factor known as rho-factor end the synthesis process. In certain viruses, RNA-dependent RNA synthesis occurs, with the viral RNA acting as a template for the synthesis of new RNA.

Judyth Sassoon, ARCS, PhD

# Roberts SC phocomelia

## Definition

Roberts SC phocomelia is a rare genetic condition that causes severe abnormalities in arm and leg bones. Other abnormalities, such as mental retardation, may also be present.

## Description

Roberts SC phocomelia was first described in the year 1919. In the past, Roberts SC phocomelia syndrome was described as two separate syndromes: Roberts syndrome, and SC or pseudo-thalidomide syndrome. More recent examination, however, indicated that they are the same disorder. The term "pseudo-thalidomide" was originally used to describe individuals with limb shortening, as the medication thalidomide is known to cause limb abnormalities in the babies of women taking it during pregnancy.

Phocomelia is a condition in which the hands and feet are present, but the arms and legs are absent. The hands and feet are attached directly to the body. Usually there is greater shortening in the arms than in the legs. People with Roberts SC phocomelia syndrome have varying degrees of hypomelia, which means that the limbs are not fully developed. Some are born without the upper bones of the arms or the legs. This is referred to as tetraphocomelia. Some people, though, have a less severe form of limb shortening.

In addition to the limb abnormalities, 80% of individuals with the syndrome have a small head (**microcephaly**). In addition, most people with the syndrome have some degree of mental retardation. Most also have facial problems affecting the development of the upper lip (**cleft lip**) and incomplete development of the palate (the roof of the mouth).

## Genetic profile

Roberts SC phocomelia is inherited in an autosomal recessive fashion. This is a pattern in which the child receives one nonfunctioning (abnormal) **gene** from each parent. When a woman and man who both carry one abnormal gene for Roberts SC phocomelia have children, there is a 25% chance that they will each pass along the gene for the syndrome. People who are termed "carriers" are not affected by the disorder, as they have only one copy of the gene that causes Roberts SC phocomelia. The chances are 50% that they will have a child who is also a carrier of the disorder. The chances are

25% that they will have a baby who is neither a carrier nor affected with Roberts SC phocomelia.

The specific gene that causes the syndrome is not yet known, and there is no direct genetic test to identify a potential carrier of the disease.

In many of the individuals who have been diagnosed with Roberts SC phocomelia, a unique feature may be observed on some of their chromosomes. The exact association of this unusual observation with the syndrome is not yet understood.

## Demographics

The exact number of people with the syndrome is not known, as some infants who die before or shortly after birth are never diagnosed or are diagnosed incorrectly. The syndrome affects males and females equally. There is no specific country or region of the world where the disorder is more common.

## Signs and symptoms

In the bones of the lower arm (radius and ulna), limb shortening or absence of limbs is evident in approximately 97% of people with the syndrome. The upper arm (humerus) is affected 77% of the time. A missing or shortened thighbone (femur) occurs in about 65% of affected individuals. The bones in the lower leg (tibia and fibula) are shortened or absent in 77% of those with the disorder.

It is often very hard to flex or bend the knees, ankles, wrists, and/or elbows. While the feet and hands are almost always present, there may be fewer than normal fingers and toes, or shortened fingers. Sometimes the fingers are fused together (syndactyly).

People with the syndrome are smaller than other babies the same age, both before and after birth. Babies with Roberts SC phocomelia syndrome may have thin hair that is often described as silvery in color. In addition, most people with Roberts SC phocomelia syndrome are born with a cleft lip (a failure of the upper lip to close completely) and **cleft palate** (an opening in the roof of the mouth). Other abnormalities that may occur include a small and underdeveloped chin, a short neck, heart and kidney problems, prominent and widely spaced eyes, and unusually shaped ears.

### Diagnosis

This disorder has been diagnosed during pregnancy at 12 weeks, through a test called an ultrasound evaluation. In these incidences, developmental problems with the growth and formation of both the arms and legs were noted. Sometimes the syndrome cannot be diagnosed by ultrasound until later in the pregnancy, when the limb shortening or absence becomes more obvious, and sometimes it cannot be diagnosed by ultrasound at all. Other abnormalities that might be seen by ultrasound include cleft lip, increased distance between the eye sockets, and extra fluid in some of the structures of the brain (**hydrocephalus**). Excess amniotic fluid levels, kidney problems, and an opening in the spine (**spina bifida**) have also been found. However, an exact diagnosis of the syndrome cannot be made by ultrasound evaluation alone.

Checking for the unusual **chromosome** feature is done through **amniocentesis**, a procedure that collects the developing fetus's cells for evaluation. But this test is not typically recommended, because not all affected individuals have this chromosome finding. In addition, the chromosome is not always evident in the cells from the amniotic fluid.

As of 2009 there was no accurate prenatal test to diagnose the syndrome during pregnancy.

After a baby is born with characteristics of Roberts SC phocomelia syndrome, a diagnosis can be made through a complete physical examination. In addition, analysis of the baby's chromosomes may also be useful. The chromosomes can be analyzed through a blood or tissue sample.

---

### QUESTIONS TO ASK YOUR DOCTOR

- What are the usual signs and symptoms associated with Roberts SC phocomelia syndrome?
- Please explain the meaning of the term "phocomelia."
- Are there prenatal tests of Roberts SC phocomelia syndrome, and under what circumstances would they be recommended?
- What is the progress for a child diagnosed with Roberts SC phocomelia syndrome?

---

### Treatment and management

At this time there is no treatment available for individuals with Roberts SC phocomelia syndrome. The shortness or absence of limbs makes it difficult for any type of limb-lengthening therapies to be useful in most instances.

### Prognosis

The majority of severely affected individuals will die in the womb, or during or shortly after birth. Those who survive will have very obvious growth deficiency as well as mental retardation. Babies who are not as severely affected, with less dramatic limb shortening and no facial cleft, have a better overall prognosis.

### Resources

#### BOOKS

Fleischer, A., et al. *Sonography in Obstetrics and Gynecology, Principles & Practice*. Stamford: 1996.

Jones, Kenneth. *Smith's Recognizable Patterns of Human Malformations*. 5th ed. Philadelphia: W.B. Saunders Company, 1997.

#### PERIODICALS

Camlibel, T. "Roberts SC Phocomelia with Isolated Cleft Palate, Thrombocytopenia, and Eosinophilia." *Genetic Counseling* 10, no. 2 (1999): 157-61.

McDaniel, L. D. "Novel Assay for Roberts Syndrome Assigns Variable Phenotypes to One Complementation Group." *American Journal of Medical Genetics* 93, no. 3 (2000): 223-9.

#### WEBSITES

"Entry 268300: Roberts syndrome; RBS." *Online Mendelian Inheritance in Man*.http://www.ncbi.nlm.nih.gov/htbin-post/Omim/dispmim?268300 .

"Limb Anomalies." *University of Kansas Medical Center*. http://www.kumc.edu/gec/support/limb.html.

Katherine Susan Hunt, MS

Roberts syndrome *see* **Roberts SC phocomelia**

Robin sequence *see* **Pierre-Robin sequence**

Robinow-Silverman-Smith syndrome *see* **Robinow syndrome**

Robinow-Sorauf syndrome *see* **Saethre-Chotzen syndrome**

Robinow dwarfism *see* **Robinow syndrome**

# Robinow syndrome

## Definition

Robinow syndrome encompasses two different hereditary disorders, both rare, with a similar pattern of physical abnormalities. Typical features of these conditions include mild to moderate short stature, distinctive facial features, skeletal abnormalities, and abnormal development of the genitalia.

## Description

A family that included several individuals with a characteristic pattern of facial features, accompanied by short stature (dwarfism), skeletal abnormalities, and underdevelopment (hypoplasia) of the external genitalia (sex organs) was first described in 1969 by Dr. Meinhard Robinow. He named the condition "Fetal face syndrome," because the facial features are similar to those of a normal fetus. Only later was Dr. Robinow's name used to identify the syndrome. Other names for the condition include Robinow dwarfism, as well as "acral dysostosis with facial and genital abnormalities."

Skeletal abnormalities of varying types and severity occur in every case of Robinow syndrome. Most people with the condition have abnormal development of specific bones of the arms and legs resulting in some degree of short stature. Spinal abnormalities are also common. Most females are fertile, but only a few males with the condition have had children.

## Genetic profile

Chromosomes are the microscopic structures inside cells that carry the genes. Each cell of the body contains 46 chromosomes in 23 pairs. The exceptions are sperm and eggs, which normally carry 23 chromosomes—one of each pair. The first 22 pairs of chromosomes in humans are known as the autosomes. An inherited condition is autosomal if the abnormal gene that causes it resides on one of the first 22 pairs of chromosomes.

Several years after Dr. Robinow's first report, it became clear that some families affected by Robinow syndrome have an autosomal dominant pattern of **inheritance**, while in other families the syndrome is inherited as an autosomal recessive trait. As of 2009, the reason for this genetic discrepancy was unknown.

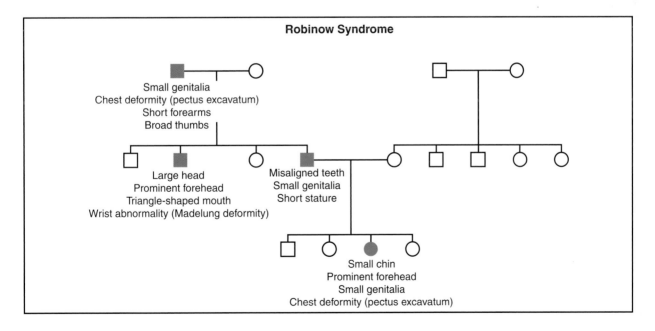

**Robinow Syndrome**

Small genitalia
Chest deformity (pectus excavatum)
Short forearms
Broad thumbs

Large head
Prominent forehead
Triangle-shaped mouth
Wrist abnormality (Madelung deformity)

Misaligned teeth
Small genitalia
Short stature

Small chin
Prominent forehead
Small genitalia
Chest deformity (pectus excavatum)

*(Gale, a part of Cengage Learning.)*

## KEY TERMS

**Acromelic**—The anatomical term used to denote the end of a limb (arm or leg). In the context of Robinow syndrome, it refers to bones of the hands and feet.

**Brachymelia**—A general medical term used to describe short limbs.

**Hypertelorism**—A wider-than-normal space between the eyes.

**Hypoplasia**—Incomplete or underdevelopment of a tissue or organ.

**Mesomelic**—The anatomical term used to describe the middle of a limb. The bones that constitute the middle of the arm are the radius and ulna, and mesomelic bones of the leg are the tibia and fibula.

**Vertebra**—One of the 23 bones which comprise the spine. *Vertebrae* is the plural form.

Dominant inheritance means that an error in only one gene of a pair is enough to produce symptoms of the disorder. In other words, the abnormally functioning gene of the pair is dominant over the normal gene. A person who carries the gene for autosomal dominant Robinow syndrome has a 50% chance of passing it on to each of his or her offspring.

In autosomal recessive inheritance, a person must have errors in both copies of a gene pair in order to be affected. Someone who carries just one copy of the disease gene has another normally functioning gene of that pair to compensate for it. Therefore, a carrier of a single recessive gene typically shows no symptoms of the disorder. If two people who both carry the gene for recessive Robinow syndrome conceive a pregnancy, there is a 25% chance that they will each contribute the Robinow syndrome gene and have an affected child.

Mutations in the ROR2 gene are responsible for recessive Robinow syndrome. As of 2009, the exact function of the protein encoded by the ROR2 gene had not been determined, and the gene responsible for dominant Robinow syndrome had not been located.

### Demographics

Both the dominant and recessive forms of Robinow syndrome are rare. Dominant Robinow syndrome does not appear to occur more frequently in any particular ethnic group. A significant proportion of recessive Robinow syndrome cases, however, have occurred in

Czechoslovakia, Turkey, and the Middle East. In addition, some children with recessive Robinow syndrome have parents who are genetically related (consanguineous), such as first cousins. Parental consanguinity is sometimes seen in rare, autosomal recessive conditions, since people who are genetically related are more likely to carry the same recessive gene(s).

### Signs and symptoms

The signs and symptoms of Robinow syndrome can be grouped into those that involve the face, those that affect the skeleton, and those affecting the genitalia. There is a good deal of overlap of symptoms between the dominant and recessive forms. In general, however, people with recessive Robinow syndrome tend to be more severely affected.

The facial features of Robinow syndrome include a flat nasal bridge, slightly upturned nose, triangular-shaped mouth, protruding forehead (frontal bossing), wide space between the eyes (hypertelorism), wide eye openings, low-set ears, long philtrum (groove from nose to upper lip), small lower jaw (micrognathia), excessive growth of the gums, and crowding of teeth.

People with Robinow syndrome have what is known as acromesomelic brachymelia. Acromesomelic refers to bones at the end (acro) and in the middle (meso) of the limbs. Brachymelia is the medical term for short limbs. Thus, short limbs in Robinow syndrome are due to shortened bones in the hands, feet, lower arms, and lower legs. Dominant Robinow syndrome is associated with normal height to borderline short stature, while recessive Robinow syndrome always results in short stature. Abnormalities of the spine often involve misshapen or fused vertebrae (so-called segmentation defects), as well as **scoliosis**. Vertebral abnormalities are more frequent and more pronounced in the recessive form of Robinow syndrome. Ribs may be fused together or abnormally shaped, and this may lead to pectus excavatum (sunken breastbone).

Males with Robinow syndrome typically have a hypoplastic penis, and may have undescended testicles (cryptorchidism). Females can have a small clitoris and hypoplastic labia. A dysfunctional sex-steroid response-and-feedback mechanism may be partly to blame for some of the signs of Robinow syndrome, particularly the genital anomalies.

Physical anomalies found less frequently in Robinow syndrome include heart defects, kidney abnormalities, cleft lip/palate, and hearing loss. Most individuals with Robinow syndrome have normal intelligence, but a few have mild mental retardation.

### Diagnosis

The diagnosis of Robinow syndrome is made by physical examination. Several other genetic syndromes have some of the same physical signs as Robinow syndrome, which can make arriving at the correct diagnosis more difficult. However, the pattern of skeletal abnormalities in Robinow syndrome has a distinct appearance when seen on x rays, which may help in confirming the diagnosis. Testing of the ROR2 gene is theoretically possible for recessive Robinow syndrome, but would only be offered on a research basis, if at all. As of 2000, there were no laboratory tests available to aid in the diagnosis of dominant Robinow syndrome.

### Treatment and management

There is no cure for either type of Robinow syndrome. Future research may help to determine if some type of hormone therapy can be used to treat the short stature and/or hypoplastic genitalia. Otherwise, no specific protocol is recommended for managing children and adults with either form of the condition. An orthopedic surgeon might be needed to address any problems that arise related to skeletal abnormalities, especially in the spine. Special educational intervention would be indicated for anyone with learning disabilities or mental retardation.

People with pronounced physical signs of the condition (short stature and facial features) may have difficulties with their self-image. Males with a hypoplastic penis can present a special problem. In those cases, added psychological and social support is particularly important. **Genetic counseling** should be offered to individuals/families affected by Robinow syndrome to help them understand the condition, its inheritance, and any testing (including prenatal) that might be available.

### Prognosis

Any one person with Robinow syndrome may have a good prognosis, depending on how well they cope with their particular symptoms. A child with recessive Robinow syndrome is more likely to have long-term difficulties than a child with the dominant form of the condition, but no blanket statements can be made. Overall, life span should not be significantly decreased in most cases of Robinow syndrome, since the majority of affected individuals do not have life-threatening complications.

### Resources

**BOOKS**

Jones, Kenneth Lyons. *Smith's Recognizable Patterns of Human Malformation*. 5th ed. Philadelphia: W.B. Saunders Company, 1997.

**OTHER**

"Robinow syndrome." National Library of Medicine (NLM). *MedlinePlus*. http://medlineplus.nlm.nih.gov/mesh/jablonski/syndromes/syndrome_cgi?index = 562.htm.

**ORGANIZATIONS**

Robinow Syndrome Foundation. PO Box 1072, Anoka, MN 55303. (612) 434-1152. http://www.robinow.org.

Scott J. Polzin, MS

Romano-Ward syndrome *see* **Long-QT syndrome**

# Rothmund-Thomson syndrome

### Definition

Rothmund-Thomson syndrome (RTS) is an extremely rare inherited disorder that appears in infancy and features skin degeneration (atrophic dermatosis), clouding of the lenses of the eyes (juvenile cataracts), skeletal abnormalities, short stature, and an increased risk of skin and bone cancers.

### Description

Rothmund-Thomson syndrome is usually first apparent between three and six months of age. This

## KEY TERMS

**Alopecia**—Loss of hair or baldness.

**Atrophic dermatosis**—Wasting away of the skin.

**Depigmentation**—Loss of pigment or skin color.

**Dysplastic**—The abnormal growth or development of a tissue or organ.

**Edema**—Extreme amount of watery fluid that causes swelling of the affected tissue.

**Frontal bossing**—A term used to describe a rounded forehead with a receded hairline.

**Hyperpigmentation**—An abnormal condition characterized by an excess of melanin in localized areas of the skin, which produces areas that are much darker than the surrounding unaffected skin.

**Hypogonadism**—Small testes in men and scarce or irregular menstruation for females.

**Keratosis**—A raised thickening of the outer horny layer of the skin.

**Microdontia**—Small teeth.

**Poikiloderma**—A condition characterized by skin atrophy, widening of the small blood vessels (telangiectasia), and pigment changes giving a mottled appearance.

**Prognathism**—A protruding lower jaw.

**Saddle nose**—A sunken nasal bridge.

**Telangiectasia**—An abnormal widening of groups of small blood vessels in the skin.

disorder is characterized by early sun sensitivity and progressive degeneration or wasting (atrophy) of the skin as well as scarring and abnormal pigmentation of the skin. Other characteristic signs include sparse hair, clouding of the lenses of the eyes (juvenile cataracts), short stature, malformations of the face and head, teeth, nails, and bone, and other physical abnormalities. In rare cases, mental retardation may be present.

The syndrome was first described in 1868 by August von Rothmund, a German ophthalmologist, and in both 1923 and 1936 by Matthew S. Thomson, a British dermatologist. Both independently noted a familial disorder with cataracts, saddle nose, and skin degeneration. It is believed that Thomson's finding was the same disease that was seen long before by Rothmund. Other names for Rothmund-Thomson syndrome include poikiloderma congenita and poikiloderma atrophicans with cataract.

### Genetic profile

Rothmund-Thomson is attributed to a mutation in a **gene** located on **chromosome** 8. Mutations in the gene RecQL4 (chromosomal locus 8q24) also called the Rothmund-Thomson gene, have been identified in four patients with Rothmund-Thomson syndrome.

Rothmund-Thomson syndrome is inherited as an autosomal recessive trait. This means that both parents have one copy of the Rothmund-Thomson gene but do not have the disease. Each of their children has a 25% chance of not having the gene, a 50% chance of having one Rothmund-Thomson gene (and, like the parents, being unaffected), and a 25% risk of having both Rothmund-Thomson genes and the disease.

### Demographics

There is no specific population group that is at greater risk for this disorder, although it is more common in women (2:1). Evidence of Rothmund-Thomson syndrome has been found to occur in all races and many nationalities. The majority of affected people are from full-term pregnancies. As of the year 2001, a total of approximately 250 cases have been reported in English-speaking medical literature. The number of carriers for Rothmund-Thomson syndrome is unknown.

### Signs and symptoms

The major characteristics of Rothmund-Thomson syndrome are skin abnormalities, short stature, juvenile cataracts, small hands, and delayed activities of the ovaries in females or testes in males. Symptoms vary from individual to individual.

Skin abnormalities usually appear in infancy, between three and six months of age. Skin changes begin as red inflamed patches, occasionally with blistering, on the cheeks along with swelling and then spread to other areas of the face, the arms and legs, and buttocks. Skin inflammation eventually subsides and a condition develops known as poikiloderma, characterized by abnormal widening (dilation) of groups of small blood vessels (telangiectasia), skin tissue degradation (atrophy), and patchy areas of abnormally decreased and/or unusually increased brown pigmentation (depigmentation and hyperpigmentation), giving the skin a mottled look. Skin that is exposed to the sun usually shows greater abnormalities. Sun sensitivity typically continues throughout the affected person's life. Those with extreme sun sensitivity can develop thickening of the skin (keratosis) of the face, hands, and feet, or cancerous skin changes later in life. Affected individuals are at increased risk of developing skin cancers (basal cell carcinoma and squamous cell carcinoma) and bone **cancer (osteosarcoma)**.

There are many other physical abnormalities that affect people with Rothmund-Thomson syndrome. Juvenile cataracts, the clouding of the lenses of the eyes, develop in almost half of the people with RTS between the ages of four and seven. Severe growth delays result in short stature throughout life. Skeletal abnormalities such as unusually small hands and feet are common. Less typical are stubby fingers and toes, underdeveloped (hypoplastic) or absent thumbs, and/ or underdeveloped (hypoplastic) or missing forearm bones (ulna and radii). Hypogonadism, the deficient activity of the ovaries in females or testes in males, causes irregular menstruation in females, and delayed sexual development and reduced fertility in both males and females. Facial skeletal abnormalities include a triangular-shaped face with a prominent forehead (frontal bossing), a sunken nasal bridge (saddle nose), and a protruding lower jaw (prognathism). Scalp hair is usually thin and fine, although alopecia (balding) occasionally occurs in early childhood. Often the eyebrows and eyelashes are sparse or absent. Dental abnormalities include excessive cavities, unusually small teeth (microdontia), or delayed or failure of teeth to erupt. Dysplastic, or abnormally developed nails are also seen in many people with Rothmund-Thomson syndrome.

## Diagnosis

A diagnosis of Rothmund-Thomson syndrome is made based on clinical examination. There are no laboratory diagnostic tests. Mutations of the RecQL4 gene have been found in a few individuals with RTS. However, as of the year 2009, **genetic testing** is still on a research basis and is not available for diagnostic purposes.

There are no published diagnostic criteria. Diagnosis is usually based on the presence of the characteristic poikilodermatous rash in childhood, along with one or more of the following features: small stature, sparse or absent hair, cataracts, cancer.

## Treatment and management

Essential management of Rothmund-Thomson syndrome includes avoiding sun exposure and diligently using sunscreen that has both UVA and UVB protection.

---

## QUESTIONS TO ASK YOUR DOCTOR

- At what age can Rothmund-Thomson syndrome be diagnosed, and how is that diagnosis made?
- How common is Rothmund-Thomson syndrome, and are there certain populations at greater risk for the disease than the general public?
- What types of treatment are recommended for Rothmund-Thomson syndrome, and what risks are associated with each kind of treatment?
- What is the prognosis for an infant diagnosed with Rothmund-Thomson syndrome?

---

An ophthalmologic evaluation for the detection and management of cataracts is recommended for affected people on an annual basis up to age 15. Surgical removal of significant cataracts may be necessary.

Because skin cancer is a risk, it is important to monitor the affected individual closely for lesions with unusual color or texture. They should also be watched carefully for any signs and symptoms of osteosarcoma, a cancerous bone tumor, including bone pain, swelling, or a growing lesion on the arms or legs.

Pulsed-dye laser therapy has been used to treat the widening of small blood vessels (telangiectases). Medications called retinoids can reduce the potential for skin cancer. Keratolytic drugs are used to cause thick skin to swell, soften, and then fall away.

## Prognosis

Individuals with Rothmund-Thomson syndrome usually have a normal life span, although an increased risk for bone and skin cancer has been found. Most affected individuals will have normal intelligence, however learning disabilities and mental retardation have been reported in a small number of patients.

### Resources

**PERIODICALS**

Hall, Judith G., et al. "Rothmund-Thomson Syndrome with Severe Dwarfism." *American Journal of Diseases of Children* 134 (1980): 165–169.

Starr D. G., et al. "Non-Dermatological Complications and Genetic Aspects of the Rothmund-Thomson Syndrome." *Clinical Genetics* 27 (1985): 102–104.

**ORGANIZATIONS**

National Organization for Rare Disorders (NORD). PO Box 8923, New Fairfield, CT 06812-8923. (203)

746-6518 or (800) 999-6673. Fax: (203) 746-6481. http://www.rarediseases.org.

**WEBSITES**

Plon, Sharon E., MD, PhD, and Lisa L. Wang, MD. (October 6, 1999). "Rothmund-Thomson syndrome." *GeneClinics*. University of Washington, Seattle. http://www.geneclinics.org/profiles/rts.

Nina B. Sherak, MS, CHES

RSH syndrome *see* **Smith-Lemli-Opitz syndrome**

RSH/SLO syndrome *see* **Smith-Lemli-Opitz syndrome**

# Rubinstein-Taybi syndrome

## Definition

Rubinstein-Taybi syndrome is a rare genetic disorder involving mental retardation, short stature, broad thumbs and great toes, and characteristic facial features. First described in 1963 by the American physicians Dr. Jack Rubinstein and Dr. Hooshang Taybi, over 550 cases have since been reported.

## Description

The clinical picture of Rubinstein-Taybi syndrome (RSTS) is highly variable. The most prominent features include mental retardation, thumb and great toe abnormalities, and distinct facial characteristics.

Rubinstein-Taybi syndrome may also be referred to as broad-thumb-hallux syndrome or Rubinstein syndrome. The abbreviation for Rubinstein-Taybi syndrome is denoted "RSTS" or "RTS," although "RSTS" is preferred so as not to be confused with other syndromes such as **Rett syndrome** and Rothmund-Thompson syndrome.

## Genetic profile

A change in a particular **gene**, known as the CREB binding protein (CBP) gene, causes RSTS. This gene is located on **chromosome** 16. Its position is denoted as 16p13.3 where p represents the short arm of the chromosome and 13.3 indicates the exact location on the arm.

CBP codes for a protein known as the human cyclic AMP regulated enhancer binding protein

(CREBBP). CREBBP has many functions within a cell. Its general role is to regulate multiple pathways and the work of other genes. It is thought that this multifunctional aspect of CREBBP is what causes the diffuse abnormalities observed in RSTS.

RSTS is thought to be autosomal dominant. Only one copy of the CBP gene must be changed or mutated for a person to have RSTS. Most cases of RSTS are sporadic. That is, the majority of affected individuals do not have a parent with RSTS, rather RSTS arose due to a new mutation in the CBP gene. Sporadic mutations in genes occur by chance. They are rare and there is nothing a person can do during a pregnancy to cause or prevent them.

## Demographics

The incidence of RSTS has been estimated at between one in 125,000 and one in 300,000 live births. Males and females are affected equally. Cases of RSTS have been observed throughout the world. Although RSTS is thought to be a rare disease, more cases are being diagnosed each year. In part, this is thought to be due to physicians' increasing awareness of the signs and symptoms involved in RSTS.

## Signs and symptoms

RSTS is a genetic disorder involving primarily physical malformations and mental retardation.

Babies with RSTS may be born small compared to other newborns. They often have trouble feeding and may need to be assisted in this area. In conjunction with feeding problems, there may be respiratory (breathing) difficulties.

As the child matures, growth remains delayed, with short stature persistent throughout life. An average height of 60 in (153 cm) in males and 58 in (147 cm) in females and an average weight of 106 lb (48 kg) in males and 120 lb (55 kg) in females has been reported.

Developmental milestones are usually delayed. Although most children with RSTS learn to walk and talk, they tend to develop these skills much later than their peers. For example, the average age at which children with RSTS learn to walk is 30 months, compared to 12 months in unaffected children.

There are several unique physical characteristics associated with RSTS. Typical facial features include down-slanting eyes, beaked nose, and the fleshy septum of the nose extending beyond the nostrils. By two to three years of age, most affected children grow into what is considered the classic physical picture of RSTS. Because of their similar facial appearances, they may resemble other children with RSTS as much as or more than they resemble family members.

The most well known features of patients with RSTS are the broad thumbs and great toes (halluces). This finding may be observed at birth although some patients with RSTS have only broad thumbs, only broad toes, or neither.

Other findings that occur on a less frequent basis include malignant (cancerous) and benign (non-cancerous) tumors, chronic ear infections, early onset of breast development in females, kidney abnormalities, high arched palate (roof of the mouth), malformed teeth (named talon cusps after their shape), heart defects, small head, and short upper lip with a pouting bottom lip.

Mental retardation of varying degrees is a constant in RSTS. Affected individuals may present mild to severe mental retardation. They have particular difficulty in expression through speech. Although affected individuals are usually able to understand what is spoken to them, they have a difficult time responding with spoken words. In general, it has been observed that many patients with RSTS do not progress beyond a first-grade level.

It has been noted that affected individuals tend to have happy, outgoing, and energetic personalities. They have been described as people who "know no strangers." People with RSTS tend to smile often, although, due to their physical differences, this smile is sometimes described as a grimace.

Not every person with RSTS will have all of the aforementioned medical, physical, and social characteristics. Although people with RSTS have much in common, it is important to remember that each person is unique with his or her own qualities and challenges.

## Diagnosis

Diagnosis is usually based on clinical findings. Laboratory techniques for definitive diagnosis by **DNA** analysis are available, but at this time are only able to identify approximately 25% of affected individuals. This is due to the considerable number of different changes within the same gene that all may lead to RSTS.

Prenatal diagnosis is available for RSTS; however, again, only approximately 25% of cases are picked up by current available techniques. Because the physical features associated with RSTS are difficult to distinguish prenatally, and the available DNA test does not identify most cases, the vast majority of individuals with RSTS are diagnosed after birth.

The age at which a person is diagnosed varies from patient to patient due to the range in severity of clinical findings. Those with a more mild presentation tend to be diagnosed later in life. Diagnosis may be more difficult in non-Caucasian persons due to the great majority of research and published data having been done on Caucasian patients.

Studies have been conducted in an effort to better identify individuals with RSTS. In 2000, the outcome of a study aimed at improving laboratory techniques for RSTS diagnosis was published. The data suggested that it soon may be possible to identify more affected individuals by DNA analysis both prenatally (before birth) and postnatally (after birth).

Misdiagnosis is sometimes made between RSTS and **Saethre-Chotzen syndrome** because of their similar clinical findings.

A correct diagnosis is important when providing a family with **genetic counseling**. A family with a child with RSTS can have many questions. Genetic counseling may be helpful in providing the family with some answers, including information about the risk of having another child with RSTS.

In general, a recurrence risk of 0.1% is given to couples that have had one child with RSTS. For individuals with RSTS there is 50% chance of passing the condition on in each pregnancy.

## Treatment and management

Treatment and management is aimed at encouraging and supporting cognitive development and alleviating medical symptoms. There is no cure for Rubinstein-Taybi syndrome.

Medical problems, such as ear and respiratory infections, are treated as they occur. Chronic ear infections may lead to hearing loss and it is therefore important to have this infection treated as quickly as possible.

Early intervention and occupational and physical therapy are encouraged along with behavioral management. It has been shown that children with mental retardation and developmental delay, due to any cause, benefit from these therapies. In particular, for children with RSTS, speech therapy and alternate forms of communication, such as sign language, have been found to be helpful. Alternative avenues of communication may help children with RSTS express their thoughts and feelings and reduce the frustration they may feel at not being understood verbally.

### Prognosis

Prognosis is variable due to the wide range of presentations among affected individuals. Mental retardation and developmental delay may range from mild to severe, with a reported average IQ of 51 (the general population average IQ is 100). Medical problems also vary in number and severity.

Most individuals with RSTS will have a normal life span. As adults, affected individuals may live in group homes or supervised apartments. Many work in sheltered workshops or in supervised employment situations.

Individuals with RSTS are capable of having children of their own. In a study of 502 individuals with RSTS, two had reproduced. In total they had three children, one affected with RSTS and two unaffected. It has also been the case that a very mildly affected woman was not diagnosed with RSTS until her child was born with the same disorder.

### Resources

#### PERIODICALS

Baxter, Garry, and John Beer. "Rubinstein-Taybi Syndrome." *Psychological Reports* 70, no. 2 (April 1992): 451–56.

#### WEBSITES

Online Rubinstein-Taybi Pamphlet. http://www.rubinstein-taybi.org/html/pamplet.html.

Rubinstein-Taybi Website. http://www.rubinstein-taybi.org.

The Arc—A National Organization on Mental Retardation. http://www.thearc.org.

#### ORGANIZATIONS

Rubinstein-Taybi Parent Support Group. c/o Lorrie Baxter, PO Box 146, Smith Center, KS 66967. (888) 447-2989. lbaxter@ruraltelnet. http://www.specialfriends.org.

Java O. Solis, MS

**Rubinstein syndrome** *see* **Rubinstein-Taybi syndrome**

# Russell-Silver syndrome

## Definition

Russell-Silver syndrome (RSS) is one of the recognized forms of intrauterine growth retardation (IUGR) diseases. It was first independently described by H. K. Silver in 1953 and by A. Russell in 1954.

## Description

Russell-Silver syndrome is one of more than 300 recognized forms of **genetic disorders** that lead to short stature. It is characterized by:

- the presence of a triangular shaped face
- an incurving fifth finger (clinodactyly)
- low birth weight and length (intrauterine growth retardation, or IUGR)
- a poor appetite in the first few years of life

This disorder is alternately known as Russell syndrome, Silver syndrome, or Silver-Russell syndrome. Some clinicians use the term Russell syndrome to indicate this disorder when the size of the sides of the body and the limbs are equal, and the term Silver syndrome to indicate this disorder when the size of the sides of the body or the length of the limbs is different (body asymmetry).

## Genetic profile

The exact genetic cause, or causes, of RSS have not been fully identified. It is currently believed that almost

## KEY TERMS

**Body asymmetry**—Abnormal development of the body in which the trunk and/or the limbs are not of equal size from one side of the body to the other.

**Clinodactyly**—An abnormal inward curving of the fingers or toes.

**Delayed bone age**—An abnormal condition in which the apparent age of the bones, as seen in x rays, is less than the chronological age of the patient.

**Hypoglycemia**—An abnormally low glucose (blood sugar) concentration in the blood.

**Intrauterine growth retardation**—A form of growth retardation occurring in the womb that is not caused by premature birth or a shortened gestation time. Individuals affected with this condition are of lower than normal birth weight and lower than normal length after a complete gestation period.

**Precocious puberty**—An abnormal condition in which a person undergoes puberty at a very young age. This condition causes the growth spurt associated with puberty to occur before the systems of the body are ready, which causes these individuals to not attain normal adult heights.

**Russell syndrome**—An alternative term for Russell-Silver syndrome. Many doctors use this term to mean a Russell-Silver syndrome affected individual who does not have body asymmetry.

**Scaphocephaly**—An abnormally long and narrow skull.

**Silver syndrome**—An alternative term for Russell-Silver syndrome. Many doctors use this term to mean an individual with Russell-Silver syndrome who also has body asymmetry.

all cases of RSS are the result of mutations on a gene, or possibly more than one gene, on **chromosome** 7.

### Demographics

RSS occurs in approximately one in every 200,000 live births. Almost all cases of RSS are sporadic, that is, they appear for the first time in individuals with no family history of RSS. However, case studies indicating all three modes of inheritance—autosomal recessive, autosomal dominant, and X-linked—have been reported.

RSS does not appear to affect any particular race or ethnic group in a greater frequency than others. It is also observed equally in males and females.

### Signs and symptoms

There are six characteristics that define Russell-Silver syndrome: a triangular shaped face; down turned corners of the mouth; inwardly curved little fingers (clinodactyly); a combination of low birth weight (intrauterine growth retardation) and short birth length after a full term gestation; a long, narrow head (scaphocephaly); and a poor appetite that causes slow growth after birth. These characteristics are commonly observed in people affected with RSS.

Several other characteristics are found in most, but not all, RSS affected individuals. These include:

- low blood sugar (hypoglycemia) in infancy and early childhood
- unequal body and limb size from one side of the body to the other (body asymmetry)
- late closure of the soft spot in the front of the skull
- a broad forehead
- a small chin and jaw
- crowding of the teeth or abnormally small teeth caused by a smaller than normal jaw
- an abnormally thin upper lip
- low-set, small, and prominent ears
- fusion or webbing of the toes (syndactyly)
- poor muscle tone (hypotonia)
- a condition in which the bones are not as mature as the bones of a typical person of the same age (delayed bone age)
- developmental delays

In males affected with RSS, undescended testicles and a misplacement of the urethral opening (**hypospadias**) on the bottom of the penis rather than on the tip of the glans is often seen.

People affected with RSS may show other symptoms on a less uniform basis. These include:

- water on the brain
- a bluish coloration of the whites of the eyes
- a highly-arched palate
- an absence of certain teeth
- frequent ear infections caused by fluid in the ear, which can lead to temporary hearing loss
- migraine headaches
- a curvature of the spine (scoliosis) or other problems with the spine, often caused by body asymmetry
- abnormalities of the kidneys
- an abnormally early onset of puberty (precocious puberty)

- irregularly colored spots on the skin (café-au-lait spots)
- high energy levels
- attention deficit disorder (ADD)
- fainting spells

## Diagnosis

Diagnosis of RSS is generally accomplished by performing a genetic test on cells grown from a skin sample. This test must be performed prior to the fifth year of life and it is not always accurate.

A diagnosis of RSS is supported by examination of the affected individual's growth curve and daily food intakes. In a child affected with RSS, these will fall well short of the mean for children of the same age.

Body measurements for asymmetry and x rays to determine the bone age versus the actual age of the patient are also useful. Additionally, a blood test indicating hypoglycemia may indicate RSS. When RSS is suspected in males, an examination of the genitals may reveal undescended testicles or a misplacement of the urethral opening.

## Treatment and management

Treatment of RSS varies on a case-by-case basis depending on the symptoms of the affected individual.

Dietary changes to increase food intake are required by all people with RSS. Many patients with RSS also require a diet high in sugars to treat hypoglycemia. When the necessary food intake can not be accomplished by dietary changes, it may be necessary to treat patients with the antihistamine periactin, which also serves as an appetite stimulant. Some patients may also benefit from a feeding pump or gastrostomy. Gastrostomy is a surgical procedure in which a permanent opening is made directly in the stomach for the introduction of food.

In cases of severe growth retardation, certain people will require the administration of an artificial form of growth hormone (recombinant growth hormone) to stimulate growth, increase the rate of growth, and to increase their final adult height.

Ear tubes may be required to improve fluid drainage from the ears of some patients affected with RSS.

In cases of body asymmetry, limb lengthening surgeries may be recommended. Alternatively, shoe lifts may be all that is necessary for the attainment of a normal gait.

Depending on the severity of physical, emotional, and psychological symptoms, some affected individuals may benefit from physical and/or occupational therapy. If ADD or other developmental problems exist, individuals with RSS may require educational assistance, such as remedial reading. In cases where the jaw is extremely small, talking may be difficult. These patients may require speech therapy.

Precocious puberty is the entrance of a child into puberty prior to the age of eight or nine. This early onset of puberty is generally accompanied by a growth spurt prior to puberty. While entering puberty before one is emotionally ready is certainly a serious problem, it is the growth spurt prior to puberty that is of major medical significance and concern.

If this growth spurt occurs prior to puberty, it is generally not as robust as if it had occurred during puberty, which causes the individual undergoing this growth spurt to grow less than a person who undergoes this process during puberty. The result is that a person who undergoes precocious puberty will generally end up much shorter in adulthood than his or her peers.

There are three hormonal therapies available in the United States to treat precocious puberty. Histrelin (trade name: Supprelin) is administered by daily injection. Leuprolide acetate (trade name: Lupron) is available as a depot formulation every four weeks. A depot formulation places medication in a tiny pump that is attached to the patient's body and releases the medication over time. Nafarelin acetate (trade name: Synarel) is administered as a nasal spray three times daily. Because of the age of people being treated, Lupron is most often the medication of choice because it is only administered once a month.

Some doctors have noticed that persons affected with RSS may have a slightly elevated chance of developing Wilm's tumor, the most common form of kidney **cancer**. Most cases of this type of cancer occur before the age of eight, and this condition is extremely rare in adults. It is important that children with RSS be screened with ultrasound every three months until the age of eight to make sure they have not developed Wilm's tumor. Wilm's tumor is quite treatable via surgery, chemotherapy, and/or radiation.

## Prognosis

With proper medical treatment to address their individual symptoms, people affected with RSS do not, in general, have a reduced quality of life relative to the remainder of the population. As these people age, the symptoms of RSS tend to become less noticeable: the triangular shape of the face tends to lessen, muscle tone and coordination improve, appetite

## QUESTIONS TO ASK YOUR DOCTOR

- Please explain the meaning of the expression "intrauterine growth retardation"?
- How I am responsible for my child's having Russell-Silver syndrome?
- What kinds of treatment will my child need because of his genetic disorder?
- What is your progress for the child's long-term development?

improves, speech improves, and learning occurs. An affected adult is generally not less happy and/or healthy than any other person.

## Resources

### WEBSITES

Parker, Brandon. "Russell-Silver Syndrome." http://www.people.unt.edu/~bsp0002/rss.htm. (February 28, 2001).

"Russell-Silver Syndrome." *Online Mendelian Inheritance in Man*.http://www.ncbi.nlm.nih.gov/entrez/dispomim.cgi?id = 180860.

"Russell-Silver Syndrome." *WebMD*. http://my.webmd.com/content/asset/adam_disease_silver_syndrome.

### ORGANIZATIONS

MAGIC Foundation for Children's Growth. 1327 N. Harlem Ave., Oak Park, IL 60302. (708) 383-0808 or (800) 362-4423. Fax: (708) 383-0899. mary@magicfoundation.org. http://www.magicfoundation.org/ghd.html.

Yahoo Groups: Russell-Silver syndrome Support Group. http://groups.yahoo.com/group/RSS-Support.

Paul A. Johnson

# S

## Saethre–Chotzen syndrome

### Definition

Saethre–Chotzen syndrome is an inherited disorder that affects one in every 50,000 individuals. The syndrome is characterized by early and uneven fusion of the bones that make the skull (cranium). This affects the shape of the head and face, which may cause the two sides to appear unequal. The eyelids are droopy; the eyes widely spaced. The disorder is also associated with minor birth defects of the hands and feet. In addition, some individuals have mild mental retardation. Some individuals with Saethre–Chotzen syndrome may require some medical or surgical intervention.

### Description

Saethre–Chotzen (say–thre chote–zen) syndrome belongs to a group of rare **genetic disorders** with **craniosynostosis**. Craniosynostosis means there is premature closure of the sutures (seams) between certain bones of the cranium. This causes the shape of the head to be tall, asymmetric, or otherwise altered in shape (acrocephaly). There is also webbing (syndactyly) of certain fingers and toes. Another name for Saethre–Chotzen syndrome is acrocephalosyndactyly type III. It is one of the more mild craniosynostosis syndromes.

The story of Saethre–Chotzen syndrome goes back to the early 1930s. It was then that a Norwegian psychiatrist, Haakon Saethre wrote about a mother and two daughters in the medical literature. Each had a low frontal hairline; long and uneven facial features; short fingers; and webbing of the second and third fingers, and second, third and fourth toes. A year later in 1931, F. Chotzen, a German psychiatrist, reported a family with similar features. However, these individuals were also quite short and had additional features of mild mental retardation and hearing loss.

### Genetic profile

Mutations in the TWIST1 **gene**, located on the short (p) arm of **chromosome** 7 at position 21.2, cause Saethre–Chotzen syndrome. It is an autosomal dominant disorder and can be inherited, and passed on, by men as well as women. Almost all genes come in pairs. One copy of each pair of genes is inherited from the father and the other copy of each pair of genes is inherited from the mother. Therefore, if a parent carries a gene mutation for Saethre–Chotzen, each of his or her children has a 50% chance of inheriting the gene mutation. Each child also has a 50% chance of inheriting the working copy of the gene, in which case they would not have Saethre–Chotzen syndrome.

The search for the gene for Saethre–Chotzen syndrome is an interesting story. The first clue as to the cause of the disorder came in 1986, with the identification of patients who had a chromosome deletion of the short arm of chromosome 7. Linkage studies in the early 1990s narrowed the region for this gene to a specific site, at 7p21. Then, in 1996, scientists at Johns Hopkins Children's Center began to study TWIST1 as the candidate gene for Saethre–Chotzen syndrome because of earlier studies that showed how this gene works in the mouse.

The mouse TWIST gene normally works in forming the skeleton and muscle of the head, face, hands, and feet. Mice lacking both copies of the gene die before birth. Many have severe birth defects, including failure of the neural tube to close. They have an abnormal head and limb defects. However, mice with just one non–working copy of the TWIST gene did not die. Closer examination of these mice showed that they had only minor hand, foot and skull defects. The features were similar to those seen in Saethre–Chotzen syndrome.

It was also known that the mouse TWIST gene was located on chromosome 12 in mice, a location that corresponds to the short arm of chromosome 7 in

## KEY TERMS

**Acrocephaly**—An abnormal cone shape of the head.

**Chromosome deletion**—A missing sequence of DNA or part of a chromosome.

**Craniosynostosis**—Premature, delayed, or otherwise abnormal closure of the sutures of the skull.

**Cranium**—The skeleton of the head, which include all of the bones of the head except the mandible.

**Exon**—The expressed portion of a gene. The exons of genes are those portions that actually chemically code for the protein or polypeptide that the gene is responsible for producing.

**Linkage**—The association between separate DNA sequences (genes) located on the same chromosome.

**Syndactyly**—Webbing or fusion between the fingers or toes.

**Transcription**—The process by which genetic information on a strand of DNA is used to synthesize a strand of complementary RNA.

**Transcription factor**—A protein that works to activate the transcription of other genes.

humans. With this evidence, the researchers went on to map and isolate the human TWIST1 gene on human chromosome 7. They showed that this gene was in the same location that was missing in some individuals with Saethre–Chotzen. The TWIST1 gene is a small gene, containing only two exons (coding regions). Upon searching for alterations (mutations) in this gene, they found five different types of mutations in affected individuals. Since none of these mutations were found in unaffected individuals, this was proof positive that the TWIST1 gene was the cause of Saethre–Chotzen syndrome.

Scientists have also used animal models and the fruit fly Drosophila to study the function of the TWIST1 gene. They have found that it takes two TWIST1 protein molecules to combine together, in order to function as a transcription factor for **DNA**. The normal function of the TWIST1 protein is to bind to the DNA helix at specific places. By doing so, it works to regulate which genes are activated or "turned on." Most of the mutations identified in the TWIST1 gene so far seem to interfere with how the protein product binds to DNA. In effect, other genes that would normally be activated during development of the embryo may in fact not be turned on.

More recent studies suggest that the TWIST1 protein may induce the activation of genes in the fibroblast growth factor receptor (FGFR) pathway. Mutations in the FGFR family of genes cause other conditions with craniosynostosis such as **Crouzon syndrome**. Crouzon syndrome, like Saethre–Chotzen syndrome, is a mild craniosynostosis disorder. There is much overlap in the features of the face and hands in each condition. In fact, some patients initially thought to have Saethre–Chotzen were given a new diagnosis of Crouzon syndrome after studying both the TWIST1 and the FGFR genes for mutations.

In all, it is thought that the TWIST1 protein most likely acts to turn on the FGFR genes. These genes, in turn, instruct various cells of the head, face, and limb structures to grow and differentiate. If the TWIST gene or other genes of the FGFR pathway are altered, an individual will have one of the craniosynostosis syndromes.

### Demographics

Saethre–Chotzen syndrome affects both males and females equally. It most likely occurs in every racial and ethnic group and is believed to be under-diagnosed. The estimated incidence of the syndrome is one in every 25,000 to 50,000 individuals, making it the most common of the craniosynostosis syndromes.

### Signs and symptoms

The cranium is made up of three main sections. The three sections are the face, the base of the cranium, and the top and sides of the head. Most of the cranium assumes its permanent shape before birth. However, the bones that make up the top and side of the head are not fixed in place, and the seams between the bones (cranial sutures) remain open. This allows the top of the head to adjust in shape, as the unborn baby passes through the narrow birth canal during labor. After birth, the cranial sutures will close, most often within the first few years of life. The shape of the cranium is then complete.

In Saethre–Chotzen, the shape of the cranium is abnormally formed. The reason is that the coronal suture closes too early, sometimes even before birth. The coronal suture separates the two frontal bones (forehead) from the parietal bones (top of the head). If the early closure is unilateral or asymmetric, then the forehead and face will form unevenly, from one side to the other. This also forces the top of the head to become more pointed, almost tower–like. The forehead looks high and wide. The face will appear uneven on each side, especially in the area of the eyes and cheeks.

There is also less space for the normal features of the face to develop. For instance, the eye sockets are more shallow, and the cheekbones are flat. This makes the eyes more prominent, and spaced further apart than normal. Adding to the unevenness of the face is drooping of the upper eyelids, and a slight down slant to the eyes. The nose may look beaked or bent slightly downward at the tip. In some individuals, the ears look small and low–set on the face.

The other main feature of the syndrome is minor abnormalities of the hands and feet. Webbing (syndactyly) commonly occurs between the second and third fingers and toes. The thumbs are short and flat. The fifth finger may be permanently curved or bent at the tip.

Each individual with Saethre–Chotzen is affected somewhat differently. The features are usually quite variable even within the same family. Most individuals are mildly affected. Their facial features may be somewhat flat and uneven, but not strikingly so. However, if more than one cranial suture closes too early (and this can happen in some individuals), there is more severe disfigurement to their face.

In addition to the physical characteristics, individuals with Saethre–Chotzen may have growth delays, leading to less than average adult height. Most individuals are of normal intelligence, although some may have mild to moderate mental retardation (IQ from 50–70). For the growth and mental delays, it becomes necessary to provide special assistance and anticipatory guidance.

## Diagnosis

For many years, there was widespread discussion among physicians (geneticists) over whether a given patient would have either Saethre–Chotzen or Crouzon syndrome. There may even be confusion with other craniosynostosis syndromes or with isolated craniosynostosis. However, the availability of direct gene testing now allows for a more definitive diagnosis for these patients. Simply using a blood sample, a direct gene test for mutations in the TWIST gene can be done. If an individual also has mental retardation or other significant birth defects, it is suggested that they be screened more fully for deletions of the TWIST gene.

## Treatment and management

Very often, the physical characteristics of Saethre–Chotzen are so mild that no surgical treatment is necessary. The facial appearance tends to improve as the child grows. However, sometimes surgery is needed to correct the early fusion of the cranial bones. A specialized craniofacial medical team, experienced with

these types of patients, should do this surgery. Surgery may also be done to release the webbing of the fingers and toes.

Some of the more severely affected individuals with Saethre–Chotzen may experience problems with their vision. There may be less space in the eye socket due to the bone abnormalities of the face. This can lead to damage of the nerves of the eye and may require corrective surgery. The tear ducts of the eye can also be missing or abnormal. Reconstructive surgery is sometimes performed to correct the drooping of the eyelids or narrowing of the nasal passage.

## Prognosis

Most individuals with Saethre–Chotzen syndrome appear to have a normal life span.

### Resources

#### BOOKS

Icon Health Publications. *Craniosynostosis —A Medical Dictionary, Bibliography, and Annotated Research Guide to Internet References.* San Diego, CA: Icon Health Publications, 2004.

#### PERIODICALS

de Heer, I. M., et al. "Clinical and genetic analysis of patients with Saethre–Chotzen syndrome." *Plastic and Reconstructive Surgery* 115, no. 7 (June 2005): 1894–1902.

Sahlin, P., et al. "Germline mutation in the FGFR3 gene in a TWIST1–negative family with saethre–chotzen syndrome and breast cancer." *Genes Chromosomes Cancer* 48, no. 3 (March 2009): 285–288.

Seto, M. L., et al. "Isolated sagittal and coronal craniosynostosis associated with TWIST box mutations." *American Journal of Medical Genetics* 143, no. 7 (April 2007): 678–686.

Touliatou, V., et al. "Saethre–Chotzen syndrome with severe developmental delay associated with deletion of chromosomic region 7p15–> pter." *Genetic Counseling* 18, no. 3 (2007): 295–301.

## ORGANIZATIONS

Children's Craniofacial Association (CCA). 13140 Coit Rd., Suite 517, Dallas, TX 75240. (800)535-3643 or (214)570-9099. Fax: (214)570-8811. Email: contactCCA@ccakids.com. http://www.ccakids.com.

March of Dimes Foundation. 1275 Mamaroneck Avenue, White Plains, NY 10605. (914)428-7100 or (888)MOD-IMES (663-4637). Fax: (914)428-8203. Email: askus@marchofdimes.com. http://www.marchofdimes.com.

National Organization for Rare Disorders (NORD). 55 Kenosia Avenue, PO Box 1968, Danbury, CT 06813-1968. (203)744-0100 or (800)999-6673. Fax: (203)798-2291. http://www.rarediseases.org.

## WEBSITES

*Saethre–Chotzen Syndrome.* Information Page, Children's Hospital Boston (May 02, 2009). http://www.childrenshospital.org/az/Site1537/mainpageS1537P0.html

*Saethre–Chotzen Syndrome.* Information Page, Madisons Foundation (May 02, 2009). http://www.madisonsfoundation.org/index.php/component/option,com_mpower/diseaseID,527/

*Saethre–Chotzen Syndrome.* Information Page, John Hopkins Medicine, December 16, 2003 (May 02, 2009). http://www.hopkinsmedicine.org/craniofacial/Education/DefinedArticle.cfm? MUArticleID = 68&Source = Family

*Saethre–Chotzen Syndrome.* Information Page, Seattle Children's Hospital (May 02, 2009). http://craniofacial.seattlechildrens.org/conditions_treated/saethre.asp

Kevin M. Sweet, MS, CGC

Sanfilippo syndrome (MPS III) *see* **Mucopolysaccharidosis (MPS)**

Sarcoma-breast-leukemia-adrenal gland (SBLA) syndrome *see* **Li-Fraumeni syndrome**

SC syndrome *see* **Roberts SC phocomelia**

Scheie syndrome (MPS I) *see* **Mucopolysaccharidosis (MPS)**

Schilder disease *see* **Adrenoleukodystrophy (ALD)**

# Schinzel-Giedion syndrome

## Definition

Schinzel-Giedion syndrome, or Schinzel-Giedion Midface-Retraction syndrome is a rare malformation syndrome characterized by skeletal anomalies, a coarse face, urogenital defects, and severe mental retardation.

## Description

In affected individuals, the ureter, or tube that carries urine from the kidney into the bladder, is obstructed causing the pelvis and kidney duct to become swollen with excess urine. This is called hydronephrosis. Other features of the syndrome include hypertrichosis or the excessive growth of hair, a flat midface, abnormal brain activity, skeletal abnormalities, and severe mental impairment.

Patients show abnormal bone maturation including broad and dense ribs and short arms and legs. Severely delayed mental and motor development is accompanied by seizures and spasticity.

## Genetic profile

Some scientists have suggested that the syndrome is inherited as an autosomal recessive trait because they observed that the syndrome appeared in two sibs of different sex, which suggested autosomal-recessive **inheritance**. However, other researchers have hypothesized that Schinzel-Giedion syndrome may be a dominant disorder with gonadal mosaicism in one parent. Gonadal mosaicism can occur when either the testes or ovaries contain some cells with an extra **chromosome**. Scientists have also postulated that the syndrome may be caused by an unbalanced structural chromosome abnormality.

## Demographics

Schinzel-Giedion syndrome is extremely rare and remains incompletely defined. About 25 to 30 well-documented cases have been reported beginning in 1978. The syndrome was originally observed in a brother, who lived less than 24 hours and a sister who survived for 16 months. Both displayed multiple skull abnormalities and profound mid-face retraction. They each had congenital heart defects, hydronephrosis, **clubfoot**, and hypertrichosis. Eight other cases, all sporadic, including two offspring of consanguineous parents were subsequently identified that year. Less than 30 cases are described in the medical literature detailing major and minor features of the syndrome. Only one case has been

## QUESTIONS TO ASK YOUR DOCTOR

- What does the term "gonadal mosaicism" mean and how is related to Schinzel-Giedion syndrome?
- Are there tests by which this genetic disorder can be detected prenatally?
- What information can a genetic counselor provide my spouse and me about Schinzel-Giedion syndrome?
- What is the prognosis for a child born with Schinzel-Giedion?

described in Japan. The other described cases have occurred in Western countries.

### Signs and symptoms

Clinical signs include a flat mid-face, low set ears, a prominent forehead, skull abnormalities including large fontanels or openings, a short broad neck, genital malformations, congenital heart defects including atrial septal defect, clubfoot, and growth retardation.

### Diagnosis

The detection of renal defects using **prenatal ultrasound** is one of the primary means of diagnosis. Clinical observation of coarse facial features, skeletal anomalies, and MRI studies aid diagnosis after birth. Serial cranial MRI studies that show a progressive neurodegenerative process affecting both gray and white matter typify Schinzel-Giedion syndrome. Clinical signs of abnormal cortical gray matter include seizures, **dementia**, and blindness in some cases. Abnormalities in the white matter can produce spasticity and hyperreflexia.

### Treatment and management

MRI studies indicate the syndrome is a progressive neurodegenerative process and patients have a limited life span. Nursing care and supportive measures are required to keep the patient comfortable.

### Prognosis

Death prior to the second year of life represents the most common outcome.

### Resources

#### BOOKS

Menkes, John H., and Harvey B. Sarnat. *Child Neurology*. 6th ed. Lippincott Williams and Wilkins, 2000.

Volpe, Joseph J. *Neurology of the Newborn*. 4th ed. Philadelphia: W.B. Saunders Company, 2001.

#### PERIODICALS

McPherson, E., et al. "Sacral Tumors in Schinzel-Giedion Syndrome." (Letter) *American Journal of Medical Genetics* 79 (1998): 62-63.

Schinzel, A., and A. Giedion. "A Syndrome of Severe Midface Retraction, Multiple Skull Anomalies, Clubfeet, and Cardiac and Renal Malformations in Sibs." *American Journal of Medical Genetics* 1 (1978): 361-375.

Shah, A.M., et al. "Schinzel-Giedion Syndrome: Evidence for a Neurodegenerative Process." *American Journal of Medical Genetics* 82 (1999): 344-347.

#### ORGANIZATIONS

National Organization for Rare Disorders (NORD). PO Box 8923, New Fairfield, CT 06812-8923. (203) 746-6518 or (800) 999-6673. Fax: (203) 746-6481. http://www.rarediseases.org.

#### WEBSITES

"Entry 269150: Schinzel-Giedion Midface-Retraction Syndrome." (Last edited 5-12-99). *OMIM—Online Mendelian Inheritance in Man*. http://www.ncbi.nlm.nih.gov/entrez/dispomim.cgi?id=269150.

Julianne Remington

## Schinzel acrocallosal syndrome *see* Acrocallosal syndrome

# Schizophrenia

## Definition

Schizophrenia is a psychotic disorder (or a group of disorders) marked by severely impaired thinking, emotions, and behaviors. Schizophrenic patients are typically unable to filter sensory stimuli and may have enhanced perceptions of sounds, colors, and other features of their environment. Most schizophrenics, if untreated, gradually withdraw from interactions with other people and lose their ability to take care of personal needs and grooming.

## Description

The course of schizophrenia in adults can be divided into three phases or stages. In the acute phase, the patient has an overt loss of contact with reality (psychotic episode) that requires intervention and treatment. In the second, or stabilization, phase, the initial psychotic symptoms have been brought under control but the patient is at risk for relapse if

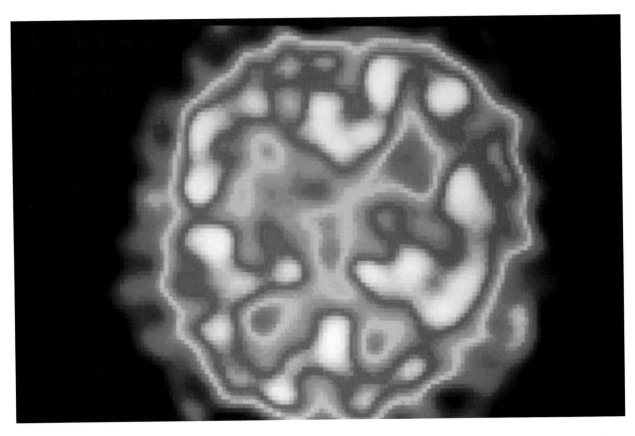

Positron emission tomograph (PET) scan showing the brain of a person with schizophrenia. *(© SPL/Custom Medical Stock Photo. Reproduced by permission.)*

treatment is interrupted. In the third, or maintenance, phase, the patient is relatively stable and can be kept indefinitely on antipsychotic medications. Even in the maintenance phase, however, relapses are not unusual and patients do not always return to full functioning.

The term schizophrenia comes from two Greek words that mean "split mind." It was observed around 1908, by a Swiss doctor named Eugen Bleuler, to describe the splitting apart of mental functions that he regarded as the central characteristic of schizophrenia.

Recently, some psychotherapists have begun to use a classification of schizophrenia based on two main types. People with type I, or positive schizophrenia, have a rapid (acute) onset of symptoms and tend to respond well to drugs. They also tend to suffer more from the "positive" symptoms, such as delusions and hallucinations. People with type II, or negative schizophrenia, are usually described as poorly adjusted before their schizophrenia slowly overtakes them. They have predominantly "negative" symptoms, such as withdrawal from others and a slowing of mental and physical reactions (psychomotor retardation).

The fourth (1994) edition of the *Diagnostic and Statistical Manual of Mental Disorders* (DSM-IV) specifies five subtypes of schizophrenia.

### Paranoid

The key feature of this subtype of schizophrenia is the combination of false beliefs (delusions) and of hearing voices (auditory hallucinations), with more nearly normal emotions and cognitive functioning (cognitive functions include reasoning, judgment, and memory). The delusions of paranoid schizophrenics usually involve thoughts of being persecuted or harmed by others or exaggerated opinions of their own importance, but may also reflect feelings of jealousy or excessive religiosity. The delusions are typically organized into a coherent framework. Paranoid schizophrenics function at a higher level than other subtypes, but are at risk for suicidal or violent behavior under the influence of their delusions.

### Disorganized

Disorganized schizophrenia (formerly called hebephrenic schizophrenia) is marked by a patient's disorganized speech, thinking, and behavior, coupled with flat or

**Affective flattening**—A loss or lack of emotional expressiveness; sometimes called blunted or restricted affect.

**Akathisia**—Agitated or restless movement, usually affecting the legs and accompanied by a sense of discomfort; a common side effect of neuroleptic medications.

**Catatonic behavior**—Behavior characterized by muscular tightness or rigidity and lack of response to the environment.

**Delusion**—A fixed, false belief that is resistant to reason or factual disproof.

**Depot dosage**—A form of medication that can be stored in the patient's body tissues for several days or weeks, thus minimizing the risk of the patient forgetting daily doses.

**Dopamine receptor antagonists (DAs)**—The older class of antipsychotic medications, also called neuroleptics, which primarily block the site on nerve cells that normally receive the brain chemical dopamine.

**Dystonia**—Painful involuntary muscle cramps or spasms.

**Extrapyramidal symptoms (EPS)**—A group of side effects associated with antipsychotic medications, including parkinsonism, akathisia, dystonia, and tardive dyskinesia.

**First-rank symptoms**—A set of symptoms designated by Kurt Schneider in 1959 as the most important diagnostic indicators of schizophrenia: delusions, hallucinations, thought insertion or removal, and thought broadcasting.

**Hallucination**—A sensory experience of something that does not exist outside the mind.

**Huntington's chorea**—A hereditary disease that typically appears in midlife, marked by gradual loss of brain function and voluntary movement; some symptoms resemble those of schizophrenia.

**Negative symptoms**—Symptoms of schizophrenia characterized by the absence or elimination of certain behaviors: affective flattening, poverty of speech, and loss of will or initiative.

**Neuroleptic**—Another name for the older type of antipsychotic medications given to schizophrenic patients.

**Parkinsonism**—A set of symptoms originally associated with Parkinson disease that can occur as side effects of neuroleptic medications: trembling of the fingers or hands, a shuffling gait, and tight or rigid muscles.

**Positive symptoms**—Symptoms of schizophrenia that are characterized by the production or presence of behaviors that are grossly abnormal or excessive, including hallucinations and thought-process disorder; DSM-IV subdivides positive symptoms into psychotic and disorganized.

**Poverty of speech**—A negative symptom of schizophrenia, characterized by brief and empty replies to questions.

**Psychotic disorder**—A mental disorder characterized by delusions, hallucinations, or other symptoms of lack of contact with reality.

**Serotonin dopamine antagonists (SDAs)**—The newer second-generation antipsychotic drugs, also called atypical antipsychotics, including clozapine (Clozaril), risperidone (Risperdal), and olanzapine (Zyprexa).

**Wilson disease**—A rare hereditary disease marked by high levels of copper deposits in the brain and liver.

**Word salad**—Speech that is so disorganized that it makes no linguistic or grammatical sense.

inappropriate emotional responses to a situation (affect). The patient may act silly or withdraw socially to an extreme extent. Most patients in this category have weak personality structures prior to their initial acute psychotic episode.

### Catatonic

Catatonic schizophrenia is characterized by disturbances of movement that may include rigidity, stupor, agitation, bizarre posturing, and repetitive imitations of the movements or speech of other people. These patients are at risk for malnutrition, exhaustion, or self-injury. This subtype is presently uncommon in Europe and the United States. Catatonia as a symptom is most commonly associated with mood disorders.

### Undifferentiated

Undifferentiated schizophrenics have the characteristic positive and negative symptoms of schizophrenia but do not meet the specific criteria for the paranoid, disorganized, or catatonic subtypes.

### Residual

Residual schizophrenia is a category used for patients who have had at least one acute schizophrenic episode but do not presently have strong positive psychotic symptoms, such as delusions and hallucinations. They may have negative symptoms, such as withdrawal from others, or mild forms of positive symptoms, which indicate that the disorder has not completely resolved.

### Schizoaffective disorder

A condition commonly diagnosed as schizophrenia is schizoaffective disorder. This relatively rare disorder is characterized by psychotic symptoms in a patient with a mood disorder, usually manic **depression**. The psychotic symptoms may or may not be present at the same time as the mood disorder. Another complicating factor, especially in younger patients, is that distinguishing between manic depression and schizophrenia can be difficult in adolescents, since psychotic features are common during manic episodes in this age group.

## Genetic profile

The risk of schizophrenia among first-degree biological relatives is 10 times greater than that observed in the general population. Furthermore, the presence of the same disorder is higher in monozygotic twins (identical twins) than in dizygotic twins (fraternal, or nonidentical, twins). The research on adoption and identical twins also supports the notion that environmental factors are important, because not all relatives who have the disorder express it. There are several chromosomes and loci (specific locations on chromosomes that contain mutated genes) have been identified. Recent research has implicated chromosomal 11 translocations in both schizophrenia and manic depression. In addition, there are now mutations of several genes that are postulated to be involved in schizophrenia, including DTNBP1, NRG1, DAO, DAOA, and RSG4. Research is actively ongoing to elucidate the causes, types, and variations of these mutations.

## Demographics

A number of studies indicate that about 1% of the world's population is affected by schizophrenia, without regard to race, social class, level of education, or cultural influences (outcome may vary from culture to culture, depending on the familial support of the patient). Most patients are diagnosed in their late teens or early 20s, but the symptoms of schizophrenia can emerge at any age in the life cycle. The male/female ratio in adults is about 1.2:1. Male patients typically have their first acute episode in their early 20s, while female patients are usually closer to age 30 when they are recognized with active symptoms.

Schizophrenia is rarely diagnosed in preadolescent children, although patients as young as five or six have been reported. Childhood schizophrenia is at the upper end of the spectrum of severity and shows a greater gender disparity. It affects one or two children in every 10,000; the male/female ratio is 2:1.

## Signs and symptoms

One of the reasons for the ongoing difficulty in classifying schizophrenic disorders is an incomplete understanding of their causes. Since 1998, it has been thought that these disorders were the end result of a combination of genetic, neurobiological, and environmental causes. A leading neurobiological hypothesis looks at the connection between the disease and excessive levels of dopamine, a chemical (neurotransmitter) that transmits signals in the brain. The genetic factor in schizophrenia has been underscored by recent findings that first-degree biological relatives of schizophrenics are 10 times as likely to develop the disorder as are members of the general population.

Prior to recent findings of abnormalities in the brain structure of schizophrenic patients, several generations of psychotherapists advanced a number of psychoanalytic and sociological theories about the origins of schizophrenia. These theories ranged from hypotheses about the patient's problems with anxiety or aggression to theories about stress reactions or interactions with disturbed parents. Psychosocial factors are now thought to influence the expression or severity of schizophrenia, rather than cause it directly.

Another hypothesis suggests that schizophrenia may be caused by a virus that attacks the hippocampus, a part of the brain that processes sense perceptions. Damage to the hippocampus would account for schizophrenic patients' vulnerability to sensory overload. Researchers are preparing to test antiviral medications on schizophrenics.

Patients with a possible diagnosis of schizophrenia are evaluated on the basis of a set or constellation of symptoms; there is no single symptom that is unique to schizophrenia. In 1959, the German psychiatrist Kurt Schneider proposed a list of so-called first-rank symptoms, which he regarded as diagnostic of the disorder. These symptoms include:

- delusions
- somatic hallucinations

- hearing voices commenting on the patient's behavior
- thought insertion or thought withdrawal

Somatic hallucinations refer to sensations or perceptions concerning body organs that have no known medical cause or reason, such as the notion that one's brain is radioactive. Thought insertion and/or withdrawal refers to delusions that an outside force (for example, the FBI, the CIA, Martians, etc.) has the power to put thoughts into one's mind or remove them.

The so-called positive symptoms of schizophrenia are those that represent an excessive or distorted version of normal functions. Positive symptoms include Schneider's first-rank symptoms as well as disorganized thought processes (reflected mainly in speech) and disorganized or catatonic behavior. Disorganized thought processes are marked by characteristics: looseness of association, in which the patient rambles from topic to topic in a disconnected way; tangentially, which means that the patient gives unrelated answers to questions; and "word salad," in which the patient's speech is so incoherent that it makes no grammatical or linguistic sense. Disorganized behavior means that the patient has difficulty with any type of purposeful or goal-oriented behavior, including personal self-care or preparing meals. Other forms of disorganized behavior may include dressing in odd or inappropriate ways, sexual self-stimulation in public, or agitated shouting or cursing.

The DSM-IV definition of schizophrenia includes three so-called negative symptoms. They are called negative because they represent the lack or absence of behaviors. The negative symptoms that are considered diagnostic of schizophrenia are a lack of emotional response (affective flattening), poverty of speech, and absence of volition or will. In general, the negative symptoms are more difficult for doctors to evaluate than the positive symptoms.

## Diagnosis

A doctor must make a diagnosis of schizophrenia on the basis of a standardized list of outwardly observable symptoms, not on the basis of internal psychological processes. There are no specific laboratory tests that can be used to diagnose schizophrenia. Researchers have, however, discovered that patients with schizophrenia have certain abnormalities in the structure and functioning of the brain compared to normal test subjects. These discoveries have been made with the help of imaging techniques, such as computed tomography (CT) scans.

When a psychiatrist assesses a patient for schizophrenia, physical conditions will be excluded that can cause abnormal thinking and some other behaviors associated with schizophrenia. These conditions include organic brain disorders (including traumatic injuries of the brain), temporal-lobe **epilepsy**, **Wilson disease**, Huntington's chorea, and encephalitis. Substance abuse disorders, especially amphetamine use, will need to be ruled out.

After ruling out organic disorders, the clinician will consider other psychiatric conditions that may include psychotic symptoms or symptoms resembling psychosis. These disorders include mood disorders with psychotic features; delusional disorder; dissociative disorder not otherwise specified (DDNOS), or multiple personality disorder; schizotypal, schizoid, or paranoid personality disorders; and atypical reactive disorders. In the past, many individuals were incorrectly diagnosed as schizophrenic. Patients who were diagnosed prior to the changes in categorization introduced by DSM-IV should have their diagnoses, and treatment, reevaluated. In children, the psychiatrist must distinguish between psychotic symptoms and a vivid fantasy life, and also identify learning problems or disorders. After other conditions have been ruled out, the patient must meet a set of criteria specified by DSM-IV, including:

- Characteristic symptoms: The patient must have two (or more) of the following symptoms during a one-month period: delusions; hallucinations; disorganized speech; disorganized or catatonic behavior; negative symptoms.
- The patient must show a decline in social, interpersonal, or occupational functioning, including self-care.
- Duration: The disturbed behavior must last for at least six months.
- Diagnostic exclusions: Mood disorders, substance abuse disorders, medical conditions, and developmental disorders have been ruled out.

## Treatment and management

The treatment of schizophrenia depends in part on the patient's stage or phase. Patients in the acute phase are hospitalized in most cases, to prevent harm to the patient or others and to begin treatment with antipsychotic medications. A patient having a first psychotic episode should be given a CT or magnetic resonance imaging (MRI) scan to rule out structural brain disease.

The primary form of treatment of schizophrenia is antipsychotic medication. Antipsychotic drugs help to control almost all the positive symptoms of the disorder. They have minimal effects on disorganized behavior and negative symptoms. Between 60–70% of schizophrenics will respond to antipsychotics. In the acute phase of the illness, patients are usually given medications by mouth or by intramuscular injection. After the patient has been stabilized, the antipsychotic drug may be given in a long-acting form called a depot dose. Depot medications last two to four weeks; they have the advantage of protecting the patient against the consequences of forgetting or skipping daily doses. In addition, some patients who do not respond to oral neuroleptics have better results with depot form. Patients whose long-term treatment includes depot medications are introduced to the depot form gradually during their stabilization period. Most people with schizophrenia are kept on antipsychotic medications indefinitely during the maintenance phase of their disorder to minimize the possibility of relapse.

The most frequently used antipsychotics has fallen into two classes: the older dopamine receptor antagonists, or DAs, and the newer serotonin dopamine antagonists, or SDAs. (Antagonists block the action of some other substance; for example, dopamine antagonists counteract the action of dopamine.) The exact mechanisms of action of these medications are not known, but it is thought that they lower the patient's sensitivity to sensory stimuli and so indirectly improve the patient's ability to interact with others.

The dopamine receptor antagonists (DAs) include the older antipsychotic (also called neuroleptic) drugs, such as haloperidol (Haldol), chlorpromazine (Thorazine), and fluphenazine (Prolixin). These drugs have two major drawbacks: it is often difficult to find the best dosage level for the individual patient, and a dosage level high enough to control psychotic symptoms frequently produces extrapyramidal side effects, or EPS. EPS include parkinsonism, in which the patient cannot walk normally and usually develops a tremor; **dystonia**, or painful muscle spasms of the head, tongue, or neck; and akathisia, or restlessness. A type of long-term EPS is tardive dyskinesia, which features slow, rhythmic, automatic movements. Schizophrenics with AIDS are especially vulnerable to developing EPS.

The serotonin dopamine antagonists (SDAs), also called atypical antipsychotics, are newer medications that include clozapine (Clozaril), risperidone (Risperdal), and olanzapine (Zyprexa). The SDAs have a better effect on the negative symptoms of schizophrenia than do the older drugs and are less likely to produce EPS than the older compounds. The newer drugs are significantly more expensive in the short term, although the SDAs may reduce long-term costs by reducing the need for hospitalization. They are also presently unavailable in injectable forms. The SDAs are commonly used to treat patients who respond

## QUESTIONS TO ASK YOUR DOCTOR

- Is schizophrenia always a genetic-based disorder, or are there other causes for the condition?
- What are the probabilities that my child will inherit schizophrenia from my spouse, who has the disorder?
- What kinds of treatment are available for dealing with schizophrenia, and how effective are those treatments?
- What factors determine the prognosis for a person with schizophrenia and, based on my spouse's current status, what is his prognosis for the disease?

poorly to the DAs. However, many psychotherapists now regard the use of these atypical antipsychotics as the treatment of first choice.

Most schizophrenics can benefit from psychotherapy once their acute symptoms have been brought under control by antipsychotic medication. Psychoanalytic approaches are not recommended. Behavior therapy, however, is often helpful in assisting patients to acquire skills for daily living and social interaction. It can be combined with occupational therapy to prepare the patient for eventual employment.

Family therapy is often recommended for the families of schizophrenic patients, to relieve the feelings of guilt that they often have as well as to help them understand the patient's disorder. The family's attitude and behaviors toward the patient are key factors in minimizing relapses (i.e., reducing stress in the patient's life), and family therapy can often strengthen the family's ability to cope with the stresses caused by the schizophrenic's illness. Family therapy focused on communication skills and problem-solving strategies is particularly helpful. In addition to formal treatment, many families benefit from support groups and similar mutual help organizations for relatives of schizophrenics.

### Prognosis

One important prognostic sign is the patient's age at onset of psychotic symptoms. Patients with early onset of schizophrenia are more often male, have a lower level of functioning prior to onset, a higher rate of brain abnormalities, more noticeable negative symptoms, and worse outcomes. Patients with later onset are more likely to be female, with fewer brain abnormalities and thought impairment, and more hopeful prognoses.

The average course and outcome for schizophrenics are less favorable than those for most other mental disorders, although as many as 30% of patients diagnosed with schizophrenia recover completely and the majority do experience some improvement. Two factors that influence outcomes are stressful life events and a hostile or emotionally intense family environment. Schizophrenics with a high number of stressful changes in their lives, or who have frequent contacts with critical or emotionally over-involved family members, are more likely to relapse. Overall, the most important component of long-term care of schizophrenic patients is complying with their regimen of antipsychotic medications.

## Resources

### BOOKS

Campbell, Robert Jean. *Psychiatric Dictionary*. New York and Oxford, UK: Oxford University Press, 1989.

Clark, R. Barkley. "Psychosocial Aspects of Pediatrics & Psychiatric Disorders." In *Current Pediatric Diagnosis & Treatment*, edited by William W. Hay Jr., et al. Stamford, CT: Appleton & Lange, 1997.

Day, Max, and Elvin V. Semrad. "Schizophrenia: Comprehensive Psychotherapy." In *The Encyclopedia of Psychiatry, Psychology, and Psychoanalysis*, edited by Benjamin B. Wolman. New York: Henry Holt and Company, 1996.

Eisendrath, Stuart J. "Psychiatric Disorders." In *Current Medical Diagnosis & Treatment 1998*, edited by Lawrence M. Tierney Jr., et al. Stamford, CT: Appleton & Lange, 1997.

Marder, Stephen R. "Schizophrenia." In *Conn's Current Therapy*, edited by Robert E. Rakel. Philadelphia: W. B. Saunders Company, 1998.

"Psychiatric Disorders: Schizophrenic Disorders." In *The Merck Manual of Diagnosis and Therapy*, Volume I, edited by Robert Berkow, et al. Rahway, NJ: Merck Research Laboratories, 1992.

"Schizophrenia and Other Psychotic Disorders." In *Diagnostic and Statistical Manual of Mental Disorders*, 4th edition. Washington, DC: The American Psychiatric Association, 1994.

Schultz, Clarence G. "Schizophrenia: Psychoanalytic Views." In *The Encyclopedia of Psychiatry, Psychology, and Psychoanalysis*, edited by Benjamin B. Wolman. New York: Henry Holt and Company, 1996.

Tsuang, Ming T., et al. "Schizophrenic Disorders." In *The New Harvard Guide to Psychiatry*, edited by Armand M. Nicholi, Jr. Cambridge, MA, and London, UK: The Belknap Press of Harvard University Press, 1988.

Wilson, Billie Ann, et al. *Nurses Drug Guide 1995*. Norwalk, CT: Appleton & Lange, 1995.

### PERIODICALS

Craddock, N., M. C. O'Donovan, and M. J. Owen. "The Genetics of Schizophrenia and Bipolar Disorder: Dissecting Psychosis." *Journal of Medical Genetics* 42 (2005): 193–204.

Klar, A. J. S. "A Genetic Mechanism Implicates Chromosome 11 in Schizophrenia and Bipolar Diseases." *Genetics* 167 (August 2004): 1833–1840.

Winerip, Michael. "Schizophrenia's Most Zealous Foe." *The New York Times Magazine*. (February 22, 1998): 26–29.

### WEB SITES

"An Introduction to Schizophrenia." The Schizophrenia Homepage. (April 22, 2005.) http://www.schizophrenia.com/family/schizintro.html.

"Schizophrenia." Internet Mental Health. (April 22, 2005.) http://www.mentalhealth.com/dis/p20-ps01.html.

Schizophrenia On-line News Articles. (April 22, 2005.) http://www2.addr.com/~y/mn/.

### ORGANIZATIONS

National Alliance for the Mentally Ill. Colonial Place Three, 2107 Wilson Blvd., Suite 300, Arlington, VA 22201. (703) 524-7600. HelpLine: (800) 950-NAMI.

Schizophrenics Anonymous. 15920 W. Twelve Mile, Southfield, MI 48076. (248) 477-1983.

Laith Farid Gulli, MD
Edward R. Rosick, DO, MPH, MS

# Schwartz–Jampel syndrome

## Definition

Schwartz–Jampel syndrome (SJS) is a rare, inherited condition of the skeletal and muscle systems that causes short stature, joint limitations, and particular facial features.

## Description

First described in 1962, SJS is now a clearly defined syndrome that is divided into two types. Type 1A is the classical form that develops in early childhood, usually between the first and third year of life. Type 1B is less common but more severe and its symptoms are present at birth. Both types of SJS involve generalized disease of the muscles called myopathy. The muscles tend to be quite stiff and are unable to relax normally. This is a condition known as myotonia. The myotonia causes many joints in the body to stay in a bent or flexed position (joint contractures).

In addition to muscle problems, the bones in the skeleton do not develop normally and this is why SJS may also be called a type of **skeletal dysplasia**. Abnormal bone shape and poor bone growth result in decreased total height, incorrect arm and leg postures, as well as curving of the spine (**scoliosis**).

Unique facial features of SJS include narrow eye openings with drooping eye lids, a small mouth, and puckered lips. These features are also due to the stiffness of the muscles that support the face and individuals with SJS appear to have a fixed facial expression.

Persons affected with SJS often have normal intelligence, although varying degrees of mental retardation may affect as many as 25% of patients. However, the myotonia may lead to poor speech articulation and drooling so that affected individuals are sometimes misdiagnosed as having mental retardation.

Respiratory and feeding difficulties are frequent with SJS Type 1B due to the more severe nature of the muscle and bone disease. These problems may be fatal in early infancy. Persons with SJS Type 1A have a much longer life expectancy, although this depends on how their disease progresses.

SJS has also been referred to as:

- myotonic myopathy, dwarfism, chrondrodystrophy, and ocular and facial abnormalities
- Schwartzndash;Jampel–Aberfeld syndrome
- Schwartz syndrome
- Aberfeld syndrome
- chrondrodystrophic myotonia
- osteochondromuscular dystrophy
- spondylo–epimetaphyseal dysplasia with myotonia

### Genetic profile

Both types of SJS are known to be inherited in an autosomal recessive manner. This was concluded after the following observations were made. SJS affects males and females alike. Parents of affected individuals

rarely show any signs or symptoms of SJS. Parents have been reported to have more than one affected child. Consanguineous relationships were seen in some families.

Genetic studies of many families revealed that all cases of SJS were linked to an area on **chromosome** one, described as 1p36.1. A gene in this region, heparan sulfate proteoglycan 2 (HSPG2), makes a protein called perlecan that plays an important role in maintaining cell membranes of the body's connective tissue (bone, cartilage, muscles, ligaments, tendons and blood vessels). As of 2009, studies have shown that perlecan helps keep cartilage and bone strong and are essential for certain chemical processes in muscle tissues. It is also thought that perlecan helps to regulate the normal growth of some cells.

Mutations in the HSPG2 gene have been found in some persons with SJS. These **gene mutations** change how the perlecan protein is made and usually prevents it from doing its normal job in the muscles and bones of the body.

The location 1p36.1 means that the gene is near the top or end of the short arm of chromosome number one. A human being has 23 pairs of chromosomes in nearly every cell of their body. One of each kind (23 total) is inherited from the mother and another of each kind (23 total) is inherited from the father, for a total of 46. One chromosome may hold hundreds to thousands of individual genes and as the chromosomes exist in pairs, so do the genes. Therefore, every person has two copies of the HSPG2 gene that makes perlecan. Individuals that have a diagnosis of SJS are thought to have a mutation in both copies of their HSPG2 gene, each of which was inherited from one of their parents. Unaffected parents of children with SJS are therefore carriers for SJS. Their one normal HSPG2 gene appears to make enough perlecan so those carriers do not show any symptoms of SJS. Most parents do not know that they are carriers for SJS until they have an affected child. When both parents are carriers for the same autosomal recessive disease such as SJS, there is a 25% chance with each and every pregnancy that they have together that their child will inherit both mutated HSPG2 genes and develop SJS.

### Demographics

SJS is a very rare genetic syndrome reported to affect males and females. It was initially described in the United States, but has also been reported in other countries. However, the exact incidence is unknown as no significant information is available on racial or sexual distribution.

## Signs and symptoms

A child born with SJS Type 1A may show no outward signs of the condition at birth. Over the following one to three years, progressive myotonia of the muscles and resulting joint contractures develop. The typical bone problems become obvious and growth in height slows down. These symptoms are evident at birth in children with SJS Type 1B. The following descriptions apply to both SJS Type 1A and Type 1B. However, each person with SJS may be affected to a different degree and their kinds of symptoms may vary.

### Head and neck

Myotonia of the muscles in the face causes a tight and fixed facial expression. The eye openings are almost always narrowed and small and the upper and lower eyelids are not joined properly at the corners of the eye (blepharophimosis). The upper eyelid may also appear droopy (ptosis). Nearsightedness (**myopia**) is present in 50% of patients and occasionally cataracts and lens dislocation may develop in the eye. The mouth is small and lips are puckered due to tight facial muscles. This may lead to speech difficulty. The chin may also be small or set back.

### Body

Hernias of the groin and navel areas are often noticed at birth. A hernia is the bulging of a tissue outside of its normal space and a simple operation can usually place it back inside. *Pectus carinatum* is a common bony deformity of the chest that causes the breast bone to protrude forward. Abnormalities in the growth and development of the bones of the spinal column (vertebrae) lead to scoliosis that usually worsens with age. Development of puberty is most often normal for persons with SJS.

### Limbs

Some babies with SJS are born with a dislocation of their hip joint. This is common in infants without SJS as well. As the muscle disease of SJS progresses, the joints become very stiff. The hips, knees and elbows in particular have very limited range of motion. These joint contractures worsen until puberty and then tend to stay the same from that point on. Eventually, a wheelchair is needed due to significant limitation of movement. The long bones in the body (i.e.: the thighbone) are bowed and shortened. This can cause a person with SJS to waddle as they walk and to stand in a crouching position. Therefore, an individual with SJS tends to be shorter than 90% of unaffected persons their age. A few have been reported

to reach average height. Typically, their arms and legs have an increased amount of body hair as well.

### Muscles

The muscles of the body show progressive myotonia, as they remain tight and are unable to relax normally. The muscle bulk may be increased in some areas, such as the thighs, and may waste away in others. As the muscles are unable to function normally, physical activity is restricted and a person may tire very easily.

### Central nervous system and behavior

Most individuals with SJS have normal intelligence, although some degree of mental retardation has been reported. Developmental language problems and attention difficulties have also been seen in some cases. Reflexes tend to be slower than normal. A high–pitched voice and drooling may be noticed due to muscle stiffness in the mouth and throat area. This may cause feeding difficulties and choking may be of concern.

## Diagnosis

The diagnosis of SJS Type 1A or Type 1B is made mainly by the presence of the symptoms described above. There is no specific biochemical or muscle testing that confirms a suspected diagnosis. Although research studies have identified mutations in the HSPG2 gene in some families, widespread **genetic testing** is not clinically available. Such genetic mutations may be unique to each family and therefore may not be found in other persons affected with SJS.

Several different studies may be performed to determine the type and severity of muscle disease when considering a diagnosis of SJS. This may include a muscle biopsy that samples a piece of muscle and examines the appearance of the muscle cells. A muscle biopsy may appear normal or it may show signs of myopathy. A particular chemical, called creatine kinase, can be measured in a person's blood. Very high levels of creatine kinase usually indicate the presence of muscle disease or wasting. An electromyogram (EMG) is a test that measures the electrical currents made within an active muscle. The EMG pattern is usually abnormal in persons with SJS. These tests will confirm the presence of muscle disease but there are no specific changes in any of them that are unique to SJS.

The following are some abnormalities of the bones that are frequently noticed on x rays:

- flat and irregularly formed vertebrae
- deformity of the upper part of the thigh bone

- a flattened joint socket where the hip and thigh bone meet
- specific changes in the development of the bones in the hand
- bowing of the long bones, especially the leg bones
- curvature of the spine that causes a hunchback appearance

Many of the symptoms of SJS are also present in other conditions and it is important to distinguish SJS from the following disorders:

- Stuve–Wiedemann syndrome (which was previously called SJS Type 2 until it was determined that they were the same condition)
- Freeman–Sheldon syndrome (also known as whistling face syndrome)
- Marden–Walker syndrome
- Kniest dysplasia
- Seckel syndrome
- myotonic dystrophy
- the mucopolysaccharidoses

### Treatment and management

There is not a cure for SJS. The treatment involves managing the symptoms of the condition as they develop and supporting the needs of the individual as the disability progresses. Several medical specialists may monitor a person with SJS for particular symptoms or complications. An orthopedic doctor manages the abnormal bone development and may offer surgical options for treatment of hip dislocation, scoliosis or bone curvature. An ophthalmologist monitors eye problems such as nearsightedness and cataracts, for which glasses and surgery may be available. Cosmetic repair of blepharophimosis by plastic surgery may also be considered.

For those with a mental deficiency, special education programs with options for activities in regular classrooms may offer the best opportunities for learning. Physical therapy may help maintain the greatest possible range of motion of the joints and speech therapy may improve speech problems due to a small and tight mouth. Physical activities of children are usually limited due to their stiff joints. As the condition progresses, persons with SJS are often wheelchair-bound by their teenage years and occupational therapy may help improve their everyday living skills. Adults who live independently may require some assistance with everyday tasks that their disability prevents them from doing, such as household chores or even bathing.

**QUESTIONS TO ASK YOUR DOCTOR**

- How do the two major types of Schwartz–Jampel syndrome differ from each other?
- What is the life expectancy of a person with each type of this disorder?
- What kinds of medical treatments are needed for each type of Schwartz–Jampel syndrome?

### Prognosis

Individuals with SJS can live well into adulthood despite progressive disability but the average life expectancy is unclear. They are usually wheelchair-bound by their teenage or young adult years. Although puberty development may be normal, no reports have been made of an individual with SJS fathering children or carrying a pregnancy.

SJS Type 1B may be fatal in the newborn period due to serious respiratory and feeding problems. As the muscles in the face and neck may be very tight, it can be difficult to place a tube down the throat (intubation) to allow a baby to breathe. Feeding may be a continuous struggle due to problems with or an inability to swallow.

Both types of SJS cause persons to be more prone to develop chest infections and pneumonia. There is also an increased risk for complications from anesthesia, specifically **malignant hyperthermia** (MH). MH is an abnormal chemical reaction in the body to the use of some anesthesia medications. It causes high fevers, breathing difficulty, rigid muscles and general serious illness. This condition may be life threatening.

### Resources

**BOOKS**

Gorlin, Robert J., et al. *Syndromes of the Head and Neck.* New York, NY: Oxford University Press, 2001.

**PERIODICALS**

Aburahma, S. K., et al. "Botulinum toxin A injections for the treatment of Schwartz–Jampel syndrome: a case series." *Journal of Child Neurology* 24, no. 1 (January 2009): 5–8.

Seto, M. L., et al. "Crying or smiling? The Schwartz–Jampel syndrome." *American Journal of Pediatrics* 148, no. 5 (May 2006): 702.

Stum, M., et al. "Spectrum of HSPG2 (Perlecan) mutations in patients with Schwartz–Jampel syndrome." *Human Mutations* 48, no. 3 (November 2006): 1082–1091.

**WEBSITES**

*Schwartz Jampel Syndrome.* Information Page, WebMD, Children's Health (May 02, 2009). http://children. webmd.com/schwartz-jampel-syndrome

*Schwartz Jampel Syndrome.* Information Page, NORD, November 26, 2008 (May 02, 2009). http://www.rare diseases.org/search/rdbdetail_abstract.html?disname= Schwartz%20Jampel%20Syndrome

**ORGANIZATIONS**

National Arthritis and Musculoskeletal and Skin Diseases Information Clearinghouse. 1 AMS Circle, Bethesda, MD 20892-3675. (3 01)495-4484 or (877)226-4267. Email: NIAMSinfo@mail.nih.gov. http://www.niams. nih.gov/Health_Info.

National Eye Institute (NEI). 2020 Vision Place, Bethesda, MD 20892-3655. (301)496-5248. http://www.nei.nih.gov.

National Organization for Rare Disorders (NORD). 55 Kenosia Avenue, PO Box 1968, Danbury, CT 06813-1968. (203)744-0100 or (800)999-6673. Fax: (203)798-2291. http://www.rarediseases.org.

Jennifer Elizabeth Neil, MS, CGC

SCIDX *see* **Severe combined immunodeficiency, X-linked**

Sclerocornea *see* **Microphthalmia with linear skin defects**

# Scleroderma

### Definition

Scleroderma is a progressive disease that affects the skin and connective tissue (including cartilage, bone, fat, and the tissue that supports the nerves and blood vessels throughout the body). There are two major forms of the disorder. The type known as localized scleroderma mainly affects the skin. Systemic scleroderma, which is also called systemic sclerosis, affects the smaller blood vessels and internal organs of the body.

### Description

Scleroderma is an autoimmune disorder, which means that the body's immune system turns against itself. In scleroderma, there is an overproduction of abnormal collagen (a type of protein fiber present in connective tissue). This collagen accumulates throughout the body, causing hardening (sclerosis), scarring (fibrosis), and other damage. The damage may affect the appearance of the skin, or it may involve only the internal organs. The symptoms and severity of scleroderma vary from person to person.

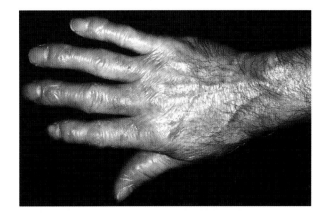

**Scleroderma results in thickening and toughening of the skin, which may also become inflamed.** *(Photo Researchers, Inc.)*

### Genetic profile

The role of **genetics** in the transmission in scleroderma is unclear. Some cases clearly run in families, but most occur in people without any family history of the disease.

### Demographics

Scleroderma occurs in all races of people all over the world, but it affects about four females for every male. Among children, localized scleroderma is more common, and systemic sclerosis is comparatively rare. Most patients with systemic sclerosis are diagnosed between ages 30 and 50. In the United States, about 300,000 people have scleroderma. Young African American women and Native Americans of the Choctaw tribe have especially high rates of the disease.

### Signs and symptoms

The cause of scleroderma is still uncertain. Although the accumulation of collagen appears to be a hallmark of the disease, researchers do not know why it occurs. Some theories suggest that damage to blood vessels may cause the tissues of the body to receive an inadequate amount of oxygen–a condition called ischemia. Some researchers believe that the resulting damage causes the immune system to overreact, producing an autoimmune disorder. According to this theory of scleroderma, the immune system gears up to fight an invader, but no invader is actually present. Cells in the immune system, called antibodies, react to the body's own tissues as if they were foreign. The antibodies turn against the already damaged blood vessels and the vessels' supporting tissues. These immune cells are designed to deliver potent chemicals in order to kill foreign invaders. Some of these cells dump

## KEY TERMS

**Autoimmune disorder**—A disorder in which the body's immune cells mistake the body's own tissues as foreign invaders; the immune cells then work to destroy tissues in the body.

**Collagen**—The main supportive protein of cartilage, connective tissue, tendon, skin, and bone.

**Connective tissue**—A group of tissues responsible for support throughout the body; includes cartilage, bone, fat, tissue underlying skin, and tissues that support organs, blood vessels, and nerves throughout the body.

**Fibrosis**—The abnormal development of fibrous tissue; scarring.

**Limited scleroderma**—A subtype of systemic scleroderma with limited skin involvement. It is sometimes called the CREST form of scleroderma, after the initials of its five major symptoms.

**Localized scleroderma**—Thickening of the skin from overproduction of collagen.

**Morphea**—The most common form of localized scleroderma.

**Raynaud phenomenon/Raynaud disease**—A condition in which blood flow to the body's tissues is reduced by a malfunction of the nerves that regulate the constriction of blood vessels. When attacks of Raynaud's occur in the absence of other medical conditions, it is called Raynaud disease. When attacks occur as part of a disease (as in scleroderma), it is called Raynaud phenomenon.

**Sclerosis**—Hardening.

**Systemic sclerosis**—A rare disorder that causes thickening and scarring of multiple organ systems.

**Telangiectasis**—Very small arteriovenous malformations, or connections between the arteries and veins. The result is small red spots on the skin known as "spider veins".

these chemicals on the body's own tissues instead, causing inflammation, swelling, damage, and scarring.

Most cases of scleroderma have no recognizable triggering event. Some cases, however, have been traced to exposure to toxic (poisonous) substances. For example, coal miners and gold miners, who are exposed to high levels of silica dust, have above-average rates of scleroderma. Other chemicals associated with the disease include polyvinyl chloride, benzine, toluene, and epoxy resins. In 1981, 20,000 people in

Spain were stricken with a syndrome similar to scleroderma when their cooking oil was accidentally contaminated. Certain medications, especially a drug used in **cancer** treatment called bleomycin (Blenoxane), may lead to scleroderma. Some claims of a scleroderma-like illness have been made by women with silicone breast implants, but a link has not been proven in numerous studies.

### Symptoms of systemic scleroderma

A condition called Raynaud's phenomenon is the first symptom in about 95% of all patients with systemic scleroderma. In Raynaud's phenomenon, the blood vessels of the fingers and/or toes (the digits) react to cold in an abnormal way. The vessels clamp down, preventing blood flow to the tip of the digit. Eventually, the flow is cut off to the entire finger or toe. Over time, oxygen deprivation may result in open ulcers on the skin surface. These ulcers can lead to tissue death (gangrene) and loss of the digit. When Raynaud's phenomenon is the first sign of scleroderma, the next symptoms usually appear within two years.

**SKIN AND EXTREMITIES.** Involvement of the skin leads to swelling underneath the skin of the hands, feet, legs, arms, and face. Swelling is followed by thickening and tightening of the skin, which becomes taut and shiny. Severe tightening may lead to abnormalities. For example, tightening of the skin on the hands may cause the fingers to become permanently curled (flexed). Structures within the skin are damaged (including those producing hair, oil, and sweat), and the skin becomes dry and scaly. Ulcers may form, with the danger of infection. Calcium deposits often appear under the skin.

In systemic scleroderma, the mouth and nose may become smaller as the skin on the face tightens. The small mouth may interfere with eating and dental hygiene. Blood vessels under the skin may become enlarged and show through the skin, appearing as purplish marks or red spots. This chronic dilation of the small blood vessels is called telangiectasis.

Muscle weakness, joint pain and stiffness, and carpal tunnel syndrome are common in scleroderma. Carpal tunnel syndrome involves scarring in the wrist, which puts pressure on the median nerve running through that area. Pressure on the nerve causes numbness, tingling, and weakness in some of the fingers.

**DIGESTIVE TRACT.** The tube leading from the mouth to the stomach (the esophagus) becomes stiff and scarred. Patients may have trouble swallowing food. The acid contents of the stomach may start to flow backward into the esophagus (esophageal reflux), causing a very uncomfortable condition known as heartburn. The esophagus may also become inflamed.

The intestine becomes sluggish in processing food, causing bloating and pain. Foods are not digested properly, resulting in diarrhea, weight loss, and anemia. Telangiectasis in the stomach or intestine may cause rupture and bleeding.

**RESPIRATORY AND CIRCULATORY SYSTEMS.** The lungs are affected in about 66% of all people with systemic scleroderma. Complications include shortness of breath, coughing, difficulty breathing due to tightening of the tissue around the chest, inflammation of the air sacs in the lungs (alveolitis), increased risk of pneumonia, and an increased risk of cancer. For these reasons, lung disease is the most likely cause of death associated with scleroderma.

The lining around the heart (pericardium) may become inflamed. The heart may have greater difficulty pumping blood effectively (heart failure). Irregular heart rhythms and enlargement of the heart also occur in scleroderma.

Kidney disease is another common complication. Damage to blood vessels in the kidneys often causes a major rise in the person's blood pressure. The blood pressure may be so high that there is swelling of the brain, causing severe headaches, damage to the retinas of the eyes, seizures, and failure of the heart to pump blood into the body's circulatory system. The kidneys may also stop filtering blood and go into failure. Treatments for high blood pressure have greatly improved these kidney complications. Before these treatments were available, kidney problems were the most common cause of death for people with scleroderma.

Other problems associated with scleroderma include painful dryness of the eyes and mouth, enlargement and destruction of the liver, and a low-functioning thyroid gland.

### Diagnosis

Diagnosis of scleroderma is complicated by the fact that some of its symptoms can accompany other connective-tissue diseases. The most important symptom is thickened or hardened skin on the fingers, hands, forearms, or face. This is found in 98% of people with scleroderma. It can be detected in the course of a physical examination. The person's medical history may also contain important clues, such as exposure to toxic substances on the job. There are a number of nonspecific laboratory tests on blood samples that may indicate the presence of an inflammatory disorder (but not specifically scleroderma). The antinuclear

antibody (ANA) test is positive in more than 95% of people with scleroderma.

Other tests can be performed to evaluate the extent of the disease. These include a test of the electrical system of the heart (an electrocardiogram), lung-function tests, and x–ray studies of the gastrointestinal tract. Various blood tests can be given to study kidney function.

### Treatment and management

At this time there is no cure for scleroderma. A drug called D-penicillamine has been used to interfere with the abnormal collagen. It is believed to help decrease the degree of skin thickening and tightening, and to slow the progress of the disease in other organs. Taking vitamin D and using ultraviolet light may be helpful in treating localized scleroderma. Corticosteroids have been used to treat joint pain, muscle cramps, and other symptoms of inflammation. Other drugs have been studied that reduce the activity of the immune system (immunosuppressants). Because these medications can have serious side effects, they are used in only the most severe cases of scleroderma.

The various complications of scleroderma are treated individually. Raynaud's phenomenon requires that people try to keep their hands and feet warm constantly. Nifedipine is a medication that is sometimes given to help control Raynaud's. Thick ointments and creams are used to treat dry skin. Exercise and massage may help joint involvement; they may also help people retain more movement despite skin tightening. Skin ulcers need prompt attention and may require antibiotics. People with esophageal reflux will be advised to eat small amounts more often, rather than several large meals a day. They should also avoid spicy foods and items containing caffeine. Some patients with esophageal reflux have been successfully treated with surgery. Acid-reducing medications may be given for heartburn. People must be monitored for the development of high blood pressure. If found, they should be promptly treated with appropriate medications, usually ACE inhibitors or other vasodilators. When fluid accumulates due to heart failure, diuretics can be given to get rid of the excess fluid.

### Prognosis

The prognosis for people with scleroderma varies. Some have a very limited form of the disease called morphea, which affects only the skin. These individuals have a very good prognosis. Other people have a subtype of systemic scleroderma called limited scleroderma. For them, the prognosis is relatively good. Limited scleroderma is characterized by limited involvement of the patient's skin and a cluster of five symptoms called the CREST syndrome. CREST stands for:

- C = Calcinosis
- R = Raynaud's disease (phenomenon)
- E = Esophageal dysmotility (stiffness and malfunctioning of the esophagus)
- S = Sclerodactyly (thick, hard, rigid skin over the fingers)
- T = Telangiectasis

In general, people with very widespread skin involvement have the worst prognosis. This level of disease is usually accompanied by involvement of other organs and the most severe complications. Although women are more commonly stricken with scleroderma, men more often die of the disease. The most common causes of death include heart, kidney, and lung diseases. About 65% of all patients survive 10 years or more following a diagnosis of scleroderma.

There are no known ways to prevent scleroderma. People can try to decrease occupational exposure to high-risk substances.

### Resources

#### BOOKS

Aaseng, Nathan. *Autoimmune Diseases*. New York: F. Watts, 1995.

Gilliland, Bruce C. "Systemic Sclerosis (Scleroderma)." In *Harrison's Principles of Internal Medicine,* ed. Anthony S. Fauci, et al. New York: McGraw-Hill, 1998.

"Systemic Sclerosis." *The Merck Manual of Diagnosis and Therapy,* ed. Mark H. Beers and Robert Berkow. Whitehouse Station, NJ: Merck Research Laboratories, 1999.

#### PERIODICALS

De Keyser, F., et al. "Occurrence of Scleroderma in Monozygotic Twins." *Journal of Rheumatology* 27 (September 2000): 2267-2269.

Englert, H., et al. "Familial Risk Estimation in Systemic Sclerosis." *Australia and New Zealand Journal of Medicine* 29 (February 1999): 36-41.

Legerton, C. W. III, et al. "Systemic Sclerosis: Clinical Management of Its Major Complications." *Rheumatic Disease Clinics of North America,* 17, no. 221 (1998).

Saito, S., et al. "Genetic and Immunologic Features Associated with Scleroderma-like Syndrome of TSK Mice." *Current Rheumatology Reports* 1 (October 1999): 34-37.

#### ORGANIZATIONS

American College of Rheumatology. 60 Executive Park South, Suite 150, Atlanta, GA 30329. (404) 633-3777. http://www.rheumatology.org.

National Organization for Rare Disorders (NORD). PO Box 8923, New Fairfield, CT 06812-8923. (203) 746-6518 or (800) 999-6673. Fax: (203) 746-6481. http://www.rarediseases.org.

Scleroderma Foundation. 12 Kent Way, Suite 101, Byfield, MA 01922. (978) 463-5843 or (800) 722-HOPE. Fax: (978) 463-5809. http://www.scleroderma.org..

Rebecca J. Frey, PhD

# Sclerosing bone dysplasias

## Definition

Sclerosing bone dysplasias are rare **genetic disorders** characterized by the creation of abnormally dense and overgrown bones. The abnormal bone formation in sclerosing bone dysplasias is caused by a defect in the replacement of old bone with new bone.

## Description

Bone consists of living cells, called osteocytes, embedded in a calcium carbonate matrix that makes up the main bone material. The calcium carbonate matrix includes inorganic mineral components like calcium and organic components, such as collagen. The replacement of old bone with new bone is mediated by two types of bone cells, osteoblasts and osteoclasts. The osteoblasts make bone, while osteoclasts resorb, or take away, bone. Problems with the ability of the osteoclasts and osteoblasts to remodel bone can result in the increased skeletal density (sclerosis) and bony overgrowth (hyperostosis) seen in the sclerosing bone dysplasias. The first description of sclerosing bone **dysplasia** occurred in 1904 when Professor Albers-Schönberg of Hamburg described a patient suffering from a benign form of thickened and very strong hard bone.

## KEY TERMS

**Bone dysplasia**—Abnormal bone development.

**Bone remodeling**—The process of breaking down old bone and building up new bone.

**Bone sclerosis**—Increased bone density and hardness.

**Diaphysis**—Primary region of ossification found in the shaft of the long bones.

**Hyperostosis**—Overgrowth of the bone.

**Metaphysis**—The growing portion of the developing long bone.

**Osteoblasts**—A bone cell that makes bone.

**Osteoclasts**—A bone cell that breaks down and reabsorbs bone.

Currently, sclerosing bone dysplasias are subdivided into types based upon the problems in bone remodeling. The three main categories of sclerosing bone dysplasias are: increased bone density without modification of bone shape; increased bone density with involvement of main body of the bone and primary region of bone formation (diaphysis); and increased bone density with involvement of the area of the developing long bone that is the growing portion of the bone (metaphysis). Although all of the sclerosing bone dysplasias share some overlapping features, it is usually possible to distinguish between these types of sclerosing bone dysplasia based on the age at which symptoms appear, the pattern of **inheritance** in the family, radiographic skeletal surveys, and genetic studies.

### Genetic profile

Although all of the genes involved in sclerosing bone dysplasias encode proteins that direct the remodeling of bone, each type of sclerosing bone dysplasia has specific symptoms and inheritance patterns caused by different **gene** defects.

Many types of sclerosing bone dysplasia are autosomal dominant genetic disorders. In autosomal dominant genetic disorders, the genes that cause a particular disorder are carried on one of the 22 pairs of numbered autosomal chromosomes, rather than on the X or Y sex chromosomes. In the case of sclerosing bone dysplasia, only one copy of the mutated, or nonworking, gene is necessary for the development of the disorder. An individual who inherits a normal gene copy from one parent and an abnormal gene copy from the other parent is likely to have symptoms of a sclerosing bone dysplasia. The children of an individual with one normal gene copy and one mutated copy have a 50% chance of inheriting the disorder. Types of sclerosing bone dysplasias inherited in an autosomal dominant pattern include: benign dominant osteopetrosis (caused by a mutation in the chloride channel 7 gene, ClCN7); progressive diaphyseal dysplasia (caused by a mutation in the beta-1 transforming growth factor gene, TGFB1); some forms of craniodiaphyseal dysplasia; Van Buchem disease, type II (caused by a mutation in the low-density lipoprotein receptor-related protein 5 gene, LRP5); and some forms of craniometaphyseal dysplasia (caused by a mutation in a multipass transmembrane protein, ANK).

Many other types of sclerosing bone dysplasia are inherited in an autosomal recessive pattern. In an autosomal recessive condition, two copies of the mutated gene are needed to develop the symptoms of the disorder. In these cases, both parents each carry one copy of a mutated gene. Individuals with only one copy of a mutated gene for a recessive condition are known as carriers and have no symptoms related to the condition. In fact, every person carries between five and 10 mutated genes for harmful, recessive conditions. However, when two people with the same mutated recessive gene for sclerosing bone dysplasia have children together, there is a 25% chance with each pregnancy for the child to inherit two mutated copies, one from each parent. That child then has no working copies of the gene and will display the signs and symptoms associated with sclerosing bone dysplasia. Sclerosing bone dysplasias that are inherited in an autosomal recessive manner include: malignant infantile osteopetrosis (caused by mutations in the ATP6i/TCIRG1, CLCN7, and GL genes); pycnodysostosis (caused by mutations in the cathepsin K gene, CATK); some forms of craniodiaphyseal dysplasia; Van Buchem disease, type I (caused by mutations in VBCH,17q11.2); sclerosteosis (caused by a mutation in the sclerostin gene, SOST); and some forms of craniometaphyseal dysplasia.

One type of sclerosing bone dysplasia, frontometaphyseal dysplasia, is caused by a mutation in the filamin A gene (FLNA) and is inherited in an X-linked recessive pattern. As opposed to genes that are carried on one of the 22 pairs of numbered autosomal chromosomes, X-linked genes are found on the sex chromosomes called X. Females have two X chromosomes, while males have a single X **chromosome** and a single Y chromosome. When a female inherits a mutated gene on the X chromosome, she is known as a carrier. Carriers most often have no symptoms related the condition because the gene on her other chromosome continues to function properly. However, males only inherit one copy of the information stored on the X chromosome. When a male inherits a mutated copy of the gene that causes an X-linked recessive condition, he will experience the symptoms associated with the disease. The chance for a carrier female to have an affected son is 50%, while the chance to have a daughter who is also a carrier for the condition is 50%. An affected male has a 100% chance of having carrier daughters and a 0% chance of having affected sons.

One type of sclerosing bone dysplasia, osteopathia striata with cranial sclerosis, is inherited in an X-linked dominant pattern. X-linked dominant inheritance occurs when the gene is located on the X chromosome, but the gene acts in a dominant manner. This means that both males and females can display the trait or disorder, while having only one copy of the gene. Furthermore, in X-linked dominant conditions, only one copy of the mutated gene is necessary for the development of the disorder. Therefore, an individual who inherits a normal gene copy from one parent and an abnormal gene copy for sclerosing bone dysplasia from the other parent is likely to have symptoms of sclerosing bone dysplasia. The children of an individual with one normal gene copy and one mutated copy have a 50% chance of inheriting a mutated sclerosing bone dysplasia gene.

## Demographics

Sclerosing bone dysplasias are rare conditions. Estimates of general population frequency range by ethnic group and type of sclerosing bone dysplasia described. Affected individuals can occur within a variety of ethnic backgrounds and cases have been found in countries, including Denmark, Egypt, the United States, Germany, Japan, Italy, Brazil, Spain, Senegal, South Africa, the Netherlands, and Cyprus. A large number of individuals affected by sclerosing bone dysplasias exist in the Afrikaner population of South Africa and the Dutch population of the Netherlands. The carrier rate for the single founder-derived mutation that causes sclerosteosis in the Afrikaner population is approximately one in 100. Van Buchem disease has been recognized predominantly in the Dutch population (±20 cases). Several of the affected families have ancestral origins on the former island of Urk in the Zuider Zee. The prevalence of later onset osteopetrosis or Albers-Schonberg is about one in 18,000 in Denmark.

## Signs and symptoms

Sclerosing bone dysplasias are rare genetic disorders characterized by increased skeletal density and excessive bone formation, or overgrowth, due to a defect in the method of replacing old bone with new bone (bone remodeling). Each of the three main categories of sclerosing bone dysplasias exhibit different symptoms, including age of onset, skeletal involvement, and prognosis.

The specific disorders in the group of sclerosing bone dysplasias that exhibits increased bone density without modification of bone shape include: osteopetrosis disorders (autosomal dominant osteopetrosis types I and II and autosomal recessive osteropetrosis); pycnodysostosis; and osteopathia striata with cranial sclerosis.

The osteopetrosis disorders are conditions that involve increased bone density without modification of bone shape. They include two forms of benign dominant conditions known as autosomal dominant osteopetrosis I (ADOI) and autosomal dominant osteopetrosis II (ADOII), and one form of malignant infantile osteopetrosis (MIOP).

Benign dominant or autosomal dominant osteopetrosis (ADO) typically presents in childhood, adolescence, or young adult life with multiple fractures, mild anomalies in head and face proportions, mild anemia, hearing loss, bone inflammation/infection, or increased bone density found on routine x-ray studies. ADO has two distinct subtypes known as types I and II that are distinguished by the location of sclerosis and presence or absence of increased bone fractures.

Autosomal dominant osteopetrosis type I (ADOI or OPTA1) is characterized by a generalized increase in the hardness, thickness, and density of bone tissue (osteosclerosis), most pronounced in the cranial vault. Patients are often asymptomatic, but some suffer from pain and hearing loss. ADOI appears to be the only type of osteopetrosis not associated with an increased fracture rate.

Autosomal dominant osteopetrosis type II (ADOII or OPTA2) is characterized by an increase in the hardness, thickness, and density of bone tissue (sclerosis) predominantly involving the spine, the pelvis, and the skull base. Fragility of bones and dental abscesses are the leading complications. Other symptoms include arthritis of the hip (hip **osteoarthritis**), bone infections (osteomyelitis), thoracic or lumbar **scoliosis**, and cranial nerve involvement responsible for hearing loss, bilateral optic atrophy, and/or facial palsy. Although other forms of osteopetrosis are considerably more severe, it has been suggested that the name benign osteopetrosis, previously used for ADOII, is probably incorrect given the complications of the condition.

Malignant infantile osteopetrosis (MIOP) is characterized by a generalized increase in bone density found at or soon after birth. The sclerosis of the bones causes a decrease in size of the bone marrow cavities, a progressively enlarging spleen, low blood iron (anemia), and blood cell production that occurs in other parts of the body (extramedullary haemopoiesis). Additionally, enlarging skull bones compress the optic nerves, auditory nerves, facial nerves, and the foramen magnum (the large hole at the base of the skull that allows passage of the spinal cord). The most frequent presentations in infancy are seizures, low calcium level, convulsions, failure of visual fixation (nystagmus), large spleen and liver (hepatosplenomegaly), and frequent broken bones.

Pycnodysostosis is characterized by an increase in bone density of the skeleton (osteosclerosis), skull deformities, short stature, short limbs, characteristic facial features, and bone fragility. Onset of the symptoms occurs around two or three years of age. Other features of the condition include: separated cranial sutures; large fontanel with delayed closure; obtuse mandibular angle; delayed teeth eruption; enamel hypoplasia; dysplastic acromial ends of the clavicles; frontal bossing; ocular proptosis; and dysplastic nails. Developmental evaluations often indicate normal motor, fine motor-adaptive, language, and personal social abilities.

Osteopathia striata with cranial sclerosis (OSCS) presents with longitudinal striations of dense bone in the long bones and formation of dense bone in the cranial and facial bones in infancy and childhood. The formation of dense bone in the head and face leads to facial disfigurement and to neurological complications, such as **deafness** due to pressure on cranial nerves. Other features include: a large head (macrocephaly); congenital heart defects, such as aortic stenosis and ventricular septal defects; scoliosis of the back; narrowed visual fields; **cleft palate**; long fingers; curving of the third to fifth fingers (clinodactyly); **clubfoot**; facial nerve palsy; and mild mental retardation.

The disorders involving increased bone density with diaphyseal involvement include: progressive diaphyseal dysplasia, or Camurati-Engelmann disease; craniodiaphyseal dysplasia; and endosteal hyperostosis disorders (Van Buchem disease (types I and II) and sclerosteosis).

Progressive diaphyseal dysplasia (PDD), or Camurati-Engelmann disease, is characterized by childhood onset of bone overgrowth (hyperostosis) and increased density (sclerosis) of the diaphyses of the long bones and the skull. Other features may include: a slender build with long limbs; angular profile; prominent bones (asthenic habitus); hearing loss; protruding eyeballs (exophthalmos); optic nerve compression; double vision (diplopia); cavities (dental caries); sclerosis of skull base; lower jaw (mandible) involvement; sclerosis of posterior part of vertebrae (body and arches); scoliosis; progressive diaphyseal widening; thickened cortices; narrowing of medullary canal; erlenmeyer flask defect of the bone; clubfoot (genu varus and valgus deformities); relative muscle weakness, especially in pelvic girdle; atrophic muscle fiber; headaches; delayed puberty; bone marrow hypoplasia; anemia; waddling gait; and leg pain. The most severely affected individuals will have progression of mild skull hyperostosis to severe skull thickening and cranial nerve compression over many years. Presentation of the disease can be very different from one individual to another.

Craniodiaphyseal dysplasia includes a wide variety of symptoms and age of onset from infancy to childhood. Facial and cranial thickening and distortion are particularly striking in this form. The characteristic facial features of craniodiaphyseal dysplasia occur from the overgrowth of bone in the face and skull that results in progressive facial anomalies, a broad nasal bridge, and wide-spaced eyes. Other symptoms of craniodiaphyseal dysplasia, like hearing loss and facial paralysis, are caused by the overgrowth of the skull as it gradually eliminates the perinasal sinuses and the large hole at the base of the skull that allows passage of the spinal cord (foramina of the skull base). Individuals with craniodiaphyseal dysplasia often are affected by mental retardation. Unlike the situation in the craniometaphyseal dysplasias, the long bones do not show metaphyseal flaring, but are shaped like a policeman's nightstick.

Endosteal hyperostosis disorders include Van Buchem disease (types I and II) and sclerosteosis. The two endosteal hyperostosis conditions include many similar features. The two disorders can be distinguished from each other via their different appearance of the bone changes on x-ray. Additionally, sclerosteosis includes the presence of asymmetric fusion (cutaneous syndactyly) of the index and middle fingers in many cases, and Van Buchem disease does not.

Van Buchem disease (or hyperostosis corticalis familiaris) is characterized by progressive enlargement of the lower jaw in childhood and symptoms, including hearing loss and facial paralysis, in adulthood caused by the overgrowth of the skull. Van Buchem disease has two distinct subtypes known as types I and II. The subtypes are distinguished by genetic cause, primary location of bone overgrowth, and phosphate levels.

The symptoms of Van Buchem disease type I begin in childhood or puberty and include features resulting from bone overgrowth. Symptoms include: cranial bone overgrowth (hyperostosis) leading to optic nerve compression; hearing loss; headaches; cranial nerve palsy; osteosclerosis; thickened cortex of long bones; and abnormally high blood levels of phosphorous (hyperphosphatasemia).

The signs and symptoms of Van Buchem disease Type II begin in childhood or puberty, and include: enlarged lower jaw bone (mandible); increased skull cap (calvarial) thickness; cranial osteosclerosis; thickened cortices of long bones; and normal alkaline phosphatase levels.

Sclerosteosis is characterized by tall stature, overgrowth of the nasal and facial bones, broad, flat nasal bridge, wide-spaced eyes (hypertelorism), and minor hand malformation, such as finger fusion (syndactyly). Other symptoms may include: small nails (nail dysplasia); square jaw due to overgrowth of the mandible; difficulties in chewing; inability to smell (anosmia); massive bone density (sclerosis) of the long tubular bones, ribs, pelvis, and skull; and multiple cranial nerve involvement resulting in optic atrophy, facial palsy, and trigeminal nerve pain episodes (neuralgia). Facial nerve paralysis may be present as early as birth or develop soon afterwards. Facial palsy and deafness as a result of cranial nerve entrapment often develop in childhood. Increased intracranial pressure may result in sudden death from impaction of the brain stem in the foramen magnum.

The disorders involving increased bone density with metaphyseal involvement include craniometaphyseal dysplasia and frontometaphyseal dysplasia.

Craniometaphyseal dysplasia involves overgrowth bone anomalies that commonly present in infancy. Some of the first indications of a craniometaphyseal dysplasia include breathing difficulties and narrowing nasal passages due to bone overgrowth. The characteristic facial features of craniometaphyseal dysplasia occur from the overgrowth of bone in the face and skull that result in progressive facial anomalies, a broad nasal bridge, and wide-spaced eyes. Other symptoms of craniometaphyseal dysplasia, like hearing loss and facial paralysis, are caused by the overgrowth of the skull as it gradually eliminates the perinasal sinuses and the large hole at the base of the skull that allows passage of the spinal cord (foramina of the skull base). The features of craniometaphyseal dysplasia are more severe than the sclerotic or hyperostotic features, except in the lower jaw where they are less severe than craniodiaphyseal dysplasia.

Frontometaphyseal dysplasia's most striking feature is a characteristic facial appearance that includes a very prominent supraorbital ridge above the eyes resulting from bone overgrowth. In many cases, the prominent ridge may be present at birth, along with a small, pointed chin, wide-spaced eyes (hypertelorism), wide nasal bridge, poor sinus development, clubfoot (coxa valga and genu valgum), and flared metaphyses. Later findings may include: progressive mixed conductive and sensorineural hearing loss; high palate; teeth issues; mitral valve prolapse; narrow trachea; winged shoulder blade (scapulae); irregular rib contours; "coat hanger" deformity of lower ribs; distended kidneys and ureters (hydronephrosis and hydroureter); scoliosis; cervical vertebral fusion; flared pelvis; elbow contractures; knee and ankle contractures; erlenmeyer-flask appearance of femur and tibia; increased density of long bone diaphyses; finger and wrist contractures; long and wide fingers; partial fusion of the bones of the feet; large feet; overgrowth of hair on the buttocks and thighs; muscle wasting (especially legs and arms); and mental retardation. The **skeletal dysplasia** and the associated clinical findings show significant variability from affected individual to individual. The syndrome has been suggested to be an allelic variant of the Melnick-Needles osteodysplasty.

### Diagnosis

Diagnosis of sclerosing bone dysplasias is most often based upon age of onset, clinical features, radiological evaluation, and family history. Radiologic examination will detect the dense bones (sclerosis) and their locations. Genetic studies may help confirm a diagnosis of a specific sclerosing bone dysplasia, but some affected individuals will not have a genetic mutation that can be identified. Not all types of sclerosing bone dysplasias have a **genetic testing** available because some forms of sclerosing bone dysplasia have not yet had a causative gene identified.

### Treatment and management

The sclerosing bone dysplasias are genetic disorders and do not have specific therapies that remove, cure, or fix all signs of the disorder. Treatment and management of the sclerosing bone dysplasias focus on treatment of specific symptoms of the condition. Management of patients with sclerosing bone dysplasias requires a comprehensive approach to characteristic clinical problems, including hematologic and metabolic abnormalities, fractures, bone deformities, back pain, bone pain, bone infection (osteomyelitis), hearing impairment, dental issues, short stature, and neurologic symptoms. Surgical intervention may be difficult and prolonged in affected individuals since standard equipment may be too short and not powerful enough to cut through the dense bone. In addition, bone regrowth occurs and may cause recurrence of symptoms after surgery.

Treatment of the hematologic issues found in the sclerosing bone dysplasias is focused on the correction of low blood iron (anemia) and low platelets. In some cases, a steroid, prednisone, may be used to treat both of these conditions. In other cases, transfusions to treat anemia and splenectomy to increase platelets may be recommended. Depending on the form of sclerosing bone dysplasia, treatment to correct hematologic issues may not be effective.

Medical treatment of sclerosis and hyperostosis in sclerosing bone dysplasias is based on efforts to stimulate host osteoclasts to break down bone or provide an alternative source of osteoclasts. Stimulation of osteoclasts has been attempted with calcium restriction and calcitrol, calcitonin therapy, steroids, parathyroid hormone therapy, and interferon. Bone marrow transplant has been used to treat infantile malignant osteopetrosis. Effective therapies for each type of sclerosing bone dysplasia need to be individualized. Many people affected by a sclerosing bone dysplasia will not respond to treatment.

Most treatments protocols for sclerosing bone dysplasias are focused upon the correction of the frequent bones fractures, using splints, casts, and braces. Orthopedic surgery may be needed to correct internal fractures.

Since hearing loss is a common feature of the sclerosing bone dysplasias, formal audiological evaluation is recommended at diagnosis. Hearing loss associated with the sclerosing bone dysplasias can be addressed through sign language, use of hearing aids, and/or surgery. Some individuals pursue exploratory tympanotomy, stapedotomy, placement of a total ossicular reconstruction prosthesis, cochlear implantation, insertion of a Wehr's prosthesis, decompression, and other surgical procedures. Widening of the external auditory canal is usually necessary to accommodate a hearing aid. Correction of hearing loss is difficult and only has limited success.

In forms of sclerosing bone dysplasias associated with short stature, most individuals make an effort to modify their environment to suit their height. For individuals who wish to treat their short stature, some progress in increasing height has been made by growth hormone (GH) supplementation in affected children. However, hormone supplementation can cause disproportionate growth, leading to longer arms and trunk and shorter legs.

Intracranial pressure is one of main features of sclerosing bone dysplasias, and the most severe. The increase in intracranial pressure caused by the increase in bone size and density often leads to headaches, hearing loss, blindness, facial paralysis, facial nerve palsies, and death. Accordingly, management of intracranial pressure includes monitoring for increased pressure, sudden onset of headaches, and blurred vision that may result in the need for decompression craniectomy or other forms of surgical decompression. Total decompression can prevent future attacks of facial paralysis in some forms of sclerosing bone dysplasias. Given the progressive nature of the sclerosing bone dysplasias, bone regrowth will occur and may cause recurrence of symptoms after surgery.

The abnormal formation of the head and skull bones impacts the form and function of the face, jaws, and remainder of the craniofacial skeleton. Surgery to correct bony overgrowth and density in the forehead, nose, and jaw bones is an option for some patients. Given the progressive nature of the sclerosing bone dysplasias, bone regrowth will occur and may cause recurrence of symptoms after surgery.

The objective of treatment for bone infection (osteomyelitis) in sclerosing bone dysplasias is to eliminate the infection and prevent the development of chronic infection. Intravenous antibiotics are started early and may later be changed, depending on culture results. Some new antibiotics can be very effective when given orally. In chronic infection, surgical removal of dead bone tissue is usually necessary.

Treatment of scoliosis depends upon the type of sclerosing bone dysplasias and the severity of the scoliosis. Treatment options may include observation, orthopedic braces, and surgery. In some cases, the progressive nature of the underlying condition makes correction of scoliosis difficult, if not impossible.

The treatment for clubfoot involves orthopedic surgery to correct the abnormal formation of the lower limbs. Correction of the abnormality may require multiple surgeries, and after care with casts, braces, and physical therapy.

Treatment of the myriad of dental issues associated with sclerosing bone dysplasias are managed best through comprehensive oral and dental care. A craniofacial team may be best suited to address the variety of issues. Mandible reduction is often performed for cosmetic reasons or if mouth closure is impaired as a result of overgrowth of the mandible. Tooth extraction may be difficult given the density of bone.

Individuals affected by sclerosing bone dysplasias may have pain from arthritis, neuralgia caused by pressure, dental pain, and other pain sources related to abnormal bone remodeling. Pain management for each of these sources is different. Severe pain resulting from nerve compression may be helped by nerve decompression surgery. Spinal cord decompression surgery may help alleviate back pain. A pain management specialist working with an individual's treatment team can determine the level of pain, determine the best medications to treat the pain, and evaluate the effectiveness of the medications.

### Prognosis

The prognosis for individuals affected by sclerosing bone dysplasia varies greatly depending upon the type of sclerosing bone dysplasia and severity of symptoms. Individuals affected by delayed or adult-onset forms of sclerosing bone dysplasia may have mild to severe symptoms that do not reduce their lifespan. Individuals who present with symptoms at birth or soon after birth, like malignant infantile osteopetrosis and sclerosteosis, have a progressive course of disease that leads to early death. Increased intracranial pressure may result from a combination of circumstances and may have led, in several instances, to sudden death from impaction of the brainstem in the foramen magnum. Surgical procedures such as total decompression may increase length and quality of life.

### Resources

**BOOKS**

De Villiers, J. C., and J. J. Du Plessis. "Neurosurgical Management of Sclerosteosis." In *Operative Neurosurgical Techniques*, edited by H.H. Scmidek, and W. H. Sweet. Philadelphia: W. B. Saunders Co., 1995.

**PERIODICALS**

Hamersma, H., J. Gardner, and P. Beighton. "The Natural History of Sclerosteosis." *Clin Genet* 63 (2003): 192–197.

Hofmeyr, L. M., and H. Hamersma. "Sclerosing Bone Dysplasias: Neurologic Assessment and Management." *Curr Opin Otolaryngol Head Neck Surg* 12, no. 5 (October 2004): 393–97.

**ORGANIZATIONS**

AboutFace International. 123 Edward Street, Suite 1003, Toronto, Ontario M5G 1E2 Canada. (800) 665-FACE (3223). Fax: (416) 597-8494. E-mail: info@aboutfaceinternational.org. (April 23, 2005.) http://www.aboutfaceinternational.org.

American Society for Deaf Children. PO Box 3355, Gettysburg, PA 17325. (800) 942-2732 (parent hotline); (717) 334-7922 (business V/TTY). Fax: (717) 334-8808. E-mail: asdc@deafchildren.org. (April 23, 2005.) http://www.deafchildren.org/home/home.html.

National Association of the Deaf. 814 Thayer Avenue, Silver Spring, MD 20910. (301) 587-1788 (voice); (301) 587-1789 (TTY). Fax: (301) 587-1791. E-mail: NADinfo@nad.org. (April 23, 2005.) http://www.nad.org.

**WEB SITES**

Geneclinics. (April 23, 2005.) http://www.geneclinics.org.

Dawn Jacob Laney, MS, CGC

## Scoliosis

### Definition

Scoliosis is a side-to-side curvature of the spine of 10 degrees or greater.

### Description

When viewed from the rear, the spine usually appears to form a straight vertical line. Scoliosis is a

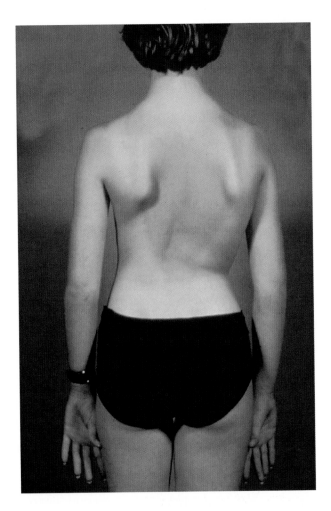

**A woman with idiopathic scoliosis.** (*Custom Medical Stock Photo, Inc.*)

## KEY TERMS

**Cobb angle**—A measure of the curvature of scoliosis, determined by measurements made on x–rays.

**Scoliometer**—A tool for measuring trunk asymmetry; it includes a bubble level and angle measure.

**Spondylosis**—Arthritis of the spine.

lateral (side-to-side) curve in the spine, usually combined with a rotation of the vertebrae. (The lateral curvature of scoliosis should not be confused with the normal set of front-to-back spinal curves visible from the side.) While a small degree of lateral curvature does not cause any medical problems, larger curves can cause postural imbalance and lead to muscle fatigue and pain. More severe scoliosis can interfere with breathing and lead to arthritis of the spine (spondylosis).

Four out of five cases of scoliosis are *idiopathic*, meaning the cause is unknown. Children with idiopathic scoliosis appear to be otherwise entirely healthy, and have not had any bone or joint disease early in life. Scoliosis is not caused by poor posture, diet, or carrying a heavy book bag exclusively on one shoulder.

Idiopathic scoliosis is further classified according to age of onset:

- Infantile. Curvature appears before age three. This type is quite rare in the United States, but is more common in Europe.

- Juvenile. Curvature appears between ages three and 10. This type may be equivalent to the adolescent type, except for the age of onset.

- Adolescent. Curvature appears between ages of 10 and 13, near the beginning of puberty. This is the most common type of idiopathic scoliosis.

- Adult. Curvature begins after physical maturation is completed.

Causes are known for three other types of scoliosis:

- Congenital scoliosis is due to congenital birth defects in the spine, often associated with other structural abnormalities.

- Neuromuscular scoliosis is due to loss of control of the nerves or muscles that support the spine. The most common causes of this type of scoliosis are cerebral palsy and muscular dystrophy.

- Degenerative scoliosis may be caused by degeneration of the discs that separate the vertebrae or arthritis in the joints that link them.

## Genetic profile

Idiopathic scoliosis has long been observed to run in families. Twin and family studies have consistently indicated a genetic contribution to the condition. However, no consistent pattern of transmission has been observed in familial cases. No genes have been identified which specifically cause or predispose to the idiopathic form of scoliosis.

There are several genetic syndromes that involve a predispostion to scoliosis, and several studies have investigated whether or not the genes causing these syndromes may also be responsible for idiopathic scoliosis. Using this *candidate gene approach*, the genes responsible for **Marfan syndrome** (fibrillin), **Stickler syndrome**, and some forms of **osteogenesis imperfecta** (collagen types I and II) have not been shown to correlate with idiopathic scoliosis.

Attempts to map a **gene** or genes for scoliosis have not shown consistent linkage to a particular **chromosome** region.

Most researchers have concluded that scoliosis is a complex trait. As such, there are likely to be multiple genetic, environmental, and potentially additional factors that contribute to the etiology of the condition. Complex traits are difficult to study due to the difficulty in identifying and isolating these multiple factors.

## Demographics

The incidence of scoliosis in the general population is 2-3%. Among adolecents, however, 10% have some degree of scoliosis (though fewer than 1% have curves which require treatment).

Scoliosis is found in both boys and girls, but a girl's spinal curve is much more likely to progress than a boy's. Girls require scoliosis treatment about five times as often. The reason for these differences is not known, but may relate to increased levels of estrogen and other hormones.

## Signs and symptoms

Scoliosis causes a noticeable asymmetry in the torso when viewed from the front or back. The first sign of scoliosis is often seen when a child is wearing a bathing suit or underwear. A child may appear to be standing with one shoulder higher than the other, or to have a tilt in the waistline. One shoulder blade may appear more prominent than the other due to rotation. In girls, one breast may appear higher than the other, or larger if rotation pushes that side forward.

Curve progression is greatest near the adolescent growth spurt. Scoliosis that begins early on is more likely to progress significantly than scoliosis that begins later in puberty.

More than 30 states have screening programs in schools for adolescent scoliosis, usually conducted by trained school nurses or gym teachers.

### Diagnosis

Diagnosis for scoliosis is done by an orthopedist. A complete medical history is taken, including questions about family history of scoliosis. The physical examination includes determination of pubertal development in adolescents, a neurological exam (which may reveal a neuromuscular cause), and measurements of trunk asymmetry. Examination of the trunk is done while the patient is standing, bending over, and lying down, and involves both visual inspection and use of a simple mechanical device called a scoliometer.

If a curve is detected, one or more x–rays will usually be taken to define the curve or curves more precisely. An x–ray is used to document spinal maturity, any pelvic tilt or hip asymmetry, and the location, extent, and degree of curvature. The curve is defined in terms of where it begins and ends, in which direction it bends, and by an angle measure known as the Cobb angle. The Cobb angle is found by projecting lines parallel to the vertebrae tops at the extremes of the curve; projecting perpendiculars from these lines; and measuring the angle of intersection. To properly track the progress of scoliosis, it is important to project from the same points of the spine each time.

Occasionally, magnetic resonance imaging (MRI) is used, primarily to look more closely at the condition of the spinal cord and nerve roots extending from it if neurological problems are suspected.

### Treatment and management

Treatment decisions for scoliosis are based on the degree of curvature, the likelihood of significant progression, and the presence of pain, if any.

Curves less than 20 degrees are not usually treated, except by regular follow-up for children who are still growing. Watchful waiting is usually all that is required in adolescents with curves of 20-25 degrees, or adults with curves up to 40 degrees or slightly more, as long as there is no pain.

For children or adolescents whose curves progress to 25 degrees, and who have a year or more of growth left, bracing may be required. Bracing cannot correct curvature, but may be effective in halting or slowing progression. Bracing is rarely used in adults, except where pain is significant and surgery is not an option, as in some elderly patients.

There are two different categories of braces, those designed for nearly 24 hour per day use and those designed for night use. The full-time brace styles are designed to hold the spine in a vertical position, while the night use braces are designed to bend the spine in the direction opposite the curve.

The Milwaukee brace is a full-time brace which consists of metal uprights attached to pads at the hips, rib cage, and neck. Other types of full-time braces, such as the Boston brace, involve underarm rigid plastic molding to encircle the lower rib cage, abdomen, and hips. Because they can be worn out of sight beneath clothing, the underarm braces are better tolerated and often leads to better compliance. The Boston brace is currently the most commonly used. Full-time braces are often prescribed to be worn for 22-23 hours per day, though some clinicians believe that recommending brace use of 16 hours leads to better compliance and results.

Night use braces bend the patient's scoliosis into a correct angle, and are prescribed for 8 hours of use during sleep. Some investigators have found that night use braces are not as effective as the day use types.

Bracing may be appropriate for scoliosis due to some types of neuromuscular disease, including **spinal muscular atrophy**, before growth is finished. **Duchenne muscular dystrophy** is not treated by bracing, since surgery is likely to be required, and since later surgery is complicated by loss of respiratory capacity.

Surgery for idiopathic scoliosis is usually recommended if:

- the curve has progressed despite bracing
- the curve is greater than 40-50 degrees before growth has stopped in an adolescent
- the curve is greater than 50 degrees and continues to increase in an adult
- there is significant pain

Orthopedic surgery for neuromuscular scoliosis is often done earlier. The goals of surgery are to correct the deformity as much as possible, to prevent further deformity, and to eliminate pain as much as possible. Surgery can usually correct 40-50% of the curve, and sometimes as much as 80%. Surgery cannot always completely remove pain.

The surgical procedure for scoliosis is called *spinal fusion*, because the goal is to straighten the spine as much as possible, and then to fuse the vertebrae together to prevent further curvature. To achieve fusion, the involved vertebra are first exposed, and then scraped to promote regrowth. Bone chips are usually used to splint together the vertebrae to increase the likelihood of fusion. To maintain the proper spinal posture before

## QUESTIONS TO ASK YOUR DOCTOR

- How do the four types of scoliosis differ from each other?
- Can scoliosis be prevented and, if so, how?
- What kinds of treatment are available for scoliosis, and how successful is each type of treatment?
- How does scoliosis affect a person's life span or the quality of life for that person?

fusion occurs, metal rods are inserted alongside the spine, and are attached to the vertebrae by hooks, screws, or wires. Fusion of the spine makes it rigid and resistant to further curvature. The metal rods are no longer needed once fusion is complete, but are rarely removed unless their presence leads to complications.

Spinal fusion leaves the involved portion of the spine permanently stiff and inflexible. While this leads to some loss of normal motion, most functional activities are not strongly affected, unless the very lowest portion of the spine (the lumbar region) is fused. Normal mobility, exercise, and even contact sports are usually all possible after spinal fusion. Full recovery takes approximately six months.

### Prognosis

The prognosis for a person with scoliosis depends on many factors, including the age at which scoliosis begins and the treatment received. Most cases of mild adolescent idiopathic scoliosis need no treatment, do not progress, and do not cause pain or functional limitations. Untreated severe scoliosis often leads to spondylosis, and may impair breathing.

### Resources

#### BOOKS

Lonstein, John, et al., eds. *Moe's Textbook of Scoliosis and Other Spinal Deformities*. 3rd ed. Philadelphia: W.B. Saunders, 1995.
Neuwirth, Michael, and Kevin Osborn. *The Scoliosis Handbook*. New York: Henry Holt & Co., 1996.

#### ORGANIZATION

National Scoliosis Foundation. 5 Cabot Place, Stoughton, MA 02072 (781) 341-6333.

Jennifer Roggenbuck, MS, CGC

## Sebastian platelet syndrome *see* **Sebastian syndrome**

# Sebastian syndrome

### Definition

Sebastian syndrome is an extremely rare genetic disease that results in impaired blood clotting function and abnormal platelet formation. Another name for Sebastian syndrome is autosomal dominant macro-thrombocytopenia with leukocyte inclusions.

### Description

Sebastian syndrome is classified as one of the inherited giant platelet disorders (IGPDs). Platelet cells are components of the blood that play a key role in blood clotting. All IGPDs are associated with bleeding disorders due to improper platelet function and increased platelet cell size. Other IGPDs include May-Hegglin anomaly, Epstein syndrome, Fechtner syndrome, and Bernard-Soulier syndrome. Sebastian syndrome is distinguished from these other IGPDs by subtle differences in the platelet and white blood cell structure and by the lack of symptoms other than bleeding abnormalities.

People affected by Sebastian syndrome have mild, non-life-threatening dysfunction of the blood related to decreased blood clotting function. They may bruise easily or be prone to nosebleeds.

### Genetic profile

Sebastian syndrome is inherited as an autosomal dominant trait. Autosomal means that the syndrome is not carried on a sex **chromosome**, while dominant means that only one parent has to pass on the **gene** mutation in order for the child to be affected with the syndrome.

Genetic studies in the year 2000 proved that Sebastian syndrome is due to a mutation in the gene that encodes a specific enzyme known as nonmuscle myosin heavy chain 9 (the MYH9 gene). The gene locus is 22q11.2, or, the eleventh band of the q arm of chromosome 22. Research has also shown that mutations in the same gene are responsible for May-Hegglin anomaly and Fechtner syndrome, two other inherited giant platelet disorders.

### Demographics

Sebastian syndrome is extremely rare and less than 10 affected families have been reported in the medical literature. Due to the very small number of cases, demographic trends for the disease have not been established. Affected individuals have been identified

## KEY TERMS

**Inherited giant platelet disorder (IGPD)**—A group of hereditary conditions that cause abnormal blood clotting and other conditions.

**Platelets**—Small disc-shaped structures that circulate in the blood stream and participate in blood clotting.

## QUESTIONS TO ASK YOUR DOCTOR

- What is an inherited giant platelet disorder, and how does Sebastian syndrome differ from other forms of this condition?
- What are the most serious medical problems that arise because of Sebastian syndrome?
- What kinds of treatments or medications are available for the control of Sebastian syndrome?
- Is it necessary to have periodic medical check-ups to monitor the progress of my Sebastian syndrome?

in Caucasian, Japanese, African-American, Spanish, and Saudi Arabian families, so there does not seem to be any clear ethnic pattern to the disease. Both males and females appear to be affected with the same probability.

### Signs and symptoms

The symptoms of Sebastian syndrome include a propensity for nosebleeds, bleeding from the gums, mildly increased bleeding time after being cut, and a tendency to bruise easily. Women may experience heavier than normal menstrual bleeding. People with Sebastian syndrome may experience severe hemorrhage after undergoing surgery for any reason. Some individuals with Sebastian syndrome may not have any observable physical signs of the disorder at all.

### Diagnosis

Diagnostic blood tests to confirm the decreased blood clotting function seen in Sebastian syndrome may include a complete blood count (CBC) to determine the number of platelets in a blood sample; blood coagulation studies; or platelet aggregation tests.

There are several other disorders, including non-genetic diseases, that can cause symptoms similar to those seen in Sebastian syndrome. A family history of easy bleeding or bruising is an important clue in diagnosing Sebastian syndrome. Once the hereditary nature of the disease is confirmed, establishing a dominant **inheritance** pattern can separate Sebastian syndrome from other inherited giant platelet disorders.

Microscopic studies of the blood can reveal the enlarged platelets and the specific shape and structure characteristics associated with Sebastian syndrome. These characteristics include a shape that is less disc-like than normal platelets. There are also bluish inclusions, or small foreign bodies, observed in the white blood cells.

Genetic sequencing to confirm the presence of a mutation on the MYH9 gene is another method to positively diagnose Sebastian syndrome, although this would rarely be performed in lieu of other methods.

### Treatment and management

No treatment is required for the majority of people affected with Sebastian syndrome. After surgery, platelet transfusion may be required in order to avoid the possibility of hemorrhage. People diagnosed with Sebastian syndrome should be made aware of the risks associated with excessive bleeding.

### Prognosis

People with Sebastian syndrome can be expected to have a normal lifespan. The main risk for some patients is the chance of severe bleeding after surgery or injury.

### Resources

#### PERIODICALS

Kunishima, Shinji, et al. "Mutations in the NMMHC-A Gene Cause Autosomal Dominant Macrothrombocytopenia with Leukocyte Inclusions (May-Hegglin Anomaly/Sebastian Syndrome)." *Blood* (February 15, 2001): 1147-9.

Mhawech, Paulette, and Abdus Saleem. "Inherited Giant Platelet Disorders: Classification and Literature Review." *American Journal of Clinical Pathology* (February 2000): 176-90.

Young, Guy, Naomi Luban, and James White. "Sebastian Syndrome: Case Report and Review of the Literature." *American Journal of Hematology* (April 1999): 62-65.

#### WEBSITES

"Sebastian Syndrome." *Online Mendelian Inheritance in Man.* http://www.ncbi.nlm.nih.gov/entrez/dispomim.cgi?id = 605249 (April 20, 2001).

ORGANIZATIONS

National Heart, Lung, and Blood Institute. PO Box 30105, Bethesda, MD 20824-0105. (301) 592-8573. nhlbiinfo@rover.nhlbi.nih.gov. http://www.nhlbi.nih.gov.

National Organization for Rare Disorders (NORD). PO Box 8923, New Fairfield, CT 06812-8923. (203) 746-6518 or (800) 999-6673. Fax: (203) 746-6481. http://www.rarediseases.org.

Paul A. Johnson

# Seckel syndrome

## Definition

Seckel syndrome is an extremely rare inherited disorder characterized by low birth weight, dwarfism, a very small head, mental retardation, and unusual characteristic facial features, including a "beak-like" protrusion of the nose, large eyes, a narrow face, low ears, and an unusually small jaw. Common signs also include abnormalities of bones in the arms and legs.

## Description

Seckel syndrome is one of the microcephalic primordial dwarfism syndromes—a category of disorders characterized by profound growth delay. It is marked by dwarfism, a small head, developmental delay, and mental retardation. Abnormalities may also be found in the cardiovascular, hematopoietic, endocrine, and central nervous systems. Children with the disorder are often hyperactive and easily distracted; about half have IQs below 50. Individuals with Seckel syndrome are able to live for an extended period of time.

Seckel syndrome is also known as "bird-headed dwarfism," Seckel type dwarfism, and nanocephalic dwarfism. The disorder was named after Helmut G.P. Seckel, a German pediatrician who came to the United States in 1936. Dr. Seckel did not discover the syndrome but he authored a publication describing the disorder's symptoms based on two of his patients.

## Genetic profile

Seckel syndrome displays an autosomal-recessive pattern of **inheritance**. This means that both parents of a child with the disorder carry a copy of the Seckel gene—but the parents appear entirely normal. When both parents carry a copy of the Seckel **gene**, their

---

### KEY TERMS

**Microcephalic primordial dwarfism syndromes—** A group of disorders characterized by profound growth delay and small head size.

---

children face a one in four chance of developing the disorder.

## Demographics

Seckel syndrome is extremely rare. Between 1960—the year that Dr. Seckel defined the disorder—and 1999, fewer than 60 cases were reported.

## Signs and symptoms

Prenatal signs of Seckel syndrome include cranial abnormalities and growth delays (intrauterine growth retardation) resulting in low birth weight. Postnatal growth delays result in dwarfism. Other physical features associated with the disorder include a very small head (often more severely affected than even the height), abnormalities of bones in the arms and legs, malformation of the hips, a permanently bent fifth finger, failure of the testes to descend into the scrotum (for males) and unusual characteristic facial features, including a "beak-like" protrusion of the nose, large eyes, a narrow face, low ears, and an unusually small jaw. Children with the disorder not only have a small head but also a smaller brain, which leads to developmental delay and mental retardation. Seizures have also been reported.

## Diagnosis

Several forms of primordial dwarfism exhibit characteristics similar to those of Seckel syndrome, and it can be challenging for physicians to differentiate true Seckel syndrome from other similar dwarfisms. Physicians do have a set of primary diagnostic criteria to follow—the criteria were first defined by Dr. Seckel in 1960 and later revised (1982) to prevent over-diagnosis of cases.

Most of the primary diagnostic features of Seckel syndrome, which include severe intrauterine growth restriction, a small head, characteristic "bird-like" facies, and mental retardation, are well suited for prenatal sonographic diagnosis. The use of ultrasound examinations to evaluate fetal growth and the careful evaluation of the fetal face and cranial anatomy have proven effective at detecting Seckel syndrome.

### Treatment and management

There is no cure for Seckel syndrome. Certain medications may be prescribed to address other symptoms associated with the disorder.

### Prognosis

Children affected with Seckel syndrome can live for an extended period of time, although they are often faced with profound mental and physical deficits.

### Resources

**WEBSITES**

Alderman, Victoria. "Seckel Syndrome: A Case Study of Prenatal Sonographic Diagnosis." *OBGYN.net Ultrasound (electronic journal)* May 1998. http://www.obgyn.net/us/cotm/9805/cotm9805.htm.

MacDonald, M.R., et al. "Microcephalic Primordial Proportionate Dwarfism, Seckel Syndrome, in a Patient with Deletion of 1q 22-1q 24.3." http://www.faseb.org/ashg97/f6229.html.

"Seckel Syndrome." *Online Mendelian Inheritance in Man.* http://www.ncbi.nlm.nih.gov/entrez/dispomim.cgi?id=210600.

**ORGANIZATIONS**

Human Growth Foundation. 997 Glen Cove Ave., Glen Head, NY 11545. (800) 451-6434. Fax: (516) 671-4055. http://www.hgf1@hgfound.org.

National Organization for Rare Disorders (NORD). PO Box 8923, New Fairfield, CT 06812-8923. (203) 746-6518 or (800) 999-6673. Fax: (203) 746-6481. http://www.rarediseases.org.

Michelle Lee Brandt

Seckel type dwarfism *see* **Seckel syndrome**

Seemanova syndrome *see* **Nijmegen breakage syndrome**

# Septo-optic dysplasia

## Definition

Septo-optic **dysplasia** (SOD) is a rare congenital disorder that includes underdevelopment of the nerves at the back of the eye(s), absence of a part of the brain called the septum pellucidum and/or corpus callosum, and dysfunction of the pituitary gland that produces hormones in the body.

## Description

SOD is also known as DeMorsier's syndrome and is commonly recognized as the association of three features: underdevelopment of the optic nerves (optic nerve hypoplasia), absence of midline structures of the brain (most often the septum pellucidum), and problems with the functioning of the pituitary gland in the brain that controls hormone production in the body. These three features of SOD most often cause partial or complete blindness and mild to severe visual problems, difficulty with coordination of mental and muscular activities, such as walking, and short stature. Individuals with SOD may have normal intelligence, or learning problems that can range from mild to severe.

## Genetic profile

Most often, SOD occurs sporadically and is not inherited. For most individuals with SOD, there is no family history of the condition. However, there have been a few familial cases reported. Benner et al., in 1990, reported a brother and sister both with features of SOD. In addition, Wales and Quarrell in 1996 reported a family in which the parents were related and had both a son and daughter with SOD. These families raise the possibility that there is a form of SOD that is inherited in an autosomal recessive pattern. In autosomal recessive **inheritance**, two unaffected parents both carry a mutation in a single copy of a **gene** for a condition. When both parents pass the mutated gene on to a child, the child with two copies of the gene mutation is affected with the condition. People who are related by blood are more likely to be carriers of mutations in the same gene since they inherit their genes from a common ancestor.

Mutations in a gene called HESX1 located on the upper short arm of **chromosome** 3 have been identified in some people with SOD. The brother and sister whose parents were related were both found to have mutations in both copies of their HESX1 genes. A 2001 study of 228 individuals with SOD or features of SOD revealed that three had a mutation in one copy

## KEY TERMS

**Computerized tomography (CT)**—A technique that uses a beam of radiation and a computerized analysis to produce an image of a body structure, often the brain.

**Corpus callosum**—A band of nerve fibers that connects the right and left hemispheres of the brain.

**Magnetic resonance imaging (MRI)**—A technique that uses a magnetic field to produce images of various body structures.

**Mutation**—A change in the DNA code of a gene that disrupts the gene from making its product, such as a protein or enzyme.

**Optic nerve**—A nerve at the back of the eyes that conducts impulses that cause sight.

**Pituitary gland**—A gland at the base of the brain that controls hormone production in the body; the hormones produced by the pituitary gland control growth, reproduction, and other bodily processes.

**Septum pellucidum**—A membrane made of nerve tissue that separates areas of fluid in the left and right sides of the brain.

of their HESX1 gene. One Japanese individual with features of SOD was also found to have a mutation in one copy of his HESX1 gene. Therefore, it is likely that HESX1 is fully or partially causative in a small subset of individuals with SOD. The product of the HESX1 gene is expressed in the brain in early development and has been shown to be involved in the development of structures that give rise to the pituitary gland. In 1998, a strain was created in mice with mutations in the HESX1 gene so that no product was made from the gene. These mice had features similar to individuals with SOD, including pituitary gland dysfunction as well as structural changes in the brain and eyes.

Other causes of SOD are thought to be related to viral infections, **diabetes**, anti-seizure medications, alcohol, and illicit drug use during pregnancy. In addition, a 2004 study suggested that amniotic bands may be responsible for SOD in some patients. Amniotic bands are formed when the inner membrane of the sac holding the fluid around a fetus tears. Pieces of the amnion may wrap around various parts of the fetus and restrict blood flow to those areas. Limb malformations have been shown to be caused by amniotic bands in some cases. However, in 2004 it was suggested that limb malformations are a recurrent

feature of SOD, rather that SOD being caused by amniotic bands.

### Demographics

The incidence of SOD is not known, but the condition is considered to be rare. SOD does not occur more often in males or females and is not known to occur more or less frequently in any racial or ethnic group. SOD may become apparent during infancy, childhood, or in adolescence.

### Signs and symptoms

A variety of changes in the structure and function of the eye(s) can occur as part of SOD. Most commonly, individuals have optic nerve hypoplasia, meaning that the nerves from the back of the eye to the brain are underdeveloped. The nerves may be small, and there are usually far fewer nerves connecting the eye to the brain than usual. The optic disk (the front surface of the optic nerve) may also be smaller than usual. Infants with SOD may have rapid, involuntary eye movements called nystagmus. Other changes in the structure of the eye may occur, such as strabismus (the eyes can not focus on the same object at the same time), **coloboma** (notch-like area of absent tissue), and micropthalmia (small openings of the eyes). The optic features of SOD may affect one or both eyes, so that an individual with the condition may have good vision in one eye, or may have decreased or no vision in both eyes.

There can also be a variety of structural changes to the brain in people with SOD. Most often, a membrane in the midline of the brain called the septum pellucidum is absent. This membrane separates the fluid-filled cavities on each side of the brain. Another midline structure, the corpus callosum, may also be absent or underdeveloped. The corpus callosum is the thick band of nerve fibers that connects the two hemispheres of the brain. In addition, the region of the brain that controls voluntary movement, the cerebellum, may be underdeveloped. Other structural brain malformations have been reported in individuals with SOD.

Additional structures in the brain that can be affected in individuals with SOD include the hypothalamus and the pituitary gland. These parts of the brain control the production and release of hormones in the body. Individuals with SOD may not produce enough growth hormone and may exhibit short stature. There may be problems with the production of hormones needed for sexual development, low blood sugar, dehydration, and seizures.

Various other conditions have been reported in individuals with SOD. These include **cleft lip** and/or palate, limb anomalies, including fusion of fingers or toes and underdevelopment of fingernails or toe nails, and apnea (difficulty breathing).

Patients affected with SOD can present at any age depending on the severity of the symptoms. Signs and symptoms, including failure to thrive, prolonged jaundice (yellow color to the skin caused by extra amounts of bile in the blood), difficulty controlling body temperature, decreased blood sugar, small genitalia, or low muscle tone, can herald the diagnosis of SOD in newborns. Older children may complain of visual difficulties, or have the inability to fixate on an object.

Many individuals with SOD have normal intelligence. However, there is a range of intelligence reported, including those with mild learning delays and those with significant mental retardation. Learning delays and mental retardation may be the result of structural changes in the brain or hormone disorders. Unrecognized visual problems or lack of education appropriate for those with visual impairment may also cause learning delays.

## Diagnosis

SOD is often suspected when a child with visual impairment also has growth delay. When a diagnosis of SOD is suspected, a person is referred to several specialists who each perform tests to verify the diagnosis. An ophthalmologist can perform vision testing and examinations of the structure of the eye for features of SOD. In individuals with SOD, the optic nerves appear small and gray or pale in color and can be surrounded by a double pigmented ring or margin. In addition, stimulation testing of the optic nerves can be performed. A neurologist (brain specialist) can perform imaging studies of the brain, such as magnetic resonance imaging (MRI) or computerized tomography (CT) scan of the brain, focusing on the visual pathways, the septum pellucidum, hypothalamus-pituitary region, and other midline structures. An endocrinologist can perform blood tests to determine if there are problems with various hormones in the body.

There has been a report of prenatal diagnosis of SOD by an ultrasound that revealed absence of the septum pellucidum. Subsequent blood and urine tests on the mother revealed low levels of the hormone estriol, indicating a problem with the fetal pituitary gland. The diagnosis was confirmed after birth.

## Treatment and management

SOD is treated symptomatically. Vision may be improved with corrective lenses, surgery or other treatment. Seizures may be controlled with medication. Hormone deficiencies are managed with hormone replacement therapy, such as growth hormones or thyroid supplements. Hormone problems may arise at different ages, so even if not present initially, a person with SOD should be followed by an endocrinologist over time. Children with SOD should receive early assessments of learning and development so that any supportive therapies, such as physical, speech, or educational therapy, can be initiated. Children with SOD may benefit from an individualized educational plan (IEP) in school, which is a plan created by a child's teachers, therapists, and other individuals who have performed developmental testing and designed techniques best suited to the child's needs. Families may consider placing a child with SOD in a school for visually impaired children. The child's pediatrician can monitor a child for any special needs and refer additional specialists as needed. Individuals and families with SOD may benefit from talking with a genetic counselor about possible patterns of inheritance and recurrence risks for SOD in the family. Families should also be introduced to the appropriate local and national support organizations, such as the American Foundation for the Blind, for further help and assistance.

## Prognosis

Prognosis is variable, depending on the number and severity of features present. Most individuals with SOD have significant visual impairment, and many are legally blind. Patients with severe visual impairment may have difficulty obtaining a driver's license or gainful employment. Lifespan is most often normal, however, cortisol deficiency can lead to life-threatening episodes brought about by infection or stress.

## Resources

### BOOKS

Jones, Kenneth. *Smith's Recognizable Patterns of Human Malformation, 5th Edition*. Philadelphia: W.B. Saunders Company, 1997.

Rimoin, D., M. Connor, and R. Pyeritz. *Emery and Rimoin's Principles and Practice of Medical Genetics, Third Edition*. New York: Pearson Professional Limited, 1997.

Swaiman, K., and S. Ashwal. *Pediatric Neurology: Principles and Practices, Volume 2, Third Edition*. St. Louis, MO: Mosby, 1999.

Tasman, W., and J. Edward. *Duane's Clinical Ophthalmology, Volume 2 and 3*. Philadelphia: Lippincott Williams & Wilkins, 2005.

### PERIODICALS

Harrison, I., et al. "Septo-Optic Dysplasia with Digital Anomalies—A Recurrent Pattern Syndrome." *American Journal of Medical Genetics* 131A (2004): 82–85.

Lepinard, C., et al. "Prenatal Diagnosis of Absence of the Septum Pellucidum Associated with Septo-Optic Dysplasia." *Ultrasound Obstet Gynecol* 25 (2005): 73–75.

Stevens, C., and W. Dobyns. "Septo-Optic Dysplasia and Amniotic Bands: Further Evidence for a Vascular Pathogenesis." *American Journal of Medical Genetics* 125A (2004): 12–16.

## ORGANIZATIONS

Focus Families. 2453 Emerald Street, San Diego, California, 92109. (866) FOCUS50. Email: Support@focusfamilies.org. (April 12, 2005.) http://www.focusfamilies.org.

The Magic Foundation. 6645 W. North Avenue, Aok Park, Illinois, 60302. (708) 383-0808, (800) 362-4423. E-mail: mary@magicfoundation.org. (April 12, 2005.) http://www.magicfoundation.org.

National Institute of Neurological Disorders and Stroke. National Institutes of Health. PO Box 5801, Bethesda, MD, 20824. (800) 352-9424. (April 12, 2005.) http://www.ninds.nih.gov.

National Organization for Rare Disorders. PO Box 1968, Danbury, CT 06813-1968. (203) 744-0100. Fax: (203) 798-2291. (800) 999-NORD. E-mail: orphan@rarediseases.org. (April 12, 2005.) http://www.rarediseases.org.

Online Mendelian Inheritance in Man, Johns Hopkins University. (April 12, 2005.) http://www.ncbi.nlm.nih.gov.

Sonja R. Eubanks, MS, CGC

Seronegative spondyloarthropathies *see* **Ankylosing spondylitis**

Severe atypical spherocytosis due to ankyrine defect *see* **Spherocytosis, hereditary**

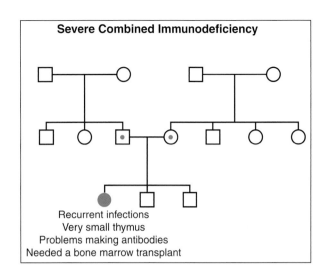

(Illustration by GGS Information Services. Gale, a part of Cengage Learning.)

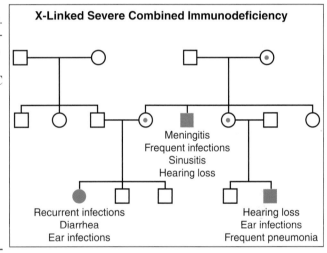

(Illustration by GGS Information Services. Gale, a part of Cengage Learning.)

# Severe combined immunodeficiency

## Definition

SCID, or severe combined immunodeficiency, is a group of rare, life-threatening diseases present at birth that impair the immune system. Without a healthy immune system the body cannot fight infections and individuals can easily become seriously ill from common infections.

## Description

SCID is one type of Primary Immunodeficiency Diseases (PID) and is considered the most severe. There are approximately 70 forms of PID. Primary immunodeficiency diseases are where a person is missing a component of the immune system—either an organ or cells of the immune system. Some deficiencies are deadly, while others are mild.

SCID is also known as the "boy in the bubble" syndrome, because living in a normal environment can be fatal. SCID initially was called Swiss agammaglobulinemia because it was first described in Switzerland in 1961. Any exposure to germs can pose a risk for infection, including bacterial, viral, and fungal. In the first few months of life, children with SCID become very ill with infections such as pneumonia (infection of the lungs which prevents oxygen from reaching the blood, making breathing difficult), meningitis (infection of the covering of the brain and spinal cord), sepsis (infection in the bloodstream) and chickenpox,

## KEY TERMS

**Amniocentesis**—A procedure performed at 16-18 weeks of pregnancy in which a needle is inserted through a woman's abdomen into her uterus to draw out a small sample of the amniotic fluid from around the baby. Either the fluid itself or cells from the fluid can be used for a variety of tests to obtain information about genetic disorders and other medical conditions in the fetus.

**Amniotic fluid**—The fluid which surrounds a developing baby during pregnancy.

**Autosomal recessive inheritance**—A pattern of genetic inheritance where two abnormal genes are needed to display the trait or disease.

**Bone marrow**—A spongy tissue located in the hollow centers of certain bones, such as the skull and hip bones. Bone marrow is the site of blood cell generation.

**Bone marrow transplant (BMT)**—A medical procedure used to treat some diseases that arise from defective blood cell formation in the bone marrow. Healthy bone marrow is extracted from a donor to replace the marrow in an ailing individual. Proteins on the surface of bone marrow cells must be identical or very closely matched between a donor and the recipient.

**Boy in the bubble**—A description for SCID since these children need to be isolated from exposure to germs, until they are treated by bone marrow transplantation or other therapy.

**Chorionic villus sampling (CVS)**—A procedure used for prenatal diagnosis at 10-12 weeks gestation. Under ultrasound guidance a needle is inserted either through the mother's vagina or abdominal wall and a sample of cells is collected from around the fetus. These cells are then tested for chromosome abnormalities or other genetic diseases.

**Failure to thrive**—Significantly reduced or delayed physical growth.

**Gene therapy**—Replacing a defective gene with the normal copy.

**Immune system**—A major system of the body that produces specialized cells and substances that interact with and destroy foreign antigens that invade the body.

**Lymphatic system**—Lymph nodes and lympatic vessels that transport infection fighting cells to the body.

**Lymphocytes**—Also called white blood cells, lymphocytes mature in the bone marrow to form B cells, which fight infection.

**Meningitis**—An infection of the covering of the brain.

**Pneumonia**—An infection of the lungs.

**Primary immunodeficiency disease (PID)**—A group of approximately 70 conditions that affect the normal functioning of the immune system.

**Sepsis**—An infection of the bloodstream.

**Severe combined immunodeficiency (SCID)**—A group of rare, life-threatening diseases present at birth, that cause a child to have little or no immune system. As a result, the child's body is unable to fight infections.

**Sporadic**—Isolated or appearing occasionally with no apparent pattern.

**Thymus gland**—An endocrine gland located in the front of the neck that houses and transports T cells, which help to fight infection.

**X-linked recessive inheritance**—The inheritance of a trait by the presence of a single gene on the X chromosome in a male, passed from a female who has the gene on one of her X chromosomes, who is referred to as an unaffected carrier.

and can die within the first year of life, since their immune system is unable to fight off these infections.

Children with SCID do not respond to medications like other children because their immune system does not function properly. They may also not have a developed thymus gland. Medication usually stimulates a person's immune system to fight infection, but in the case of SCID, the immune system is unable to respond. The immune system is a complex network of cells and organs that protect the body from infection. The thymus and lymphatic system (lymph nodes and lymphatic vessels) house and transport two very important cells that fight infection: the B and T cells. The bone marrow (center of bones) produces cells that become blood cells as well as cells for the immune system. One type of cell, called lymphocytes or white blood cells, mature in the bone marrow to form "B" cells, while others mature in the thymus to become "T" cells. B and T cells are the two major groups of lymphocytes that recognize and attack infections. Children with SCID have either abnormal or absent B and T cells.

Other infections can be seen in children with SCID including skin infections, yeast infections in the mouth and diaper area, diarrhea, and infection of the liver. Children with SCID fail to gain weight and grow normally. Treatment for SCID is available, however, many children with SCID are not diagnosed in time and die before their first birthday.

A diagnosis of SCID, besides being painful, frightening, and frustrating, needs to be made quickly since common infections can prove fatal. In addition, permanent damage can result in the ears, lungs, and other organs.

### Genetic profile

SCID is a group of inherited disorders with about half inherited by a **gene** on the X **chromosome** called IL2RG, 15% inherited by an autosomal recessive gene called ADA, and the remaining 35% caused by either an unknown autosomal recessive gene or are the result of a new mutation.

Genetic information is carried in tiny packages called chromosomes. Each chromosome contains thousands of genes and each gene contains the information for a specific trait. All human cells (except egg and sperm cells) contain 23 pairs of chromosomes for a total of 46 chromosomes. One of each pair of chromosomes is inherited from the mother and the other is inherited from the father. SCID is usually inherited in one of two ways: X-linked recessive or autosomal recessive. Autosomal recessive means that the gene for the disease or trait is located on one of the first 22 pairs of chromosomes, which are also called autosomes. Males and females are equally likely to have an autosomal recessive disease or trait. Recessive means that two copies of the gene are necessary to express the condition. Therefore, a child inherits one copy of the gene from each parent, who are called carriers (because they have only one copy of the gene). Since carriers do not express the gene, parents usually do not know they carry the SCID gene until they have an affected child. Carrier parents have a 1-in-4 chance (or 25%) with each pregnancy, to have a child with SCID.

The last pair of human chromosomes, either two X's (female) or one X and one Y (male)—determines gender. X-linked means the gene causing the disease or trait is located on the X chromosome. The term "recessive" usually infers that two copies of a gene—one on each of the chromosome pair—are necessary to cause a disease or express a particular trait. X-linked recessive diseases are most often seen in males, however, because they only have a one X chromosome. Therefore, if a male inherits a particular gene on the X, he expresses the gene, even though he only has a single copy of it. Females, on the other hand, have two X chromosomes, and therefore can carry a gene on one of their X chromosomes yet not express any

symptoms. (Their second X chromosome works normally). A mother usually carries the gene for SCID unknowingly, and has a 50/50 chance with each pregnancy to transmit the gene. If the child is male, he will have SCID; if the child is female, she will be a carrier for SCID like the mother.

New mutations—alterations in the **DNA** of the gene—can cause disease. In these cases, neither parent has the disease-causing mutation. This may occur because the mutation in the gene happened for the first time only in the egg or sperm for that particular pregnancy. New mutations are thought to happen by chance and are therefore referred to as "sporadic", meaning, by chance.

### Demographics

It is estimated that about 400 children a year are born with some type of primary immunodeficiency disease. Approximately one in 100,000 children are born with SCID each year, regardless of the part of the world the child is from, or the ethnic background of the parents. This disease can affect both males and females depending on its mode of **inheritance**.

### Signs and symptoms

Babies with SCID fail to thrive, are frail, and do not grow well. They have numerous, serious, life-threatening infections that usually begin in the first few months of life. Because they do not respond to medications like other children, they may be on antibiotics for 1–2 months with no improvement before a physician considers a diagnosis of SCID. The types of infections typically include chronic (developing slowly and persisting for a long period of time) skin infections, yeast infections in the mouth and diaper area, diarrhea, infection of the liver, pneumonia, meningitis, and sepsis. They can also have serious sinus and ear infections, as well as a swollen abdomen. Sometimes deep abscesses occur, which are pockets of pus that form around infections in the skin or in the body organs.

### Diagnosis

About half of children who see a doctor for frequent infections are normal; another 30% may have allergies, 10% have some other type of serious disorder, and 10% have a primary or secondary immunodeficiency. A diagnosis of SCID is usually made based on a complete medical history and physical examination, in addition to multiple blood tests and chest x–rays. The gene in X-linked recessive SCID is called the interleukin receptor gamma chain gene or IL2RG. The autosomal recessive forms of SCID are caused by a variety of different genes; one of the more common is called the adenosine deaminase gene or ADA. Since newborns do not routinely have a test to count white blood cells, SCID is not usually suspected and then diagnosed until the child develops their first infection. A pattern of recurrent infections suggests an immunodeficiency.

Once a couple has had a child with SCID, and they have had the genetic cause identified by DNA studies (performed from a small blood sample), prenatal testing for future pregnancies may be considered on a research basis for some types of SCID. (Note that prenatal testing may not be possible if a mutation cannot be identified). Prenatal diagnosis is available via either CVS (chorionic villus sampling) or **amniocentesis**. CVS is a biopsy of the placenta performed in the first trimester or the first 12 weeks of pregnancy under ultrasound guidance. Ultrasound is the use of sound waves to visualize the locations of the developing baby and the placenta. The genetic makeup of the placenta is identical to the fetus (developing baby) and therefore the presence or absence of one of the SCID genes can be determined from this tissue. Amniocentesis is a procedure performed under ultrasound guidance where a long thin needle is inserted into the mother's abdomen, into the uterus, to withdraw a couple of tablespoons of amniotic fluid (fluid surrounding the developing baby) to study. The SCID gene can be studied using cells from the amniotic fluid. Other genetic tests, such as a chromosome analysis, may also be performed on either a CVS or amniocentesis. A small risk of miscarriage is associated with amniocentesis and CVS.

### Treatment and management

The best treatment for SCID is a bone marrow transplant (BMT). A bone marrow transplant involves taking cells that are normally present in bone marrow (the center of bones that produce and store blood cells), and giving them back to the child with SCID or to another person. The goal of BMT is to infuse healthy bone marrow cells into a person after their own unhealthy bone marrow has been eliminated. BMT helps to strengthen a child with SCID's immune system.

Other treatment for SCID includes treating each infection promptly and accurately. Injections are also available to help boost a child's immune system.

In the year 2000, **gene therapy** was first reported to be successful in two French patients with SCID. The idea behind gene therapy is to replace an abnormal gene with a normal copy. In SCID, bone marrow is removed to isolate the patients' stem cells. Stem cells are special cells in the bone marrow that produce lymphocytes. In a laboratory, the normal gene is added to the abnormal stem cells. The genetically altered stem cells now have the normal gene and are transplanted back into the patient. Once the functioning stem cells

with the normal gene enter the bone marrow, they reproduce quickly and replace stem cells that have the abnormal gene. So, ultimately, the patient with SCID produces B and T cells normally and can fight off infections without antibiotics or other treatment. The long-term effects of gene therapy are unknown, since the children treated are still very young.

### Prognosis

When SCID is diagnosed early, successful bone marrow transplantation usually corrects the problem and the child lives a normal life. This means children can go to school, mix with playmates, and take part in sports. However, the quality of life for individuals with severe cases of SCID can be greatly impaired if they do not receive a bone marrow transplant. Children with SCID may not live long if they do not receive the proper treatment or if their disease goes undiagnosed.

### Resources

#### PERIODICALS

Buckley, Rebecca H. "Gene Therapy for Human SCID: Dreams Become Reality." *Nature Medicine* 6 (June 2000): 623.

Stephenson, Joan. "Gene Therapy Trials Show Efficacy." *Journal of the American Medical Association* 283 (February 2, 2000): 589.

#### WEBSITES

International Patient Organization for Patients with Primary Immunodeficiencies. www.ipopi.org.

Pediatric Primary ImmuneDeficiency. www.pedpid.com.

Severed Combined ImmuneDeficiency Homepage. www.scid.net.

#### ORGANIZATIONS

Immune Deficiency Foundation. 40 W. Chesapeake Ave., Suite 308, Towson, MD 21204. (800) 296-4433. Fax: (410) 321-9165. http://www.primaryimmune.org.

National Organization for Rare Disorders (NORD). PO Box 8923, New Fairfield, CT 06812-8923. (203) 746-6518 or (800) 999-6673. Fax: (203) 746-6481. http://www.rarediseases.org.

Catherine L. Tesla, MS, CGC

# Short-rib polydactyly

## Definition

Short-rib **polydactyly** (SRP) syndromes are a group of skeletal dysplasias consisting of short ribs, short limbs, extra fingers or toes, and various internal organ abnormalities present at birth. There are four

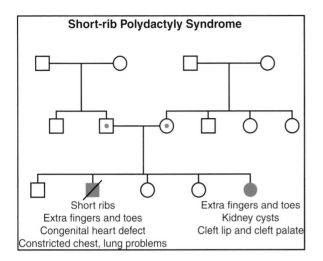

**Short-rib Polydactyly Syndrome**

Short ribs
Extra fingers and toes
Congenital heart defect
Constricted chest, lung problems

Extra fingers and toes
Kidney cysts
Cleft lip and cleft palate

*(Illustration by GGS Information Services. Gale, a part of Cengage Learning.)*

types of SRP and all are fatal shortly after birth due to underdevelopment of the lungs.

## Description

In 1972, R. M. Saldino and C. D. Noonan first described two siblings with a dwarfism syndrome and symptoms of extremely shortened limbs, short ribs, small chest, abnormal bone formation, extra fingers, and internal organ damage. Since then, three additional SRP subtypes have been identified, all named after those who first described them. The subtypes are: SRP type I (Saldino-Noonan), SRP type II (Majewski), SRP type III (Verma-Namauf), and SRP type IV (Beemer-Langer). While each subtype has distinguishing features, there is a great amount of overlap between them. There is still debate about whether the different types are caused by different genetic changes or if they result from the same genetic change and are variable between patients. Some people believe that the subtypes are different expressions of a single syndrome.

The SRP syndromes also overlap with two other dwarfism syndromes, asphyxiating thoracic **dysplasia** (Jeune syndrome) and Ellis van Creveld syndrome. These syndromes, like the SRP types, have shortened limbs and ribs, small chest and extra fingers or toes. These syndromes may all be genetically related.

The exact cause of these syndromes is unknown but they all result in abnormal bone development and growth prenatally. This causes shortened bones in the arms, legs, and ribcage. The ribcage is also constricting, leaving very little room for the lung growth. Development can also be abnormal in the internal organs,

including the heart, kidneys, liver, and pancreas. The cause of death for these newborns is usually inability to breathe due to severely underdeveloped lungs.

## Genetic profile

Even though the exact genetic cause of the SRP syndromes is unknown, it is well-documented that they are inherited as autosomal recessive conditions. This is because babies with SRP are born to unaffected parents and many parents have had more than one affected child. Parents of an affected child are assumed to be carriers. Those parents have a 25% chance of having another affected child with each pregnancy.

The **gene** (or genes) involved in the SRP syndromes has not yet been identified but is suspected to be on **chromosome** 4. Some researchers feel that the SRP gene is near the region of the gene for Ellis van Creveld syndrome on chromosome 4. The gene for another dwarfism syndrome, **thanatophoric dysplasia**, is also located in this area. Research is still being done to find the SRP gene (or genes) and learn more about its role during early development.

## Demographics

Approximately 2-3 births per 10,000 are affected with some type of **skeletal dysplasia**. The SRP syndromes account for a small percentage of these. Due to the rarity of the SRP syndromes, an exact incidence is unknown.

## Signs and symptoms

There is much overlap of symptoms between the SRP subtypes and it is often difficult to distinguish between them. They all have extremely shortened bones of the arms, legs, and ribs. They all also have a small, constricted chest.

Saldino-Noonan (type I) is considered the most severe type. Features reported with this type include spur formation on the bones, abnormal vertebrae (bones of the spinal column), and decreased ossification (hardening of the bones). Heart defects are common. Cysts are often seen on the kidneys and pancreas. Extra fingers and/or toes (polydactyly) are a classic feature and are usually on the same side of the hand/foot as the "pinkie" finger/little toe (postaxial). Sex reversal has also been reported. This means that the baby is genetically male but has visible female genitalia.

Majewski (type II) also has cystic kidneys and postaxial polydactyly. This type can also have preaxial polydactyly where the extra fingers/toes are on the same side of the hand/foot as the thumb/big toe. Other distinguishing features include **cleft lip and palate** and liver damage. The tibia (one of the bones of the lower leg) is often oval shaped and shorter than the fibula (the other bone of the lower leg). The ends of the bones may also appear smooth on an x–ray.

Verma-Namauf (type III) has much overlap with Saldino-Noonan (type I) and may be a milder variant. Internal organ involvement is less common. The ends of the bones may appear jagged and widened on an x–ray. The vertebrae are often small and flat. Polydactyly is also common in this type. Visible genitalia may be ambiguous (not clearly male or female).

Beemer-Langer (type IV), like Majewski, can have cleft lip and palate and liver damage. Cysts on the kidneys and pancreas are common. Polydactyly is usually absent but has been reported. A distinguishing feature of this type is bowed or curved bones.

### Diagnosis

Diagnosis of the SRP syndromes can be difficult. A careful examination of internal organs and x–ray evaluation is needed to distinguish SRP syndromes from Jeune syndrome and Ellis van Creveld syndrome. When SRP syndrome is suspected, x–rays and internal organ involvement can also help to determine the particular type.

The main features of SRP syndromes (short bones, short ribs, small chest) can be seen on **prenatal ultrasound**. This is the only method of prenatal diagnosis for at-risk families. **Genetic testing** for the SRP syndromes is not available.

### Treatment and management

There is no treatment or cure for the SRP syndromes. The abnormal prenatal bone development is irreversible. The chest is usually too small to allow for lung growth after birth. Internal organs with cysts may not be functional.

Infants born with SRP syndromes are given minimum care for warmth and comfort. Due to the poor prognosis, extreme measures to prolong life are rarely taken.

---

## QUESTIONS TO ASK YOUR DOCTOR

- What are the four types of short-rib polydactyly, and how does the prognosis for the four types differ from each other?
- Can short-rib polydactyly be diagnosed prenatally and, if so, what are the risks and benefits from having such a test?
- Are that treatments available that will extend the life of an infant born with short-rib polydactyly?
- Where can I read more about this genetic disorder?

---

### Prognosis

The prognosis for infants born with SRP syndromes is quite poor. These babies usually die within hours or days of birth due to underdeveloped lungs.

### Resources

**PERIODICALS**

Sarafoglou, K., et al. "Short-rib Polydactyly: More Evidence of a Continuous Spectrum." *Clinical Genetics* 56 (1999):145-148.

**WEBSITES**

"Short Rib-Polydactyly Syndrome, Type 1." *Online Mendelian Inheritance in Man.* http://ncbi.nlm.nih.gov/entrez/dispomim.cgi?id = 263530.

**ORGANIZATIONS**

SRPS Family Network. http://www.srps.net.

Amie Stanley, MS

---

# Shprintzen-Goldberg craniosynostosis syndrome

### Definition

Shprintzen-Goldberg **craniosynostosis** syndrome (SGS) is a disorder of the connective tissue, featuring craniosynostosis and marfanoid body type.

### Description

SGS, also known as marfanoid craniosynostosis syndrome, is one of a group of disorders characterized by craniosynostosis and marfanoid body type. It is a condition that involves craniofacial, skeletal, and

## KEY TERMS

**Aortic root**—The location where the aorta (main heart blood vessel) inserts in the heart. Enlargement of the aortic root can cause it to rupture.

**Craniosynostosis**—Premature, delayed, or otherwise abnormal closure of the sutures of the skull.

**Marfanoid**—Term for body type which is similar to people with Marfan syndrome. Characterized by tall, lean body with long arms and long fingers.

other abnormalities. SGS is caused by genetic mutations (changes affecting the structure and function of the **gene**) in a gene that contributes to the formation of connective tissue.

### Genetic profile

SGS is associated with abnormalities of the elastic fibers of connective tissue. Elastic fibers are complex in structure and are composed of at least 19 different proteins. Mutations in three of the genes that encode the majority of these 19 proteins cause abnormalities in several body systems, including the skeletal system, blood vessels, and eye.

SGS shares characteristics with the Marfan syndrome, which is an inherited genetic disorder of the connective tissue which involves the eye, heart, aorta, and skeletal system. Marfan syndrome is caused by mutations in the fibrillin-1 (FBN1) gene, which is located on **chromosome** 15. Since SGS is similar in many ways to Marfan syndrome, studies of the FBN1 gene were conducted on SGS patients to see if they also had mutations in this gene. There were indeed abnormalities found in the FBN1 genes of persons with SGS. Researchers think that these mutations predispose a person to develop SGS, but that other factors are required in addition to the mutation in the gene to develop the disease. The other factors may be genetic mutations, environmental influences, or a combination of these, but they are not well-understood at this time.

The mutations appear to be sporadic in nature (not inherited), and are autosomal dominant (only one mutation is necessary to be predisposed to the disease). Sporadic genetic mutations in the sperm occur (in any gene, not just FBN1) at a higher rate in older men (over 45 years) and there is in fact one case report of a child with SGS in which the father was 49 years old. The father of another child with SGS reportedly had chemotherapy and radiation treatment prior to conception

of the child. The recurrence risk for siblings is probably low, although such data is not available.

### Demographics

There are 15 reported cases as of 2000, with the first case being described in 1981. The ratio of females to males is 10:5, making females affected twice as often as males. Ethnicities would be expected to be affected equally with sporadic mutations, although data regarding SGS specifically is limited.

### Signs and symptoms

Findings in SGS include skeletal abnormalities, **hydrocephalus**, and mental retardation. Most babies have been born well-nourished and had a relatively long birth length. The most frequently described craniofacial features of SGS include abnormal head shape (dolichocephaly), a high, prominent forehead, bulging eyes (ocular proptosis), wide spaced eyes (hypertelorism), downslanting eyes, strabismus (wandering eye), small jaw (maxillary hypoplasia), high narrow palate (roof of the mouth), and low-set ears.

The main skeletal findings in persons with SGS include long, thin fingers (arachnodactyly—or spider-like fingers), flat feet (pes planus), "bird" chest deformity (pectus deformity), **scoliosis** (curvature of the spine), and joint hypermobility (loose joints).

Other features can include **clubfoot**, enlarged aortic root, mitral valve prolapse (floppy heart valve which allows flow of blood back into the chamber of the heart that it came from), low muscle tone (hypotonia), developmental delay, mental retardation, very little body fat, and small penis in males. **Myopia** (nearsightedness) and abdominal wall defects (developmental problem that occurs during formation of the fetus where parts of the intestine or other organs can protrude outside of the body; usually surgically correctable) can also occur.

Radiologic findings include hydrocephalus (water on the brain), certain brain malformations (Chiari-I malformation or dilatation of the lateral ventricles), abnormalities in the first and second cervical vertebrae (vertebrae in the neck), square shaped vertebrae, thin ribs, thinning of the bones, and craniofacial abnormalities.

### Diagnosis

There are more than 75 syndromes associated with craniosynostosis. There are also a number of different syndromes associated with both craniosynostosis and marfanoid body type. X-ray evaluation can be helpful in determining whether a person has SGS, as they tend to have abnormal first and second cervical vertebrae, hydrocephalus (water on the brain), and certain brain abnormalities.

SGS must be differentiated from other syndromes with craniosynostosis and marfaniod body type. Two such syndromes include Idaho syndrome II and Antley-Bixler syndrome. Idaho syndrome II has less severe craniofacial problems than SGS and has abnormal leg bones and absent patellae (knee caps). Antley-Bixler syndrome is an inherited syndrome with craniofacial abnormalities, abnormal arm and leg bones, and fractures in the femurs (thigh bones). These characteristics are different from SGS. A clinical geneticist is a physician who has special training in recognizing and diagnosing rare genetic conditions and is a good resource for differentiating among these complicated and similar conditions.

### Treatment and management

Cardiology evaluation is important since several children have been reported to have severe cardiac disease with SGS. Aortic root must be evaluated and measured routinely to minimize the risk for rupture. Enlarged aortic roots may need to be surgically repaired.

Patients should have an ophthalmologic evaluation, since mutations in the FBR1 gene are associated with abnormalities in the eyes.

Surgical correction of craniofacial problems or pectus are sometimes necessary or desirable. Shunting (surgical placement of a shunt to drain the accumulated fluid in the brain to the abdominal cavity to relieve pressure) may be required for patients with hydrocephalus. Orthopedic devices may be required for scoliosis or other bone deformities.

Special education for mentally retarded individuals or individuals with developmental delay is recommended.

**Genetic counseling** is recommended for persons with relatives diagnosed with SGS.

### Prognosis

SGS does not alter life span, although complications from associated abnormalities such as mental retardation or respiratory problems can cause problems.

### Resources

#### BOOKS

Gorlin, R.J., M.M. Cohen, and L.S. Levin. "Marfaniod Features and Craniosynostosis (including Shprintzen-Goldberg Syndrome)." In *Syndromes of the Head and Neck*. New York: Oxford University Press, 1990.

#### PERIODICALS

Furlong, J., T.W. Kurczynski, and J.R. Hennessy. "New Marfanoid Syndrome with Craniosynostosis." *American Journal of Medical Genetics* 26 (1987): 599-604.

Greally, M.T., et al. "Shprintzen-Goldberg Syndrome: A Clinical Analysis." *American Journal of Medical Genetics* 76 (1998): 202-212.

Lee, Y.C., et al. "Marfanoid Habitus, Dysmorphic Features, and Web Neck." *Southerna Medical Journal* 93 (2000): 1197-1200

#### WEBSITES

National Organization for Rare Diseases (NORD). www.rarediseases.org.

"Shprintzen-Goldberg Craniosynostosis Syndrome." *Online Mendelian inheritance in Man (OMIM)*. http://www.ncbi.nlm.nig.gov/entrez/dispomim.cgi?id = 182212.

#### ORGANIZATIONS

Coalition for Heritable Disorders of Connective Tissue (CHDCT). 382 Main Street, Port Washington, NY 11050. (516) 883-8712. http://www.chdct.org.

Hydrocephalus Association. 870 Market St. Suite 705, San Francisco, CA 94102. (415) 732-7040 or (888) 598-3789. Fax: (415) 732-7044. hydroassoc@aol.com. http://www.hydroassoc.org.

Amy Vance, MS, CGC

Sialidoses types I and II *see* **Neuraminidase deficiency**

# Sickle cell disease

## Definition

Sickle cell disease describes a group of inherited blood disorders characterized by chronic anemia, painful events, and various complications due to associated tissue and organ damage.

## Description

The most common and well-known type of sickle cell disease is sickle cell anemia, also called SS disease. All types of sickle cell disease are caused by a genetic change in hemoglobin, the oxygen-carrying protein inside the red blood cells. The red blood cells of affected individuals contain a predominance of a structural variant of the usual adult hemoglobin. This variant hemoglobin, called sickle hemoglobin, has a tendency to develop into rod-like structures that alter the shape of the usually flexible red blood cells. The cells take on a shape that resembles the curved blade of the sickle, an agricultural tool. Sickle cells have a shorter life span than normally-shaped red blood cells. This results in chronic anemia characterized by low levels of hemoglobin and decreased numbers of red blood cells. Sickle cells are also less flexible and more sticky than normal red blood cells, and can become trapped in small blood vessels preventing blood flow. This compromises the delivery of oxygen, which can result in pain and damage to associated tissues and organs. Sickle cell disease presents with marked variability, even within families.

## Demographics

Carriers of the sickle cell **gene** are said to have sickle cell trait. Unlike sickle cell disease, sickle cell trait does not cause health problems. In fact, sickle cell trait is protective against malaria, a disease caused by blood-borne parasites transmitted through mosquito bites. According to a widely accepted theory, the genetic mutation associated with the sickle cell trait occurred thousands of years ago. Coincidentally, this mutation increased the likelihood that carriers would survive malaria infection. Survivors then passed the mutation on to their offspring, and the trait became established throughout areas where malaria was common. As populations migrated, so did the sickle cell trait. Today, approximately one in 12 African Americans has sickle cell trait.

Worldwide, it has been estimated that one in every 250,000 babies is born annually with sickle cell disease. Sickle cell disease primarily affects people of African, Mediterranean, Middle Eastern, and Asian Indian ancestry. In the United States, sickle cell disease is most often seen in African Americans, in whom the disease occurs in one out of every 400 births. The disease has been described in individuals from several different ethnic backgrounds and is also seen with increased frequency in Latino Americans—particularly those of Caribbean, Central American, and South American ancestry. Approximately one in every 1,000-1,400 Latino births are affected.

## Genetic profile

Humans normally make several types of the oxygen-carrying protein hemoglobin. An individual's stage in development determines whether he or she makes primarily embryonic, fetal, or adult hemoglobins. All types of hemoglobin are made of three components: heme, alpha (or alpha-like) globin, and beta (or beta-like) globin. Sickle hemoglobin is the result of a genetic change in the beta globin component of normal adult hemoglobin. The beta globin gene is

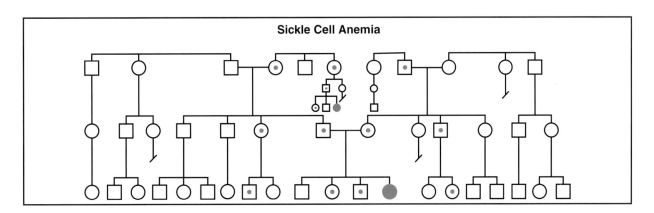

**Sickle Cell Anemia**

(Illustration by GGS Information Services. Gale, a part of Cengage Learning.)

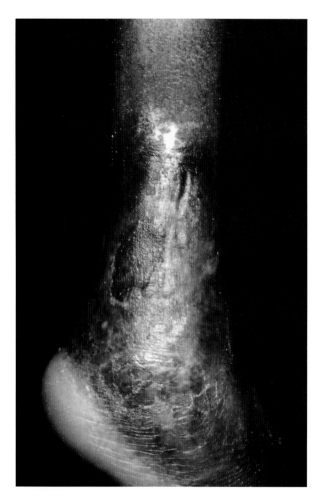

**The lower leg of this woman has ulcerated, necrotic tissue, resulting from sickle cell anemia.** *(Custom Medical Stock Photo, Inc.)*

located on **chromosome** 11. The sickle cell form of the beta globin gene results from the substitution of a single **DNA** nucleotide, or genetic building-block. The change from adenine to thymine at codon (position) 6 of the beta globin gene leads to insertion of the amino acid valine—instead of glutamic acid—at this same position in the beta globin protein. As a result of this change, sickle hemoglobin has unique properties in comparison to the usual type of adult hemoglobin.

Most individuals have two normal copies of the beta globin gene, which make normal beta globin that is incorporated into adult hemoglobin. Individuals who have sickle cell trait (called sickle cell carriers) have one normal beta globin gene and one sickle cell gene. These individuals make both the usual adult hemoglobin and sickle hemoglobin in roughly equal proportions, so they do not experience any health problems as a result of having the

trait. Although traces of blood in the urine and difficulty in concentrating the urine can occur, neither represents a significant health problem as a result of sickle cell trait. Of the millions of people with sickle cell trait worldwide, a small handful of individuals have experienced acute symptoms. In these very rare cases, individuals were subject to very severe physical strain.

When both members of a couple are carriers of sickle cell trait, there is a 25% chance in each pregnancy for the baby to inherit two sickle cell genes and have sickle cell anemia, or SS disease. Correspondingly, there is a 50% chance the baby will have sickle cell trait and a 25% chance that the baby will have the usual type of hemoglobin.

Other types of sickle cell disease include SC disease, SD disease, and S/beta **thalassemia**. These conditions are caused by the co-inheritance of the sickle cell gene and another altered beta globin gene. For example, one parent may have sickle cell trait and the other parent may have hemoglobin C trait (another hemoglobin trait that does not cause health problems). For this couple, there would be a 25% chance of SC disease in each pregnancy.

## Signs and symptoms

Normal adult hemoglobin transports oxygen from the lungs to tissues throughout the body. Sickle hemoglobin can also transport oxygen. However, once the oxygen is released, sickle hemoglobin tends to polymerize (line-up) into rigid rods that alter the shape of the red blood cell. Sickling of the red blood cell can be triggered by low oxygen, such as occurs in organs with slow blood flow. It can also be triggered by cold temperatures and dehydration.

Sickle cells have a decreased life span in comparison to normal red blood cells. Normal red blood cells survive for approximately 120 days in the bloodstream; sickle cells last only 10-12 days. As a result, the bloodstream is chronically short of red blood cells and hemoglobin, and the affected individual develops anemia.

Sickle cells can create other complications. Due to their shape, they do not fit well through small blood vessels. As an aggravating factor, the outside surfaces of sickle cells may have altered chemical properties that increase the cells' 'stickiness'. These sticky sickle cells are more likely to adhere to the inside surfaces of small blood vessels, as well as to other blood cells. As a result of the sickle cells' shape and stickiness, blockages form

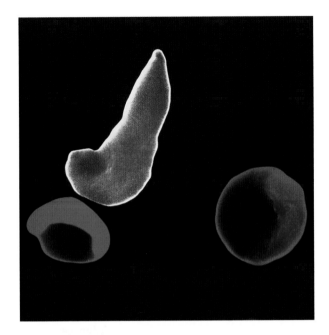

Scanning electron micrograph (SEM) of red blood cells taken from a person with sickle cell anemia. The red blood cells at the bottom are normal; the diseased, sickle-shaped cell appears at the top. *(Photo Researchers, Inc.)*

in small blood vessels. Such blockages prevent oxygenated blood from reaching areas where it is needed, causing pain as well as organ and tissue damage.

The severity of symptoms cannot be predicted based solely on the genetic **inheritance**. Some individuals with sickle cell disease develop health- or life-threatening problems in infancy, but others may have only mild symptoms throughout their lives. Individuals may experience varying degrees of health at different stages in the lifecycle. For the most part, this clinical variability is unpredictable, and the reasons for the observed variability can not usually be determined. However, certain types of sickle cell disease (i.e. SC disease) tend to result in fewer and less severe symptoms on average than other types of sickle cell disease (i.e. SS disease). Some additional modifying factors are known. For example, elevated levels of fetal hemoglobin in a child or adult can decrease the quantity and severity of some symptoms and complications. Fetal hemoglobin is a normally occurring hemoglobin that usually decreases from over 90% of the total hemoglobin to under 1% during the first year of life. This change is genetically determined, although some individuals may experience elevated levels of fetal hemoglobin due to variation in the genes that control fetal hemoglobin production. Such individuals often experience a reduction in their symptoms and complications due to the ability of fetal hemoglobin to prevent the polymerization of sickle hemoglobin, which leads to sickling of the red blood cell.

There are several symptoms that warrant immediate medical attention, including the following:

- Signs of infection (fever 101°F or 38.3°C, coughs frequently or breathing trouble, unusual crankiness, feeding difficulties)
- Signs of severe anemia (pale skin or lips, yellowing of the skin or eyes, very tired, very weak)
- Signs indicating possible dehydration (vomiting, diarrhea, fewer wet diapers)
- Other signs (pain or swelling in the abdomen, swollen hands or feet, screams when touched).

These can be signs of various complications that occur in sickle cell disease.

### Infections and effects on the spleen

Children with sickle cell disease who are under age three are particularly prone to life-threatening bacterial infections. *Streptococcus pneumoniae* is the most common offending bacteria, and invasive infection from this organism leads to death in 15% of patients. The spleen, an organ that helps to fight bacterial infections, is particularly vulnerable to the effects of sickling. Sickle cells can impede blood flow through the spleen, causing organ damage, which usually results in loss of spleen function by late childhood. The spleen can also become enlarged due to blockages and/or increased activity of the spleen. Rapid enlargement of the spleen may be a sign of another complication called *splenic sequestration*, which occurs mostly in young children and can be life-threatening. Widespread sickling in the spleen prevents adequate blood flow from the organ, removing increasing volumes of blood from the circulation and leading to accompanying signs of severe anemia.

### Painful events

Painful events, also known as *vaso-occlusive events*, are a hallmark symptom of sickle cell disease. The frequency and duration of the pain can vary tremendously from person to person and over an individual's lifecycle. Painful events are the most common cause of hospitalizations in sickle cell disease. However, only a small portion of individuals with sickle cell disease experience frequent and severe painful events. Most painful events can be managed at home. Pain results when small blood vessel blockages prevent oxygen from reaching tissues. Pain can affect any area of the body, although the extremities, chest, abdomen, and bones are frequently affected sites. There is some evidence that cold temperatures or infection can trigger a painful event, but

**Amino acid**—Organic compounds that form the building blocks of protein. There are 20 types of amino acids (eight are "essential amino acids" which the body cannot make and must therefore be obtained from food).

**Anemia**—A blood condition in which the level of hemoglobin or the number of red blood cells falls below normal values. Common symptoms include paleness, fatigue, and shortness of breath.

**Bilirubin**—A yellow pigment that is the end result of hemoglobin breakdown. This pigment is metabolized in the liver and excreted from the body through the bile. Bloodstream levels are normally low; however, extensive red cell destruction leads to excessive bilirubin formation and jaundice.

**Bone marrow**—A spongy tissue located in the hollow centers of certain bones, such as the skull and hip bones. Bone marrow is the site of blood cell generation.

**Bone marrow transplantation**—A medical procedure used to treat some diseases that arise from defective blood cell formation in the bone marrow. Healthy bone marrow is extracted from a donor to replace the marrow in an ailing individual. Proteins on the surface of bone marrow cells must be identical or very closely matched between a donor and the recipient.

**Globin**—One of the component protein molecules found in hemoglobin. Normal adult hemoglobin has a pair each of alpha-globin and beta-globin molecules.

**Heme**—The iron-containing molecule in hemoglobin that serves as the site for oxygen binding.

**Hemoglobin**—Protein-iron compound in the blood that carries oxygen to the cells and carries carbon dioxide away from the cells.

**Hemoglobin A**—Normal adult hemoglobin that contains a heme molecule, two alpha-globin molecules, and two beta-globin molecules.

**Hemoglobin electrophoresis**—A laboratory test that separates molecules based on their size, shape, or electrical charge.

**Hemoglobin S**—Hemoglobin produced in association with the sickle cell trait; the beta-globin molecules of hemoglobin S are defective.

**Hydroxyurea**—A drug that has been shown to induce production of fetal hemoglobin. Fetal hemoglobin has a pair of gamma-globin molecules in place of the typical beta-globins of adult hemoglobin. Higher-than-normal levels of fetal hemoglobin can prevent sickling from occurring.

**Impotence**—The inability to have a penile erection, which can be due to tissue damage resulting from sickling within the penis (priapism).

**Iron overload**—A side effect of frequent blood transfusions in which the body accumulates abnormally high levels of iron. Iron deposits can form in organs, particularly the heart, and cause life-threatening damage.

**Jaundice**—Yellowing of the skin or eyes due to excess of bilirubin in the blood.

**Magnetic resonance imaging (MRI)**—A technique that employs magnetic fields and radio waves to create detailed images of internal body structures and organs, including the brain.

**Mutation**—A permanent change in the genetic material that may alter a trait or characteristic of an individual, or manifest as disease, and can be transmitted to offspring.

**Narcotics**—Strong, prescription medication that can be effective in treating pain, but have the potential to be habit-forming if their use is not supervised correctly.

**Nucleic acid**—A type of chemical used as a component for building DNA. The nucleic acids found in DNA are adenine, thymine, guanine, and cytosine.

**Ophthalmology**—The medical specialty of vision and the eye.

**Placenta**—The organ responsible for oxygen and nutrition exchange between a pregnant mother and her developing baby.

**Red blood cell**—Hemoglobin-containing blood cells that transport oxygen from the lungs to tissues. In the tissues, the red blood cells exchange their oxygen for carbon dioxide, which is brought back to the lungs to be exhaled.

**Screening**—Process through which carriers of a trait may be identified within a population.

**Sickle cell**—A red blood cell that has assumed a elongated shape due to the presence of hemoglobin S.

most events occur for unknown reasons. The hand-foot syndrome, or *dactylitis*, is a particular type of painful event. Most common in toddlers, dactylitis results in pain and swelling in the hands and feet, sometimes accompanied by a fever.

### Anemia

Sickle cells have a high turnover rate leading to a deficit of red blood cells in the bloodstream. Common symptoms of anemia include fatigue, paleness, and a shortness of breath. A particularly severe form of anemia—aplastic anemia—occurs following infection with parvovirus. Parvovirus causes extensive destruction of the bone marrow, bringing production of new red blood cells to a halt. Bone marrow production resumes after seven to 10 days; however, given the short lives of sickle cells, even a brief shut-down in red blood cell production can cause a rapid decline in hemoglobin concentrations.

### Delayed growth

The energy demands of the bone marrow for red blood cell production compete with the demands of a growing body. Children with sickle cell anemia may have delayed growth and reach puberty at a later age than normal. By early adulthood, they catch up on growth and attain normal height; however, weight typically remains below average.

### Stroke

Children with sickle cell disease have a significantly elevated risk of having a stroke, which can be one of the most concerning complications of sickle cell disease. Approximately 11% of individuals with sickle cell disease will have a recognizable stroke by the age of 20. Magnetic resonance imaging studies have found that 17% of children with sickle cell anemia have evidence of a previous stroke or clinically 'silent' stroke-like events called *transient ischemic events*. Stroke in sickle cell disease is usually caused by a blockage of a blood vessel, but about one fourth of the time may be caused by a hemorrhage (or rupture) of a blood vessel.

Strokes result in compromised delivery of oxygen to an area of the brain. The consequences of stroke can range from life-threatening, to severe physical or cognitive impairments, to apparent or subtle learning disabilities, to undetectable effects. Common stroke symptoms include weakness or numbness that affects one side of the body, sudden behavioral changes, loss of vision, confusion, loss of speech or the ability to understand spoken words, dizziness, headache, seizures, vomiting, or even coma.

Approximately two-thirds of the children who have a stroke will have at least one more. Transfusions have been shown to decrease the incidence of a second stroke. A recent study showed that children at highest risk to experience a first stroke were 10 times more likely to stroke if untreated when compared to high-risk children treated with chronic blood transfusion therapy. High-risk children were identified using transcranial doppler ultrasound technology to detect individuals with increased blood flow speeds due to constricted intracranial blood vessels.

### Acute chest syndrome

Acute chest syndrome (ACS) is a leading cause of death for individuals with sickle cell disease, and recurrent attacks can lead to permanent lung damage. Therefore, rapid diagnosis and treatment is of great importance. ACS can occur at any age and is similar but distinct from pneumonia. Affected persons may experience fever, cough, chest pain, and shortness of breath. ACS seems to have multiple causes including infection, sickling in the small blood vessels of the lungs, fat embolisms in the lungs, or a combination of factors.

### Priapism

Males with sickle cell anemia may experience priapism, a condition characterized by a persistent and painful erection of the penis. Due to blood vessel blockage by sickle cells, blood is trapped in the tissue of the penis. Priapism may be short in duration or it may be prolonged. Priapism can be triggered by low oxygen (hypoxemia), alcohol consumption, or sexual intercourse. Since priapism can be extremely painful and result in damage to this tissue causing impotence, rapid treatment is essential.

### Kidney disease

The environment in the kidney is particularly prone to damage from sickle cells. Signs of kidney damage can include blood in the urine, incontinence, and enlarged kidneys. Adults with sickle cell disease often experience insufficient functioning of the kidneys, which can progress to kidney failure in a small percentage of adults with sickle cell disease.

### Jaundice and gallstones

Jaundice is indicated by a yellow tone in the skin and eyes, and alone it is not a health concern. Jaundice may occur if bilirubin levels increase, which can occur with high levels of red blood cell destruction. Bilirubin is the final product of hemoglobin degradation, and is typically removed from the bloodstream by the liver. Therefore, jaundice can also be a sign of a poorly functioning liver, which may also be evidenced by an enlarged liver. Increased bilirubin also leads to increased chance for gallstones in children with sickle cell disease. Treatment, which may include removal of the gall bladder, may be selected if the gallstones start causing symptoms.

### Retinopathy

The blood vessels that supply oxygen to the retina—the tissue at the back of the eye—may be blocked by sickle cells, leading to a condition called retinopathy. This is one of the only complications that is actually more common in SC disease as compared to SS disease. Retinopathy can be identified through regular ophthalmology evaluations and effectively treated in order to avoid damage to vision.

### Joint problems

Avascular necrosis of the hip and shoulder joints, in which bone damage occurs due to compromised blood flow due to sickling, can occur later in childhood. This complication can affect an individual's physical abilities and result in substantial pain.

## Diagnosis

Inheritance of sickle cell disease or trait cannot be prevented, but it may be predicted. Screening is recommended for individuals in high-risk populations. In the United States, African Americans and Latino Americans have the highest risk of having the disease or trait. Sickle cell is also common among individuals of Mediterranean, Middle Eastern, and Eastern Indian descent.

A complete blood count (CBC) will describe several aspects of an individual's blood cells. A person with sickle cell disease will have a lower than normal hemoglobin level, together with other characteristic red blood cell abnormalities. A *hemoglobin electrophoresis* is a test that can help identify the types and quantities of hemoglobin made by an individual. This test uses an electric field applied across a slab of gel-like material. Hemoglobins migrate through this gel at various rates and to specific locations, depending on their size, shape, and electrical charge. Although sickle hemoglobin (Hb S) and regular adult hemoglobin (called Hb A) differ by only one amino acid, they can be clearly separated using hemoglobin electrophoresis. *Isoelectric focusing* and *high-performance liquid chromatography (HPLC)* use similar principles to separate hemoglobins and can be used instead of or in various combinations with hemoglobin electrophoresis to determine the types of hemoglobin present.

Another test, called the 'sickledex' can help confirm the presence of sickle hemoglobin, although this test cannot provide accurate or reliable diagnosis when used alone. When Hb S is present, but there is an absence or only a trace of Hb A, sickle cell anemia is a likely diagnosis. Additional beta globin DNA testing, which looks directly at the beta globin gene, can be performed to help confirm the diagnosis and establish the exact genetic type of sickle cell disease. CBC and hemoglobin electrophoresis are also typically used to diagnosis sickle cell trait and various other types of beta globin traits.

Diagnosis of sickle cell disease can occur under various circumstances. If an individual has symptoms that are suggestive of this diagnosis, the above-described screening tests can be performed followed by DNA testing, if indicated. Screening at birth using HPLC or a related technique offers the opportunity for early intervention. More than 40 states include sickle cell screening as part of the usual battery of blood tests done for newborns. This allows for early identification and treatment. Hemoglobin trait screening is recommended for any individual of a high-risk ethnic background who may be considering having children. When both members of a couple are found to have sickle cell trait, or other related hemoglobin traits, they can receive **genetic counseling** regarding the risk of sickle cell disease in their future children and various testing options.

Sickle cell disease can be identified before birth through the use of prenatal diagnosis. Chorionic villus sampling (CVS) can be offered as early as 10 weeks of pregnancy and involves removing a sample of the placenta made by the baby and testing the cells. CVS carries a risk of causing a miscarriage that is between one-half to one percent.

**Amniocentesis** is generally offered between 16 and 18 weeks of pregnancy, but can sometimes be offered earlier. Two to three tablespoons of the fluid surrounding the baby is removed. This fluid contains fetal cells that can be tested. This test carries a risk of causing a miscarriage, which is less than 1%. Pregnant woman and couples may choose prenatal testing in order to prepare for the birth of a baby that may have sickle cell disease.

Preimplantation genetic diagnosis (PGD) is a relatively new technique that involves in-vitro fertilization followed by **genetic testing** of one cell from each developing embryo. Only the embryos unaffected by sickle cell disease are transferred back into the uterus. PGD is currently available on a research basis only, and is relatively expensive.

## Treatment and management

There are several practices intended to prevent some of the symptoms and complications of sickle cell disease. These include preventative antibiotics, good hydration, immunizations, and access to comprehensive care. Maintaining good health through adequate nutrition, avoiding stresses and infection, and getting proper rest is also important. Following these guidelines is intended to improve the health of individuals with sickle cell disease.

### Penicillin

Infants are typically started on a course of penicillin that extends from infancy to age six. Use of this antibiotic is meant to ward off potentially fatal infections. Infections at any age are treated aggressively with antibiotics. Vaccines for common infections, such as *pneumococcal pneumonia*, are also recommended.

### Pain management

Pain is one of the primary symptoms of sickle cell anemia, and controlling it is an important concern. The methods necessary for pain control are based on individual factors. Some people can gain adequate pain control through over-the-counter oral painkillers (analgesics). Other individuals, or painful events, may require stronger methods which can include administration of narcotics. Alternative therapies may be useful in avoiding or controlling pain, including relaxation, hydration, avoiding extremes of temperature, and the application of local warmth.

### Blood transfusions

Blood transfusions are not usually given on a regular basis but are used to treat individuals with frequent and severe painful events, severe anemia, and other emergencies. In some cases blood transfusions are given as a preventative measure, for example to treat spleen enlargement or prevent a second stroke (or a first stroke in an individual shown to be at high risk).

Regular blood transfusions have the potential to decrease formation of hemoglobin S, and reduce associated symptoms. However, there are limitations and risks associated with regular blood transfusions, including the risk of blood-borne infection and sensitization to proteins in the transfused blood that can make future transfusions very difficult. Most importantly, chronic blood transfusions can lead to iron overload. The body tends to store excess iron, such as that received through transfusions, in various organs. Over time, this iron storage can cause damage to various tissues and organs, such as the heart and endocrine organs.

Some of this damage can be prevented by the administration of a medication called *desferoxamine* that helps the body to eliminate excess iron through the urine. Alternately, some individuals receive a new, non-standard treatment called *erythrocytapheresis*. This involves the automated removal of sickle cells and is used in conjunction with a reduced number of regular transfusions. This treatment helps to reduce iron overload.

### Hydroxyurea

Emphasis is being placed on developing drugs that treat sickle cell anemia directly. The most promising of these drugs since the late 1990s has been hydroxyurea, a drug that was originally designed for anticancer treatment. Hydroxyurea has been shown to reduce the frequency of painful crises and acute chest syndrome in adults, and to lessen the need for blood transfusions. Hydroxyurea, and other related medications, seem to work by inducing a higher production of fetal hemoglobin. The major side effects of the drug include decreased production of platelets, red blood cells, and certain white blood cells. The effects of long-term hydroxyurea treatment are unknown.

### Bone marrow transplantation

Bone marrow transplantation has been shown to cure sickle cell anemia in some cases. This treatment is reserved primarily for severely affected children with a healthy donor whose marrow proteins match those of the recipient, namely a brother or sister who has inherited the same tissue type. Indications for a bone marrow transplant are stroke, recurrent acute chest syndrome, and chronic unrelieved pain.

Bone marrow transplantations tend to be the most successful in children; adults have a higher rate of transplant rejection and other complications. There is approximately a 10% fatality rate associated with bone marrow transplants done for sickle cell disease. Survivors face potential long-term complications, such as chronic graft-versus-host disease (an immune-mediated attack by the donor marrow against the recipient's tissues), infertility, and development of some forms of **cancer**. A relatively recent advance in transplantation involves the use of donor stem cells obtained from *cord blood*, the blood from the placenta that is otherwise discarded following the birth of a new baby. Cord blood cells, as opposed to fully mature bone marrow cells, appear to be less likely to result in graft-versus-host disease in the recipient. This increases the safety and efficacy of the transplant procedure.

### Surgery

Certain surgical interventions are utilized in the treatment of specific sickle cell-related complications. Removal of a dysfunctioning gallbladder or spleen can often lead to improvements in health. Investigations are currently underway to establish the efficacy of hip coring surgery, in which a portion of affected bone is removed to treat avascular necrosis of the hip. The hope is that this may provide an effective treatment to alleviate some pain and restore function in the affected hip.

### Psychosocial support

As in any lifelong, chronic disease, comprehensive care is important. Assistance with the emotional, social, family-planning, economic, vocational, and other consequences of sickle cell disease can enable affected individuals to better access and benefit from their medical care.

## Prognosis

Sickle cell disease is characteristically variable between and within affected individuals. Predicting the course of the disorder based solely on genes is not possible. Several factors aside from genetic inheritance determine the prognosis for affected individuals, including the frequency, severity, and nature of specific complications in any given individual. The availability and access of comprehensive medical care also plays an important role in preventing and treating serious, acute complications, which cause the majority of sickle cell-related deaths. For those individuals who do not experience such acute events, life-expectancy is probably substantially greater than the average for all people with sickle cell disease. The impact of recent medical advances supports the hypothesis that current life-expectancies may be significantly greater than those estimated in the early 1990s. At that time, individuals with SS disease lived to the early- to mid-40s, and those with SC disease lived into the upper 50s on average. With early detection and comprehensive medical care, most people with sickle cell disease are in fairly good health most of the time. Most individuals can be expected to live well into adulthood, enjoying an improved quality of life including the ability to choose a variety of education, career, and family-planning options for themselves.

## Resources

### BOOKS

Beutler, Ernest. "The Sickle Cell Diseases and Related Disorders." In *Williams Hematology,* edited by Ernest Beutler, et al. 5th ed. New York: McGraw-Hill, 1995.

Bloom, Miriam. *Understanding Sickle Cell Disease.* Jackson, MS: University Press of Mississippi, 1995.

Embury, Stephen H., et al., eds. *Sickle Cell Disease: Basic Principles and Clinical Practice.* New York: Raven Press, 1994.

Reid, C.D., S. Charache, and B. Lubin, eds. *Management and Therapy of Sickle Cell Disease.* 3rd ed. National Institutes of Health Publication No. 96-2117, 1995.

### PERIODICALS

Adams, R.J., et al. "Prevention of a First Stroke by Transfusions in Children with Sickle Cell Anemia and Abnormal Results on Transcranial Doppler Ultrasonography." *New England Journal of Medicine* 339 (1998): 5-11.

Davies, Sally C. "Management of Patients with Sickle Cell Disease." *British Medical Journal* 315 (September 13, 1997): 656.

Golden, C., L. Styles, and E. Vichinsky. "Acute Chest syndrome and Sickle Cell Disease." *Current Opinion in Hematology* 5 (1998): 89-92.

Hoppe, C., L. Styles, and E. Vichinsky. "The Natural History of Sickle Cell Disease." *Current Opinion in Pediatrics* 10 (1998): 49-52.

Kinney, T.R., et al. "Safety of Hydroxyurea in Children with Sickle Cell Anemia: Results of the HUG-KIDS Study, A Phase I/II Trial." *Blood* 94 (1999): 1550-1554.

Platt, O., et al. "Mortality in Sickle Cell Disease: Life Expectancy and Risk Factors for Early Death." *New England Journal of Medicine* 330 (1994): 1639-1644.

Reed, W., and E.P. Vichinsky. "New Considerations in the Treatment of Sickle Cell Disease." *Annual Review of Medicine* 49 (1998): 461.

Schnog, J.B., et al. "New Concepts in Assessing Sickle Cell Disease Severity." *American Journal of Hematology* 58 (1998): 61-66.

Serjeant, Graham R. "Sickle-Cell Disease." *The Lancet* 350 (September 6, 1997): 725.

Singer, S.T., et al. "Erythrocytapheresis for Chronically Transfused Children with Sickle Cell Disease: An Effective Method for Maintaining a Low Hemoglobin S Level and Reducing Iron Overload." *Journal of Clinical Apheresis* 14 (1999): 122-125.

Xu, K., et. al. "First Unaffected Pregnancy Using Preimplantation Genetic Diagnosis for Sickle Cell Anemia." *Journal of the American Medical Association* 281 (1999): 1701-1706.

### ORGANIZATIONS

Sickle Cell Disease Association of America, Inc. 200 Corporate Point Suite 495, Culver City, CA 90230-8727. (800) 421-8453. Scdaa@sicklecelldisease.org. http://sicklecell disease.org/.

Jennifer Bojanowski, MS, CGC

Siewert syndrome *see* **Kartagener syndrome**

Silver-Russell syndrome *see* **Russell-Silver syndrome**

# Simpson-Golabi-Behmel syndrome

### Definition

Simpson-Golabi-Behmel syndrome (SGBS) is a rare X-linked recessive inherited condition. It causes general overgrowth in height and weight. Individuals with SGBS also have characteristic facial features in childhood which tend to become less obvious in adulthood.

### Description

SGBS is also known as Simpson dysmorphia syndrome (SDYS), bulldog syndrome, Golabi-Rosen syndrome, and **dysplasia** gigantism syndrome X-linked (DGSX). SGBS is a rare X-linked recessive inherited condition. Individuals with this condition have increased height and weight for their age; a broad, stocky appearance; a large protruding jaw; a short, broad nose; incomplete closure of the roof of the mouth (**cleft palate**); and broad, short hands and fingers. Individuals with SGBS are usually taller than average. The characteristic features usually become less apparent in adulthood. There are at least two genes for SGBS. Both genes are located on the X **chromosome**.

### Genetic profile

SGBS is caused by an alteration (mutation) in one of two genes on the X chromosome. Chromosomes are units of hereditary material passed from a parent to a child through the egg and sperm. The information on the chromosomes is organized into units called genes. Genes contain information necessary for normal

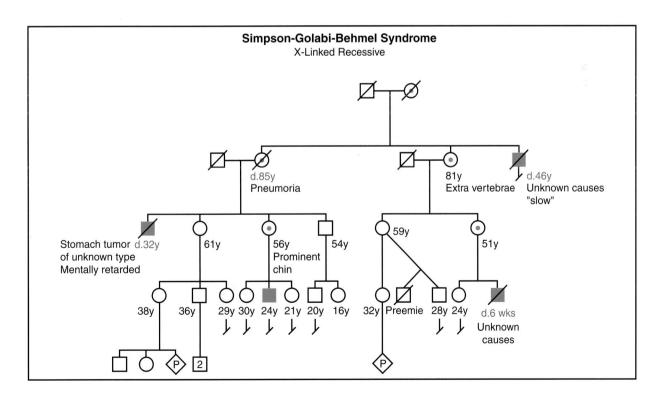

*(Illustration by GGS Information Services. Gale, a part of Cengage Learning.)*

## KEY TERMS

**Amniocentesis**—A procedure performed at 16-18 weeks of pregnancy in which a needle is inserted through a woman's abdomen into her uterus to draw out a small sample of the amniotic fluid from around the baby. Either the fluid itself or cells from the fluid can be used for a variety of tests to obtain information about genetic disorders and other medical conditions in the fetus.

**Chorionic villus sampling (CVS)**—A procedure used for prenatal diagnosis at 10-12 weeks gestation. Under ultrasound guidance a needle is inserted either through the mother's vagina or abdominal wall and a sample of cells is collected from around the early embryo. These cells are then tested for chromosome abnormalities or other genetic diseases.

**Chromosome**—A microscopic thread-like structure found within each cell of the body and consists of a complex of proteins and DNA. Humans have 46 chromosomes arranged into 23 pairs. Changes in either the total number of chromosomes or their shape and size (structure) may lead to physical or mental abnormalities.

human growth and development. Each cell in the body usually contains 46 chromosomes, arranged as 23 pairs. Twenty-two pairs of chromosomes are the same in males and females. The twenty-third pair is the sex chromosomes: females have two X chromosomes and males have an X and a Y chromosome. There are two genes on the X chromosome that can cause SGBS. The first gene is responsible for making a protein called glypican-3 (GPC3). The exact role of GPC3 is not known but it is thought to play a role in growth and development. When the gene for GPC3 is altered, the signs and symptoms of SGBS result. A second candidate gene, which causes a more severe form of SGBS, is also located on the X chromosome. The function of this second gene is not known. Generally, individuals who have SGBS due to a gene alteration in the GPC3 gene are said to have SGBS type 1 (SGBS1) and individuals who have SGBS due to an alteration in the second gene on the X chromosome are said to have SGBS type 2 (SGBS2).

SGBS is inherited as an X-linked recessive condition. With X-linked recessive conditions, males are usually more severely affected than females. Females have two copies of the SGBS gene (because they have two X chromosomes) while males have one copy of SGBS gene(because they have one X chromosome). Females who have an alteration in one copy of the SGBS gene are said to be carriers of SGBS. Generally, carriers show minimal or no effects of the altered gene because they have a second normal copy of the gene that is able to compensate for the altered copy. Since males have only one working copy of the SGBS gene to start, if that gene is altered, they will develop SGBS. When carrier females have children, they are at risk to have a child with SGBS. In each pregnancy, carrier females have a 25% chance of having a child (always a son) with SGBS and a 25% chance of having a child (always a daughter) whom is a carrier of SGBS. Males who are affected with SGBS cannot pass this condition to their sons (because their sons inherit the Y chromosome); however, all daughters of a male affected with SGBS will be carriers for the condition.

### Demographics

SGBS is a rare inherited condition that primarily affects males from all ethnic groups. Female carriers for SGBS may show subtle features of the condition. It is not known precisely how many individuals are affected with SGBS.

### Signs and symptoms

The spectrum of clinical features in SGBS is broad, ranging from very mild forms in carrier females to forms that are lethal in the newborn male. SGBS affects the face, hands, chest, abdomen, genitals, internal organs and overall growth.

Individuals with SGBS are larger than average at birth in height, weight, and head size. This overgrowth continues into adulthood with affected males being taller than average. Final height in males ranges from 74 in to 83 in (188 cm to 210 cm). There are typical facial characteristics in affected males including widely spaced eyes, short nose, large mouth, large tongue, a groove in the lower lip, and teeth that do not align properly. Incomplete closure of the lip (**cleft lip**) and/or the roof of the mouth (cleft palate) can also occur. The large tongue and improperly aligned teeth can be a cause of speech difficulties.

The hands and feet of males with SGBS tend to be short and broad. Other hand abnormalities such as small nails, webbing of the skin between the fingers, and extra fingers/toes, is also common. Males with SGBS have extra nipples and some may have undescended testicles.

The internal organs are larger than average, particularly the liver, spleen, and kidneys. The kidneys may also have many cysts on them. A few individuals have been known to have lung and diaphragm abnormalities. Heart abnormalities can also occur in SGBS1 and have been a cause of death in several individuals under two years of age. These include conduction defects causing arrythmias. The stomach and intestines can also be affected, which may cause digestive problems. The bones may also be affected. Some individuals have an abnormal curving and twisting of the spine (**scoliosis**), extra ribs, and/or problems with the structure of the bones of the spine. The bony changes can be seen on x–ray but may not cause any symptoms.

Despite their large size, newborns with SGBS tend to be floppy babies with decreased muscle tone. Due to this low muscle tone, there are several features that can result such as mouth breathing, a deformity of the chest wall (pectus excavatum), shoulders that droop, hernias, and undescended testicles.

There is an increased risk to develop tumors of the kidney (Wilms tumor) in SGBS in early childhood. This risk appears to be greatest in individuals under two years of age.

Most individuals with SGBS are of average intelligence, although some degree of mental impairment has been observed in males who are more severely affected. Individuals with SGBS may have psychological difficulties dealing with their distinctive facial appearance and speech difficulties, which often give the false impression that they are mentally impaired.

## Diagnosis

The diagnosis of SGBS is based on the presence of certain clinical features and in some cases may be confirmed through **genetic testing**. Not all affected individuals will have all of the features associated with SGBS. SGBS should be considered in an individual who is large in height, weight, and head circumference both before and after birth. Features of the condition that are almost always present include overgrowth; extra nipples; chest deformity; low muscle tone; and characteristic facial features including widely spaced eyes, short nose, large tongue and mouth, central groove of the lower lip, and improperly aligned teeth.

It may be possible to confirm the diagnosis of SGBS through genetic testing. Genetic testing for mutations in the GPC3 gene causing SGB1 is available. Genetic testing involves obtaining a blood sample from the affected individual in order to look for the specific disease-causing mutation in the GPC3 gene. Since not all individuals with SGBS have mutations in the GPC3 gene, it may not be possible to confirm the diagnosis through genetic testing in all individuals suspected of having this condition. Genetic testing for the SGBS can be done on the developing baby before birth through **amniocentesis** or chorionic villus sampling if a mutation in the gene for GPC3 is first identified in an affected family member. Prenatal testing for parents of an affected individual should only be undertaken after the SGBS carrier status of the parents has been confirmed and the couple has been counseled regarding the risks of recurrence.

## Treatment and management

The heart function of individuals with SGBS should be carefully monitored because it can be a cause of early death. Individuals with SGBS should be regularly followed by a heart specialist (cardiologist).

Individuals with SGBS are at increased risk to develop kidney tumors. They should be screened for possible kidney tumor development or other tumors of infancy for at least the first five years of life. Screening usually involves an ultrasound (sound wave picture) of the abdomen, including the kidneys.

The large tongue and improperly aligned teeth may lead to speech difficulties. Some individuals may require surgery to reduce the size of the tongue to aid with speech development or for cosmetic reasons. Individuals with speech difficulties may benefit from speech therapy.

Individuals with SGBS may benefit from psychological support and social support to help them reach an adequate level of self-esteem. They may also benefit from **genetic counseling**, which may provide them with further information on the condition itself and recurrence risks for future pregnancies.

## Prognosis

The spectrum of clinical manifestations in SGBS is broad, varying from very mild forms in carrier females to infantile lethal forms in affected males. As many as 50% of males affected with SGBS die in the newborn period. The cause of this high mortality is not known but may be related to heart defects. In one reported family with a severe form of SGBS causing death in the newborn period, the responsible gene was not glypican-3 but the second candidate gene on the X chromosome.

QUESTIONS TO ASK YOUR DOCTOR

- What signs and symptoms are characteristic of Simpson-Golabi-Behmel syndrome?
- What information about Simpson-Golabi-Behmel syndrome can a genetic counselor provide me?
- What is the projected life span for a newborn infant diagnosed with Simpson-Golabi-Behmel syndrome, and what factors affect that prognosis?
- Where can I obtain additional information about this genetic disorder?

### Resources

#### PERIODICALS

Hughes-Benzie, R.M., et al. "Simpson-Golabi-Behmel Syndrome: Genotype/Phenotype Analysis of 18 Affected Males From 7 Unrelated Families." *American Journal of Medical Genetics* 66 (1996): 227-234.

Neri, Giovanni, et al. "Clinical and Molecular Aspects of the Simpson-Golabi-Behmel Syndrome." *American Journal of Medical Genetics* 79 (1998): 279-283.

#### WEBSITES

"Simpson-Golabi-Behmel Syndrome, type 1." *Online Mendelian Inheritance in Man*.http://www.ncbi.nlm.nih.gov/entrez/dispomim.cgi?id=312870. (March 9, 2001)

#### ORGANIZATIONS

Beckwith-Wiedemann Support Network. 2711 Colony Rd., Ann Arbor, MI 48104. (734) 973-0263 or (800) 837-2976. http://www.beckwith-wiedemann.org.

National Organization for Rare Disorders (NORD). PO Box 8923, New Fairfield, CT 06812-8923. (203) 746-6518 or (800) 999-6673. Fax: (203) 746-6481. http://www.rarediseases.org.

Nada Quercia, MS, CGC, CCGC

## Simpson dysmorphia syndrome (SDYS) *see* Simpson-Golabi-Behmel syndrome

# Sirenomelia

### Definition

Sirenomelia is a lethal birth defect of the lower body characterized by apparent fusion of the legs into a single lower limb. Other birth defects are always associated with sirenomelia, most commonly abnormalities of the kidneys, large intestines, and genitalia.

KEY TERMS

**Aorta**—The main artery located above the heart which pumps oxygenated blood out into the body. Many congenital heart defects affect the aorta.

**Autosomal dominant**—A pattern of genetic inheritance where only one abnormal gene is needed to display the trait or disease.

**Iliac arteries**—Arteries that supply blood to the lower body including the pelvis and legs.

**Imperforate anus**—Also known as anal atresia. A birth defect in which the opening of the anus is absent or obstructed.

**Mermaid syndrome**—Alternate name for sirenomelia, often used in older references.

**Mutation**—A permanent change in the genetic material that may alter a trait or characteristic of an individual, or manifest as disease, and can be transmitted to offspring.

**Oligohydramnios**—Reduced amount of amniotic fluid. Causes include non–functioning kidneys and premature rupture of membranes. Without amniotic fluid to breathe, a baby will have underdeveloped and immature lungs.

**Stillborn**—The birth of a baby who has died sometime during the pregnancy or delivery.

**Teratogenic**—Any agent that can cause birth defects or mental retardation in a developing fetus. Common teratogens are medications or other chemicals but they also include infections, radiation, maternal medical condition, and other agents.

**Ultrasound**—An imaging technique that uses sound waves to help visualize internal structures in the body.

### Description

This pattern of birth defects is associated with abnormal umbilical cord blood vessels. The normal fetus develops two umbilical arteries, which pump blood from the fetus to the placenta, and one umbilical vein, which returns blood from the placenta to the fetus. The umbilical arteries branch off the iliac arteries in the pelvis. The iliac arteries supply the legs and pelvic organs such as the genitalia. Most babies with sirenomelia have only one umbilical artery and one vein. Rarely a baby with sirenomelia can have the typical two arteries and one vein with occlusion (blockage) of one artery.

In sirenomelia, the one functional artery is larger than normal and branches from the aorta high in the abdomen. Below this umbilical artery, the aorta becomes abnormally narrow. This type of single umbilical artery is known as a vitelline artery because it is thought to arise from the primitive vitelline arteries early in the life of the embryo. The vitelline arteries normally fuse a few weeks after conception to form the arteries that supply the gastrointestinal system and genitourinary system (superior mesenteric, inferior mesenteric, and celiac arteries). If the normal umbilical arteries do not form correctly as branches from the iliac arteries, then a vitelline artery might persist.

The vitelline umbilical artery steals blood and nutrition from the lower body and diverts it to the placenta. This results in a small aorta and variable absence of the arteries that supply the kidneys, large intestine, and genitalia (renal, inferior mesenteric, and celiac arteries). Because of the loss of nutrition and blood flow, the lower limbs fail to form as separate limbs, the kidneys do not form or are malformed, the large intestine ends blindly in the abdominal cavity, the anus is imperforate, and the internal and external genitalia are absent or malformed.

The typical malformation of the lower limbs seen in babies with sirenomelia consists of apparent fusion of the legs. There is a spectrum of severity with severe cases having one lower limb that tapers to a point with the absence of foot structures. In these severe cases there are only two bones present in the entire limb (a femur and presumably a tibia). On the mild end of the spectrum are babies with fusion of the skin of the lower limbs only. In these infants the feet may be fully formed with fusion at the ankles. All bones are fully formed and separate. Normally there are three bones in each leg—the femur in the upper leg (thigh) and the tibia and fibula in the lower leg (calf).

Other birth abnormalities of the upper body involving the heart, lungs, spine, brain, and arms can also be seen in this syndrome, however, not in every affected individual. It is unknown at this time why a single umbilical artery could cause these changes.

Single umbilical artery occurs in about 1% of all live–born infants. In most of these infants the one umbilical artery is normally formed and not of vitelline origin. In these cases, the risk of other birth defects is low (about 8%). All infants born with a vitelline umbilical artery will have other malformations, the most common being sirenomelia.

## Genetic profile

All cases of sirenomelia have occurred in families as isolated cases, and there is no known genetic cause.

It is possible that sirenomelia is an autosomal dominant condition and because it is lethal, all cases represent a new mutation. Alternatively, it might be a multifactorial trait where multiple genes and environmental factors come together to cause this pattern of malformations. The fact that all cases have been isolated does not support this possibility. Sirenomelia is more common in twin pregnancies. This may be indicative of an environmental cause.

## Demographics

Sirenomelia is very rare, estimated to occur once in every 100,000 births. While the exact incidence in different populations is not known, sirenomelia has been reported worldwide in a variety of ethnic groups. It is known to be more common in twin pregnancies and in babies born to mothers with **diabetes** mellitus.

## Signs and symptoms

Abnormalities associated with sirenomelia include:

- absence of the kidneys or malformed nonfunctioning kidneys
- blind ending colon and imperforate anus
- Small, absent, fused, or poorly formed pelvic bones
- small, absent, or poorly formed internal and external genitalia
- fusion of the lower limbs along the inner leg, from skin only to complete fusion with the appearance of only one leg
- death from underdeveloped and immature lungs caused by oligohydramnios
- birth defects in the upper body sometimes occur and include abnormalities in the heart, lungs, arms, spine, and brain

## Diagnosis

The diagnosis is obvious at birth on examination of a baby, but prenatal diagnosis often occurs in the second trimester (weeks 13 through 26 of a pregnancy) by an ultrasound.

## Treatment and management

Babies born alive with functioning kidneys may survive with appropriate surgical management. Operations to reconstruct the urinary and gastrointestinal outlet tracts are almost always needed. Other procedures and treatments depend of the extent of other birth defects. It appears that if a baby does survive, he or she will not have any mental delays.

## Prognosis

Because of the birth defects involving the gastrointestinal tract and kidneys, sirenomelia is almost always fatal. About 50% of babies are stillborn (the baby has died before delivery) and 50% are live–born with survival lasting a few minutes to a few days. There have been at least two reported cases of sirenomelia that have survived beyond the first month of life. These infants had normal functioning kidneys during their development.

## Resources

### BOOKS

Chen, Harold. *Atlas of Genetic Diagnosis and Counseling.* New York, NY: Humana Press, 2006.

### PERIODICALS

Bruce, J. H., et al. "Caudal dysplasia syndrome and sirenomelia: are they part of a spectrum?" *Fetal and Pediatric Pathology* 28, no. 3 (2009): 109–131.

Guven, M. A., et al. "A prenatally diagnosed case of sirenomelia with polydactyly and vestigial tail." *Genetic Counseling* 19, no. 4 (2008): 419–424.

Sawhney, S., et al. "Sirenomelia: MRI appearance." *Journal of Postgraduate Medicine* 52, no. 3 (July–September 2006): 219–220.

Taori, K. B., et al. "Sirenomelia sequence (mermaid) : Report of three cases." *Indian Journal of Radiological Imaging* 12, no. 3 (2002): 399–401.

### WEBSITES

*Sirenomelia Sequence.* Information Page, NORD, November 26, 2008 (May 02, 2009). http://www.rarediseases.org/search/rdbdetail_abstract.html?disname=Sirenomelia%20Sequence

*Sirenomelia Syndrome.* Information Page, Madisons Foundation, August 14, 2005 (May 02, 2009). http://www.madisonsfoundation.org/index.php/component/option,com_mpower/Itemid,49/diseaseID,631

### ORGANIZATIONS

National Institute of Child Health and Human Development (NICHD). P.O. Box 3006, Rockville, MD 20847. (800)370-2943. Fax : (866)760-5947. Email: NICHDInformationResourceCenter@mail.nih.gov. http://www.nichd.nih.gov

National Organization for Rare Disorders (NORD). 55 Kenosia Avenue, PO Box 1968, Danbury, CT 06813-1968. (203)744-0100 or (800)999-6673. Fax: (203)798-2291. http://www.rarediseases.org.

Randall Stuart Colby, MD

# Sjögren-Larsson syndrome

## Definition

Sjögren-Larsson syndrome is an inherited disorder characterized by **ichthyosis** (scaly skin), speech abnormalities, mental retardation, and spasticity (a state of increased muscle tone with heightened reflexes). Severity is variable.

## Description

Sjögren-Larsson syndrome is a rare genetic disorder inherited in an autosomal recessive fashion. First characterized by Swedish psychiatrist Torsten Sjögren in 1956 (and by Sjögren and Tage Larsson in 1957), they suggested that all Swedes with the syndrome are descended from one ancestor in whom a mutation (a genetic change) occurred about 600 years ago. The highest incidence of the disease occurs in northern Sweden.

In infancy, development of various degrees of scaling and reddened skin occurs, often accompanied by hyperkeratosis (thickening of the skin) on the outer skin layer. After infancy, skin on the arms, legs and abdomen often is dark, scaly, and lacking redness. Seizures and speech abnormalities may accompany skin symptoms. About half of children affected with the syndrome experience degeneration of the pigment in the retina of the eye.

Sjögren-Larsson syndrome is also sometimes known as SLS; congenital ichthyosis-mental retardation-spasticity syndrome; ichthyosis-spastic neurologic disorder-oligophrenia syndrome; fatty aldehyde dehydrogenase deficiency (FALDH deficiency); fatty aldehyde dehydrogenase 10 deficiency (FALDH10 deficiency); or disorder of cornification 10 (Sjögren-Larsson Type). Sjögren-Larsson syndrome is not to be confused with Sjögren syndrome; it is sometimes called the T. Sjögren syndrome to distinguish it from Sjögren syndrome (characterized by dry eyes and mouth), which was described by Swedish ophthalmologist Henrick Sjögren.

## Genetic profile

**Inheritance** of Sjögren-Larsson syndrome is autosomal recessive. In autosomal recessive inheritance, a single abnormal **gene** on one of the autosomal chromosomes (one of the first 22 "non-sex" chromosomes) from both parents can cause the disease. Both of the parents must be carriers in order for the child to inherit the disease since recessive genes are expressed only when both copies in the pair have the same recessive instruction. Neither of the parents has the disease (since it is recessive).

A child with both parents who carry the disease has a 25% chance having the disease; a 50% chance of being a carrier of the disease (but not affected by the disease, having both one normal gene and one gene with the mutation for the disorder); and a 25% chance of receiving both normal genes, one from each parent, and being genetically normal for that particular trait.

The gene for the Sjögren-Larsson syndrome, FALDH, is located on **chromosome** number 17 in band 17p11.2. The gene mutation that is responsible for the disorder is located near the center of the chromosome and is strongly associated the gene markers called D17S805 and ALDH10.

## Demographics

Sjögren-Larsson syndrome is a rare disorder. The highest incidence occurs in northern Sweden. The mutation responsible for the disease is present in approximately 1% of the population in northern Sweden. All Swedes with the syndrome are believed to be descendents of one ancestor in whom a genetic change occurred about 600 years ago. (The phenomenon wherein everyone is descended from one person within what was once a tiny group of people is called founder effect.) The disease also occurs in members of families of other European, Arabic, and native American descent, but is less prevalent. Sjögren-Larsson syndrome affects both males and females.

## Signs and symptoms

There are several signs and symptoms of Sjögren-Larsson syndrome. The major features of the disorder are the following:

- Skin: In infancy, development of various degrees of scaling and reddened skin occurs (ichthyosis), often accompanied by hyperkeratosis (thickening of the skin) on the outer skin layer. After infancy, skin on the arms, legs, and abdomen is often dark and scaly and lacking redness. Bruises are present at birth or soon after.

- Hair: Hair may be brittle.

- Extremities: Joint contracture and hypertonia cause resistance of joints to movement and of muscles to stretching. Most individuals with the syndrome never walk.

- Eyes: About half of the individuals with this syndrome have retinitis pigmentosa (pigmentary degeneration of the retina). Glistening white or yellow-white dots on the retina (ocular fundus) are characteristic. They may be an early sign of the disease, presenting at age 1–2, and may increase with age.

- Nervous system: Spastic diplegia or tetraplegia (paralysis) affecting arms and/or legs. About half of the individuals with this disorder have seizures.

- Urogenital system: Kidney diseases may be associated with this syndrome.

- Growth and development: Individuals with the disorder tend to be unusually short in stature. Mental retardation is characteristic. Speech disorders may be present.

Speech abnormalities, mental retardation, and seizures usually occur during the first two or three years of life.

## Diagnosis

The clinical features of Sjögren-Larsson syndrome are often distinctive, and a pattern of anomalies may suggest the diagnosis. In addition to ichthyosis and spasticity at birth, glistening white or yellow-white dots on the retina may be an early sign of the disease, presenting in the first or second year of life. If they occur, speech abnormalities, mental retardation, and seizures present during the first two or three years of life.

Laboratory findings are important in diagnosing Sjögren-Larsson syndrome. A laboratory test for deficiency of an enzyme (a protein that catalyzes chemical reactions in the human body) called fatty aldehyde dehydrogenase 10 (FALDH10) will determine presence of the disease. Sjögren-Larsson is due to a deficiency of FALDH10, and the gene for the Sjögren-Larsson syndrome is the same as the FALDH10 gene.

Positive laboratory results for Sjögren-Larsson will include the following findings:

- Hexadeconal elevated in fibroblasts.
- Fatty alcohol NAD+ deficient in Sjögren-Larsson syndrome fibroblasts.
- Fatty aldehyde dehydrogenase (FALDH) deficiency.

### Genetic counseling

Individuals with a family history of Sjögren-Larsson syndrome may benefit from **genetic counseling** to learn about the condition including treatments, inheritance, testing, and options available to them so that they can make informed decisions appropriate to their families. A child with both parents who carry the Sjögren-Larsson gene mutation has a 25% chance having the disorder. Couples who have had one affected child have a 25% risk of having another child with the disorder in each pregnancy.

### Prenatal testing

Families at risk to have a child with Sjögren-Larsson syndrome may have the option of prenatal diagnosis. **DNA** can be extracted from fetal cells obtained by either chorionic villus sampling (usually done until 12 weeks gestation) or **amniocentesis** (usually done at 16–18 weeks gestation) and tested to determine if the altered gene in the family is present. These techniques usually require that the alteration in the gene has been identified previously in an affected family member.

Chorionic villus sampling is a procedure to obtain chorionic villi tissue for testing. Chorionic villi are microscopic, finger-like projections that emerge from the chorionic membrane and eventually form the placenta. The cells of the chorionic villi are of fetal origin so laboratory analysis can identify a number of genetic abnormalities of the fetus. Because the villi are attached to the uterus, however, there is a chance that maternal tissue may be analyzed rather than the fetal cells. If the

sample is too small, it may be necessary to repeat the procedure. In addition, the quality of the chromosome analysis is usually not as good with chorionic villus sampling as with amniocentesis. The chromosomes may not be as long, and so it may not be possible to identify some of the smaller bands on the chromosomes.

Amniocentesis is a procedure that involves inserting a thin needle into the uterus, into the amniotic sac, and withdrawing a small amount of amniotic fluid (a liquid produced by the fetal membranes and the fetus that surrounds the fetus throughout pregnancy). DNA can be extracted from the fetal cells contained in the amniotic fluid and tested for the specific mutation known to cause Sjögren-Larsson syndrome.

### Treatment and management

Individuals with Sjögren-Larsson syndrome should be under routine health supervision by a physician who is familiar with the disorder, its complications, and its treatment. Supportive resources for individuals with Sjögren-Larsson syndrome and their families should be provided. Some clinical improvement has been reported to occur with fat restriction in the diet and supplementation with medium-chain triglycerides.

Other treatment of the disorder is generally symptomatic.

- For dermatologic symptoms, various skin softening ointments are useful in reducing symptoms. Plain petroleum jelly may be effective, especially when applied while the skin is still moist, such as after bathing. Salicylic acid gel may also be effective. When using the ointment, skin is covered at night with an airtight, waterproof dressing. Lactate lotion is another effective treatment for the dermatologic symptoms.

- For ocular symptoms, regular care from a qualified ophthalmologist is important.

- To control seizures, anti-convulsant medications may be helpful.

- Speech therapy and special education services may be helpful.

### Prognosis

Prognosis is variable depending upon the severity of the disease. Sjögren-Larsson does not generally lead to shortened life span.

### Resources

**BOOKS**

*Medical Genetics,* edited by Lynn B. Jorde, et al. 2nd ed. St. Louis: Mosby, 1999.

**PERIODICALS**

Rizzo, W.B. "Inherited Disorders of Fatty Alcohol Metabolism." *Molecular Genetics and Metabolism* (1998) 65: 63-73.

Rizzo, W.B., G. Carney, and Z. Lin. "The Molecular Basis of Sjögren-Larsson Syndrome: Mutation Analysis of the Fatty Aldehyde Dehydrogenase Gene." *American Journal of Human Genetics* 65(December 1999): 1547-60.

Willemsen, M.A., et al. "Sjögren-Larsson Syndrome." *Journal of Pediatrics* 136(February 2000): 261.

**ORGANIZATIONS**

Arc (a National Organization on Mental Retardation). 1010 Wayne Ave., Suite 650, Silver Spring, MD 20910. (800) 433-5255. http://www.thearclink.org.

Foundation for Ichthyosis and Related Skin Types. 650 N. Cannon Ave., Suite 17, Landsdale, PA 19446. (215) 631-1411 or (800) 545-3286. Fax: (215) 631-1413. http://www.scalyskin.org.

National Institute of Arthritis and Musculoskeletal and Skin Diseases. National Institutes of Health, One AMS Circle, Bethesda, MD 20892. http://www.nih.gov/niams.

**WEBSITES**

*Online Mendelian Inheritance in Man.*http://www.ncbi.nlm.nih.gov:80/entrez/query.fcgi?db=OMIM.

Jennifer F. Wilson, MS

# Skeletal dysplasia

## Definition

Skeletal dysplasias are a group of congenital abnormalities of the bone and cartilage that are characterized by short stature.

## Description

Skeletal **dysplasia**, sometimes called dwarfism, is a disorder of short stature defined as height that is three or more standard deviations below the mean height for age, race, and gender. Although all skeletal dysplasias involve disproportionately short stature, there are many other associated conditions.

Skeletal dysplasia may also have additional skeletal abnormalities, including:

- short arms and truck, bowlegs, and a waddling gait
- skull malformations, such as a large head, cloverleaf skull, craniosynostosis (premature fusion of the bones in the skull), and wormian bones (abnormal thread-like connections between the skull bone)
- anomalies of the hands and feet, including polydactyly (extra fingers), "hitchhiker" thumbs, and abnormal finger and toe nails
- chest anomalies, such as pear-shaped chest and narrow thorax

Other anomalies that may be present in individuals with skeletal dysplasia include:

- anomalies of the eyes, mouth, and ears, such as congenital cataract, myopia (nearsightedness), cleft palate, and deafness
- brain malformations, such as hydrocephaly, porencephaly, hydranencephaly, and agenesis of the corpus callosum
- heart defects, such as atrial septal defect (ASD), patent ductus arteriosus (PDA), and transposition of the great vessels (TGV)
- developmental delays and mental retardation

Skeletal dysplasia encompasses more than 200 different specific diagnoses. A list of some of the more common types of skeletal dysplasia includes **achondrogenesis**, **achondroplasia**, acrodystosis, acromesomelic dysplasia, atelosteogenesis, **diastrophic dysplasia, chondrodysplasia punctata,** fibrochondrogenesis hypochondrodysplasia, Kniest syndrome, Langer-type mesomelic dysplasia, micromelia, **metaphyseal dysplasia,** metatrophic dysplasia, Morquio syndrome, osteochondrodysplasia, **osteogenesis imperfecta,** Reinhardt syndrome, Roberts syndrome, **Robinow syndrome, spondyloepiphyseal dysplasia** congenital, spondyloepimetaphyseal dysplasia, and **thanatophoric dysplasia.**

## Genetic profile

With more than 200 distinct skeletal dysplasias currently recognized, naming and categorizing these disorders is a significant task. In 1997, a standardized method for naming and classifying the skeletal

**Agenesis of the corpus callosum**—An absence of the structure in the brain that connects the two hemispheres of the brain.

**Atrial septal defect (ASD)**—An abnormal opening between the two upper chambers of the heart (atria).

**Autosomal**—Genetic trait found on a chromosome that is not involved in determining sex.

**Calcification**—The process by which tissue becomes hardened by the depositing of calcium in the tissue.

**Cleft palate**—An abnormal opening, or cleft, between the roof of the mouth and the nasal cavity.

**Cloverleaf skull**—An abnormal, or cloverleaf, appearance to the skull caused by premature fusion of the bones in the skull of an infant.

**Computed tomography (CT) scan; 3D CT scan**—A diagnostic imaging procedure in which x-ray and computer technology are used to generate slices or cross-sectional images of the body; 3D CT scan produces three-dimensional images.

**Congenital cataract**—Clouding of the lens in the eye that is present at birth.

**Congenital**—Present at birth.

**Craniosynostosis**—An abnormal premature fusion of the bones of the skull in an infant.

**Developmental delay**—Not reaching the milestones of childhood development as expected.

**Dominant**—A genetic trait that is expressed when only one copy of it is present.

**Echocardiogram (ECHO)**—A diagnostic procedure that uses sound waves to produces images of the heart.

**Epiphyses**—Areas at the tip of the long bones that allow them to grow.

**Gene mutation**—A permanent change in genetic material that is transmittable.

**Histological studies**—Laboratory tests performed on tissue samples and cells.

**"Hitchhiker" thumbs**—A congenital anomaly of the thumb in which it is abnormally positioned at a right angle to the first joint.

**Hydranencephaly**—Congenital enlargement of the head and brain.

**Hydrocephaly**—An increase of cerebrospinal fluid in the brain.

**Hypoplasia/hypoplastic**—Small.

**Kyphosis**—Anomaly of the spine in which it curves backwards.

**Long bones**—The femur in the leg and the humerus in the arm.

**Lordosis**—An abnormal curvature of the spine in which the lumbar, or lower section, is excessively curved.

**Magnetic resonance imaging (MRI)**—A diagnostic procedure that uses a combination of high-powered magnets, radio frequencies, and computers to generate detailed images of structures within the body.

**Molecular analysis**—Evaluation of molecules, tests that may identify single gene mutations.

**Myopia**—Nearsightedness.

**Patent ductus arteriosus (PDA)**—A congenital anomaly of the heart occurring when the ductus arteriosus (the temporary fetal blood vessel that connects the aorta and the pulmonary artery) does not close at birth.

**Polydactyly**—Extra fingers or toes.

**Porencephaly**—A congenital anomaly of the brain in which there are abnormal holes or cavities in the brain.

**Prenatal ultrasound**—An imaging test using high-frequency sound waves to create images of internal organs. Prenatal indicates the test is preformed to on fetus while still in the womb.

**Recessive**—A genetic trait that is only expressed when another identical recessive gene is present.

**Scapula**—Shoulder blade.

**Scoliosis**—Abnormal curvature of the spine in which the spine curves to the side.

**Short stature**—Height of less than three standard deviations from the mean for age, race, and gender.

**Short trunk**—An abnormally short torso or body.

**Sleep apnea**—A potentially life-threatening condition in which the individual has episodes during sleep in which breathing temporarily stops.

**Thorax**—Chest cavity.

**Transposition of the great vessels (TGV)**—A congenital heart defect in which the major vessels of the heart are attached to the wrong chambers of the heart.

**Wormian bones**—A condition of the bones and cartilage in which growing bones are abnormally connected by thin string-like structures.

**X-linked**—A genetic trait that is carried on the X chromosome.

**X ray**—An imaging test that uses beams of energy to create images of structures within the body.

dysplasias was proposed using information about the etiology of each disorder based on the genetic mutation or protein defect involved. Disorders that originate from similar or identical **gene mutations** were grouped together, and other categories were renamed in an attempt to create a more logical classification system. With so many unique disorders, categorizing the skeletal dysplasias will continue to evolve as new genetic mutations are identified.

Skeletal dysplasia refers to a group of disorders characterized by abnormalities of bone and cartilage with similar modes of transmission: autosomal dominant and recessive and X-linked dominant and recessive.

The following is a list of skeletal dysplasias with known genetic causes:

- Achondroplasia group: These dysplasias are caused by mutations in the fibroblast growth factor 3 gene (FGFR3).

- Diastrophic dysplasia group: This group is caused by mutations in the diatrophic dysplasia sulfate transporter gene (DTDST).

- Type II collagenopathies: These are caused by mutations in the procollagen II gene (COL2A1).

- Type XI collagenopathies: These dysplasias are caused by mutations in the procollagen XI genes (COL11A1 and COL11A2).

- Multiple epiphyseal dysplasias and pseudoachondroplasia: These groups are caused by mutations in the cartilage oligomatrix protein gene (COMP).

- Chondrodysplasia punctata: This complex group of skeletal dysplasias has several different types, each of which is caused by a unique genetic mutation. Chondrodysplasia punctata is caused by one of the following genetic mutations: arylsulfatase E gene (ARSE), X-linked dominant chondrodysplasia punctata gene (CPXD), X-linked recessive chondrodysplasia (CPDR), and genes responsible for production of the peroxisomal factors (PEX).

- Metaphyseal dysplasias: Three different genetic mutations are responsible for the three types of this dysplasia: adenosine deaminase gene (ADA), the procollagen X gene (COL10A1), and the gene responsible for producing the parathyroid hormone/parathyroid hormone-related polypeptide receptor (PTHR).

- Acromelic and acromesomelic dysplasias: These disorders are caused by genetic mutations in the genes responsible for encoding the cartilage-derived morphogenic protein-1 gene (CDMP 1) and the guanine nucleotide-binding protein of the edenylate cyclase a-subunit (GNAS1).

- Dysplasia with prominent membranous bone involvement: This group is caused by a mutation of the transcription core binding a1-subunit gene (CBFA1).

- Bent-bone dysplasia group: This group of dysplasias is caused by mutations in the SRY-box 9 protein (SOX9).

- Dysplasia with defective mineralization: This dysplasia is caused by the following gene mutations: the liver alkaline phosphatase gene (ALPL), the parathyroid calcium-sensing receptor gene (CASR), and the X-linked hypophsphatemia gene (PHEX).

- Increased bone density without modification of bone shape: Mutations in the carbonic anhydrase II gene (CA2) and the cathepsin K (CTSK) cause these dysplasias.

- Disorganized development of cartilaginous and fibrous components of the skeleton: These dysplasias are caused by several mutations, including abnormalities of the bone morphogenic protein 4 gene (BMP4), the guanine nucleotide-binding protein a-subunit gene (CNAS1), and exostosis genes (EXT1, EXT2, and EXT3).

### Demographics

Skeletal dysplasia is usually diagnosed at birth; however, some dysplasias may not be detected until much later. For this reason, it is difficult to determine the true incidence. The reported rate in the United States is one per every 4,000–5,000 births.

No one race is more likely to have skeletal dysplasia. The X-linked recessive disorders affect males almost exclusively, and X-linked dominant types are often lethal in males. Autosomal recessive and dominant transference affects males and females equally.

### Signs and symptoms

The primary sign of skeletal dysplasia is abnormally shortened long bones in the legs and arms, short trunk, and abnormalities of the skull.

In addition to the skeletal system, skeletal dysplasia disorders may also affect the heart, the face, extremities, and joints.

Some forms are lethal, and a significant number of fetuses with skeletal dysplasia die in utero.

### Diagnosis

Many skeletal dysplasias can be diagnosed prenatally during routine **prenatal ultrasound**. If skeletal dysplasia is suspected, assessment and careful measurement of the extremities, thorax, spine, and facial structure can detect signs of the condition. Fetal movement may be decreased, and associated congenital heart and renal heart defects may be observed as well.

After birth, x–rays are the most effective diagnostic tool for evaluating the skeleton. A skeletal study includes views of the long bone, hands and feet, skull, chest, spine, and pelvis.

Abnormal x-ray results that may indicate a skeletal dysplasia include:

- dumbbell-shaped long bones
- bowing of the arms and legs
- oval-shaped translucencies in the femur and humerus
- scapula hypoplasia (small shoulder blades)
- abnormal pelvis
- vertebral abnormalities
- rib abnormalities, including cupping of the ends or shortening of the entire rib and stippled or spotted appearance to the cartilage
- epiphyses (growth centers of the long bones) abnormalities, including cone shape, stippled appearance, or an absence of calcification centers
- long bone fractures

Computed tomography (CT) scan and magnetic resonance imaging (MRI) are useful in assessing concurrent brain anomalies. MRI is useful in determining the extent and type of spinal abnormalities and compression present.

Three-dimension CT scan is used to evaluate craniofacial anomalies prior to reconstructive surgery. MRI of the spine is also helpful in pre-surgical planning prior to surgical treatment of spinal and pelvic abnormalities.

**Chromosome** analysis may be performed to help determine the type of skeletal dysplasia an individual has. This is important so that other associated conditions can be diagnosed and treated as well.

Other diagnostic procedures that may be performed, including molecular analysis to identify single **gene** mutations, sleep studies to evaluate potentially life-threatening sleep apnea that is often a problem for individuals with skeletal dysplasia, histological studies to examine specific types of cells that identify some skeletal dysplasia forms, and an echocardiogram (ECHO) to evaluate the heart for defects.

### Treatment and management

Treatment and management of children with skeletal dysplasia begins, in some cases, at birth. Neonatal resuscitation may be necessary for infant with certain more severe types of skeletal dysplasia in which the thoracic cavity is extremely small. This intervention can be life-saving.

The medical management of children with skeletal dysplasia begins at birth and continues into adulthood. Careful monitoring of height, weight, and head circumference is essential. Obesity is a risk for those with skeletal dysplasia. Excess weight can cause serious complications, including breathing difficulties such as sleep apnea, and may aggravate other spinal cord compression and joint instability found in many types of skeletal dysplasia.

Surgical treatment of skeletal dysplasia varies depending on the specific type present and the associated conditions. Sleep apnea may be treated by removal of the adenoids.

Spinal abnormalities, such as spinal cord compression, **scoliosis**, kyphosis, and lordosis, may be treated surgically. A spinal column fusion can relieve the stress on the spinal cord caused by malformations of the spinal column. In a spinal fusion, two or more vertebrae are fused together using bone grafts or metal rods.

In some individuals with short-limbed types of skeletal dysplasia, bone growth may be induced by a surgical bone-lengthening procedure. This procedure involves several surgeries and an extensive recovery period. The bone to be lengthened is cut. Leaving a narrow gap between the two pieces of bone, metal pins are inserted into the bone and the skin is closed. An external frame is attached to the pins and, gradually, the bone is pulled apart just enough to provide a small gap for the bone to grow into. As the bone grows, the space is widened and more bone grows. After the bone has healed, the pins are surgically removed. In some cases, as much as 6 in (15 cm) has been added to leg length using this procedure.

### Prognosis

While some skeletal dysplasias are lethal, most individuals with skeletal dysplasia have a normal life expectancy. The associated conditions may require medical and surgical treatment; however, these treatments are highly effective. Intelligence is usually normal. Most people with skeletal dysplasia have an excellent prognosis.

### Resources

**BOOKS**

Rimoin, David, Ralph Lachman, and Shelia Unger. "Chrondfrodysplasia." In *Emery and Rimion's Principles and Practice of Medical Genetics*, 4th edition, edited by David L. Rimoin, J. Michael Connor, Reed Pyeritz, and Bruce R. Korf. London: Churchill Livingstone, 2002.

**PERIODICALS**

Committee on Genetics. "Health Supervision for Children with Achondroplasia." *Pediatrics* 95 (March 1995): 443–451.

Savarirayan, Ravi, and David L. Rimoin. "Skeletal Dysplasia." *Advances in Pediatrics* 51 (2004): 1–21.

Unger, Sheila. "A Genetic Approach to the Diagnosis of Skeletal Dysplasia." *Clinical Orthopedics and Related Research* 401 (2002): 32–38.

**WEB SITES**

Rhizomelic Chondrodysplasia Punctata (RCP) Family Support Group. (Accessed April 1, 2005; April 13, 2005.) http://www.angelfire.com/in/sassyshideout/RCP.html.

**ORGANIZATIONS**

Little People of America. 5289 NE Elam Young Parkway, Suite F-100, Hillsboro, OR 97124. (888) LPA-2001 (English and Spanish), (503) 846-1562. Fax: (503) 846-1590. (April 13, 2005.) http://www.lpaonline.org/index.html.

March of Dimes. 1275 Mamaroneck Ave., White Plains, NY 10605. (April 13, 2005.) http://www.marchofdimes.com.

Human Growth Foundation. 997 Glen Cove Ave., Suite 5, Glen Head, NY, 11545. (800) 451-6434. (April 13, 2005.) http://www.hgfound.org.

Deborah L. Nurmi, MS

Skeletal dysplasia *see* **Larsen syndrome**

Sly syndrome (MPS VII) *see* **Mucopolysaccharidosis (MPS)**

# Smith–Fineman–Myers syndrome

## Definition

Smith–Fineman–Myers syndrome (SFMS) is a rare and severe type of X–linked inherited mental retardation.

## Description

Smith–Fineman–Myers syndrome is also known as Smith–Fineman–Myers type mental retardation and Smith–Fineman–Myers type X–linked mental retardation. SFMS results in severe mental retardation along with characteristic facial features and skeletal differences.

## Genetic profile

Smith–Fineman–Myers syndrome is an X–linked disease. X–linked diseases map to the human X **chromosome**, a sex chromosome. Females have two X chromosomes, whereas males have one X chromosome and

one Y chromosome. Because males have only one X chromosome, they require only one copy of an abnormal X–linked **gene** to display disease. Because females have two X chromosomes, the effect of one X–linked recessive disease gene is masked by the disease gene's normal counterpart on her other X chromosome.

In classic X–linked **inheritance** males are affected, presenting full clinical symptoms of the disease. Females are not affected. Affected fathers can never pass X–linked diseases to their sons. However, affected fathers always pass X–linked disease genes to their daughters. Females who inherit the faulty gene but do not show the disease are known as carriers. Female carriers of SFMS have a 50% chance to pass the disease–causing gene to each of their children. Each of a female carrier's sons has a 50% chance to display the symptoms of SFMS. None of a female carrier's daughters would display symptoms of SFMS.

Some patients with SFMS have been found to have a mutation in the ATRX gene, on the X chromosome at position Xq13.3. ATRX is also the disease gene for several other forms of X–linked mental retardation, such as X–linked Alpha–thalassemia/mental retardation syndrome, **Carpenter syndrome**, Juberg–Marsidi syndrome, and X–linked mental retardation with spastic paraplegia. A 2008 report mapped the causative gene in a large Chinese family with SFMS to Xq25.

## Demographics

SFMS affects only males and is very rare. As of 2009, only 12 cases have been reported in the medical literature. SFMS has been reported in brothers of affected boys.

## Signs and symptoms

SFMS visibly affects the skeletal and nervous systems and results in an unusual facial appearance. The genitals may also show effects ranging from mild (e.g. undescended testes) to severe (leading to female gender assignment).

### Skeletal features

Boys with SFMS have short stature and a thin body build. Their heads are small and may also be unusually shaped. **Scoliosis** and chest abnormalities have been reported to occur with SFMS. X–rays may show that their bones have characteristics of the bones of people younger than they are. Hands are often short with unusual palm creases and short, unusually shaped fingers. Fingernails may be abnormal. Foot abnormalities and shortened or fused toes have also been reported.

### Neurological features

Boys with SFMS exhibit severe mental retardation. Restlessness, behavior problems, seizures, and severe delay in language development are common. Boys with SFMS may be self–absorbed with reduced ability to socialize with others. Affected boys show reduced muscle tone as infants and young children. Later, muscle tone and reflexes are abnormally increased causing spasticity.

Boys with SFMS may display cortical atrophy, or degeneration of the brain's outer layer, on brain imaging studies. Cortical atrophy is commonly found in older unaffected people. When cortical atrophy is found in younger people it is typically due to a serious brain injury. Brain biopsies of two patients with SFMS have been normal.

### Facial features

SFMS is associated with unusual facial features including a large mouth with a drooping lower lip, prominent upper jaw and front teeth, and an under-developed chin. **Cleft palate** has been reported in one set of affected twins. Eyes are widely spaced with drooping eyelids. Skin may be lightly pigmented with multiple freckles.

## Diagnosis

Assessment for any type of mental retardation should include a detailed family history and thorough physical exam. Brain and skeletal imaging through CT scans or x–rays may be helpful. A chromosome study and certain other genetic and biochemical tests help to rule out other possible causes of mental retardation.

Diagnosis of SFMS has traditionally been based on the visible and measurable symptoms of the disease. Until 2000, SFMS was not known to be associated with any particular gene. Scientists do not yet know if other genes may be involved in some cases of this rare

## QUESTIONS TO ASK YOUR DOCTOR

- I recently read about a child with Smith–Fineman–Myers syndrome. How common is this disease?
- Other than mental retardation, what symptoms are associated with this disorder?
- What is the life span of an individual with Smith–Fineman–Myers syndrome?
- Why do there not seem to be any clinical trials for the treatment of Smith–Fineman–Myers syndrome?

disease. Genetic analysis of the ATRX gene may, however, prove to be helpful in diagnosis of SFMS.

## Treatment and management

Treatment for SFMS is based on the symptoms each individual displays. Seizures are controlled with anticonvulsants. Medications and behavioral modification routines may help to control behavioral problems.

## Prognosis

Retardation is severe, but it does not seem to get worse with age. Lifespan does not appear to be shortened.

### Resources

#### BOOKS

Smith, Moyra. *Mental Retardation and Developmental Delay: Genetic and Epigenetic Factors.* New York, NY: Oxford University Press, 2005.

#### PERIODICALS

Cilliers, D. D., et al. "A new X–linked mental retardation (XLMR) syndrome with late–onset primary testicular failure, short stature and microcephaly maps to Xq25–q26." *European Journal of Medical Genetics* 50, no. 3 (May–June 2007): 216–223.

Stephenson, L. D., et al. "Smith–Fineman–Myers syndrome: Report of a third case." *American Journal of Medical Genetics* 22, no. 2 (June 2005): 301–304.

Villard, L., et al. "Identification of a mutation in the XNP/ATR–X gene in a family reported as Smith–Fineman–Myers syndrome." *American Journal of Medical Genetics* 19, no. 4 (March 2000): 83–85.

#### WEBSITES

*Mental Retardation Smith Fineman Myers Type.* Information Page, GARD (May 02, 2009). http://

raredisseases.info.nih.gov/GARD/Disease.aspx?Pa-
geID = 4& DiseaseID = 3521&expand = NLMGateway

ORGANIZATIONS

Genetic Alliance. 4301 Connecticut Ave. NW, Suite 404,
Washington, DC 20008-2369. (202)966-5557. Fax:
(202)966-8553. E-mail: info@geneticalliance.org.
http://www.geneticalliance.org
National Organization for Rare Disorders (NORD). 55
Kenosia Avenue, PO Box 1968, Danbury, CT 06813-
1968. (203)744-0100 or (800)999-6673. Fax: (203)798-
2291. http://www.rarediseases.org.

Judy C. Hawkins, MS

## Smith-Fineman-Myers type X-linked mental retardation *see* **Smith-Fineman-Myers syndrome**

# Smith-Lemli-Opitz syndrome

## Definition

Smith-Lemli-Opitz syndrome (SLOS) is a syndrome characterized by **microcephaly** (small head size), mental retardation, short stature, and major and minor malformations. It is caused by an abnormality in cholesterol metabolism.

## Description

SLOS was first characterized by David W. Smith, John M. Opitz, and Luc Lemli in 1964. The syndrome has variable characteristics marked mainly by short stature, mental retardation, microcephaly, postaxial **polydactyly** (an extra digit on the little finger side of the hand or the little toe side of the foot), **cleft palate**, cardiovascular defects, genital malformations and other abnormalities associated with abnormal cholesterol metabolism. In 1993, scientists discovered that children with SLOS have a metabolic disorder that prevents cholesterol from being made in amounts sufficient for normal growth and development.

Sometimes the severe form of the disease is called SLOS type II. But laboratory testing has shown that type II is not biochemically distinct. Rather it represents the more severe expression of the SLOS **phenotype**.

SLOS is also known as Smith syndrome, RSH syndrome, and RSH/Smith-Lemli-Opitz (RSH/SLO) syndrome. The designation RSH represents initials of

the surnames of the first three patients in whom the syndrome was first observed.

## Genetic profile

SLOS is inherited in an autosomal recessive manner. In autosomal recessive **inheritance**, a single abnormal **gene** on one of the autosomal chromosomes (one of the first 22 "non-sex" chromosomes) from both parents can cause the disease. Both of the parents must be carriers in order for the child to inherit the disease since recessive genes are expressed only when both copies in the pair have the same recessive instruction. Neither of the parents has the disease (since it is recessive).

A child with both parents who carry the disease has a 25% chance having the disease; a 50% chance of being a carrier of the disease (having both one normal gene and one gene with the mutation for the disorder but not affected by the disease); and a 25% chance of receiving both normal genes, one from each parent, and being genetically normal for that particular trait.

The gene for SLOS, DHCR7, encodes 7-dehydrocholesterol (7-DHC) reductase, the enzyme that is deficient in SLOS. DHCR7 is on the long arm of **chromosome** 11 at locus 11q12-q13.

## Demographics

SLOS occurs in approximately one in 20,000 to 30,000 births in populations of northern and central European background. Evidence suggests that there is a higher frequency of SLOS in people of northern European ancestry and a lower frequency in people of Asian or African background.

Because of the presence of recognizable genital abnormalities, males are more likely than females to be evaluated for a diagnosis of SLOS. Therefore, the occurrence of the disease among females is less certain.

## Signs and symptoms

The following are features of the congenital multiple anomaly syndrome.

- Nearly 90% of people with SLOS have microcephaly.
- Nearly all people with SLOS have moderate to severe mental retardation.
- Other neurologic findings are less common. These include seizures and muscle hypotonia.
- Characteristic facial features include narrowing at the temples, epicanthal folds (skin fold of the upper eyelid covering the inner corner of the eye), downslanting eyes, drooping upper eyelids, anteverted nares (nostrils that tilt forward), and abnormal smallness of the jaw (micrognathia). Cleft palate is present in 40–50% of people with SLOS, and about 20% have congenital cataracts. Strabismus, poor tracking, opsoclonus (impairment of eye movements), and optic nerve demyelination (deterioration) are other possible ophthalmologic manifestations.
- Cardiac abnormalities are present in about 35–40% of patients with SLOS. Increased incidence of atrioventricular canal defects and anomalous pulmonary venous return is seen in people with SLOS.
- Urogenital anomalies are frequent. Kidney hypoplasia (smaller than normal) or dysplasia (abnormal development) occurs in about 40% of people with SLOS. Genital anomalies of variable severity may include hypospadias and/or bilateral cryptorchidism, which occur in about half of reported cases, and small penis. Many 46,XY individuals with severe manifestations of SLOS have undermasculinization of the external genitalia, resulting in female external genitalia (sex reversal). Abnormalities in the uterus and vagina have been noted in 46,XX females.
- Syndactyly of the second and third toes occurs frequently. Postaxial polydactyly is present in 25–50% of all cases. Other abnormalities affecting the hands and feet may be present.
- Short stature is common. Limbs and neck are shorter than normal.

In addition, a child with SLOS will often show failure to thrive, have abnormal sleep patterns, and have photosensitivity. The hair of children with SLOS is blonde.

Growth may be retarded prenatally. Neonates frequently have poor suck, irritability, and failure to thrive.

## Diagnosis

The clinical features of SLOS are often distinctive, and a pattern of **congenital anomalies** suggests the diagnosis. Features that are most commonly seen are microcephaly, postaxial polydactyly, 2–3 syndactyly of the toes, growth and mental retardation, cleft palate, and **hypospadias** in males.

The diagnosis of SLOS relies on clinical suspicion and detection of abnormally elevated serum concentration of 7-dehydrocholesterol (7-DHC) or an elevated 7-dehydrocholesterol:cholesterol ratio. Serum concentration of cholesterol is usually low, with cholesterol levels less than 50 mg/dl (normal is greater than 100 mg/dl). Cholesterol is an essential building block of all cell membranes and the white matter of the brain, and SLOS appears to be caused by abnormally low levels of the enzyme 7-DHC-reductase, which converts 7-DHC into cholesterol. Children with SLOS with the lowest cholesterol levels tend to have the most severe forms of the disorder and often die at birth or in the first few months. In about 10% of patients, cholesterol is in the normal range, so it is an unreliable marker for screening and diagnosis.

Molecular **genetic testing** of the DHCR7 gene is not generally available. But since the molecular structure of the DHCR7 has been identified, the possibility now exists for DNA-based testing for diagnosis and **genetic counseling**. Currently, such testing is available on a research basis only.

### Genetic counseling

Carrier detection is problematic using biochemical testing. In carriers, 7-DHC and cholesterol levels are usually normal. Carrier testing is now possible, although not generally available, by measurement of 7DHC or enzyme levels in cultured cells. More accurate **DNA** testing for DHCR7 mutations is not currently available, but it is anticipated in the near future. Couples who have had one affected child have a 25% risk of having a child with SLOS in each pregnancy.

### Prenatal testing

For couples known to be at 25% risk for having a baby with SLOS, testing is available to assist in prenatal diagnosis. Prior testing of family members is usually necessary for prenatal testing.

Either chorionic villus sampling (CVS) or **amniocentesis** may be performed for prenatal testing. CVS is a procedure to obtain chorionic villi tissue for testing. Abnormal levels of 7-dehydrocholesterol in amniotic fluid or chorionic villus samples is diagnostic of SLOS. Chorionic villus sampling can be performed at 10–12 weeks gestation.

Amniocentesis is a procedure that involves inserting a thin needle into the uterus, into the amniotic sac, and withdrawing a small amount of amniotic fluid. SLOS can be diagnosed from biochemical testing performed on the amniotic fluid. DNA can also be extracted from the fetal cells contained in the amniotic fluid and tested. Amniocentesis is performed at 16–18 weeks gestation.

Abnormal concentration of 7-dehydrocholesterol levels in tissue obtained from CVS or in amniotic fluid is diagnostic.

For low-risk pregnancies, in which there is no family history of SLOS, certain findings in the fetus might prompt consideration of SLOS. The combination of low unconjugated estriol levels, low HCG, and low alpha-fetoprotein on routine maternal serum testing at 16–18 weeks gestation might suggest the possible diagnosis of SLOS. Findings on ultrasound examination such as cardiac defects, cleft palate, genital abnormalities, or growth retardation might be suggestive, prompting consideration of a 7-dehydrocholesterol assay of amniotic fluid.

Low uE3 levels alone may be an indication of further investigation, especially if it is associated with abnormal ultrasonographic findings suggestive of SLOS.

## Treatment and management

It is not known what role the elevated levels of 7-DHC and other sterol precursors—not usually present in significant concentrations in the plasma—play in the pathogenesis of SLOS. Children with SLOS should be under routine health supervision by a physician who is familiar with SLOS, its complications, and its treatment.

Since a common complication of the syndrome is pneumonia, it should be treated with appropriate antibiotics when it occurs.

Special education services and physical therapy may be recommended as needed.

## QUESTIONS TO ASK YOUR DOCTOR

- Please explain the genetic basis of Smith-Lemli-Opitz syndrome.
- What are the most serious medical consequences of this genetic disorder?
- What is the prognosis for Smith-Lemli-Opitz syndrome?
- Where can I find additional information about this genetic disorder?

### Infant care

A physician familiar with the range of problems seen in infants with SLOS is important for appropriate health supervision and anticipatory guidance. Poor feeding and problems with weight gain are common in infants with SLOS. Many infants have difficulties with suck and/or swallow and may require alternative feeding. A diagnosis of **pyloric stenosis** (caused by a thickening and spasm of the stomach outlet) should be considered for those with frequent vomiting or apparent gastroesophageal reflux. Particular attention should also be given to the stooling pattern, abdominal distention, or other signs of possible obstruction, particularly in children with more severe phenotype, since these may indicate **Hirschsprung disease** (absent nerves in colon).

### Surgical treatment

Surgical management of congenital anomalies such as cleft palate, **congenital heart disease**, and genital anomalies for the more severely affected infants need to be considered as they would in any other infant with a severe, usually lethal disorder. Even with vigorous intervention, children with multiple major manifestations of SLOS are believed to have decreased survival. Reassignment of sex of rearing for 46,XY infants with female genitalia may not always be appropriate because most will have early death. The process of gender reassignment can be disruptive to a family already coping with the difficult issues of having a child with a genetic disorder that has life-threatening medical complications.

### Dietary supplementation

Because SLOS is a cholesterol deficiency syndrome, research trials have recently included dietary cholesterol supplementation. An increase in total caloric intake and an increase in cholesterol intake hold promise for treatment of SLOS, but the research is still preliminary. Benefits reported in preliminary studies include improved growth in children with SLOS, possible enhanced developmental progress, reduced dermatologic problems (rashes, photosensitivity), and improved behavior. No harmful side effects of cholesterol supplementation have been documented.

### Prognosis

Prognosis is variable depending upon the severity of the disease. Children with SLOS who have multiple major malformations are believed to have decreased survival, even with vigorous intervention.

### Resources

#### BOOKS

Jorde, Lynn B., et al., eds. *Medical Genetics.* 2nd ed. St. Louis: Mosby. 1999.

#### PERIODICALS

Kelley, R.I., and R.C. Hennekam. "The Smith-Lemli-Opitz Syndrome." *Medical Genetics* 37 (2000): 321–35.

Porter, F.D. "RSH/Smith-Lemli-Opitz Syndrome: A Multiple Congenital Anomaly/Mental Retardation Syndrome Due to an Inborn Error of Cholesterol Biosynthesis." *Molecular Genetics and Metabolism* 71 (2000): 163–74.

#### WEBSITES

Online Mendelian Inheritance in Man. http://www.ncbi.nlm. nih.gov:80/entrez/query.fcgi?db=OMIM.

#### ORGANIZATIONS

March of Dimes Birth Defects Foundation. 1275 Mamaroneck Ave., White Plains, NY 10605. (888) 663-4637. resourcecenter@modimes.org. http://www.modimes.org.

National Organization for Rare Disorders (NORD). PO Box 8923, New Fairfield, CT 06812-8923. (203) 746-6518 or (800) 999-6673. Fax: (203) 746-6481. http://www.rarediseases.org.

Smith-Lemli-Opitz Advocacy and Exchange (RSH/SLO). 2650 Valley Forge Dr., Boothwyn, PA 19061. (610) 485-9663. http://members.aol.com/slo97/index.html.

Jennifer F. Wilson, MS

Smith-Magenis chromosome region *see* Smith-Magenis syndrome

# Smith-Magenis syndrome

## Definition

Smith-Magenis syndrome (SMS) is a relatively rare genetic disorder characterized by a specific pattern of physical, behavioral, and developmental features.

## KEY TERMS

**Brachycephaly**—An abnormal thickening and widening of the skull.

**Brachydactyly**—Abnormal shortness of the fingers and toes.

**Chromosome**—A microscopic thread-like structure found within each cell of the body and consists of a complex of proteins and DNA. Humans have 46 chromosomes arranged into 23 pairs. Changes in either the total number of chromosomes or their shape and size (structure) may lead to physical or mental abnormalities.

**Contiguous gene syndrome**—Conditions that occur as a result of microdeletions or microduplications involving several neighboring genes.

**FISH (fluorescence *in situ* hybridization)** —Technique used to detect small deletions or rearrangements in chromosomes by attempting to attach a fluorescent (glowing) piece of a chromosome to a sample of cells obtained from a patient.

**Melatonin**—A sleep-inducing hormone secreted by the pineal gland.

**Phenotype**—The physical expression of an individuals genes.

**Scoliosis**—An abnormal, side-to-side curvature of the spine.

First described in 1982 by Ann C.M. Smith (a **genetics** counselor) and Ellen Magenis (a physician and **chromosome** expert), the syndrome results from a deletion on chromosome 17, specifically referred to as deletion 17p11.2.

## Description

Until the mid 1990s, SMS was not a well-known disorder, even among genetics experts; the chromosome deletion is small (a microdeletion) and difficult to detect. Most individuals are not diagnosed until they receive specialized genetic tests, usually in midchildhood or adulthood.

Smith-Magenis syndrome causes multiple birth defects (congenital abnormalities) as well as moderate to severe mental retardation. The clinical manifestations of SMS vary. However, a number of characteristic physical features, developmental delays, and behavioral problems occur in all patients with the disorder. According to some researchers, the extent of the chromosomal deletion may account for the variable severity of symptoms.

The most common and clinically recognizable features of those with SMS include mild to moderate brachycephaly (short, wide head), flat mid-face, mental retardation, and short, broad hands. Common but less consistent physical abnormalities include prominent forehead, protruding jaw, and low-set ears. The major clinical features and the specific abnormalities of SMS are the most obvious diagnostic clues to the disorder. Some experts believe that with more research on this syndrome, SMS may be determined to be a relatively common cause of mental retardation.

### Genetic profile

Although SMS is caused by a deletion of genetic material from a portion of chromosome 17, the syndrome usually does not run in families. In most cases, the deletion occurs accidentally at conception when an abnormal sperm or egg from one parent unites with a normal sperm or egg from the other parent. The abnormal sperm or egg contains the missing chromosomal material. These abnormal sperm or eggs are present in everyone; however, the risk of an abnormal conception increases significantly with the parents' ages.

Research has shown a random parental origin of deletion, suggesting that SMS is likely a contiguous **gene** deletion syndrome. Contiguous gene syndromes are conditions that occur as a result of microdeletions or microduplications involving several neighboring genes.

### Demographics

Although the exact incidence of SMS is not known, the disorder is rare and estimated to occur in approximately one in 25,000-50,000 live births. Only about 150 cases have been identified worldwide from a diversity of ethnic groups. The ages of those affected ranges from neonates to individuals in their 70s. About an equal number of males and females are affected by the disorder.

### Signs and symptoms

Although there are many features associated with SMS, not every individual exhibits all of these features. The following is a common list of traits that have been reported:

- Distinct facial features: brachycephaly, flat mid-face area, prominent forehead, eyelid folds, broad nasal bridge, protruding jaw, and low-set ears

- brachydactyly (short fingers and toes)
- short stature
- hoarse, deep voice
- speech delay
- learning disabilities
- chronic ear infections
- mental retardation (typically in the 50-60 range for IQ)
- poor muscle tone and/or feeding problems in infancy
- eye disorders
- sleep disturbances
- insensitivity to pain
- behavioral problems: hyperactivity, head banging, hand/nail biting, skin picking, pulling off fingernails and toenails, explosive outbursts, tantrums, destructive and aggressive behavior, excitability, arm hugging/squeezing when excited
- engaging and endearing personality

    Less common symptoms include:

- heart abnormalities
- scoliosis (curvature of the spine)
- seizures
- urinary tract abnormalities
- abnormalities of the palate, cleft lip
- hearing impairment

### Diagnosis

Although SMS is generally believed to be under-diagnosed, with increased professional awareness and improved methods of testing, the number of individuals identified increases annually. In diagnosing the disorder, the characteristic behavioral features of SMS are usually recognized before the facial features, often leading to a delay in diagnosis.

#### Phenotype (physical features) identification

Facial abnormalities evolve over time and are more subtle in early childhood. Thus, diagnosis of SMS at birth or in infancy is infrequent and is usually made by chance when abnormal facial features suggest a diagnosis of **Down syndrome** (a more commonly known congenital abnormality caused by an extra chromosome 21) and chromosome testing reveals the SMS 17p11.2 deletion.

The phenotypic overlap of SMS with Down syndrome, particularly in early life, can be striking. Both conditions share a number of features, including brachycephaly, upward-slanting eyes, a short and broad nose, mid-face flattening, eye disorders, short stature, small hands and feet, and poor muscle tone. However, age evolves the somewhat coarse appearance of the face, and by young adulthood, the **phenotype** of the disorder is well developed and striking. Familiarity with the clinical manifestations of both **genetic disorders** improves the likelihood of early diagnosis and intervention.

### High resolution chromosome analysis

The diagnosis of SMS is often confirmed through a blood test called a high resolution chromosome analysis, which is generally performed for the evaluation of developmental delays or congenital abnormalities. In the case of microdeletions, the chromosome deletions are so small that often they cannot be detected by chromosome analysis alone. In the older child, however, the phenotype is distinctive enough for a clinical diagnosis to be made by an experienced clinician prior to the chromosome analysis.

### FISH analysis

If chromosome analysis is inconclusive, FISH (fluorescence in situ hybridization) is the test of choice to document the SMS deletion because its high degree of accuracy. In FISH analysis, which has become a standard molecular test, denatured **DNA** (DNA altered by a process that separates the complimentary strands within the DNA double helix structure) is kept in place in the chromosome and is then hybridized (mixed) with **RNA** or DNA (extracted from another source) to which a fluorescent tag has been attached. The advantage of maintaining the DNA in the chromosome is that the specific chromosome (or chromosomes) containing the gene of interest can be identified by observing, under a microscope, the location of the fluorescence. Combining FISH and standard chromosome analysis can characterize the structural rearrangements and marker chromosomes.

In SMS, predictive or prenatal screening is an unlikely outcome of identifying the flawed gene because the disease is so rare and does not run in families. Instead, researchers hope to determine how the extent of the microdeletion on chromosome 17 is related to the various signs and symptoms of SMS.

### Treatment and management

There is no cure for SMS because the disorder is so complex and has received relatively little research attention. Therefore, managing symptoms becomes a priority in those diagnosed with the disorder.

A child with SMS typically displays self-injurious behavior as well as attention-seeking outbursts and aggressive behavior. Medications such as carbamazapine (an anticonvulsant) may be prescribed for severe behavioral problems associated with SMS. However, in most cases, drugs to help control or modify behavior or increase attention span have been found to be minimally effective. Any pharmacologic treatment of SMS remains individual, and several drugs may need to be tested to optimize results.

In addition to behavioral problems, children with SMS tend to have speech delays. Therefore, speech therapy, starting as early as possible, is typically beneficial. Most children learn to communicate verbally, either with sign language or gestures.

Since children with SMS are often easily distracted, they tend to do better in small, focused classroom settings in which there are no more than five to seven children. If the classroom is larger, competition for the teacher's attention increases, along with the probability of behavioral problems. These children also seem to respond to consistency, structure, and routines; changes in routine can provoke behavioral outbursts and tantrums.

Children with SMS have problems with sequential processing, which makes counting, mathematical skills, and multi-step tasks especially difficult. They tend to learn best with visual cues (such as pictures illustrating tasks). Also, since they have a fascination with electronics, the use of computers and other technology may be effective teaching tools in these children. Generally very responsive to affection, praise, and other positive emotions, children with SMS usually enjoy interacting with adults. A parent or teacher's positive response can often motivate a child to learn.

More than half of children with SMS have sleep disturbances such as daytime sleepiness, difficulty falling asleep at night, nocturnal awakening, decreased sleep time, and abnormalities in REM (rapid eye movement) sleep. These disturbances are due to abnormal melatonin metabolism. Melatonin is a sleep-inducing hormone secreted by the pineal gland in the brain. Therefore, a locking mechanism on the door may be helpful in preventing the child from wandering out of his or her bedroom at night. Also, a night-time dose of melatonin has been recommended for some children and adults with SMS.

Some experts have suggested that every individual with SMS have annual examinations for thyroid function, **scoliosis**, and eye problems. If any of these tests is abnormal, intervention and further clinical evaluation is appropriate.

### Prognosis

Although there is no medical prevention or cure for SMS, early diagnosis gives parents time to learn about and prepare for the challenges of the disease. Although there is insufficient data regarding the average life expectancy of those diagnosed with SMS, some individuals have lived well into their 70s.

### Resources

#### BOOKS

Cohen, Michael, Jr. *The Child With Multiple Birth Defects.* 2nd ed. New York: Oxford University Press, 1997.

Harris, Jacqueline L. *Hereditary Diseases (Bodies in Crisis).* Twenty First Century Books, 1995.

#### PERIODICALS

Hirsch, David. "Identifying Smith-Magenis Syndrome." *Exceptional Parent* 27 (July 1997): 72-73.

Hodapp, R.M., D.J. Fidler, and A.C.M. Smith. "Stress and Coping in Families of Children With Smith-Magenis Syndrome." *Journal of Intellectual Disability Research.* 42 (October 1, 1998): 331-340.

McBride, Gail. "Melatonin Disrupts Sleep in Smith-Magenis Syndrome."*Lancet* 354 (November 6, 1999): 1618.

#### WEBSITES

Baylor College of Medicine, Smith-Magenis Research. http://www.imgen.bcm.tmc.edu/molgen/lupski/sms/Index-SMS.htm.

Smith-Magenis Mailing List. http://www.egroups.com/group/sms-list.

Special Child: For Parents of Children With Disabilities. http://www.specialchild.com.

#### ORGANIZATIONS

National Organization for Rare Disorders (NORD). PO Box 8923, New Fairfield, CT 06812-8923. (203) 746-6518 or (800) 999-6673. Fax: (203) 746-6481. http://www.rarediseases.org.

Genevieve T. Slomski, PhD

Smith syndrome *see* **Smith-Lemli-Opitz syndrome**

# Sotos syndrome

### Definition

Sotos syndrome is a genetic condition causing excessive growth and a distinctive head and facial appearance. It has in the past been known as cerebral gigantism. It is often accompanied by delayed development, low muscle tone, and impaired speech.

### Description

Sotos syndrome was first described in 1964 and is primarily classified as an overgrowth syndrome, which means that the individual affected with it experiences rapid growth. A number of different symptoms occur in Sotos syndrome, however, it primarily results in rapid growth beginning in the prenatal period and continuing through the infancy and toddler years and into the elementary school years. It is also strongly associated with the bones developing and maturing more quickly (advanced bone age), in a distinctive appearing face, and in developmental delay.

The excessive prenatal growth often results in the newborn being large with respect to length and head circumference; weight is usually average. The rapid growth continues through infancy and into the youth years with the child's length/height and head circumference often being above the 97th percentile, meaning that out of 100 children of the same age, the child is longer/taller and has a larger head than 97 of the children. The rate of growth appears to decrease in later childhood and adolescence and final heights tend to be within the normal ranges.

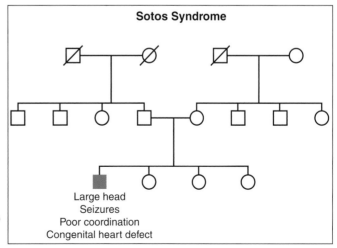

(Illustration by GGS Information Services. Gale, a part of Cengage Learning.)

The facial features of individuals with Sotos syndrome change over time. In infants and toddlers, the face is round with the forehead being prominent and the chin small. As the child grows older and becomes an adolescent, the face becomes long with the chin being more prominent, usually with a pointed or square shape. In adults, faces are usually long and thin. The head remains large from birth through adulthood.

Hypotonia is present at birth in nearly every child with Sotos syndrome. Hypotonia means that there is significantly less tone in the muscles. Bodies with hypotonia are sometimes referred to as "floppy". Muscle tone improves as the child grows older but even in adults, it is still present to some degree. Hypotonia affects many aspects of the baby's development. It can cause difficulty in sucking and swallowing and many babies are diagnosed with failure to thrive in the newborn period. This, however, usually lasts for about three to four months and then goes away. Hypotonia makes attaining fine motor skills (grasping, playing with toys, babbling) and gross motor skills (rolling, crawling, walking) difficult and these developmental milestones are usually delayed. Speech is also affected by hypotonia but as the child grows older and the hypotonia resolves or goes away, speech improves. Although the child may have delayed development, intellect typically is borderline to normal. Special attention may be needed in certain subjects, such as reading comprehension and arithmetic. Severe mental retardation is rarely seen.

There are a number of other features that have been associated with Sotos syndrome including jaundice in the newborn period, coordination problems and a tendency for clumsiness. Behavioral problems and emotional immaturity are commonly reported. About half of the children with Sotos syndrome will experience a seizure associated with fever. Dental problems such as early eruption of teeth, excessive wear, discoloration, and gingivitis are common. Teeth may also be aligned incorrectly due to changes in the facial structure.

Infections tend to develop in the ear, upper respiratory tract and urinary tract. In some children, hearing may be disrupted due to recurrent ear infections and in these situations, a referral to an otolaryngologist (a doctor specializing in the ear, nose and throat) may be necessary for assessment of hearing. Urinary tract infections occur in about one out of five children with Sotos syndrome. These have been associated with structural problems of the bladder and ureters; consequently, if urinary tract infections occur, the child should undergo further evaluations.

Congenital heart problems and development of tumors have been reported in individuals with Sotos syndrome. However, the information regarding the actual risks of these problems is not definitive and medical screening for these conditions is not routinely recommended.

### Genetic profile

Sotos syndrome is for the most part a sporadic condition, meaning that a child affected by it did not inherit it from a parent. In a very few families, autosomal dominant **inheritance** has been documented, which means that both a parent and his/her child is affected by Sotos syndrome. The cause of Sotos syndrome is not known and the gene(s) that are involved in it have not been identified.

### Demographics

Sotos syndrome is described by different groups as being both "fairly common" and "rare". A 1998 article in the *American Journal of Medical Genetics* states that over 300 cases of Sotos syndrome have been published and probably many more are unpublished. Incidence numbers have not been determined. Sotos syndrome occurs in both males and females and has been reported in several races and countries.

### Signs and symptoms

A variety of clinical features are associated with Sotos syndrome.

- Newborns are large with respect to length and head circumference; weight is usually average. The rapid growth continues through infancy and into childhood with the child's length/height and head circumference often being above the 97th percentile. The rate of growth appears to decrease in later childhood and adolescence.

- Respiratory and feeding problems (due to hyoptonia) may develop in the neonatal period.
- Infants have a round face with prominent forehead and small chin. As the child grows into adolescence and then adulthood the face becomes long and thin, and the chin becomes more prominent.
- Hypotonia is present at birth. This affects the development of fine and gross motor skills, and developmental milestones are usually delayed. Speech is also affected by hypotonia but as the child grows older and the hypotonia resolves or goes away, speech improves.
- Intellect typically is borderline to normal.
- Behavioral problems and emotional immaturity are commonly reported.
- Dental problems such as early eruption of teeth, excessive wear, discoloration, and gingivitis are common.

## Diagnosis

Diagnosis of Sotos syndrome is based upon clinical examination, medical history and x–ray data. There are no laboratory tests that can provide a diagnosis. The clinical criteria that are considered to be diagnostic for Sotos syndrome are excessive growth during the prenatal and postnatal period, advanced bone age, developmental delay, and a characteristic facial appearance. It should be noted that although features suggestive of Sotos syndrome may be present at birth or within 6-12 months after birth, making a diagnosis in infancy is not clear cut and may take multiple evaluations over several years.

There are many conditions and genetic syndromes that cause excessive growth, consequently, a baby and/or child who has accelerated growth needs to be thoroughly examined by a physician knowledgeable in overgrowth and genetic syndromes. The evaluation includes asking about health problems in the family as well as asking about the growth patterns of the parents and their final height. In some families, growth patterns are different and thus may account for the child's excessive growth. The child will also undergo a complete physical examination. Additional examination of facial appearance, with special attention paid to the shape of the head, width of the face at the level of the eyes, and the appearance of the chin and forehead is necessary as well. Measurement of the head circumference, arm length, leg length, and wing span should be taken. Laboratory testing such as **chromosome** analysis (**karyotype**) may be done along with testing for another genetic syndrome called fragile-X.

## QUESTIONS TO ASK YOUR DOCTOR

- Please describe the progress of Sotos syndrome from the time it first appears in a fetus.
- What specific signs and symptoms are typically associated with Sotos syndrome?
- What do parents need to do to manage a child's health as she or he matures with Sotos syndrome?
- In what respects will a child with Sotos syndrome be able or not be able to live a normal life?

A bone age will also be ordered. Bone age is determined by x–rays of the hand. If the child begins to lose developmental milestones or appears to stop developing, metabolic testing may be done to evaluate for a metabolic condition.

### Treatment and management

There is no cure or method for preventing Sotos syndrome. However, the symptoms can be treated and managed. In the majority of cases, the symptoms developed by individuals with Sotos syndrome are treated and managed the same as in individuals in the general population. For example, physical and occupational therapy may help with muscle tone, speech therapy may improve speech, and behavioral assessments may assist with behavioral problems.

Managing the health of a child with Sotos syndrome includes regular measurements of the growth parameters, i.e. height, head circumference and weight, treatment of excessive growth is not treated. Regular eye and dental examinations are also recommended. Medical screening for congenital heart defects and tumors is not routinely recommended, although it has been noted that symptoms should be evaluated sooner rather than later.

### Prognosis

With appropriate treatment, management and encouragement, children with Sotos syndrome can do well. Adults with Sotos syndrome are likely to be within the normal range for height and intellect. Sotos syndrome is not associated with a shortened life span.

## Resources

### BOOKS

Anderson, Rebecca Rae, and Bruce A. Buehler. *Sotos Syndrome: A Handbook for Families.* Omaha, NB: Meyer Rehabilitation Institute, 1992.

Cole, Trevor R.P. "Sotos Syndrome." In *Management of Genetic Syndromes,* edited by Suzanne B. Cassidy and Judith E. Allanson. New York: Wiley-Liss, 2001, pp.389-404.

### PERIODICALS

*Sotos Syndrome Support Association Quarterly Newsletter.*

### WEBSITES

Genetic and Rare Conditions Site. http://www.kumc.edu/gec/support/.

The Family Village. http://www.familyvillage.wisc.edu/index.htmlx.

### ORGANIZATIONS

Sotos Syndrome Support Group. Three Danda Square East #235, Wheaton, IL 60187. (888) 246-SSSA or (708) 682-8815. http://www.well.com/user/sssa/.

Cindy L Hunter, CGC

# Spastic cerebral palsy

## Definition

Spastic **cerebral palsy** (CP) is a disorder in which brain damage results in a movement disability.

## Description

Cerebral palsy is a nonprogressive disorder of movement and/or posture caused by a brain abnormality. It is evident before the age of two. There are several types of CP, but spastic CP is the most common—about 60%. The term "spasticity" refers to increased muscle tone (stiffness), leading to uncontrolled, awkward movements.

## Genetic profile

Only about 2% of cases of CP are believed to result from genetic causes. Most cases of CP are associated with risk factors such as low birth weight, premature birth, and lack of oxygen at birth. Multiple births (such as twins or triplets) also have an increased risk. A genetic cause is more likely if these risk factors are not present. If the paralysis and spasticity are symmetrical—that is, if both sides of the body are similarly affected—then the condition is more likely to be genetic in nature. Mental retardation is usually, but

---

**KEY TERMS**

**Cerebral palsy**—Movement disability resulting from nonprogressive brain damage.

**Spasticity**—Increased muscle tone, or stiffness, which leads to uncontrolled, awkward movements.

not always, associated with genetic forms. Researchers have not yet found which gene is associated with the disease.

## Demographics

CP has an overall incidence of one in 250 to 1,000 births. Most forms of CP that are genetic have an autosomal recessive pattern of **inheritance**. This means that in order for a child to have the disorder, they must inherit one altered copy of the causative gene from each parent. A person who has only one altered copy of the disease gene is called a carrier. Two carriers have a 25% chance of having a child with CP with each pregnancy. As studied in the British Pakistani population, a consanguineous marriage—marriage between relatives—appears to increase the prevalence of a genetic form of spastic CP.

## Signs and symptoms

CP may not be noticed immediately after birth. Children with CP are slow to meet developmental motor milestones, which are expected ages at which certain mobility skills are achieved. These milestones include reaching for toys, sitting, and walking. People with CP also have abnormal muscle tone (increased in spastic CP), abnormal or uncontrolled movements, and abnormal reflexes. The spasticity may not be present at birth but usually develops during the first two years of life. Many children with spastic CP have normal intelligence, but mental retardation does occur, especially in inherited forms of the disease. Depending on the severity and extent of the paralysis, some affected individuals can walk (often late and with crutches or walkers), while others with more severe disability cannot walk at all. Seizures are not uncommon in individuals with CP.

## Diagnosis

A diagnosis of spastic CP is based on delay in or lack of meeting developmental motor milestones, along with the presence of abnormal muscle tone, movements, and reflexes. Since the exact gene causing some cases of symmetric spastic CP has not yet been identified, molecular testing is not available at this time. Since

---

Miller, Freeman, and Steven J. Bachrach. *Cerebral Palsy: A Complete Guide for Caregiving.* Baltimore: Johns Hopkins University Press, 1995.

**PERIODICALS**

McHale, D.P., et al. "A Gene for Autosomal Recessive Symmetrical Spastic Cerebral Palsy Maps to Chromosome 2q24-25." *American Journal of Human Genetics* 64 (1999): 526-532.

**ORGANIZATIONS**

United Cerebral Palsy Association, Inc. (UCP). 1660 L St. NW, Suite 700, Washington, DC 20036-5602. (202)776-0406 or (800)872-5827. http://www.ucpa.org.

Toni I. Pollin, MS, CGC

**Sphingomyelin lipidosis** *see* **Niemann-Pick disease**

**Sphingomyelinease deficiency** *see* **Niemann-Pick disease**

**Spielmeyer-Vogt-Sjögren-Batten disease** *see* **Batten disease**

# Spina bifida

### Definition

Spina bifida is a serious birth abnormality, termed a neural tube defect, in which the spinal cord is malformed and lacks its usual protective skeletal and soft tissue coverings.

### Description

Spina bifida is a lesion that may appear in the midline of the body anywhere from the neck to the buttocks. It is caused by the failure of the vertebrae to form properly in fetal development, leaving the spinal cord some degree of vulnerability or exposure to the environment. Spina bifida occurs in multiple forms of varying exposure of the spinal cord.

#### Spina bifida occulta

This form of spina bifida usually involves the deformation of a single vertebra in the cervical, lumbar, or sacral regions. The spinal cord and nerves are usually normal with no neurological symptoms. There is usually skin covering the vertebral abnormality, which is typically indicated visually by a dimple with a tuft of hair. Clinical symptoms are absent in the majority of cases.

---

## QUESTIONS TO ASK YOUR DOCTOR

- What bodily changes are characteristic of a child with spastic cerebral palsy?
- What kind of home care will a child with spastic cerebral palsy require as he or she grows older?
- What physical, mental, and emotional problems is a child with spastic cerebral palsy likely to experience?
- What organizations provide advice and support for parents of a child with spastic cerebral palsy?

---

CP-like symptoms can be found in other genetic conditions, **chromosome** testing and molecular testing for other suspected conditions may help determine the cause of the CP-like symptoms. Testing may also enable other family members to see if they carry the condition, and allow a fetus to be diagnosed prenatally. Prenatal diagnosis of known genetic conditions can be accomplished using procedures such as chorionic villi sampling, in which cells from the placenta are studied; and **amniocentesis**, in which skin cells from the fluid surrounding the fetus are studied.

### Treatment and management

Treatment of spastic CP is focused on maximizing mobility through physical therapy, and/or providing necessary physical support using devices such as splints, walkers, and wheelchairs. Speech and occupational therapy are sometimes useful as well. Certain types of surgery of the bone, nerves, tendon, and brain tissue can correct abnormalities, improve mobility, and reduce spasticity. Orthodontic work on the teeth is often indicated in children with CP. Some level of special educational services is usually required.

### Prognosis

Spastic CP is not a progressive condition, so living into old age is possible. However, complications such as reduced mobility, mental retardation, feeding difficulties, and respiratory infections can reduce the life span. More severe disabilities are associated with greater decreases in life expectancy, but at least half of people with CP live to at least age 35.

### Resources

**BOOKS**

Geralis, Elaine, ed. *Children with Cerebral Palsy: A Parents' Guide.* Bethesda, MD: Woodbine House, 1991.

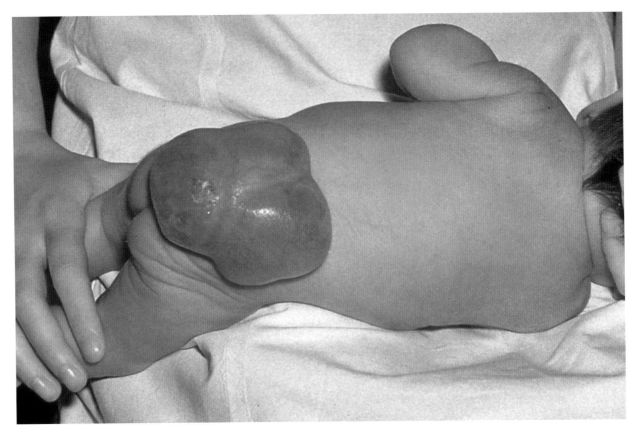

**An infant with spina bifida. The large fluid-filled sac at the base of the spinal cord contains the meninges and possibly part of the spinal cord.** *(Photo Researchers, Inc.)*

### Spina bifida cystica

Spina bifida cystica is a term used to describe several severe forms of spina bifida. The spinal cord protrudes outward through an open defect in the vertebrae, forming a cyst-like sac on the outside of the body filled with cerebrospinal fluid. When the sac includes the meninges, a protective three-layered membrane that covers the spinal cord, the condition is said to involve a meningocele. When the actual spinal cord or nerve roots are included in the sac, the condition is described as involving a meningomyelocele. This is a more common form of spina bifida cystica. Neurological deficits occur because nervous tissue is integrated in the wall of the sac, disrupting their function. Both types of spina bifida cystica are most common in the lumbar and sacral regions.

### Rachischisis and spina bifida with myeloschisis

The most severe type of spina bifida is caused by the failure of the neural folds to fuse. The entire spinal canal is open, exposing the spinal nerves completely. The spinal cord is only developed into a flattened mass of nervous tissue.

Spina bifida is usually readily apparent at birth because of the malformation of the back and clinical symptoms associated with most forms of the abnormality. There are varying degrees of neurological deficit present, depending on the position and degree of the abnormality. There is usually a loss of sensation to the skin, with varying skeletal muscle paralysis in the region below the lesion. Paralysis of the urinary bladder or anal sphincters is also common.

## Genetic profile

Spina bifida may occur as an isolated defect or associated with other malformations, such as partial absence of the brain. As an isolated abnormality, spina bifida is caused by a combination of genetic factors and environmental influences. The most important factor that causes **neural tube defects** such as spina bifida is a maternal folic acid deficiency during early pregnancy. Folic acid levels are dependent on dietary intake. During pregnancy, the requirement for folic acid is increased, and is difficult to meet with an average contemporary diet. Mothers of children with neural tube defects may have reduced blood folate levels, along

## KEY TERMS

**Allele**—One of two or more different genes that encode specific and inheritable characteristics that occupy corresponding locations on a pair of chromosomes.

**Amnion**—The thin, protective sac that suspends the fetus in a protective amniotic fluid.

**Cerebrospinal fluid**—Fluid that bathes and supports the brain and the spinal cord, protecting it from physical impact.

**Chiari II anomaly**—A structural abnormality of the lower portion of the brain (cerebellum and brainstem) associated with spina bifida; the lower structures of the brain are crowded and may be forced into the foramen magnum, the opening through which the brain and spinal cord are connected.

**Hydrocephalus**—The excess accumulation of cerebrospinal fluid around the brain, often causing enlargement of the head.

**Neural folds and tube**—Portions of the developing embryo from which the brain and spinal cord arise.

**Vertebral divisions**—The human vertebral regions are divided into cervical, thoracic, lumbar, and sacral from the neck to the tailbone.

with a defect in the recycling pathway for digested folic acid. This defect can be caused by a genetic mutation in the enzyme 5,10-methylenetetrahydrofolate reductase (MTHFR). The mutation in the gene for MTHFR causes an unstable enzyme that cannot function properly in the metabolism of folic acid. The mutant allele for unstable MTHFR is very common in many populations. Between 5–15% of the population may have both alleles for MTHFR in a mutated form. Research has demonstrated that mothers of infants with neural tube defects are twice as likely to have all mutant alleles of the gene for MTHFR. A folic acid deficiency may be caused by other genetic defects or by dietary deprivation alone. A small percentage of neural tube defects such as spina bifida can be narrowed down to other specific causes, such as the early rupture of the amnion-forming fibrous amniotic bands that disrupt vertebral development. Exposure to some teratogens, chemicals that produce abnormal fetal development, may cause spina bifida. Other causes may include separate single **gene mutations**, **chromosomal abnormalities**, environmental insults such as maternal **diabetes** mellitus, or prenatal exposure to certain anticonvulsant drugs. The recurrence risk varies with each of these specific causes.

## Demographics

Spina bifida occurs worldwide, but there has been a steady decrease in occurrence rates over the past 50–70 years, due to dietary supplementation with folic acid. Before folic acid fortification, approximately 2,500–3,000 births in the United States were affected annually by some form of neural tube defect. In 2001, there was a 24% decline in spina bifida in the United States from folic acid fortification of enriched grain products and other folic acid initiatives. The highest prevalence rates, about one in 200 pregnancies, have been reported from northern provinces in China. High prevalence rates of approximately one in 1,000 pregnancies have also been found in Central and South America. The lowest prevalence rates, less than one in 2,000 pregnancies, have been found in the European countries. Regionally, the highest prevalence in the United States occurs in the southeast, in approximately one in 500 pregnancies. A study performed by the CDC in North Carolina between 1995 and 1999 demonstrated a 32% decline in the incidence of spina bifida. The decline in incidence was not uniform across the population, but was dependent on geographic region as correlated with maternal sociodemographic characteristics. Populations with higher income and education have afforded the greatest decline in spina bifida. Although the use of multivitamins has played a role in this population, much of the recent decline in neural tube defects in the United States has been a result of the mandatory government fortification program of enriched grain products.

## Signs and symptoms

In most cases, spina bifida is obvious at birth because of the malformation of the spinal column and associated neurological deficits. The spinal cord may be completely exposed, appearing as a mass on the back covered by the meningeal membranes or skin. Although spina bifida may occur anywhere from the base of the skull to the buttocks, about 75% of cases occur in the lumbar region. When the defect is covered by skin, it may include a dimple or depression, a port wine-colored birthmark, or a bulge with a tuft of hair.

Along with the malformations, the neurological deficit is also obvious. The level of anesthesia of the skin depends on which dermatomes are affected. Dermatomes are patches of skin innervated by specific spinal nerves. The spinal nerves leave the spinal cord to innervate structures in descending order. The higher the lesion of spina bifida is located on the vertebral column, the more spinal nerves may be affected. Skeletal muscle may also be paralyzed in the same fashion, over the entire pelvic area and lower extremity. Saddle anesthesia is the term used to refer to the entire loss of sensation to the area of the body that touches the saddle during horseback riding. Saddle anesthesia is a symptom often seen when paralysis of urinary bladder and anal sphincters is present. A lack of response to touch, lack of leg movement or resistance to passive-elicited movement, severe flaccidity, and lack of anal reflex (reflex of musculature in response to touch) in an infant are signs that neurological deficits in the lower region are present.

There are other complications that sometimes develop in association with spina bifida. Some infants develop hydrocephaly, an accumulation of excess fluid in the four cavities of the brain. At least one of every seven cases develops findings of Chiari II malformation, a condition in which the lower part of the brain is crowded and may be forced into the upper part of the spinal cavity. A lipomeningocele or lipomyelomeningocele may occur in the lumbar or sacral back area. In these conditions, a tumor of fatty tissue becomes isolated among the nerves below the spinal cord, which may result in tethering of the spinal cord and complications similar to those with open spina bifida.

## Diagnosis

A mother carrying a fetus with spina bifida will not experience any unusual signs or symptoms in early pregnancy. Spina bifida is often discovered prenatally by initial signs and symptoms in the maternal amniotic fluid. During **amniocentesis** obstetricians may screen for high levels of a protein called alphafetoprotein (AFP). High AFP is a general indicator that the fetus may have a defect. The AFP test is not indicative of spina bifida specifically, but alerts the obstetrician that a detailed ultrasonogram (use of ultrasound) may be necessary. Spina bifida may cause elevated levels of AFP because it is an open fetal defect that allows high levels of the AFP of the fetus to travel into maternal amniotic fluid and smaller amounts to enter maternal blood serum. A prenatal diagnosis of spina bifida may be made with ultrasonograpic examination. Malformations may be detected via ultrasonogram as early as 12–14 weeks of pregnancy. Postnatally, the diagnosis is usually obvious, based on external lesions. In addition to the characteristic malformations, paralysis below the level of the lesion may be part of the diagnosis. In cases in which there are no external indicators, the diagnosis may not become evident until neurological abnormalities develop weeks, months, or years following birth.

## Treatment and management

Prevention of spina bifida and other neural tube defects is improved with the use of folic acid vitamin supplements for several months prior to and following conception. The Centers for Disease Control and Prevention (CDC) recommend an intake of 400 mcg of synthetic folic acid per day for all women of childbearing years to prevent neural tube defects.

Open fetal surgery has been performed for spina bifida during the several months of pregnancy. After direct closure of the spine malformation, the fetus is returned to the womb. By preventing chronic intrauterine exposure to mechanical and chemical trauma, prenatal surgery improves neurological function and leads to fewer complications after birth. Fetal surgery is considered experimental, and results have been mixed.

Postnatally, aggressive surgical and medical management have improved the survival and function of infants with spina bifida. Initial surgery on the spinal column defect may be performed in the first days of life, providing protection against injury and infection. Subsequent surgery is often necessary to protect against excessive curvature of the spine. When spina bifida occurs in conjunction with hydrocephaly, surgery is performed to implant a mechanical shunt to decrease the pressure and amount of cerebrospinal fluid in the cavities of the brain. Because of weakness or paralysis below the level of the spinal defect, most children will require physical therapy, bracing, and other orthopedic assistance to enable them to walk. A variety of approaches, including periodic bladder catheterization, surgical diversion of urine, and antibiotics, is used to protect urinary function.

Although most individuals with spina bifida have normal intellectual function, learning disabilities or mental impairment may occur. This may result, in part, from hydrocephaly and/or infections of the nervous system. Children so affected may benefit from early educational intervention, physical therapy, and occupational therapy. Counseling to improve self-image and lessen barriers to socialization becomes important in late childhood and adolescence.

## Prognosis

More than 80% of infants born with spina bifida survive with surgical and medical management. Although complications from paralysis, hydrocephaly, Chiari II malformation, and urinary tract deterioration threaten the well-being of the survivors, the outlook for normal intellectual function is good.

## Resources

### BOOKS

Moore, Keith L., and T. V. N. Persaud. *The Developing Human, Clinically Oriented Embryology, Seventh Edition.* St. Louis, MO: Elsevier Science, 2003.

*Thompson & Thompson Genetics in Medicine, Sixth Edition.* St. Louis, MO: Elsevier Science, 2004.

### PERIODICALS

Sells, C. J., and J. G. Hall, guest eds. "Neural Tube Defects." *Mental Retardation and Developmental Disabilities Research Reviews.* Volume 4, Number 4. New York: Wiley-Liss, 1998.

### WEB SITES

*Medline.* (April 7, 2005.) http://medlineplus.gov/.

*Prevalence of Spina Bifida at Birth—United States, 1983–1990: A Comparison of Two Surveillance Systems.* CDC Surveillance Summaries. (April 7, 2005.) http://www.cdc.gov/mmwr/preview/mmwrhtml/00040954.htm.

*Sociodemographic Patterns in Spina Bifida Birth Prevalence Trends—North Carolina, 1995–1999.* CDC Recommendations and Reports. (April 7, 2005.) http://www.cdc.gov/mmwr/preview/mmwrhtml/rr5113a4.htm.

*Spina Bifida and Anencephaly Prevalence—United States, 1991–2001.* CDC Recommendations and Reports. (April 7, 2005.) http://www.cdc.gov/mmwr/preview/mmwrhtml/rr5113a3.htm.

*NINDS Spina Bifida Information Page.* (April 7, 2005.) http://www.ninds.nih.gov/disorders/spina_bifida/spina_bifida.htm.

*Surveillance for Anencephaly and Spina Bifida and the Impact of Prenatal Diagnosis—United States, 1985–1994.* (April 7, 2005.) http://www.cdc.gov/mmwr/preview/mmwrhtml/00038567.htm.

### ORGANIZATIONS

March of Dimes Birth Defects Foundation. 1275 Mamaroneck Ave., White Plains, NY 10605. (888) 663-4637. resourcecenter@modimes.org. (April 7, 2005.) http://www.modimes.org.

National Birth Defects Prevention Network. Atlanta, GA (770) 488-3550. (April 7, 2005.) http://www.nbdpn.org/NBDPN.

Shriners Hospitals for Children. International Shrine Headquarters, 2900 Rocky Point Dr., Tampa, FL 33607-1460. (813) 281-0300. (April 7, 2005.) http://www.shrinershq.org.

Spina Bifida Association of America. 4590 MacArthur Blvd. NW, Suite 250, Washington, DC 20007-4226. (800) 621-3141 or (202) 944-3285. Fax: (202) 944-3295. http://www.sbaa.org.

Maria Basile, PhD

**Spinal and bulbar muscular atrophy** *see* **Kennedy disease**

# Spinal muscular atrophy

## Definition

Spinal muscular atrophy (SMA) is a disease characterized by degradation of the anterior horn cells of the spinal cord and has similar characteristics to Spinobulbar muscular atrophy (SBMA). SBMA differs from SMA in its mode of **inheritance**, the disease-determining **gene**, the mutational events that trigger disease and the cellular specificity of the disease pathology.

## Description

The anterior horn cells control the voluntary muscle contractions from large muscle groups such as the arms and legs. For example, if an individual wants to move his/her arm, electrical impulses are sent from the brain down the anterior horn cells to the muscles of the arm, which then stimulates the arm muscles to contract allowing the arm to move. Degradation is a rapid loss of functional motor neurons. Loss of motor neurons results in progressive symmetrical atrophy of the voluntary muscles. Progressive symmetrical atrophy refers to the loss of function of muscle groups from both sides of the body. For example, both arms and both legs are equally effected to similar degrees of muscle loss and the inability to be controlled and used properly. Progressive loss indicates that muscle loss is not instantaneous, rather, muscle loss occurs consistently over a period of time. These muscle groups include those skeletal muscles that control large muscle groups such as the arms, legs and torso. The weakness in the legs is generally greater than the weakness in the arms.

## KEY TERMS

**Anterior horn cells**—Subset of motor neurons within the spinal cord.

**Atrophy**—Wasting away of normal tissue or an organ due to degeneration of the cells.

**Degradation**—Loss or diminishing.

**Dorsal root ganglia**—The subset of neuronal cells controlling impulses in and out of the brain.

**Intragenic**—Occuring within a single gene.

**Motor neurons**—Class of neurons that specifically control and stimulate voluntary muscles.

**Motor units**—Functional connection with a single motor neuron and muscle.

**Sensory neurons**—Class of neurons that specifically regulate and control external stimuli (senses: sight, sound).

**Transcription**—The process by which genetic information on a strand of DNA is used to synthesize a strand of complementary RNA.

**Voluntary muscle**—A muscle under conscious control, such as arm and leg muscles.

Spinal muscular atrophy (SMA) arises primarily from degradation of the anterior horn cells of the spinal cord, resulting in proximal weakness and atrophy of voluntary skeletal muscle. Proximal weakness effects the limbs positioned closer to the body, such as arms and legs, rather than more distant body parts such as hands, feet, fingers, or toes.

Spinal muscular atrophy only affects the motor neurons of the spinal cord and voluntary muscles of the limb and trunk. Patients do not display sensory loss, heart problems, or mental retardation. There are numerous secondary complications seen in SMA, including bending of the legs and arms and pneumonia. SMA development involves an initial substantial loss of motor units, followed by a stabilization of the surviving motor units. Motor units refer to an entire motor neuron and the connections within a muscle required for neuronal function.

### Clinical subgroups

The childhood form of SMA is subdivided into three main clinical subgroups, Type I, II, and III, depending upon the age of onset and severity. A fourth subgroup, Type O, was recently discovered in London.

### Type I

Type I SMA, or Werdnig-Hoffmann disease, is the acute or severe form, characterized by severe muscle atrophy. Guido-Werdig, an Austrian doctor, first identified the disease in 1891. He described two brothers displaying progressive muscle weakness from the age of 10 months, starting in the legs and progressing to the back and arms. The first brother died at the age three years with respiratory problems. The second brother survived to the age of six years.

Symptoms emerge in the first three months of life with the affected children never gaining the ability to sit, stand or walk. Swallowing and feeding may be difficult and the child may show difficulties with their own secretions. There is general weakness in the intercostals and accessory respiratory muscles (the muscles situated between the ribs). The chest may appear concave (sunken in) due to the diaphragmatic (tummy) breathing.

### Type II

Type II SMA was first described in 1964. It is less severe than type I, with clinical symptoms emerging between three and 15 months of age. Most patients can sit but are unable to stand or walk unaided. Feeding and swallowing problems are uncommon in patients with Type II SMA. Again, as with patients diagnosed with type I SMA, the intercostal muscles are affected, with diaphragmatic breathing a main characteristic of children with type II. Most patients will survive beyond the age of four years and, depending upon how their respiratory system is affected, may live through adolescence.

### Type III

The chronic form of SMA, Type III (Kugelberg-Welander disease) was first described in 1956. The clinical symptoms manifest after the age of four. It produces proximal muscle weakness, predominantly in the lower body. Affected individuals can walk unaided and have a normal life span depending upon the extent of respiratory muscles loss.

### Type O

Clinicians in London have recently identified a fourth form of the childhood disease; Type 0 SMA. This form appears to have a fetal-onset in that affected individuals display reduced movement within the uterus and are born with severe muscular atrophy with massive motor neuronal cell death. Therefore, these patients have very few functional motor neurons and motor units.

## Diagnosis

One of the main diagnostic tools is electromyography (EMG). Contraction of voluntary muscle is controlled by electrical impulses originating from the brain. These impulses pass down the motor neurons of the spinal cord to the connecting muscles, where it triggers the contraction. The EMG records this electrical impulse and determines whether the electric current is the same as in normal individuals. Metal needles are inserted into the arms and thigh and the electrical impulse is recorded.

In addition, the speed at which the electric impulse passes down the motor neuron can also be used as a diagnostic test. In SMA patients, both the nerve conduction velocity (NVC) and the EMG readings are reduced.

The third test is an invasive procedure called a muscle biopsy. This involves a surgeon removing a small section of muscle. This is then tested for signs of degradation.

## Genetic profile

All forms of childhood SMA are autosomal recessive, with both parents needing to be carriers to pass the disease on. If both parents are carriers, there is a 25% chance of their child being affected.

All three forms are caused by a decrease in the production of a protein, termed Survival of Motor Neuron (SMN). The SMN protein is encoded by two nearly identical genes located on **chromosome** 5; SMN-1 and SMN-2 (previously referred to as telomeric and centomeric SMN, respectively). Remarkably, only mutations or deletions of SMN-1 result in disease development.

In most individuals who do not have SMA, each chromosome (maternal and paternal) contains one copy of SMN-1 and one copy of SMN-2. Therefore, in most unaffected individuals, there are two SMN-1 and two SMN-2 genes. Importantly, a subset of SMA-causing mutations are intragenic SMN-1 single amino acid substitutions. Intragenic indicates that mutations are within an otherwise intact SMN gene, but that there is a small and very subtle mutation that is only found within the SMN gene. This is in contrast to large genomic deletions that can delete the SMN gene and also neighboring genes. The intragenic or small mutations thereby confirms SMN-1 as the SMA-determining gene.

## Signs and symptoms

Research shows that, in SMA, the reduced SMN protein levels result in motor neuronal cell degradation. How, and why this occurs is still not known.

## Demographics

Approximately, one in 10,000 live births are affected with SMA, which is slightly lower than expected since the carrier frequency is between one in 40 and one in 50. Since this is a recessive disease, meaning two copies of the abnormal gene must be present for the disease to occur, carriers are unaffected because only one copy of the abnormal gene is present.

The genomic SMN region is remarkably unstable, and *de novo* mutations (mutations that are new and not inherited from the parents) are quite frequent, accounting for nearly 2% of all SMA cases. In 90% of patients, death occurs before the age of two due to respiratory failure. In North America and Europe, type I SMA accounts for one in every 25,000 infant mortalities. SMA is the leading genetic cause of infantile death and is the second most common autosomal recessive disorder behind **cystic fibrosis**. Carrier frequencies and disease frequencies are similar throughout the world, although slight variations can exist. Asian populations have a slightly reduced carrier frequency although it is not known why this discrepancy has occurred.

## Treatment and management

To date, there is no treatment for childhood SMA. However, there are possible mechanisms through which treatment could be developed. **Gene therapy** could be used for SMA to replace the abnormal SMN-1 gene. Such treatment is not yet available or possible at this time though.

## Prognosis

In Type I SMA, eating and swallowing can become difficult as the muscles of the face are affected. Due to the degradation of the respiratory muscles breathing can also be labored. It is therefore essential for patients to undergo chest physiotherapy (CPT). CPT is a standard set of procedures designed to trigger and aid coughing in patients. Coughing is important as it clears the patients lungs and throat of moisture and prevents secondary problems, such as pneumonia.

As symptoms progress, patients may require a ventilator to aid breathing. There are two main forms of ventilation systems. Negative Pressure Ventilation can be achieved by placing the patient in a Port-A-Lung. This machine ensures that the air pressure around the patient is lower than the air pressure within the patient's lungs, enabling easier breathing. The pressure can be raised or lowered if the patients ventilation rate increases or decreases.

The second method is called Bi-Pap (Biphasic Positive Airway Pressure). This procedure involves the insertion of a small tube down the nose into the patient's lungs, through which oxygen is pumped into the lungs and waste carbon dioxide is removed. This system allows maximum inspiration and expiration levels to be reached.

Of all the forms of childhood SMA, Type II is the most diverse. It is therefore hard to tell when muscle weakness will occur and how severe the disease will be. With the aid of leg braces and walking devices, some children may gain the ability to stand. Unlike Type I SMA, not all children with Type II are affected by respiratory weakness. The main cause of death in patients with Type II is respiratory failure resulting from a respiratory infection. It is therefore important to ensure that mucus does not build up in patients respiratory tracts as this could aid viral and bacterial infections.

### Resources

#### PERIODICALS

Crawford, T. O., and C. A. Pardo. "The neurobiology of childhood spinal muscular atrophy." *Neurobiology of Disease* 3 (1996): 97-110.

#### WEBSITES

Families of Spinal Muscular Atrophy. http://www.fsma.org.

The Andrew's Buddies web site. *FightSMA.com* http://www.andrewsbuddies.com/news.html.

#### ORGANIZATIONS

Muscular Dystrophy Association. 3300 East Sunrise Dr., Tucson, AZ 85718. (520) 529-2000 or (800) 572-1717. http://www.mdausa.org.

Philip J. Young
Christian L. Lorson, PhD

# Spinocerebellar ataxia

## Definition

The spinocerebellar ataxias (SCAs) are a group of inherited conditions that affect the brain and spinal cord, causing progressive difficulty with coordination. Some types of SCA also involve impairment of speech and eye movement.

## Description

The SCAs are named for the parts of the nervous system that are affected in this condition. *Spino* refers to the spinal cord and *cerebellar* refers to the cerebellum, or back part of the brain. The cerebellum is the area of the brain that controls coordination. In people with SCA, the cerebellum often becomes atrophied or smaller. Symptoms of SCA usually begin in the 30s or 40s, but onset can be at any age. Onset from childhood through the 70s has been reported.

At least 25 different types of SCA have been described. This group is numbered 1–26, and each is caused by mutations, or changes, in a different **gene**. Although the category of SCA9 has been reserved, there is no described condition for SCA9 and no gene has been found. Spinocerebellar ataxia has also been called olivopontocerebellar atrophy, Marie's ataxia, and cerebellar degeneration. SCA3 is sometimes called **Machado-Joseph disease**, named after two of the first families described with this condition. All affected people in a family have the same type of SCA.

## Genetic profile

Although each of the SCAs is caused by mutations in different genes, the types of mutations are the same in all of the genes that have been found. Most genes come in pairs; one member of a pair comes from a person's mother and the other one comes from their father. The genes are made up of **deoxyribonucleic acid (DNA)**, which is made up of chemical bases that are represented by the letters C, T, G, and A. This is the DNA alphabet. The letters are usually put together in three-letter words. The arrangement of the words are what give the gene its meaning, and therefore tells the body how to grow and develop.

In each of the genes that cause SCA, there is a section of the gene where a three-letter DNA word is repeated a certain number of times. In most of the types of SCA, the DNA word that is repeated is CAG. So there is a part of the gene that reads CAGCAGCAG-CAGCAG...and so on. In people who have SCA, this DNA segment is repeated too many times, making this

## KEY TERMS

**Anticipation**—Increasing severity in disease with earlier ages of onset, in successive generations; a condition that begins at a younger age and is more severe with each generation

**Ataxia**—A deficiency of muscular coordination, especially when voluntary movements are attempted, such as grasping or walking.

**Calcification**—The addition of calcium deposits.

**Trinucleotide repeat expansion**—A sequence of three nucleotides that is repeated too many times in a section of a gene.

section of the gene too big. This is called a trinucleotide repeat expansion. In SCA8, the DNA word that is repeated is CTG. In SCA10, the repeated DNA word is five DNA letters long and is ATTCT. This is called a pentanucleotide expansion. The actual number of DNA repeats that is normal or that causes SCA is different in each type of SCA.

In each type of SCA, there are a certain range or number of repeats that still fall within the normal range. People who have repeat numbers in the normal range will not develop SCA and cannot pass it to their children. There are also a certain number of repeats that cause SCA (the affected range). People who have repeat numbers in the affected range will go on to develop SCA sometime in their lifetime, if they live long enough. People with repeat numbers in the affected range can pass SCA onto their children. Between the normal and affected ranges, there is a gray range. People who have repeat numbers in the gray range may or may not develop SCA in their lifetime. Why some people with numbers in the gray zone develop SCA and others do not is not known. People with repeat numbers in the gray range can also pass SCA onto their children.

In general, the more repeats in the affected range that someone has, the earlier the age of onset of symptoms and the more severe the symptoms. However, this is a generalized rule. It is not possible to look at a person's repeat number and predict at what age they will begin to have symptoms or how their condition will progress.

Sometimes when a person who has repeat numbers in the affected or gray range has children, the DNA expansion grows larger during the passing on of genes. This is called anticipation. Anticipation can result in an even earlier age of onset in children than in their affected parent. Anticipation does not occur in SCA6.

However, significant anticipation can occur in SCA7. It is not unusual for a child with SCA7 to be affected before their parent or even grandparent begins to show symptoms. In most types of SCA, anticipation happens more often when a father passes SCA on to his children then when a mother passes it. However, in SCA8, the opposite is true; anticipation happens more often when a mother passes SCA8 to her children. Occasionally, repeat sizes stay the same or even get smaller when they are passed to a person's children.

The SCAs are passed on by autosomal dominant **inheritance**. This means that males and females are equally likely to be affected. It also means that only one gene in the pair needs to have the mutation in order for a person to become affected. Since a person only passes one copy of each gene on to their children, there is a 50%, or one in two, chance that a person who has SCA will pass it on to each of their children. A person who has repeat numbers in the gray range also has a 50%, or one in two, chance of passing the gene onto each of their children. However, whether or not their children will develop SCA depends on the number of their repeats. A person who has repeat numbers in the normal range cannot pass SCA onto their children.

Usually a person with SCA has a long family history of the condition. However, sometimes a person with SCA appears to be the only one affected in the family. This can be due to a couple of reasons. First, it is possible that one of their parents is or was affected, but died before they began to show symptoms. It is also possible that their parent had a mutation in the gray range and was not affected, but the mutation expanded into the affected range when it was passed on. Other family members may also have SCA but have been misdiagnosed with another condition or are having symptoms, but have no definitive diagnosis. It is also possible that a person has a new mutation for SCA. New mutations are changes in the gene that happen for the first time in an affected person. Although a person with a new mutation may not have other affected family members, they still have a 50%, or one in two, chance of passing it on to their children.

### Demographics

SCA has been found in people from all over the world. However, some of the types of SCA are more common in certain areas and ethnic groups. SCA types 1, 2, 3, 6, 7, and 8 are the most commonly documented autosomal dominant SCA. SCA1 accounts for at least 25% of SCA cases in South Africa and Italy. SCA2 accounts for 25% of SCA cases in Singapore, India, and Italy. SCA3 appears to be the most common type and was first described in families from Portugal.

SCA3 accounts for almost 100% of SCA cases in Brazil. SCA3 also accounts for the majority of SCA cases in Portugal, the Netherlands, Germany, China, and Singapore, and a significant proportion in Japan. SCA6 accounts for a significant proportion of SCA cases in the Netherlands, Germany, and Japan. In the United States, SCA2, SCA3, and SCA6 account for the majority of documented cases; these three types also account for 51% of worldwide cases. SCA1, SCA7, and SCA8 each account for less than 10% of SCA cases worldwide.

SCA types 4, 5, and 10 through 26 are rare and have each only been described in a few families. The first family described with SCA5 may have been distantly related to President Abraham Lincoln and was first called Lincoln ataxia. SCA10 has only been described in Mexican families, SCA13 and 25 have each only been described in single French families, SCA14 and 16 have each only been described in single families from Japan, and SCA19 and 23 have each only been described in single Dutch families.

### Signs and symptoms

Although different genes cause each of the SCAs, they all have similar symptoms. All people with SCA have ataxia or a lack of muscle coordination. Walking is affected, and eventually the coordination of the arms and hands and of the speech and swallowing is also affected. One of first symptoms of SCA is often problems with walking and difficulties with balance. The muscles that control speech and swallowing usually become affected. This results in dysarthria, or slurred speech, and difficulties with eating. Choking while eating can become a significant problem and can lead to a decrease in the number of calories a person can take in. The age of the onset of symptoms can vary greatly—anywhere from childhood through the seventh decade have been reported. The age of onset and severity of symptoms can also vary between people in the same family.

As the condition progresses, walking becomes more difficult and it is necessary to use a cane, walker, and often a wheelchair. Because of the uncoordinated walking that develops, it is not uncommon for people with SCA to be mistaken for being intoxicated. Carrying around a note from their doctor explaining their medical condition can often be helpful.

Some of the SCA types can also have other symptoms, although not all of these are seen in every person with that particular type. SCA2 may have slower eye movements; this does not usually interfere with a person's sight. People with SCA1 and 3 may develop problems with the peripheral nerves, which carry information to and from the spinal cord. This can lead to decreased sensation and weakness in the hands and feet. In SCA3, people may also have twitching in the face and tongue, and bulging eyes. SCA4 may cause a loss of sensation, but affected individuals often have a normal lifespan. SCA5 often has an adult onset, and is slowly progressive, not affecting the lifespan. SCA6 often has a later onset, progresses very slowly, and does not shorten the lifespan. SCA7 involves progressive visual loss that eventually leads to blindness. SCA8 may cause sensory loss, but people have a normal lifespan. SCA10 may cause affected individuals to develop seizures. SCA11 is a relatively mild type, resulting in a normal lifespan for the affected person. SCA12 cases often develop a tremor as the first noticeable symptom and the people may eventually develop **dementia**. SCA13 may cause individuals to be shorter than average and have mild mental retardation. SCA14 may have an early onset, between 12 and 42 years of age, with an average of 28 years of age. SCA15 and 22 may be slow to progress, with SCA22 sometimes being early onset. SCA16 may involve tremors, SCA17 may involve mental deterioration, and SCA19 may involve both. SCA20 may result in calcification of some brain areas that shows up on brain imaging tests. SCA21 can be early onset, but involve only mild cognitive impairment. SCA23 is late onset and may involve sensory loss. SCA25 may also cause sensory loss. SCA26 may involve irregular eye movements.

### Diagnosis

Genetic forms of ataxia must be distinguished from non-genetic causes of ataxia that may have their own, individual treatment. Non-genetic causes of ataxia are not types of SCA, and include **alcoholism**, vitamin deficiencies, **multiple sclerosis**, vascular disease, and some cancers. The genetic forms of ataxia, such as SCA, are diagnosed by family history, physical examination, and brain imaging.

An initial workup of people who are having symptoms of ataxia will include questions about a person's medical history and a physical examination. Magnetic resonance imaging (MRI) of the brain in people with SCA will usually show degeneration, or atrophy, of the cerebellum and may be helpful in suggesting a diagnosis of SCA. A thorough family history should be taken to determine if others in the family have similar symptoms and the inheritance pattern in the family.

Since there is so much overlap between symptoms in the different types of SCA, it is not usually possible to tell the different types apart based on clinical symptoms. The only way to definitively diagnose SCA and determine a specific subtype is by **genetic testing**, which involves drawing a small amount of blood. The DNA in the blood cells is then examined, and the number of CAG repeats in each of the SCA genes is counted. Clinical testing is available to detect the mutations that cause SCA1, 2, 3, 6, 7, 8, 10, 12, 14, and 17. These tests may be offered as two sequential groups based on population frequency. Testing is often first performed for the more common ataxias, SCA1 through SCA7. Testing for the less common hereditary ataxias are often individualized as appropriate. Factors that may indicate testing for less common SCA types may include factors, such as ethnic background (SCA10 in the Mexican population), or specific symptoms, such as the presence of a tremor (SCA12). In these cases, testing can be performed for a single disease. If genetic testing is negative for the available testing, it does not mean that a person does not have SCA. It could mean that they have a type of SCA for which genetic testing is not yet available.

It is possible to test someone who is at risk for developing SCA before they are showing symptoms to see whether they inherited an expanded trinucleotide repeat. This is called predictive testing. Predictive testing cannot determine the age of onset that someone will begin to have symptoms, or the course of the disease. The decision to undergo this testing is a very personal decision. Some people choose to have testing so that they can make decisions about having children or about their future education, career, or finances. Protocols for predictive testing have been developed, and only certain centers perform this testing. Most centers require that the diagnosis of SCA has been confirmed by genetic testing in another family member.

A person who is interested in testing will be seen by a team of specialists over the course of a few visits. Often they will meet a neurologist who will perform a neurological examination to see if they may be showing early signs of the condition. If a person is having symptoms, testing may be performed to confirm the diagnosis. The person will also meet with a genetic counselor to talk about SCA, how it is inherited, and what testing can and cannot tell someone. They will also explore reasons for testing and what impact the results may have on their life, their family, their job, and their insurance. Most centers also require a person going through predictive testing to meet a few times with a psychologist. The purpose of these visits is to make sure that the person has thought through the decision to be tested and is prepared to deal with whatever the results may be.

If a child is having symptoms, it is appropriate to perform testing to confirm the cause of their symptoms. However, testing will not be performed on children who are at risk for developing SCA, but are not having symptoms. Children can make their own choice whether to know this information when they are old enough to make a mature decision. Testing a child who does not have symptoms could lead to possible problems with their future relationships, education, career, and insurance.

Testing a pregnant woman to determine whether an unborn child is affected is possible if genetic testing in a family has identified a certain type of SCA. This can be done between 10 and 12 weeks gestation by a procedure called chorionic villus sampling (CVS) that involves removing a tiny piece of the placenta and examining the cells. It can also be done by **amniocentesis** after 16 weeks gestation by removing a small amount of the amniotic fluid surrounding the fetus and analyzing the cells in the fluid. Each of these procedures has a small risk of miscarriage associated with it. Continuing a pregnancy that is found to be affected is like performing predictive testing on a child. Therefore, couples interested in these options should have **genetic counseling** to carefully explore all of the benefits and limitations of these procedures.

There is also another procedure, called preimplantation diagnosis, that allows a couple to have a child that is unaffected with the genetic condition in their family. This procedure is experimental and not widely available.

### Treatment and management

Although there is a lot of ongoing research to learn more about SCA and develop treatments, no cure currently exists for the SCAs. Although vitamin supplements are not a cure or treatment for SCA, they may be recommended if a person is taking in fewer calories because of feeding difficulties. Different types of therapy might be useful to help people maintain as independent a lifestyle as possible. An occupational therapist may be able to suggest adaptive devices to make the activities of daily living easier. Canes, walkers, and wheelchairs are often useful. A speech therapist may recommend devices that may make communication easier as speech progressively becomes affected. As swallowing becomes more difficult, a special swallow evaluation may lead to better strategies for eating and to help lessen the risk of choking.

Genetic counseling helps people and their families make decisions about their medical care, genetic testing, and having children. It can also help people

Yu–Wai–Man, P., et al. "Vertigo and vestibular abnormalities in spinocerebellar ataxia type 6." *Journal of Neurology* 256, no. 1 (January 2009): 78–82.

**WEBSITES**

*Ataxia.* Information Page, We Move, December 7, 2008 (May 02, 2009). http://www.wemove.org/ataxia/

*Ataxias and Cerebellar or Spinocerebellar Degeneration.* Information Page, NINDS, April 24, 2009 (May 02, 2009). http://www.ninds.nih.gov/disorders/ataxia/ataxia.htm

*Spinocerebellar Ataxia.* Information Page, Genes and Disease (May 02, 2009). http://www.ncbi.nlm.nih.gov/books/bv.fcgi?rid = gnd.section.218

**ORGANIZATIONS**

National Ataxia Foundation (NAF). 2600 Fernbrook Lane, Suite 119, Minneapolis, MN 55447-4752. (763)553-0020. Fax: (763)553-0167. Email: naf@ataxia.org. http://www.ataxia.org.

National Organization for Rare Disorders (NORD). 55 Kenosia Avenue, PO Box 1968, Danbury, CT 06813-1968. (203)744-0100 or (800)999-6673. Fax: (203)798-2291. http://www.rarediseases.org.

We Move. 204 West 84th St., New York, NY 10024. Email: wemove@wemove.org. http://www.wemove.org.

Maria Basile, PhD

Spinocerebellar atrophy I *see* **Spinocerebellar ataxia**

# Spondyloepiphyseal dysplasia

## Definition

Spondyloepiphyseal **dysplasia** is a rare hereditary disorder characterized by growth deficiency, spinal malformations, and, in some cases, ocular abnormalities.

## Description

Spondyloepiphyseal dysplasia is one of the most common causes of short stature. There are two forms of spondyloepiphyseal dysplasia. Both forms are inherited and both forms are rare.

### Congenital spondyloepiphyseal dysplasia

Congenital spondyloepiphyseal dysplasia is primarily characterized by prenatal growth deficiency and spinal malformations. Growth deficiency results in short stature (dwarfism). Abnormalities of the eyes may be present, including nearsightedness (**myopia**) and retina (the nerve–rich membrane lining the eye) detachment in

---

### QUESTIONS TO ASK YOUR DOCTOR

- A distant relative was once diagnosed with spinocerebellar ataxia. Is there any way of knowing if I am at risk for this condition?
- What are the most common symptoms associated with this disorder?
- At what age does spinocerebellar ataxia first manifest?
- What is the prognosis for spinocerebellar ataxia once it has been diagnosed?

---

to deal with the medical and emotional issues that arise when there is a genetic condition diagnosed in the family.

## Prognosis

Most people with the SCAs do have progression of their symptoms that leads to fulltime use of a wheelchair. The duration of the disease after the onset of symptoms is about 10–30 years, but can vary depending in part to the number of trinucleotide repeats and age of onset. In general, people with a larger number of repeats have an earlier age of onset and more severe symptoms. Choking can be a major hazard because, if food gets into the lungs, a life-threatening pneumonia can result. As the condition progresses, it can become difficult for people to cough and clear secretions. Most people die from respiratory failure or pulmonary complications.

## Resources

**BOOKS**

Brice, Alexis, and Stefan–M. Pulst. *Spinocerebellar Degenerations: The Ataxias and Spastic Paraplegias.* Oxford, UK: Butterworth–Heinemann, 2007.

Fernandez, Hubert H. *A Practical Approach to Movement Disorders: Diagnosis, Medical and Surgical Management.* New York, NY: Demos Medical Publishing, 2007.

**PERIODICALS**

Globas, C., et al. "Early symptoms in spinocerebellar ataxia type 1, 2, 3, and 6." *Movement Disorders* 23, no. 15 (November 2008): 2232–2238.

Labauge, P., et al. "Beta–mannosidosis: a new cause of spinocerebellar ataxia." *Clinical Neurology and Neurosurgery* 111, no. 1 (January 2009): 109–110.

Lee, Y. C., et al. "The 'hot cross bun' sign in the patients with spinocerebellar ataxia." *European Journal of Neurology* 16, no. 4 (April 2009): 513–516.

## KEY TERMS

**Cleft palate**—A congenital malformation in which there is an abnormal opening in the roof of the mouth that allows the nasal passages and the mouth to be improperly connected.

**Coxa vara**—A deformed hip joint in which the neck of the femur is bent downward.

**Dysplasia**—The abnormal growth or development of a tissue or organ.

**Hypotonia**—Reduced or diminished muscle tone.

**Kyphoscoliosis**—Abnormal front–to–back and side–to–side curvature of the spine.

**Lumbar lordosis**—Abnormal inward curvature of the spine.

**Malar hypoplasia**—Small or underdeveloped cheekbones.

**Myopia**—Nearsightedness. Difficulty seeing objects that are far away.

**Ochronosis**—A condition marked by pigment deposits in cartilage, ligaments, and tendons.

**Ossification**—The process of the formation of bone from its precursor, a cartilage matrix.

**Retina**—The light–sensitive layer of tissue in the back of the eye that receives and transmits visual signals to the brain through the optic nerve.

approximately half of individuals with the disorder. Congenital spondyloepiphyseal dysplasia is inherited as an autosomal dominant genetic trait.

Congenital spondyloepiphyseal dysplasia is also known as SED, congenital type; SED congenita; and SEDC.

### Spondyloepiphyseal dysplasia tarda

Spondyloepiphyseal dysplasia tarda primarily affects males. It is characterized by dwarfism and hunched appearance of the spine. The disorder doesn't become evident until five to 10 years of age. Spondyloepiphyseal dysplasia tarda is an X–linked recessive inherited disorder.

Spondyloepiphyseal dysplasia tarda is also known as SEDT; spondyloepiphyseal dysplasia, late; and SED tarda, X–linked.

### Genetic profile

Both forms of the disorder are inherited, however they are inherited differently.

### Congenital spondyloepiphyseal dysplasia

Congenital spondyloepiphyseal dysplasia is thought to probably always result from abnormalities in the COL2A1 **gene**, which codes for type II collagen. Collagen is a protein that is a component of bone, cartilage, and connective tissue. A variety of abnormalities (such as deletions and duplications) involving the COL2A1 gene may lead to the development of the disorder.

It is one of a group of skeletal dysplasias (dwarfing conditions) caused by changes in type II collagen. These include **hypochondrogenesis**; spondyloepimetaphyseal dysplasia, Strudwick (SEMD); and **Kniest dysplasia**. Type 2 collagen is the major collagen of a component of the spine called the nucleus pulposa, of cartilage, and of vitreous (a component of the eye). All of these conditions have common clinical and radiographic findings including spinal changes resulting in dwarfism, myopia, and retinal degeneration.

Congenital spondyloepiphyseal dysplasia is inherited as an autosomal dominant genetic trait. In autosomal dominant **inheritance**, a single abnormal gene on one of the autosomal chromosomes (one of the first 22 "non–sex" chromosomes) from either parent can cause the disease. One of the parents will have the disease (since it is dominant) and is the carrier. Only one parent needs to be a carrier in order for the child to inherit the disease. A child who has one parent with the disease has a 50% chance of also having the disease.

Autosomal recessive inheritance of congenital spondyloepiphyseal dysplasia has been considered in cases when a child with the disorder is born to parents who are not affected by the disorder. It considered more likely that in these cases the disorder resulted from germline mosaicism in the collagen Type II gene of the parent. Germline mosaicism occurs when the causal mutation, instead of involving a single germ cell, is carried only by a certain proportion of the germ cells of a given parent. Thus, the parent carries the mutation in his or her germ cells and therefore runs the risk of generating more than one affected child, but does not actually express the disease.

### Spondyloepiphyseal dysplasia tarda

Spondyloepiphyseal dysplasia tarda is caused by mutations in the TRAPPC2 (also called SEDL) gene, which is located on the X **chromosome** at locus Xp22.2–p22.1. This gene provides instructions for producing the protein sedlin, believed to be part of a large molecule called the trafficking protein particle (TRAPP) complex, known to plays a role in the transport of proteins between various cell compartments.

Spondyloepiphyseal dysplasia tarda is inherited as an X–linked disorder. The following concepts are important to understanding the inheritance of an X–linked disorder. All humans have two chromosomes that determine their gender: females have XX, males have XY. X–linked recessive, also called sex–linked, inheritance affects the genes located on the X chromosome. It occurs when an unaffected mother carries a disease–causing gene on at least one of her X chromosomes. Because females have two X chromosomes, they are usually unaffected carriers. The X chromosome that does not have the disease–causing gene compensates for the X chromosome that does. For a woman to show symptoms of the disorder, both X chromosomes would have the disease–causing gene. That is why women are less likely to show such symptoms than males.

If a mother has a female child, the child has a 50% chance of inheriting the disease gene and being a carrier who can pass the disease gene on to her sons. On the other hand, if a mother has a male child, he has a 50% chance of inheriting the disease–causing gene because he has only one X chromosome. If a male inherits an X–linked recessive disorder, he is affected. All of his daughters will be carriers, but none of his sons.

### Demographics

Spondyloepiphyseal dysplasia is rare and its incidence is unknown. As of 2008, some 175 cases of congenital spondyloepiphyseal dysplasia had been reported. As for spondyloepiphyseal dysplasia tarda, its incidence is estimated at 1 in 150,000 to 200,000 people worldwide.

Congenital spondyloepiphyseal dysplasia affects both males and females. Spondyloepiphyseal dysplasia tarda affects mostly males.

### Signs and symptoms

#### Congenital spondyloepiphyseal dysplasia

Congenital spondyloepiphyseal dysplasia is characterized by these main features:

- Prenatal growth deficiency occurs prior to birth, and growth deficiencies continue after birth and throughout childhood, resulting in short stature (dwarfism). Adult height ranges from approximately 36–67 in (91–170 cm).
- Spinal malformations include a disproportionately short neck and trunk and a hip deformity wherein the thigh bone is angled toward the center of the body (coxa vara). Abnormal front–to–back and side–to–side curvature of the spine (kyphoscoliosis) may

occur, as may an abnormal inward curvature of the spine (lumbar lordosis). Spinal malformations are partially responsible for short stature.

- Hypotonia (diminished muscle tone), muscle weakness, and/or stiffness is exhibited in most cases.
- Progressive nearsightedness (myopia) may develop and/or retinal detachment. Retinal detachment, which can result in blindness, occurs in approximately 50% of cases.
- An abnormally flat face, underdevelopment of the cheek bone (malar hypoplasia), and/or cleft palate may present in some individuals with congenital spondyloepiphyseal dysplasia.
- Additional associated abnormalities may include underdevelopment of the abdominal muscles; a rounded, bulging chest (barrel chest) with a prominent sternum (pectus carinatum); diminished joint movements in the lower extremities; the heel of the foot may be turned inward toward body while the rest of the foot is bent downward and inward (clubfoot); and rarely, hearing impairment due to abnormalities of the inner ear may occur.

The hypotonia, muscle weakness, and spinal malformations may result in a delay in affected children learning to walk. In some cases, affected children may exhibit an unusual "waddling" gait.

#### Spondyloepiphyseal dysplasia tarda

Symptoms of spondyloepiphyseal dysplasia tarda are not usually apparent until five to 10 years of age. At that point, a number of symptoms begin to appear:

- abnormal growth causes mild dwarfism,
- spinal growth appears to stop and the trunk is short,
- the shoulder may assume a hunched appearance,
- the neck appears to become shorter,
- the chest broadens (barrel chest),
- additional associated abnormalities may include unusual facial features such as a flat appearance to the face. Progressive degenerative arthritis may affect hips and other joints of the body.

Spine and hip changes become evident between 10 and 14 years of age. In adolescence, various skeletal abnormalities may cause pain in the back, hips, shoulders, knees and ankles, a large chest cage, and relatively normal limb length. In adulthood, height usually ranges from 52 to 62 inches; hands, head and feet appear to be normal size.

## Diagnosis

X–rays may be used to diagnose spondyloepiphyseal dysplasia when it is suspected.

### Congenital spondyloepiphyseal dysplasia

Individuals with congenital spondyloepiphyseal dysplasia have characteristic x–rays that show delayed ossification of the axial skeleton with ovoid vertebral bodies. With time, the vertebral bodies appear flattened. There is delayed ossification of the femoral heads, pubic bones, and heel. The coxa vara deformity of the hip joint is common.

It should be noted that x–rays of individuals with spondyloepimetaphyseal dysplasia type Strudwick are virtually identical to congenital spondyloepiphyseal dysplasia. In early childhood, irregularity in the region beneath the ends of bones (metaphyseal) and thickening of the bones (sclerosis) are noted in spondyloepimetaphyseal dysplasia type Strudwick. Also, there is platyspondyly (flattened vertebral bodies) and odontoid hypoplasia.

### Spondyloepiphyseal dysplasia tarda

Radiologic diagnosis cannot be established before 4–6 years of age. Symptoms usually begin to present between five and 10 years of age. Symptomatic changes in the spine and hips usually present between 10 and 14 years of age.

In adults, vertebral changes especially in the lumbar region, may be diagnostic. Ochronosis (pigment deposits in cartilage, ligaments, and tendons) is suggested by apparent intervertebral disc calcification, and the vertebral bodies are malformed and flattened with most of the dense area part of the vertebral plate.

### Genetic counseling

**Genetic counseling** may be of benefit for patients and their families.

In congenital spondyloepiphyseal dysplasia, only one parent needs to be a carrier in order for the child to inherit the disorder. A child has a 50% chance of having the disorder if one parent has the disorder and a 75% chance of having the disease if both parents have congenital spondyloepiphyseal dysplasia.

In spondyloepiphyseal dysplasia tarda, if a mother has a male child, he has a 50% chance of inheriting the disease–causing gene. A male who inherits an X–linked recessive disorder is affected, and all of his daughters will be carriers, but none of his sons.

### Prenatal testing

Prenatal testing may be available to couples at risk for bearing a child with spondyloepiphyseal dysplasia. Testing for the genes responsible for congenital spondyloepiphyseal dysplasia and spondyloepiphyseal dysplasia tarda is possible. Congenital spondyloepiphyseal dysplasia testing may be difficult, however, since although the gene has been located, there is variability in the mutations in the gene amongst persons with the disorder.

Either chorionic villus sampling (CVS) or **amniocentesis** may be performed for prenatal testing. CVS is a procedure to obtain chorionic villi tissue for testing. Examination of fetal tissue can reveal information about the defects that lead to spondyloepiphyseal dysplasia. Chorionic villus sampling can be performed at 10–12 weeks gestation.

Amniocentesis is a procedure that involves inserting a thin needle into the uterus, into the amniotic sac, and withdrawing a small amount of amniotic fluid. **DNA** can be extracted from the fetal cells contained in the amniotic fluid and tested. Amniocentesis is performed at 16–18 weeks gestation.

## Treatment and management

Individuals with spondyloepiphyseal dysplasia should be under routine health supervision by a physician who is familiar with the disorder, its complications, and its treatment.

### Congenital spondyloepiphyseal dysplasia

Treatment is mostly symptomatic, and may include:

- Orthopedic care throughout life. Early surgical interventional may be needed to correct clubfoot and/or cleft palate. Hip, spinal, and knee complications may occur, and hip replacement is sometimes warranted in adults. Additionally, arthritis may develop due to poorly developed type II collagen. Spinal fusion may be indicated if evaluation of the cervical vertebrae C1 and C2 detects odontoid hypoplasia. If the odontoid is hypoplastic or small, it may predispose to instability and spinal cord compression in congenital spondyloepiphyseal dysplasia).

- Ophthalmologic examinations are important for the prevention of retinal detachment and treatment of myopia and early retinal tears if they occur.

- Hearing should be checked and ear infections should be closely monitored. Tubes may need to be placed in the ear.

- Due to neck instability, persons with SEDC should exercise caution to avoid activities/sports that could result in trauma to the neck or head.

Individuals with congenital spondyloepiphyseal dysplasia should be closely monitored during anesthesia and for complications during a respiratory infection. In particular, during anesthesia, special attention is required to avoid spinal injury resulting from lax ligaments causing instability in the neck. This condition may also result in spinal injury in contact sports and car accidents. Chest constriction may also cause decreased lung capacity.

### Spondyloepiphyseal dysplasia tarda

Treatment is mostly symptomatic, and may include:

- Physical therapy to relieve joint stiffness and pain.

- Orthopedic care may be needed at different times throughout life. Bone changes of the femoral head often lead to secondary osteoarthritis during adulthood and some patients require total replacement of the hip before the age of 40 years.

Some individuals with short stature resulting from spondyloepiphyseal dysplasia may consider limb-lengthening surgery. This is a controversial surgery that lengthens leg and arm bones by cutting the bones, constructing metal frames around them, and inserting pins into them to move the cut ends apart. New bone tissue fills in the gap. While the surgery can be effective in lengthening limbs, various complications may occur.

### Prognosis

Prognosis is variable dependent upon severity of the disorder. Generally, congenital spondyloepiphyseal dysplasia is more symptomatic than spondyloepiphyseal dysplasia tarda. Neither form of the disorder generally leads to shortened life span. Cognitive function is generally normal.

### Resources

**BOOKS**

Parker, Philip M. *Spondyloepiphyseal Dysplasia Congenita —A Bibliography and Dictionary for Physicians, Patients, and Genome Researchers.* San Diego, CA: Icon Health Publications, 2007.

Stevenson, Roger E., and Judith G. Hall, editors. *Human Malformations and Related Anomalies,* 2nd edition, New York, NY: Oxford University Press, 2006.

**PERIODICALS**

Bal, S., et al. "Spondyloepiphyseal dysplasia tarda: four cases from two families." *European Journal of Neurology* 29, no. 6 (April 2009): 699–702.

Cui, Y. X., et al. "Rapid molecular prenatal diagnosis of spondyloepiphyseal dysplasia congenita by PCR–SSP assay." *Genetic Testing* 12, no. 4 (December 2008): 533–536.

Xia, X., et al. "A first familial G504S mutation of COL2A1 gene results in distinctive spondyloepiphyseal dysplasia congenita." *Clinica Chimica Acta* 382, no. 1–2 (July 2007): 148–150.

**WEBSITES**

*Congenital Spondyloepiphyseal Dysplasia.* Information Page, Rare Diseases in Sweden, March 3, 2009 (May 17, 2009). http://www.socialstyrelsen.se/en/rarediseases/Congenital+spondyloepiphyseal+dysplasia.htm

*Dwarfism.* Health Topic, Medline Plus, May 18, 2009 (May 17, 2009). http://www.nlm.nih.gov/medlineplus/dwarfism.html

*Late–Onset Spondyloepiphyseal dysplasia.* Information Page, Rare Diseases in Sweden, March 3, 2009 (May 17, 2009). http://www.socialstyrelsen.se/en/rarediseases/Late-onset+spondyloepiphyseal+dysplasia.htm

*Spondyloepiphyseal Dysplasia Congenita.* Information Page, Madisons Foundation, 2009 (May 17, 2009). http://www.madisonsfoundation.org/index.php/component/option,com_mpower/Itemid,49/diseaseID,625

*Spondyloepiphyseal Dysplasia, Congenital.* Information Page, NORD, November 26, 2008 (May 17, 2009). http://www.rarediseases.org/search/rdbdetail_abstract.html?disname=Spondyloepiphyseal+Dysplasia,+Congenital

*Spondyloepiphyseal Dysplasia Tarda.* Information Page, NORD, November 26, 2008 (May 17, 2009). http://www.rarediseases.org/search/rdbdetail_abstract.html?disname=Spondyloepiphyseal+Dysplasia+Tarda

*Spondylo–Epiphyseal Dysplasia.* Information Page, Nemours Foundation, October 2, 2007 (May 17, 2009). http://www.nemours.org/hospital/de/aidhc/service/skeletal/disorder/spondylo-epiphyseal.html

## ORGANIZATIONS

Human Growth Foundation. 997 Glen Cove Ave., Glen Head, NY 11545. (516)671-4041 or (800)451-6434. E-mail: hgf1@hgfound.org. http://www.hgfound.org.

Little People of America. 250 El Camino Real, Suite 201, Tustin, CA 92780. (888)LPA-2001 or (714)368-3689. Fax: (714)368-3367. Email: info@lpaonline.org. http://www.lpaonline.org.

National Organization for Rare Disorders (NORD). 55 Kenosia Avenue, PO Box 1968, Danbury, CT 06813-1968. (203)744-0100 or (800)999-6673. Fax: (203)798-2291. http://www.rarediseases.org.

Jennifer F. Wilson, MS

# I Spondyloepiphyseal dysplasia congenita

## Definition

**Spondyloepiphyseal dysplasia** congenita (SEDC) is a form of dwarfism (**achondroplasia**) that is caused by a **gene** mutation interfering with prenatal bone development. People with SEDC have a short physique, misshaped bones and a flattened face. The name for this condition was derived from the Greek words spondylos (referring to the spine) and epiphyseal (referring to the formative areas of the bones). The Greek word **dysplasia** refers to abnormal tissue formation.

## Demographics

This condition is most often caused by a sporadic mutation; therefore, it is very rare. It is estimated that it is observed in only 1 out of 100,000 births. Since it is a recently discovered disorder, the exact number is not yet established. The gene responsible for this disorder has been determined to be autosomal dominant. This means that it is not sex related; men and women are equally affected. Because most cases are due to a sporadic mutation, there are no racial trends in its occurrence, as is true for most cases of achondroplasia.

## Description

This disorder is caused by a mutation on the gene responsible for producing collagen II. Collagen II is an organic gel that influences the transformation of cartilage into bone. It is also essential in developing the lubricants of the joints and the eyes. People with SEDC are affected mostly in the development and structure of their bones. Almost half suffer from **myopia**, or near sightedness. There is no effect on intellectual function.

SEDC is distinguished from other forms of achondroplasia by its onset at birth and by the mutation causing it. Spondyloepiphyseal dysplasia tarda is not observable until later in life. The most notable feature of SEDC is the short stature of those affected. Other observable features a skeletal framework being that is not properly aligned and that has an abnormal shape. The chest is barrel shaped and the trunk and the neck are unusually short.

Some of the expected characteristics of people with SEDC include the following:

- Shortened limbs
- Average-sized hands and feet
- Abnormal spine curvature
- Vertebral instability in the neck
- Flattened vertebrae
- Bow legs
- Early onset of arthritis
- Flattened face

Other characteristics may include:

- Clubfoot in one or both feet
- Moderate hearing loss
- Lack of muscle tone
- Cleft palate

Some of the common deformities that continue to cause problems throughout person's life include hip and knee irregularities that may cause pain in the joints and contribute to abnormal walking patterns. Many people with SEDC suffer from spinal deformities that contribute to breathing and standing problems. Most have a curvature of the spine to some degree. Spinal deformities contribute to a rigid posture and uncontrollable spasms throughout the skeletal system. Spinal cord compression can result from these deformities, creating even more complications.

## Causes and symptoms

The skeletal disorder SEDC is caused by a mutations in the COL2A1 gene on **chromosome** 12. This gene is responsible for producing collagen II, which is essential in the development of the lubricants for the bones and eyes. It is also involved in the prenatal development of bone from cartilage. Any mutation in the COL2A1 gene interferes with proper development of bones and, more generally, the skeletal system. Because the mutation produces an autosomal dominant trait, only one gene with the mutation is necessary for the condition to occur. Most observed

## QUESTIONS TO ASK YOUR DOCTOR

- What corrective surgery should I expect?
- How do other people with SEDC cope with daily living skills?
- Is genetic counseling important for my situation?
- What are the chances that a child of mine will be born with SEDC?
- How often should I be physically evaluated per year?
- What do I do when conditions get worse?

cases are from sporadic mutations, which means that the parents had normal genes that for some reason mutated. However, a person with the mutation could pass it on to offspring who would then have a 50% chance of developing the condition, given that both parents do not have the disorder.

The siblings of affected individuals have no chance of passing the trait on to their children. If both parents have the mutated genes, there is a 50% chance that either one will pass on the gene to the child who will then develop SEDC. There is a 25% chance that neither parent will pass on the gene; the child will grow normally. However, there is a 25% chance that both will pass on the gene; in this case, the child is not likely to survive the first few years of life.

### Diagnosis

There are signs of this form of achondroplasia that are observable from birth. However, ascertaining that this condition is actually SEDC with its accompanying complications is only possible through a blood test. Unlike other congenital forms of achondroplasia, babies with SEDC show signs of the disorder; they tend to have a flattened spine and a flattened face because of poorly developed facial muscle. The short stature, along with the disproportionate ratio of head to body and trunk to body, indicates that the baby has some form of achondroplasia; the face and spine indicate that it is very likely SEDC.

Because these characteristics are observed at birth, the question arises, "Why are they not observable through the prenatal ultrasound?" Most ultrasound images of the developing fetus are not powerful enough to detect the subtle features that would suggest achondroplasia, or more specifically SEDC.

As the child with SEDC grows, development must be constantly assessed. Normal scale of development, particularly motor development, may indicate delays. However, there should be normal development expected for cognitive and language development. All areas of motor and skeletal development should be constantly assessed, including signs for spinal cord compression, motor weakness, problems with walking and a lack of physical endurance. The prevalent curvature of the spine is expected to increase with age and should be continuously assessed as it tends to lead to problems with flexibility in the hips. Any deformation observed at birth or with later development has a strong likelihood of contributing to later deterioration of any part of the skeletal system. Particular attention should be given to problems of the hips.

### Treatment

Although there are some forms of achondroplasia that respond well to growth therapies, the treatment for SEDC and most forms of achondroplasia is not focused on increasing physical stature. Because SEDC is not a result of growth hormone deficiency, growth therapies would not be appropriate. The various treatments for SEDC are concerned with easing associated disabilities and delaying any perceived deterioration.

#### Traditional treatment

The usual treatment for children with any form of achondroplasia is continuous evaluations by a team of specialists. This is especially true for the child with SEDC who has to face the strong possibility of deterioration in sight, hearing, breathing, and motor function. Orthopedic surgery is a certainty; however, physical therapy and adaptive devices may reduce the number of operations necessary. Some of the more common adaptive devices include leg braces, forearm crutches, and orthopedic footwear.

Some of the purposes of orthopedic surgery include procedures to help steer growing bones into the appropriate direction. Another procedure designed for straightening out a crooked bone involves breaking the bone and then resetting it as straight. Metal plates are inserted to hold it in the corrected position. Surgery to correct the curved spine is common, as well as surgery to offset spinal compression.

In recent years there have been experiments to lengthen the limbs of people with achondroplasia. This procedure is controversial because it means having the child undergo surgery and does not resolve the underlying problems of SEDC and undergoing the procedure implies that there is something wrong with short height. In this surgical procedure, a bone is broken and the two parts of the bone are attached to a metal rod. The bone is expected to grow around the rod and the limb is expected to stretch to accommodate the new length. However, the deficiency of collagen II still exists for the person undergoing this surgery. The bone cannot grow at a normal or predictable rate. The deterioration and lack of lubrication in the joints will still continue.

## Prognosis

The first point in considering the prognosis for a person born with SEDC is that there is no cure. The baby born with SEDC will still have the condition into adulthood. For the most part life expectancy is no different for someone born with SEDC than for the general population. There are two exceptions. The first exception is that the child who inherits the mutated gene from both parents is not likely to live past the third birthday. However, since most cases are due to sporadic mutations, this situation is very rare. The other exception is that neck injuries pose a greater threat for the person with SEDC. Thus, children with the disorder must be extremely careful in situations that could cause neck injuries.

## Prevention

Because most cases are unpredictable due to a spontaneous mutation, it is not easy to detect SEDC before birth. The differences suggesting SEDC are too subtle in the developing fetus to detect in the womb by ultrasound. However, recent research conducted by at the Clinical School of Medical College, Nanjing University in China has demonstrated that detection through analysis of amniotic fluid is possible. Detecting the mutation for SEDC is not usually a goal of typical **amniocentesis** because the condition is so rare. Prenatal counseling is recommended for a couple when one or both are carriers of the mutated gene. It is also recommended when the father is over 56 years of age, because more mutations take place in the sperm of older men.

## Resources

### BOOKS

Parker, Philip M. *Spondyloepiphyseal Dysplasia Congenita - A Bibliography and Dictionary for Physicians, Patients, and Genome Researchers* . San Diego: Icon Group International, 2007.

Castriota-Scanderbeg, Alessandro, and Bruno Dallapiccola. *Abnormal Skeletal Phenotypes: From Simple Signs to Complex Diagnoses* New York: Springer, 2005.

### PERIODICALS

Ying-Xia Cui, et al. Rapid Molecular Prenatal Diagnosis of Spondyloepiphyseal Dysplasia Congenita by PCR-SSP Assay *Genetic Testing* 12(2008):533–536.

### WEB SITES

Madisons Foundation. http://www.madisonsfoundation.org/index.php/component/option,com_mpower/Itemid,49/diseaseID,625.

Mayo Clinic. Dwarfism: Treatments and Drugs. *http://www.mayoclinic.com/health/dwarfism/DS01012/DSECTION=treatments-and-drugs*

### ORGANIZATIONS

Shital Parikh, Alvin H. Crawford, and Preeti Batra. Spondyloepiphyseal Dysplasia *http://emedicine.medscape.com/article/1260836-overview*

Human Growth Foundation, 997 Glen Cove Avenue, Suite 5, Glen Head, NY, 11545, 800-451-6434, www.hgfound.org.

Little People of America, Inc., 250 El Camino Real, Suite 201, Tustin, CA, 92780, (888)572-2001, www.lpaonline.org.

Ray F Brogan, PhD

# SRY (sex determining region Y)

## Definition

The sex determining region Y (SRY) **gene** is located on the Y **chromosome**. SRY is the main genetic switch for the sexual development of the human male. If the SRY gene is present in a developing embryo, typically it will become male.

## Description

The development of sex in a human depends on the presence or absence of an Y chromosome. Chromosomes are the structures in our cells that contain genes. Genes instruct the body on how to grow and develop by making proteins. For example, genes (and the proteins they make) are responsible for what color hair or eyes a person may have, how tall they will be, and what color skin they will have. Genes also direct the development of organs, such as the heart and brain. Genes are constructed out of **DNA, deoxyribonucleic acid**. DNA is found in the shape of a double helix, like a twisted ladder. The DNA contains the "letters" of the genetic code that make up the "words" or genes that govern the development of the

**Flow chart of human sex differentiation**

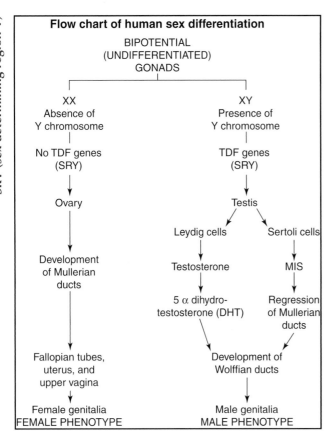

Flow chart of male and female sex differentiation from conception through development. *(Gale, a part of Cengage Learning.)*

body. The genes are found in the "books" or chromosomes in the cells.

Normally, there are 46 chromosomes, or 23 pairs, in each cell. The first 22 pairs are the same in men and women and are called the autosomes. The last pair, the sex chromosomes, consists of two X chromosomes in females (XX) and an X and an Y chromosome in males (XY). These 23 pairs of chromosomes contain approximately 35,000 genes.

Human males differ from human females in the fact that they have an Y chromosome and females do not. Scientists thought there must be a gene on the Y chromosome that is responsible for determining maleness. The gene for determining maleness was called TDF for testis determining factor. In 1990, the SRY gene was found and scientist believed it was the TDF gene they had been looking for. The evidence scientists had to show SRY was indeed TDF included the fact that is was located on the Y chromosome. When SRY was found in individuals with two X chromosomes

(normally females) these individuals had male physical features. Furthermore, some individuals with XY sex chromosomes that had female physical features had mutations or alterations in their SRY gene. Finally, experiments were done on mice that showed a male mouse would develop when SRY was put into a chromosomally female embryo. This evidence proved that SRY is the TDF gene that triggers the pathway of a developing embryo to become male. While the SRY gene triggers the pathway to the development of a male, it is not the only gene responsible for sexual development. Most likely, the SRY gene serves to regulate the activity of other genes in this pathway.

## Genetic profile

Men and women both have 23 pairs of chromosomes—22 pairs of autosomes and one pair of sex chromosomes (either XX in females or XY in males). The SRY gene is located on the Y chromosome. When a man and woman have a child, it is the man's chromosomes that determine if the baby will be male or female. This is because the baby inherits one of its sex chromosomes from the mother and one from the father. The mother has only X chromosomes to pass on, while the father can pass on either his X chromosome or his Y chromosome. If he passes on his X chromosome, the baby will be female. If he passes on his Y chromosome (with the SRY gene) the baby will be male. Statistically, each pregnancy has a 50% chance of being female and a 50% chance of being male. The Y chromosome is the smallest human chromosome and the SRY region contains a very small number of genes.

## Signs and symptoms

Individuals with point mutations or deletions of the SRY gene have a condition known as gonadal dysgenesis, XY female type, also called Swyer syndrome. At birth the individuals with the XY female type of gonadal dysgenesis appear to be normal females (with female inner and outer genitalia), however, they do not develop secondary sexual characteristics at puberty, do not menstruate, and have "streak" (undeveloped) gonads. They have normal stature and an increased incidence of certain neoplasms (gonadoblastoma and germinoma).

### Normal development

In normal human sexual development, there are two stages called determination and differentiation. Determination occurs at conception when a sperm from a man fertilizes an egg from a woman. If the sperm has an Y chromosome, the conception will eventually become male. If no Y chromosome is present, the conception will become female.

Though the determination of sex occurs at conception, the differentiation of the developing gonads (future ovaries in the female and testes in the males) does not occur until about seven weeks. Until that time, the gonads look the same in both sexes and are called undifferentiated or indifferent. At this point in development, the embryo has two sets of ducts: the Mullerian ducts that form the fallopian tubes, uterus and upper vagina in females and the Wolffian ducts that form the epididymis, vas deferens, and seminal vesicles in males.

In embryos with SRY present, the undifferentiated gonads will develop into the male testes. The testes produce two hormones that cause the differentiation into maleness. Mullerian inhibiting substance (MIS), also called anti-mullerian hormone (AMH), causes the Mullerian ducts to regress and the Wolffian ducts develop into the internal male structures. Testosterone also helps with the development of the Wolffian ducts and causes the external genitals to become male.

When SRY is not present, the pathway of sexual development is shifted into female development. The undifferentiated gonads become ovaries. The Mullerian ducts develop into the internal female structures and the Wolffian ducts regress. The external genitals do not masculinize and become female.

### SRY and male development

How the SRY gene causes an undifferentiated gonad to become a testis and eventually determine the maleness of a developing embryo is not completely understood. What scientists believe happens is that SRY is responsible for "triggering" a pathway of other genes that cause the gonad to continue to develop into a testis. The SRY protein is known to go into the nucleus of a cell and physically bend the DNA. This bending of DNA may allow other genes to be turned on that are needed in this pathway. For example, anti-Mullerian hormone is thought to be indirectly turned on by SRY.

It is also thought that a threshold exists that must be met at a very specific time for SRY to trigger this pathway. This means that enough SRY protein must be made early in development (before seven weeks) to turn an undifferentiated gonad into a testis. If enough SRY is not present or if it is present too late in development, the gonad will shift into the female pathway.

### Other genes in sex development

Several other genes have been found that are involved in the development of human sex, including the gene SOX9. Mutations or alterations in this gene can cause a condition called camptomelic **dysplasia**. People with camptomelic dysplasia have bone and cartilage changes. SOX9 alterations also cause male to female sex reversal in most affected individuals (male chromosomes and female features). It is not known how SRY, SOX9, and other genes in the sexual developmental pathway interact to turn an undifferentiated gonad into a testis or an ovary.

## Resources

### PERIODICALS

Zenteno, J.C., et al. "Clinical Expression and SRY Gene Analysis in XY Subjects Lacking Gonadal Tissue."

*American Journal of Medical Genetics* 99 (March 15, 2001): 244-47.

**WEBSITES**

"Sex-determining Region Y." *Online Mendelian Inheritance in Man*. http://www.ncbi.nlm.nih.gov/entrez/dispomim. cgi?id = 480000.

Carin Lea Beltz, MS

# Stargardt disease

## Definition

Stargardt disease (STGD) is an inherited vision disorder with macular degeneration that typically affects younger people.

## Description

STGD is the most common form of inherited macular degeneration (or dystrophy), a disorder of the retina, that affects younger people. The condition is also known as Stargardt macular dystrophy, juvenile macular degeneration, macular dystrophy with flecks, and fundus flavimaculatus.

Common symptoms of STGD include progressive loss of central vision, problems identifying and differentiating colors, and difficulty seeing fine details clearly.

## Genetic profile

There are different types of STGD. The most common form is Type 1, which is associated with autosomal recessive **inheritance**. In this type, there may be no family history of the condition, and it usually affects only one generation. A couple has a 25% chance of having another affected son or daughter once a child is diagnosed with STGD Type 1. This type of STGD is associated with mutations in the ABCA4 (or ABCR) gene, which is located on **chromosome** 1. This gene is involved in moving vitamin A compounds naturally to and from cells in the retina; these cells are often impaired in STGD.

Other rarer forms of macular dystrophy with symptoms nearly identical to STGD have been called Stargardt-like macular dystrophy types 2, 3, and 4. These are associated with autosomal dominant inheritance. In these types, a family history of the condition is quite common and STGD may be present in several generations of a family tree. A parent with these macular dystrophies has a 50% chance of having an affected son or daughter. Some of these individuals

---

**KEY TERMS**

**Dystrophy**—Progressive abnormal changes in a tissue or organ.

**Fluorescein angiography**—Procedure to look at the blood vessel system of the eye. Fluorescein, a dye, is injected and photographs are taken as the dye passes through the eye's blood vessels.

**Fundus**—The interior back wall of the eyeball.

**Macular degeneration**—Progressive condition that affects the macula, a small portion of the retina at the back of the eye.

**Mutation**—Small change in the sequence of a gene.

**Photoreceptor**—Cells at the back of the eye that process the light that hit them; examples are cone and rod cells.

**Retina**—Structure at the back of the eye with multiple layers, containing different types of cells.

---

have been found to have mutations in the ELOVL4 gene on chromosome 6.

## Demographics

STGD is found worldwide, affecting males and females equally. The incidence for Type 1 is estimated to be between one in 1,600 and one in 15,000 individuals. In all, it accounts for 7% of all retinal dystrophies.

STGD Type 1 is usually diagnosed in individuals under the age of 20 when decreased central vision is the first problem noticed. In contrast, Stargardt-like macular dystrophies and age-related macular degeneration typically first show up in adulthood.

## Signs and symptoms

Each person with STGD experiences their symptoms differently. STGD affects the macula, a specialized portion of the retina that is highly responsible for the ability to see straight in front, notice colors, and see fine details. The macula is normally full of photoreceptors called cone cells. Cone cells help process the light rays that naturally hit the retina. In STGD, these cone cells slowly begin to die and lose function. In addition, the macula's appearance may begin showing abnormal yellow-white flecks that are shaped irregularly in people who have STGD.

Problems with central vision may be an early sign of STGD. The progression of this varies from person to person, and is impossible to predict. In addition, one's ability to see clearly (visual acuity) becomes progressively worse over time. This can progress from near-normal visual acuity to legal blindness. By the age of 50 years, about half of people with STGD have visual acuity equal to or worse than that of legal blindness. Unfortunately, the reduced visual acuity in STGD cannot usually be corrected with prescription eyeglasses or contact lenses.

In later stages of STGD, color vision can be impacted. People may have trouble identifying colors or distinguishing them from one another. Rarely, people may experience difficulty with brightly lit conditions, blind spots in their vision, and problems with adjusting to dark environments.

## Diagnosis

A diagnosis is most commonly made based on a person's symptoms. However, **genetic testing** is available to those suspected to have the condition. A few laboratories offer molecular testing of the ABCA4 and ELOVL4 genes on a clinical basis. Still others offer testing of these genes as part of a research study.

A young person who complains of problems with their central vision or has poor visual acuity that cannot be corrected should be tested for STGD. A combination of various visual investigations can help rule out other diagnoses and identify visual problems that are consistent with STGD.

A detailed eye examination with an ophthalmologist can help determine one's visual acuity and general eye health. The physician may want to track the visual acuity over time to determine whether it can be corrected with prescription eyeglasses or contact lenses. The ophthalmologist may also order visual tests to get more information about a diagnosis.

Testing of the visual fields can determine how much is being seen from left to right, and up and down. The full field of vision is studied to identify any blind spots or clarify whether the central vision is affected.

Fluorescein angiography (FA) can be helpful to determine whether blood flow is normal throughout the back of the eye. These detailed photographs of the eye's blood vessels can help identify any circulatory problems at the back of the eye, as well as changes in the retina's structure.

Fundus photographs can be taken to document changes in the eye structure, shape, and color. In STGD, this can sometimes show the yellowish-white flecks on the retina, which may actually fade with time.

Sometimes there are other color changes in the retina of people with STGD as well.

An electroretinogram (ERG) tests how well the photoreceptors in the retina are functioning. Specifically for STGD, this test is very good at identifying how well the cone cells are working. It can also show how a person with STGD progressively loses their working cone cells.

An electro-oculogram is similar to an ERG in that it studies retinal function and health. However, it is also meant to study the natural connection that exists between the eye and brain. This pathway must function normally in order for people to recognize an image that their eye sees. For STGD, this type of test can further document the cone cell abnormalities or loss.

STGD should not be confused with age-related macular degeneration (AMD), a relatively common condition in individuals often past the age of 50 years. Though the symptoms may be very similar, AMD has not been found to be associated with mutations in the ABCA4 or ELOVL4 genes.

## Treatment and management

There is no cure for STGD, or known way to stop the disease progression altogether. However, some things can help maintain good retinal function and health.

It is felt that a diet rich in leafy green vegetables and fish may be good for the retina. In addition, certain fish contain omega-3 fatty acids, such as docosahexanoic acid (DHA) that is naturally found in the retina in very high concentrations. Eating a diet of fish like salmon, tuna, mackerel, or whitefish twice a week should naturally provide good DHA levels. Otherwise, good fish oil capsules containing DHA and other omega fatty acids can be obtained with a prescription or purchased at specialty health stores.

Multivitamins containing vitamins A, E, and C may be useful. These have antioxidant properties, which may be protective for the eyes. However, large doses of certain vitamins may be toxic, and affected individuals should speak to their doctors before taking supplements.

Protecting the eyes from harmful ultraviolet rays is essential to cone cell health. People with STGD should wear good sunglasses outdoors and especially when over water or near snow on a bright, sunny day.

Smoking has been associated with deteriorating retinal health. Even quitting smoking late in life can make a positive impact on eye health.

Low vision aids can be helpful for those in school or at work. Binocular lens and magnifying screens, large-print reading materials, closed-circuit television, and other tools can be helpful and are often available from organizations supporting those with vision loss.

Living with a chronic vision problem makes a significant impact on a person's life and family. It is often helpful for families to have a social worker connect them to helpful resources. Others may find **genetic counseling**, psychotherapy, or meeting other individuals with STGD through support groups helpful.

### Prognosis

Life expectancy is normal in STGD. A person's vision loss is progressive, but the rate of this is unpredictable. Research and future treatments continue to offer hope for those with this type of macular dystrophy.

### Resources

**WEB SITES**

Genetic Alliance. 2005 (March 16, 2005). http://www.geneticalliance.org.

Online Mendelian Inheritance in Man. (March 16, 2005.) http://www.ncbi.nlm.nih.gov/entrez/query.fcgi?db = OMIM.

**ORGANIZATIONS**

The Canadian National Institute for the Blind. National Office, 1929 Bayview Avenue, Toronto, ON M4G 3E8. Phone: (416) 486-2500. Fax: (416) 480-7677. http://cnib.ca/.

The Foundation Fighting Blindness. 11435 Cronhill Drive, Owings Mills, MD 21117-2220. Local phone: (410) 568-0150. Local TDD: (410) 363-7139. Toll-free phone: (888) 394-3937. Toll-free TDD: (800) 683-5555. Email: info@blindness.org. http://www.blindness.org/.

The Foundation Fighting Blindness–Canada. 60 St. Clair Ave., East Suite 703, Toronto, ON, Canada M4T 1N5. Phone: (416) 360-4200. Toll-free phone: (800) 461-3331. Fax: (416) 360-0060. Email: info@ffb.ca. http://www.ffb.ca/.

Deepti Babu, MS, CGC

Stein-Leventhal syndrome *see* **Polycystic ovary syndrome**

Steinert disease *see* **Myotonic dystrophy**

# Stickler syndrome

### Definition

Stickler syndrome is a disorder caused by a genetic malfunction in the tissue that connects bones, heart, eyes, and ears.

### Description

Stickler syndrome, also known as hereditary arthro-ophthalmopathy, is a multisystem disorder that can affect the eyes and ears, skeleton and joints, and craniofacies. Symptoms may include **myopia**, cataract, and retinal detachment; hearing loss that is both conductive and sensorineural; midfacial underdevelopment and **cleft palate**; and mild **spondyloepiphyseal dysplasia** and/or arthritis. The collection of specific symptoms that make up the syndrome were first documented by Stickler et al., in a 1965 paper published in *Mayo Clinic Proceedings* titled "Hereditary Progressive Arthro-Opthalmopathy." The paper associated the syndrome's sight deterioration and joint changes. Subsequent research has redefined Stickler syndrome to include other symptoms.

### Genetic profile

Stickler syndrome is associated with mutations in three genes: COL2A1 (chromosomal locus 12q13), COL11A1 (chromosomal locus 1p21), and COL11A2 (chromosomal locus 6p21). It is inherited in an autosomal dominant manner. The majority of individuals with Stickler syndrome inherited the abnormal allele from a parent, and the prevalence of new **gene mutations** is unknown. Individuals with Stickler syndrome have a 50% chance of passing on the abnormal gene to each offspring.

The syndrome can manifest itself differently within families. If the molecular genetic basis of Stickler syndrome has been established, molecular **genetic testing** can be used for clarification of each family member's genetic status and for prenatal testing.

A majority of cases are attributed to COL2A1 mutations. All COL2A1 mutations known to cause Stickler syndrome result in the formation of a premature termination codon within the type-II collagen gene. Mutations in COL11A1 have only recently been described, and COL11A2 mutations have been identified only in patients lacking ocular findings.

Although the syndrome is associated with mutations in the COL2A1, COL11A1, and COL11A2 genes, no linkage to any of these three known loci can be

## KEY TERMS

**Cleft palate**—A congenital malformation in which there is an abnormal opening in the roof of the mouth that allows the nasal passages and the mouth to be improperly connected.

**Dysplasia**—The abnormal growth or development of a tissue or organ.

**Glossoptosis**—Downward displacement or retraction of the tongue.

**Micrognathia**—Small lower jaw with recession of lower chin.

**Mitral valve prolapse**—A heart defect in which one of the valves of the heart (which normally controls blood flow) becomes floppy. Mitral valve prolapse may be detected as a heart murmur but there are usually no symptoms.

**Otitis media**—Inflammation of the middle ear, often due to fluid accumulation secondary to an infection.

**Phenotype**—The physical expression of an individuals genes.

**Spondyloepiphyseal dysplasia**—Abnormality of the vertebra and epiphyseal centers that causes a short trunk.

established in some rare cases with clinical findings consistent with Stickler syndrome. It is presumed that other, as yet unidentified, genes mutations also account for Stickler syndrome.

### Genetically related disorders

There are a number of other phenotypes associated with mutations in COL2A1. **Achondrogenesis** type I is a fatal disorder characterized by absence of bone formation in the vertebral column, sacrum, and pubic bones, by the shortening of the limbs and trunk, and by prominent abdomen. **Hypochondrogenesis** is a milder variant of achondrogenesis. Spondyloepiphyseal **dysplasia** congenita, a disorder with skeletal changes more severe than in Stickler syndrome, manifests in significant short stature, flat facial profile, myopia, and vitreoretinal degeneration. Spondyloepimetaphyseal dysplasia Strudwick type is another skeletal disorder that manifests in severe short stature with severe protrusion of the sternum and **scoliosis**, cleft palate, and retinal detachment. A distinctive radiographic finding is irregular sclerotic changes, described as dappled, which are created by alternating zones of osteosclerosis and ostopenia in the metaphyses

(ends) of the long bones. Spondyloperipheral dysplasia is a rare condition characterized by short stature and radiographic changes consistent with a spondyloepiphyseal dysplasia and **brachydactyly**. Kneist dysplasia is a disorder that manifests in disproportionate short stature, flat facial profile, myopia and vitreoretinal degeneration, cleft palate, backward and lateral curvature of the spine, and a variety of radiographic changes.

Other phenotypes associated with mutations in COL11A1 include **Marshall syndrome**, which manifests in ocular hypertelorism, hypoplasia of the maxilla and nasal bones, flat nasal bridge, and small upturned nasal tip. The flat facial profile of Marshall syndrome is usually evident into adulthood, unlike Stickler syndrome. Manifestations include radiographs demonstrating hypoplasia of the nasal sinuses and a thickened calvarium. Ocular manifestations include high myopia, fluid vitreous humor, and early onset cataracts. Sensorineural hearing loss is common and sometimes progressive. Cleft palate is seen both as isolated occurrence and as part of the **Pierre-Robin sequence** (micrognathia, cleft palate, and glossoptosis). Other manifestations include short stature and early onset arthritis, and skin manifestations that may include mild hypotrichosis and hypohidrosis.

Other phenotypes associated with mutations in COL11A2 include autosomal recessive oto-spondylo-meta-epiphyseal dysplasia, a disorder characterized by flat facial profile, cleft palate, and severe hearing loss. Anocular Stickler syndrome caused by COL11A2 mutations is close in similarity to this disorder. Weissenbach-Zweymuller syndrome has been characterized as neonatal Stickler syndrome but it is a separate entity from Stickler syndrome. Symptoms include midface hypoplasia with a flat nasal bridge, small upturned nasal tip, micrognathia, sensorineural hearing loss, and rhizomelic limb shortening. Radiographic findings include vertebral coronal clefts and dumbbell-shaped femora and humeri. Catch-up growth after age two or three is common and the skeletal findings become less apparent in later years.

### Demographics

No studies have been done to determine Stickler syndrome prevalence. An approximate incidence of Stickler syndrome among newborns is estimated based on data on the incidence of Pierre-Robin sequence in newborns. One in 10,000 newborns have Pierre-Robin sequence, and 35% of these newborns subsequently develop signs or symptoms of Stickler syndrome. These data suggest that the incidence of Stickler syndrome among neonates is approximately one in 7,500.

## Signs and symptoms

Stickler syndrome may affect the eyes and ears, skeleton and joints, and craniofacies. It may also be associated with coronary complications.

### Ocular symptoms

Near-sightedness is a common symptom of Stickler syndrome. High myopia is detectable in newborns. Common problems also include astigmatism and cataracts. Risk of retinal detachment is higher than normal. Abnormalities of the vitreous humor, the colorless, transparent jelly that fills the eyeball, are also observed. Type 1, the more common vitreous abnormality, is characterized by a persistence of a vestigial vitreous gel in the space behind the lens, and is bordered by a folded membrane. Type 2, which is much less common, is characterized by sparse and irregularly thickened bundles throughout the vitreous cavity. These vitreous abnormalities can cause sight deterioration.

### Auditory symptoms

Hearing impairment is common, and some degree of sensorineural hearing loss is found in 40% of patients. The degree of hearing impairment is variable, however, and may be progressive. Typically, the impairment is high tone and often subtle. Conductive hearing loss is also possible. It is known that the impairment is related to the expression of type II and IX collagen in the inner ear, but the exact mechanism for it is unclear. Hearing impairment may be secondary to the recurrent ear infections often associated with cleft palate, or it may be secondary to a disorder of the ossicles of the middle ear.

### Skeletal symptoms

Skeletal manifestations are short stature relative to unaffected siblings, early-onset arthritis, and abnormalities at ends of long bones and vertebrae. Radiographic findings consistent with mild spondyloepiphyseal dysplasia. Some individuals have a physique similar to **Marfan syndrome**, but without tall stature. Young patients may exhibit joint laxity but it diminishes or even resolves completely with age. Early-onset arthritis is common and generally mild, mostly resulting in joint stiffness. Arthritis is sometimes severe, leading to joint replacement as early as the third or fourth decade.

### Craniofacial findings

Several facial features are common with Stickler syndrome. A flat facial profile referred to as a "scooped out" face results from underdevelopment of the maxilla and nasal bridge, which can cause telecanthus and epicanthal folds. Flat cheeks, flat nasal bridge, small upper jaw, pronounced upper lip groove, small lower jaw, and palate abnormalities are possible, all in varying degrees. The nasal tip may be small and upturned, making the groove in the middle of the upper lip appear long. Micrognathia is common and may compromise the upper airway, necessitating tracheostomy. Midfacial hypoplasia is most pronounced in infants and young children, and older individuals may have a normal facial profile.

### Coronary findings

Mitral valve prolapse may be associated with Stickler syndrome, but studies are, as yet, inconclusive about the connection.

## Diagnosis

Stickler is believed to be a common syndrome in the United States and Europe, but only a fraction of cases are diagnosed since most patients have minor symptoms. Misdiagnosis may also occur because symptoms are not correlated as having a single cause. More than half of patients with Stickler syndrome are originally misdiagnosed according to one study.

While the diagnosis of Stickler syndrome is clinically based, clinical diagnostic criteria have not been established. Patients usually do not have all symptoms attributed to Stickler syndrome. The disorder should be considered in individuals with clinical findings in two or more of the following categories:

- Ophthalmologic. Congenital or early-onset cataract, myopia greater than -3 diopters, congenital vitreous anomaly, rhegmatogenous retinal detachment. Normal newborns are typically hyperopic ( + 1 diopter or greater), and so any degree of myopia in an at-risk newborn, such as one with Pierre-Robin sequence or an affected parent, is suggestive of the diagnosis of Stickler syndrome. Less common ophthalmological symptoms include paravascular pigmented lattice degeneration and cataracts.
- Craniofacial. Midface hypoplasia, depressed nasal bridge in childhood, anteverted nares (tipped or bent nasal cavity openings), split uvula, cleft hard palate, micrognathia, Pierre-Robin sequence.
- Audiologic. Sensorineural hearing loss.
- Joint. Hypermobility, mild spondyloepiphyseal dysplasia, precocious osteoarthritis.

It is appropriate to evaluate at-risk family members with a medical history and physical examination and ophthalmologic, audiologic, and radiographic assessments. Childhood photographs may be helpful in the evaluation of adults since craniofacial findings may become less distinctive with age.

### *Molecular genetic testing*

Mutation analysis for COL2A1, COL11A1, and COL11A2 is available. Detection is performed by mutation scanning of the coding sequences. Stickler syndrome has been associated with stop mutations in COL2A1 and with missense and splicing mutations in all of the three genes. Because the meaning of a specific missense mutation within the gene coding sequence may not be clear, mutation detection in a parent is not advised without strong clinical support for the diagnosis.

Clinical findings can influence the order for testing the three genes. In patients with ocular findings, including type 1 congenital vitreous abnormality and mild hearing loss, COL2A1 may be tested first. In patients with typical ocular findings including type 2 congenital vitreous anomaly and significant hearing loss, COL11A1 may be tested first. In patients with hearing loss and craniofacial and joint manifestations but without ocular findings, COL11A2 may be tested first.

### *Prenatal testing*

Before considering prenatal testing, its availability must be confirmed and prior testing of family members is usually necessary. Prenatal molecular genetic testing is not usually offered in the absence of a known disease-causing mutation in a parent. For fetuses at 50% risk for Stickler syndrome, a number of options for prenatal testing may exist. If an affected parent has a mutation in the gene COL2A1 or COL11A1, molecular genetic testing may be performed on cells obtained by chorionic villus sampling at 10–12 weeks gestation or **amniocentesis** at 16–18 weeks gestation. Alternatively, or in conjunction with molecular genetic testing, ultrasound examination can be performed at 19–20 weeks gestation to detect cleft palate. For fetuses with no known family history of Stickler syndrome in which cleft palate is detected, a three-generation pedigree may be obtained, and relatives who have findings suggestive of Stickler syndrome should be evaluated.

### Treatment and management

Individuals diagnosed with Stickler syndrome, and individuals in whom the diagnosis cannot be excluded, should be followed for potential complications.

Evaluation by an ophthalmologist familiar with the ocular manifestations of Stickler syndrome is recommended. Individuals with known ocular complications may prefer to be followed by a vitreoretinal specialist. Patients should avoid activities that may lead to traumatic retinal detachment, such as contact sports. Patients should be advised of the symptoms associated with a retinal detachment and the need for immediate evaluation and treatment when such symptoms occur. Individuals from families with Stickler syndrome and a known COL2A1 or COL11A1 mutation who have not inherited the mutant allele do not need close ophthalmologic evaluation.

A baseline audiogram to test hearing should be performed when the diagnosis of Stickler syndrome is suspected. Follow-up audiologic evaluations are recommended in affected persons since hearing loss can be progressive.

Radiological examination may detect signs of mild spondyloepiphyseal dysplasia. Treatment is symptomatic, and includes over-the-counter anti-inflammatory medications before and after physical activity. No preventative therapies currently exist to minimize joint damage in affected individuals. In an effort to delay the onset of arthropathy, physicians may recommend avoiding physical activities that involve high impact to the joints, but no data support this recommendation.

Infants with Pierre-Robin sequence need immediate attention from otolaryngology and pediatric critical care specialists. Evaluation and management in a comprehensive craniofacial clinic that provides all the necessary services, including otolaryngology, plastic surgery, oral and maxillofacial surgery, pediatric dentistry, and orthodontics is recommended. Tracheostomy may be required, which involves placing a tube in the neck to facilitate breathing.

Middle ear infections (otitis media) may be a recurrent problem secondary to the palatal abnormalities, and ear tubes may be required. Micrognathia (small jaw) tends to become less prominent over time in most patients, allowing for removal of the tracheostomy. In some patients, however, significant micrognathia persists and causes orthodontic problems. In these patients, a mandibular advancement procedure may be required to correct jaw misalignment.

Cardiac care is recommended if complaints suggestive of mitral valve prolapse, such as episodic tachycardia and chest pain, are present. While the prevalence of mitral valve prolapse in Stickler syndrome is unclear, all affected individuals should be screened since individuals with this disorder need antibiotic prophylaxis for certain surgical procedures.

### Prognosis

Prognosis is good under physician care. It is particularly important to receive regular vision and hearing exams. If retinal detachment is a risk, it may be advisable to avoid contact sports. Some craniofacial symptoms may improve with age.

**Resources**

PERIODICALS

Bowling, E. L., M. D, Brown, and T. V. Trundle. "The Stickler Syndrome: Case Reports and Literature Review." *Optometry* 71 (March 2000): 177+.

MacDonald, M. R., et al. "Reports on the Stickler Syndrome, An Autosomal Connective Tissue Disorder." *Ear, Nose & Throat Journal* 76 (October 1997): 706.

Snead, M. P., and J. R. Yates. "Clinical and Molecular Genetics of Stickler Syndrome." *Journal of Medical Genetics* 36 (May 1999): 353+.

Wilkin, D. J., et al. "Rapid Determination of COL2A1 Mutations in Individuals with Stickler Syndrome: Analysis of Potential Premature Termination Codons." *American Journal of Medical Genetics* 11 (September 2000): 141+.

WEBSITES

Robin, Nathaniel H., and Matthew L. Warman. "Stickler Syndrome." *GeneClinics*. University of Washington, Seattle. http://www.geneclinics.org/profiles/stickler.

"Stickler Syndrome." *NORD—National Organization for Rare Disorders*. http://www.rarediseases.org.

ORGANIZATIONS

Stickler Involved People. 15 Angelina, Augusta, KS 67010. (316) 775-2993. http://www.sticklers.org.

Stickler Syndrome Support Group. PO Box 371, Walton-on-Thames, Surrey KT12 2YS, England. 44-01932 267635. http://www.stickler.org.uk.

Jennifer F. Wilson, MS

# Sturge-Weber syndrome

## Definition

Sturge-Weber syndrome (SWS) is a condition involving specific brain changes that often cause seizures and mental delays. It also includes port-wine

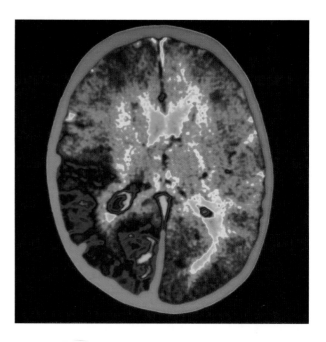

This magnetic resonance image of the brain shows a patient affected with Sturge-Weber syndrome. The front of the brain is at the top. Green colored areas indicate fluid-filled ventricles. The blue area is where the brain has become calcified. *(Photo Researchers, Inc.)*

colored birthmarks (or "port-wine stains"), usually found on the face.

## Description

The brain finding in SWS is leptomeningeal angioma, which is a swelling of the tissue surrounding the brain and spinal cord. These angiomas cause seizures in approximately 90% of people with SWS. A large number of affected individuals are also mentally delayed.

Port-wine stains are present at birth. They can be quite large and are typically found on the face near the eyes or on the eyelids. Vision problems are common, especially if a port-wine stain covers the eyes. These vision problems can include **glaucoma** and vision loss.

Facial features, such as port-wine stains, can be very challenging for individuals with SWS. These birthmarks can increase in size with time, and this may be particularly emotionally distressing for the individuals, as well as their parents. A state of unhappiness about this is more common during middle childhood and later than it is at younger ages.

## Genetic profile

The **genetics** behind Sturge-Weber syndrome are still unknown. Interestingly, in other genetic conditions involving changes in the skin and brain (such as

## KEY TERMS

**Calcification**—A process in which tissue becomes hardened due to calcium deposits.

**Choroid**—A vascular membrane that covers the back of the eye between the retina and the sclera and serves to nourish the retina and absorb scattered light.

**Computed tomography (CT) scan**—An imaging procedure that produces a three-dimensional picture of organs or structures inside the body, such as the brain.

**Glaucoma**—An increase in the fluid eye pressure, eventually leading to damage of the optic nerve and ongoing visual loss.

**Leptomeningeal angioma**—A swelling of the tissue or membrane surrounding the brain and spinal cord, which can enlarge with time.

**Magnetic resonance imaging (MRI)**—A technique that employs magnetic fields and radio waves to create detailed images of internal body structures and organs, including the brain.

**Port-wine stain**—Dark-red birthmarks seen on the skin, named after the color of the dessert wine.

**Sclera**—The tough white membrane that forms the outer layer of the eyeball.

neurofibromatosis and tuberous sclerosis) the genetic causes are well described. It is known that most people with SRS are the only ones in their family with the condition; there is usually not a strong family history of the disease. However, gene known to cause SRS is still not known. For now, SWS is thought to be caused by a random, sporadic event.

### Demographics

Sturge-Weber syndrome is a sporadic disease that is found throughout the world, affecting males and females equally. The total number of people with Sturge-Weber syndrome is not known, but estimates range between one in 400,000 to one in 40,000.

### Signs and symptoms

People with SWS may have a larger head circumference (measurement around the head) than usual. Leptomeningeal angiomas can progress with time. They usually only occur on one side of the brain, but can exist on both sides in up to 30% of people with SWS. The angiomas can also cause great changes within the brain's white matter. Generalized wasting,

or regression, of portions of the brain can result from large angiomas. Calcification of the portions of the brain underlying the angiomas can also occur. The larger and more involved the angiomas are, the greater the expected amount of mental delays in the individual. Seizures are common in SWS, and they can often begin in very early childhood. Occasionally, slight paralysis affecting one side of the body may occur.

Port-wine stains are actually capillaries (blood vessels) that reach the skin's surface and grow larger than usual. As mentioned earlier, the birthmarks mostly occur near the eyes; they often occur only on one side of the face. Though they can increase in size over time, port-wine stains cause no direct health problems for the person with SWS.

Vision loss and other complications are common in SWS. The choroid of the eye can swell, and this may lead to increased pressure within the eye in 33-50% of people with SWS. Glaucoma is another common vision problem seen in SWS, and is more often seen when a person has a port-wine stain that is near or touches the eye.

In a 2000 study about the psychological functioning of children with SRS, it was noted that parents and teachers report a higher incidence of social problems, emotional distress, and problems with compliance in these individuals. Taking the mental delays into account, behaviors associated with attention-deficit hyperactivity disorder (ADHD) were noted; as it turns out, about 22% of people with SWS are eventually diagnosed with ADHD.

### Diagnosis

Because no **genetic testing** is available for Sturge-Weber syndrome, all diagnoses are made through a careful physical examination and study of a person's medical history.

Port-wine stains are present at birth, and seizures may occur in early childhood. If an individual has both of these features, SWS should be suspected. A brain MRI or CT scan can often reveal a leptomeningeal angioma, brain calcifications, as well as any other associated white matter changes.

### Treatment and management

Treatment of seizures in SWS by anti-epileptic medications is often an effective way to control them. In the rare occasion that an aggressive seizure medication therapy is not effective, surgery may be necessary. The general goal of the surgery is to remove the portion of brain that is causing the seizures, while keeping the normal brain tissue intact. Though most patients with SWS only have brain surgery as a final attempt to treat seizures, some physicians favor earlier surgery because this may prevent some irreversible damage to the brain (caused by the angiomas).

Standard glaucoma treatment, including medications and surgery, is used to treat people with this complication. This can often reduce the amount of vision loss.

There is no specific treatment for port-wine stains. Because they contain blood vessels, it could disrupt blood flow to remove or alter the birthmarks.

### Prognosis

The prognosis for people with SWS is directly related to the amount of brain involvement for the leptomeningeal angiomas. For those individuals with smaller angiomas, prognosis is relatively good, especially if they do not have severe seizures or vision problems.

### Resources

**BOOKS**

Charkins, Hope. *Children with Facial Difference: A Parent's Guide.* Bethesda, MD: Woodbine House, 1996.

**WEBSITES**

"Sturge-Weber Syndrome." *Family Village.* http://www.familyvillage.wisc.edu/lib_stur.htm.
Sturge-Weber Syndrome Support Group of New Zealand. http://www.geocities.com/HotSprings/Spa/1563/.

**ORGANIZATIONS**

The Sturge-Weber Foundation. PO Box 418, Mount Freedom, NJ 07970. (800) 627-5482 or (973) 895-4445. Fax: (973) 895-4846. swfoffice@aol.com. http://www.sturgeweber.com/.

Deepti Babu, MS

Summitt syndrome *see* **Carpenter syndrome**
Surdicardiac syndrome *see* **Jervell and Lange-Nielsen syndrome**

# Sutherland-Haan syndrome

### Definition

Sutherland-Haan syndrome is an inherited X-linked disorder characterized by mental retardation, small head circumference, small testes, and spastic diplegia. Grant Sutherland and co-workers first described the syndrome in 1988. At present, it has only been fully described in one single, large, Australian family. Thus, it is unknown if the disorder occurs worldwide or only in certain ethnic and racial groups. Since the responsible **gene** is located on the X **chromosome**, Sutherland-Haan syndrome is exclusively found in males. As the gene is unknown and only one family has been described (although there are families suspected of having Sutherland-Haan) the prevalence is unknown.

### Description

Sutherland-Haan syndrome is among the group of **genetic disorders** known as **X-linked mental retardation** (XLMR) syndromes. Manifestations in males may be present prior to birth, as intrauterine growth appears to be mildly impaired since birth weight is below normal. Similarly, postnatal growth is slow with the head circumference being quite small (**microcephaly**) and height being rather short. Affected males exhibit poor feeding during infancy. Additionally, affected males have small testes after puberty.

The diagnosis is very difficult especially if there is no family history of mental retardation. If there is a family history of mental retardation and if the **inheritance** pattern is consistent with X-linkage, then the diagnosis is possible based on the presence of the above clinical findings and localization to Xp11.3 to Xq12.

### Genetic profile

Sutherland-Haan syndrome is caused by an alteration in an unknown gene located in the pericentric region (area flanking the centromere) of the X chromosome. The altered gene in affected males is most likely inherited from a carrier mother. As males have only one X chromosome, a mutation in

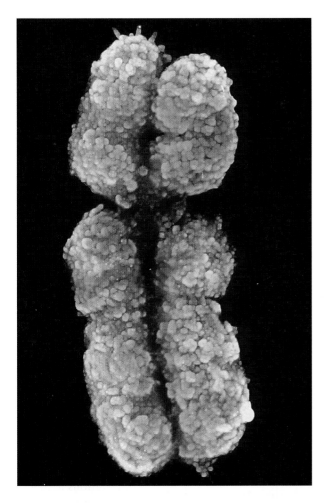

**Sutherland-Haan syndrome is a form of mental retardation linked to a gene abnormality on the X chromosome.** *(Photo Researchers, Inc.)*

### Signs and symptoms

Evidence of Sutherland-Haan syndrome is present at birth as affected males have below normal birth weight. This may reflect mildly impaired intrauterine growth. Postnatal growth is also slow. Head circumference is smaller than normal (microcephaly) and affected males tend to be short. Small testes are also present after puberty.

There are some somatic manifestations present in most of the males with Sutherland-Haan syndrome. These include mild to moderate spastic diplegia (increased muscular tone with exaggeration of tendon reflexes of the legs), upslanting of the eye openings, brachycephaly (disproportionate shortness of the head), and a thin body build. Additionally, a few of the affected males may have anal abnormalities.

Mental impairment is mild to moderate with IQ ranging from 43 to 60. One male was reported to have an IQ in the 63-83 range (borderline).

### Diagnosis

The diagnosis of Sutherland-Haan can only be made on the basis of the clinical findings in the presence of a family history consistent with X-linked inheritance of mental retardation and segregation of X chromosome markers in Xp11.2-Xq12. Unfortunately, there are no laboratory or radiographic changes that are specific for Sutherland-Haan syndrome.

**Renpenning syndrome**, another X-linked mental retardation syndrome, also has microcephaly, short stature, small testes, and upslanting of the eye openings. Furthermore, this syndrome is localized to Xp11.2-p11.4, which overlaps with the localization of

an X-linked gene is fully expressed in males. On the other hand, as carrier females have a normal, second X-chromosome, they do not exhibit any of the **phenotype** associated with Sutherland-Haan syndrome.

Female carriers have a 50/50 chance of transmitting the altered gene to a daughter or a son. A son with the altered gene will be affected but will likely not reproduce.

### Demographics

Only males are affected with Sutherland-Haan syndrome. Carrier females exhibit none of the phenotypic features. Although Sutherland-Haan has only been reported in a single Australian family, there is no reason to assume it is not present in other racial/ethnic groups.

Sutherland-Haan. However, males with Renpenning syndrome lack spasticity of the legs, brachycephaly, and a thin appearance. It is possible these two syndromes have different mutations in the same gene.

Chudley-Lowry syndrome also has microcephaly, short stature, and small testes. However, males have distinct facial features, similar to those of XLMR-hypotonic facies, and obesity. As with Renpenning syndrome, this syndrome may result from a different mutation in the same gene responsible for Sutherland-Haan syndrome.

Two other X-linked mental retardation syndromes (XLMR-hypotonic facies and X-linked hereditary bullous dystrophy) have microcephaly, short stature, and small testes. However, these conditions have different somatic features and are not localized to Xp11.2-Xq12.

### Treatment and management

There is neither treatment nor cure available for Sutherland-Haan syndrome. Early educational intervention is advised for affected males. Some affected males may require living in a more controlled environment outside the home.

### Prognosis

Life threatening concerns usually have not been associated with Sutherland-Haan syndrome. However, two affected males were found to have anal abnormalities, which required some form of surgery.

## QUESTIONS TO ASK YOUR DOCTOR

- What physical traits are typically associated with Sutherland-Haan syndrome?
- How is a diagnosis for Sutherland-Haan syndrome made if no confirmatory tests are available?
- Are there any organizations that can provide information to a family with a Sutherland-Haan child?
- What is the prognosis for a child with Sutherland-Haan syndrome, and how likely is that prognosis to change over time?

**Resources**

**PERIODICALS**

Gedeon, A., J. Mulley, and E. Haan. "Gene Localization for Sutherland-Haan Syndrome (SHS:MIM309470)." *American Journal of Medical Genetics* 64 (1996): 78-79.

Sutherland, G.R., et al. "Linkage Studies with the Gene for an X-linked Syndrome of Mental Retardation, Microcephaly, and Spastic Diplegia (MRX2)." *American Journal of Medical Genetics* 30 (1988): 493-508.

Charles E. Schwartz, PhD

Swedish-type porphyria *see* **Porphyrias**

Systemic elastorrhexis *see* **Pseudoxanthoma elasticum**

Systemic sclerosis *see* **Scleroderma**

Talipes *see* **Clubfoot**

# Tangier disease

## Definition

Tangier disease is a rare autosomal recessive condition characterized by low levels of high density lipoprotein cholesterol (HDL-C)in the blood, accumulation of cholesterol in many organs of the body, and an increased risk of arteriosclerosis.

## Description

Donald Fredrickson was the first to discover Tangier disease. He described this condition in 1961 in a five-year-old boy from Tangier Island who had large, yellow-orange colored tonsils that were engorged with cholesterol. Subsequent tests on this boy and his sister found that they both had virtually no high density lipoprotein cholesterol (HDL-C) in their blood stream. Other symptoms of Tangier disease such as an enlarged spleen and liver, eye abnormalities, and neurological abnormalities were later discovered in others affected with this disease.

It was not until 1999 that the **gene** for Tangier disease, called the ABCA1 gene, was discovered. This gene is responsible for producing a protein that is involved in the pathway by which HDL removes cholesterol from the cells of the body and transports it to the liver where it is digested and removed from the body.

Cholesterol is transported through the body as part of lipoproteins. Low density lipoproteins (LDL) and high density lipoproteins (HDL) are two of the major cholesterol transporting lipoproteins. Cholesterol attached to LDL (LDL-C) is often called bad cholesterol since it can remain in the blood stream for a long time, and high levels of LDL-C can increase the risk of clogging of the arteries (arteriosclerosis) and heart disease. Cholesterol attached to HDL is often called good cholesterol since it does not stay in the blood stream for a long period of time, and high levels are associated with a low risk of arteriosclerosis.

Research as of 2001 suggests that the ABCA1 protein helps to transport cholesterol found in the cell to the surface of the cell where it joins with a protein called ApoA-1 and forms an HDL-C complex. The HDL-C complex transports the cholesterol to the liver where the cholesterol is digested and removed from the body. This process normally prevents an excess accumulation of cholesterol in the cells of the body and can help to protect against arteriosclerosis.

## Genetic profile

Changes in the ABCA1 gene, such as those found in Tangier disease, cause the gene to produce abnormal ABCA1 protein. The abnormal ABCA1 protein is less able to transport cholesterol to the surface of the cell, which results in an accumulation of cholesterol in the cell. The accumulation of cholesterol in the cells of the body causes most of the symptoms associated with Tangier disease. The decreased efficiency in removing cholesterol from the body can lead to an increased accumulation of cholesterol in the blood vessels, which can lead to a slightly increased risk of arteriosclerosis and ultimately an increased risk of heart attacks and strokes. The ABCA1 protein defect also results in decreased amounts of cholesterol available on the surface of the cell to bind to ApoA-1 and decreased cholesterol available to form HDL-C. This in turn results in the rapid degradation of ApoA-1 and reduced levels of ApoA-1 and HDL-C in the bloodstream. It also leads to lower levels of LDL-C in the blood.

The ABCA1 gene is found on **chromosome** 9. Since we inherit one chromosome 9 from our mother and one chromosome 9 from our father, we also inherit two ABCA1 genes. People with Tangier disease have

**Anemia**—A blood condition in which the level of hemoglobin or the number of red blood cells falls below normal values. Common symptoms include paleness, fatigue, and shortness of breath.

**Arteriosclerosis**—Hardening of the arteries that often results in decreased ability of blood to flow smoothly.

**Autosomal recessive**—A pattern of genetic inheritance where two abnormal genes are needed to display the trait or disease.

**Biochemical testing**—Measuring the amount or activity of a particular enzyme or protein in a sample of blood, urine, or other tissue from the body.

**Cholesterol**—A fatty-like substance that is obtained from the diet and produced by the liver. Cells require cholesterol for their normal daily functions.

**Chromosome**—A microscopic thread-like structure found within each cell of the body that consists of a complex of proteins and DNA. Humans have 46 chromosomes arranged into 23 pairs. Changes in either the total number of chromosomes or their shape and size (structure) may lead to physical or mental abnormalities.

**Deoxyribonucleic acid (DNA)**—The genetic material in cells that holds the inherited instructions for growth, development, and cellular functioning.

**DNA testing**—Analysis of DNA (the genetic component of cells) in order to determine changes in genes that may indicate a specific disorder.

**Gene**—A building block of inheritance, which contains the instructions for the production of a particular protein, and is made up of a molecular sequence found on a section of DNA. Each gene is found on a precise location on a chromosome.

**Hemolytic anemia**—Anemia that results from premature destruction and decreased numbers of red blood cells.

**High density lipoprotein (HDL)**—A cholesterol carrying substance that helps remove cholesterol from the cells of the body and deliver it to the liver where it is digested and removed from the body.

**Low density lipoproteins (LDL)**—A cholesterol carrying substance that can remain in the blood stream for a long period of time.

**Lymph node**—A bean-sized mass of tissue that is part of the immune system and is found in different areas of the body.

**Mucous membrane**—Thin, mucous covered layer of tissue that lines organs such as the intestinal tract.

**Prenatal testing**—Testing for a disease such as a genetic condition in an unborn baby.

**Protein**—Important building blocks of the body, composed of amino acids, involved in the formation of body structures and controlling the basic functions of the human body.

**Spleen**—Organ located in the upper abdominal cavity that filters out old red blood cells and helps fight bacterial infections. Responsible for breaking down spherocytes at a rapid rate.

**Thymus gland**—An endocrine gland located in the front of the neck that houses and transports T cells, which help to fight infection.

**Ureters**—Tubes through which urine is transported from the kidneys to the bladder.

---

inherited one changed ABCA1 gene from their father and one changed ABCA1 gene from their mother, making Tangier disease an autosomal recessive condition.

Parents who have a child with Tangier disease are called carriers, since they each possess one changed ABCA1 gene and one unchanged ABCA1 gene. Carriers for Tangier disease do not have any of the symptoms associated with the disease, except for increased levels of HDL-C in their blood stream and a slightly increased risk of arteriosclerosis. The degree of risk of arteriosclerosis is unknown, and is dependent on other genetic and environmental factors, such as diet. Each child born to parents who are both carriers of Tangier disease has a 25% chance of having Tangier disease, a 50% chance of being a carrier, and a 25% chance of being neither a carrier nor affected with Tangier disease.

### Demographics

Tangier disease is a very rare disorder with less than 100 cases diagnosed worldwide. Tangier disease affects both males and females.

### Signs and symptoms

The symptoms of Tangier disease are quite variable but the most common symptoms of Tangier disease are enlarged, yellow-colored tonsils, an enlarged spleen, accumulation of cholesterol in the mucous membranes of the intestines, abnormalities in the nervous system (neuropathy), and an increased risk of arteriosclerosis. Less commonly seen symptoms are an enlarged liver, lymph nodes and thymus, and hemolytic anemia. Cholesterol accumulation has been seen in other organs such as the bone marrow, gall bladder, skin, kidneys, heart valves, ureters, testicles, and the cornea of the eye.

### Symptoms involving the tonsils, intestines and spleen

The unusual appearance of the tonsils is due to an accumulation of cholesterol. Even when the tonsils are removed, small yellow patches at the back of the throat may be evident. The accumulation of cholesterol in the mucous membranes of the intestines results in the appearance of orange-brown spots on the rectum, and can occasionally result in intermittent diarrhea and abdominal pain. The enlargement of the spleen can result in anemia and decreased numbers of certain blood cells called platelets.

### Nervous system abnormalities

Cholesterol can accumulate in the nerve cells which can result in nervous system abnormalities and symptoms such as loss of heat and pain sensation, weakness, increased sweating, burning prickling sensations, loss of feeling, eye muscle spasms, double vision, drooping eyelids, and decreased strength and reflexes. These symptoms can be mild to severe, and can be temporary or permanent. Most people with Tangier disease have some nervous system dysfunction, but in many cases the symptoms are mild and may be undetectable. Occasionally patients with Tangier disease experience progressive and debilitating nervous system abnormalities.

### Arteriosclerosis

Since so few people are known to be affected with Tangier disease it is difficult to precisely predict their risk of developing arteriosclerosis and heart disease. Depending on their age, people with Tangier disease appear to have approximately four to six times increased risk for arteriosclerosis leading to heart disease. People over the age of 30 appear to have a six-fold increased risk. It is possible that Tangier patients are protected from higher risks of arteriosclerosis by lower than average levels of LDL-C in their blood stream.

### Diagnosis

Tangier disease is diagnosed through assessment of clinical symptoms and biochemical testing. A diagnosis of Tangier disease should be considered in anyone with deposits of cholesterol on the cornea, an unexplained enlarged spleen or liver, or neurological abnormalities. Examination of the throat and tonsils and rectal mucous membrane should be performed on those suspected to have Tangier disease. Measurements of the total cholesterol, HDL-C, LDL-C, ApoA-1 and triglycerides should also be performed. Patients with Tangier disease have virtually no HDL-C in their bloodstream and ApoA-1 levels are reduced to one to three percent of normal. LDL-C levels are also reduced to approximately 40% of normal and triglyceride levels can be mildly elevated. As of 2001, **DNA** testing for Tangier disease is not available through clinical laboratories, although DNA testing on a clinical basis should be available in the future. Some laboratories may identify ABCA1 gene changes in patients as part of their research. Prenatal testing is only available if ABCA1 gene changes are identified in the parents.

### Treatment and management

There is no treatment for Tangier disease and treatment of decreased HDL-C with medication is usually ineffective. Occasionally organs such as the spleen and tonsils are removed because of extensive accumulation of cholesterol. Arteriosclerosis may be treated through angioplasty or bypass surgery. Angioplasty involves inserting a small, hollow tube called a catheter with a deflated balloon through the groin or arm and into a clogged artery. The balloon is then inflated which enlarges the artery and compresses the blockage. Coronary artery disease can also be treated through bypass surgery, which is performed by taking a blood vessel from another part of the body and constructing an alternate path around the blocked part of the artery.

### Prognosis

In most cases the prognosis for Tangier is disease is quite good. People who develop heart disease may, however, have a decreased life span depending on the severity of the disease and the quality of medical treatment.

### Resources

**BOOKS**

Scriver, C.R., et al., eds. *The Metabolic and Molecular Basis of Inherited Disease*. New York: McGraw-Hill, 1995.

**ORGANIZATIONS**

National Tay-Sachs and Allied Diseases Association. 2001 Beacon St., Suite 204, Brighton, MA 02135. (800) 906-8723. ntasd-Boston@worldnet.att.net. http://www.ntsad.org.

**PERIODICALS**

Brooks-Wilson, A., et al. "Mutations in ABCA1 in Tangier Disease and Familial High-density Lipoprotein Deficiency."*Nature Genetics* 22, no. 4 (August 1999): 336-345.

Oram, John. "Tangier Disease and ABCA1." *Biochimica et Biophysica Acta* 1529 (2000): 321-330.

**WEBSITES**

"High Density Lipoprotein Deficiency, Tangier Type 1; HDLDT1." *Online Mendelian Inheritance in Man*. http://www.ncbi.nlm.nih.gov/entrez/dispomim.cgi?id = 271900 (December 8, 1999).

Lisa Maria Andres, MS, CGC

# TAR syndrome

## Definition

Thrombocytopenia-absent radius (TAR) syndrome is a rare condition that is apparent at birth. Affected infants are born with incomplete or missing forearms. Typically, the bone on the thumb side of the forearm (radius) is absent, but other bones may be missing or abnormally formed. TAR syndrome also causes life-threatening bleeding episodes due to low levels of platelets in the blood (thrombocytopenia). It is inherited in an autosomal recessive manner.

## Description

Dr. S. Shaw first wrote about two siblings (a brother and a sister) with missing forearms and bleeding problems in 1956. Thirteen years later, Dr. Judith Hall gave

the name and acronym of TAR syndrome to the disorder. She described three families containing nine individuals. TAR syndrome has also been called the tetraphocomelia-thrombocytopenia syndrome.

The forearm is comprised of two bones. The radius is the long bone on the thumb side of the forearm. The ulna is the long bone on the little finger side. In TAR syndrome, the radius is missing on each forearm. Many times the ulna may also be missing or shorter than normal.

As these bone deficiencies are quite obvious at birth, the forearms will look very short. In fact, the hand looks as if it comes directly from the elbow. In more severe cases, the bone of the upper arm is also missing, with the hand connected to the shoulder. Approximately 50% of the time there are other skeletal abnormalities, particularly in the lower limbs.

Each individual seems to be affected somewhat differently. For instance, some individuals with TAR syndrome might have one arm longer than the other arm; another might have both arms short, and bones missing in the feet; a third person might have all four limbs severely affected. The one constant feature is the absence of the radius bone. The forearm defects cause the hands to be bent inwards towards the body. However, the four fingers and thumb usually look normal.

The other main feature of the syndrome is thrombocytopenia. Thrombocytopenia means abnormally low levels of platelets in the blood. Platelets are made from cells called megakaryocytes. The megakaryocytes are formed in the red bone marrow, lungs and spleen. In TAR syndrome, the megakaryoctyes are either absent, decreased in number or not formed properly. Therefore, the platelets are not properly made. The exact reason remains unknown.

When injury occurs, platelets are needed so that the blood can clot. The process is called blood coagulation. The platelets help initiate this process by attaching to the injured tissue, and clumping together, almost like a temporary patch. The platelets then release an enzyme called thromboplastin. Thromplastin acts to cleave a particle called fibrinogen (also in the blood) to fibrin. Fibrin is a hard substance that attaches to the injured area, and forms a meshwork (a blood clot). Along with other clotting factors, this permanently stops the bleeding.

In TAR syndrome, the normal process of making platelets is defective. The effect of this is excessive bleeding and bruising. These individuals have frequent nosebleeds and their skin bruises more easily. The platelet problem makes them more prone to bleeding inside the body, such as in the kidney or lungs. Bleeding can also occur inside the brain (intracranial hemorrhage), and be so severe that these infants die from the internal bleeding.

### Genetic profile

There have been numerous instances of siblings, each with TAR syndrome. The parents were not affected. A few families have also been seen where the parents were said to be closely related (i.e. may have shared the same altered **gene** within the family). For these reasons, TAR syndrome is most likely an autosomal recessive disorder. Autosomal means that both males and females can have the condition. Recessive means that both parents would be carriers of a single copy of the responsible gene. Autosomal recessive disorders occur when a person inherits a particular pair of genes which do not work correctly. The chance that this would happen to children of carrier parents is 25% (1 in 4) for each pregnancy.

It is known that the limbs (arms, legs), the heart and the precursors of the blood system form between the fourth and eighth week of pregnancy. The birth defects seen in TAR syndrome must occur during this crucial period of development. As of 2001, the genetic cause remains unknown.

### Demographics

TAR syndrome affects both males and females equally. It most likely occurs in every racial and ethnic group. It is estimated that one in every 250,000 infants are born with TAR syndrome. In all, more than 200 individuals with this disorder have been described in the medical literature.

### Signs and symptoms

Aside from the limb deficiencies and the thrombocytopenia, the heart can also be affected. Around one-third of these infants are born with heart defects. These are usually found at birth. The heart problems include holes in the atrial chamber of the heart (atrial septal defect) and tetralogy of Fallot. The name tetralogy of Fallot means there are four different defects of the heart. Because of the high risk for excessive bleeding to occur, these infants are not good candidates for heart surgery. Some of them have died from heart failure.

### Diagnosis

Diagnosis of TAR syndrome is made with the use of x rays of the bones, and by testing for low platelet levels in the blood at birth. TAR syndrome can be diagnosed during pregnancy. By using ultrasound (sound waves) at around 16-20 weeks of pregnancy, the shortening of the arms can be seen. A second test is then done called cordocentesis. In this procedure, using ultrasound guidance, a thin needle is introduced through the mother's abdomen into the amniotic sac. A blood sample is taken directly from the umbilical cord. With this blood sample, a count of the platelets can be done. If the platelet count is low, along with the short arms (absent radii), the diagnosis of TAR syndrome is made.

### Prognosis

About 40% of these individuals die in infancy, usually due to severe bleeding episodes. Cow's milk allergy or intolerance is a common problem. Stomach infections seem particularly threatening to these infants, and can also trigger the bleeding episodes. The thrombocytopenia is treated with platelet transfusions, which may or may not control the bleeding, and death may occur.

The thrombocytopenia seen in TAR syndrome does improve with age. If these individuals survive the first two years of life, they appear to have a normal life span. However, the easy bruising continues throughout life. Many females with TAR syndrome also have abnormal menstrual periods, possibly related to the thrombocytopenia.

Surgery is sometimes done in an attempt to straighten and improve the use of their hands. They may wear corrective braces for the forearms. Many of these individuals develop arthritis, especially of the wrists and knees as they get older. This may further limit the use of their hands and legs. However, most individuals with TAR syndrome learn to adapt well to their disability, and lead productive lives.

### Resources

**PERIODICALS**

Hall, Judith. "Thrombocytopenia with Absent Radius (TAR)." *Medicine* (1969): 411-439.

**WEBSITES**

The Association for Children with Hand or Arm Deficiency. http://www.reach.org.uk.htm.

**ORGANIZATIONS**

T.A.R.S.A. Thrombocytopenia Abset Radius Syndrome Association. 212 Sherwood Drive, Linwood, NJ 08324-7658. (609) 927-0418.

Kevin M. Sweet, MS, CGC

# ▌TAY–Sachs disease

### Definition

Tay–Sachs disease is a genetic disorder caused by a missing enzyme that results in the accumulation of a fatty substance in the nervous system. This results in disability and death.

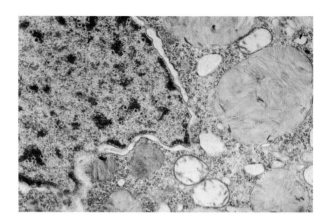

**Section of brain tissue from patient with Tay-Sachs disease.** *(Custom Medical Stock Photo, Inc.)*

### Demographics

Tay–Sachs disease is very rare in the general American population but particularly common among Jewish people of Eastern European and Russian (Ashkenazi) origin. About one out of every 3,600 babies born to Ashkenazi Jewish couples will have the disease. Tay–Sachs is also more common among certain French–Canadian and Cajun French families.

### Description

Gangliosides are a fatty substance necessary for the proper development of the brain and nerve cells (nervous system). Under normal conditions, gangliosides are continuously broken down, so that an appropriate balance is maintained. In Tay–Sachs disease, the enzyme necessary for removing excess gangliosides is missing. This allows gangliosides to accumulate throughout the brain, and is responsible for the disability associated with the disease.

#### Risk factors

People at highest risk for Tay–Sachs are those who have a family history of the condition and who are of Jewish or French–Canadian ancestry (from the St. Lawrence River Valley of Quebec) or members of the Cajun population in Louisiana.

### Causes and symptoms

Tay–Sachs is caused by a defective HEXA **gene**, located on **chromosome** 15. The HEXA gene provides instructions for making an enzyme called beta–hexosaminidase A. Without this enzyme, gangliosides cannot be degraded. They build up within the brain, interfering with nerve functioning. Because it is a recessive disorder, only people who receive two defective genes (one from the mother and one from the father) will actually have the disease. People who have only one defective gene and one normal gene are called carriers. They carry the defective gene and thus the possibility of passing the gene and/or the disease onto their offspring.

When a carrier and a non–carrier have children, none of their children will actually have Tay–Sachs. It is likely that 50% of their children will be carriers themselves. When two carriers have children, their children have a 25% chance of having normal genes, a 50% chance of being carriers of the defective gene, and a 25% chance of having two defective genes. The two defective genes cause the disease itself.

Classic Tay–Sachs disease strikes infants around the age of six months. Up until this age, the baby will appear to be developing normally. When Tay–Sachs begins to show itself, the baby will stop interacting with other people, and develop a staring gaze. Normal levels of noise will startle the baby to an abnormal degree. By about one year of age, the baby will have very weak, floppy muscles, and may be completely blind. The head will be quite large. Patients also present with loss of peripheral (side) vision, inability to breathe and swallow, and paralysis as the disorder progresses. Seizures become a problem between ages one and two, and the baby usually dies by about age four.

A few variations from this classical progression of Tay–Sachs disease are possible:

- Juvenile hexosaminidase A deficiency. Symptoms appear between ages two and five; the disease progresses more slowly, with death by about 15 years of age.
- Chronic hexosaminidase A deficiency. Symptoms may begin around age five, or may not occur until age 20–30. The disease is milder. Speech becomes slurred. The individual may have difficulty walking due to weakness, muscle cramps, and decreased coordination of movements. Some individuals develop mental illness. Many have changes in intellect, hearing, or vision.

## Diagnosis

### Examination

Examination of the eyes of a child with Tay–Sachs disease will reveal a very characteristic cherry–red spot at the back of the eye (in an area called the retina).

### Tests

Prenatal tests such as **amniocentesis** and chorionic villus sampling (CVS) can diagnose the disease before

---

birth. Amniocentesis usually is done between the 15th and 20th week of pregnancy. In this test, the doctor draws a sample of the fluid that surrounds the fetus. The fluid contains fetal cells, which are tested to see if they contain hexosaminidase A. A carrier will have about half of the normal level of hexosaminidase A present, while a patient with the disease will have none..

## Treatment

Providing good, supportive care and treating the symptoms as they arise is the only way to treat Tay–Sachs; there is no way to treat the disease itself. Researchers are investigating whether stem cell transplants could help babies with Tay–Sachs. However, as of 2009, stem cell transplantation has not yet been successful in stopping or reversing brain damage, and the treatment also carries a high risk of death.

## Prognosis

Children born with infantile Tay–Sachs, even with the best available care, usually die before the age of five. Children born with juvenile Tay–Sachs usually die before the age of 15.

## Prevention

Prevention involves identifying carriers of the disease and providing them with appropriate information concerning the chance of their offspring having Tay–Sachs disease. When the levels of hexosaminidase A are half the normal level a person is a carrier of the defective gene. Blood tests of carriers reveals reduction of hexosaminidase A.

## Resources

### BOOKS

Freedman, Jeri. *Tay–Sachs Disease*. New York, NY: Chelsea House Publications, 2009.

Parker, Philip. *Tay–Sachs Disease —A Bibliography and Dictionary for Physicians, Patients, and Genome Researchers*. San Diego, CA: ICON Health Publications, 2007.

Walker, Julie. *Tay–Sachs Disease*. New York, NY: Rosen Publishing Group, 2006.

## ORGANIZATIONS

March of Dimes Foundation, 1275 Mamaroneck Avenue, White Plains, NY, 10605, (914) 428-7100, (888) MOD-IMES, (914) 428-8203, askus@marchofdimes.com, http://www.marchofdimes.com.

National Organization for Rare Disorders (NORD), 55 Kenosia Avenue, Danbury, CT, 06813-1968, (203) 744-0100, (800) 999-NORD, (203) 798-2291, orphan@rarediseases.org, http://www.rarediseases.org.

National Tay–Sachs and Allied Diseases Association, 2001 Beacon Street, Suite 204, Brighton, MA, 02135, (617) 277-4463, (800) 90-NTSAD, (617) 277-0134, info@ntsad.org, http://www.ntsad.org.

## OTHER

"Tay–Sachs Disease." *Medline Plus.* Health Topic. http://www.nlm.nih.gov/medlineplus/taysachsdisease.html (accessed October 25, 2009)

"Tay–Sachs Disease." *Genetics Home Reference.* Information Page. http://ghr.nlm.nih.gov/condition = taysachsdisease (accessed October 25, 2009)

"Tay–Sachs Disease." *Mayo Clinic.* Information Page. http://www.mayoclinic.org/Tay–Sachs-disease/ (accessed October 25, 2009)

"Tay–Sachs Disease." *Chicago Center for Jewish Genetic Diseases.* Information Page. http://www.jewishgenetics.org/?q = content/Tay–Sachs-disease (accessed October 25, 2009)

## PERIODICALS

Elstein, D., et al. "Neurocognitive testing in late–onset Tay–Sachs disease: a pilot study." *Journal of Inherited Metabolic Disease* 31, no. 4 (August 2008): 518–523

Fernandez Filho, J. A., and B. E. Shapiro. "Tay–Sachs disease." *Archives of Neurology* 61, no. 9 (September 2004): 1466–1468.

Shapiro, B. E., et al. "Late–onset Tay–Sachs disease: adverse effects of medications and implications for treatment." *Neurology* 67, no. 5 (September 2006): 875–877

Laith Farid Gulli, MD
Tish Davidson, AM

# Teratogen

## Definition

A teratogen is any environmental influence that adversely affects the normal development of the fetus.

## Description

Abnormal fetal development may result from exposure to a teratogen. There are four different teratogen categories: physical agents (radiation and hyperthermia),

---

metabolic conditions affecting the mother, infection, and drugs (like thalidomide) and alcohol.

## Physical agents

### Hyperthermia

Women whose body temperature is raised while pregnant may have abnormalities result in their fetus. The rise in body temperature can be caused by infection or by spending time in hot areas such as a sauna or hot tub.

### Ionizing radiation–mutagens versus teratogens

Any outside agent (like radiation) interfering with the process of development is considered a teratogen. Development is the process in which a tiny mass of undifferentiated cells (the embryo) multiplies and differentiates into the kidney, liver, heart, bone, muscles, and so on. Mutagens, however, are agents that directly affect and disrupt **DNA**, the genetic blueprint of an organism. Some agents, like radiation, are mutagens and teratogens. Ionizing radiation can cause defects either in development or it can damage DNA directly.

## Metabolic disease

Infants of women with metabolic disorders have increased risks for abnormalities. Diabetic women, for example, are three to four times more likely to have fetuses with congenital abnormalities than infants of mothers without **diabetes**. The metabolic disease of the mother can have genetic or other causes.

## Infection

There are a number of known infectious organisms which are teratogenic to the fetus, some of which cause damage directly, and some of which damage the fetus by causing a fever and raising the temperature of the mother.

### Alcohol and drugs

#### Thalidomide

A dramatic example of a teratogen is thalidomide. In the early 1960s it was shown that more than 7,000 women who took the anti-nausea drug thalidomide during their pregnancy had children with very short or absent arms and legs. Other abnormalities were also seen in the children, such as the absence of ears, as well as heart and intestinal malformations. Affected infants were born to women who took thalidomide during the critical time period, also known as the period of susceptibility.

#### Period of susceptibility: The example of thalidomide

Thalidomide also teaches the importance of timing in the action of teratogens. Only a small amount of thalidomide was necessary to cause birth defects, but it had to be taken between 34 and 50 days after conception in order to harm the embryo. The time when teratogens can act, in this case from day 34 to day 50 after conception, is called the period of susceptibility. Since organ development in the unborn child occurs at different times, it was shown that taking thalidomide on different days caused the infants to have a variety of defects (heart vs. ears vs. limb formation). Drugs very often affect specific parts of the process of development. Before, or after, the processes take place, the drug will have no effect. Of course many teratogens, like thalidomide, work on a number of different developmental processes at different times (sometimes they are consecutive times, or they may be non-consecutive: for example from days 16 to 20 and days 24 to 48). The period of susceptibility of the fetus to most teratogens is between the third and eighth week after conception.

#### Dose and duration: The example of alcohol

The most common teratogen, alcohol, illustrates the important concept that the dose of a teratogen (for example, the number of alcoholic drinks a mother has) and duration of exposure to a teratogen (for example, the number of days a mother drinks alcohol) both play an important role in the effect of a teratogen. Alcohol can have a wide range of effects on a fetus, from no mental change or very mild mental changes (usually a small dose of alcohol) to full-blown **fetal alcohol syndrome**, in which the infant is severely retarded. Even two glasses of alcohol can be teratogenic to a fetus, but the mental retardation and characteristic facial changes seen in full-blown fetal alcohol syndrome generally requires the mother to drink 2-3 oz of alcohol per day for a sustained period of time (the exact amount of time is not known) during pregnancy. Thus, dose and duration help determine the severity of a teratogen's effects.

#### Other factors that affect teratogens

Although the dose and duration are important in determining how much of an effect alcohol will have on the fetus, other factors have an impact, too. When normal mice and mutant mice are given the same dose of a particular teratogen, the mutant mice are affected much more severely. This means that in humans, the genetic makeup of the fetus helps determine to what extent the teratogen will affect the fetus. A fetus with one particular set of genes might be severely affected by the mother drinking one glass of alcohol, while another fetus may be unaffected by the first or even second glass of alcohol. The outcome of teratogens probably depends on a combination of factors: the mother's condition (genetic or otherwise), the genetic background of the fetus, and the dose and duration of the teratogen. However, the importance of each factor probably varies greatly from teratogen to teratogen and from individual to individual.

Although the discussion of these teratogenic concepts has revolved around examples from the category of drugs and alcohol, the concepts may be applied to any of the categories of teratogens.

### Demographics

Exact numbers of infants affected by teratogens are difficult to estimate. *Langman's Medical Embryology* states 4-6% of all infants will have major developmental or genetic abnormalities. This source estimates that of the children with major abnormalities, 10% can be attributed to teratogens, 20-25% can be attributed to genetic and environmental influences, and 40-60% of the abnormalities are due to unknown causes (possibly teratogenic). That means as many as 95% of all major birth disorders may involve teratogens.

### Diagnosis

The diagnosis varies from teratogen to teratogen. Some genetic diseases and teratogens can present with the same abnormalities and symptoms. If the gene causing the disorder has been isolated and is well understood, the difference between a genetic and a teratogenic disorder may be established. Many abnormalities in children go unexplained. In these cases, teratogen exposure should be considered.

## Treatment, prevention, and the period of susceptibility

Treatment options and how well they work vary widely according to the teratogen. The best course is to prevent teratogen exposure, or reduce the exposure as much as possible. Prevention is complicated because very often women may not realize they are pregnant until the middle of the period of susceptibility. Substances that are not harmful to an adult, like the derivatives of retinoic acid found in a number of skin creams, alcohol, and many prescription drugs, can be extremely harmful to the fetus. Retinoic acid, for example, has a period of susceptibility from days 20-35 after conception—a time when many women might not realize they are pregnant.

Thus, women who are engaging in activities that can lead to pregnancy and want to avoid any potential damage to their fetus should attempt to avoid teratogenic substances (including a large number of over-the-counter, prescription, and illegal drugs). Alternatively, women can also prevent most damage to the fetus by closely monitoring their pregnancy status and avoiding teratogens as soon as pregnancy occurs.

## Partial list of teratogens

*Drugs and chemicals*:

- alcohol
- aminoglycosides
- aminopterin
- antithyroid agents
- bromine
- cortisone
- diethylstilbesterol (DES)
- diphenylhydantoin
- heroin
- lead
- methylmercury
- penicillamine
- retinoic acid (Isoretinoin, Accutane)
- tetracycline
- thalidomide
- trimethadione
- valproic acid
- warfarin

*Physical agents*:

- hyperthermia (fever, sauna)
- ionizing radiation (x rays)

*Infectious organisms*:

- Coxsackie virus
- Cytomegalovirus
- Herpes simplex virus
- Parvovirus
- Rubella
- Toxoplasma gondii
- Treponema pallidum (syphilis)

*Metabolic conditions in the mother*:

- autoimmune disease
- diabetes
- malnutrition
- phenylketonuria

### Resources

#### BOOKS

Gilbert, Scott F. *Developmental Biology*. Sunderland, MA: Sinauer Associates, 1994, pp. 633-645.

Sadler, T.W. *Langman's Medical Embryology*. Baltimore, Williams and Williams, 1995, pp. 122-143.

#### PERIODICALS

Incardona, J.P., and H. Roelink. "The Role of Cholesterol in Shh Signaling and Teratogen-induced Holoprosencephaly." *Cellular and Molecular Life Sciences* 57, no.12 (November 2000): 1709-19.

Machado, A.F., et al. "Teratogenic Response to Arsenite During Neurulation: Relative Sensitivities of C57BL/6J and SWV/Fnn Mice and Impact of the Splotch Allele." *Toxicological Sciences* 51, no. 1 (September 1999): 98-107.

Sampson, P.D., et al. "On Categorization in Analyses of Alcohol Teratogenesis." *Environmental Health Perspectives* 108, Supplement 3 (June 2000): 421-428.

#### WEBSITES

Organization of Teratology Information Services. http://www.otispregnancy.org/index.html.

Michael V. Zuck, PhD

Testicular feminization syndrome *see*
**Androgen insensitivity syndrome**

# Thalassemia

### Definition

Thalassemia describes a group of genetic blood disorders characterized by absent or reduced production of hemoglobin, the oxygen–carrying protein inside the red blood cells. There are two basic groups of thalassemia disorders: alpha thalassemias and beta

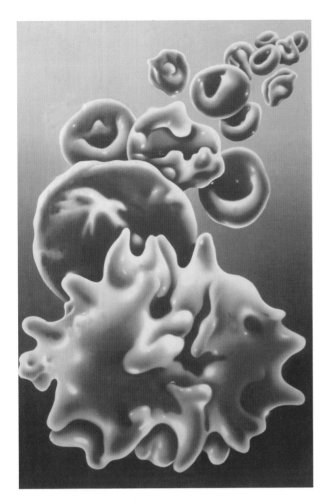

Illustration depicting the various abnormal red blood cells of thalassemia. The red blood cells rapidly break up as they move through the body due to poor hemoglobin production. *(Photo Researchers, Inc.)*

thalassemias. These conditions cause varying degrees of anemia, which can range from mild to life–threatening.

## Description

Normal adult hemoglobin consists of four protein chains: two alpha and two beta globins. Each chain carries a group called a heme, a ring–like molecule that contains the iron that binds the oxygen. Thalassemias are classified according to the globin that is affected, hence the names *alpha* and *beta* thalassemia. Although both classes of thalassemia affect the same protein, the alpha and beta thalassemias are distinct diseases that affect the body in different ways.

### Alpha thalassemias

People whose hemoglobin does not produce enough alpha globin have alpha thalassemia. The condition is the result of changes in the genes that code for making alpha chains in hemoglobin. There are four types of alpha thalassemias:

- Hemoglobin H disease (HHD): This thalassemia causes severe anemia and serious health problems such as an enlarged spleen, and bone deformities.

- Alpha thalassemia major: this is the most severe type of alpha thalassemia. It is also called hydrops fetalis and most individuals affected by this condition die before or shortly after birth.

- Alpha thalassemia minor: individuals affected by this thalassemia have smaller red blood cells and display mild anemia. It is often misdiagnosed as iron deficiency anemia.

- Alpha thalassemia silent carrier: this thalassemia is difficult to detect because it usually does not cause symptoms, hence its name.

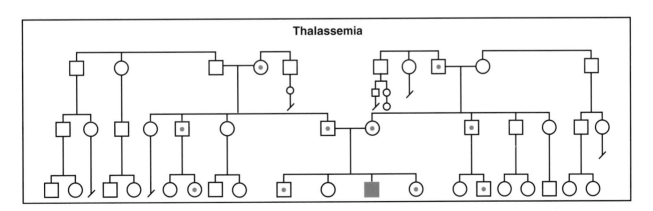

**Thalassemia**

*(Gale, a part of Cengage Learning.)*

**Anemia**—A blood condition in which the level of hemoglobin or the number of red blood cells falls below normal values. Common symptoms include paleness, fatigue, and shortness of breath.

**Bilirubin**—A yellow pigment that is the end result of hemoglobin breakdown. This pigment is metabolized in the liver and excreted from the body through the bile. Bloodstream levels are normally low; however, extensive red cell destruction leads to excessive bilirubin formation and jaundice.

**Bone marrow**—A spongy tissue located in the hollow centers of certain bones, such as the skull and hip bones. Bone marrow is the site of blood cell generation.

**Bone marrow transplantation**—A medical procedure used to treat some diseases that arise from defective blood cell formation in the bone marrow. Healthy bone marrow is extracted from a donor to replace the marrow in an ailing individual. Proteins on the surface of bone marrow cells must be identical or very closely matched between a donor and the recipient.

**Desferoxamine**—The primary drug used in iron chelation therapy. It aids in counteracting the life–threatening buildup of iron in the body associated with long–term blood transfusions.

**Globin**—Protein chains found in hemoglobin. Normal adult hemoglobin has two alpha globin chains and two beta globin chains.

**Heme**—The iron–containing molecule in hemoglobin that serves as the site for oxygen binding. Each of the four hemoglobin chains has one heme.

**Hemoglobin**—Tetrameric protein in the blood that carries oxygen to the cells and carries carbon dioxide away from the cells. Hemoglobin consists of four chains, each containing a heme.

**Hemoglobin A (HbA)**—Normal adult hemoglobin consists of two alpha globins and two beta globins.

**Hemoglobin electrophoresis**—A laboratory test that separates molecules based on their size, shape, or electrical charge.

**Hemoglobin F (HbF)**—Fetal hemoglobin consists of two alpha and two gamma globins. HbF is produced by the fetus in utero and until about 48 weeks after birth. At this stage, the production of HbA rapidly increases while that of HbF drops off.

**Hepatomegaly**—An abnormally large liver.

**HLA type**—Refers to the unique set of proteins called human leukocyte antigens. These proteins are present on each individual's cells and allow the immune system to recognize 'self' from 'foreign'. HLA type is particularly important in organ and tissue transplantation.

**Hydroxyurea**—A drug that has been shown to induce production of fetal hemoglobin. HbF has a pair of gamma– –globin molecules instead of the beta–globins of HbA. Higher–than–normal levels of HbF can alleviate some of the symptoms of thalassemia.

**Iron deficiency anemia**—A decrease in the number of red cells in the blood caused by too little iron in the diet, poor absorption of iron by the body, or loss of blood.

**Iron overload**—A side effect of frequent blood transfusions in which the body accumulates abnormally high levels of iron. Iron deposits can form in organs, particularly the heart, and cause life–threatening damage.

**Jaundice**—Yellowing of the skin or eyes due to excess of bilirubin in the blood.

**Mutation**—A permanent change in the genetic material that may alter a trait or characteristic of an individual, or manifest as disease, and can be transmitted to offspring.

**Placenta**—The organ responsible for oxygen and nutrition exchange between a pregnant mother and her developing baby.

**Red blood cell**—Hemoglobin–containing blood cells that transport oxygen from the lungs to tissues. In the tissues, the red blood cells exchange their oxygen for carbon dioxide, which is brought back to the lungs to be exhaled.

**Screening**—Process through which carriers of a trait may be identified within a population.

**Splenomegaly**—Enlargement of the spleen.

**Tetramer**—Protein that consists of four amino acid chains.

---

*Beta thalassemias*

People whose hemoglobin does not produce enough beta protein have **beta thalassemia**. The condition is the result of changes in the genes that code for making beta globins in hemoglobin. There are three major types of beta thalassemias:

• Beta thalassemia major: this condition is the most severe form of beta thalassemia, characterized by complete lack of beta chains in the hemoglobin. Also called Cooley's anemia, it causes a life–threatening anemia that requires regular blood transfusions.

- Beta thalassemia minor: individuals affected by this thalassemia simply carry the genetic trait for thalassemia and commonly experience no health problems other than a possible mild anemia.

- Beta thalassemia intermedia: with this condition, the lack of beta chains in the hemoglobin is significant enough to cause a moderately severe anemia and significant health problems, including bone deformities and spleen enlargement. However, the condition has a wide range of severity, from mild to moderately severe.

Beta thalassemias can be classified based on clinical symptoms. Beta thalassemia major usually causes severe anemia that can occur within months after birth. If left untreated, severe anemia can result in insufficient growth and development, as well as other characteristic physical complications that can lead to a dramatically decreased life expectancy. Fortunately, in developed countries, beta thalassemia is usually identified by screening in the newborn period, before symptoms have developed. Children who are identified early can be started on ongoing blood transfusion therapy as needed. Although transfusion therapy prevents many of the complications of severe anemia, the body is unable to eliminate the excess iron contained in the transfused blood. Over time, this excess iron deposits in tissues and organs, resulting in damage and organ failure. Another medication must be administered to help the body eliminate the excess iron and prevent iron–overload complications. Individuals with beta thalassemia intermedia usually have moderate anemia that only requires blood transfusions intermittently, if at all.

### Demographics

The thalassemias are among the most common genetic diseases worldwide, with more than 100,000 babies worldwide born each year with severe forms of thalassemia, resulting in some 15 million people having thalassemic disorders. Both alpha and beta thalassemia have been described in individuals of almost every ancestry, but the conditions are more common among certain ethnic groups. Unaffected carriers of all types of thalassemia traits do not experience health problems. In fact, thalassemia trait protects against malaria, a disease caused by blood-borne parasites transmitted through mosquito bites. According to a widely accepted theory, most genetic mutations that cause thalassemia occurred multiple generations ago. Coincidentally, these mutations increased the likelihood that carriers would survive malaria infection. Survivors passed the mutation onto their offspring, and the trait became established throughout areas where malaria is common. As populations migrated, so did the thalassemia traits.

Beta thalassemia trait is seen most commonly in people with the following ancestry: Mediterranean (including North African, and particularly Italian and Greek), Middle Eastern, Indian, African, Chinese, and Southeast Asian (including Vietnamese, Laotian, Thai, Singaporean, Filipino, Cambodian, Malaysian, Burmese, and Indonesian). Alpha thalassemia trait is seen with increased frequency in the same ethnic groups. However, there are different types of alpha thalassemia traits within these populations. The frequency of hemoglobin H disease and alpha thalassemia major depends on the type of alpha thalassemia trait. The populations in which alpha thalassemia diseases are most common include Southeast Asians and Chinese (particularly Southern Chinese).

It is difficult to obtain accurate prevalence figures for the various types of thalassemia within different populations. This is due to testing limitations in obtaining exact genetic diagnoses, and to the fact that many studies have focused on small, biased hospital populations. It is known, however, that there has been an increase in the incidence of thalassemia in North America in the last ten years, primarily due to immigration from Southeast Asia. According to the Federal Census of 2000, 10.2 million Asians were in the United States, almost three times the number reported in the 1980 Census count. The various thalassemias affecting this population is very high and increasing in California due to the large number of Asian immigrants in that state.

Determining prevalence figures for alpha thalassemia is even more difficult due to increased limitations in diagnostic testing. All types of alpha thalassemia disease are most common among people of Southeast Asian and Chinese descent, for reasons that become clearer with an understanding of the underlying **genetics** of alpha thalassemia. For example, one study of 500 pregnant women in Northern Thailand estimated a frequency of one in 500 pregnancies affected by alpha thalassemia major. Prevalence of alpha thalassemia disease is significantly lower in the United States owing primarily to immigration patterns. However, at least one state, California, has observed growing hemoglobin H disease incidence rates that are high enough to justify universal newborn screening for the condition.

## Genetic profile

Humans normally make several types of hemoglobin. An individual's stage in development determines whether he or she makes primarily embryonic, fetal, or adult hemoglobins. Normal adult hemoglobin (HbA) is a tetrameric protein consisting of four chains: two alpha globins, and two beta globins, each chain also containing a heme. It is the major hemoglobin component of red blood cells (95%). Additionally, red blood cells contain other minor hemoglobin forms: hemoglobin A2 (HbA2) consisting of two alpha chains and two delta chains (~3%) and hemoglobin F (HbF), consisting of two alpha chains and two gamma chains (~2%). If a person can't produce enough of either alpha or beta globins, the red blood cells do not form normally and cannot carry oxygen properly, resulting in anemia. All thalassemias are caused by deletions or modifications in the genes that control globin production. These genes are located on **chromosome** 16 (alpha globin genes) and chromosome 11 (beta, gamma, and delta genes). Mutations modify the amount of alpha globin relative to that of the other globins being produced, leading to an abnormal hemoglobin ratio and decreased hemoglobin production. The globin that is produced in normal amounts over the other globin accumulates and forms aggregates that damage the red blood cell membrane.

The thalassemias are recessively inherited, meaning that a genetic change must be inherited from both the mother and the father. The severity of the disease is influenced by the exact thalassemia mutations inherited, as well as other genetic and environmental factors. There are rare exceptions, notably with beta thalassemia, where globin **gene mutations** exhibit a dominant pattern of **inheritance** in which only one gene needs to be altered in order to see disease expression.

### Beta thalassemia

In beta thalassemia, alpha globins are produced in excess over the beta globins, which leads to the formation of alpha globin tetramers that accumulate and interfere with red blood cell production (erythropoiesis). These mutations occur in the HBB gene that provides instructions for making beta hemoglobin. As of 2009, approximately 200 genetic mutations have been described that cause beta thalassemia, designated as either beta0 or beta+ mutations. No beta globin is produced with a beta0 mutation, and only a small fraction of the normal amount of beta globin is produced with a beta+ mutation.

An individual having one normal HBB gene and one with a beta thalassemia mutation is said to carry the beta thalassemia trait. Beta thalassemia trait, like other hemoglobin traits, is protective against malaria infection. Trait status is generally thought not to cause health problems, although some women with beta thalassemia trait may have an increased tendency toward anemia during pregnancy.

When two members of a couple carry the beta thalassemia trait, there is a 25% chance that each of their children will inherit beta thalassemia disease by inheriting two beta thalassemia mutations, one from each parent. The clinical severity of the beta thalassemia disease—whether an individual has beta thalassemia intermedia or beta thalassemia major—will depend largely on whether the mutations inherited are beta0 or beta+ thalassemia mutations. Two beta0 mutations generally lead to beta thalassemia major, and two beta+ thalassemia mutations generally lead to beta thalassemia intermedia. Inheritance of one beta0 and one beta+ thalassemia mutation tends to be less predictable.

Although relatively uncommon, there are other thalassemia-like mutations that can affect the beta globin gene. Hemoglobin E is the result of a substitution of a single nucleotide. This change results in a structurally altered hemoglobin that is produced in decreased amounts. Therefore, hemoglobin E is unique in that it is both a quantitative (i.e. thalassemia-like) and qualitative trait. When co-inherited with a beta thalassemia trait, it causes a disease that is almost indistinguishable from beta thalassemia disease. Large deletions around and including the beta globin gene can lead to delta/beta thalassemia or hereditary persistence of fetal hemoglobin (HPFH). Interestingly, delta/beta thalassemia trait behaves very similarly to beta thalassemia trait clinically. However, HPFH trait does not tend to cause hemoglobin disease when co-inherited with a second thalassemia or other beta globin mutation.

### Alpha thalassemia

In alpha thalassemia, beta globins are produced in excess over the alpha globins, which leads to the formation of beta globin tetramers that also accumulate and interfere with erythropoiesis. Most individuals have four normal copies of the alpha globin gene, two copies on each chromosome 16. These genes make the alpha globin component of HbA. Alpha globin is also a component of HbF and HbA2. Mutations of the alpha globin genes are usually deletions of the gene, resulting in absent production of alpha globin. Since there are four genes (instead of the usual two) to consider when looking at alpha globin gene inheritance, there are several alpha globin types that are possible.

Absence of one alpha globin gene leads to a condition known as silent alpha thalassemia trait. This condition causes no health problems and can be detected only by special **genetic testing**. Alpha thalassemia trait occurs when two alpha globin genes are missing. This can occur in two ways. The genes may be deleted from the same chromosome, causing the 'cis' type of alpha thalassemia trait. Alternately, they may be deleted from different chromosomes, causing the 'trans' type of alpha thalassemia trait. In both instances, there are no associated health problems, although the trait status may be detected by more routine blood screening.

Hemoglobin H disease results from the deletion of three alpha globin genes, such that there is only one functioning gene. Typically, this can occur when one parent carries the silent alpha thalassemia trait, and the other parent carries the 'cis' type of the alpha thalassemia trait. In this situation, there is a 25% chance for hemoglobin H disease in each of such a couple's children.

Hemoglobin H disease–like symptoms can also be a part of a unique condition called alpha thalassemia mental retardation syndrome. Alpha thalassemia mental retardation syndrome can be caused by a deletion of a significant amount of chromosome 16, affecting the alpha globin genes. This is usually not inherited, but rather occurs sporadically in the affected individual. Affected individuals have mild hemoglobin H disease, mild–to–moderate mental retardation, and characteristic facial features. This syndrome can also occur as a sex–linked form in which a mutation is inherited in a particular gene on the X chromosome. This gene influences alpha globin production, as well as various other developmental processes. Individuals affected with this form of the syndrome tend to have more severe mental retardation, delayed development, nearly absent speech, characteristic facial features, and genital–urinary abnormalities.

Alpha thalassemia major results from the deletion of all four alpha globin genes, such that there are no functioning alpha globin genes. This can occur when both parents carry the 'cis' type of the alpha thalassemia trait. In this situation, there is a 25% chance for alpha thalassemia major in each of such a couple's children.

### Diagnosis

Thalassemia may be suspected if an individual shows signs that are suggestive of the disease. In all cases, however, laboratory diagnosis is essential to confirm the exact diagnosis and to allow for the provision of accurate **genetic counseling** about recurrence risks and testing options for parents and affected individuals. Screening is likewise recommended to determine trait status for individuals of high–risk ethnic groups.

The following tests are used to screen for thalassemia disease and/or trait:

- Complete blood count
- Hemoglobin electrophoresis with quantitative hemoglobin A2 and hemoglobin F
- Free erythrocyte–protoporphyrin (or ferritin or other studies of serum iron levels)

A complete blood count will identify low levels of hemoglobin, small red blood cells, and other red blood cell abnormalities that are characteristic of a thalassemia diagnosis. Since thalassemia trait can sometimes be difficult to distinguish from iron deficiency, tests to evaluate iron levels are important. A hemoglobin electrophoresis is a test that can help identify the types and quantities of hemoglobin made by an individual. This test uses an electric field applied across a slab of gel–like material. Hemoglobins migrate through this gel at various rates and to specific locations, depending on their size, shape, and electrical charge. Isoelectric focusing and high–performance liquid chromatography (HPLC) use similar principles to separate hemoglobins and can be used instead of or in various combinations with hemoglobin electrophoresis to determine the types and quantities of hemoglobin present. Hemoglobin electrophoresis results are usually within the normal range for all types of alpha thalassemia. However, hemoglobin A2 levels and sometimes hemoglobin F levels are elevated when beta thalassemia disease or trait is present. Hemoglobin electrophoresis can also detect structurally abnormal hemoglobins that may be co–inherited with a thalassemia trait to cause thalassemia disease (i.e., hemoglobin E) or other types of hemoglobin disease (i.e., sickle hemoglobin). Sometimes **DNA** testing is needed in addition to the above screening tests. This can be performed to help confirm the diagnosis and establish the exact genetic type of thalassemia.

Diagnosis of thalassemia can occur under various circumstances and at various ages. Several states offer thalassemia screening as part of the usual battery of blood tests done for newborns. This allows for early identification and treatment. Thalassemia can be identified before birth through the use of prenatal diagnosis. Chorionic villus sampling (CVS) can be offered as early as 10 weeks of pregnancy and involves removing a sample of the placenta made by the baby and testing the cells. **Amniocentesis** is generally offered between 15 and 22 weeks of pregnancy, but can sometimes be offered earlier. Two to three tablespoons of the fluid surrounding the baby is removed. This fluid contains fetal cells that can be tested. Pregnant woman and couples may choose prenatal testing in order to prepare for the birth of a baby that may have thalassemia. Alternately, knowing the diagnosis during pregnancy allows for the option of pregnancy termination. Preimplantation genetic diagnosis (PGD) is a relatively new technique that involves in–vitro fertilization followed by genetic testing of one cell from each developing embryo. Only the embryos unaffected by **sickle cell disease** are transferred back into the uterus. PGD is currently available on a research basis only and is relatively expensive.

## Signs and symptoms

### Beta thalassemia

Beta thalassemia major is characterized by severe anemia that can begin months after birth. In the United States and other developed countries beta thalassemia is identified and treated early and effectively. Therefore, the following discussion of symptoms applies primarily to affected individuals in the past and unfortunately in some underdeveloped countries now. If untreated, beta thalassemia major can lead to severe lethargy, paleness, and growth and developmental delay. The body attempts to compensate by producing more blood, which is made inside the bones in the marrow. However, this is ineffective without the needed genetic instructions to make enough functioning hemoglobin. Instead, obvious bone expansion and changes occur that cause characteristic facial and other changes in appearance, as well as increased risk of fractures. Severe anemia taxes other organs in the body—such as the heart, spleen, and liver—which must work harder than usual. This can lead to heart failure, as well as enlargement and other problems of the liver and spleen. When untreated, beta thalassemia major generally results in childhood death usually due to heart failure. Fortunately, in developed countries diagnosis is usually made early, often before symptoms have begun. This allows for treatment with blood transfusion therapy, which can prevent most of the complications of the severe anemia caused by beta thalassemia major. Individuals with beta thalassemia intermedia have a more moderate anemia that may only require treatment with transfusion intermittently, such as when infections occur and stress the body. As a person with beta thalassemia intermedia gets older, however, the need for blood transfusions may increase to the point that they are required on a regular basis. When this occurs their disease becomes more similar to beta thalassemia major. Other genetic and environmental factors can influence the course of

the disease as well. For example, co–inheritance of one or two alpha thalassemia mutations can tend to ameliorate some of the symptoms of beta thalassemia disease, which result in part from an imbalance in the amount of alpha and beta globin present in the red blood cells.

### Hemoglobin H disease

Absence of three alpha globin genes causes an imbalance of alpha and beta globin proteins in the red blood cells. The excess beta globin proteins tend to come together to form hemoglobin H, which is unable to release oxygen to the tissues. In addition, hemoglobin H tends to precipitate out in the cells, causing damage to the red blood cell membrane. When affected individuals are exposed to certain drugs and chemicals known to make the membrane more fragile, the cells are thought to become vulnerable to breakdown in large numbers, a complication called hemolytic anemia. Fever and infection are also considered to be triggers of hemolytic anemia in hemoglobin H disease. This can result in fatigue, paleness, and a yellow discoloration of the skin and whites of eyes called jaundice. Usually, the anemia is mild enough not to require treatment. Severe anemia events may require blood transfusion, however, and are usually accompanied by other symptoms such as dark feces or urine and abdominal or back pain. These events are uncommon in hemoglobin H disease, although they occur more frequently in a more serious type of hemoglobin H disease called hemoglobin H/Constant Spring disease. Individuals effected with this type of hemoglobin H disease are also more likely to have enlargement of and other problems with the spleen.

### Alpha thalassemia major

Because alpha globin is a necessary component of all major hemoglobins and some minor hemoglobins, absence of all functioning alpha globin genes leads to serious medical consequences that begin even before birth. Affected fetuses develop severe anemia as early as the first trimester of pregnancy. The placenta, heart, liver, spleen, and adrenal glands may all become enlarged. Fluid can begin collecting throughout the body as early as the start of the second trimester, causing damage to developing tissues and organs. Growth retardation is also common. Affected fetuses usually miscarry or die shortly after birth. In addition, women carrying affected fetuses are at increased risk of developing complications of pregnancy and delivery. Up to 80% of such women develop toxemia, a disturbance of metabolism that can potentially lead to convulsions and coma. Other maternal complications include premature delivery and increased rates of cesarean section, as well as hemorrhage after delivery.

## Treatment and management

### Beta thalassemia

Individuals with beta thalassemia major receive regular blood transfusions, usually on a monthly basis. This helps prevent severe anemia and allows for more normal growth and development. Transfusion therapy does have limitations, however. Individuals can develop reactions to certain proteins in the blood—called a transfusion reaction. This can make locating appropriately matched donor blood more difficult. Although blood supplies in the United States are very safe, particularly relative to the past and other areas of the world, there remains an increased risk of exposure to blood–borne infection such as hepatitis. Additionally, the body is not able to get rid of the excess iron that accompanies each transfusion. An additional medication called desferoxamine is administered, usually five nights per week over a period of several hours using an automatic pump that can be used during sleep or taken anywhere the person goes. This medication is able to bind to the excess iron, which can then be eliminated through urine. If desferoxamine is not used regularly or is unavailable, iron overload can develop and cause tissue damage and organ damage and failure. The heart, liver, and endocrine organs are particularly vulnerable. Desferoxamine itself may rarely produce allergic or toxic side effects, including hearing damage. Signs of desferoxamine toxicity are screened for and generally develop in individuals who overuse the medication when body iron levels are sufficiently low. Overall, however, transfusion and desferoxamine therapy has increased the life expectancy of individuals with the most severe types of beta thalassemia major to the fourth or fifth decade. This can be expected to improve with time and increased developments in treatment, as well as for those with more mild forms of the disease.

Other treatments offer additional options for some individuals with beta thalassemia major. There are various medications that target the production of red blood cells (i.e., erythropoeitin) or HbF (i.e., hydroxyurea and butyrate). Their effectiveness in alleviating the severity of beta thalassemia is currently being investigated. Another promising treatment is bone marrow transplantation, in which the bone marrow of an affected individual is replaced with the bone marrow of an unaffected donor. If successful, this treatment can provide a cure. However, there is an approximately 10–15% chance the

procedure could be unsuccessful (i.e., the thalassemia returns), result in complications (i.e., graft–versus–host disease), or result in death. The risk for specific individuals depends on current health status, age, and other factors. Because of the risks involved and the fact that beta thalassemia is a treatable condition, transplant physicians require a brother or sister donor who has an identically matched tissue type, called HLA type. HLA type refers to the unique set of proteins present on each individual's cells, which allows the immune system to recognize "self" from "foreign." HLA type is genetically determined, so there is a 25% chance for two siblings to be a match. Transplant physicians and researchers are also investigating ways to improve the safety and effectiveness of bone marrow transplantation. Using newborn sibling umbilical cord blood—the blood from the placenta that is otherwise discarded after birth but contains cells that can go on to make bone marrow—seems to provide a safer and perhaps more effective source of donor cells. Donors and recipients may not have to be perfect HLA matches for a successful transplant using cord blood cells. Trials are also underway to determine the effectiveness of "partial transplants," in which a safer transplant procedure is used to replace only a percentage of the affected individual's bone marrow. Other possible treatments on the horizon may include **gene therapy** techniques aimed at increasing the amount of normal hemoglobin the body is able to make.

### Hemoglobin H disease

Hemoglobin H disease is a relatively mild form of thalassemia that may go unrecognized. It is not generally considered a condition that will reduce one's life expectancy. Education is an important part of managing the health of an individual with hemoglobin H disease. It is important to be able to recognize the signs of severe anemia that require medical attention. It is also important to be aware of the medications, chemicals, and other exposures to avoid due to the theoretical risk they pose of causing a severe anemia event. When severe anemia occurs, it is treated with blood transfusion therapy. For individuals with hemoglobin H disease, this is rarely required. For those with the hemoglobin H/Constant Spring form of the disease, the need for transfusions may be intermittent or ongoing, perhaps on a monthly basis and requiring desferoxamine treatment. Individuals with this more severe form of the disease may also have an increased chance of requiring removal of an enlarged and/or overactive spleen.

### Alpha thalassemia major

Because alpha thalassemia major is most often a condition that is fatal in the prenatal or newborn period, treatment has previously been focused on identifying affected pregnancies in order to provide appropriate management to reduce potential maternal complications. Pregnancy termination provides one form of management. Increased prenatal surveillance and early treatment of maternal complications is an approach that is appropriate for mothers who wish to continue their pregnancy with the knowledge that the baby will most likely not survive. In recent years, there have been a handful of infants with this condition who have survived long–term. Most of these infants received experimental treatment including transfusions before birth, early delivery, and even bone marrow transplantation before birth, although the latter procedure has not yet been successful. For those infants that survive to delivery, there seems to be an increased risk of developmental problems and physical effects, particularly heart and genital malformations. Otherwise, their medical outlook is similar to a child with beta thalassemia major, with the important exception that ongoing, life–long blood transfusions begin right at birth.

### Clinical trials

Clinical trials on thalassemias are currently sponsored by the National Institutes of Health (NIH) and other agencies. As of 2009, NIH was reporting 53 on–going and completed studies.

Examples include:

- The evaluation of the amount of liver fibrosis and iron storage in a patient's liver before transplant (bone marrow/stem cell) from an unrelated donor. (NCT00578292)

- A study to collect information on complications among people who currently have or previously had thalassemia. (NCT00661804)

- The evaluation of how pain varies during the blood transfusion cycle in people with thalassemia who are treated with regular blood transfusions. (NCT00872833)

- The evaluation of the genetic factors which influence the severity of beta thalassemia. (NCT00159042)

Clinical trial information is constantly updated by NIH and the most recent information on thalassemia trials can be found at: http://clinicaltrials.gov/search/

### Prognosis

The prognosis for individuals with the most serious types of thalassemia has improved drastically in the last several years following recent medical advances in transfusion, chemotherapy, and transplantation therapy. Advances continue and promise to improve the life expectancy and quality of life further for affected individuals.

### Resources

**BOOKS**

Bridges, Kenneth, and Howard A. Pearson. *Anemias and Other Red Cell Disorders.* New York, NY: McGraw–Hill, 2008.

Garrison, Cheryl. *The Iron Disorders Institute Guide to Anemia.* Nashville, TN: Cumberland House Publishing, 2009.

Parker, Philip M. *Beta Thalassemia —A Bibliography and Dictionary for Physicians, Patients, and Genome Researchers.* San Diego, CA: Icon Health Publications, 2007.

Steinberg, Martin H., et al., editors. *Disorders of Hemoglobin: Genetics, Pathophysiology and Clinical Management.* New York, NY: Cambridge University Press, 2001.

**PERIODICALS**

Bedair, E. M., et al. "Review of radiologic skeletal changes in thalassemia." *Pediatric Endocrinology Reviews* 6, suppl. 1 (October 2008): 123–126.

Bukvic, N., et al. "Coexistence of beta–thalassemia and hereditary hemochromatosis in homozygosity: a possible synergic effect?" *Hemoglobin* 33, no. 2 (2009): 155–157.

Burdick, C. O. "Separating thalassemia trait and iron deficiency by simple inspection." *American Journal of Clinical Pathology* 131, no. 3 (March 2009): 444.

Cianciulli, P. "Treatment of iron overload in thalassemia." *Pediatric Endocrinology Reviews* 6, suppl. 1 (October 2008): 208–213.

Di Matteo, R., et al. "Bone and maxillofacial abnormalities in thalassemia: a review of the literature." *Journal of*

*Biological Regulators and Homeostatic Agents* 22, no. 4 (October–December 2008): 211–216.

Geffner, M. E., and H. Karlsson. "Use of recombinant human growth hormone in children with thalassemia." *Hormone Research* 71, suppl. 1 (January 2009): 46–50.

Giordano, P. C., et al. "Frequency of alpha–globin gene triplications and their interaction with beta–thalassemia mutations." *Hemoglobin* 33, no. 2 (2009): 124–131.

Maggio, A., et al. "A critical review of non invasive procedures for the evaluation of body iron burden in thalassemia major patients." *Pediatric Endocrinology Reviews* 6, suppl. 1 (October 2008): 193–203.

Ribeiro, D. M., and M. F. Sonati. "Regulation of human alpha–globin gene expression and alpha–thalassemia." *Genetics and Molecular Research* 7, no. 4 (October 2008): 1045–1053.

Skordis, N., et al. "Hormonal dysregulation and bones in thalassaemia—an overview." *Pediatric Endocrinology Reviews* 6, suppl. 1 (October 2008): 107–115.

**WEBSITES**

*Learning About Thalassemia.* Information Page, NHGRI, April 10, 2009 (May 17, 2009). http://www.genome.gov/page.cfm?pageID=10001221

*Beta Thalassemia.* Information Page, Genetics Home Reference, February, 2007 (May 17, 2009). http://ghr.nlm.nih.gov/condition=betathalassemia

*Thalassemia.* Medical Encyclopedia, Medline Plus, May 4, 2009 (May 17, 2009). http://www.nlm.nih.gov/medlineplus/ency/article/000587.htm

*Thalassemia.* Information Page, Iron Disorders Institute, November 3, 2006 (May 17, 2009). http://www.irondisorders.org/Disorders/Thalassemia.asp

*Thalassemia.* Information Page, March of Dimes Foundation, 2009 (May 17, 2009). http://www.marchofdimes.com/professionals/14332_1229.asp

*Thalassemia.* Information Page, Mayo Clinic, February 4, 2009 (May 17, 2009). http://www.mayoclinic.com/print/thalassemia/DS00905/METHOD=print&DSECTION=all

*What Are Thalassemias?* Information Page, NHLBI, January 2008 (May 17, 2009). http://www.nhlbi.nih.gov/health/dci/Diseases/Thalassemia/Thalassemia_WhatIs.html

*What Is Thalassemia?* Information Page, Cooley's Anemia Foundation, 2009 (May 17, 2009). http://www.thalassemia.org/index.php?option=com_content&view=article&id=19&Itemid=27

**ORGANIZATIONS**

Cooley's Anemia Foundation. 330 Seventh Ave., #900, New York, NY 10001. (800)522-7222. Fax: 212-279-5999. http://www.thalassemia.org.

March of Dimes Foundation. 1275 Mamaroneck Avenue, White Plains, NY 10605. (914)428-7100 or (888)MODIMES (663-4637). Fax: (914)428-8203. Email: askus@marchofdimes.com. http://www.marchofdimes.com.

National Heart, Lung, and Blood Institute (NHLBI). PO Box 30105, Bethesda, MD 20824-0105. (301)592-8573.

Email: nhlbiinfo@rover.nhlbi.nih.gov. http://www.nhlbi.nih.gov.

Northern California Thalassemia Center at Children's Hospital Oakland. 747 52nd St., Oakland, CA 94609. (510)428-3885 x 4398. http://www.thalassemia.com.

Thalassemia Foundation of Canada. 340 Falstaff Ave., North York, ON M6L 2E8, Canada. (416)242-8425. Email: info@thalassemia.ca. http://www.thalassemia.ca.

Jennifer Bojanowski, MS, CGC
Monique Laberge, PhD

# Thalidomide embryopathy

## Definition

The term thalidomide embryopathy (TE) is used to describe a specific pattern of birth defects caused by a mother's use of the drug thalidomide during her pregnancy. The drug is able to cross the placenta and reaches the developing embryo, causing parts of the embryo's body to form abnormally. The most common birth defects observed in infants with TE include structural abnormalities of the arms, legs, ears, and eyes, although other organs may also be affected. The most harmful time to use thalidomide is during the first three to six weeks of pregnancy.

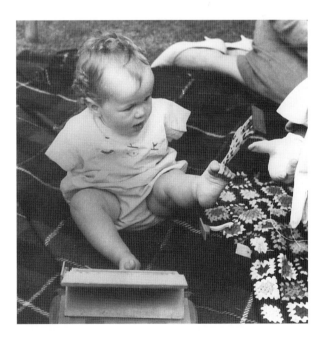

**Thomas Yendell, a baby affected by thalidomide, picks up a toy with his feet.** *(AP Images.)*

## KEY TERMS

**Cataract**—A clouding of the eye lens or its surrounding membrane that obstructs the passage of light resulting in blurry vision. Surgery may be performed to remove the cataract.

**Embryo**—The earliest stage of development of a human infant, usually used to refer to the first eight weeks of pregnancy. The term *fetus* is used from roughly the third month of pregnancy until delivery.

**Erythema nodosum leprosum**—A complication of leprosy characterized by development of painful small swellings due to inflammation of a blood or lymph vessel. It is often accompanied by inflammation of a nerve or nerves, causing decreased function of the affected area.

**Glaucoma**—An increase in the fluid eye pressure, eventually leading to damage of the optic nerve and ongoing visual loss.

**Immunologic**—Related to immunology, the study of how the body's immune system fights disease. Many immunologic disorders are characterized by the body's use of antibodies.

**Insomnia**—An inability to either fall or stay asleep, particularly at a time of day when sleep is expected. A number of medications are available, and may be used, for treatment.

**Leprosy**—A chronic, contagious skin and nervous system disease that leads, in the more serious form, to numbness, muscle weakness, and paralysis. Leprosy is sometimes referred to as Hansen's disease.

**Placenta**—The organ responsible for oxygen and nutrition exchange between a pregnant mother and her developing baby.

**Sedative**—Medication that has a soothing or tranquilizing effect.

**Strabismus**—An improper muscle balance of the ocular muscles resulting in crossed or divergent eyes.

## Description

Thalidomide was originally marketed in Germany in October 1957 as a safe, inexpensive, and effective sedative. Its use was later expanded to include treatment of insomnia, anxiety, upset stomach, and morning sickness during pregnancy. Prior to its release onto the market, thalidomide had been tested in rodents and had been deemed safe; human studies were not performed. It was made available in at least 46 countries.

However, the drug was never approved for marketing in the United States due to concerns about the medication's potential side effects, one of which, peripheral neuropathy, was first recognized in 1960. Symptoms of peripheral neuropathy, or nerve damage, include burning, numbness, or tingling in the arms, legs, hands, or feet. The damage may not be reversible even after stopping the medication. Early in the 1960s, an increased number of infants with severe abnormalities of the arms and legs were observed in Germany, Great Britain, and Australia. Once it became clear that the mothers of these infants had taken thalidomide while pregnant, a connection was made between the drug and the birth defects. In 1961, the drug was withdrawn from the worldwide market. It has since become known as a powerful human **teratogen**, a drug or other agent proven to cause birth defects. The experience with thalidomide also led to greater overall attention to the potential effects of drug and other environmental exposures on a developing fetus, and to improved legislation regarding testing requirements before a new drug is released to the public.

Although the use of thalidomide decreased dramatically after 1961, it remained available in the United States and other countries on a "compassionate use" basis: physicians could obtain special permission to treat ill patients they believed could significantly benefit from the drug. Over time, it became clear that thalidomide is effective in the treatment of a number of medical conditions. This surprising resurgence of thalidomide has, in turn, led to concern over the possibility of another generation of children born with thalidomide-related birth defects. The manufacturer of thalidomide, Celgene Corporation, is working in close partnership with the U.S. Food and Drug Administration (FDA) to tightly control the use of the drug and to maintain close follow-up on all individuals to whom it is prescribed. The drug is marketed under the brand name Thalomid.

Limb abnormalities are the most readily identified, and most well known, type of birth defect caused by prenatal thalidomide exposure. However, other types of physical problems may also occur in an exposed infant. In addition to limb abnormalities, TE may include abnormalities of the ears, eyes, kidneys, heart, intestinal tract, and nervous system. Mental retardation has been reported in approximately 5% of older individuals with TE.

## Genetic profile

TE is not an inherited medical condition. However, thalidomide is a known teratogen. Therefore, women who use this medication while pregnant are at risk of having infants with physical, and possibly mental, birth defects. A woman who does not use thalidomide during pregnancy cannot have a child with TE. It is still not entirely clear how thalidomide causes birth defects. One hypothesis is that the drug prevents formation of new blood vessels. Research is continuing in this area.

## Demographics

It is estimated that 10,000-12,000 infants were born with birth defects consistent with TE following its initial period of use in the late 1950s to early 1960s. According to the Teratology Society 1998 Public Affairs Symposium, approximately 40%, or roughly 5,000, of the affected individuals survived.

In July 1998, the FDA approved the use of thalidomide in the United States, under a very tightly controlled protocol, for the treatment of erythema nodosum leprosum (ENL), a painful skin complication of leprosy. The drug has been available in South America, an area where leprosy is more common than in the United States. Reports of thalidomide-affected South American infants were published as recently as 1996.

Medical researchers are studying whether or not thalidomide may be effective in the treatment of other medical conditions, including certain skin and immunologic disorders, certain complications associated with human immunodeficiency virus (HIV) infection, and certain cancers. Although pregnancies among female patients with any of these conditions may be rare, unintended pregnancies will occur and will be at risk for fetal abnormalities if the mothers are taking thalidomide.

## Signs and symptoms

TE includes a spectrum of physical abnormalities, all of which may occur at various levels of severity. An affected individual may not have every type of birth defect. All affected infants, however, have been exposed to thalidomide in early pregnancy, a time when the organs and body of an embryo are rapidly developing. Although use of thalidomide at any point in pregnancy is strongly discouraged, women who use the drug during the first six weeks of pregnancy are at the greatest risk of having children with birth defects. Rigorous control of the drug is necessary since many pregnancies are unplanned and may go unrecognized until after the drug exposure has occurred.

The clinical features of TE include:

### Limb defects

The most well known type of abnormality is referred to as phocomelia. Phocomelia occurs when most of the bones in the arms or legs are missing, and the hand or foot is attached directly to the body, similar to a flipper. Radial aplasia, or absence of the thumb and connecting bone in the forearm (radius), is another common abnormality. Abnormalities of the digits include a triphalangeal thumb (three small bones in the thumb, rather than two, such that the thumb looks like a finger), or an absent (hypoplastic) thumb only. Similar defects of the legs may also occur. Frequently, affected infants have abnormalities on both sides of their bodies, involving all four extremities.

### Ears

Malformations of the ears are common. These range from complete absence of the ear (severe microtia, also sometimes referred to in the medical literature as anotia) to mild changes in the appearance of the external ear. Abnormalities of the inner ear frequently cause **deafness**. Inner ear malformations may occur even if the external ear appears normal.

### Eyes

A range of eye abnormalities have been reported, including a very small eye (microphthalmos), **glaucoma**, strabismus, cataract, and abnormal production of tears.

### Other

• Structural heart defects.
• Kidney malformations, most often an absent or misplaced kidney.
• Abnormalities of the intestinal system.
• Structural defects of the spine and chest.
• Central nervous system abnormalities, such as mental handicap, described in a small percentage of older individuals with TE.
• Paralysis of the nerves of the face on either one side, both sides equally, or both sides but asymmetrically.
• An increased risk for early infant death, particularly among those infants with severe abnormalities of their internal organs.

## Diagnosis

Exposure to thalidomide during the first six weeks of pregnancy poses a significantly increased risk of having a child with TE. It is important to note that the exact dosage of the drug during this period is irrelevant.

Thalidomide is rapidly broken down in the mother's body and is therefore able to reach her developing embryo quickly. There is no direct genetic test to accurately diagnose all thalidomide-related birth defects before delivery. However, **prenatal ultrasound** examinations may be used to identify major structural abnormalities, such as those involving the limbs, heart, kidneys, and intestinal tract. A careful physical examination by a knowledgeable and experienced physician(s) is warranted after birth to document the nature and severity of any thalidomide-induced birth defects. Additional studies, such as hearing evaluations, are also indicated.

### Treatment and management

Management of the individual with TE is primarily symptomatic. Specialized medical care, such as heart surgery, may be necessary in certain situations, and should be determined on a case-by-case basis. Deaf individuals may require hearing aids and/or will need to learn sign language. Severe limb abnormalities may lead to the use of a wheelchair or other device to assist in mobility.

In order to try to minimize the number of future children born with TE, the drug manufacturer and the FDA implemented the System for Thalidomide Education and Prescribing Safety (S.T.E.P.S.) program in 1998. The goals of the program are three-fold: (1) to limit the risk of fetal exposure to thalidomide; (2) to enforce universal compliance of patients, physicians, and pharmacists with the designated components of the program; and, (3) to support appropriate, controlled use of the drug. To achieve this, the S.T.E.P.S. program requires informed consent from all patients to whom the drug will be given. Face-to-face counseling, a patient information booklet, and videotape are all used to review the potential benefits and side effects of the medication. Plans for birth control (contraception) and/or abstinence from sexual intercourse are also discussed. All women of childbearing age must agree to a pregnancy test prior to receiving their medication and at frequent intervals during treatment. Two methods of birth control are additionally required. Physicians who will be prescribing thalidomide must be registered in the S.T.E.P.S. program and must agree to follow each step of the program. Prescriptions may only be filled at registered pharmacies. No more than a one-month supply of the medication may be provided at one time; there are no automatic refills. It is recommended that women receive only a one-week supply, particularly during the first four weeks of treatment. Weekly refills are granted only with proof from a physician of a negative pregnancy test. In the event that a woman becomes pregnant, or suspects that she may be pregnant, an immediate referral is made for medical evaluation. Follow-up care is provided, and a database of all patients taking thalidomide is maintained.

Despite this unprecedented level of strict control, the S.T.E.P.S. program is unlikely to completely prevent the birth of *every* child in the United States with TE. Other countries in which the drug has been approved for use have been encouraged to develop similar methods to follow outcomes of pregnancies exposed to thalidomide. In the meantime, research is continuing to find drugs that will be as effective as thalidomide without the same dangers to embryonic development.

### Prognosis

There is no data addressing long-term survival rates among individuals with TE. Nonetheless, the presence and severity of thalidomide-related birth defects, particularly those involving the heart, would be expected to have the greatest impact on longevity. Severe heart malformations that cannot be corrected by surgery are likely to lead to early death. In the absence of such abnormalities, a normal life span is anticipated.

### Resources

#### PERIODICALS

Calabrese, Leonard, and Alan B. Fleischer. "Thalidomide: Current and Potential Clinical Applications." *American Journal of Medicine* 108 (April 15, 2000): 487-495.

Friedman, J.M., and C.A. Kimmel. "Teratology Society 1998 Public Affairs Committee Symposium." *Teratology* 59 (1999): 120-123.

Miller, Marilyn T., and Kerstin Stromland. "Teratogen Update: Thalidomide: A Review, With a Focus on Ocular Findings and New Potential Uses." *Teratology* 60, no. 5 (November 1999): 306-321.

---

## QUESTIONS TO ASK YOUR DOCTOR

- Is my child a candidate for a hearing aid or or devices to assist with mobility?
- Could my child be helped by physical or occupational therapy?
- If I do not take thalidomide again, is there a continued risk of having another child with TE?
- How long does it take for thalidomide to be completely out of my system?

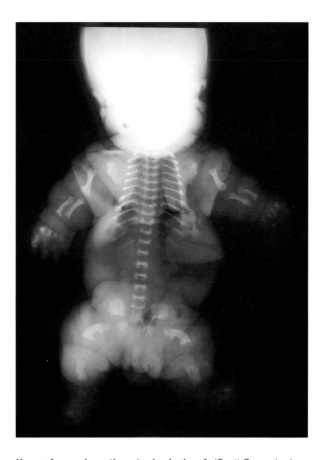

Public Affairs Committee. "Teratology Society Public Affairs Committee Position Paper: Thalidomide." *Teratology* 62, no. 3 (September 2000): 172-173.

**WEBSITES**

"Thalidomide (Systemic)." *MEDLINEplus Health Information.*http://www.nlm.nih.gov/medlineplus/druginfo/thalidomidesystemic202692.html.

"Thalidomide Information." http://www.fda.gov/cder/news/thalinfo/thalidomide.htm.

"Thalidomide." http://www.modimes.org.healthlibrary2/factsheets/Thalidomide.htm.

**ORGANIZATIONS**

Food and Drug Administration. 5600 Fishers Lane, Rockville, MD 20857. (888) 463-6332. http://www.fda.gov.

March of Dimes Birth Defects Foundation. 1275 Mamaroneck Ave., White Plains, NY 10605. (888) 663-4637. resourcecenter@modimes.org. http://www.modimes.org.

Terri A. Knutel, MS, CGC

# Thanatophoric dysplasia

## Definition

Thanatophoric **dysplasia** is one of the most common and most severe forms of dwarfism. Affected infants have marked shortening of their arms and legs, a small chest, and a relatively large head. Most die within a few days after birth; longer-term survivors have been reported but are rare.

## Description

Thanatophoric dysplasia (TD) was first described in 1967 to refer to infants with a severe form of dwarfism who died within the first hours of life. The word "thanatophoric" is derived from the Greek word, *thanatophorus,* which means "death-bringing." The term thanatophoric dwarfism is occasionally used. However, over time, the word dysplasia, which refers to any disorder in growth, has become the preferred terminology.

Two distinct types of TD were delineated in 1987. Affected infants are divided based on their particular combination of physical features and skeletal findings. While all individuals with TD have micromelia, or abnormally small or short arms and legs, differences in the length and shape of the femurs, the bones of the thigh, can be used to distinguish between TD types 1 (TD1) and 2 (TD2). Infants with TD1 have curved, "telephone-receiver"-like femurs. In contrast, the femurs of infants with TD2 are longer and straighter.

**X ray of a newborn thanatophoric dwarf.** *(Scott Camazine/ Photo Researchers, Inc)*

The presence of skull abnormalities is another important distinction between the two types: infants with TD2 typically have a severe abnormality of the bones of the skull, referred to as cloverleaf skull or kleeblattschadel anomaly. The skull of a normal infant is composed of several segments of bone, some of which are completely joined together, or fused, by the time of delivery. Their lines of fusion are referred to as sutures. Some sutures are only partially fused, leaving soft, skin-covered openings that will gradually close over the first year of life. Premature closure of these sutures leads to a condition called **craniosynostosis**. Craniosynostosis often leads to an abnormal skull shape and, if not eventually corrected by surgery, prevents normal growth of the brain. The most extreme form of craniosynostosis, as seen in infants with TD2, causes a severely abnormal skull whose shape resembles that of a cloverleaf. Although milder forms of craniosynostosis may be found in infants with TD1, cloverleaf skull is not typically present.

Other bone abnormalities occur in both TD types 1 and 2, including an abnormal shape of and spacing between the bones in the spine (vertebrae), shortened

## KEY TERMS

**Acondroplasia**—An autosomal dominant form of dwarfism caused by a defect in the formation of cartilage at the ends of long bones. Affected individuals typically have short limbs, a large head with a prominent forehead and flattened profile, and a normal-sized trunk.

**Amniocentesis**—A procedure performed at 16-18 weeks of pregnancy in which a needle is inserted through a woman's abdomen into her uterus to draw out a small sample of the amniotic fluid from around the baby. Either the fluid itself or cells from the fluid can be used for a variety of tests to obtain information about genetic disorders and other medical conditions in the fetus.

**Chorionic villus sampling (CVS)**—A procedure used for prenatal diagnosis at 10-12 weeks gestation. Under ultrasound guidance a needle is inserted either through the mother's vagina or abdominal wall and a sample of cells is collected from around the fetus. These cells are then tested for chromosome abnormalities or other genetic diseases.

**Hypochondroplasia**—An autosomal dominant form of dwarfism whose physical features are similar to those of achondroplasia but milder. Affected individuals have mild short stature and a normal facial appearance.

ribs, and small pelvic bones. Most of the other organs of the body, with the exception of the brain, are normal, although occasional abnormalities of the kidneys have been reported. A variety of abnormal changes in the structure of the brain have been described. The small number of children with TD who have survived past infancy have been severely mentally and physically handicapped.

The most common cause of death among individuals with TD is respiratory insufficiency. The small chest and, consequently, limited growth of the lungs, are the primary reasons for the breathing problems. However, associated abnormalities of the central nervous system are most likely also involved since these interfere with the body's ability to regulate normal breathing.

### Genetic profile

Both types of thanatophoric dysplasia occur as sporadic, autosomal dominant conditions. Only one copy of the altered **gene** causing TD needs to be present

in order for the condition to occur. Males and females are equally likely to be affected. The parents of an affected child do not have TD and are normal. Thus, it is believed that, in most cases, a new genetic mutation, or change, causing TD occurred in either the egg or sperm cell that gave rise to that particular pregnancy. Such a mutation cannot be made to happen; it occurs simply by chance. A very low risk of recurrence, or chance of another affected child in a future pregnancy, would be expected. Unfortunately, families have been described with more than one child with TD. The most likely explanation in these families is gonadal mosaicism.

Gonadal mosaicism occurs when a normal adult has a mixed population of cells in his or her gonads (testes or ovaries). All of the other cells in that individual's body are presumably normal. Most sperm or egg cells from these gonads would be normal and would not have a TD mutation; however, an unknown percentage would carry the mutation. As a result, even though the parent would be normal, he or she could, with the same or a different partner, have another child with TD. It is virtually impossible to prove whether or not a parent has gonadal mosaicism. Even so, all parents of an affected child are counseled that gonadal mosaicism in one of them is a possibility.

Thanatophoric dysplasia is caused by mutations in the fibroblast growth factor receptor 3 gene (FGFR3), located on the short arm of **chromosome** 4 at band 16.3 (abbreviated as 4p16.3). The fibroblast growth factors are a family of important proteins in the human body. They are involved in the production of new cells and new blood vessels as well as in the healing of wounds. Mutations in each of the fibroblast growth factor genes (FGFR1, 2, and 3) have been linked to a variety of genetic conditions. The FGFR3 protein is primarily found in cartilage and the central nervous system. Different mutations in the FGFR3 gene have been associated with other skeletal dysplasias, most notably **achondroplasia** and **hypochondroplasia**.

As might be expected, different mutations in FGFR3 have been found in patients with TD1 versus those with TD2. A wider variety of mutations have been identified among infants with TD1. One predominant mutation has been present in nearly all cases of TD2 studied so far. Regardless of the specific mutation, the net effect of each of the mutations in both TD1 and TD2 is the same: the linear growth of bone is prevented, resulting in very short, small bones.

### Demographics

Thanatophoric dysplasia is the most common lethal **skeletal dysplasia**, with an estimated incidence of one in 35,000–50,000 births. It has been described in all races and ethnic groups.

## Signs and symptoms

Infants with TD are typically identified either during pregnancy or at the time of birth. Affected pregnancies are often complicated by polyhydramnios, or excess amniotic fluid around the fetus. As a result, the mother often appears more pregnant than she actually is. It is common for a **prenatal ultrasound** examination to be performed to rule out a fetal birth defect as the cause. The serious limb abnormalities typical of TD are often identified in this way. Polyhydramnios may also lead to an increased chance of early labor and premature delivery. The pregnant woman may require more intensive monitoring of her pregnancy.

At birth, newborns with TD typically have a very large head with a prominent forehead, a flattened bridge of the nose, and prominent, bulging eyes. Their limbs are extremely short and are often held extended out from the rest of the body. The neck is short, the chest is narrow, and the belly appears unusually large, giving an overall resemblance to a pear. The shape of the skull may be abnormal due to either cloverleaf skull or a milder form of craniosynostosis. Newborns are often rather floppy, or hypotonic, with poor muscle tone and absent primitive neurologic reflexes. Breathing is very difficult due to the small chest and lungs, often leading to the use of a ventilator to prolong survival.

The physical appearance of individuals with TD who survive the neonatal period does not dramatically change over time. Affected children remain very small and have limited potential to walk or move about unaided. Mental retardation due to structural brain malformations has been reported. Seizures and hearing loss frequently develop.

## Diagnosis

Prenatal diagnosis of TD is possible based on ultrasound examination, usually during the second half of pregnancy. However, it is important to realize that many of the physical abnormalities seen in fetuses with TD, such as an enlarged head and shortened long bones, may also be found in fetuses with other forms of skeletal dysplasia. Consequently, while ultrasound may suggest a diagnosis of a skeletal dysplasia, it may not be possible to confirm a diagnosis of TD until after birth.

Upon delivery, a careful examination of the infant should be performed to look for many of the more obvious external features of TD. Radiologic studies are extremely important, particularly to distinguish between TD1 and TD2. X ray will confirm the marked

shortening of the long bones, identify curved or straight femurs, document the shape and appearance of the spinal vertebrae, and reveal the extent of craniosynostosis. An autopsy, including x rays, is highly recommended on any stillborn infant with TD to confirm the diagnosis.

Mutation studies by analysis of the FGFR3 gene are being used more often to confirm a diagnosis of TD and to determine TD type. Perhaps the greatest benefit of direct **genetic testing** is for those parents who have been told by a prenatal ultrasound examination that their unborn child has a serious bone dysplasia. An **amniocentesis** for additional genetic studies may be offered. Further clarification of the diagnosis allows for more refined counseling regarding the infant's likely prognosis. Termination of the pregnancy may be an option for some couples. For those couples wishing to continue an affected pregnancy, plans can be made for the remaining prenatal care, especially given the risk for polyhydramnios and/or early labor and delivery. Careful consideration may be given as to the level of intervention and medical care desired for the infant after birth.

Knowledge of the specific TD mutation is also helpful in planning care for any future pregnancy. Despite the sporadic nature of TD, a couple with a history of one affected child has a small risk of having a second affected child due to the possibility of gonadal mosaicism. Prenatal testing in a new pregnancy, such as chorionic villus sampling or amniocentesis, may be offered to look for a TD mutation. However, in order for this to be possible, the TD mutation in the previous child must have been determined.

Studies are ongoing to assess whether or not three-dimensional ultrasound, in contrast to the current, much more widely available, two-dimensional ultrasound, may be used to accurately prenatally diagnose TD and other skeletal dysplasias. If effective, additional prenatal studies could become less common. However, early results have shown no significant improvement in the detection or diagnosis of TD and related disorders. The present standard of care therefore remains a prenatal ultrasound examination, if available, physical evaluations after delivery, and identification of the underlying genetic mutation, whenever possible.

## Treatment and management

The treatment and care of an infant with TD is mainly supportive. The poor prognosis associated with TD should be discussed. Infants who survive the newborn period will require intensive, ongoing medical care.

## Prognosis

Nearly all infants with TD, both types 1 and 2, die either at the time of delivery or shortly thereafter due to severe respiratory distress. Aggressive medical treatment after birth has not always helped affected infants live even a short amount of time. Prolonged survival, including one child who, as of 1997, was still alive at the age of nine years, has been reported but is highly unusual. Survival is associated with poor growth and development and with continuing, serious respiratory problems.

## Resources

### BOOKS

"Disorders Involving Transmembrane Receptors." In *Nelson Textbook of Pediatrics,* edited by Richard E. Behrman, Robert M. Kleigman, and Hal B. Jenson. 16th ed. Philadelphia: W.B. Saunders, 2000, pp. 2120-2122.

*Smith's Recognizable Patterns of Malformations,* edited by Kenneth L. Jones. 5th ed. Philadelphia: W.B. Saunders, 1997, p. 338.

### PERIODICALS

Baker, Kristin M., et al. "Long-term Survival in Typical Thanatophoric Dysplasia Type 1." *American Journal of Medical Genetics* 70, no. 4 (June 27, 1997): 427-436.

Cohen, M. Michael, Jr. "Achondroplasia, Hypochondroplasia, and Thanatophoric Dysplasia: Clinically Related Skeletal Dysplasias That Are Also Related at the Molecular Level." *International Journal of Oral and Maxillofacial Surgery* 27, no. 6 (December 1998): 451-455.

Garjian, Kareen V., et al. "Fetal Skeletal Dysplasias: Three-dimensional Ultrasound—Initial Experience." *Radiology* 214, no. 3 (March 2000): 717-723.

Wilcox, William R., et al. "Molecular, Radiologic, and Histopathologic Correlations in Thanatophoric Dysplasia." *American Journal of Medical Genetics* 78, no. 3 (July 7, 1998): 274-281.

### WEBSITES

Dwarfism.org. http:www.dwarfism.org.&gt;

*OMIM—Online Mendelian Inheritance in Man.*http:// www.ncbi.nlm.nih.gov.

### ORGANIZATIONS

Greenberg Center for Skeletal Dysplasias. 600 North Wolfe Street, Blalock 1012C, Baltimore, MD 21287-4922. (410) 614-0977. http://www.med.jhu.edu/Greenberg. Center/Greenbrg.htm.

Terri A. Knutel, MS, CGC

# Thrombasthenia of Glanzmann and Naegeli

## Definition

Thrombasthenia of Glanzmann and Naegeli is an extremely rare inherited disorder in which there is abnormal function of a component of the blood called the platelets, leading to abnormalities in blood clotting and increased bleeding.

## Description

Blood clotting, or coagulation, is the process by which several factors in the blood stick together to form a physical barrier that prevents bleeding. In response to a disruption in blood flow or bleeding because of injury, several factors in the blood stick together at the site of injury, sealing off the blood vessel and stopping blood loss in a process called hemostasis. If any of the factors that contribute to the process of coagulation and hemostasis are abnormal, dangerous bleeding conditions can result.

One of the factors involved in hemostasis is called the platelet. Platelets are small disc-shaped structures that circulate in the blood stream in an inactive state. When an injury occurs, platelets become activated and stick to fibrous proteins, called fibrinogen, that are also circulating in the blood stream. Because there are multiple sites on the fibrinogen proteins for platelets to bind and vice versa, a cross-linked net or mass called a "platelet plug" is formed which seals off the injury and prevents further bleeding. Next, the platelet mass actively contracts to form an even more solid mass in a process called "clot retraction." Over time, repair cells can use this mass as a scaffolding to lay down new tissue and thereby effect a permanent repair of the injury.

Platelets attach to fibrinogen through the use of specialized sugar- proteins (glycoproteins) that are present on the platelet surface. There are two specific glycoproteins that form a complex responsible for the

## KEY TERMS

**Autosomal dominant**—A pattern of genetic inheritance where only one abnormal gene is needed to display the trait or disease.

**Autosomal recessive**—A pattern of genetic inheritance where two abnormal genes are needed to display the trait or disease.

**Carrier**—A person who possesses a gene for an abnormal trait without showing signs of the disorder. The person may pass the abnormal gene on to offspring.

**Coagulation**—The process by which a liquid becomes a solid, as in blood clotting.

**Fibrinogen**—A fibrous protein that circulates in blood and participates in blood clotting by attaching to platelets.

**Glycoprotein IIb/IIIa (GP IIb/IIIa)**—Sugar-proteins on the surface of platelets that bind to the fibrous protein, fibrinogin. These sugar-proteins are defective in Glanzmann's thrombasthenia.

**Hemostasis**—The arrest of bleeding by blood coagulation.

**Mutant**—A change in the genetic material that may alter a trait or characteristic of an individual or manifest as disease.

**Platelets**—Small disc-shaped structures that circulate in the blood stream and participate in blood clotting.

**Transfusion**—The injection of a component of the blood from a healthy person into the circulation of a person who is lacking or deficient in that same component of the blood.

platelet-fibrinogen interaction: glycoprotein IIb, and glycoprotein IIIa.

The platelet disorder thrombasthenia of Glanzmann and Naegeli (TGN) results from an inherited defect in the glycoprotein IIb/IIIa complex (GP IIb/IIIa). As a result of this glycoprotein defect, platelets fail to stick to fibrinogen, leading to defective hemostasis and prolonged bleeding. TGN is sometimes subdivided into different groups: type I, in which there is no functional GP IIb/IIIa; type II, in which small amounts of working GP IIb/IIIa can be detected; and variant thrombasthenia, in which the amount of working GP IIb/IIIa may vary. Thrombasthenia of Glanzmann and Naegeli has also been referred to by other names including Glanzmann's thrombasthenia, diacyclothrombopathia IIb-IIIa, Glanzmann disease, and glycoprotein complex IIb/IIIa deficiency.

TGN was first described by the Swiss physician, Edward Glanzmann in 1918. Glanzmann used the term, "thrombasthenia," meaning "weak platelets," because clots from patients with the disorder did not retract well. Although the disease is exceedingly rare, platelets taken from people with the disease have been very useful in the research that first discovered how normal platelets function.

### Genetic profile

TGN is a genetic condition and can be inherited or passed on in a family. The disorder results from any number of different mutations that can occur in either the gene for glycoprotein IIb or the gene for glycoprotein IIIa (both located on **chromosome** 17, locus 17q21.32), with defects split equally between the two genes.

In the majority of cases, it appears that the genetic abnormality for the disorder is inherited as an autosomal recessive trait, meaning that two abnormal genes are needed to display the disease. A person who carries one abnormal gene does not display the disease and is called a carrier. A carrier has a 50% chance of transmitting the gene to his or her children, who must inherit one abnormal gene from each parent to display the disease. People who are carriers of the abnormal gene appear to have only half-normal amounts of working GP IIb/IIIa, which is still sufficient for normal platelet function.

There are reports of a few families in which the defect is inherited in an autosomal dominant fashion. In this pattern of **inheritance**, only one abnormal gene is needed to display the disease, and the chance of passing the gene to offspring is 50%.

### Demographics

TGN is exceedingly rare, with less than 1,000 cases identified between 1962 and 2000. There are several groups in which the majority of cases of thrombasthenia have been discovered, including Iraqi Jews, Arabs living in Israel and Jordan, populations of south India, and French Gypsies of the Manouche tribe.

### Signs and symptoms

Most people with TGN will have a major bleeding event before the age of five. Common manifestations of the disease include nose bleeds, bleeding from the gums, or skin rashes caused by bleeding into the skin (known as purpura or petechiae). Larger amounts of bleeding into underlying tissue may result in diffuse black bruises, usually seen on the arms and the legs. Normal handling of infants can cause superficial bruises and may be mistaken for abuse. As a result of chronic bleeding, patients may have lower amounts of red blood cells in their blood (anemia) and suffer from iron deficiencies. Rarely, there may be bleeding into the joints, causing disfiguration. Bleeding after traumatic accidents or after surgical operations and dental procedures may be profuse and require vigorous medical treatment. Prolonged untreated or unsuccessfully treated bleeding associated with TGN may be life-threatening. For reasons which are unclear, severity of bleeding events appears to decrease with increasing age.

There are other concerns when TGN is diagnosed in a woman. Because of the platelet disorder, women may experience particularly heavy menstrual bleeding. In fact, the first occurrence of menstrual bleeding in a young woman may be so severe that it requires prompt medical attention and treatment. Further, pregnancy and delivery represent severe bleeding risks and may not always be manageable with medical treatment.

### Diagnosis

TGN is diagnosed through a combination of medical history, physical examination, and laboratory testing. Bleeding episodes and physical manifestations of the disease (as described above) may prompt an investigation for the underlying cause. The presence of a bleeding disorder in more than one close or distant relative is especially important, as it may indicate that a genetic cause of the condition is involved.

Blood tests will reveal normal amounts of platelets. Tests performed with substances that stimulate platelet clumping though GP IIb/IIIa will show minimal effects as a result of the platelet defect. Conversely, tests performed using a different substance, ristocetin, which causes platelet clumping through different mechanisms, will provoke a brisk and appropriate platelet response. Other blood tests will reveal a longer than normal bleeding time, poor clot retraction, and may demonstrate low numbers of red blood cells and iron deficiency.

The diagnosis of TGN is ultimately confirmed by investigating the GP IIb/IIIa glycoprotein complex. Antibodies that are specifically designed to distinguish between normal and abnormal GP IIb/IIIa can be used in a technique known as immunofluorescence (in which the antibody is attached to a fluorescent dye) or a test called a Western blot (in which proteins are first separated by size and then exposed to antibodies). These methods can also be used to detect people who are carriers of a mutant gene for TGN by demonstrating only half-normal amounts of GP IIb/IIIa. Prenatal diagnosis may also be possible but is not recommended as sampling of the blood in an affected fetus may lead to uncontrollable bleeding that could prove fatal.

### Treatment and management

Several medications can aid in the treatment of TGN, while others should be avoided. Some patients will demonstrate shortening of their bleeding time with DDAVP, a medication that improves the function of platelets. Women who have heavy bleeding may benefit from birth control pills to prevent their menstrual periods. Nutritional iron supplements may alleviate or prevent the development of iron deficiency and will aid in restoring normal levels of red blood cells. Medications to be avoided are those which interfere with platelet function and predispose to bleeding, including aspirin, ibuprofen and ibuprofen-like drugs, heparin, warfarin, ticlopidine, clopidogrel, abciximab, streptokinase, urokinase, or tissue plasminogen activator.

The treatment of choice for stopping active bleeding is through transfusion of normal platelets that are obtained from donors without the disease. Studies have shown that most people (approximately 85%) with the disorder will require platelet transfusions during their lifetime. For individuals with TGN, transfusion with one unit of platelets for every 11-22 lbs (5-10 kg) of body weight will correct the defect in blood clotting and may be life-saving. Pre-emptive transfusions are especially important before surgical operations or dental procedures. Transfusions should be continued until wound healing is complete.

Over time, platelet transfusion may become less effective. Platelets obtained from donors and given to a patient with TGN are recognized by the immune system as foreign cells. The immune system, in turn, generates antibodies that attach to the donor platelets and impair their function, ultimately leading to their destruction. Because of this unfortunate effect, platelet transfusions are best reserved for life-threatening bleeding or before procedures in which bleeding is likely. Using platelets from donors closely related to the patient may delay the immune response and extend the benefits of transfusion therapy.

Patients with TGN should be followed closely by a hematologist and should be vaccinated against the hepatitis B virus, because of the high risk of exposure to the virus with ongoing blood-product transfusions. Patients should also been seen regularly by a dentist to prevent gum disease that could result in profuse bleeding.

## QUESTIONS TO ASK YOUR DOCTOR

- Which tecnique do you recommend to confirm the diagnosis?
- Should family members be tested to see if they are appropriate platelet donors?
- How often are dental checkups recommended?
- What are the risks of bone marrow transplant?

**Genetic counseling** can be offered to affected individuals or couples with a family history of the disorder.

Bone marrow transplantation is currently the only curative form of treatment for patients with TGN. However this is generally considered more hazardous than the disease itself, except in exceptional circumstances. In 2000, a multidisciplinary team of scientists, led by a researcher at the Medical College of Wisconsin, was able to correct the GP IIb/IIIa defect in bone marrow cells taken from patients with TGN using advanced **gene therapy** techniques. The researchers are now focusing on applying the technique to lab animals with a form of TGN, but these positive early results give hope for an eventual cure in humans.

### Prognosis

Although there is no cure, the prognosis for people with TGN is quite good. Despite the fact that the majority of people with this disorder will require medical treatment to control bleeding, patients rarely die of massive blood loss. Interestingly, the severity of bleeding appears to decrease with increasing age. Barring any catastrophic accident which results in uncontrollable bleeding, life span is approximately the same as the general population.

### Resources

#### BOOKS

Cotran R. S. *Robbins Pathologic Basis of Disease.* Philadelphia:W.B. Saunders, 1999.

"Disorders of the platelet and vessel wall." *Harrison's Principles of Internal Medicine,* edited by A.S. Fauci. New York: McGraw-Hill, 1998.

"Disorders of the platelets and the blood vessels." *Nelson Textbook of Pediatrics,* edited by R.E. Behrman. Philadelphia: W.B. Saunders, 2000, pp. 1520-1525.

"Hereditary Disorders of Platelet Function." *Wintrobe's Clinical Hematology,* edited by R. Lee. Philadelphia: Lippincott Williams & Wilkins, 1999, pp. 1662- 1669.

#### PERIODICALS

French, D.L., and U. Seligsohn. "Platelet Glycoprotein IIb/IIIa Receptors and Glanzmann's Thrombasthenia." *Arteriosclerosis Thrombosis and Vascular Biology* 20 (March 2000): 607- 610.

Tomiyama, Y. "Glanzmann Thrombasthenia: Integrin Alpha IIb Beta 3 Deficiency." *International Journal of Hematology* 72 (December 2000): 448-454.

#### WEBSITES

"Glanzmann Thrombasthenia." *Online Mendelian Inheritance in Man.*http://www.ncbi.nlm.nih.gov/entrez/dispomim. cgi?id = 187800.

#### ORGANIZATIONS

Glanzmann's Thrombasthenia Support Group. 28 Duke Rd., Newton, Hyde, SK14 4JB. UK 0161-368-0219

Oren Traub, MD, PhD

**Thrombocytopenia absence of radius syndrome** *see* **TAR syndrome**

# Tomaculous neuropathy

### Definition

Tomaculous neuropathy is a rare disease that, for most of those affected, is rather benign. It is characterized by swelling of the myelin sheath that leads to irritation of the nerves, particularly in the arms and legs. Many people who have the condition are unaware that they have it. Those that do experience the irritation or numbness are treated according to the symptoms rather than according to the underlying condition. For a small percentage of affected people, tomaculous neuropathy can be painful and debilitating.

The word *tomaculous* refers to the sausage-like appearance of the affected nerve cells. The term *neuropathy* refers to any abnormality of the nerve cells. This condition is more commonly known as hereditary neuropathy with liability to pressure palsies. It is also referred to as **compression neuropathy**, **entrapment neuropathy**, familial pressure sensitive neuropathy, or a number of other terms emphasizing the fact that it is inherited.

### Demographics

Tomaculous neuropathy is such a rare disorder that as of 2009 there were no established ratios for prevalence or incidence. It is an autosomal dominant trait. Therefore, it can affect male and female equally. The estimated age range for observed symptoms is from

8 through 72 years. Most occurrences of observed symptoms take place during the affected person's twenties and thirties.

## Description

The common characteristic shared by all people affected with tomaculous neuropathy is a deletion of a protein in **gene** PMP-22. This protein is responsible for myelination, which is the production and maintenance of the myelin sheath (insulation for the axon of the nerve cell). While the **genotype** (genetic makeup) is shared, the **phenotype** (symptoms experienced) is widely diverse. Most people who are affected will only show symptoms after adolescence. Most of the episodes occur for a short period of time. The symptoms of these episodes are numbness in the area and a weakness in the affected limb. The episodes are recurrent but do fade over time. However, there are two extremes from this normal situation. Some people with the gene for this disorder never show symptoms, which has led genetic researchers to speculate that it is more common than was observed as of 2009. Another extreme can occur when too many episodes happen. This condition can develop into a permanent disability. The severity of the disability varies a lot among cases.

The main symptom of this disorder is a localized, temporary paralysis of the nerve. It is brought on by too much pressure or exertion in the affected area. During this paralysis, the area affected has no feeling and is weak. The paralysis can last from less than an hour to over a month.

## Causes and symptoms

The cause of tomaculous neuropathy is a mutation that eliminates an important protein on gene PMP-22 on **chromosome** 17. The effect of this mutation is the swelling of the myelin sheath of the nerve cells in the peripheral nervous system. The myelin sheath serves as insulation for the axon, which is the cable of the nerve cell through which neurotransmitters run with messages from the brain to the muscular-skeletal system and from the muscular-skeletal system to the brain. Without the tight insulation of the myelin sheath, the neurotransmitters running through the axon are not contained, which interferes with effective neural communication. How this neurological problem is manifested depends on the metabolism of the person affected and the severity of the event generating the emergence. Although one nerve cell is tomaculous, it may not be the one that experiences the symptoms. When the symptoms are recurrent, the symptoms are not usually manifested in the same nerves as in previous episodes.

## KEY TERMS

**Carpal tunnel syndrome**— A condition in which the median nerve is compressed at the wrist, leading to numbness and pain in the hand.

**Myelination**—Production and maintenance of the myelin sheath.

**Neuropathy**—A general term for disorders of the nerves of the peripheral nervous system.

**Neurotransmitters**—Chemicals that relay signals between a neuron and another cell.

**Paralysis**—Complete loss of muscle function for one or more muscle groups, often with loss of feeling and mobility in the affected area.

The usual symptoms are numbness, pain, weakness, or paralysis. Some of those affected experience carpal tunnel syndrome.

Genetic researchers are particularly interested in tomaculous neuropathy because of its relationship with another, more common disorder. **Charcot-Marie-Tooth disease** (CMT) is caused by a duplication of the PMP-22 gene, whereas tomaculous neuropathy is caused by a deletion on that gene. The two disorders sometimes share symptoms and are often mistaken for each other.

## Diagnosis

The diagnosis of tomaculous neuropathy begins with observing a patient who has recurring episodes characterized by numbness, pain, weakness, paralysis, or a combination of these. The diagnosis would also be dependent on a search of the family history for evidence that the condition may have been inherited.

The only sure diagnosis would be a genetic test detecting the chromosome 17 abnormality, which is the deletion on gene PMP-22.

## Treatment

The main goal of treatment is to relieve the irritation of the nerve damage. Adaptive equipment such as wrist splints, protective pads for elbows and knee, and ankle-foot orthoses (braces) can relieve episodes. Prevention of the nerve pressure is the best treatment for those who have been diagnosed. Pacing is an important habit to develop as it relieves pressure. Avoiding repetitive movements as well as staying in one position for any prolonged period is recommended.

**PERIODICALS**

Chance, P. F. "Inherited Focal, Episodic Neuropathies: Hereditary Neuropathy with Liability to Pressure Palsies and Hereditary Neuralgic Amyotrophy." *Neuromolecular Medicine*. 2006. 8: 159-174.

**OTHER**

Bird, Thomas D. Hereditary Neuropathy with Liability to Pressure Palsies. GeneReviews. http://www.ncbi.nlm.nih.gov/bookshelf/br.fcgi?book = gene&part = hnpp

**ORGANIZATIONS**

Neuropathy Association , 60 East Forty-second Street, Suite 942, New York, NY, 10165, 212-692-0662, http://www.neuropathy.org.

Ray F. Brogan, PHD

---

## QUESTIONS TO ASK YOUR DOCTOR

- What are the chances that I will have continuous troublesome episodes?
- What adaptive equipment is best for me?
- How often do people with my condition end up disabled?
- Would surgery help my condition?
- How do other people with my level of tomaculous neuropathy adapt their lifestyles?
- Should I have relatives tested for tomaculous neuropathy?

---

Under extreme conditions, surgery to remove the compression on the nerve may be recommended. However, it is controversial. Many cases of tomaculous neuropathy experience spontaneous remission where the condition wanes without treatment. In such cases, surgery is unnecessary. Furthermore, surgery does not always bring results, and when it does, the results do not always hold.

### Prognosis

There is no cure for tomaculous neuropathy. However, with conscientious maintenance, most affected people do not have any prolonged periods of troublesome episodes. Nerves destroyed in an episode eventually repair themselves. However, with increase episodes the nerves take longer to repair.

### Prevention

Many people with tomaculous neuropathy avoid any episode through maintaining good physical fitness. Once diagnosed the tomaculous neuropathy individuals must avoid the activities and conditions that could put undue pressure on the nerves. Activities that could become repetitive can be interchanged with other activities to reduce repetitive motion. People can avoid remaining in one position too long by getting up and stretching or pacing.

### Resources

**BOOKS**

Amato, Anthony, and James Russell. *Neuromuscular Disorders*. New York: McGraw-Hill Professional, 2008.

Cros, Didier. *Peripheral Neuropathy: A Practical Approach to Diagnosis and Management*. Philadelphia: Lippincott Williams & Wilkins, 2001.

# Tourette syndrome

## Definition

Tourette syndrome (TS) is an inherited disorder of the nervous system, characterized by a variable expression of unwanted movements and noises (tics).

## Description

The first references in the literature to what might today be classified as Tourette syndrome largely described individuals who were wrongly believed to be possessed by the devil. In 1885, Gilles de la Tourette, a French neurologist, provided the first formal description of this syndrome. He described the disorder as an inherited neurological condition characterized by motor and vocal tics.

Although vocal and motor tics are the hallmark of Tourette syndrome, other symptoms such as the expression of socially inappropriate comments or behaviors, obsessive compulsive disorder, attention deficit disorder, self injuring behavior, **depression**, and anxiety also appear to be associated with Tourette syndrome. Most research suggests that Tourette syndrome is an inherited disorder, although a **gene** responsible for Tourette syndrome has not yet been discovered.

## Genetic profile

The cause of Tourette syndrome is unknown although some studies suggest that the tics associated with Tourette syndrome are caused by an increased amount of a neurotransmitter called dopamine. A neurotransmitter is a chemical found in the brain that helps to transmit information from one brain cell to another.

## KEY TERMS

**Attention deficit disorder (ADD)**—Disorder characterized by a short attention span, impulsivity, and, in some cases, hyperactivity.

**Autosomal dominant**—A pattern of genetic inheritance where only one abnormal gene is needed to display the trait or disease.

**Coprolalia**—The involuntary expression of obscene words or phrases.

**Copropraxia**—The involuntary display of unacceptable/obscene gestures.

**Decreased penetrance**—Individuals who inherit a changed disease gene, but do not develop symptoms.

**Dysphoria**—Feelings of anxiety, restlessness, and dissatisfaction.

**Echolalia**—Involuntary echoing of the last word, phrase, or sentence that is spoken by someone else or by sounds in the environment.

**Echopraxia**—The imitation of the movement of another individual.

**Linkage analysis**—A type of genetic study used to identify genes that cause specific diseases.

**Neurotransmitter**—Chemical in the brain that transmits information from one nerve cell to another.

**Obsessive compulsive disorder (OCD)**—Disorder characterized by persistent, intrusive, and senseless thoughts (obsessions) or compulsions to perform repetitive behaviors that interfere with normal functioning.

**Phalilalia**—Involuntary echoing of the last word, phrase, sentence, or sound vocalized by oneself.

**Tic**—Brief and intermittent involuntary movement or sound.

Other studies suggest that the defect in Tourette syndrome involves another neurotransmitter called serotonin, or involves other chemicals required for normal functioning of the brain.

It is clear that genetic factors are involved in the occurrence of Tourette syndrome because studies of identical twins (twins who share all the same genes) show that about 85% of the time that one is affected, the other is also affected. One theory is that Tourette syndrome is an autosomal dominant disorder with decreased penetrance. This theory has not been proven and may not be true in all families. An autosomal dominant disorder results from a change in one copy of a pair of genes. Individuals with an autosomal dominant disorder have a 50% chance of passing on the changed gene to their children. Decreased penetrance means that not all people who inherit the changed gene will develop symptoms. There is some evidence that females who inherit the Tourette syndrome gene have a 70% chance of exhibiting symptoms and males have a 99% chance of having symptoms.

Other theories about the cause of Tourette syndrome include the presence of a single gene in combination with other genetic or environmental changes that cause the condition. Some studies have indicated that it is unlikely that there is one genetic change alone that is responsible for causing Tourette syndrome. It is possible that Tourette syndrome has different causes in different individuals. Linkage analysis has been performed by several researchers to identify genes that may be associated with Tourette syndrome. In linkage analysis, researchers determine if people with Tourette syndrome have more markers (identifiable **DNA** sequences) associated with particular genes in common than would be expected by chance. These studies have indicated several chromosomal locations of interest, including locations on **chromosome** 2, 4, 5, 7, 8, 10, 11, 13, 17, and 19. In addition, individuals with Tourette syndrome features from different families have been reported to have chromosomal rearrangements that involve chromosome breaks in chromosomes 2, 6, 8, 7, and 18q. The areas where the chromosome broke in these families are under further investigation. More research is needed to establish the cause of Tourette syndrome.

Researchers are also interested in determining if the sex of the parent passing on a particular genetic change for Tourette syndrome influences the occurrence or severity of symptoms. Researchers also want to determine how having a family history of Tourette syndrome in both parents affects the chance for and the severity of the condition in their children.

### Demographics

Tourette syndrome is found in all populations and all ethnic groups, but is three to four times more common in males than females and is more common in children than adults. The exact frequency of Tourette syndrome is unknown, but estimates range from 1–10 in 1,000 children or adolescents.

### Signs and symptoms

#### Motor and vocal tics

The principal symptoms of Tourette syndrome include simple and complex motor and vocal tics.

Simple motor tics are characterized by brief muscle contractions of one or more limited muscle groups. An eye twitch is an example of a simple motor tic. Complex motor tics tend to appear more complicated and purposeful than simple tics and involve coordinated contractions of several muscle groups. Some examples of complex motor tics include the act of hitting oneself and jumping. Copropraxia, the involuntary display of unacceptable/obscene gestures, and echopraxia, the imitation of the movement of another individual, are other examples of complex motor tics.

Vocal tics are actually manifestations of motor tics that involve the muscles required for vocalization. Simple vocal tics include stuttering, stammering, abnormal emphasis of part of a word or phrase, and inarticulate noises such as throat clearing, grunts, and high-pitched sounds. Complex vocal tics typically involve the involuntary expression of words. Perhaps the most striking example of this is coprolalia, the involuntary expression of obscene words or phrases, which occurs in less than one-third of people with Tourette syndrome. The involuntary echoing of the last word, phrase, sentence, or sound vocalized by oneself (phalilalia) or of another person or sound in the environment (echolalia) are also classified as complex tics.

The type, frequency, and severity of tics exhibited vary tremendously between individuals with Tourette syndrome. Tourette syndrome has a variable age of onset, and tics can start anytime between infancy and age 18. Initial symptoms usually occur before the early teens, and the mean age of onset for both males and females is approximately seven years of age. Most individuals with symptoms initially experience simple muscle tics involving the eyes and the head. These symptoms can progress to tics involving the upper torso, neck, arms, hands, and occasionally the legs and feet. Complex motor tics are usually the latest onset muscle tics. Vocal tics usually have a later onset then motor tics. In some rare cases, people with Tourette syndrome suddenly present with multiple, severe, or bizarre symptoms.

Not only is there extreme variability in clinical symptoms between individuals with Tourette syndrome, but individuals commonly experience a variability in type, frequency, and severity of symptoms within the course of their lifetime. Adolescents with Tourette syndrome often experience unpredictable and variable symptoms, which may be related to fluctuating hormone levels and decreased compliance in taking medications. Adults often experience a decrease in symptoms or a complete end to symptoms.

A number of factors appears to affect the severity and frequency of tics. Stress appears to increase the frequency and severity of tics, while concentration on another part of the body that is not taking part in a tic can result in the temporary alleviation of symptoms. Relaxation, following attempts to suppress the occurrence of tics, may result in an increased frequency of tics. An increased frequency and severity of tics can also result from exposure to drugs such as steroids, cocaine, amphetamines, and caffeine. Hormonal changes such as those that occur prior to the menstrual cycle can also increase the severity of symptoms.

### Other associated symptoms

People with Tourette syndrome are more likely to exhibit non-obscene, socially inappropriate behaviors such as expressing insulting or socially unacceptable comments or socially unacceptable actions. It is not known whether these symptoms stem from a more general dysfunction of impulse control that might be part of Tourette syndrome.

Tourette syndrome appears to also be associated with attention deficit disorder (ADD). ADD is a disorder characterized by a short attention span and impulsivity and, in some cases, hyperactivity. Researchers have found that 21–90% of individuals with Tourette syndrome also exhibit symptoms of ADD, whereas 2–15% of the general population exhibit symptoms of ADD.

People with Tourette syndrome are also at higher risk for having symptoms of obsessive-compulsive disorder (OCD). OCD is a disorder characterized by persistent, intrusive, and senseless thoughts (obsessions) or compulsions to perform repetitive behaviors that interfere with normal functioning. A person with OCD, for example, may be obsessed with germs and may counteract this obsession with continual hand washing. Symptoms of OCD are present in 1.9–3% of the general population, whereas 28–50% of people with Tourette syndrome have symptoms of OCD.

Self-injurious behavior (SIB) is also seen more frequently in those with Tourette syndrome. Approximately 34–53% of individuals with Tourette syndrome exhibit some form of self-injuring behavior. The SIB is often related to OCD, but can also occur in those with Tourette syndrome who do not have OCD.

Symptoms of anxiety and depression are also found more commonly in people with Tourette syndrome. It is not clear, however, whether these symptoms are symptoms of Tourette syndrome or occur as a result of having to deal with the symptoms of moderate to severe Tourette syndrome.

People with Tourette syndrome may also be at increased risk for having learning disabilities and personality disorders and may be more predisposed to behaviors such as aggression, antisocial behaviors, severe temper outbursts, and inappropriate sexual behavior. Further controlled studies need to be performed, however, to ascertain whether these behaviors are symptoms of Tourette syndrome. Individuals with Tourette syndrome are more likely to get migraine headaches and to have sleep disorders, such as difficulty falling asleep, staying asleep, or having unusual movements during sleep.

## Diagnosis

Tourette syndrome cannot be diagnosed through a blood test. The diagnosis is made through observation and interview of the patient and discussions with other family members. The diagnosis of Tourette syndrome is complicated by a variety of factors. The extreme range of symptoms of this disorder makes it difficult to differentiate Tourette syndrome from other disorders with similar symptoms. Diagnosis is further complicated by the fact that some tics appear to be within the range of normal behavior. For example, an individual who only exhibits tics such as throat clearing and sniffing may be misdiagnosed with a medical problem such as allergies. In addition, bizarre and complex tics such as coprolalia may be mistaken for psychotic or "bad" behavior. Diagnosis is also confounded by individuals who attempt to control tics in public and in front of health care professionals and deny the existence of symptoms. Although there is disagreement over what criteria should be used to diagnosis Tourette syndrome, one aid in the diagnosis is the *Diagnostic and Statistical Manual of Mental Disorders* (DSM-IV). The DSM-IV outlines suggest diagnostic criteria for a variety of conditions, including Tourette syndrome, such as:

- Presence of both motor and vocal tics at some time during the course of the illness.
- The occurrence of multiple tics nearly every day through a period of more than one year, without a remission of tics for a period of greater than three consecutive months.
- Symptoms cause distress or impairment in functioning.
- Age of onset prior to 18 years of age.
- The symptoms are not due to medications or drugs and are not related to another medical condition.

Some physicians critique the DSM-IV criteria, citing that they do not include the full range of behaviors and symptoms seen in Tourette syndrome. Others criticize the criteria since they limit the diagnosis to those who experience a significant impairment, which may not be true for individuals with milder symptoms. For this reason, many physicians use their clinical judgment as well as the DSM-IV criteria as a guide to diagnosing Tourette syndrome.

## Treatment and management

There is no cure for Tourette syndrome, and treatment involves the control of symptoms through educational and psychological interventions, behavioral training, and/or medications. The treatment and management of Tourette syndrome vary from patient to patient and should focus on the alleviation of the symptoms that are most bothersome to the patient or that cause the most interference with daily functioning.

### Psychological and educational interventions

Psychological treatments such as counseling are not generally useful for the treatment of tics, but can be beneficial in the treatment of associated symptoms such as obsessive-compulsive behavior and attention deficit disorder. Counseling may also help individuals to cope better with the symptoms of this disorder and to have more positive social interactions. Psychological interventions may also help people cope better with stressors that can normally be triggers for tics and negative behaviors. The education of family members, teachers, and peers about Tourette syndrome can be helpful and may foster acceptance and prevent social isolation.

### Behavioral training

A variety of behavioral training techniques has been suggested and tried in people with Tourette syndrome. Some of these include conditioning techniques (training a person to respond to a particular stimulus with a particular behavior), awareness training, biofeedback training (learning how to control one's involuntary nervous system), and habit reversal. Relaxation therapies have been tried with short-term success. The effectiveness of behavioral training as a whole is not clear.

### Medications

Many people with mild symptoms of Tourette syndrome never require medications. Those with severe symptoms may require medications for all or part of their lifetime. The most effective treatment of tics associated with Tourette syndrome involves the use of drugs such as Haloperidol, pimozide, sulpiride, and tiapride, which decrease the amount of dopamine in the body. Unfortunately, the incidence of side effects, even at low dosages, is quite high. The short-term side effects can include sedation, dysphoria, weight gain, movement abnormalities, depression, and poor school performance. Long-term side effects can include phobias, memory difficulties, and personality changes. These drugs are therefore better candidates for short-term rather than long-term therapy.

Tourette syndrome can also be treated with other drugs such as clonidine, clonazepam, and risperidone, but the efficacy of these treatments is unknown. In many cases, treatment of associated conditions such as ADD and OCD is often more of a concern than the tics themselves. Clonidine used in conjunction with stimulants such as Ritalin may be useful for treating people with Tourette syndrome who also have symptoms of ADD. Stimulants should be used with caution in individuals with Tourette syndrome since they can sometimes increase the frequency and severity of tics. OCD symptoms in those with Tourette syndrome are often treated with drugs such as Prozac, Luvox, Paxil, and Zoloft.

In many cases, the treatment of Tourette syndrome with medications can be discontinued after adolescence. Trials should be performed through the gradual tapering off of medications and should always be done under a doctor's supervision.

### Surgical treatments

Several areas of the brain have been targeted for surgical approaches to the treatment of severe tic disorders. In addition, deep brain stimulation (using sound waves to stimulate certain areas of the brain) has been suggested as treatment, as there has been some success with this treatment in other movement disorders. Clinical trials are needed to determine the effectiveness and safety of this treatment for possible use in the future.

### Prognosis

The prognosis for Tourette syndrome in individuals without associated psychological conditions is often quite good, and only approximately 10% of people with Tourette syndrome experience severe tic symptoms. Approximately 46% of individuals with Tourette syndrome will experience a decrease in the frequency and severity of tics, and another 26% will experience a complete end of symptoms by late adolescence. Fourteen percent will have no change and 14% will have an increase in symptoms. There does not appear to be a definite correlation between the type, frequency, and severity of symptoms and the eventual prognosis. Patients with severe tics may experience social difficulties and may isolate themselves from others for fear of shocking and embarrassing them. People with Tourette syndrome who have other symptoms such as obsessive

---

**QUESTIONS TO ASK YOUR DOCTOR**

- Would my child benefit from psychotherapy?
- What side effects could result from taking Ritalin and Clonidine?
- Are there early signs of medication side effects?
- What educational interventions do you recommend?

---

compulsive disorder, attention deficit disorder, and self-injurious behavior usually have a poorer prognosis.

### Resources

**BOOKS**

Goldstein, Sam, and Cecil Reynolds. *Handbook of Neurodevelopmental and Genetic Disorders in Children.* New York, NY: The Guilford Press, 1999.

Haerle, Tracy, ed., and Jim Eisenreich. *Children with Tourette Syndrome: A Parent's Guide.* Bethesda, MD: Woodbine House, 1992.

Leckman, James, and Donald Cohen. *Tourette's Syndrome: Tics, Obsessions, Compulsions: Development, Psychopathology and Clinical Care.* New York: John Wiley & Sons, 1999.

Rimoin, David, Michael Connor, and Reed Pyeritz. *Emery and Rimoin's Principles and Practice of Medical Genetics, Third Edition.* Stoke-on-Trent, England: Pearson Professional Limited, 1997.

**PERIODICALS**

Alsobrook, J. P. II, and D.L. Pauls. "The Genetics of Tourette Syndrome." *Neurologic Clinics* 15 (May 1997): 381–393.

Chappell, P. B., L. D. Scahill, and J. F. Leckman. "Future Therapies of Tourette Syndrome." *Neurologic Clinics* 15 (May 1997): 429–450.

Cuker, Adam, et al. "Candidate Locus for Gilles de la Tourette Syndrome/Obsessive Compulsive Disorder/Chronic Tic Disorder at 18q22." *American Journal of Medical Genetics* 130A (2004): 37–39.

Diaz-Amzaldua, Adriana, et al. "Association Between 7q31 Markers and Tourette Syndrome." *American Journal of Medical Genetics* 127A (2004): 17–20.

Eidelberg, D., et al. "The Metabolic Anatomy of Tourette's Syndrome." *Neurology* 48 (April 1997): 927–934.

Freeman, R. D. "Attention Deficit Hyperactivity Disorder in the Presence of Tourette Syndrome." *Neurologic Clinics* 15 (May 1997): 411–420.

Lichter, D. G., and L. A. Jackson. "Predictors of Clonidine Response in Tourette Syndrome: Implications and Inferences." *Journal of Child Neurology* 11 (March 1997): 93–97.

Paschou, P., et al. "Indications of Linkage and Association of Gilles de la Tourette Syndrome in Two Independent Family Samples: 17q25 Is a Putative Susceptibility Region." *American Journal of Human Genetics* 75 (2004): 545–560.

Pauls, David. "An Update on the Genetics of Gilles de la Tourette Syndrome." *Journal of Psychosomatic Research* 55 (2003): 7–12.

Robertson, Mary. "Tourette Syndrome, Associated Conditions and the Complexities of Treatment." *Brain* 123 (2000): 425–462.

Singer, Harvey. "Tourette Syndrome: From Behavior to Biology." *Lancet Neurology* 4 (2005): 149–159.

Hu, Chun, et al. "Evaluation of the Genes for the Adrenergic Receptors alpha2A and alpha1C and Gilles de la Tourette syndrome" *American Journal of Medical Genetics part B (Neuropsychiatric Genetics)* 119B (2003): 54–59.

**OTHER**

"About Tourette Syndrome." Tourette Help. (April 2, 2005.) http://www.tourettehelp.com/pages/patient/about.html.

"Tourette's Disorder." Internet Mental Health. (April 2, 2005.) http://www.mentalhealth.com/fr20.html.

"Online Mendelian Inheritance in Man." (April 2, 2005.) http://www.ncbi.nlm.nih.gov.

**ORGANIZATIONS**

National Institute of Neurological Disorders and Stroke. 31 Center Drive, MSC 2540, Bldg. 31, Room 8806, Bethesda, MD 20814. (301) 496-5751 or (800) 352-9424. (April 2, 2005.) http://www.ninds.nih.gov.

Tourette Syndrome Association, Inc. 42-40 Bell Blvd.,Suite 205, Bayside, NY 11361-2820. (718) 224-2999. Fax: (718) 279-9596. (April 2, 2005.) http://www.tsa-usa.org.

Tourette Syndrome Foundation of Canada. 194 Jarvis Street, #206, Toronto, ONT M5B 2B7. Canada. (800) 361-3120. tsfc.org@sympatico.ca. (April 2, 2005.) http://www.tourette.ca.

Sonja Rene Eubanks, MS, CGC

Translation *see* **Chromosomal abnormalities**

# Treacher Collins syndrome

## Definition

Treacher Collins syndrome (TCS) is a genetic disorder involving abnormal facial development. Individuals with TCS have underdevelopment of the jawbone, cheekbones, ears, and eye area. These features range widely from mild to severe. Intelligence and life span are usually normal.

## Description

TCS was first described by E. Treacher Collins in 1900 after observation of two individuals with similar facial abnormalities. In 1940, Franceschetti and Klein gave TCS another name, mandibulofacial dysostosis. TCS is also sometimes called Franceschetti-Klein syndrome or Franceschetti syndrome.

The features of TCS result from a problem in early embryonic development. After an embryo forms, there are cells that are unspecialized and have the ability to develop into any type of cell in any part of the body (neural crest cells). Early in development, the neural crest cells travel to different areas of the embryo and specialize to become a specific type of cell for a specific organ or body part. The branchial arches is the area where neural crest cells specialize to develop the bone structure and features of the face. In individuals with TCS there is thought to be an error in the movement of the neural crest cells to the branchial arches or in the specialization of those cells once they reach the branchial arches. The result is underdevelopment of the facial bones, eyes, and ears.

Individuals with mild features of TCS may go undiagnosed. Sometimes adults do not know they have TCS until they have a child with more noticeable features. This can cause feelings of guilt for the parent. Children with more moderate to severe features of TCS look strikingly different and may be teased or shunned. These children are at risk for psychological stress and low self-esteem. Even adults with TCS who are productive and successful may battle issues of social stigma and low self-esteem regarding their facial differences.

## Genetic profile

TCS is an autosomal dominant condition. Children of an affected parent have a 50% chance of inheriting the disorder. Males and females are affected equally. The severity of symptoms ranges widely, even among members of the same family. Therefore, the severity of a child's features cannot be predicted by the features of the affected parent.

About 40% of babies born with TCS have one affected parent. The other 60% are assumed to have a new, sporadic **gene** mutation (alteration). If a child has a new mutation (one that is not carried by the parents) then his or her siblings will have an extremely low chance of also having TCS. When a baby with TCS is born to seemingly normal parents, it is important to examine both parents carefully for mild features of TCS in order to give them accurate recurrence risks.

The gene for TCS is on **chromosome** 5 and is called TCOF1. This gene produces a protein that has been named treacle. Disease-causing TCOF1 mutations result in absent or inactive treacle. The exact role of treacle is not known but it is thought to be involved in early embryo neural crest cell movement or specialization in the branchial arches.

## Demographics

TCS is rare and affects an estimated one in 25,000 to 50,000 live births.

## Signs and symptoms

TCS is described as a craniofacial condition because its features are all related to the head and face. The overall head size may be smaller than average (**microcephaly**). The outer corners of the eyes slant downward. There may be colobomas on the lower eyelids, giving the lids a droopy appearance. The bridge of the nose is usually wide. Most individuals with TCS have underdeveloped cheekbones (malar bones) which give that area of the face a flat or sunken appearance. The lower jaw and chin are usually small and retroverted (jawbone points downward toward the neck instead of pointing out perpendicular to the neck). Many individuals also have a large mouth. **Cleft palate** (with or without **cleft lip**) is seen in one-quarter to one-third of patients with TCS.

Ear abnormalities are also common in TCS. The ears may be low-set, small, misshapen, or absent. For this reason, hearing loss or **deafness** is a common feature of TCS. The hearing loss is usually due to abnormalities in the middle ear structures rather than the outer ear structures.

Infants with moderate or severe malar bone underdevelopment may have compressed airways. These babies can have problems breathing after birth and may need a respirator or tracheostomy. A small, retroverted jaw and chin can cause feeding problems that may warrant a feeding tube.

The severity of features present at birth remains constant throughout life. TCS does not get progressively better or worse as an individual ages.

## Diagnosis

The diagnosis of TCS is usually made by physical examination and identification of the typical facial features. Computerized tomography (CT scans) can be used to determine the degree of underdevelopment of the facial bone structure.

There are other syndromes that have facial appearances that resemble TCS. A complete physical examination of other body systems can help to establish a diagnosis of TCS. TCS can be distinguished from Nager syndrome and Miller syndrome if no abnormalities are present in the hands or arms. TCS can be distinguished from oculoauriculovertebral (OAV) conditions (for example, Goldenhar syndrome) because facial involvement is bilateral (affecting both sides of the face) and the spinal column is normal.

If there are several people in a family with TCS, genetic linkage studies can be performed. Linkage studies require blood samples from many family members, both affected and unaffected. Markers on the TCOF1 gene are analyzed and compared to determine which gene version is shared by affected family members. The disease-causing gene should be present in all affected family members and absent from all unaffected members. Linkage studies can be performed on an unborn baby to determine if the baby inherited the family's disease-causing gene. **Prenatal ultrasound** can also be used to look for facial features of TCS. While there have been reports of prenatal diagnosis of TCS with ultrasound only, babies with mild features may appear normal. Detection may also depend on the skill of the physician performing the ultrasound and his or her experience with features of TCS.

## Treatment and management

Newborn infants with severe TCS may require a ventilator, tracheostomy, or feeding tube if life-threatening breathing or feeding problems exist. A cleft palate can be repaired with surgery. Hearing aids can help individuals with hearing loss.

For most individuals, the problems of TCS are largely cosmetic. Plastic surgery can help to rebuild the bone structure of the face, which may improve appearance as well as breathing and feeding. Surgeons can use bone grafts to build up the underdeveloped cheekbones.

The jawbone can be "lengthened" and its angle repositioned. The bridge of the nose can be narrowed. Ears can be reconstructed using cartilage from the ribcage. Surgery can also be performed on the eye area.

This reconstruction may take multiple surgeries at different ages. Each individual must be evaluated for his or her unique features and needs. Surgeries are timed with facial growth and emotional needs and maturity of the patient.

### Prognosis

A small percentage of newborns with TCS will have life-threatening breathing difficulties, and infant deaths can occur. However, the majority of individuals with TCS have a normal life span.

### Resources

#### PERIODICALS

Dixon, M.J. "Treacher Collins Syndrome." *Journal of Medical Genetics* 32 (1995): 806–08.

Posnick, J.C., and R.L. Ruiz. "Treacher Collins Syndrome: Current Evaluation, Treatment, and Future Directions." *Cleft Palate-Craniofacial Journal* 37, no. 5 (September 2000): 483 +.

#### ORGANIZATIONS

FACES: The National Craniofacial Association. PO Box 11082, Chattanooga, TN 37401. (423) 266-1632 or (800) 332-2373. faces@faces-cranio.org. http://www.faces-cranio.org/.

Treacher Collins Foundation. Box 683, Norwich, VT 05055. (800) 823-2055.

#### WEBSITES

"A Guide to Understanding Treacher Collins Syndrome." *Children's Craniofacial Association.* http://www.cca-kids.com/srvSyndBklt.stm.

Amie Stanley, MS

# Trichorhinophalangeal syndrome

### Definition

Trichorhinophalangeal syndrome, or Langer-Giedion syndrome (LGS), is characterized by skeletal abnormalities and dysmorphic (distinctive) facial features. Most people with LGS also have mental retardation.

### Description

LGS affects mostly the skeletal system and facial structure. Since the features include abnormalities in the hair (tricho), nose shape (rhino), and fingers and toes (phalangeal), the technical name for LGS is trichorhinophalangeal syndrome.

### Genetic profile

LGS is not usually passed through generations in a family. However, the condition is considered a contiguous-gene syndrome. This means that it is caused by the loss of functional copies of two genes near each other on **chromosome** 8. Research suggests that another gene may be involved. **Genetic counseling** is suggested for anyone considering pregnancy who has a relative with this condition.

### Demographics

About 50 cases of Langer-Giedion syndrome have been reported in the literature. Males are affected three times more often than females.

### Signs and symptoms

Craniofacial features associated with Langer-Giedion syndrome include a bulbous, pear-shaped nose; a small jaw; a thin upper lip; and large ears. The hair is usually sparse, and the head is small in 60% of individuals with LGS. Mild to severe mental retardation is present in 70% of people; it often affects speech more than other skills.

Skeletal features include exostoses—spiny growths on the bone—which occur before age five and usually increase in number until the skeleton matures. Compression of nerves or blood vessels, asymmetric limb growth, and limitation of movement are problems that can result from the exostoses. Scoliosis—a curvature of the spine—is found in some people, as well as thin ribs. Short stature is often seen as a result of epiphyses—cone-shaped bone ends. Longitudinal bone growth

## KEY TERMS

**Contiguous gene syndrome**—A genetic syndrome caused by the deletion of two or more genes located next to each other.

**Craniofacial**—Relating to or involving both the head and the face.

**Epiphysis**—The end of long bones, usually terminating in a joint.

**Exostose**—An abnormal growth (benign tumor) on a bone.

**Mental retardation**—Significant impairment in intellectual function and adaptation in society. Usually associated with an intelligence quotient (IQ) below 70.

**Philtrum**—The center part of the face between the nose and lips that is usually depressed.

**Short stature**—Shorter than normal height, can include dwarfism.

appears to be slowed. Short and/or curved fingers are common. Loose skin often occurs, but that tends to improve with age.

Features of LGS that are less commonly seen include loose joints and low muscle tone. Others are wandering eye (exotropia), droopy eyelid, widely spaced eyes, fractures in the bones, birthmarks that increase with age, hearing loss, heart or genito-urinary abnormalities, and webbing of the fingers.

### Diagnosis

The criteria for diagnosis of LGS are a bulbous, pear-shaped nose, and epiphyses and exostoses. These signs are probably all related to abnormal bone growth, but researchers do not yet understand the link to mental retardation and hair abnormalities. The distinctive facial features may be recognized at birth. Changes in the epiphyses are recognizable through x ray by age three, and exostoses are visible by age five. Chromosome analysis will likely reveal an abnormality in a certain region of chromosome 8.

There are no reports of prenatal diagnosis of this condition. To provide accurate genetic counseling regarding prognosis and risk of recurrence, it is important to distinguish this condition from others that are similar to it, such as tricho-rhino-phalangeal syndrome, type 1.

### Treatment and management

The treatment for LGS is tailored to each person. Exostoses may need to be surgically removed if they are causing problems with nerves or blood vessels. If the two leg lengths are different, corrective shoes may be helpful. Orthopedic devices such as braces or, more rarely, surgery may be indicated in severe cases of skeletal abnormality. Plastic surgery to alter specific features, such as the ears or nose, has been chosen by some people.

The risk of **cancer** at the site of the exostoses is not known but may be higher.

Special education for mentally retarded individuals is indicated. A focus on speech development may be appropriate.

### Prognosis

Langer-Giedion syndrome does not alter life span. Complications from associated abnormalities such as mental retardation, however, can cause problems. Asymmetry of the limbs can interfere with their function and cause pain. Psychological effects due to physical abnormalities may also be experienced.

### Resources

**BOOKS**

"Tricho-rhino-phalangeal Syndrome, Type II." *Birth Defects Encyclopedia,* ed. Mary Louise Buyse. Boston: Blackwell Scientific Publications, 1990.

Goodman, Richard M., and Robert J. Gorlin. "Langer-Giedion Syndrome." *The Malformed Infant and Child.* New York: Oxford University Press, 1983.

**PERIODICALS**

Moroika, D., and Y. Hosaka. "Aesthetic and Plastic Surgery for Trichorhinophalangeal Syndrome." *Aesthetic Plastic Surgery* 24 (2000): 39-45.

**WEBSITES**

*NORD—National Organization for Rare Diseases.*http://www.rarediseases.org.

*OMIM—Online Mendelian Inheritance in Man.*http://www.ncbi.nlm.nig.gov.

**ORGANIZATIONS**

Langer-Giedion Syndrome Association. 89 Ingham Ave., Toronto, Ontario M4K 2W8, Canada. (416) 465-3029. kinross@istar.ca.

National Institute on Deafness and Other Communication Disorders. 31 Center Dr., MSC 2320, Bethesda, MD 20814. (301) 402-0900. nidcdinfo@nidcd.nih.gov. http://www.nidcd.nih.gov.

Amy Vance, MS, CGC

# Triose phosphate isomerase deficiency

## Definition

Triose phosphate isomerase (TPI) deficiency is a rare non-sex-linked (autosomal) disorder that is a result of an insufficient amount of the enzyme triose phosphate isomerase. This disorder is inherited as a dominant trait and it is known to be caused by more than one different mutation in the same **gene** (allelic variants).

## Description

Triose phosphate isomerase is an enzyme involved in the breakdown of glucose into the energy required to sustain cellular metabolism. Glucose is first converted into the chemical pyruvate. Pyruvate then enters the tricarboxylic acid cycle (TCA cycle) to produce ATP, the chemical form of energy used by the cells. Glucose is broken down to the chemical pyruvate via a chemical pathway that involves 10 enzymes. TPI is the fifth enzyme in this reaction chain. The two major products of the reaction proceeding the TPI reaction are D-glyceraldehyde-3-phosphate (GAP) and dihydroxyacetone phosphate (DHAP). These two chemicals are isomers, which means that they have the same chemical formulas but different chemical structures. TPI is the enzyme that converts DHAP into GAP. This conversion (isomerization) is important because it is only GAP that is used in the

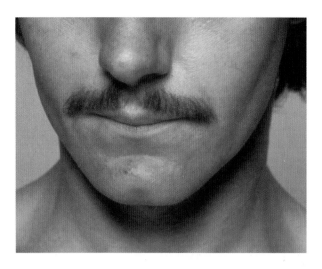

Malformations of the red blood cells in triose phosphate isomerase deficiency cause the liver, the organ responsible for cleaning the blood, to become overworked. This results in jaundice, an abnormal yellowing of the skin and the whites of the eyes. *(Custom Medical Stock Photo, Inc.)*

subsequent steps in the reaction pathway to the essential pyruvate molecules.

Under normal physiological conditions, DHAP is produced in much greater quantities than GAP (approximately 20:1). Therefore, it is essential that TPI convert the DHAP to GAP to increase the overall efficiency of pyruvate production from glucose. Individuals affected with TPI deficiency have extremely low levels of TPI activity because the enzyme that they do produce is not properly formed and, thus, it is highly inefficient.

## Genetic profile

The gene that is responsible for the production of TPI has been localized to a region on **chromosome** 12. There are at least five mutations in this gene that lead to TPI deficiency. In every case, very slight changes in the chemical structure of TPI occur such that the TPI produced is less effective than a normal TPI molecule, especially when the body is hot, either from the weather or from exercise.

## Demographics

TPI deficiency is extremely rare. In 1998, there were only 13 people known to be living with TPI deficiency, eleven children and two adult Hungarian brothers affected with an extremely mild form of the disease. Since 1998, at least five of these children have passed away. The documented rarity of this disorder does not seem to coincide with the observed frequency of reduced TPI activity in the population.

In a 1996 study of unselected individuals of Caucasian and Japanese descent, a Japanese researcher found that approximately five out of every 1,000 individuals had TPI activity that was only half of the normal TPI activity. In a separate study, it was estimated that nine in 1,713 Caucasians and seven in 168 African-Americans showed these low levels of TPI activity. One possible explanation is that complete TPI deficiency is an embryo-lethal condition. In other words, if complete TPI deficiency is inherited at conception, this embryo is miscarried before the mother even knows that conception had occurred.

All of the mutations in the gene responsible for the production of TPI are expressed as dominant traits. This means that a child can inherit this condition from just one of his or her parents. Also, if one child has been born affected with TPI deficiency, the likelihood that a second child, of the same parents, will also be affected is 50%. This likelihood is increased to 75% if both parents carry the defective gene.

## Signs and symptoms

TPI deficiency affects primarily the circulatory and nervous systems. Disorders of the circulatory system include at least four separate forms of anemia (a lack of properly functioning red blood cells) that cause a lack of oxygen transport to the tissues and organs of the body. Disorders of the nervous system include developmental retardation and degenerative neurologic disorder with spasticity, a condition in which the nervous system progressively degenerates and the affected person suffers from spasticity similar to that seen in people with **multiple sclerosis**.

Because of the malformations of the red blood cells in TPI deficiency affected individuals, the liver, the organ that is responsible for cleaning the blood, often becomes overworked. This causes jaundice (an abnormal yellowing of the skin and the whites of the eyes). Heart failure is also quite common and is often the cause of death in TPI deficiency patients.

People affected with TPI deficiency are generally highly susceptible to recurrent infections. This tendency is believed to be due to a **depression** of the immune system caused by improper blood function.

## Diagnosis

If a family history of the disease leads to suspicion, TPI deficiency can be detected prenatally by a test of umbilical cord blood. A device recognized by the U. S. Food and Drug Administration is available to measure the activity of TPI on red blood cells taken in a sample. This device provides a definitive test for TPI deficiency. A blood test indicating extremely elevated levels of DHAP is also indicative of TPI deficiency.

Another blood test that can be performed is an autohemolysis test. This test allows TPI deficiency to be differentially diagnosed from certain other enzymatic deficiencies. In this test, samples of blood are drawn and incubated at body temperature for 48 hours. After this time, the amount of breakdown of the red blood cells is recorded. One sample is left untreated, one sample has added glucose, and a third sample has added ATP. If the untreated sample shows higher than normal breakdown of the red blood cells, but those samples treated with glucose or ATP show a lessened breakdown of red blood cells, this is indicative of TPI deficiency. If glucose, but not ATP, slows the breakdown of the red blood cells, this indicates a diagnosis of G6PD deficiency. If ATP, but not glucose, slows the breakdown of the red blood cells, this indicates a diagnosis of **pyruvate kinase deficiency**. G6PD and pyruvate kinase are two other enzymes involved in the breakdown of glucose to pyruvate to ATP.

## Treatment and management

No treatment is currently available for TPI deficiency. Studies are ongoing to determine the feasibility of bone marrow transplants and enzyme replacement therapies. In 1999, TPI deficiency was corrected in a four-year-old boy by an enzyme replacement blood transfusion treatment. However, due to the temporary nature of the observed corrections in the biochemistry, it was concluded that a sustained reversal of the symptoms of TPI deficiency would require a continuous delivery of an active form of the TPI enzyme.

## Prognosis

There are only two reported cases of TPI deficiency affected individuals living beyond the age of six. These are a set of Hungarian brothers, one who did not develop neurological symptoms of TPI deficiency until 1980, at the age of 12, and an older brother, who was 30 in 2001, who has no neurological symptoms but does have anemia. Enzyme replacement therapy and/or bone marrow transplantation may eventually prove to be effective means of treating TPI deficiency, and improve survival rates for this rare genetic disorder.

### Resources

#### PERIODICALS

Ationu, A. "Toward Enzyme-replacement Treatment in Triosephosphate Isomerase Deficiency." *Lancet* (April 1999): 1155-56.

Humphries, A., et al. "Ancestral Origin of Variation in the Triosephosphate Isomerase Gene Promoter." *Human Genetics* (June 1999): 486-91.

Pekrun, A., et al. "Triosephosphate Isomerase Deficiency: Biochemical and Molecular Genetic Analysis for Prenatal Diagnosis." *Clinical Genetics* (April 1995): 175-9.

Watanabe, M., B. Zingg, and H. Mohrenweiser. "Molecular Analysis of a Series of Alleles in Humans with Reduced Activity at the Triosephosphate Isomerase Locus." *American Journal of Human Genetics* (February 1996): 308-16.

#### WEBSITES

James Stewardson TPI Trust. http://members.gconnect.com/users/tpi/top.htm (February 23, 2001).

"Triosephosphate Isomerase 1." *OMIM—Online Mendelian Inheritance in Man.*http://www.ncbi.nlm.nih.gov/entrez/dispomim.cgi?id=190450 (February 23, 2001).

#### ORGANIZATIONS

National Organization for Rare Disorders (NORD). PO Box 8923, New Fairfield, CT 06812-8923. (203) 746-6518 or (800) 999-6673. Fax: (203) 746-6481. http://www.rarediseases.org.

Paul A. Johnson

# Triple X syndrome

### Definition

Triple X syndrome is a chromosomal disorder resulting from the presence of an extra X **chromosome** that can cause mild learning disabilities, tall statures

and psychiatric problems in some women with this disorder. Many women with triple X syndrome have no symptoms or complications from this condition.

### Demographics

Approximately 1 in 1,000 women has triple X syndrome. This condition is underdiagnosed because of a lack of identifiable physical features. Only women are affected by triple X syndrome.

### Description

Triple X syndrome is also called triplo-X syndrome, trisomy X, XXX syndrome and 47,XXX syndrome. Many women with this syndrome have no physical characteristics or intellectual differences because of it. Others have very mild differences, and a small minority of women with triple X syndrome can have more pronounced symptoms and signs of this condition.

The symptoms of this condition include:

- Tall stature
- Learning disabilities
- Motor delays
- Speech and language delay
- Premature ovarian failure
- Psychological problems

Learning disabilities are more common in girls with triple X than in the general population. Women with triple X syndrome have an average IQ in the 85-90 range, compared to normal IQ of about 100. However, there is considerable variability in cognitive abilities, including IQs above normal for some affected girls. Many children with triple X require speech therapy in childhood, and they may reach both speech and motor milestones slightly later than their unaffected siblings. In adolescence, psychological problems such as **depression** or conduct disorder may be somewhat more common in girls with triple X, although this may be due to environment in which the girls live more than the physical effects of triple X syndrome.

Triple X is not associated with abnormal physical characteristics, although girls with triple X are slightly taller (by approximately 4 inches, on average) than their siblings. Triple X is associated with normal puberty and fertility, and women with this condition are not at an increased risk above to have children with chromosome abnormalities. Premature ovarian failure has been reported in some women with triple X syndrome.

## Causes and symptoms

### Genetic profile

Triple X syndrome is caused by the presence of an extra X chromosome. Chromosomes are packages of genetic information that are present in every cell of the body. They come in pairs and humans have a total of 46 chromosomes, arranged into 23 pairs. The first 22 pairs of chromosomes are called "autosomes" and are numbered 1 to 22, from largest to smallest. The 23rd pair is called the "sex chromosomes." Females typically have two X chromosomes (46,XX), and males have one X chromosome and one Y chromosome (46,XY).

Triple X syndrome results from an extra copy of the X chromosome in each of a female's cells. As a result of the extra X chromosome, each cell has a total of 47 chromosomes (47,XXX) instead of the usual 46. Women with triple X syndrome have three X chromosomes for a total of 47 chromosomes. Triple X syndrome occurs when there is an error in chromosome division, called nondisjunction, that occurs before conception in either the mother's egg or the father's sperm. This error occurs randomly; Triple X syndrome is not an inherited disorder.

## Diagnosis

### Tests

Triple X syndrome is diagnosed by **karyotype** testing. A karyotype is a chromosome analysis that can be

done on a blood sample or tissue obtained via prenatal diagnosis testing. A karyotype looks at the structure and number of a person's chromosomes. The diagnosis of triple X syndrome is made if an extra X chromosome is present.

Most cases of triple X syndrome are diagnosed during pregnancy in mothers who have elected to have prenatal testing such as **amniocentesis** or chorionic villus sampling for reasons unrelated to triple X syndrome. Prospective parents should meet with a geneticist or genetic counselor to discuss the diagnosis of triple X syndrome if this condition is diagnosed during a pregnancy. Because of its lack of physical findings and mild symptoms, triple X syndrome is underdiagnosed in the general population.

## Treatment

### Traditional

There is no cure for triple X syndrome and treatment is based upon symptoms. The therapies for the symptoms of triple X syndrome are no different than the therapies that someone without triple X syndrome, but with the same symptoms, would receive. Individuals with symptoms due to triple X syndrome may receive speech therapy for speech delay, physical therapy for motor problems, and treatment for learning disabilities. In addition, they may receive treatment and counseling for psychiatric conditions if they develop this complication.

## Prognosis

The prognosis for women with triple X syndrome is very good. They live a normal lifespan and there are no physical abnormalities or mental retardations associated with this condition.

## Prevention

Because of the possible psychiatric issues and learning disabilities children with triple X syndrome may experience, it is important that girls with triple X syndrome be raised in a stable and supportive environment. The symptoms of this condition—especially learning disabilities and psychiatric problems — should be treated promptly.

### Resources

#### PERIODICALS

Otter M., C.T. Schrander-Stumpel, L.M. Curfs. "Triple X Syndrome: A Review of the Literature" *European Journal of Human Genetics* (2009): 1–7.

#### ORGANIZATIONS

Triple X Support Group, 32 Francemary Rd.,LondonBrockley, England, SE4 1JS, (020) 869-09445, helenclements@ hotmail.com, http://www.triplo-x.org.

UNIQUE - Rare Chromosome Disorder Support Group, PO Box 2189, CaterhamSurrey, United Kingdom, CR3 5GN, + 44 (0)1883 330766, , info@rarechromo.org, http://www.rar echromo.org/html/home.asp.

Kathleen A Fergus, M.S., C.G.C.

# Triploidy

## Definition

Triploidy is a rare lethal **chromosome** abnormality caused by the presence of an entire extra set of chromosomes. A fetus with triploidy has 69 chromosomes, rather than 46. The majority of fetuses with triploidy are spontaneously miscarried during pregnancy. Those that survive until birth will have severe growth retardation and multiple birth defects.

## Description

Triploidy is a condition caused by having a full extra set of chromosomes. This extra set of chromosomes causes a variety of serious birth defects, placental problems, and severe growth problems in a fetus. In fact, most pregnancies in which the fetus has triploidy end in a spontaneous miscarriage. Very few infants with triploidy survive to term. Of those that do, most are stillborn and those that are born alive usually die shortly after birth. Infants with this lethal condition are generally small due to severe intrauterine growth retardation (IUGR) and they have multiple birth defects, including facial abnormalities, such as **cleft lip**, heart defects, **neural tube defects** (**spina bifida**), and other serious birth defects. The exact pattern of abnormalities depends on whether the extra set of chromosomes was inherited from the mother or from the father. Unfortunately, there is nothing that can be done to treat or cure triploidy.

## Genetic profile

Triploidy is a chromosomal disorder. Chromosomes are the structures that contain all of the body's genes (the basic unit of **inheritance**). Humans have 46 chromosomes in every cell of their body, with the exception of their sperm and eggs cells, which contain only 23 chromosomes. When a sperm and an egg unite at conception, the resulting fertilized egg will have 46 chromosomes: half from the mother and half from the father. This fertilized egg will continue to develop and grow into a fetus and, eventually, into a live-born infant with 46 chromosomes in every cell of their body.

Of these 46 chromosomes, 22 pairs (or 44 chromosomes) are called autosomes (or non-sex chromosomes) and the twenty-third pair is the sex chromosomes. Women have two X chromosome (46,XX) and men have an X and Y chromosome (46,XY). Fetuses with triploidy can be 69,XXX (female), 69,XXY (male), or 69,XYY (male). Twenty-three chromosomes (or one set) is referred to as a haploid set of chromosomes, 46 chromosomes (or two sets) is referred to as a diploid set of chromosomes, and 69 chromosomes (or three sets) is referred to a triploid set of chromosomes. A fetus with triploidy has three haploid sets of chromosomes.

Triploidy occurs in several different ways. The extra set of chromosomes can be inherited from the father (paternal inheritance) or they can be from the mother (maternal inheritance). The most common mechanism for triploidy is the fertilization of a single egg by two sperm. This results in a triploid egg with two sets of paternal chromosomes and one set of maternal chromosomes. This accounts for about 60% of cases of triploidy. The other mechanism is an error in cell division in which an egg cell ends up with 46 chromosomes instead of 23. This egg with 46 chromosomes is fertilized by a sperm with 23 chromosomes, resulting in a fertilized egg with 69 chromosomes, which then has two sets of maternal chromosomes and one set of paternal chromosomes. This mechanism is responsible for about 40% of cases of triploidy. The physical effects of triploidy differ depending on whether the extra set of chromosomes was inherited from the mother (maternally inherited) or from the father (paternally inherited).

In pregnancies in which the extra set of chromosomes is maternally inherited, the fetuses tend to be well-formed, with a small head (**microcephaly**). The placenta in these pregnancies is generally enlarged and cystic (filled with cysts). This type of placenta is often referred to as a hydatiform mole and the pregnancy as a whole may be referred to as a partial molar pregnancy. In pregnancies in which the extra set of

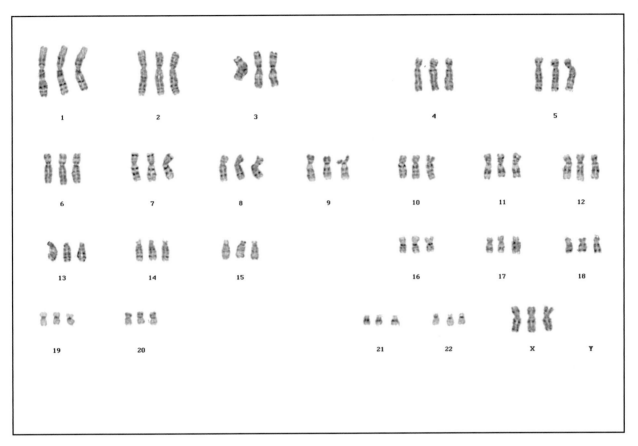

**Human karyotype showing three copies of each chromosome as opposed to the normal pairs, an occurrence known as triploidy. Triploidy is not compatible with life and is often associated with spontaneous abortion.** *(Illustration by Argosy Publishing. Reproduced by permission of Gale, a part of Cengage Learning.)*

chromosomes is paternally inherited, the fetuses have severe growth retardation, a large head, and a small, non-cystic placenta.

The physical birth defects seen in triploidy are variable. All fetuses will have some of these birth defects, but very few will have all of them. The birth defects most commonly seen are heart defects, cleft lip, neural tube defects, kidney malformation, abnormal genitalia (males), and defects in the abdominal wall. Regardless of the presence or absence of these birth defects, triploidy is incompatible with life.

Triploidy is a sporadic (or accidental) event. It is not caused by anything that a parent may or may not have done. Unlike some other chromosome abnormalities (trisomy 21 or Down syndrome), triploidy is not associated with a mother's age. This means that there is not an increased risk for triploidy for an older mother to have a pregnancy. Because triploidy is an accidental event, there is no increased recurrence risk in future pregnancies. A woman who has had one triploid pregnancy is not at any increased risk to have a second one.

## Demographics

Triploidy occurs in about 1–2% of all conceptions, but most of these pregnancies end in early spontaneous miscarriage. Very few pregnancies with a triploid infant go to term. Only one in 10,000 infants is born with triploidy, and it is estimated that for every live-born infant with triploidy, 1,200 have been lost as miscarriages. Most infants with triploidy are either stillborn or die shortly after birth. The longest recorded lifespan of an infant with full triploidy is 10 months, although this length of survival is extremely rare.

There is a milder form of triploidy that is the result of mosaicism, which is the presence of two separate types of cells within the same individual. Infants with mosaic triploidy have both a normal cell line (46,XX or 46,XY) and a triploid cell line (69,XXX or 69,XXY or 69,XYY). These infants can survive to be live born,

## KEY TERMS

**Diploid**—Two sets of chromosomes; in humans, this is 46 chromosomes.

**Haploid**—One single set of chromosomes; in humans, this is 23 chromosomes.

**Triploid**—Three sets of chromosomes; in humans, this is 69 chromosomes.

but they generally have growth retardation, growth asymmetry (their limbs may be different sizes), some of the other birth defects seen in full triploidy, and severe mental retardation. It is thought that the presence of the normal cell line aids in survival.

### Signs and symptoms

Triploidy manifests itself in many different ways. It can be diagnosed both prenatally and at birth.

The diagnosis of triploidy is often made prenatally or during the course of a pregnancy. The diagnosis is often suspected because of an abnormal sonogram or because of an abnormal maternal serum screening test.

A sonogram, or ultrasound, is a common test done during pregnancy that uses sound waves to examine the fetus. There is no known risk to the fetus from an ultrasound. However, a fetus affected with triploidy will often show abnormalities that will warrant further testing to confirm the diagnosis of triploidy. Some of the most common abnormalities seen on a sonogram of a fetus with triploidy include severe growth problems or intrauterine growth retardation (IUGR), an abnormal placenta, and limb abnormalities.

Not every fetus with triploidy will have all of these findings, but most will show some signs that can be detected by sonogram. Abnormal sonogram findings include:

- severe early-onset intrauterine growth retardation (detected as early as 12–14 weeks)
- brain abnormalities, including isolated ventriculomegaly (enlarged ventricles), Arnold-Chiari malformation, holoprosencephaly, and agenesis of the corpus callosum
- cleft lip and possible cleft palate
- limb abnormalities, such as clubfoot or syndactyly (webbing of the fingers and toes)
- heart defects
- kidney abnormalities

- abdominal wall defects, such as an omphalocele (an opening in the abdominal wall, which causes the intestines to be located outside the body)
- neural tube defects, such as spina bifida (an opening in the spinal cord)
- oligohydramnios (a decrease amount of amniotic fluid)
- placental abnormalities, including an enlarged placenta or a cystic placenta

In addition to detection by prenatal sonogram, many fetuses with triploidy are detected by an abnormal maternal serum screening test. A maternal serum screening test is a voluntary blood test usually performed in the second trimester of pregnancy. It is not specifically designed to detect triploidy, but often does because of some of the abnormalities seen in triploidy. The blood test measures the amount of certain proteins in the mother's blood. These proteins, alpha-fetoprotein, human chorionic gonadotropin (hCG), and estriol, are all made either by the fetus or by the placenta. These proteins cross the placenta and get into the mother's blood system. By looking at the amount of these proteins present in the mother's blood system, it is possible to screen for certain genetic abnormalities. Because fetuses with triploidy often have abnormal placentas, too much or too little of these proteins are leaked into the mother's system and the blood test results are often abnormal. If a maternal serum screening test is abnormal, the patient should be offered a detailed ultrasound and **amniocentesis**.

Both prenatal sonograms and maternal serum screening testing are screening tests. They can pick out individuals with a higher risk to have a fetus with a specific disorder, but they cannot actually give a specific diagnosis. Because of this, if an individual has an abnormal screening test, further diagnostic testing is indicated.

The only way to definitively diagnose triploidy is to have a chromosome analysis (**karyotype**) done and actually count the number of chromosomes present. In order to do a chromosome analysis during pregnancy, it is necessary to obtain some tissue from the fetus. This is commonly done through either a chorionic villi sampling (CVS) test or through an amniocentesis. During a chorionic villi test, a catheter is used to remove a small piece of tissue from the placenta. Since the placenta and fetus have come from the same fertilized egg, the chromosomes in the placenta are the same as the chromosomes in the fetus. A CVS test is usually done between 10 and 12 weeks of pregnancy. If a patient is further along in the pregnancy when an abnormality is suspected, an amniocentesis may be performed. This test is usually done between 15 and 20 weeks of pregnancy. It involves using a needle to remove some of the amniotic fluid from around the fetus. The amniotic fluid contains fetal skin cell, which can then be cultured (grown) and analyzed. The results from these tests can take between one and two weeks. By doing a fetal karyotype (counting the number of chromosome the fetus has), it is possible to definitely diagnose triploidy. A newer technique, **fluorescent in situ hybridization** (FISH), is available in some laboratories and results may be available in as little as 24 hours. It is always wise to do a complete karyotype in addition to FISH testing.

Very few fetuses survive to be born to term with triploidy. Those infants that survive do show a very specific pattern of birth defects. Almost all of these infants will have growth retardation and characteristic facial features, including wide-set eyes (hypertelorism), low-set ears, and limb abnormalities, such as **clubfoot** and syndactyly (webbing of the fingers and toes). Other anomalies include heart defects, kidney malformations, and genital malformations (particularly in males). Once triploidy is suspected in an infant, a blood chromosome analysis (a karyotype) should be performed to confirm the diagnosis. Additionally, the newer technique, FISH, is advised.

### Diagnosis

The diagnosis is often suspected in pregnancies due to abnormal growth parameters, abnormalities seen on a sonogram, an abnormal screening test, or an abnormal CVS or amniocentesis result.

The diagnosis in infants is made by physical examination shortly after birth. Severe growth retardation, an abnormal placenta and physical birth defects first raise the suspicion of triploidy. This diagnosis is then confirmed through a chromosome analysis (karyotype) which is blood test performed on the infant. A karyotype is a picture of an individuals chromosomes and in this case will show an abnormal number of chromosomes (69 instead of 46).

The diagnosis in infants with the rare mosaic form of triploidy (one normal cell line and one abnormal cell line) may be suspected shortly after birth due to the presence of growth retardation, asymmetrical growth of the limbs, and other physical birth defects. The diagnosis is then confirmed through a chromosome analysis (karyotype), which, in this case, will show the presence of two cell lines: one normal cell line with 46 chromosomes and an abnormal cell line with 69 chromosomes.

### Treatment and management

There is no cure and no treatment for triploidy. Infants that survive to term should receive palliative care, including warmth, nourishment, and comfort, until the parents have a chance to incorporate the diagnosis and make decisions about care options. Surgical correction of birth defects is not indicated given the lethal nature of this diagnosis.

If triploidy is detected during a pregnancy, patients have the option to terminate a pregnancy based upon the lethality of this condition. This is a very personal decision and should be made following complete counseling about the nature and outcome of this diagnosis. If the pregnancy continues, then the mother should be monitored for pre-eclampsia and hyperthyroidism. There is no need for special interventions, such as fetal monitoring or a caesarean section, based solely on the diagnosis of triploidy given the inevitability of the outcome.

Once the diagnosis has been firmly establish, there is no need for heroic measures given the established lethality of the conditions. Infants should be provided with basic supportive care until the family can make decisions.

This diagnosis is devastating for families. The bleak prognosis and lack of treatment can be very shocking. Families should be reassured that there is nothing that they did or did not do that could have prevented the outcome. While grieving is inevitable and appropriate, the family needs time to incorporate the information about the diagnosis. Many families find it helpful to have reminders of their baby, including footprints, photographs, and locks of hair, and the neonatal staff can aid in collecting these materials following the birth of the infant. Parents also need to understand the genetic diagnosis and its implications for future pregnancies. It is important to make sure that they understand the sporadic nature of this diagnosis and that it is unlikely to recur in a future pregnancy.

### Prognosis

The prognosis for a fetus or infant with full (non-mosaic) triploidy is very bleak. Many pregnancies end in spontaneous abortion, and those that go to term often result in a stillborn infant or one that dies shortly after birth. The longest recorded survival of an infant with triploidy is 10 months, although this length of survival is exceedingly rare.

Infants with mosaic triploidy (two cell lines: one normal and one with triploidy) often survive pregnancy but generally have multiple birth defects, severe growth abnormalities, and severe mental retardation. Their life expectancy is often dependant on the severity of their associated birth defects.

## Resources

### BOOKS

Ilse, Sherokee. *Empty Arms: Coping After Miscarriage, Stillbirth and Infant Death.* Maple Plain, MN: Wintergreen Press, 2000.

### WEB SITES

Bulletin Board for Triploidy Support. (April 13, 2005.) http://bbs.babycenter.com/board/pregnancy/pregnancygrief/1143151.

Help After Neonatal Death. (April 13, 2005.) http://www.handonline.org/resources/groups/index.html.

### ORGANIZATIONS

Compassionate Friends. P. O. Box 3696, Oak Brook, IL 60522-3696. (877) 969-0010. E-mail: nationaloffice@compassionatefriends.org.

UNIQUE—Rare Chromosome Disorder Support Group. P. O. Box 2189, Caterham, Surrey, Intl CR3 5GN, England. Telephone: 4401883 330766. Fax: 4401883 330766. E-mail: info@rarechromo.org. (April 13, 2005.) http://www.rarechromo.org.

Kathleen A. Fergus, MS, CGC

# Trismus-pseudocamptodactyly syndrome

## Definition

Trismus-pseudocamptodactyly syndrome is a rare genetic condition characterized by the inability to completely open the mouth (trismus), difficulty chewing, short stature, and abnormally short muscle-tendon units in the fingers that cause the fingers to curve or bend when the hand is bent back at the wrist (pseudocamptodactyly).

## Description

Trismus-pseudocamptodactyly syndrome was first described by the pediatrician/geneticist Frederick Hecht and the orthopedist Rodney K. Beals of the Oregon Health Sciences University in 1969 as inability-to-open-the-mouth-fully syndrome. Explaining the first descriptive name for the syndrome, individuals affected by trismus-pseudocamptodactyly syndrome cannot fully open the mouth (trismus). In addition, affected individuals are unable to bend their fingers when their wrist is extended (pseudocamptodactyly). The muscles and tendons in the forearms and/or the legs may also be abnormally short, resulting in limited movements and various deformities of the feet, including **clubfoot**, hammer and claw toes, and tightening of the muscles of the posterior

part of the leg, producing other multiple foot abnormalities. The severity of the physical findings in trismus-pseudocamptodactyly syndrome varies from individual to individual.

Trismus-pseudocamptodactyly syndrome is also known as inability-to-open-the-mouth-fully syndrome, Dutch-Kennedy syndrome, camptodactyly-limited jaw excursion, Hecht syndrome, inability to open mouth completely and short finger-flexor, Hecht-Beals-Wilson syndrome, distal arthrogryposis, and Hecht-Beals syndrome.

## Genetic profile

Trismus-pseudocamptodactyly syndrome is a rare condition inherited in an autosomal dominant pattern. In an autosomal dominant condition, only one copy of the mutated, or nonworking, **gene** for a particular condition is necessary for a person to experience the symptoms associated with the condition. Accordingly, most individuals with an autosomal dominant condition have one working copy and one nonworking copy of the gene for the disorder. Individuals contribute only half of their genetic information to their children and pass on only one copy of each gene. As a result, there is a 50% chance for a person with trismus-pseudocamptodactyly syndrome to pass on the nonworking gene for that condition and have a child affected with trismus-pseudocamptodactyly syndrome. There is also a 50% chance that a person with trismus-pseudocamptodactyly syndrome will pass on the working gene and have a child unaffected by trismus-pseudocamptodactyly syndrome. Individuals in the same family who inherit a copy of the nonworking copy of the gene causing trismus-pseudocamptodactyly syndrome can be affected in different manners and with different symptoms. Symptoms of trismus-pseudocamptodactyly syndrome present in a variety of mild to severe features (variable expressivity). However, in trismus-pseudocamptodactyly syndrome, a high percentage of individuals who inherit the abnormal gene will have some sign of the disorder (high penetrance).

The genetic cause of trismus-pseudocamptodactyly syndrome is not yet fully understood. In 2004, several families with members affected by complex variant conditions associated with trismus pseudocamptodactyly were examined, and it was determined that affected members of two families had a mutation in the MYH8 gene (perinatal myosin heavy-chain gene) on the short arm of **chromosome** 17 (17q13.1). The same mutation was also identified in affected members of a large Caucasian Belgian family affected by trismus-pseudocamptodactyly syndrome alone. Based on these studies, it appears that many cases of trismus-pseudocamptodactyly syndrome are caused by a mutation in MYH8; however, it is still unclear if trismus-pseudocamptodactyly syndrome is caused by mutations in other genes as well.

## Demographics

Trismus-pseudocamptodactyly syndrome is a rare condition affecting both men and women equally. It was originally described in a Dutch family and believed to only occur in Dutch families or the descendants of Dutch families in West Virginia. Since the original families were identified, families of other ethnic backgrounds, including Canadians, Taiwanese, and Japanese, have been found to be affected. Accordingly, it is believed that trismus-pseudocamptodactyly syndrome can occur in any race or ethnic background.

## Signs and symptoms

Individuals affected by trismus-pseudocamptodactyly syndrome classically present with two main features: limited excursion of the mandible (trismus) and flexion deformity of the fingers that occurs with wrist extension (pseudocamptodactyly). At birth, trismus-pseudocamptodactyly syndrome may be diagnosed based on the infant's clenched fists and inability to fully open its mouth. Additional features include short stature and foot malformations caused by short muscle-tendon units, which prevent normal growth and development. The forms of foot abnormalities caused by short muscle-tendons in the hamstrings, calves, and feet include malformations that occur when the foot is turned inward and downward (equinovarus or talipes equinovarus), inward bending for the front half of the foot (metatarsus varus), and angling foot at the heel with the toes pointing upward and outward (calcaneovalgus deformity). Different family members who have inherited the same mutated,

or nonworking, gene can have symptoms that range from very mild to very severe.

## Diagnosis

Diagnosis of trismus-pseudocamptodactyly syndrome is made through a detailed physical exam, medical history, and family history most often performed by a medical **genetics** team. Clinical **genetic testing** is not available at this time; however, research testing for MYH8 at 17p13.1 may be available through a genetic clinic.

## Treatment and management

The treatment and management of trismus-pseudocamptodactyly syndrome depends on the severity of the symptoms. Most individuals are treated with a combination of physical therapy, speech therapy, occupational therapy, and surgery.

An infant's inability to fully open its mouth can cause severe difficulties with feeding, adequate calorie intake, speech development, and dental care. Speech and physical therapy are recommended to help address jaw issues. Jaw surgery may be necessary to open infants' jaws for nourishment. The clenched fists found in many infants affected by trismus-pseudocamptodactyly syndrome can cause difficulties in learning to crawl and grasp items. Often infants will learn to crawl on their knuckles. The clenched fists involved with pseudocamptodactyly may also impair manual dexterity and cause occupational disability that requires physical and occupational therapy or surgery. Contractures due to the short muscle-tendons may result in foot abnormalities that, like clenched fists, may delay milestones. Affected infants may require surgical correction of contractures and foot abnormalities in order to walk.

Adults affected by trismus-pseudocamptodactyly syndrome continue to have issues with inability to open their mouths fully, short muscle-tendons, and foot anomalies. Although many individuals pursue surgical options, there is no consensus on the optimal treatment. In one report, endoscopic surgery to release the jaw in one patient resulted in recurrence three months postoperatively. Another technique that had some success was a passive stretching of the mouth with tongue blades. Early treatment of trismus can prevent or minimize many of the conditions. Passive motion, applied several times per day, has been shown to be more effective than static stretching for keeping short muscle-tendons supple. Recent research has shown that passive motion provides significant reduction in inflammation and pain. Ongoing physical therapy and stretching of contractures caused by short muscle-tendons may help maintain optimal muscle length over time, allowing improved range of motion and preventing relapse after surgery.

General anesthesia and muscle relaxants do not relieve the trismus or increase the jaw's opening. Since an open mouth is necessary to intubate in the traditional manner, general anesthesia for any surgery can be difficult and hazardous. Several reports on intubation techniques are found in the anesthesia literature that recommend techniques, such as avoiding muscle relaxants and using fiberoptic-assisted nasotracheal intubation, blind nasotracheal intubation, or mask anesthesia with spontaneous ventilation to assess the delivery of anesthesia and surgery. During all surgical procedures, it is recommended that a surgeon experienced in obtaining an emergency surgical airway be available.

### Prognosis

Most individuals with trismus-pseudocamptodactyly syndrome can achieve a mouth opening large enough for food and speech and a sufficient range of motion in their affected joints to live healthy, complete lives. In many individuals, physical therapy and stretching of contractures caused by short muscle-tendons may help maintain optimal muscle length, allowing improved range of motion and quality of life. However, the severe contractures and pseudocamptodactyly that appear in some individuals affected by trismus-pseudo-camptodactyly syndrome may impair manual dexterity and cause occupational disability that places physical restrictions.

### Resources

#### PERIODICALS

Lefaivre, J. F., and M. J. Aitchison. "Surgical Correction of Trismus in a Child with Hecht Syndrome." *Ann Plast Surg.* 2003 Mar; 50(3): 310–4.

#### WEB SITES

On-line Mendelian Inheritance in Man (OMIM). (April 13, 2005.) http://www.ncbi.nlm.nih.gov/entrez/dispomim. cgi?id=158300.

Trismus information. (April 13, 2005.) http://www.oralcancerfoundation.org/dental/trismus.htm.

#### ORGANIZATIONS

Avenues-Arthrogryposis Multiplex Congenita. P. O. Box 5192, Sonora, CA 95370. (209) 928-3688. E-mail: avenues@sonnet.com. (April 13, 2005.) http://sonnet1. sonnet.com/avenues/.

Genetic Alliance. 4301 Connecticut Avenue NW, Washington, DC 20008-2304. (202) 966-5557, (800) 336-4363. E-mail: information@geneticalliance.org.

National Institute of Arthritis and Musculoskeletal and Skin Diseases. 1 AMS Circle, Bethesda, MD 20892-3675. (301) 496-8188, (877) 226-4267. E-mail: NAMSIC@ mail.nih.gov. (April 13, 2005.) http://www.nih.gov/ niams/.

Dawn Jacob Laney

Trisomy *see* **Chromosomal abnormalities**

# Trisomy 8 mosaicism syndrome

### Definition

Trisomy 8 is defined as the presence of three full copies of **chromosome** 8 in all of a person's cells. Mosaic trisomy 8 describes the situation that occurs when only a portion of these cells contains three copies of chromosome 8, while others contain the usual two copies of that chromosome. For example, people with mosaic trisomy 8 may have cells in their blood and other tissues with the normal chromosome number, but may have cells in their skin with trisomy 8.

### Description

The condition is sometimes also referred to as trisomy 8 mosaicism syndrome (T8mS) and mosaic Warkany syndrome. Common characteristics of T8mS are distinct facial features, including low-set or abnormally shaped ears and a bulbous-tipped nose, eye abnormalities like strabismus and corneal clouding, bone and tissue abnormalities, various structural heart problems, palate abnormalities, hydronephrosis, cryptorchidism, mild to moderate mental delays, and deep hand and feet creases. These characteristics tend to vary widely from person to person.

### Genetic profile

The presence of three copies of a chromosome typically arises from a process called nondisjunction. This happens during the very complex process of cell division. It can occur during meiosis, the process of cell division within the sperm and eggs prior to fertilization. It can also happen during mitosis, the process of cell division in the **zygote** after fertilization.

A fertilized human zygote usually has 46 chromosomes in total. In mitosis, the zygote's cells divide and duplicate themselves evenly, keeping the chromosome number the same in all of the duplicated cells. If

## KEY TERMS

**Amniocentesis**—A procedure involving removal of a small amniotic fluid sample during pregnancy to obtain fetal chromosome results.

**Chorionic villus sampling (CVS)**—A procedure involving removal of a small placenta sample during pregnancy to obtain fetal chromosome results.

**Chromosome**—The structures in most cells that contain genes, the instructions for various traits and characteristics.

**Cryptorchidism**—Failure of one or both testes to descend into the scrotal sacs in the developing male fetus.

**Epicanthic folds**—Folds of skin of the upper eyelid continued over the inner edge of the eye.

**Hydronephrosis**—An accumulation of urine in the kidney, usually caused by a blockage in the urinary tract that leads to it.

**Optic disc**—Circular area at the back of the eyeball where the optic nerve connects to the retina.

**Strabismus**—Improper aligning of an eye, resulting in a crossed-eye appearance.

**Zygote**—Egg, after it has been fertilized by a sperm.

nondisjunction occurs, a pair of chromosomes does not divide evenly. This can result in too few chromosomes in some cells, which is called monosomy. It also results in too many chromosomes in other cells. If nondisjunction involves chromosome 8, it can lead to trisomy 8.

When nondisjunction happens during mitosis and causes trisomy 8, it only causes trisomy 8 in a portion of that individual's cells. A single cell then has trisomy 8, and these continue to duplicate themselves in certain organs and tissues. At the same time, cells with the normal number of chromosomes duplicate themselves in other organs and tissues. In the end, the affected person has a combination of cells with the normal chromosome number and those with trisomy 8, which is T8mS. This may occur in varying different tissues of that person and the exact ones cannot be predicted. Depending on when the nondisjunction happened, the person may have few or many cells with trisomy 8.

Nondisjunction is a cell division error that occurs by chance. Thus, no parent has control over this process and cannot influence the number of chromosomes their child receives at, or after, conception. In turn, T8mS is considered an unpredictable event that

typically carries a very low recurrence risk for that person's parents and family. Unlike other conditions involving nondisjunction, like **Down syndrome**, T8mS has not been strongly associated with a mother's or father's age at conception.

Most people with T8mS do not have a family history of the condition, since it usually occurs by chance.

### Demographics

Full trisomy 8 occurs in about 0.7% of spontaneous miscarriages. It is estimated to occur in about 0.1% of recognized pregnancies. When seen at birth, it is almost always due to mosaic trisomy 8 as opposed to full trisomy 8. The exact incidence of live-born children with T8mS was not known as of 2005, but a study by Nielsen, et al., in 1991 found one child with the condition among 34,910 newborns.

T8mS has been reported worldwide, being slightly more common in males than in females.

### Signs and symptoms

Characteristics of T8mS vary. In other chromosome mosaicism conditions, more severe symptoms and a worse prognosis are associated with a larger proportion of cells with an abnormal chromosome number being present. Interestingly, that does not seem to be the case in T8mS. The percentage of cells with trisomy 8 does not appear to correlate with the types of symptoms the affected person experiences.

The creases on the palms and soles of people with T8mS are the most unique characteristic of the condition. On the palms there may be more arches than usual on the fingertips and a single crease running across the palm. The creases are often deep and vertical, with a furrowed appearance, on the soles of the feet.

People with T8mS often have distinct facial characteristics. This can include a wide upturned nose, thicker and downturned lower lip, and low-set and prominent ears that may not be shaped in the usual way. They may also have abnormalities of the palate, including a cleft (opening) or highly arched palate.

Mental retardation can occur with the condition, and the degree of mental delays varies from mild to moderate.

Other findings in T8mS can include those of the bone and tissues. These may be narrow shoulders, absent knee caps, abnormally shaped toes, tighter joints, slender palms, extra or missing ribs, and curving of the spine.

Eye abnormalities are seen in T8mS, and the two most common findings are corneal clouding and strabismus where an eye turns in. These may or may not cause significant vision problems and require treatment. More rare eye problems can include a smaller eye size, smaller eye openings, droopy eyelids, wide-set eyes, tilted optic discs, nearsightedness, retinal abnormalities, and epicanthic folds.

Occasional other characteristics can include structural heart problems, hydronephrosis, underdeveloped genitalia, **cancer**, and testes that have not descended into the scrotal sacs.

### Diagnosis

Suspicions about T8mS are usually based on a child being born with unique characteristics, since there usually is no reason one would suspect it, such as a family history of the condition. Blood chromosome testing is widely available to diagnose chromosome abnormalities. If enough cells are carefully analyzed in the laboratory, T8mS can often be found in a blood sample.

In situations where a child with multiple characteristics has normal blood chromosome results, other tissues like the skin can be studied for its chromosome makeup. A trained physician can do a brief procedure called a skin biopsy to obtain a small skin sample. During this, the physician takes a pencil eraser-sized piece of skin from a child's arm or back. Sometimes this testing reveals the presence of **trisomy 18** in skin cells, which would confirm a diagnosis of T8mS.

Many characteristics of T8mS will not be seen during a pregnancy. However, a woman may be offered a routine prenatal chromosome testing for other reasons, such as her age or family history. A chorionic villus sampling (CVS) or **amniocentesis** procedure, done in the first two trimesters of pregnancy, can usually identify trisomy 8. Depending on the number of cells that are carefully studied, T8mS may also be identified.

In about 1-2% of CVS procedures that are performed, chromosomal mosaicism is found. However, this is confined to the placenta and does not represent the chromosomal status of the fetus. Additionally, a few babies reported in the literature were born with T8mS whose mothers had completely normal amniocentesis chromosome results during their pregnancies. For an unknown reason, amniocentesis may not provide the most accurate results with respect to T8mS. This makes it difficult when counseling and providing information to couples during pregnancy with respect to T8mS.

Individuals with T8mS can also be formally assessed by a medical geneticist and genetic counselor to aid in diagnosis, discussion of testing options, and interpretation of test results.

### Treatment and management

There is no cure for T8mS. Therefore, treatments are based on a person's signs and symptoms.

A **cleft palate** can be repaired through stages with surgery, often first occurring in the first year of life. This usually requires a multidisciplinary team consisting of a plastic surgeon, pediatric dentist, pediatric anesthesiologist, nurses, dietician/feeding specialist, and social worker.

Hydronephrosis, if severe enough, can warrant surgery shortly after birth. The goal is to open the blocked area of the urinary tract and clear the obstruction into the kidney. Surgery may involve a team approach, including a pediatric urologist, pediatric nephrologist, nurses, and surgery technicians.

Congenital heart defects, if severe enough, can require surgery. Surgery varies depending on the problem and may involve a team, including a pediatric cardiologist, pediatric cardiovascular surgeon, pediatric anesthesiologist, pediatric cardiovascular radiologist, nurses, and surgery technicians.

Strabismus can often be treated with patching therapy or surgery. This may require a team involving a pediatric ophthalmologist, pediatric anesthesiologist, orthoptist, nurses, and surgery technicians. Severe corneal clouding may lead to vision problems, and can sometimes be treated with surgery, laser therapy, or corneal transplants.

Undescended testicles or testes can be brought down to the proper location in the scrotal sacs by a brief surgical procedure. This can involve a team, including a pediatric urologist, pediatric anesthesiologists, and nurses.

Some characteristics of T8mS do not necessitate treatment as they cause no medical harm. Examples of these include facial features, hand/foot creases, and some tissue and bone changes.

Mental delays and retardation may be assessed by a child development team or early childhood program. Extra assistance is sometimes available through early intervention programs and special education in schools. Social workers are useful to connect families to helpful resources.

## Prognosis

People with T8mS have a prognosis that is entirely dependent upon the symptoms they experience. Someone born with a severe congenital heart defect may have a poorer prognosis for survival, growth, and development based on this. The average lifespan for someone with the T8mS is estimated to be near normal in the literature. Medical treatments and surgeries continue to offer hope.

## Resources

### WEB SITES

Chromosomal Mosaicism. Medical Genetics department at University of British Columbia. December 31, 2003 (March 15, 2005). http://www.medgen.ubc.ca/wrobin son/mosaic/.

Genetic Alliance. 2005 (March 15, 2005). http://www. geneticalliance.org.

The Human Genome Organization–Chromosome 8. (March 15, 2005.) http://gdbwww.gdb.org/hugo/chr8/.&gt;

### ORGANIZATIONS

Chromosome Deletion Outreach, Inc. P.O. Box 724, Boca Raton, FL 33429-0724. Phone/Fax: (561) 395-4252. Email: info@chromodisorder.org. www.chromodisorder. org.

UNIQUE Rare Chromosome Disorder Group. P.O. Box 2189, Caterham, Surrey CR3 5GN, UK. Phone/Fax: (44)(0)1883 330766. Email: info@rarechromo.org. www. rarechromo.org.

Deepti Babu, MS, CGC

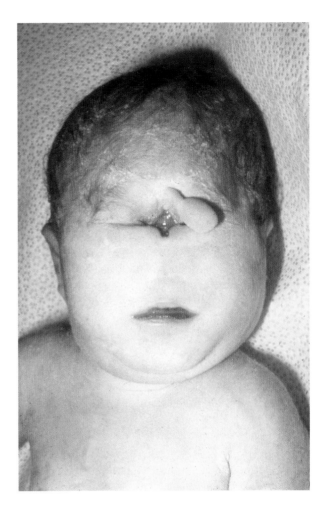

A severe complication that may be present in infants with trisomy 13 is synopthamia, in which the eyes are fused together in the center of the face. *(Photo Researchers, Inc.)*

# Trisomy 13

## Definition

Trisomy 13, also called Patau syndrome, is a congenital (present at birth) disorder associated with the presence of an extra copy of **chromosome** 13. The extra chromosome 13 causes numerous physical and mental abnormalities, especially heart defects. Dr. Klaus Patau reported the syndrome and its association with trisomy in 1960.

## Description

Children normally inherit 23 chromosomes from each parent, for a total of 46 chromosomes. A typical human being has 46 chromosomes: 22 pairs of non-sex linked chromosomes and one pair of sex-linked chromosomes that determine the child's sex. Sometimes a child may end up with more than 46 chromosomes

because of problems with the father's sperm or the mother's egg; or, because of mutations that occurred after the sperm and the egg fused to form the embryo (conception).

Normally, there are two copies of each of the 23 chromosomes: one from each parent. A condition called trisomy occurs when three, instead of two, copies of a chromosome are present in a developing human embryo. An extra copy of a particular chromosome can come either from the egg or sperm, or because of mutations that occur after conception.

The most well-known trisomy-related disorder is **Down syndrome** (trisomy 21), in which the developing embryo has an extra copy of chromosome 21. In trisomy 13, the developing embryo has three copies of chromosome 13.

An extra copy of chromosome 13 is not the only cause of trisomy 13. Other changes in the chromosome,

**Aminocentesis**—A procedure performed at 16-18 weeks of pregnancy in which a needle is inserted through a woman's abdomen into her uterus to draw out a small sample of the amniotic fluid from around the baby. Either the fluid itself or cells from the fluid can be used for a variety of tests to obtain information about genetic disorders and other medical conditions in the fetus.

**Chorionic villus sampling (CVS)**—A procedure used for prenatal diagnosis at 10-12 weeks gestation. Under ultrasound guidance a needle is inserted either through the mother's vagina or abdominal wall and a sample of cells is collected from around the fetus. These cells are then tested for chromosome abnormalities or other genetic diseases.

**Chromosome**—A microscopic thread-like structure found within each cell of the body and consists of a complex of proteins and DNA. Humans have 46 chromosomes arranged into 23 pairs. Changes in either the total number of chromosomes or their shape and size (structure) may lead to physical or mental abnormalities.

**Karyotyping**—A laboratory procedure in which chromosomes are separated from cells, stained and arranged so that their structure can be studied under the microscope.

**Mosaicism**—A genetic condition resulting from a mutation, crossing over, or nondisjunction of chromosomes during cell division, causing a variation in the number of chromosomes in the cells.

**Translocation**—The transfer of one part of a chromosome to another chromosome during cell division. A balanced translocation occurs when pieces from two different chromosomes exchange places without loss or gain of any chromosome material. An unbalanced translocation involves the unequal loss or gain of genetic information between two chromosomes.

**Trisomy**—The condition of having three identical chromosomes, instead of the normal two, in a cell.

**Ultrasound**—An imaging technique that uses sound waves to help visualize internal structures in the body.

such as mispositioning (translocation), can also result in the characteristics associated with the disorder. In these cases, an error occurs that causes a portion of chromosome 13 to be exchanged for a portion of another chromosome. There is no production of extra chromosomes; but a portion of each affected chromosome is "misplaced" (translocated) to another chromosome.

Trisomy 13 causes serious physical and mental abnormalities including heart defects; incomplete brain development; unusual facial features such as a sloping forehead, a smaller than average head (**microcephaly**), small or missing eyes, low set ears, and **cleft palate** or hare lip; extra fingers and toes (**polydactyly**); abnormal genitalia; spinal abnormalities; seizures; gastrointestinal hernias, particularly at the navel (**omphalocele**); and mental retardation. Due to the severity of these conditions, fewer than 20% of those affected survive beyond infancy.

### Genetic profile

When an extra copy (trisomy) of a chromosome is made, it may either be a total trisomy (in which an extra copy of the entire chromosome is made), or partial trisomy (in which only one part of the chromosome is made an extra time).

In most cases of trisomy, errors in chromosome duplication occur at conception because of problems with the egg or the sperm that are coming together to produce an offspring. In these cases, every cell in the body of the offspring has an extra copy of the affected chromosome. However, errors in chromosome duplication may also occur during the rapid cell division that takes place immediately after conception. In these cases, only some cells of the body have the extra chromosome error. The condition in which only some of the cells in the body have the extra chromosome is called mosaicism.

Seventy-five to 80% of the cases of trisomy 13 are caused by a trisomy of chromosome 13. Some of these cases are the result of a total trisomy, while others are the result of a partial trisomy. Partial trisomy generally causes less severe physical symptoms than full trisomy. Ten percent of these cases are of the mosaic type, in which only some of the body's cells have the extra chromosome. The physical symptoms of the mosaic form of trisomy 13 depends on the number and type of cells that carry the trisomy.

Most cases of trisomy are not passed on from one generation to the next. Usually they result from a malfunction in the cell division (mitosis) that occurs after conception. At least 75% of the cases of trisomy 13 are caused by errors in chromosome replication that occur after conception. The remaining 25% are caused by the **inheritance** of translocations of chromosome 13 with other chromosomes within the parental chromosomes. In these cases, a portion of another chromosome switches places with a portion of chromosome 13. This leads to errors in the genes on both chromosome 13 and the chromosome from which the translocated portion originated.

### Demographics

Trisomy 13 occurs in approximately one in 10,000 live births. In many cases, miscarriage occurs and the fetus does not survive to term. In other cases, the affected individual is stillborn. As appears to be the case in all trisomies, the risk of trisomy 13 seem to increase with the mother's age, particularly if she is over 30 when pregnant. Male and female children are equally affected, and the syndrome occurs in all races.

### Signs and symptoms

The severity and symptoms of trisomy 13 vary with the type of chromosomal anomaly, from extremely serious conditions to nearly normal appearance and functioning. Full trisomy 13, which is present in the majority of the cases, results in the most severe and numerous internal and external abnormalities. Commonly, the forebrain fails to divide into lobes or hemispheres (**holoprosencephaly**) and the entire head is unusually small (microcephaly). The spinal cord may protrude through an opening in the vertebrae of the spinal column (myelomeningocele). Children who survive infancy have profound mental retardation and may experience seizures.

Incomplete development of the optic (sight) and olfactory (smell) nerves often accompany the brain abnormalities described above. The eyes may be unusually small (microphthalmia) or one eye may be absent (anophthalmia). The eyes are sometimes set close together (hypotelorism) or even fused into a single structure. Incomplete development of any structures in the eye (**coloboma**) or failure of the retina to develop properly (retinal **dysplasia**) will also produce vision problems. Individuals with trisomy 13 may be born either partially or totally deaf and many are subject to recurring ear infections.

The facial features of many individuals with trisomy 13 appear flattened. The ears are generally malformed and lowset. Frequently, children with the disorder have a **cleft lip**, a cleft palate, or both. Other physical characteristics include loose folds of skin at the back of the neck, extra fingers or toes (polydactyly), permanently

flexed (closed) fingers (camptodactyly), noticeably prominent heels, "rocker-bottom foot," and missing ribs. Genital malformations are common and include undescended testicles (cryptorchidism), an abnormally developed scrotum, and **ambiguous genitalia** in males, or an abnormally formed uterus (bicornuate uterus) in females.

In nearly all cases, affected infants have respiratory difficulties and heart defects, including atrial and ventricular septal defects (holes between chambers of the heart); malformed ducts that cause abnormal direction of blood flow (**patent ductus arteriosus**); holes in the valves of the lungs and the heart (pulmonary and aortic valves); and misplacement of the heart in the right, rather than the left side of the chest (dextrocardia). The kidneys and gastrointestinal system may also be affected with cysts similar to those seen in **polycystic kidney disease**. These abnormalities are frequently severe and life-threatening.

Partial trisomy of the distal segment of chromosome 13 generally results in less severe, but still serious, symptoms and a distinctive facial appearance including a short upturned nose, a longer than usual area between the nose and upper lip (philtrum), bushy eyebrows, and tumors made up of blood capillaries on the forehead (frontal capillary hemangiomata). Partial trisomy of the proximal segment of chromosome 13 is much less likely to be fatal and has been associated with a variety of facial features including a large nose, a short upper lip, and a receding jaw. Both forms of partial trisomy also result in severe mental retardation.

Beyond one month of age, other symptoms include: feeding difficulties and constipation, reflux disease, slow growth rates, curvature of the spine (**scoliosis**), irritability, sensitivity to sunlight, low muscle tone, high blood pressure, sinus infections, urinary tract infections, and ear and eye infections.

### Diagnosis

Trisomy 13 is detectable during pregnancy through the use of ultrasound imaging, **amniocentesis**, and chorionic villus sampling (CVS). At birth, the newborn's numerous malformations indicate a possible chromosomal abnormality. Trisomy 13 is confirmed by examining the infant's chromosomal pattern through karyotyping or another procedure. Karyotyping involves the separation and isolation of the chromosomes present in cells taken from an individual. These cells are generally extracted from cells found in a blood sample. The 22 non-sex-linked chromosomes are identified by size, from largest to smallest, as chromosomes 1 through 22. The sex-determining chromosomes are also identified. Trisomy 13 is confirmed by the presence of three, rather than the normal two, copies of chromosome 13.

## Treatment and management

Some infants born with trisomy 13 have severe and incurable birth defects. However, children with better prognoses require medical treatment to correct structural abnormalities and associated complications. For feeding problems, special formulas, positions, and techniques may be used. Tube feeding or the placement of a gastric tube (gastrostomy) may be required. Structural abnormalities such as cleft lip and cleft palate can be corrected through surgery. Special diets, hearing aids, and vision aids can be used to mitigate symptoms. Physical therapy, speech therapy, and other types of developmental therapy will help the child reach his or her potential.

Since the translocation form of trisomy 13 is genetically transmitted, **genetic counseling** for the parents should be part of the management of the disease.

## Prognosis

Approximately 45% of infants with trisomy 13 die within their first month of life; up to 70% in the first six months; and more than 70% by one year of age. Survival to adulthood is very rare. Only one adult is known to have survived to age 33.

Most survivors have profound mental and physical disabilities; however, the capacity for learning in affected children varies from patient to patient. Older children may be able to walk with or without a walker. They may also be able to understand words and phrases, follow simple commands, use a few words or signs, and recognize and interact with others.

### Resources

**BOOKS**

Gardner, R. J. McKinlay, and Grant R. Sutherland. *Chromosome Abnormalities and Genetic Counseling.* New York: Oxford University Press, 1996.

Jones, Kenneth Lyons. *Smith's Recognizable Patterns of Human Malformation.* 5th ed. Philadelphia: W.B. Saunders Company, 1997.

**PERIODICALS**

Baty, Bonnie J., Brent L. Blackburn, and John C. Carey. "Natural History of Trisomy 18 and Trisomy 13: I. Growth, Physical Assessment, Medical Histories, Survival, and Recurrence Risk." *American Journal of Medical Genetics* 49 (1994): 175–87.

Baty, Bonnie J., et al. "Natural History of Trisomy 18 and Trisomy 13: II. Psychomotor Development." *American Journal of Medical Genetics* 49 (1994): 189–94.

Delatycki, M. and Gardner, R. "Three cases of trisomy 13 mosaicism and a review of the literature." *Clinical Genetics* (June 1997): 403–7.

**WEBSITES**

Pediatric Database (PEDBASE) Homepage. [cited February 9, 2001]. http://www.icondata.com/health/pedbase/files/TRISOMY1.HTM.

"Trisomy 13." *WebMD* [cited February 9, 2001]. http://my.webmd.com/content/asset/adam_disease_trisomy_13.

**ORGANIZATIONS**

Rainbows Down Under—A Trisomy 18 and Trisomy 13 Resource. SOFT Australia, 198 Oak Rd., Kirrawee, NSW 2232. Australia 02-9521-6039. http://members.optushome.com.au/karens.

Support Organization for Trisomy 18, 13, and Related Disorders (SOFT). 2982 South Union St., Rochester, NY 14624. (800) 716-SOFT. http://www.trisomy.org.

Paul A. Johnson

# Trisomy 18

## Definition

Trisomy 18 is a genetic syndrome of multiple **congenital anomalies** and severe to profound mental retardation. It is caused by the presence of an extra **chromosome** 18 in some or all of the cells of the body. Babies with the condition usually do not survive past their first

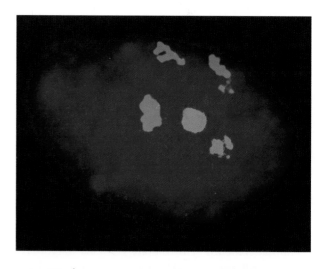

FISH (Fluorescent In Situ Hybridization) micrograph of trisomy 18 chromosomes (green) in the nucleus of a cell (blue). In this image, the three copies of chromosome 18 are visible. *(Photo Researchers, Inc.)*

## KEY TERMS

**Aneuploidy**—An abnormal number of chromosomes in a cell. Trisomy 18 and trisomy 13 are examples of aneuploid conditions.

**Chromosome translocation**—The exchange of genetic material between chromosomes, which can lead to extra or missing genetic material.

**Geneticist**—A specialist (M.D. or Ph.D.) who has training and certification in diagnosing, managing, and counseling individuals/families with genetic disorders. Genetic counselors hold a master's degree in medical genetics, and provide many of the same services as geneticists.

**Meiosis**—The process in which a cell in the testes or ovaries undergoes chromosome separation and cell division to produce sperm or eggs.

**Mitosis**—The process by which a somatic cell—a cell not destined to become a sperm or egg—duplicates its chromosomes and divides to produce two new cells.

**Mosaicism**—A genetic condition resulting from a mutation, crossing over, or nondisjunction of chromosomes during cell division, causing a variation in the number of chromosomes in the cells.

**Neonatologist**—A physician (pediatrician) who has special training in the care of newborns (neonates).

**Nondisjunction**—Non-separation of a chromosome pair, during either meiosis or mitosis.

**Perinatologist**—A physician (obstetrician) who has special training in managing difficult pregnancies. Some prenatal tests, such as chorionic villus sampling and level II ultrasound, are performed primarily by perinatologists.

**Trisomy**—The condition of having three identical chromosomes, instead of the normal two, in a cell.

several months. Trisomy 18 in the embryo/fetus is also a common chromosomal cause of pregnancy loss.

### Description

Chromosomes are the microscopic structures inside cells that carry the genes. The genetic material inside each cell contains all of the instructions the body needs to develop and function normally. Humans have 23 different pairs of chromosomes. Chromosomes 1-22 are numbered from largest to smallest, and as a group are known as the autosomes. The last pair of chromosomes are designated X and Y, and are known as the sex chromosomes—females have two X chromosomes and males have one X and one Y. Other than sperm and eggs, each cell in the body normally has 46 chromosomes—a pair of each of the autosomes plus two sex chromosomes. In order for normal development and functioning to occur, chromosomes and genes must be present in the correct quantity and in the correct proportion to each other. Too much or too little genetic material usually causes serious problems.

The term euploid means "good set," and is used to designate a full set of 46 chromosomes. A cell is aneuploid ("not a good set") if it has any number of chromosomes other than 46. A trisomy is one type of aneuploidy, and refers to a cell that contains three of the same chromosome. Trisomy 18, then, refers to three chromosomes 18. After **Down syndrome** (trisomy 21), trisomy 18 is the most common autosomal aneuploid condition seen in live-born babies. Trisomy 18 is also known as Edwards syndrome.

Edwards syndrome is comprised of a specific but broad pattern of multiple congenital anomalies and mental retardation. Babies with Edwards syndrome tend to have similar physical features and medical problems because they all have the same genetic imbalance—an extra copy of the genes on chromosome 18. The physical anomalies associated with Edwards syndrome involve nearly every organ and system of the body. However, some anomalies occur more often than others, such as those of the heart, kidney, brain, skeleton, and craniofacial (head and face) area. The birth defects are typically serious and, combined with the large number of anomalies possible, result in a high mortality rate. About 60% of newborns with Edwards syndrome die within the first week, and 80% do not survive past the first month. Even those with Edwards syndrome who live longer will have severe to profound mental retardation and chronic medical problems, necessitating involved care and monitoring throughout their lives.

### Genetic profile

Edwards syndrome occurs in three different forms: full trisomy 18, mosaic trisomy 18, and partial trisomy 18. Before each of these is described, however, it is helpful to review the basics of normal reproduction and early embryonic development. As noted, cells in the body normally contain 46 chromosomes in 23 pairs, except sperm in males and eggs in females, which contain one chromosome of each pair, or 23 total. Meiosis is the process by which sperm and eggs, collectively known as gametes, are produced. In normal meiosis, the 46 chromosomes line up in pairs in the middle of a cell, and the cell divides down the middle separating each pair of chromosomes. When a sperm fertilizes an egg at conception, the 23 chromosomes from each gamete combine. A process of repeated chromosome duplication followed by cell division, known as mitosis, then begins. A cell that goes through mitosis produces two new cells, each with 46 chromosomes. A developing human is called an embryo during the eight weeks after conception, and a fetus for the remainder of pregnancy.

### Full trisomy 18

Occasionally, chromosomes of a single pair do not separate during meiosis, an abnormal process known as nondisjunction. The result is one gamete with 24 chromosomes and another with 22. If a gamete with 24 chromosomes results in conception with a normal counterpart, an embryo with 47 chromosomes is produced. In most cases, all cells in the body will then have 47 chromosomes, a condition known as full trisomy 18 (when referring to an individual with the disorder, unless otherwise specified, the term "trisomy 18" implies a full trisomy, whereas Edwards syndrome may refer to any of the forms).

Nondisjunction of two chromosomes 18 during the formation of an egg or sperm is by far the most common cause of Edwards syndrome. Nondisjunction is a chance occurrence, with no known causative or preventive factors. The incidence of nondisjunction does increase, however, as men and women age. For anyone who has a fetus or child diagnosed with trisomy 18, the risk for a chromosomal disorder of any type in subsequent offspring is about 1%, the exception being women over age 35, who face their age-related risk.

### Mosaic trisomy 18

If the body contains a mixture of cells, some with trisomy 18 and some with a normal chromosome count, the condition is called mosaic trisomy 18. A small percentage of Edwards syndrome cases are due to mosaic trisomy 18.

Mosaic trisomy 18 occurs in one of two ways. The first involves mitotic (rather than meiotic) nondisjunction of chromosomes 18, in which a cell undergoing mitosis in a chromosomally normal embryo produces one cell with trisomy 18 and another with monosomy 18. The cell with monosomy 18 cannot survive, but if the trisomic cell survives, all cells in the body derived from it will have trisomy 18. These trisomic cells, combined with the normal cells that continue to develop, result in mosaic trisomy 18. The other cause of mosaicism involves an embryo with full trisomy 18. In this case, however, one cell loses its extra chromosome during mitosis. The result is a euploid cell, which in turn produces a euploid cell line in addition to the original trisomic cell line. Since mitotic nondisjunction appears to be the cause in most cases, and is due purely to chance, the recurrence risk for subsequent offspring after the diagnosis of mosaic trisomy 18 is less than 1%.

Because they have some normal cells, individuals with mosaic trisomy 18 tend to be less severely affected than those with full trisomy 18, but not always. Much of the prognosis depends on the total percentage of trisomic cells in the body and/or the proportion of trisomic cells in specific tissues and organs. There is no way to determine exact percentages of cells, and therefore no way to provide an accurate prognosis.

### Partial trisomy 18

A third cause of Edwards syndrome is a rearrangement, or translocation, of genetic material between chromosome 18 and another chromosome. An unbalanced chromosome translocation (extra and/or missing genetic material) may result in an embryo that has an extra piece of chromosome 18, known as partial trisomy 18. If cells are trisomic for a portion of chromosome 18, the result could be a form of Edwards syndrome. However, translocations between chromosomes can be complicated, and some cases of partial trisomy 18 may result in a pattern of anomalies that does not resemble Edwards syndrome.

Unbalanced translocations can occur in an embryo for the first time (*de novo*), or they can be inherited from a healthy parent who is a carrier of the translocation in a balanced state (no missing or extra genetic material). Normal blood chromosome tests on both parents implies the translocation was *de novo*, which means no increased risk for subsequent offspring. Detection of a balanced translocation in one parent, however, presents an increased risk for unbalanced translocations in subsequent offspring, as well as an increased risk for pregnancy loss. In cases of partial trisomy 18, **genetic counseling** is critical to help determine risks and available options. Chromosome translocations resulting in partial trisomy 18 make up a small percentage of Edwards syndrome cases.

### Demographics

The incidence of Edwards syndrome is about one in 5,000 births. Two-thirds of all newborns with the condition are female, probably because males with trisomy 18 are more likely to be miscarried. The condition is not known to occur more frequently in any ethnic group or in any part of the world. Increased parental age is the only factor known to result in a greater risk for trisomy 18. In the United States, parents of babies with trisomy 18 average about 32 years-of-age, while 26 is the average age for parents of children without a chromosomal disorder. The risk increases with age in both sexes, but begins earlier and is more pronounced in women.

Increasing maternal age elevates the risk for chromosomal disorders due to nondisjunction in general, not just trisomy 18. For instance, a 20-year-old woman has about a one in 10,000 chance of having a child with trisomy 18, while the risk of having a child with *any* chromosomal disorder at that age is one in 800. By age 35, those same risks have risen to one in 2,000 and one in 200 respectively, and increase to one in 600 and one in 65 at age 40. Other common chromosomal disorders caused by nondisjunction that result in live birth include trisomy 21 (Down syndrome), **trisomy 13** (Patau syndrome), and several conditions caused by aneuploidy of the sex chromosomes.

### Signs and symptoms

Many physical anomalies and medical complications are associated with Edwards syndrome. In fact, well over 100 different anomalies have been reported in the medical literature. The more common findings are categorized and described below.

#### Prenatal anomalies

The majority of pregnancies in which the embryo/fetus has trisomy 18 will result in miscarriage or stillbirth. Some physical anomalies of the heart, skeleton, brain, kidneys, and body walls have the best chance of being detected by **prenatal ultrasound**. Other, pregnancy-related findings include intrauterine growth restriction (IUGR) of the fetus, a single umbilical artery (also called two vessel cord), and too much (polyhydramnios) or too little (oligohydramnios) amniotic fluid. While detection of fetal anomalies by ultrasound may lead to suspicion of Edwards syndrome, the diagnosis can only be confirmed by chromosome testing. Women carrying a fetus with Edwards syndrome sometimes report they feel little movement. Cesarean sections are more common due to abnormal fetal position or fetal distress near term.

#### General anomalies

Of those babies with Edwards syndrome that are live-born, two-thirds are delivered several weeks earlier or later than their expected due date. Low birth weight is common, as are low Apgar scores (measurements of a newborn's activity just after birth).

Newborns are frail, and tend to have a weak cry and difficulty feeding. Muscles may be poorly developed, and often become tight and contracted (hypertonic). Extra hair (hirsutism) on the forehead and back is sometimes seen, as is loose, redundant skin.

Abnormalities of the lungs, kidneys, pancreas, spleen, and gastrointestinal system are associated with Edwards syndrome. The thyroid, thymus, and adrenal glands may be affected. Anomalies of the breastbone, radius (bone in the forearm), ribs, pelvis, and the spine (**scoliosis**) are the more frequent skeletal findings. An abdominal wall defect (**omphalocele**) or hernia in the abdominal region may be present. Genital (sex organ) anomalies in both males and females have been described.

#### Heart anomalies

Ninety percent of babies with Edwards syndrome have one or more heart defects. Ventricular septal defects (VSD) and atrial septal defects (ASD), holes between the lower and upper chambers of the heart respectively, are the most common cardiac problems. Patent ductus arteriosis (open connection between the pulmonary artery and aorta) and abnormal heart valves are also typical.

#### Craniofacial anomalies

Small head size (**microcephaly**) and a prominent occiput (back of the skull) are variations in skull shape typical of Edwards syndrome. Common facial features include widely spaced and/or slanted eyes, skin folds at the inner eyelid (epicanthal folds), ptosis (drooping) of the eyelids, low-set malformed ears, a small oral opening, narrow palate or cleft lip/palate, and a small jaw (micrognathia).

#### Hand and foot anomalies

A specific pattern of hand and foot anomalies is seen in most infants with Edwards syndrome. Clenched hands, with the index finger overlapping the third and the fifth finger overlapping the fourth, are a classic sign. Abnormal dermatoglyphics (finger print pattern), underdeveloped nails, outward or inward deviation of the hand, underdeveloped or absent thumbs, and a single crease across the palm are other frequent anomalies of the hands. Abnormalities affecting the feet include so-called "rocker-bottom feet" and **clubfoot**.

#### Central nervous system anomalies

Probably the most medically significant abnormal development that occurs in Edwards syndrome involves the brain. Some anomalies, such as a small cerebellum or **hydrocephalus** (increased fluid within the brain), can be visualized by ultrasound or other imaging techniques. However, some neurologic problems may only be noticed through their physical effects. For example, difficulties in feeding and breathing, hypertonic muscles, a diminished response to sound, seizures, and severe mental retardation all indicate serious neurologic deficits. **Spina bifida** (open spine) is an infrequent but serious problem affecting the spinal cord. Babies with spina bifida usually have some degree of paralysis below the point on the back where the spine failed to close.

## Diagnosis

### Prenatal

Two screening and two diagnostic procedures for trisomy 18 are available to women during pregnancy. Following are brief explanations of each of the prenatal testing alternatives.

Maternal serum alpha-fetoprotein (MSAFP)-Plus, also known as the "triple screen," is a routine maternal blood test offered to women at 15-20 weeks of pregnancy. It screens for open defects (such as spina bifida), Down syndrome, and trisomy 18. However, the screen's sensitivity for trisomy 18 is not as well established as it is for the other conditions. Test results provide a risk adjustment only, not a diagnosis of any condition in the fetus. Any woman who has a result showing an increased risk for trisomy 18 in the fetus is offered follow-up testing such as **amniocentesis** or a detailed (level II) ultrasound.

Ultrasound, also called sonography, visualizes structures inside the body using high frequency sound waves. During a prenatal ultrasound, a technician or doctor moves an instrument (transducer) back-and-forth across the skin of a pregnant woman's lower abdomen. The transducer emits and receives harmless high frequency sound waves, which the ultrasound machine then converts into images of the fetus. Today's sophisticated ultrasound machines, used by skilled technicians and doctors, can detect a number of different physical anomalies in the fetus. An ultrasound screen for trisomy 18 has good (but not absolute) sensitivity, and presents no risk to the mother or fetus. Ultrasound becomes more sensitive for trisomy 18 the later in pregnancy it is performed. A level II ultrasound is performed after 20 weeks of pregnancy by a specialist (perinatologist). An abnormal ultrasound suggesting trisomy 18 would lead to the option of amniocentesis to confirm the diagnosis.

Chorionic villus sampling (CVS) is a method used to obtain tissue (chorionic villi) from the edge of the developing placenta. CVS is typically performed at 10-12 weeks of pregnancy. Chorionic villi come from the fetal side of the placenta, and thus are chromosomally the same as cells in the fetus. Guided by ultrasound, a physician inserts a needle through either the abdomen or the cervix, into the placenta, and removes a small sample of tissue. Cells from the sample are analyzed under the microscope and a chromosome count is obtained. CVS carries a minimal risk for miscarriage and appears to have a very small risk of causing certain types of limb defects in the fetus as well. In about 3% of cases, CVS produces results that are difficult to interpret, which may lead to a follow-up amniocentesis.

Amniocentesis is the most widely used procedure to obtain fetal cells for **genetic testing**. The procedure can be performed anytime after about 15 weeks of pregnancy. Under ultrasound guidance, a physician passes a thin needle through the lower abdomen into the amniotic sac and removes a small amount of amniotic fluid. Fetal skin cells that normally float in the fluid are then extracted for genetic analysis. Diagnosis of chromosomal disorders by this method is highly accurate. Amniocentesis causes a miscarriage in about one in 300 women who have the procedure, but poses no other serious risk to the fetus.

The benefit of CVS and amniocentesis is their accuracy at detecting trisomy 18, while the drawback is their risk to the pregnancy. The procedures are typically not offered unless the risk for a chromosomal disorder in the fetus is greater than the risk of the procedure, such as in pregnant women who are 35 or older, a couple with a previous child with trisomy 18, and any woman who carries, or whose partner carries, a balanced chromosome translocation. Detection of fetal anomalies by ultrasound or an abnormal MSAFP-Plus screen would lead to the option of amniocentesis.

The benefit of ultrasound and MSAFP-Plus is their lack of risk to the pregnancy, while the drawback is that neither procedure is diagnostic. Women who wish to first modify their risk for a fetal chromosomal disorder (and spina bifida) may choose screening. In any case, prenatal testing, whether screening or diagnostic, is never mandatory. Careful consideration must always be given to what action might be taken after an abnormal result, and how reassuring a normal result might be.

### Postnatal

A newborn with typical signs of Edwards syndrome can sometimes be diagnosed from a physical examination alone, especially by a physician who is familiar with the condition such as a geneticist or neonatologist. However, chromosome testing is the only method to confirm the diagnosis, and should always be performed if Edwards syndrome is suspected.

Chromosome analysis helps to determine whether the underlying cause is full, mosaic, or partial trisomy 18, and may exclude other syndromes with similar signs and symptoms. Fetuses and newborns with Edwards syndrome sometimes die before chromosome analysis can be performed. In those cases, the diagnosis unfortunately cannot be confirmed, and an accurate cause and recurrence risk cannot be given.

Chromosome testing will detect full trisomy 18 with near 100% accuracy. Likewise, a translocation of chromosome 18 that produces signs of Edwards syndrome should be detected in virtually every case. Mosaic trisomy 18 presents more of a problem for chromosome analysis. The likelihood of confirming mosaic trisomy 18 depends on the percentage of trisomic cells in the particular tissue examined. Mosaicism, if present, can be confirmed by chromosome testing, and usually is. However, normal chromosome tests do not rule out the possibility of trisomic cells elsewhere in the body.

### Treatment and management

Medical management of an infant with Edwards syndrome depends on the number and severity of anomalies present. In order to make the best-informed and most appropriate decisions for their child, parents must establish a close working relationship with the treating physicians.

Regardless of the medical procedures that might be performed, most babies with Edwards syndrome will not survive. Nearly all will be transferred to the neonatal intensive care unit (NICU) after birth. In some cases, parents elect not to have any life-prolonging, heroic measures taken should their child experience cardiac or respiratory failure. They may also elect not to have certain types of surgery performed if other complicating medical problems make it unwise.

A more medically stable, less severely affected infant with Edwards syndrome will likely require various medical procedures and treatments. Surgical repair of certain physical anomalies, ventilator (breathing) support, medications, and/or placement of a feeding tube into the stomach are common. A baby may go home and remain there after some length of hospital stay, or may need to be readmitted one or more times. For those children that show some possibility of longer-term survival (more than 6 months), a plan for their medical care, both in the hospital and at home, must be established. Parents should also be informed of the various educational and support services available to them, including the Support Organization For Trisomy 18, 13, and Related Disorders (S.O.F.T.). Genetic counseling, to discuss the cause, prognosis, and recurrence risks

for their child's type of trisomy 18, can be of great help to parents.

There is no way to prevent the occurrence of trisomy 18. The technology now exists to test multiple embryos conceived by in vitro fertilization for certain chromosome anomalies, but this is very expensive and is only performed at several centers in the world.

### Prognosis

The prognosis for a baby born with trisomy 18 is poor. On average, about 40% of newborns with trisomy 18 survive the first week, 20% are alive at one month, 6% at six months, and about 5% live past their first birthday. Survival rates are somewhat higher for children with mosaic or partial trisomy 18. As is the case before birth, males with trisomy 18 have a higher mortality rate than females, with about one-third as many males as females surviving infancy.

The outlook for trisomy 18 is not likely to change much in the coming years. Surgery to repair various birth defects has improved dramatically over the years. However, most babies with trisomy 18 do not die from repairable anomalies. For those parents whose babies are expected to survive some length of time, connecting them with support groups and providing them with accurate information as soon as possible is important.

### Resources

#### PERIODICALS

Baty, Bonnie J., Brent L. Blackburn, and John C. Carey. "Natural History of Trisomy 18 and Trisomy 13: I. Growth, Physical Assessment, Medical Histories, Survival, and Recurrence Risk." *American Journal of Medical Genetics* 49 (1994): 175-88.

Baty, Bonnie J., Brent L. Blackburn, and John C. Carey. "Natural History of Trisomy 18 and Trisomy 13: II. Psychomotor Development." *American Journal of Medical Genetics* 49 (1994): 189-94.

Matthews, Anne L. "Chromosomal Abnormalities: Trisomy 18, Trisomy 13, Deletions, and Microdeletions." *Journal of Perinatal and Neonatal Nursing* 13 (1999): 59-75.

#### ORGANIZATIONS

Chromosome 18 Registry and Research Society. 6302 Fox Head, San Antonio, TX 78247. (210) 567-4968. http://www.chromosome18.org.

National Society of Genetic Counselors. 233 Canterbury Dr., Wallingford, PA 19086-6617. (610) 872-1192. http://www.nsgc.org/GeneticCounselingYou.asp.

Support Organization for Trisomy 18, 13 and Related Disorders (SOFT). 2982 South Union St., Rochester, NY 14624. (800) 716-SOFT. http://www.trisomy.org.

Scott J. Polzin, MS

### Trisomy 21 *see* **Down syndrome**

# Tuberous sclerosis complex

## Definition

Tuberous sclerosis complex (TSC) is a genetic condition that affects many organ systems including the brain, skin, heart, kidneys, eyes, and lungs. Benign (non-cancerous) growths or tumors called hamartomas form in various parts of the body, disrupting their normal functions.

## Description

The term tuberous sclerosis refers to the small, knoblike growths in the brain of patients with TSC that were found in patients upon autopsy and, today, can be viewed using computed tomography (also called a CT scan). The condition is also referred to as tuberose sclerosis or simply tuberous sclerosis. The designation tuberous sclerosis complex is used to distinguish this condition from another genetic condition called **Tourette syndrome** that is abbreviated TS.

Persons with TSC have a variety of symptoms ranging from very mild to severe. Affected individuals may experience no serious health problems and, in the absence of a thorough clinical examination, may go through life without knowing that they are affected.

**A common sign of tuberous sclerosis is skin lesions called hypomelanotic macules. These are white or light patches of skin sometimes in an ash-leaf shape and called Ash-leaf spots.** *(Custom Medical Stock Photo, Inc.)*

Conversely, patients with TSC may have problems with behavioral, mental, and emotional functions as well as with their kidneys, heart, and eyes. In addition, specific skin abnormalities, often medically insignificant, are among the most common symptoms of TSC.

## Genetic profile

TSC is an autosomal dominant genetic disorder caused by a single change or alteration in a **gene** called a mutation in either the TSC1 gene, located on **chromosome** 9, or the TSC2 gene, located on chromosome 16. Approximately two-thirds (66%) of patients with TSC have it as the result of a new change in one of the TSC genes; that is, it was not inherited from one of their parents. When a new change occurs, it most commonly occurs in the TSC2 gene. An individual must have a mutation in one of these two copies of a TSC-causing gene in order to develop the condition. In addition, a person who has been diagnosed with TSC and who, therefore, has a genetic mutation in one of the TSC genes, has a 50% chance of passing on the genetic mutation to his or her offspring. Laboratory testing for changes in the TSC genes is not currently available.

TSC is a condition that can be caused by a change in either one of two separate genes. In addition, people who have the same change in the same gene may have very different medical problems and symptoms.

TSC1 is responsible for producing the protein hamartin and TSC2, tuberin. Both genes are known as tumor suppressor genes meaning that their normal function is to prevent the growth of tumors. Conversely, when gene function is altered, tumor growth results. Research on how the disruption of either protein results in the clinical condition of TSC is ongoing.

It is currently believed that every person who inherits or develops a mutation in either the TSC1 or TSC2 gene will develop some form of TSC. However, the severity of the disease, with its wide range of symptoms and complications, cannot accurately be predicted by identifying the specific gene mutation.

Germline mosaicism can explain the rare occurrence of unaffected parents having more than one child with TSC. Germline refers to the gonadal cells (sperm in males and eggs in females) and mosaicism refers to the presence of different cell lines in any given individual. A person with germline mosaicism for either the TSC1 or TSC2 gene is not affected with TSC but may have an affected child. Unaffected parents of a child with TSC are quoted a 2-3% chance of having additional affected children. Typical **genetic testing** methods are performed on somatic (non-germline) tissues such as blood or skin and, therefore, will not detect germline mosaicism.

**Bone cysts**—Fluid- or air-filled space within the bones.

**Cardiac rhabdomyoma**—Benign (non-cancerous) tumor of the heart muscle.

**Cerebral white matter migration lines**—Pattern of defects found in the cerebral cortex of the brain probably caused by abnormal migration of neurons during brain formation.

**Confetti skin lesions**—Numerous light or white spots seen on the skin that resemble confetti.

**Cortical tuber**—Round (nodular) growth found in the cortex of the brain.

**Dental pits**—Small, shallow holes or crevices in the tooth enamel.

**Facial angiofibromas**—Benign (non-cancerous) tumors of the face.

**Forehead plaque**—Flat, fibrous skin growth on the forehead.

**Gingival fibromas**—Fibrous growths found on the gums.

**Hamartomatous rectal polyps**—Benign (non-cancerous) growths found in the rectum.

**Hypomelanotic macules**—Patches of skin lighter than the surrounding skin.

**Lymphangiomyomatosis**—Serious lung disease characterized by the overgrowth of an unusual type of muscle cell resulting in the blockage of air, blood, and lymph vessels to and from the lungs.

**Nonrenal hamartoma**—Benign (non-cancerous) tumor-like growths not found in the kidneys that often disrupt the normal function of a particular organ system.

**Nontraumatic ungual or periungual fibroma**—Fibrous growth that appears around the fingernails and/or toenails

**Renal angiomyolipoma**—Benign (non-cancerous) tumors in the kidney that are made up of vascular tissue (angio), smooth muscle (myo), and fat (lipoma).

**Renal cysts**—Fluid or air-filled spaces within the kidneys.

**Retinal achromic patch**—Defect in the coloration of the retina.

**Retinal hamartomas**—Benign (non-cancerous) tumor found on the retina.

**Shagreen patch**—Area of tough and dimpled skin.

**Subependymal giant cell astrocytoma**—Benign (non-cancerous) tumor of the brain comprised of star-shaped cells (astrocytes).

**Subependymal nodule**—Growth found underneath the lining of the ventricles in the brain.

## Demographics

Although tuberous sclerosis complex is considered to be a rare condition, estimates of the prevalence of the disorder have increased as clinical testing methods have improved. In the United States, as many as one child in 6,000 born is affected with TSC and about 50,000 people are currently living in the U.S. with the disease. TSC is seen in all ethnic groups and populations and, worldwide, there are between one and two million cases.

## Signs and symptoms

The basic underlying cause for illness and, less often, death due to tuberous sclerosis complex, is the development of growths called hamartomas throughout the body. Hamartoma is a general term used to describe tumor-like growths that are not cancerous and are composed of cells usually found in that site but poorly developed. While these growths are typically benign (i.e., not cancerous), their presence often disrupts the normal functions of a particular organ system. The various hamartomas found in TSC patients can be further distinguished and classified by their location and their histological properties—that is, their physical composition and characteristic appearance under a microscope. As each hamartoma is comprised of different cellular elements, each one has a particular name. For example, while both are hamartomas, a fibroma is comprised of connective tissue whereas a lipoma is made up of fat cells.

While the organs affected vary from person to person, most people with TSC have some type of skin irregularities called lesions. Some of the most commonly seen skin lesions are hypomelanotic macules—white or light patches sometimes in an ash-leaf shape and called Ash-leaf spots. Many people in the general population have one or two light areas of skin. However, the presence of three or more such macules in any one individual is considered a major diagnostic finding of TSC. A second major diagnostic feature of the condition is the appearance of small, red bumps called fibromas, either on the face (facial angiofibromas) or around or under the finger- or toenails (ungual fibromas). In addition, rough patches of skin termed Shagreen patches are highly specific to a diagnosis of TSC. Finally, groups of small light circles called Confetti spots are considered a minor feature of the disorder.

In contrast to skin lesions, brain lesions tend to be serious and are responsible for the neurological symptoms and cognitive impairment seen in severely affected individuals. There are four primary abnormalities that can be detected by magnetic resonance imaging (MRI) or computer tomography (CT) scanning, the first of which are cortical tubers—nodular growths found in the cortex of the brain—and give tuberous sclerosis (literally "hard growths") its name. Subependymal nodules are growths found underneath the lining of the ventricles in the brain and may cause no problems for the patient unless they grow or begin to block the flow of the cerebral spinal fluid. In contrast, subependymal giant cell astrocytomas, non-cancerous brain tumors comprised of star-shaped cells and found in about 5% of patients with TSC, can, if untreated, result in blindness, **hydrocephalus** (fluid on the brain), and even death. Finally, cerebral white matter migration lines may be seen through radiographic (x ray) studies and are considered a minor diagnostic feature of TSC.

About 85% of affected individuals will develop epileptic seizures at some point in their lifetime, most beginning by the first year of life. Research suggests that early control of **epilepsy** by medication will decrease the chance of a child developing serious mental complications. People with TSC have a range of mental abilities from normal to mild or moderate developmental delays and learning disabilities, to servere mental retardation. **Autism, attention deficit hyperactivity disorder** (ADHD), and other behavioral problems are seen in affected individuals.

Fatty kidney tumors, known as renal angiomyolipomas, are one of the most common findings in TSC patients, affecting 70-80% of older children and adults, and often cause serious renal malfunction. In addition, the presence of multiple renal cysts (fluid filled areas within the kidneys) is suggestive of the condition. In addition to these benign growths, malignant kidney tumors may also develop.

The most common cardiac symptom is one or more tumors (cardiac rhabdomyomas) in the heart. These tumors are almost exclusively seen in infants and young children and usually spontaneously disappear by late childhood, thereby avoiding the need for surgery. About 47-67% of infants and children with TSC have heart tumors and some females develop the rhabdomyomas when they reach puberty.

Tuberous sclerosis complex affects the eyes in the form of retinal nodular hamartomas—multiple growths on the retina. A discoloration on the retina (retinal achromic patch) is also considered a minor feature of the condition.

In addition to the above, symptoms of TSC may include dental pits in the teeth, growths in the rectum (hamartomatous rectal polyps), bone cysts, growths on the gums (gingival fibromas) and other non-specific growths (nonrenal hamartomas). Women with TSC may develop lymphangiomyomatosis—a serious lung disease. Furthermore, all individuals with TSC are at a higher risk over the general population for developing specific cancers, with 2% of patients developing a malignant tumor in one of the affected body tissues such as kidney or brain.

### Diagnosis

When a person exhibits signs of TSC or has a family history of the condition, an evaluation by a medical geneticist, neurologist or other qualified professional is recommended to confirm (or rule out) the diagnosis and to recommend screening and management options for the individual. In addition, speaking with a genetic counselor may help families understand the **genetics** behind the disorder, their recurrence risks (chances for having another affected family member) and the practical and psychosocial implications of the disease on their personal situation.

Detection of hypomelanotic macules (light patches on the skin) can be performed quickly and easily using a special ultraviolet lamp called a Wood's lamp. This light emphasizes the lightened areas on the skin that may otherwise be difficult to see using normal light. Other skin lesions called fibromas are easily visible and identifiable due to their characteristic smooth form, red color, and their even distribution on the face and/or their protrusions among the nails on the fingers and toes. Radiographic imaging using ultrasound, MRI, or CT technology can detect growths present in the brain, kidneys, heart, and eyes.

As basic understanding of and testing methods for tuberous sclerosis complex have improved, criteria used for confirming a diagnosis of tuberous sclerosis complex have been revised. The National Institutes of Health (NIH) held a consensus conference on TSC in

1998 and published the following diagnostic criteria in 2000:

Major features:

- facial angiofibromas or forehead plaque
- nontraumatic ungual or periungual fibroma
- hypomelanotic macules (more than three)
- shagreen patch
- multiple retinal hamartomas
- cortical tuber
- subependymal nodule
- subependymal giant cell astrocytoma
- cardiac rhabdomyoma (one or more)
- lymphangiomyomatosis
- renal angiomyolipoma

Minor features:

- multiple randomly distributed dental pits
- hamartomatous rectal polyps
- bone cysts
- cerebral white matter migration lines
- gingival fibromas
- nonrenal hamartoma
- retinal achromic patch
- confetti skin lesions
- multiple renal cysts

A confirmed diagnosis of TSC requires that a patient display either two major features or one major and two minor features, a suspected diagnosis one major and one minor feature, and a possible diagnosis one major or two minor features in any one individual.

### Treatment and management

Optimal treatment for TSC is dependent upon proper disease management. The following should be performed on all patients with TSC at the time of diagnosis to confirm a diagnosis of the disease as well as obtain baseline medical data for future evaluations:

- dermatologic (skin) examination
- fundoscopic (eye) examination
- renal (kidney) imaging study
- cardiac electrocardiogram (ECG) and echocardiogram (ECHO)
- brain magnetic resonance imaging (MRI)

Since the characteristic feature of tuberous sclerosis complex is the growth of benign tumors, treatments are often focused on appropriate surgical interventions to arrest tumor growth or remove tumors whose growth has resulted in or may lead to medical complications especially in the kidney or brain. Regular brain MRI studies should be performed in children and adults with previous findings as clinically indicated and every one to three years in children and, less frequently, in adults without symptoms. In addition, periodic brain electroencephalogram (EEG) studies are recommended for both children and adult patients when clinically indicated.

Children without previous kidney findings should be offered renal imaging studies using ultrasound, MRI, or CT scanning every three years until they reach adolescence and then, every one to three years as adults. Likewise, asymptomatic adults should have imaging of their kidneys every one to three years. Both children and adults who have kidney symptoms should be monitored using imaging studies every six months to one year until the tumor growth stabilizes or decreases.

Any child with cardiac rhabdomyomas should be monitored every six months to one year until the tumor stabilizes or regresses completely. Adults with previous findings of cardiac tumors should be monitored as clinically recommended by their treating physician. While monitoring is important, cardiac rhabdomyomas, as well as retinal lesions and gingival fibromas, usually do not require treatment. In contrast to these benign tumors, cancerous tumors that develop in patients with TSC should be treated by an oncologist as appropriate.

Facial angiofibromas and peri- and subungual fibromas on the nails are common symptoms in TSC patients. While they are generally not medically significant, they can cause skin irritations or be a cosmetic concern to the individual. Special techniques involving dermabrasion or laser therapy can be performed by a dermatologist or plastic surgeon to remove such growths.

Patients with seizure disorders are prescribed specific medications to control seizures. As of 2001, a new anti-epileptic drug (vigabatrin) have been shown to be an effective medication in infants with seizures and has been shown to improve long-term outcomes in behavioral and intellectual areas. In addition to controlling seizures, early intervention programs that include special education, behavior modification, physical and occupational therapies, and speech therapy is often recommended for individuals with learning disabilities, developmental delays, mental retardation, autism, and other mental and emotional disorders.

Neurodevelopmental testing is appropriate at the time of diagnosis for all children and should be performed every three years until adolescence and for any

*Molecular Studies*. New York: The New York Academy of Sciences, 1991.

## QUESTIONS TO ASK YOUR DOCTOR

- How often should brain and MRI studies be performed?
- What are the risks and benefits of vigabratin therapy?
- How early should we begin physical and occupational therapies?
- What developmental milestones should I look for in my child?

adult diagnosed with TSC who displays signs of impairment. Subsequent evaluations should be done on both children and adults with previous findings of developmental delays or problems.

While present in only 1% of patients with TSC, almost exclusively in females, lung complications can be serious and even fatal. Symptoms may include spontaneous pneumothorax (air in the chest cavity), dyspnea (difficult breathing), cough, hemoptysis (spitting of blood), and pulmonary failure. Therefore, a computed tomography (CT) scan of the lungs is recommended for any TSC patient who has symptoms of lung disease or complications and for all female TSC patients at the age of 18. Clinical trials involving Tamoxifen and progesterone treatments have shown positive results in some patients with lung disease.

### Prognosis

The life span of individuals with TSC varies with the severity of the condition in any one person. Many affected people have normal life expectancies and a high quality of life, relatively free of symptoms or complication of the disease. Conversely, severely affected or disabled individuals may experience a shortened life span and a high rate of illness and medical complications. Therefore, proper disease management, diagnostic monitoring, and follow-up are critical to achieving and maintaining optimal health in patients with TSC.

### Resources

#### BOOKS

Gomez, Manuel R., ed. *Tuberous Sclerosis*. New York: Raven Press, 1988.

Gomez, Manuel R., Julian R. Sampson, and Vicky H. Whittemore, (eds). *Tuberous Sclerosis Complex*. Oxford: Oxford University Press, 1999.

Johnson, William G., and Manuel R. Gomez, eds. *Tuberous Sclerosis and Allied Disorders: Clinical, Cellular, and*

#### PERIODICALS

Arbuckle, H. Alan, and Joseph G. Morelli. "Pigmentary Disorders: Update on Neurofibromatosis-1 and Tuberous Sclerosis." *Current Opinion in Pediatrics* 12 (2000): 354-358.

Hyman, Mark H., and Vicky H. Whittemore. "National Institutes of Health Consensus Conference: Tuberous Sclerosis Complex." *Archives of Neurology* 57 (May 2000): 662-665.

Jambaque, I., et al. "Mental and Behavioural Outcome of Infantile Epilepsy Treated by Vigabatrin in Tuberous Sclerosis Patients." *Epilepsy Research* 38 (2000): 151-160.

O'Callaghan, Finbar J., and John P. Osborne. "Advances in the Understanding of Tuberous Sclerosis." *Archives of Disease in Childhood* 83 (August 2000): 140-142.

Sparagana, Steven P., and E. Steve Roach. "Tuberous Sclerosis Complex." *Current Opinion in Neurology* 13 (2000): 115-119.

#### WEBSITES

Australasian Tuberous Sclerosis Society. http://www.net space.net.au/~atss/.

Global Tuberous Sclerosis Information Link. http://memb ers.aol.com/gtsil/ts/index.htm.

Tuberous Sclerosis Alliance. http://www.tsalliance.org.

The Tuberous Sclerosis Association. http://www.tuberous-sclerosis.org/.

#### ORGANIZATIONS

Tuberous Sclerosis Alliance. 801 Roeder Rd., Suite 750, Silver Spring, MD 20910. (800) 225-6872. http://www.tsalliance.org.

Pamela E. Cohen, MS, CGC

Turcot syndrome *see* **Familial adenomatous polyposis**

# Turner syndrome

### Definition

Turner syndrome is a chromosomal disorder affecting females wherein one of the two X chromosomes is defective or completely absent.

### Description

Chromosomes are structures in the nucleus of every cell in the human body. Chromosomes contain the genetic information necessary to direct the growth and normal functioning of all cells and systems of the body. A normal individual has a total of 46

# Urea cycle disorders

## Definition

Urea cycle disorders are inborn errors in metabolism that can lead to brain damage and death. They involve a deficiency in one of the enzymes required by the urea cycle that removes ammonia from the blood.

## Description

Ammonia accumulates in toxic levels if the urea cycle does not convert nitrogen from protein metabolism into urea for excretion into the urine. A series of biochemical reactions are necessary to complete the urea cycle. When an enzyme is missing or deficient, the cycle is interrupted and nitrogen accumulates in the form of ammonia. It cannot be excreted from the body and enters the bloodstream, damaging nervous tissues, including the brain.

Seizures, poor muscle tone, respiratory distress, and coma follow if an affected infant is not treated. Acute neonatal symptoms are most frequently seen in boys with ornithine transcarbamylase, or OTC, deficiency. Mental retardation and even death may follow. People with partial deficiencies may not discover the problem until childhood or adulthood. Children may avoid meat or other protein foods. As ammonia levels rise in the body, individuals begin to show lethargy and delirium. Left untreated they may suffer a coma or death.

Sometimes young people with urea cycle disorders, who go undiagnosed, begin to show behavioral and eating problems. Those with partial enzyme deficiencies may experience episodes of high ammonia levels in the blood. This can occur after suffering from viral illnesses including chicken pox, or after eating high-protein meals, or even after significant physical exertion.

The incidence of adults with urea cycle disorders is increasing. Recent evidence has indicated that some people have survived undiagnosed into adulthood. They can suffer stroke-like symptoms, lethargy, and delirium. Without proper diagnosis and treatment, adults are at risk for permanent brain damage, coma, and death. Symptoms can appear after giving birth or after contracting a virus, and some adults have shown deficiencies after using the medication valproic acid (an anti-epileptic drug). Adult onset is more common in women with OTC deficiency.

Different enzymes may be lacking in the various forms of urea cycle disorders. The six major disorders of the urea cycle include:

- CPS–Carbamyl Phosphate Synthetase
- NAGS–N-Acetylglutamate Synthetase
- OTC–Ornithine Transcarbamylase
- ASD–Argininosuccinic Acid Synthetase (Citrullinemia)
- ALD–Argininosuccinase Acid Lyase (Argininosuccinic Aciduria)
- AG–Arginase

## Genetic profile

All of these disorders are inherited as autosomal recessive traits except for ornithine transcarbamylase (OTC) deficiency. It is inherited as an X-linked trait, from the mother.

## Demographics

It is estimated the incidence of urea cycle disorders is about one in 30,000 births. Males and females are affected equally, except for the OTC deficiency which is more prevalent in males due to the fact that it is an X-linked disorder.

## Signs and symptoms

In severe urea cycle disorders, rising ammonia levels cause irritability, vomiting and lethargy within the first 24–72 hours of life. Seizures, poor muscle tone, respiratory distress, and coma follow if the infant is not

## QUESTIONS TO ASK YOUR DOCTOR

- What specific dietary recommendations to you have?
- Can you recommend a dietitian?
- How often should blood tests be performed?
- What symptoms should I report immediately?

treated. Acute neonatal symptoms are most frequently seen in boys with ornithine transcarbamylase or OTC deficiency. However, patients with mild or moderate urea cycle enzyme deficiencies may not show symptoms until early childhood.

### Diagnosis

Early detection through blood testing is essential to prevent irreversible brain damage in severe cases of urea cycle disorders.

### Treatment and management

Therapy consists of eating a diet that provides enough protein so the body gets the essential amino acids needed for growth, but not so much that toxic levels of ammonia are formed. Treatment may entail a protein restricted diet together with medications that provide alternative pathways for the removal of ammonia from the blood. These medications tend to be unpalatable and may be given by way of tube feedings. Blood tests are needed to monitor levels of ammonia, and hospitalizations may become necessary if levels rise to high.

### Prognosis

With early detection and proper diet restrictions, individuals can lead relatively normal lives. However, irreversible brain damage can develop quickly in severe cases that go undetected.

### Resources

#### ORGANIZATIONS

National Organization for Rare Disorders (NORD). PO Box 8923, New Fairfield, CT 06812-8923. (203) 746-6518 or (800) 999-6673. Fax: (203) 746-6481. http://www.rarediseases.org.

National Urea Cycle Disorders Foundation. 4841 Hill St., La Canada, CA 91001. (800) 38-NUCDF.

Julianne Remington

# Urogenital adysplasia syndrome

### Definition

Urogenital adysplasia syndrome is a rare disorder characterized by anomalies of the kidneys, urinary tract, and/or reproductive system.

### Description

The development of urogenital adysplasia syndrome resulted from the combined work of multiple physicians examining several families. The first report of siblings born with both kidneys missing (bilateral **renal agenesis**) was made by H. Madisson in 1934. However, the term hereditary renal adysplasia was not coined until 1973 when R. M. Buchta combined the terms aplasia, the complete absence of one or both kidneys, and **dysplasia**, developmental anomalies of the kidneys, to form the term adysplasia to apply to familial, bilateral kidney anomalies. In 1980, R. N. Schimke and C. R. King suggested that the developmental defects in certain family's reproductive and urinary tracts (mesonephric and mullerian ducts) may have a common genetic basis and that the designation hereditary urogenital adysplasia should be used as a descriptive syndrome name.

Urogenital adysplasia syndrome is an autosomal dominant inherited condition. The symptoms of urogenital adysplasia syndrome are variable. Affected individuals within families may have features of the disease that include one or two missing kidneys (renal agenesis), one or two malformed kidneys (renal dysplasia), bladder anomalies, ureter abnormalities, hypertension, vaginal anomalies, uterine anomalies, fallopian tube anomalies, lack of a menstrual period (amenorrhea), and cysts of the seminal vesicle. Fetuses that have two missing or very abnormal kidneys are often born with a condition called Potter's sequence,

## KEY TERMS

**Adysplasia**—A term referring to the combination of renal agenesis (complete absence of one or both kidneys) and renal dysplasia (developmental anomaly of the kidney).

**Amniotic fluid**—Fluid contained in a sac within the uterus that surrounds and protects the fetus during its development.

**Mesonephric duct**—Embryonic structure that in the male becomes the vas deferens, and in both sexes gives rise to the ureters leading to the kidney.

**Mullerian duct**—Two embryo structures that in the female develop into vagina, uterus, and oviducts, and in the male disappear except for the vestigial vagina masculina and the appendix testis.

**Oligohydramnios**—A condition characterized by insufficient amniotic fluid surrounding a developing fetus during pregnancy.

**Renal agenesis**—Complete absence of one or both kidneys.

**Renal dysplasia**—A developmental anomaly of the kidney.

or syndrome. Potter's sequence occurs when the fetal kidneys cannot produce enough amniotic fluid to surround the fetus as it develops. Features of Potter's sequence include wide-set eyes, squashed nose, small and receding chin, low-set ears, deformities of the hands and feet, and incompletely formed lungs (lung hypoplasia).

Urogenital adysplasia syndrome is also referred to as hereditary renal adysplasia (HRA), renal agenesis, and bilateral renal agenesis (BRA). The age of diagnosis for affected individuals often is determined by the symptoms they exhibit. Individuals affected by urogenital adysplasia syndrome may be diagnosed prenatally based on two (bilateral) missing kidneys, at birth based on the features of Potter's syndrome, or not until adulthood with the findings of reproductive problems or one missing kidney.

### Genetic profile

The genetic cause of urogenital adysplasia syndrome is not fully understood. Studies in 1995, 1997, 2000, and 2001 found evidence that nonworking, or mutated, genes on the long arm of **chromosome** 10 (10q) result in the abnormal development of the urogenital tract. However, it is still unclear if the features

of urogenital adysplasia syndrome are caused by a single mutation in one gene on chromosome 10q or by mutations in multiple genes found in this and other chromosomal locations.

Although the genetic location and mutations that cause urogenital adysplasia syndrome have not yet been determined, family studies have found that the syndrome is inherited as an autosomal dominant condition. In an autosomal dominant condition, only one mutated copy of a gene is necessary for a person to experience symptoms of the condition. If a parent has an autosomal dominant condition, there is a 50% chance for each of his or her children to have the same or a similar condition. However, in an autosomal condition with variable expressivity and incomplete penetrance like urogenital adysplasia syndrome, individuals inheriting the same mutated copy of a gene in the same family can have very different symptoms.

### Demographics

Urogenital adysplasia syndrome is a genetic condition that has been found in individuals descended from a variety of ethnic backgrounds. Although the exact frequency of urogenital adysplasia syndrome is unknown, it can be estimated based upon past family studies. Family studies also indicate that disease symptoms are more severe in males than in females. Between one in 3,000 and 10,000 newborns are born with two severely malformed or missing kidneys (bilateral renal agenesis or dysplasia). It is suggested that urogenital adysplasia syndrome is currently underdiagnosed due to its variability of symptoms within families.

### Signs and symptoms

The signs and symptoms of urogenital adysplasia syndrome vary from individual to individual (variable expressivity). Most people diagnosed with urogenital adysplasia syndrome have anomalies in their urinary and reproductive tract. The most common findings include missing kidneys and uterine abnormalities. Specific features may include any of the following:

- one or two missing kidneys (renal agenesis)
- one or two malformed kidneys (dysplastic kidneys)
- bladder anomalies
- hypertension
- vaginal anomalies
- uterine anomalies
- fallopian tube anomalies
- lack of a menstrual period (amenorrhea)
- cysts of the seminal vesicle

Additionally, since Potter's sequence occurs when the fetal kidneys cannot produce enough amniotic fluid to cushion the fetus as it develops, the features of Potter's sequence can suggest a diagnosis of urogenital adysplasia syndrome in a baby with wide-set eyes, squashed nose, small and receding chin, low-set ears, deformities of the hand and feet, and incompletely formed lungs (lung hypoplasia).

## Diagnosis

Diagnosis of urogenital adysplasia syndrome is usually made by physical examination by a medical geneticist or other physician, an ultrasound of the kidneys and the urinary and reproductive tracts, and a detailed medical family history.

Prenatal diagnosis of severe cases can sometimes be made using targeted ultrasound imaging during pregnancy to provide pictures of the fetal kidneys, bladder, and amniotic fluid levels. Ultrasound results that may indicate urogenital adysplasia syndrome include low amniotic fluid levels (oligohydramnios) combined with missing or abnormally formed kidneys (renal agenesis or adysplasia). Ultrasonographic screening for parents and siblings of infants born with agenesis or adysplasia of the kidneys is recommended since the diagnosis of urogenital adysplasia syndrome can have implications for their health and medical care. Diagnostic prenatal or postnatal molecular **genetic testing** is not available as of 2009.

## Treatment and management

Urogenital adysplasia syndrome is a genetic condition that has no specific treatment that can remove, cure, or fix its underlying genetic error. Treatment for urogenital adysplasia syndrome is limited to the management of specific symptoms. Individuals with one only kidney should be followed by a nephrologist who can evaluate their need for antihypertensive agents and/or a kidney transplant. Individuals affected by urinary tract anomalies should be followed by an urologist. Individuals with reproductive anomalies can consult an obstetrician/gynecologist who specializes in pelvic reproductive reconstructive surgery for infertility, endometriosis, pelvic pain, and **congenital anomalies**. Medical geneticists and genetic counselors are available to discuss **inheritance** patterns of the syndrome and reproductive options with affected individuals. Pregnant women whose fetuses are at risk for urogenital adysplasia syndrome should be evaluated by a perinatalogist or maternal fetal medicine specialist. Other specialists and/or surgeons may be added to an individual's medical team to address specific individual concerns.

## Prognosis

Since urogenital adysplasia syndrome results in a variety of different physical symptoms, the prognosis for each affected individual is very different.

Individuals who have one normal kidney and one malformed have an excellent prognosis, and most live normal lives. Individuals who have only one functional kidney may have issues with hypertension and proteinuria.

Individuals with reproductive anomalies may be infertile or have fertility issues. An obstetrician/gynecologist who specializes in pelvic reproductive reconstructive surgery for infertility, endometriosis, pelvic pain, and congenital anomalies may be able, in some cases, to correct some anomalies and restore fertility.

On the most severe end of the spectrum, babies found prenatally to have low amniotic fluid (oligohydramnios) and two missing kidneys (bilateral agenesis or adysplasia) might be miscarried, stillborn, or die after birth due to combined health implications of incompletely formed lungs and missing kidneys.

### Resources

#### BOOKS

Greenburg, Arthur, ed. *Primer on Kidney Diseases*, 4th Edition. San Diego: Academic Press, 2005.

#### PERIODICALS

McPherson, E., et al. "Dominantly Inherited Renal Adysplasia." *American Journal of Medical Genetics* 1987 Apr. 26(4): 863–72.

#### WEB SITES

Surgical Management of Mullerian Duct Anomalies. (Last updated: February 19, 2003; April 7, 2005.) http://www.emedicine.com/med/topic3521.htm.

#### ORGANIZATIONS

National Potters Syndrome Support Group (NPSSG). 225 Louisiana Street, Dyess AFB, TX 79607. (915) 692-0831. Wright01@Camalott.com. (April 7, 2005.) http://www.geocities.com/Heartland/Meadows/5586/syndrome.htm.

American Association of Kidney Patients. 3505 E. Frontage Rd., Ste. 315 Tampa, FL, 33607-1796. (800) 749-2257. (813) 636-8100. Fax: (813) 636-8122. info@aakp.org. (April 7, 2005.) http://www.aakp.org/.

Kidney and Urology Foundation of America, Inc. 1250 Broadway, Suite 2001, New York, NY 10001. (212) 629-9770 or (800) 633-6628. Fax: (212) 629-5652. info@kidneyurology.org. (April 7, 2005.) http://www.kidneyurology.org/homepage.htm.

National Kidney Foundation. 30 East 33rd Street, New York, NY 10016. (800) 622-9010. (April 7, 2005.) http://www.kidney.org/.

Dawn Jacob Laney

# Usher Syndrome

## Definition

Usher syndrome is an inherited condition that causes hearing loss and a form of vision loss, called **retinitis pigmentosa** (RP), which worsens over time. Some people with Usher syndrome also have difficulties with balance and/or psychological problems. Although the symptoms of Usher syndrome were first described in 1858 by an ophthalmologist named Albrecht von Graefe, it was not until 1914 that it was well documented and recognized to be a genetic condition by another ophthalmologist, Charles Usher. There are three forms of Usher syndrome: type I, type II, and type III. Genetic research has shown there are many genes located on different chromosomes, all of which can lead to one of the types of Usher syndrome if they are altered.

## Description

Usher syndrome is sometimes called hereditary deafness—retinitis pigmentosa, or retinitis pigmentosa and congenital **deafness**. Usher syndrome causes a specific type of hearing impairment called sensorineural

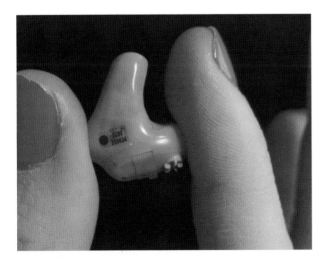

**Hearing aids are medical devices that amplify sound for individuals experiencing hearing loss.** *(Custom Medical Stock Photo, Inc.)*

hearing loss (SNHL). In order to understand how SNHL occurs, it is important to first understand how normal hearing works. The ear can be divided into three main parts: the outer ear, the middle ear and the inner ear. The parts of the outer ear include the pinna (the visible portion of the ear), the ear canal and eardrum. The pinna directs sound waves from the environment through the ear canal, toward the eardrum. The eardrum vibrates, and causes tiny bones (called ossicles), which are located in the middle ear, to move. This movement causes pressure changes in fluids surrounding the parts that make up the inner ear. The main structures of the inner ear are the cochlea and the vestibular system. These structures send information regarding hearing and balance to the brain. The cochlea is shaped like a snail shell, and it contains specialized sensory cells (called hair cells) that change the sound waves into electrical messages. These messages are then sent to the brain through a nerve (called the auditory nerve) that allows the brain to "hear" sounds from the environment. The vestibular system is a specialized organ that helps people maintain their balance. The vestibular system contains three structures called semi-circular canals, which send electrical messages to the brain about movement and body position. This allows people to maintain their balance when moving by sensing changes in their direction and speed.

Sensorineural hearing loss occurs when parts of the inner ear (including the cochlea and/or auditory nerve) do not work correctly. The amount (or degree) of hearing loss can be described by measuring the hearing threshold (the sound level that a person can just barely hear) in decibels (dB). The greater a person's dB hearing level, the louder the sound must be to just barely be heard. Hearing loss is often defined as mild, moderate, severe, or profound. For people with mild hearing loss (26-45 dB), understanding conversations in a noisy environment, at a distance, or with a soft-spoken person is difficult. Moderate hearing loss (46-65 dB) causes people to have difficulty understanding conversations, even if the environment is quiet. People with severe hearing loss (66-85 dB) have difficulty hearing conversation unless the speaker is nearby or is talking loudly. Profound hearing loss (85 dB) may prevent people from hearing sounds from their environment or even loud conversation. People with Usher syndrome generally have moderate, severe or profound SNHL, depending upon the type (I, II, or III) diagnosed.

Usher syndrome also causes a specific type of vision loss called retinitis pigmentosa (RP). In order to understand how RP occurs, it is helpful to first understand how normal vision works. The eye is made up of many different types of cells and tissues that all work together

## KEY TERMS

**Central vision**—The ability to see objects located directly in front of the eye. Central vision is necessary for reading and other activities that require people to focus on objects directly in front of them.

**Cochlea**—A bony structure shaped like a snail shell located in the inner ear. It is responsible for changing sound waves from the environment into electrical messages that the brain can understand, so people can hear.

**Genetic heterogeneity**—The occurrence of the same or similar disease, caused by different genes among different families.

**Peripheral vision**—The ability to see objects that are not located directly in front of the eye. Peripheral vision allows people to see objects located on the side or edge of their field of vision.

**Photoreceptors**—Specialized cells lining the innermost layer of the eye that convert light into electrical messages so that the brain can perceive the environment. There are two types of photoreceptor cells: rod

cells and cone cells. The rod cells allow for peripheral and night vision. Cone cells are responsible for perceiving color and for central vision.

**Retina**—The light-sensitive layer of tissue in the back of the eye that receives and transmits visual signals to the brain through the optic nerve.

**Retinitis pigmentosa**—Progressive deterioration of the retina, often leading to vision loss and blindness.

**Sensorineural hearing loss (SNHL)**—Hearing loss that occurs when parts of the inner ear, such as the cochlea and/or auditory nerve, do not work correctly. It is often defined as mild, moderate, severe, or profound, depending upon how much sound can be heard by the affected individual.

**Vestibular system**—A complex organ located inside the inner ear that sends messages to the brain about movement and body position. It allows people to maintain their balance when moving by sensing changes in their direction and speed.

to send images from the environment to the brain, similar to the way a camera records images. When light enters the eye, it passes through the lens and lands on the retina, a very thin tissue lining the inside of the eye. The retina is actually made up of 10 different layers of specialized cells, which allow the retina to function similarly to film in a camera, by recording images. There is a small, yellow-pigmented area called the macula, located in the back of the eye in the center of the retina. The retina contains many specialized cells called photoreceptors, which sense light coming into the eye and convert it into electrical messages that are then sent to the brain through the optic nerve. This allows the brain to "see" the environment.

The retina contains two types of photoreceptor cells: rod cells and cone cells. Rod cells are located primarily outside of the macula and they allow for peripheral (side) and night vision. Most of the photoreceptor cells inside of the macula, however, are the cone cells, which are responsible for perceiving color and for viewing objects directly in front of the eye (central vision). If the retina is diseased, as in RP, night vision and peripheral vision are altered. This happens in RP because the rod and cone cells degenerate (breakdown) and die over time, resulting in night blindness and decreased peripheral vision (also called "tunnel vision"). People with Usher syndrome develop RP at different ages depending upon the type (I, II, or

III) diagnosed. Although most people with Usher syndrome have fairly good vision before they reach their 30s, it worsens slowly over time and approximately 75% of people in their 70s are blind.

### Usher syndrome type I

People with Usher syndrome type I are born with profound SNHL that occurs in both ears. As a result, they do not learn to speak, and typically learn to use sign language to communicate with others. Hearing aids usually are not very helpful, due to the amount of hearing loss present. However, some individuals benefit from a procedure called cochlear implantation, in which a small electronic device is surgically placed behind the ear (underneath the skin) and is attached to a wire that stimulates the inner ear, allowing people to hear useful sounds.

Usher syndrome type I also causes vestibular areflexia, which means affected individuals have balance problems because they cannot sense changes in direction or speed when they are moving. This causes children to develop certain skills that involve motion (such as walking) more slowly, to be clumsier, and to have a hard time with activities that require good balance (such as riding a bicycle). As affected people age, they tend to have an ataxic gait, which means they tend to stumble and shuffle their feet when walking.

The visual problems caused by RP usually develop during childhood among people with this type of Usher syndrome, and they gradually worsen over time. Usually the rod cells in the peripheral retina are affected first, causing night blindness and tunnel vision during childhood. Cone cells may eventually be affected, causing blind spots to develop. Eventually, vision loss worsens and affected people can have vision problems during the day. Cataracts (cloudiness in the lens of the eye) may also develop and cause decreased central vision. Although most people with this type of Usher syndrome do not become completely blind, worsening vision may make communication via sign language and lip reading difficult.

Mental retardation and psychiatric problems (such as **depression**, **bipolar disorder**, and psychosis) have been diagnosed in a number of people with Usher syndrome type I as well. Although some authors believe that the stress of losing both hearing and vision may lead to psychological problems, at least one study has suggested that these problems may be due to an overall smaller brain size that has been measured in some affected individuals.

### Usher syndrome type II

People with Usher syndrome type II are born with mild to severe SNHL for low frequency sound that occurs in both ears. The SNHL is profound for higher frequency sounds. The amount of hearing loss is different between affected individuals, even those within the same family, although the ability to hear low frequency sound is often maintained. While hearing problems may worsen very slowly over time, speech therapy and the use of hearing aids are often helpful. Unlike people with type I, the vestibular (balance) system is not affected in people with Usher syndrome type II. Thus, they learn to walk on time as children (i.e. at approximately one year) and do not have problems with clumsiness. Although the symptoms of RP do occur among individuals with type II, they generally occur later in life (teenage years or later), compared to people with type I. Symptoms are similar, including night blindness, tunnel vision, blind spots, cataracts, and generally decreased vision. In addition, mental retardation, psychiatric problems, and decreased brain size have been seen in some people with Usher syndrome type II.

### Usher syndrome type III

People with Usher syndrome type III may be born with normal hearing or mild hearing loss. However, their hearing loss is progressive, which means that it tends to worsen over time. The vestibular system causes mild balance problems that worsen over time

among individuals with Usher syndrome type III. Older affected people may have balance problems similar to those seen in type I. There is a broad age range when the symptoms of RP occur among people with type III, although usually they happen later in life (late teens to early adult years). Vision problems also worsen over time. In addition, mental retardation and psychiatric problems also have been seen in some people with Usher syndrome type III.

People with Usher syndrome and their families often experience emotional and psychological distress. Depression, anger, and grief are common among affected teenagers and adults. The vision and hearing problems create ongoing challenges for people, in terms of their ability to receive information from the world and to effectively communicate with others. Affected people have to continually learn new skills, such as Braille or tactile sign language (i.e. using their hands to physically feel the signs), to adapt to their gradually worsening vision.

### Genetic profile

Usher syndrome is inherited in an autosomal recessive manner. "Autosomal" means that males and females are equally likely to be affected. "Recessive" refers to a specific type of **inheritance** in which both copies of a person's **gene** pair (i.e. both alleles) need to have a change or "mutation" in order for the disease to develop. In this situation, an affected individual receives a mutated copy of the same gene from each parent. If the parents are not affected, they each have one working copy of the gene and one non-working (mutated) copy, and are only "carriers" for Usher syndrome. The chance that two carrier parents will have a child affected with Usher syndrome is 25% for each pregnancy. They also have a 50% chance to have an unaffected child who is simply a carrier, and a 25% chance to have an unaffected child who is not a carrier, with each pregnancy. In the United States, as many as one in every 70 people may be carriers of a mutation that can lead to Usher syndrome.

Although there are three recognizable types of Usher syndrome (I, II, and III), genetic research has shown that there are numerous genes, located on different chromosomes, that can all lead to Usher syndrome. This indicates that there is genetic heterogeneity among different families with Usher syndrome, meaning that different genes can lead to the same or similar disease among different families. As of February 2001, researchers have identified six different subtypes of Usher syndrome type I (USH1A, USH1B, USH1C, USH1D, USH1E, and USH1F), four subtypes of Usher syndrome type II (USH 2A, USH2B, USH2C, and USH2D), and one type of Usher syndrome type III (USH3). Although specific genes have been identified for only four of the 11 subtypes, the other seven have been linked to specific chromosomal regions.

Genetic Classification of Usher syndrome - February, 2001

- USH1A - Located on chromosome 14q32. Specific gene unknown.
- USH1B - Located on chromosome 11q13.5. Specific gene called myosin VIIA.
- USH1C - Located on chromosome 11p15.1. Specific gene called harmonin.
- USH1D - Located on chromosome 10q21-22. Specific gene called CDH23.
- USH1E - Located on chromosome 21q21. Specific gene unknown.
- USH1F - Located on chromosome 10. Specific gene unknown.
- USH2A - Located on chromosome 1q41. Specific gene called usherin.
- USH2B - Located on chromosome 3p23-24.2. Specific gene unknown.
- USH2C - Located on chromosome 5q14.3-21.3. Specific gene unknown.
- USH2D - Chromosome location unknown. Specific gene unknown.
- USH3 - Located on chromosome 3q21-25. Specific gene unknown.

Although specific genes have been identified for some of the Usher syndrome subtypes (i.e. myosin VIIA, harmonin, CDH23, and usherin), not all mutations in these genes lead specifically to Usher syndrome. For example, although mutations in CDH23 can lead to Usher syndrome type 1D, some people who have certain types of mutations in both of their CDH23 gene copies have a form of autosomal recessive deafness (called DFNB12) in which affected individuals have profound SNHL at birth, but do not have balance or vision changes that are typically seen in Usher syndrome.

### Demographics

It is estimated that 2.5-4.5 per 100,000 people are affected with Usher syndrome in various countries, including the United States, Denmark, Sweden, Norway, Finland, and Columbia, although it has been diagnosed in other parts of the world as well. There are some areas where Usher syndrome seems to be more common, including communities in northern Sweden and among the French Acadians in Louisiana. Certain types of Usher syndrome are more common in certain areas of the world as well. For example, among affected people in Finland, approximately 40% have type III. However, in the United States, types I and II are most common and occur with nearly equal frequency, while type III is very rare.

### Signs and symptoms

Symptoms of Usher syndrome type I:

- Profound hearing loss at birth, causing lack of speech
- Lack of vestibular function at birth, leading to delayed ability to walk and increased clumsiness
- Retinitis pigmentosa in childhood, causing night blindness, tunnel vision and decreased vision over time
- May cause mental retardation or psychiatric problems in some people

Symptoms of Usher syndrome type II:

- Mild to severe hearing loss (for low-frequency sound) and profound hearing loss (for high-frequency sound) at birth
- Normal vestibular function, resulting in normal ability to maintain balance
- Retinitis pigmentosa in teens or early adult years, causing night blindness, tunnel vision and decreased vision over time
- May cause mental retardation or psychiatric problems in some people

Symptoms of Usher syndrome type III:

- Normal hearing or mild hearing loss at birth that worsens over time
- Abnormal vestibular function, causing mild balance problems that worsen over time
- Retinitis pigmentosa by teenage or early adult years, causing night blindness, tunnel vision and decreased vision over time
- May cause mental retardation or psychiatric problems in some people

### Diagnosis

As of 2009, **genetic testing** is not readily available for people with Usher syndrome to look for their specific mutations (and thus confirm their diagnosis), in spite of the fact that a number of important genes have been identified. Some families do participate in genetic research studies by providing blood samples, with the hope that useful information may be learned about their genetic mutations, as well as Usher syndrome in general.

The diagnosis of Usher syndrome is based on the results from a variety of tests that measure hearing, vision, and balance. Sometimes the diagnosis is not made until a person with SNHL reaches adolescence and develops vision problems. A follow-up eye examination may allow an eye care specialist to detect changes seen in RP, thus confirming the diagnosis of Usher syndrome. Specialized testing of an affected person's vestibular system can be done to help determine the type of Usher syndrome as well.

## Treatment and management

As of 2001, there is no cure for Usher syndrome. However, there are a number of ways to treat various symptoms.

### Treatment and management of SNHL

Regular hearing exams are important to check for changes in hearing ability, especially for people with type II or type III Usher syndrome. Among people with milder forms of hearing loss, hearing aids and speech therapy are often useful. Sign language training for people with profound SNHL and their families provides a method of communication, although these skills need to be modified into tactile sign language as vision decreases. Some people with severe to profound forms of hearing loss may have cochlear implants placed in an effort to improve their perception of sound.

### Treatment and management of RP

People with night blindness, tunnel vision and decreasing vision may benefit from a variety of techniques that help them cope with their ever-changing vision. The use of walking canes, guide dogs, magnifying lenses, flashlights, and Braille may be helpful. Specialized filtering lenses may decrease glare and make the eye more comfortable. Some people also find it useful to meet with low-vision specialists who can help them adapt to new lifestyle changes that help with daily living. Regular eye exams are important and allow early detection of cataracts, which may be treated with surgery.

Although there is no way to completely halt the symptoms of RP, studies published in the 1990s found that 15,000 IU of vitamin A palmitate can slow the course of the retinal changes among people with Usher syndrome type II. This therapy has not been recommended for people under 18 years of age, and women who may become pregnant need to discuss with their doctor the potential harms that vitamin A can cause for a developing baby. People who want to take the vitamin should speak with their doctor first and have regular blood tests to check vitamin levels as well as to rule out liver problems caused by the supplement.

---

**QUESTIONS TO ASK YOUR DOCTOR**

- When should hearing evaluations begin and how often should they be repeated?
- Do you recommend vitamin A?
- What are the signs of vitamin A toxicity?
- What measures or resources do you recommend to improve quality of life?

---

There are a number of support groups available that provide education, support, and helpful advice to help people cope with the symptoms of Usher syndrome.

## Prognosis

Usher syndrome generally does not cause a shortened life span for affected individuals. Although people live for many years with Usher syndrome, the physical symptoms and emotional side effects change over time. The vision problems usually worsen slowly over the years, forcing people to adapt their lifestyles, habits, and sometimes change professions. Regular eye exams can help diagnose cataracts that may be removed in an effort to maintain the best vision possible. Regular monitoring of hearing may be helpful for people with mild, moderate, and/or severe hearing loss, so that they can receive appropriate hearing aids. As vision problems (and sometimes hearing and/or balance problems) worsen, people are more likely to suffer emotionally, due to decreasing quality of life and independence. However, many low-vision devices, lifestyle modifications, and various support groups often provide much needed assistance to help maintain and/or improve quality of life for affected individuals.

## Resources

### BOOKS

Duncan, Earlene, et al. *Usher's Syndrome: What It Is, How to Cope, and How to Help.* New York: Charles C. Thomas Publisher, 1988.

Gorlin, R.J., H.V. Toriello, and M.M. Cohen. "Retinitis Pigmentosa and Sensorineural Hearing Loss (Usher Syndrome)." *Hereditary Hearing Loss and Its Syndromes.* Oxford Monographs on Medical Genetics, no. 28. New York and Oxford: Oxford University Press, 1995.

Stiefel, Dorothy H., and Richard A. Lewis. *The Madness of Usher's: Coping With Vision and Hearing Loss/Usher Syndrome Type II.* Business of Living Publishing, 1991.

**PERIODICALS**

Keats, Bronya J.B., and David P. Corey. "The Usher Syndromes." *American Journal of Medical Genetics* 89, no. 3 (September 24, 1999): 158-166.

Kimberling, William J., Dana Orten, and Sandra Pieke-Dahl. "Genetic Heterogeneity of Usher Syndrome." *Advances in Oto-rhino-laryngology* 56 (December 2000): 11-18.

Miner, I.D. "People with Usher Syndrome, Type II: Issues and Adaptations." *Journal of Visual Impairment & Blindness* 91, no. 6 (November/December 1997): 579-590.

Miner, I.D. "Psychosocial Implications of Usher Syndrome, Type I, Throughout the Life Cycle." *Journal of Visual Impairment & Blindness* 89, no.3 (May/June 1995): 287-297.

Steel, Karen P. "New Interventions in Hearing Impairment." *British Medical Journal* 7235 (March 4, 2000): 622-626.

**WEBSITES**

Sense homepage. http://www.sense.org.uk/homepage.html.

**ORGANIZATIONS**

American Council of the Blind. 1155 15th St. NW, Suite 720, Washington, DC 20005. (202) 467-5081 or (800) 424-8666. http://www.acb.org.

Boys Town National Research Hospital. 555 N. 30th St., Omaha, NE 68131. (402) 498-6749. http://www.boystown.org/Btnrh/Index.htm.

DB-LINK, Teaching Research. 345 N. Monmouth Ave., Monmouth, OR 97361. (800) 438-9376. http://www.tr.wou.edu/dblink/about.htm.

Foundation Fighting Blindness Executive Plaza 1, Suite 800, 11350 McCormick Rd., Hunt Valley, MD 21031. (888) 394-3937. http://www.blindness.org.

Helen Keller National Center for Deaf-Blind Youths and Adults. 111 Middle Neck Rd., Sands Point, NY 11050. (516) 944-8900. http://www.helenkeller.org/national/index.htm.

Usher Family Support. 4918 42nd Ave. South, Minneapolis, MN 55417. (612) 724-6982.

Vestibular Disorders Association. PO Box 4467, Portland, OR 97208-4467. (800) 837-8428. http://www.vestibular.org.

Pamela J. Nutting, MS, CGC

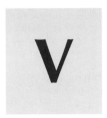

VACTERL *see* **VATER association**

# Van der Woude syndrome

## Definition

Van der Woude syndrome (VWS) is a condition affecting the lips, palate and teeth. Depressions or pits typically are present on the lower lip at birth and **cleft lip** and/or **cleft palate** may also be present. Less commonly, certain teeth may not develop. VWS has previously been known as the lip pit syndrome.

## Description

Van der Woude syndrome primarily involves pits developing on the lower lip, clefting of the lip and/or palate, and the absence of certain teeth. More than 80% or more than eight out of 10 individuals with VWS will develop pits near the center of the lower lip and about 60–70% (six to seven people out of 10) will have a cleft lip and/or palate at birth. About half to two–thirds of the individuals will have both lower lip pits and a cleft of the lip and/or palate. In some cases, a cleft palate is present but is not immediately noticeable; this is called a submucosal cleft palate. The least common feature in VWS, missing teeth, is seen in about 10–20% (one to two people out of 10) of individuals with VWS. The teeth most commonly affected are the second incisors and the second molars.

Van der Woude syndrome is related to another condition called popliteal pterygium syndrome (PPS). Popliteal pterygium syndrome is similar to VWS in that both conditions cause lip pits and cleft lip and/or palate to develop. Popliteal pterygium syndrome differs from VWS in that popliteal pterygium webs are present at birth. Pterygium means webbed skin. Popliteal refers to the back of the legs. Popliteal pterygium

means that there is webbed skin on the back of the legs, usually on the back of the knees. Individuals with PPS may also have underdevelopment of the genitals, webbing between the fingers, adhesion of the lower and upper eyelids, and fibrous bands attaching the lower and upper jaws.

Some families have features consistent with both VWS and PPS. In other words, within a family, some family members have features that are entirely consistent with VWS and other family members have features consistent with PPS. Since the gene(s) causing VWS and PPS have not been identified, it is not known why these families have features of both diseases.

## Genetic profile

Mutations in the interferon regulatory factor 6 (IRF6) **gene** cause van der Woude syndrome. This gene, located on **chromosome** 1 at position 1q32.3–q41, provides instructions for making a protein that plays an important role in early development, particularly in cells associated with the growth of tissues in the head and face. A shortage of the IRF6 protein impairs the maturation of these tissues, resulting in the symptoms of van der Woude syndrome. The syndrome follows autosomal dominant **inheritance**, indicating that every individual affected by VWS has a 50% (1 in 2) chance of passing on the condition to each of his/her children. Every individual inheriting the VWS gene will develop at least one feature of VWS. However, family members may develop different features, and some may develop very minor features whereas another family member may have more severe problems. In some cases, a family member's features may be so mild that he or she is initially thought to be unaffected. Apparently unaffected parents of a newborn with VWS should undergo a thorough examination since it is possible that one of the parents is very mildly affected. If such a parent is determined to be affected, all of his or her children will have a 50% chance of inheriting VWS.

### Demographics

According to the Office of Rare Diseases (ORD), van der Woude syndrome is a rare condition, meaning that it affects less than 200,000 people in the United States. Prevalence in the general European population is estimated at around 1 in 60,000.

### Signs and symptoms

The primary symptom associated with VWS is the development of pits near the center of the lower lip (present in more than 80% of cases). In addition, 60–70% of individuals with VWS also have cleft lip and/or cleft palate. A few individuals (about 10–20%) with VWS are missing teeth, most commonly the second incisors and the second molars.

### Diagnosis

As of 2009, diagnosis of VWS relies solely upon physical examination and whether or not the characteristic features of VWS are present or absent. The family history may also have an important role in determining the diagnosis. For example, if lower lip pits and a cleft palate are present in a newborn and no popliteal webs or other feature of PPS is present, then the child has VWS. If a newborn is born with a cleft palate only but has a family history of VWS, then the child most likely has inherited VWS.

As cleft lip and/or palate occurs in other genetic conditions as well as by itself, a newborn with this birth defect needs to be fully evaluated to ensure that the reason for the cleft is correctly determined. Likewise, lower lip pits may be seen in VWS, in PPS and rarely, in a third genetic condition called orofaciodigital syndrome, type 1; consequently, a baby born with lower lips pits needs to be fully evaluated.

Prenatal diagnosis for VWS can be attempted through ultrasound examination of unborn babies at risk for the condition. Cleft lip and very rarely cleft palate can be identified on ultrasound examination. However, as some clefts are small and some individuals with VWS do not have clefts at all, a normal ultrasound examination cannot completely rule out the chance the baby has inherited VWS. An ultrasound examination with high resolution, or a level 2 ultrasound, and an experienced technician may increase the chance of seeing cleft lips or palate. Lip pits cannot be seen on ultrasound examination, even with a higher resolution ultrasound. As of 2009, **genetic testing** of the unborn baby is not available as the gene(s) causing VWS have not been identified.

### Treatment and management

An individual with VWS will be treated and followed according to the features he or she has developed. The lip pits seen in VWS rarely cause problems. Occasionally, saliva may ooze from the pits and if so, a fistula may have developed. A fistula is an abnormal passageway or opening that develops, and in VWS, a fistula may develop between a salivary gland located under the lip and the lip surface. The pits and fistulas may be surgically removed.

If a cleft lip and/or palate is present, surgery will be necessary to correct this problem. The treatment and management of cleft lips and palates in individuals with VWS is no different from cleft lips and palates occurring in other genetic conditions or by themselves. The child will need to be followed closely for ear and sinus infections and hearing problems. The child may need speech therapy and should be followed by a dentist and orthodontist. Counseling may be needed as the child grows up to address any concerns about speech and/or appearance.

### Prognosis

Overall, individuals with VWS do well. If a cleft lip and/or palate is present at birth, there may be some feeding difficulties in the newborn period and in the following three to six months, until the cleft is corrected. However, once surgery repairing the cleft is completed, the child typically does well. Van der Woude syndrome is not associated with a shorter life span.

## QUESTIONS TO ASK YOUR DOCTOR

- How is van der Woude symptom diagnosed in a newborn child?
- What procedures are typically used for the treatment of this disorder?
- Does van der Woude symptom result in serious mental or physical abnormalities later in life?
- How common is van der Woude symptom in the United States?

## Resources

### BOOKS

Berkowitz, Samuel, editor. *Cleft Lip and Palate: Diagnosis and Management.* New York, NY: Springer, 2005.

Reuss, Alexander. *Analysis of Speech Disorders in Children with Cleft Lip and Palate.* Saarbrücken, Germany: VDM Verlag Dr. Mueller e.K., 2008.

Wyszynski, Diego F, editor. *Cleft Lip and Palate: From Origin to Treatment.* New York, NY: Oxford University Press, 2002.

### PERIODICALS

Brookes, J. T., and J. W. Canady. "Surgical correction of congenital lower lip sinuses in Van der Woude syndrome." *Cleft Palate–Craniofacial Journal* 44, no. 5 (September 2007): 555–557.

Krauel, L., et al. "Van der Woude Syndrome and lower lip pits treatment." *Journal of Oral and Maxillofacial Surgery* 66, no. 3 (March 2008): 589–592.

Little, H. J., et al. "Missense mutations that cause Van der Woude syndrome and popliteal pterygium syndrome affect the DNA–binding and transcriptional activation functions of IRF6." *Human Molecular Genetics* 18, no. 3 (February 2009): 535–545.

Nopoulos, P. Et al. "Abnormal brain structure in adults with Van der Woude syndrome." *Clinical Genetics* 71 no. 6 (June 2007): 511–517.

Tan, E. C., et al. "Identification of IRF6 gene variants in three families with Van der Woude syndrome." *International Journal of Molecular Medicine* 21, no. 6 (June 2008): 747–751.

### WEBSITES

*Cleft Lip and Palate.* Health Topics, Medline Plus, November 1, 2008 (May 17, 2009). http://www.nlm.nih.gov/medlineplus/cleftlipandpalate.html

*Van der Woude Syndrome.* Information Page, Genetics Home Reference, April, 2008 (May 17, 2009). http://ghr.nlm.nih.gov/condition = vanderwoudesyndrome

*Van der Woude Syndrome.* Information Page, Seattle Children's (May 17, 2009). http://craniofacial.seattlechildrens.org/conditions_treated/vanderwoude.asp

*Van der Woude Syndrome (VWS).* Information Page, University of Iowa Children's Hospital, June 30, 2008 (May 17, 2009). http://www.uihealthcare.com/topics/medicaldepartments/pediatrics/vanderwoudesyndrome/index.html

### ORGANIZATIONS

American Cleft Palate–Craniofacial Association,Cleft Palate Foundation. 1504 East Franklin St., Suite 102, Chapel Hill, NC 27514-2820. (919)933-9044. Fax: (919)933-9604. http://www.cleftline.org.

National Organization for Rare Disorders (NORD). 55 Kenosia Avenue, PO Box 1968, Danbury, CT 06813-1968. (203)744-0100 or (800)999-6673. Fax: (203)798-2291. http://www.rarediseases.org.

Cindy L. Hunter, CGC

# VATER association

## Definition

VATER association describes a pattern of related birth defects in the same infant involving three or more of the following: vertebrae (spine), anus and rectum, heart, trachea (windpipe), esophagus, radius (bone of the arm), and kidneys. Infants can have any combination of features and there is a wide range of severity. Survival and medical complications depend on the extent and severity of features in each case.

## Description

Quan and Smith first developed the term VATER association in 1973 to describe a similar pattern of birth defects in more than one infant. The problems at birth did not represent a certain syndrome but appeared to be associated since they were present in several babies. VATER is an acronym or abbreviation representing the first letter of each feature in the association: *V*ertebral (spine) abnormalities, *A*nal atresia (partial absence of the anus or unusual connection between anus and rectum), *T*racheo-*E*sophageal fistula (connection between the windpipe and the tube carrying food from mouth to stomach), and *R*adial (bone of the forearm) or *R*enal (kidney) differences.

In the 1970s some researchers expanded the VATER abbreviation to VACTERL. It was expanded to include *c*ardiac (heart) abnormalities, and *l*imb differences in general (differences in the arms and hands). In the expanded VACTERL, "L" includes radial differences and "R" represents kidney differences only. Both

VATER and VACTERL are used to describe the same association of birth defects.

The exact cause of VATER is unknown. This is because VATER is rare and because the features vary from patient to patient. Many researchers agree that the cause of VATER occurs very early in the development of the embryo in order to affect so many organ systems. It is unknown whether VATER has a single cause or multiple causes during this early development process.

In the first couple of weeks after conception, a human embryo is a clump of cells that are unspecialized and full of potential. In the third week of pregnancy the embryo undergoes a process called gastrulation. This is when the cells of the embryo begin to group together in different areas. The different cell groups begin to specialize and prepare to form different organs and body parts. The mesoderm is the group of cells that organizes and eventually forms the baby's bones, muscles, heart, blood, kidneys, and reproductive organs. In the third week of pregnancy, the notochord also develops. The notochord is the future spinal cord and gives the early embryo a center and stability. It may also have a role in organizing other cell groups. The primitive gut also organizes in the fourth week. The primitive gut undergoes more specialization and division into zones called the foregut, midgut, and hindgut. The esophagus (tube from mouth to stomach) and trachea (windpipe) develop from the foregut. The anus and rectum develop from the hindgut. The constant cell movement, grouping, and specialization is a precise process. Any interruption or damage in this early stage can affect multiple organs and body structures.

Some researchers believe the cause of VATER is a problem with gastrulation. Other researchers believe the error occurs when mesoderm cells begin to move to areas to begin specialization. Another theory is that the mesoderm receives abnormal signals and becomes disorganized. Other researchers believe more than one error occurs in more than one area of the early embryo to produce VATER. Some also believe an abnormality of the notochord is involved in the development of VATER.

One group of researchers has discovered that pregnant rats that are given a toxic drug called adriamycin have offspring with birth defects very similar to those seen in humans with VATER. This has allowed the researchers to study normal and abnormal development of the early embryo. The study of rats showed abnormal notochord development in offspring with connections of the trachea and esophagus. In those offspring, the notochord was thickened and connected unusually to the foregut. More research of this animal model will answer many questions about the development and cause of the features of VATER.

### Genetic profile

The exact genetic cause of VATER association is unknown. Most cases are sporadic and do not occur more than once in the same family. This was determined by studies of families with an affected individual. Since cases are rare and most are isolated in a family, studies to find a genetic cause have been unsuccessful. Parents of a child with VATER association have a 1% or less chance of having another baby with the same condition. There have been a few reports of affected individuals with a parent or sibling showing a single feature of the VATER spectrum. There has only been one reported case of a parent and child both affected with multiple VATER features.

Most individuals with VATER association have a normal **chromosome** pattern. However, a few cases of chromosome differences have been reported in individuals with VATER. One child with VATER had a deletion (missing piece) on the long arm of chromosome 6. Another male infant had a deletion on the long arm of chromosome 13. There have been other children reported with a chromosome 13 deletion and VATER-like features. This infant was the first reported with the deletion to have all of the VACTERL main features. He was also the first with this chromosome deletion to have a connection between his trachea and esophagus. Another child with VATER association had an extra marker chromosome. This is a fragment of chromosomal material present in the cell in addition to the usual 46 chromosomes. This child's marker was found to contain material from chromosome 12. These cases have not led to the discovery of a **gene** involved in VATER.

There has only been one VATER case reported in which a genetic change was identified. That female infant died one month after birth because of kidney failure. Her mother and sister later were diagnosed with a mitochondrial disease. Mitochrondria are the structures in the cell that create energy by chemical reactions. The mitochrondria have their own set of

DNA and a person inherits mitochondrial DNA from the mother only. Stored kidney tissue from the deceased infant was analyzed and she was found to have the same genetic change in her mitochondrial DNA as her mother and sister. The researchers could not prove that the gene change caused the infant's features of VATER.

There are two subtypes of VACTERL that seem to be inherited. Both types have the typical VACTERL features in addition to hydrocephaly (excess water in the brain). They are abbreviated VACTERL-H. The first subtype was described in 1975 by David and O'Callaghan and is called the David-O'Callaghan subtype. It appears to be an autosomal recessive condition. Parents of an affected child are carriers of a normal gene and a gene that causes VACTERL-H. When both parents are carriers there is a 25% chance for an affected child with each pregnancy. The second subtype is called Hunter-MacMurray and appears to be an X-linked recessive condition. In X-linked conditions, the disease-causing gene is located on the X chromosome, one of the sex-determining chromosomes. Females have two X chromosomes and males have an X chromosome and a Y chromosome. A female who carries a disease-causing gene on one of her X chromosomes shows no symptoms. If a male inherits the gene he will show symptoms of the condition. A woman who carries the VACTERL-H X-linked gene has a 25% chance of having an affected son with each pregnancy. Both of these subtypes are rare and account for a small number of VACTERL cases.

### Demographics

VATER is rare, but has been reported worldwide. Exact incidence can be difficult to determine because of different criteria for diagnosis. Some studies consider two or more VATER features enough to make the diagnosis. Other studies require at least three features to diagnose VATER. Also, infants with features of VATER may have other genetic syndromes such as **trisomy 13**, **trisomy 18**, **Holt-Oram syndrome**, **TAR syndrome**, and **Fanconi anemia**. VATER does appear to be more frequent in babies of diabetic mothers. It is also more frequent in babies of mothers taking certain medications during pregnancy, including estroprogestins, methimazole, and doxorubicin.

### Signs and symptoms

VATER has six defining symptoms. "V" represents vertebral abnormalities. Approximately 70% of individuals with VATER have some type of spine difference such as **scoliosis** (curvature of the spine), hemivertebrae

(unusually aligned, extra, or crowded spinal bones), and sacral absence (absence of spinal bones in the pelvic area). Vertebral differences are usually in the lumbrosacral area (the part of the spine in the small of the back and pelvis). "A" represents anal atresia which is present in about 80% of individuals with VATER. This is an unusual arrangment or connection of the anus and rectum. Imperforate anus is also common, in which the anal opening does not form or is covered. Babies with this problem cannot pass bowel movements out of the body. "TE" stands for tracheo-esophageal fistula. About 70% of babies with VATER have this problem. This is a connection between the two tubes of the throat - the esophagus (carries food from mouth to stomach) and the trachea (windpipe). This connection is dangerous because it causes breathing problems. These babies can also get food into their windpipe and choke. Lung infections are also common with this connection. Some infants may be missing part of their esophagus, causing problems with choking and feeding. These babies spit up their food because the food cannot get to the stomach.

In the original VATER association, "R" stood for radial differences and renal (kidney) problems. The radius is the forearm bone that connects to the hand on the side of the thumb. Radial differences can include an absent or underdeveloped radius. This often results in a twisted, unusual position of the arm and hand. The thumb can also be small, misplaced, or absent. Kidney problems are present in about half of individuals with VATER. These can include missing kidneys, kidney cysts, or fluid buildup in the kidneys. Some individuals also have an abnormal position of the urethra (the tube that carries urine out of the body).

The expanded VACTERL includes "C" for cardiac (heart) problems and "L" for limb differences. The heart problems are usually holes or other structural abnormalities. Limb differences usually involve the arms rather than the legs. The term includes more general differences such as extra fingers, shortened or missing fingers, and underdeveloped humerus (the bone of the upper arm). These differences often cause unusual arm or hand positions (bent or twisted) and fingers that are short, absent, or misplaced.

Many people have proposed an expanded VACTERL pattern to include differences of the reproductive system and absent sacrum. Small or ambiguous (not clearly male or female) genitalia, or misplaced reproductive parts are common in VACTERL. They tend to occur more frequently in infants with anal and kidney abnormalities. They are seen less often with esophagus and arm features. Absence of the bones of the sacrum (spine in the pelvis area) is also commonly seen in VACTERL.

Individuals with VATER have an average of seven to eight features or differences at birth. About two-thirds of features involve the lower body (intestines, genitals, urinary system, pelvis, and lower spine). One-third of features involve the upper body (arms, hands, heart, esophagus, and trachea). In addition to the typical VATER features, infants may have problems with the intestines or excess water in the brain. Intestinal problems (such as missing sections of intestine) are more common in individuals with anal or esophagus features.

Shortly after birth, infants with VATER often have failure to thrive. This involves feeding problems and difficulty gaining weight. Their development is often slow. Infants with visible signs of VATER should immediately be checked for internal signs. Quick detection of problems with the trachea, esophagus, heart, and kidneys can lead to earlier treatment and prevention of major illness. Most individuals with VATER have normal mental development and mental retardation is rare.

### Diagnosis

Some features of VATER can be seen on **prenatal ultrasound** so that the diagnosis may be suspected at birth. Ultrasound can see differences of the vertebrae, heart, limbs, limb positions, kidneys, and some reproductive parts. Other problems that are associated with VATER on ultrasound are poor fetal growth, excessive fluid in the womb, absent or collapsed stomach, and one artery in the umbilical cord instead of the usual two. VATER features that cannot be seen on ultrasound are differences of the anus, esophagus, and trachea.

Even if VATER is suspected before birth, an infant must be examined after birth to determine the extent of features. The entire pattern of internal and external differences will determine if the infant has VATER association, another multiple birth defect syndrome, or a genetic syndrome (such as Holt-Oram syndrome, **TAR syndrome**, or Fanconi anemia). Since VATER overlaps with some genetic syndromes, some infants may fit the VATER pattern and still have another diagnosis. VATER only describes the pattern of related birth defects. Since the genetic causes of VATER are unknown, **genetic testing** is not available. A family history focusing on VATER features can help to determine if an infant has a sporadic case or a rare inherited case.

### Treatment and management

Treatment for VATER involves surgery for each separate feature. Holes in the heart can be closed by surgery. Structural problems of the heart can also{\hskip 0.7pt}often be repaired. Prognosis is best for infants with small or simple heart problems. Some

vertebral problems may also need surgery. If the vertebral differences cause a problem for the individual's posture, braces or other support devices may be needed.

Problems with the trachea and esophagus can also be repaired with surgery. Before surgery the infant usually needs a feeding tube for eating. This will stop the choking and spitting up. The infant may also need oxygen to help with breathing. If the trachea and esophagus are connected, the connection is separated first. Once separated, the two trachea ends and esophagus ends can be sealed together. When part of the esophagus is missing, the two loose ends are connected. If the gap between the loose ends is too big, surgery may be delayed until the esophagus grows. Some infants still have problems after surgery. They may have a difficult time swallowing or food may get stuck in their throat. They may also have **asthma** and frequent respiratory infections.

Surgery can also repair problems of the anus and rectum. Before surgery, a temporary opening is made from the small intestine to the abdomen. This allows the infant to have bowel movements and pass stool material. An anal opening is created with surgery. The intestines and rectum are adjusted to fit with the new anal opening. The temporary opening on the abdomen may be closed immediately after surgery or it may be closed weeks or months later. Surgeons must be very careful not to damage the nerves and muscles around the anus. If they are damaged, the individual may lose control of their bowel movements.

Differences of the hands and arms can also be improved with surgery. Infants with underdeveloped or absent radius may have a stiff elbow, stiff wrist, or twisted arm. Surgery can loosen the elbow and wrist to allow for movement. The arm can also be straightened. If needed, muscles from other parts of the body can be put into the arm. This may also improve movement. Even after surgery, individuals may not have completely normal function of the muscles and tendons of the arms and hands.

### Prognosis

Prognosis for individuals with VATER association depends on the severity of features. Infants with complex heart problems or severe abnormalities of the anus, trachea, or esophagus have a poorer prognosis. Infants with several features that require surgery have a higher death rate than infants that need minor surgery or no surgery. Survival also depends on how quickly internal problems are discovered. The sooner problems with the heart, anus, trachea, and esophagus are found and repaired, the better the outlook for the infant. One study estimated that infants with VATER have a death rate 25 times higher than healthy infants. Another study estimated that up to 30% of individuals with VATER die in the newborn period.

## Resources

### PERIODICALS

Beasley, S.W., et al. "The Contribution of the Adriamycin-induced Rat Model of the VATER Association to Our Understanding of Congenital Abnormalities and Their Embryogenesis." *Pediatric Surgery International* 16 (2000): 465-72.

Botto, Lorenzo D., et al. "The Spectrum of Congenital Anomalies of the VATER Association: An International Study." *American Journal of Medical Genetics* 71 (1997): 8-15.

Rittler, Monica, Joaquin E. Paz, and Eduardo E. Castilla. "VATERL: An Epidemiologic Analysis of Risk Factors." *American Journal of Medical Genetics* 73 (1997): 162-69.

Rittler, Monica, Joaquin E. Paz, and Eduardo E. Castilla. "VACTERL Association, Epidemiologic Definition and Delineation." *American Journal of Medical Genetics* 63 (1996): 529-36.

### ORGANIZATIONS

VACTRLS Association Family Network. 5585 CY Ave. Casper, WY 82604. http://www.homestead.com/VAFN/VAFN.html.

VATER Connection. 1722 Yucca Lane, Emporia, KS 66801. (316) 342-6954. http://www.vaterconnection.org.

VATER Connection. 1722 Yucca Lane, Emporia, KS 66801. (316) 342-6954. http://www.vaterconnection.org.

### WEBSITES

"Vater Association." *Online Mendelian Inheritance in Man.*http://www.ncbi.nlm.nih.gov/entrez/dispomim.cgi?id = 192350.

Amie Stanley, MS

Velocardiofacial syndrome *see* **Deletion 22q1 syndrome**
Ventriculomegaly *see* **Hydrocephalus**

# Von Hippel-Lindau syndrome

## Definition

Von Hippel-Lindau (VHL) syndrome is an inherited condition characterized by tumors that arise in multiple locations in the body. Some of these tumors cause **cancer** and some do not. Many of the tumors seen in VHL are vascular, meaning that they have a rich supply of blood vessels.

## Description

In the mid-1800s, ophthalmologists described vascular tumors in the retina, the light-sensitive layer that lines the interior of the eye. These tumors, called *angiomas*, were not cancerous but were associated with vision loss. In 1904, a German ophthalmologist named Eugen von Hippel noted that these retinal angiomas seemed to run in families. Twenty-three years later, Arvid Lindau, a Swedish pathologist, reported a connection between these retinal angiomas and similar tumors in the brain, called *hemangioblastomas*. Like angiomas, hemangioblastomas are vascular tumors as well. After Lindau noted this association, there were many more reports describing families in which there was an association of retinal angiomas and central nervous system (CNS) hemangioblastomas. Other findings were found to be common in these families as well. These findings included cysts and/or tumors in the kidney, pancreas, adrenal gland, and various other organs. In 1964, Melmon and Rosen wrote a review of the current knowledge of this condition and named the disorder von Hippel-Lindau disease. More recently, the tumors in the retina were determined to be identical to those in the CNS. They are now referred to as *hemangioblastomas*, rather than angiomas.

There are four distinct types of VHL, based on the manifestations of the disorder. Type 1 is characterized by all VHL-related tumors except those in the adrenal gland. Type 2 includes tumors of the adrenal gland and is subdivided into type 2A (without kidney tumors or cysts in the pancreas), type 2B (with kidney tumors and cysts in the pancreas), and type 2C (adrenal gland tumors only).

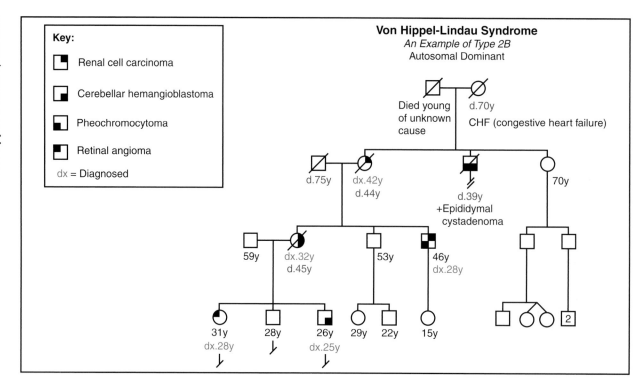

**Von Hippel-Lindau Syndrome**
*An Example of Type 2B*
Autosomal Dominant

Key:
- Renal cell carcinoma
- Cerebellar hemangioblastoma
- Pheochromocytoma
- Retinal angioma

dx = Diagnosed

(Gale, a part of Cengage Learning.)

## Genetic profile

VHL is inherited in an autosomal dominant manner. This means that an affected person has a 50% chance of passing the disease on to each of his or her children. Nearly everyone who carries the mutation in the VHL **gene** will show signs of the disorder, usually by the age of 65.

VHL is caused by a change or *mutation* in the VHL gene. This gene is located on **chromosome** 3 and produces the VHL protein. The VHL protein is a tumor suppressor, meaning that it controls cell growth. When the VHL gene is changed, the VHL protein does not function correctly and allows cells to grow out of control. This uncontrolled cell growth forms tumors and these tumors may lead to cancer.

People without VHL have two working copies of the VHL gene, one on each chromosome 3. Each of these copies produces the VHL protein. People affected with VHL inherit one working copy and one non-working copy of the gene. Thus, one gene does not make the VHL protein but the corresponding gene on the other chromosome continues to make the functional protein. In this case, cell growth will still be controlled because the VHL protein is available. However, as this person lives, another mutation may occur in the working gene. If this happens, the VHL protein can no longer be

made. Cell growth cannot be controlled and tumors develop. Mutations like this occur in various organs at various times, leading to multiple tumors forming in distinct parts of the body over a period of time.

The majority of patients with VHL syndrome inherited the mutation from one of their parents. In approximately 1–3% of cases, there is no family history of the disorder and VHL occurs because of a new mutation in the affected individual. If a person appears to be an isolated case, it is important that the parents have **genetic testing**. It is possible that a parent could carry the mutation in the VHL gene but have tumors that do not cause any noticeable symptoms. If a parent is affected, each of his or her future children would have a 50% of being affected with VHL. If both parents test negative for the VHL gene mutation, each future child has a 5% risk of inheriting VHL. This small risk is to account for the rare possibility that one parent carries the mutation in his or her sex cells (egg or sperm) but does not express the disorder in any of the other cells of the body.

## Demographics

VHL occurs in approximately one in 36,000 live births. It is seen in all ethnic groups and both sexes are affected equally.

**Adrenal gland**—A triangle-shaped endocrine gland, located above each kidney, that synthesizes aldosterone, cortisol, and testosterone from cholesterol. The adrenal glands are responsible for salt and water levels in the body, as well as for protein, fat, and carbohydrate metabolism.

**Angioma**—A benign tumor composed of blood vessels or lymph vessels.

**Benign**—A non-cancerous tumor that does not spread and is not life-threatening.

**Bilateral**—Relating to or affecting both sides of the body or both of a pair of organs.

**Broad ligament**—The ligament connecting the ovaries to the uterus.

**Computed tomography (CT) scan**—An imaging procedure that produces a three-dimensional picture of organs or structures inside the body, such as the brain.

**Cyst**—An abnormal sac or closed cavity filled with liquid or semisolid matter.

**Epididymus**—Coiled tubules that are the site of sperm storage and maturation for motility and fertility. The epididymis connects the testis to the vas deferens.

**Hemangioblastoma**—A tumor of the brain or spinal cord arising in the blood vessels of the meninges or brain.

**Hormone**—A chemical messenger produced by the body that is involved in regulating specific bodily functions such as growth, development, and reproduction.

**Magnetic resonance imaging (MRI)**—A technique that employs magnetic fields and radio waves to create detailed images of internal body structures and organs, including the brain.

**Mutation**—A permanent change in the genetic material that may alter a trait or characteristic of an individual, or manifest as disease, and can be transmitted to offspring.

**Pancreatic islet cell**—Cells located in the pancreas that serve to make certain types of hormones.

**Pheochromocytoma**—A small vascular tumor of the inner region of the adrenal gland. The tumor causes uncontrolled and irregular secretion of certain hormones.

**Renal cell carcinoma**—A cancerous tumor made from kidney cells.

**Retina**—The light-sensitive layer of tissue in the back of the eye that receives and transmits visual signals to the brain through the optic nerve.

## Signs and symptoms

There are several characteristic features of VHL but no single, unique finding. Thus, it is necessary that many different specialties be involved in the diagnosis and management of the disease. This approach will ensure proper, thorough care for these patients.

VHL is characterized by *hemangioblastomas*, tumors that arise in the blood vessel. These tumors are found in the central nervous system, or the brain and spinal cord. They most commonly present between the ages of 25 and 40 years and are the first symptom of VHL in 40% of cases. It is common to see multiple tumors. They may appear at the same time or at different times. These tumors generally grow slowly but, in some cases, may enlarge more rapidly. Hemangioblastomas seen in VHL are *benign* (non-cancerous) but may produce symptoms depending on their size, site, and number. Hemangioblastomas in the brain may lead to headache, vomiting, slurred speech, or unsteady and uncoordinated movements. These symptoms are usually due to the tumors disrupting brain function or causing increased pressure in the brain. Hemangioblastomas of the spine are usually accompanied by pain and can lead to loss of sensation and motor skills. Some of these tumors may fail to cause any observable symptoms.

In patients with VHL, hemangioblastomas also appear in the retina, the light-sensitive layer that lines the interior of the eye. These tumors occur in approximately half the cases of VHL and may be the first sign that a person is affected. It is common to see numerous retinal hemangioblastomas develop throughout a person's lifetime. They often can be found in both eyes. These tumors have been detected as early as the age of four years but are more typically found between the ages of 21 and 28 years. They often occur without symptoms, but can be detected on a routine eye exam. If untreated or undetected, they may cause the retina to detach from the eye. This condition is accompanied by bleeding and leads to vision loss and possibly blindness.

Approximately 50–70% of individuals with VHL also have numerous *cysts* on their kidneys. Cysts are sacs or closed cavities filled with liquid. In VHL, these cysts are vascular and frequently occur in both kidneys; however, they rarely result in noticeable symptoms. In some cases, these cysts may develop into *renal cell carcinomas*. These are cancerous tumors that are composed of kidney cells. Seventy percent of people affected with VHL will develop this type of kidney tumor during their lifetime. This type of cancer is generally diagnosed between the ages of 41 and 45 years. By the time this condition produces symptoms, it is likely that the cancer has already spread to other parts of the body. If this is the case, the tumors will respond poorly to chemotherapy and radiation, two common cancer treatments.

VHL can also cause multiple cysts in the pancreas. These occur at the average age of 41 years and are vascular in nature. Pancreatic cysts rarely cause problems and tend to grow fairly slowly. *Pancreatic islet cell tumors* can occur as well but are unrelated to the cysts. Islet cells in the pancreas produce *hormones*. Hormones are substances that are produced in one organ and then carried through the bloodstream to another organ where they perform a variety of functions. When tumors occur in the islet cells of the pancreas, these cells secrete too many hormones. This increase in hormones rarely leads to recognizable symptoms. Pancreatic islet cell tumors grow slowly and are non-cancerous.

Additionally, tumors in the adrenal gland, called *pheochromocytomas*, are common in VHL. The adrenal glands are located on top of each kidney. They secrete various hormones into the bloodstream. Pheochromocytomas are made of cells from the inner region of the adrenal gland. These tumors are benign but can be numerous and are often located in both adrenal glands. They can be confined to the inside of the adrenal gland or they can travel and appear outside of it. Some do not cause any observable symptoms. Others can lead to high blood pressure, sweating, and headaches.

In approximately 10% of cases, tumors can also be found in the inner ear. Most often, these tumors occur in both ears. They may lead to hearing loss of varying severity. This hearing loss may be one of the first signs that an individual is affected with VHL. Less commonly, a person may complain of dizziness or a ringing in the ear due to these inner ear tumors.

Men with VHL commonly have tumors in the *epididymus*. The epididymus is a structure that lies on top of the testis and serves as the site for sperm storage and maturation for motility and fertility. If these tumors occur bilaterally, they can lead to infertility. However, as a general rule, they do not result in any health problems. The equivalent tumor in females is one that occurs in the broad ligament. This ligament connects the ovaries to the uterus. These tumors, however, are much less common than those in the epididymus.

It is important to note that wide variation exists amoung all individuals affected with VHL in regards to the age of onset of the symptoms, the organ systems involved, and the severity of disease.

### Diagnosis

VHL can be diagnosed clinically, without genetic testing, in some cases. If a person has no family history of the disorder, a diagnosis of VHL can be made if one of the following criteria are met:

- the patient has two or more hemangioblastomas of the retina or CNS
- the patient has a single hemangioblastoma along with one of the other tumors or cysts that are commonly associated with the disorder.

A diagnosis of VHL can also be established in a person who has a positive a family history of the disorder if they show one or more of the following before the age of 60:

- retinal hemangioblastoma
- CNS hemangioblastoma
- pheochromocytoma
- multiple pancreatic cysts
- tumor of the epididymus
- multiple renal cysts
- renal cell carcinoma

Several tests are available that can assist in the diagnosis of VHL. They can also determine the extent of symptoms if the diagnosis has already been made. A computed tomography (CT) scan or magnetic resonance imaging (MRI) are often utilized for these purposes. These procedures serve to produce images of various soft tissues in the body, such as the brain and abdominal area. In someone with VHL, they are used to assess for the presence of CNS hemangioblastomas and other tumors associated with the disorder, such as pheochromocytomas and inner ear tumors. Pheochromocytomas may also cause abnormal substances to be released into the urine. A urinalysis can detect these substances and, therefore, suggest the existence of these tumors. Additionally, ultrasound examination can assist in evaluating the epididymus, broad ligament, and kidneys. Ultrasound examination involves the use of high frequency sound waves. These sound waves are directed into the body and the echoes of reflected sound are used to form an electronic image of various internal structures.

VHL can also be diagnosed via examination of the VHL gene on the molecular level. This type of testing detects approximately 100% of people who are affected with the disorder and is indicated for confirmation of the diagnosis in cases of suspected or known VHL. Molecular genetic testing examines the VHL gene and detects any mutations, or changes in the gene. Most often, in this disorder, the gene change involves a deletion of a part of the gene or a change in one of the bases that makes up the genetic code.

Since molecular testing is so accurate, it is recommended even in cases where the clinical criteria for diagnosis are not met. It is possible that the tumors associated with VHL are present but are not causing any observable symptoms. Thus, even if a person does not meet the diagnostic criteria mentioned above, molecular testing can be used as a means of "ruling out" VHL with a high degree of certainty. For patients with numerous, bilateral pheochromocytomas or for those who have a family history of these tumors, molecular testing is strongly suggested since these tumors may be the only signs of the disorder in those with VHL type 2C.

VHL can be diagnosed at various ages, ranging from infancy to the seventh decade of life or later. The age of diagnosis depends on the expression of the condition within the family and whether or not asymptomatic lesions are detected.

### Treatment and management

There is no treatment for VHL because the genetic defect cannot be fixed. Management focuses on routine surveillance of at-risk and affected individuals for early detection and treatment of tumors.

For at-risk relatives of individuals diagnosed with VHL, molecular genetic testing is recommended as part of the standard management. If a person tests negative for the mutation, costly screening procedures can be avoided. If an at-risk relative has not been tested for the mutation, surveillance is essential for the early detection of signs of VHL.

The following groups of people should be routinely monitored by a physician familiar with VHL:

- individuals diagnosed with VHL
- individuals who are asymptomatic but who have tested positive for a mutation in the VHL gene
- individuals who are at-risk due to a family history of the disorder but have not undergone molecular testing

For these groups of people, annual physical examinations are recommended, along with neurologic evaluation for signs of brain or spinal cord tumors. Additionally, an eye exam should be completed annually, beginning around the age of five years. These exams can detect retinal hemangioblastomas, which often produce no clinical symptoms until serious damage occurs. When a person reaches the age of 16, an abdominal ultrasound should be completed annually as well. Any suspicious findings should be followed up with a CT scan or MRI. If pheochromocytomas are in the family history, blood pressure should be monitored annually. A urinalysis should be completed annually as well, beginning at the age of five. Although the majority of tumors associated with VHL are benign in nature, they all have a small possibility of becoming cancerous. For this reason, surveillance and early detection is very important to the health of those affected with VHL.

If any tumors are identified by the above surveillance, close monitoring is necessary and surgical intervention may be recommended. Hemangioblastomas of the brain or spine may be removed before they cause symptoms. They may also be followed with yearly imaging studies and removed only after they begin to cause problems. Most of these tumors require surgical removal at some point and results are generally good. Retinal hemangioblastomas can be treated with various techniques that serve to decrease the size and number of these tumors.

Early surgery is recommended for renal cell carcinoma. Extreme cases may require removal of one or both kidneys, followed by a transplant. Additionally, pheochromocytomas should be surgically removed if they are causing symptoms. Inner ear tumors, however, generally are slow-growing. The benefit of removing one of these tumors must be carefully compared to the risk of **deafness**, which may result from the surgery. Epididymal and broad ligament tumors generally do not require surgery.

### Prognosis

The average life expectancy of an individual with VHL is 49 years. Renal cell carcinoma is the leading cause of death for affected individuals. If an affected person is diagnosed with renal cell carcinoma, their average life expectancy decreases to 44.5 years. CNS hemangioblastomas are responsible for a significant proportion of deaths in affected individuals as well, due to the effects of the tumor on the brain.

## Resources

### BOOKS

*The VHL Handbook: What You Need to Know About VHL.* Brookline, MA: VHL Family Alliance, 1999.

### PERIODICALS

Couch, Vicki, et al. "Von Hippel-Lindau Disease." *Mayo Clinic Proceedings* 75 (March 2000): 265-272.

Friedrich, Christopher A. "Von Hippel-Lindau Syndrome: A Pleiomorphic Condition." *Cancer* 86, no. 11 Supplement (December 1, 1999): 2478-2482.

### WEBSITES

Schimke, R. Neil, Debra Collins, and Catharine A. Stolle. "Von Hippel-Lindau Syndrome." *GeneClinics.*http://www.geneclinics.org/profiles/vhl/index.html.

"Von Hippel-Lindau Syndrome." *Genes and Disease.*http://www.ncbi.nlm.nih.gov/disease/VHL.html.

### ORGANIZATIONS

VHL Family Alliance. 171 Clinton Ave., Brookline, MA 02455-5815. (800) 767-4VHL. http://www.vhl.org.

Mary E. Freivogel, MS

# von Recklinghausen's neurofibromatosis

## Definition

von Recklinghausen's **neurofibromatosis** is also called von Recklinghausen disease, or simply neurofibromatosis (NF)1. It is an autosomal dominant hereditary disorder. NF is the most common neurological disorder caused by a single **gene**. Patients develop multiple soft tumors (neurofibromas) and very often skin spots (freckling AND café au lait spots). The tumors occur under the skin and throughout the nervous system. The disease is named for Friedrich Daniel von Recklinghausen (1833–

1910), a German pathologist, although cases of it have been described in European medical publications since the sixteenth century.

## Description

There are three types of neurofibromatosis, although some researchers have proposed as many as eight categories. The two main types of neurofibromatosis are neurofibromatosis 1 (NF1), which affects about 85% of patients diagnosed with neurofibromatosis, and neurofibromatosis 2 (NF2), which accounts for another 10% of patients. NF1 affects approximately 1 in 2,000 to 1 in 5,000 births worldwide. NF2 affects 1 in 35,000 to 1 in 40,000 births worldwide. Recently, schwannomatosis has been recognized as a rare form of NF. Since NF is the most common neurological disorder, NF is more prevalent than the number of people affected by **cystic fibrosis**, hereditary **muscular dystrophy**, Huntington's disease, and **Tay-Sachs disease** combined. In addition to skin and nervous system tumors and skin freckling, NF can lead to disfigurement, blindness, **deafness**, skeletal abnormalities, loss of limbs, malignancies, and learning disabilities. The degree a person is affected with a form of neurofibromatosis may vary greatly between patients.

## Causes and symptoms

A defective gene causes NF1 and NF2. NF1 is due to a defect on **chromosome** 17q. NF2 results from a defect on chromosome 22. Both neurofibromatosis disorders are inherited in an autosomal dominant fashion. In an autosomal dominant disease, one copy of a defective gene will cause the disease. However, family pattern of NF is only evident for about 50% to 70% of all NF cases. The remaining cases of NF are due to a spontaneous mutation (a change in a person's gene rather than a mutation inherited from a parent). As with an inherited mutated gene, a person with a spontaneously mutated gene has a 50% chance of passing the spontaneously mutated gene to any offspring.

NF1 has a number of possible symptoms:

- Five or more light brown skin spots (café au lait spots, a French term meaning "coffee with milk"). The skin spots measure more than 0.2 inches (5 millimeters) in diameter in patients under the age of puberty or more than 0.6 inches (15 millimeters) in diameter across in adults and children over the age of puberty. Nearly all NF1 patients display café au lait spots.

- Multiple freckles in the armpit or groin area.

**Audiometry**—Testing a person's hearing by exposing ear to sounds in a soundproof room.

**Autosomal dominant**—Genetic information on a single non-sex chromosome that is expressed with only one copy of a gene. Child of an affected parent has a 50% chance of inheriting an autosomal dominant gene.

**Cancer**—Abnormal and uncontrolled growth of cells that can invade surrounding tissues and other parts of the body. Although some cancers are treatable, recurrence and death from cancer can occur.

**Cataract**—Lens of eye loses transparency and becomes cloudy. Cloudiness blocks light rays entering the eye that may lead to blindness.

**Chromosome**—A structure within the nucleus of every cell, that contains genetic information governing the organism's development. There are 22 non-sex chromosomes and one sex chromosome.

**Ependymoma**—Tumor that grows from cells that line the cavities of brain ventricles and spinal cord.

**Gamma knife**—A type of highly focused radiation therapy.

**Gene**—Piece of information contained on a chromosome. A chromosome is made of many genes.

**Magnetic resonance imaging**—Magnetic resonance imaging (MRI) measures the response of tissues to magnetic fields to produce detailed pictures of the body, including the brain.

**Meningioma**—Tumor that grows from the protective brain and spinal cord membrane cells (meninges).

**Mutation**—A permanent change to the genetic code of an organism. Once established, a mutation can be passed on to offspring.

**Neurofibroma**—A soft tumor usually located on a nerve.

**Radiation therapy**—Exposing tumor cells to controlled doses of x-ray irradiation for treatment. Although tumor cells are susceptible to irradiation, surrounding tissues will also be damaged. Radiation therapy alone rarely cures a tumor, but can be useful when used in conjunction with other forms of therapy or when a patient cannot tolerate other forms of therapy.

**Schwannoma**—Tumor that grows from the cells that line the nerves of the body (Schwann cells).

**Tinnitus**—Noises in the ear that can include ringing, whistling or booming.

**Tumor**—An abnormally multiplying mass of cells. Tumors that invade surrounding tissues and other parts of the body are malignant and considered a cancer. Non-malignant tumors do not invade surrounding tissues and other parts of the body. Malignant and non-malignant tumors can cause severe symptoms and death.

- Ninety percent of patients with NF1 have tiny tumors in the iris (colored area of the eye) called Lisch nodules (iris nevi).

- Two or more neurofibromas distributed over the body. Neurofibromas are soft tumors and are the hallmark of NF1. Neurofibromas occur under the skin, often located along nerves or within the gastrointestinal tract. Neurofibromas are small and rubbery, and the skin overlying them may be somewhat purple in color.

- Skeletal deformities, such as a twisted spine (scoliosis), curved spine (humpback), or bowed legs.

- Tumors along the optic nerve, which cause visual disturbances in about 20% of patients.

- The presence of NF1 in a patient's parent, child, or sibling.

There are very high rates of speech impairment, learning disabilities, and attention deficit disorder in children with NF1. Other complications include the development of a seizure disorder, or the abnormal accumulation of fluid within the brain (**hydrocephalus**). A number of cancers are more common in patients with NF1. These include a variety of types of malignant brain tumors, as well as leukemia, and cancerous tumors of certain muscles (rhabdomyosarcoma), the adrenal glands (pheochromocytoma), or the kidneys (Wilms' tumor). Symptoms are often visible at birth or during infancy, and almost always by the time a child is about 10 years old.

In contrast to patients with NF1, patients with NF2 have few, if any, café au lait spots or tumors under the skin. Patients with NF2 most commonly have tumors (schwannomas) on the eighth cranial nerve (one of 12 pairs of nerves that enter or emerge from the brain), and occasionally on other nerves. The location of the schwann cell derived tumors determines the effect on the body. The characteristic symptoms of NF2 include dysfunction in hearing, ringing in the ears (tinnitus), and body balance. The common

## QUESTIONS TO ASK YOUR DOCTOR

- How can I tell if I have neurofibromatosis?
- Which type of neurofibromatosis do I have?
- Will I develop tumors? Will they be cancerous?
- Is my neurofibromatosis genetic?
- What medical tests are important?
- What treatments are available for neurofibromatosis?
- Will I die from neurofibromatosis?

characteristic symptoms of NF2 are due to tumors along the acoustic and vestibular branches of the eighth cranial nerve. Tumors that occur on neighboring nervous system structures may cause weakness of the muscles of the face, headache, dizziness, numbness, and weakness in an arm or leg. Cloudy areas on the lens of the eye (called cataracts) frequently develop at an early age. As in NF1, the chance of brain tumors developing is unusually high. Symptoms of NF2 may not begin until after puberty.

Multiple schwannomas on cranial, spinal, and peripheral nerves characterize schwannomatosis. People with schwannomatosis usually have greater problems with pain than with neurological disability. The first symptom of schwannomatosis is usually pain in any part of the body without any source. It can be several years before a tumor is found. About 1/3 of patients with schwannomatosis have tumors in a single part of the body, such as an arm, leg or segment of spine. People with schwannomatosis do not develop vestibular tumors, any other kinds of tumors (such as meningiomas, ependymomas, or astrocytomas), do not go deaf, and do not have learning disabilities.

### Diagnosis

Diagnosis of a form of neurofibromatosis is based on the symptoms outlined above. Although a visual inspection may be sufficient for inspection of tumors for a clinical diagnosis of neurofibromatosis, magnetic resonance imaging (MRI) is the most useful type of imaging study for early diagnosis of tumors while CT scans are better for detecting skeletal abnormalities. Diagnosis of NF1 requires that at least two of the above listed symptoms are present. A slit lamp is used to visualize the presence of any Lisch nodules in a person's eye. A person with a parent, sibling, or child with NF1 is another tool used to diagnose a person with NF1.

NF2 can be diagnosed three different ways and with symptoms different from NF1 symptoms:

- The presence of bilateral cranial eighth nerve tumors.
- A person who has a parent, sibling, or child with NF2 and a unilateral eighth nerve tumor (vestibular schwannoma or acoustic neuroma).
- A person who has a parent, sibling, or child with NF2 and any two of the following: glioma, meningioma, neurofibroma, schwannoma, or an early age cataract.

The presence of multiple schwannomas may be a symptom of NF2 or schwannomatosis. An older person with multiple schwannomas and no hearing loss probably does not have NF2. A high-quality MRI scan should be used to detect any possible vestibular tumors to differentiate between NF2 and schwannomatosis in a younger person with multiple schwannomas or any person with hearing loss and multiple schwannomas.

In prepubertal children a yearly assessment including blood pressure measurement, eye examination, development screening, and neurologic examination is recommended.

Monitoring the progression of neurofibromatosis involves careful testing of vision and hearing (audiometry). X-ray studies of the bones are frequently done to watch for the development of deformities. CT scans and MRI scans are performed to track the development/progression of tumors in the brain and along the nerves. Auditory evoked potentials (the electric response evoked in the cerebral cortex by stimulation of the acoustic nerve) may be helpful to determine involvement of the acoustic nerve, and EEG (electroencephalogram, a record of electrical currents in the brain) may be needed for patients with suspected seizures.

### Treatment

There are no cures for any form of neurofibromatosis. To some extent, the symptoms of NF1 and NF2 can be treated individually. Skin tumors can be surgically removed. Some brain tumors, and tumors along the nerves, can be surgically removed, or treated with drugs (chemotherapy) or x-ray treatments (radiation therapy, including gamma knife therapy). Twisting or curving of the spine and bowed legs may require surgical treatment or the wearing of a special brace.

### Prognosis

Prognosis varies depending on the types of tumors which an individual develops. In general, however, patients with neurofibromatosis have a shortened life expectancy; the average age at death is 55–59 years, compared with 70–74 years for the general United States population. As tumors grow, they begin to destroy surrounding nerves and structures. Ultimately, this destruction can result in blindness, deafness, increasingly poor balance, and increasing difficulty with the coordination necessary for walking. Deformities of the bones and spine can also interfere with walking and movement. When cancers develop, prognosis worsens according to the specific type of **cancer**.

## Clinical Trials

As of 2004 the National Cancer Institute (NCI) is sponsoring one clinical trial for children with neurofibromatosis type 1. The trial is an evaluation of tipifarnib (Zarnestra), a drug that inactivates certain proteins that encourage tumor growth. It is hoped that tipifarnib may prove to be an effective drug treatment for the disorder, as surgery is presently considered the only standard treatment.

The use of an auditory brainstem implant (ABI) as part of hearing rehabilitation in patients with NF2 has been tested in Europe and the United States.

## Prevention

There is no known way to prevent the cases of NF that are due to a spontaneous change in the genes (mutation). Since genetic tests for NF1 and NF2 are available, new cases of inherited NF can be prevented with careful **genetic counseling**. A person with NF can be made to understand that each of his or her offspring has a 50% chance of also having NF. When a parent has NF, and the specific genetic defect causing the parent's disease has been identified, prenatal tests can be performed on the fetus during pregnancy. **Amniocentesis** and chorionic villus sampling are two techniques that allow small amounts of the baby's cells to be removed for examination. The tissue can then be examined for the presence of the parent's genetic defect. Some families choose to use this information in order to prepare for the arrival of a child with a serious medical problem. Other families may choose not to continue the pregnancy. **Genetic testing** may also be useful for evaluating individuals with a family history of neurofibromatosis, who do not yet show symptoms.

## Resources

### BOOKS

Beers, Mark H., MD, and Robert Berkow, MD, editors. "Disorders of the Peripheral Nervous System." Section 14, Chapter 183 In*The Merck Manual of Diagnosis and Therapy*. Whitehouse Station, NJ: Merck Research Laboratories, 2002.

### PERIODICALS

Bance, M., and R.T. Ramsden. "Management of Neurofibromatosis Type 2." *Ear Nose & Throat Journal* 78, no. 2 (1999): 91–4.

Evans, D.G. "Neurofibromatosis Type 2: Genetic and Clinical Features." *Ear Nose & Throat Journal* 78, no. 2 (1999): 97–100.

Gillespie, J.E. "Imaging in Neurofibromatosis Type 2: Screening Using Magnetic Resonance Imaging." *Ear Nose & Throat Journal* 78, no. 2 (1999): 102–9.

Huson, S.M. "What Level of Care for the Neurofibromatoses?" *Lancet* 353, no. 9159 (1999): 1114–6.

Khan, Ali Nawaz, MBBS, and Ian Turnbull, MD. "Neurofibromatosis Type 1." *eMedicine* February 10, 2004. http://emedicine.com/radio/topic474.htm.

Laszig, R., et al. "Central Electrical Stimulation of the Auditory Pathway in Neurofibromatosis Type 2." *Ear Nose & Throat Journal* 78, no. 2 (1999): 110–7.

Lynch, H. T., T. G. Shaw, and J. F. Lynch. "Inherited Predisposition to Cancer: A Historical Overview." *American Journal of Medical Genetics, Part C: Seminars in Medical Genetics* 129 (August 15, 2004): 5–22.

Rasmussen, S.A., and J.M. Friedman. "NF1 Gene and Neurofibromatosis." *American Journal of Epidemiology* 151, no. 1 (2000): 33–40.

### ORGANIZATIONS

Acoustic Neuroma Association. 600 Peachtree Parkway, Suite 108, Cumming, GA, 30041-6899. (770) 205-8211. http://www.anausa.org.

March of Dimes Birth Defects Foundation. National Office, 1275 Mamaroneck Ave., White Plains, NY 10605. http://www.modimes.org.

Massachusetts General Hospital Neurofibromatosis Clinic. Harvard Medical School, Massachusetts General Hospital, Boston, MA 02114. (617) 724-7856. http://neurosurgery.mgh.harvard.edu/NFclinic.htm.

National Cancer Institute. Information Office, Building 31, Room 10A03, 9000 Rockville Pike, Bethesda, MD, 20892-2580. (800) 4-CANCER. http://cancernet.nci.nih.gov.

National Institute of Child Health and Human Development. Building 31, Room 2A32, MSC 2425, 31 Center Dr., Bethesda, MD, 20892. (800) 370-2943. http://www.nichd.nih.gov.

National Institute of Neurological Disorders and Stroke. Office of Communications and Public Liaison, PO Box 5801, Bethesda, MD, 20824. (800) 352-9424. http://www.ninds.nih.gov. National Organization focused on neurological biomedical research.

The National Neurofibromatosis Foundation, Inc.(NNF). 95 Pine St., 16th Floor, New York, NY 10005. (800) 323-7938. http://www.nf.org.

Neurofibromatosis Association (NFA). 82 London Road, Kingston upon Thames, Surrey KT2 6PX. 0208 547 1636. e-mail: nfa@zetnet.co.uk. http://www.nfa.zetnet.co.uk.

Neurofibromatosis, Inc. 8855 Annapolis Rd., #110, Lanham, MD 20706-2924. (800) 942-6825. http://www.nfinc.org.

Rosalyn S. Carson-DeWitt, M.D.
Laura Ruth, Ph.D.
Rebecca J. Frey, Ph.D.

# von Willebrand disease

## Definition

von Willebrand disease is caused by a deficiency or an abnormality in a protein called von Willebrand factor and is characterized by prolonged bleeding.

## Description

The Finnish physician Erik von Willebrand was the first to describe von Willebrand disease (VWD). In 1926 Dr. von Willebrand noticed that many male and female members of a large family from the Aland Islands had increased bruising (bleeding into the skin) and prolonged episodes of bleeding. The severity of the bleeding varied between family members and ranged from mild to severe and typically involved the mouth, nose, genital and urinary tracts, and occasionally the intestinal tract. Excessive bleeding during the menstrual period was also experienced by some of the women in this family. What differentiated this bleeding disorder from classical **hemophilia** was that it appeared not to be associated with muscle and joint bleeding and affected women and men rather than just men. Dr. von Willebrand named this disorder *hereditary pseudohemophilia*.

Pseudohemophilia, or von Willebrand disease (VWD) as it is now called, is caused when the body does not produce enough of a protein called von Willebrand factor (vWF) or produces abnormal vWF. vWF is involved in the process of blood clotting (coagulation). Blood clotting is necessary to heal an injury to a blood vessel. When a blood vessel is injured, vWF enables blood cells called platelets to bind to the injured area and form a temporary plug to seal the hole and stop the bleeding. vWF is secreted by platelets and by the cells that line the inner wall of the blood vessels (endothelial cells). The platelets release other chemicals, called factors, in response to a blood vessel injury, which are involved in forming a strong permanent clot. vWF binds to and stabilizes factor VIII, one of the factors involved in forming the permanent clot.

A deficiency or abnormality in vWF can interfere with the formation of the temporary platelet plug and also affect the normal survival of factor VIII, which can indirectly interfere with the production of the permanent clot. Individuals with

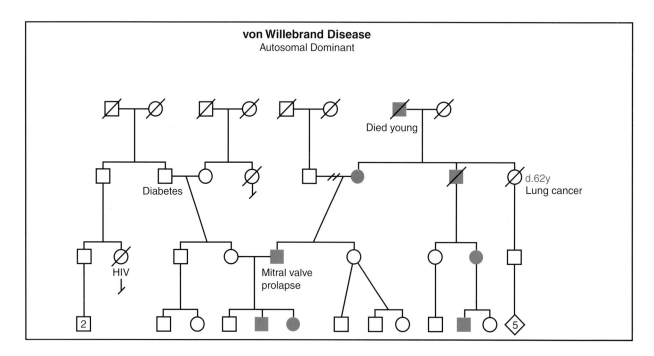

*(Gale, a part of Cengage Learning.)*

**Amniocentesis**—A procedure performed at 16-18 weeks of pregnancy in which a needle is inserted through a woman's abdomen into her uterus to draw out a small sample of the amniotic fluid from around the baby. Either the fluid itself or cells from the fluid can be used for a variety of tests to obtain information about genetic disorders and other medical conditions in the fetus.

**Autosomal dominant**—A pattern of genetic inheritance where only one abnormal gene is needed to display the trait or disease.

**Autosomal recessive**—A pattern of genetic inheritance where two abnormal genes are needed to display the trait or disease.

**Biochemical testing**—Measuring the amount or activity of a particular enzyme or protein in a sample of blood or urine or other tissue from the body.

**Carrier**—A person who possesses a gene for an abnormal trait without showing signs of the disorder. The person may pass the abnormal gene on to offspring.

**Chorionic villus sampling (CVS)**—A procedure used for prenatal diagnosis at 10-12 weeks gestation. Under ultrasound guidance a needle is inserted either through the mother's vagina or abdominal wall and a sample of cells is collected from around the fetus. These cells are then tested for chromosome abnormalities or other genetic diseases.

**Chromosome**—A microscopic thread-like structure found within each cell of the body that consists of a complex of proteins and DNA. Humans have 46 chromosomes arranged into 23 pairs. Changes in either the total number of chromosomes or their shape and size (structure) may lead to physical or mental abnormalities.

**Deoxyribonucleic acid (DNA)**—The genetic material in cells that holds the inherited instructions for growth, development, and cellular functioning.

**Desmopressin (DDAVP)**—A drug used in the treatment of von Willebrand's disease.

**Diagnostic testing**—Testing performed to determine if someone is affected with a particular disease.

**DNA testing**—Analysis of DNA (the genetic component of cells) in order to determine changes in genes that may indicate a specific disorder.

**Endothelial cells**—The cells lining the inner walls of the blood vessels.

**Factor VIII**—A protein involved in blood clotting that requires vWF for stability and long-term survival in the bloodstream.

**Gene**—A building block of inheritance, which contains the instructions for the production of a particular protein, and is made up of a molecular sequence found on a section of DNA. Each gene is found on a precise location on a chromosome.

**Mutation**—A permanent change in the genetic material that may alter a trait or characteristic of an individual, or manifest as disease, and can be transmitted to offspring.

**Platelets**—Small disc-shaped structures that circulate in the bloodstream and participate in blood clotting.

**Prenatal testing**—Testing for a disease such as a genetic condition in an unborn baby.

**Protein**—Important building blocks of the body, composed of amino acids, involved in the formation of body structures and controlling the basic functions of the human body.

**Skin hematoma**—Blood from a broken blood vessel that has accumulated under the skin.

**von Willebrand factor (vWF)**—A protein found in the blood that is involved in the process of blood clotting.

---

VWD, therefore, have difficulty in forming blood clots and as a result they may bleed for longer periods of time. In most cases the bleeding is due to an obvious injury, although it can sometimes occur spontaneously.

VWD is classified into three basic types: type 1, 2, and 3 based on the amount and type of vWF that is produced. Type 1 is the most common and mildest form and results when the body produces slightly decreased amounts of typically normal vWF. Type 2 can be classified into five subtypes (A, B, M, N) and results when the body produces an abnormal type of vWF. Type 3 is the rarest and most severe form and results when the body does not produce any detectable vWF.

### Genetic profile

The **genetics** of VWD are complex and involve a gene that produces vWF and is found on **chromosome** 12. Since individuals inherit two of each type of chromosome, they inherit two vWF genes. There are different types of changes in the vWF gene that can affect the production of vWF. Some types of changes can cause the vWF gene to produce decreased amounts of normal vWF, while other changes can cause the gene to produce abnormal vWF. Most of the gene changes are significant enough that a change in only one vWF gene is sufficient to cause VWD. Some gene changes only cause VWD if both genes are changed, which often leads to more severe symptoms. Type 1 VWD is called an autosomal dominant condition since it is caused by a change in only one vWF gene. Since type 1 VWD results in only a slight decrease in the amount of vWF produced, the symptoms are often mild and even nonexistent in some patients. Most cases of Type 2 VWD are autosomal dominant since they are caused by a change in only one vWF gene that results in the production of an abnormal protein. An autosomal dominant form of VWD can be inherited from either parent or can occur spontaneously in the embryo that is formed when the egg and sperm cells come together during fertilization.

Some cases of type 2 VWD and all cases of type 3 VWD are autosomal recessive since they are caused by changes in both vWF genes. A person with an autosomal recessive form of VWD has inherited a changed gene from his or her mother and a changed gene from his or her father. Parents who have a child with an autosomal recessive form of VWD are called carriers, since they each possess one changed vWF gene and one unchanged vWF gene. Many carriers for the autosomal recessive forms of type 2 VWD and type 3 VWD do not have any symptoms, although some people with type 3 VWD are born to parents who have type 1 VWD and may have symptoms. Each child born to parents who are both carriers for VWD has a 25% chance of having VWD, a 50% chance of being a carrier, and a 25% chance of being neither a carrier nor affected with VWD disease. A person with an autosomal dominant form of VWD has a 50% chance of passing the changed gene on to his or her children who may or may not have symptoms.

## Demographics

Approximately one out of 100 people are affected with VWD, making it the most common inherited bleeding disorder (hemophilia). VWD affects people of all ethnic backgrounds. Approximately 70–80% of people with VWD have type 1 and close to 20–30% have type 2. Type 3 is very rare and occurs in less than one percent of people with VWD.

## Signs and symptoms

VWD is usually a relatively mild disorder characterized by easy bruising, recurrent nosebleeds, heavy menstrual periods, and extended bleeding after surgeries and invasive dental work. There is a great deal of variability in the severity of symptoms, which can range from clinically insignificant to life threatening. Even people within the same family who are affected with the same type of VWD may exhibit different symptoms. An individual with VWD may exhibit a range of symptoms over the course of his or her lifetime and may experience an improvement in symptoms with age. The severity of the disease is partially related to the amount and type of vWF that the body produces, but is also influenced by other genetic and nongenetic factors.

### Type 1

Type 1, the mildest form of VWD, is usually associated with easy bruising, recurrent nosebleeds, heavy menstrual periods, and prolonged bleeding after surgeries and invasive work. Many people with type 1 VWD do not have any noticeable symptoms or only have prolonged bleeding after surgery or significant trauma. The amount of vWF produced by the body increases during pregnancy, so prolonged bleeding during delivery is uncommon in people with type 1 VWD.

### Type 2

People with type 2 VWD usually have symptoms from early childhood and symptoms may even be present at birth. They usually experience prolonged bleeding from cuts, easy bruising, nose bleeds, skin hematomas, and prolonged bleeding from the gums following teeth extraction and minor trauma. More than 50% of women with type 2 VWD experience heavy periods that may require a blood transfusion. Gastrointestinal bleeding is rare but can be life-threatening. Some women with type 2 VWD exhibit prolonged bleeding during delivery.

### Type 3

Type 3 VWD can be quite severe and is associated with bruising and bleeding from the mouth, nose, intestinal, genital and urinary tracts. Type 3 is also associated with spontaneous bleeding into the muscles and joints, which can result in joint deformities. Some women with type 3 VWD experience prolonged bleeding during delivery.

## Diagnosis

### Diagnostic testing

Many people with VWD have mild symptoms or symptoms that can be confused with other bleeding disorders making it difficult to diagnose VWD on the basis of clinical symptoms. VWD should be suspected in any person with a normal number of platelets in their blood and bleeding from the mucous membranes such as the nose, gums and gastrointestinal tract. Testing for an individual with suspected VWD often includes the measurement of:

- how long it takes for the bleeding to stop after a tiny cut is made in the skin (the bleeding time)
- the amount of vWF (vWF antigen measurement)
- the activity of vWF (ristocetin co-factor activity)
- the amount of factor VIII (factor VIII antigen measurement)
- activity of factor VIII

People with type 1 VWD usually have an increased bleeding time but they may have an intermittently normal bleeding time. They also have a decreased amount of vWF, decreased vWF activity, and usually have slightly decreased factor VIII levels and activity. People with type 2 VWD have a prolonged bleeding time, decreased activity of vWF, and may have decreased amounts of vWF and factor VIII, and decreased factor VIII activity. Type 3 individuals have undetectable amounts of vWF, negligible vWF activity, factor VIII levels of less than 5–10%, and significantly reduced factor VIII activity. The activity of vWF is reduced for all types of VWD, making it the most sensitive means of identifying all three types of VWD. Patients with borderline results should be tested two to three times over a three month period.

Once a patient is diagnosed with VWD, further testing such as vWF multimer analysis and ristocetin-induced platelet aggregation (RIPA) may need to be performed to determine the subtype. Multimer analysis evaluates the structure of the vWF, and RIPA measures how much ristocetin is required to cause the clumping of platelets in a blood sample. The vWF multimer analysis is able to differentiate people with a structurally normal vWF (type 1) from people with a structurally abnormal vWF (type 2) and is often able to identify the subtype of patients with type 2 VWD. People with type 1 VWD usually have normal to decreased RIPA concentrations. Depending on the subtype, patients with type 2 VWD either have increased or decreased RIPA. RIPA is usually absent and the multimer analysis shows undetectable vWF in people with type 3 VWD.

In some cases **DNA** testing can be a valuable adjunct to biochemical testing. The detection of gene alteration(s) can confirm a diagnosis and can determine the type and subtype of VWD. It can also help to facilitate prenatal testing and testing of other family members. Unfortunately, as of 2001, many people with VWD possess DNA changes that are not detectable through DNA testing. A person who has a mother, father, or sibling diagnosed with VWD should undergo biochemical testing for VWD. If the relative with VWD possesses a detectable gene change, then DNA testing should also be considered.

### Prenatal testing

If one parent has been diagnosed with an autosomal dominant form of VWD or both parents are carriers for an autosomal recessive form of VWD, then prenatal testing can be considered. If the parent with an autosomal dominant form of VWD possesses a detectable gene change or both parents who are carriers for an autosomal recessive form of VWD possess detectable mutations, then DNA testing of their fetus would be available. DNA testing can be performed through **amniocentesis** or chorionic villus sampling. If the DNA change in the parent(s) is unknown then prenatal testing can sometimes be performed through biochemical testing of blood obtained from the fetal umbilical cord, which is less accurate and is associated with a higher risk of pregnancy loss.

## Treatment and management

VWD is most commonly treated by replacement of vWF through the administration of blood products that contain vWF or through treatment with desmopressin (DDAVP, 1-deamino-8-D-arginine vasopressin). DDAVP functions by increasing the amount of factor VIII and vWF in the bloodstream. Treatment with blood products or DDAVP may be started in response to uncontrollable bleeding or may be administered prior to procedures such as surgeries or dental work. The type of treatment chosen depends on the type of VWD and a patient's response to a preliminary treatment trial.

### Treatment with desmopressin

DDAVP is the most common treatment for people with type 1 VWD. About 80% of people with type 1 VWD respond to DDAVP therapy. Treatment with DDAVP can also be used to treat some people with type 2 VWD. Patients with Type 2B VWD should not be treated with this medication since DDAVP can induce dangerous platelet clumping. Type 3 VWD should not be treated with DDAVP since this medication does not increase the level of vWF in type 3 patients. DDAVP should only be used in people who have been shown to be responsive through a pre-treatment trial transfusion with this medication.

DDAVP can be administered intravenously or through a nasal inhaler. DDAVP has relatively few side effects although some people may experience facial flushing, tingling sensations, and headaches after treatment with this medication. Often treatment with this medication is only required prior to invasive surgeries or dental procedures.

### Treatment with blood products

Patients who are unable to tolerate or are unresponsive to drug-based treatments are treated with concentrated factor VIII obtained from blood products. Not all factor VIII concentrates can be used since some do not contain enough vWF. The concentrate is treated to kill most viruses, although caution should be used since not all types of viruses are destroyed. If the factor VIII concentrates are unable to manage a severe bleeding episode, then blood products called cryoprecipitates, which contain concentrated amounts of vWF, or platelet concentrates should be considered. Caution should be used when treating with these blood products since they are not treated to kill viruses.

### Other treatments and precautions

Medications called fibrinolytic inhibitors can be helpful in the control of intestinal, mouth, and nose bleeding. Estrogens such as are found in oral contraceptives increase the synthesis of vWF and can sometimes be used in the long-term treatment of women with mild to moderate VWD. Estrogens are also sometimes used prior to surgery in women with type 1 VWD. Some topical agents are available to treat nose and mouth bleeds. Patients with VWD should avoid taking aspirin, which can increase their susceptibility to bleeding and people with severe forms of VWD should avoid activities that increase their risk of injury such as contact sports.

### Prognosis

The prognosis for VWD disease is generally fairly good and most individuals have a normal life span. The prognosis can depend, however, on accurate diagnosis and appropriate medical treatment.

## QUESTIONS TO ASK YOUR DOCTOR

- What are the risks and benefits of DDAVP therapy?
- In DDAVP therapy, do you recommend the intravenous or nasal inhaler mode of treatment?
- How can nasal and mouth bleeding be managed?
- In addition to avoiding aspirin, should other drugs be avoided?

### Resources

**BOOKS**

Handin, Robert I. "Disorders of the Platelet and Vessel Wall." *Harrison's Principles of Internal Medicine.* Ed. Anthony S. Fauci, et al. New York: McGraw-Hill, 1998.

Sadler, J.E. "Von Willebrand Disease." *The Metabolic and Molecular Basis of Inherited Disease.* Ed. C.R. Scriver, et al. New York: McGraw Hill, 1995.

**PERIODICALS**

Ginsburg, David. "Molecular Genetics of von Willebrand Disease." *Thrombosis and Haemostasis* 82, no. 2 (1999): 585–591.

Nichols, William C., and David Ginsburg. "Von Willebrand's Disease." *Medicine* 76 (Jan. 1997): 1.

Voelker, Rebecca. "New Focus on von Willebrand's Disease." *Journal of the American Medical Association* 278 (October 8, 1997): 1137.

**OTHER**

Mannucci, Pier. "Desmopressin (DDAVP) in the Treatment of Bleeding Disorders: The First Twenty Years." *The Treatment of Hemophilia Monograph Series* no. 11 (1998). http://www.wfh.org/InformationAboutHemophilia/Publications/Monographs/Treatment_Series/TOH_PDF/TOH11_DDAVP.pdf.

Paper, Renee. "Gynecological Complications in Women with Bleeding Disorders." *The Treatment of Hemophilia Monograph Series* no. 5 (1996). http://www.wfh.org/InformationAboutHemophilia/Publications/Monographs/Treatment_Series/TOH_PDF/TOH5_VWD.pdf.

World Federation of Hemophilia. "Protocols for the Treatment of Hemophilia and von Willebrand Disease." No. 14 (1998). http://www.wfh.org/InformationAboutHemophilia/Publications/Monographs/Treatment_Series/TOH_PDF/TOH14_Protocols_Treatment.pdf.

**ORGANIZATIONS**

Canadian Hemophilia Society. 625 President Kennedy, Suite 1210, Montreal, QUE H3A 1K2. Canada (514) 848-0503. Fax: (514) 848-9661. chs@hemophilia.ca. http://www.hemophilia.ca/english/index.html.

Haemophelia Society—Von Willebrand Support Services. Chesterfield House, 385 Euston Road, London, NW1 3AU. UK 0171 380 0600. Fax: 0171 387 8220. melissa@haemophilia-soc.demon.co.uk. http://www.haemophilia-soc.demon.co.uk/vwd%20services1.html.

National Hemophilia Foundation. Soho Building, 110 Greene Street, Suite 406, New York, NY 10012. (212) 219-8180. http://www.hemophilia.org/home.htm.

Lisa Maria Andres, MS, CGC

## Vrolik type of osteogenesis imperfecta *see* Osteogenesis imperfecta

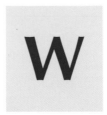

# Waardenburg syndrome

## Definition

Waardenburg syndrome (WS) encompasses several different hereditary disorders, the main features of which variably include abnormal pigmentation, hearing loss, and a subtle difference in facial features. Certain other physical anomalies occur less frequently in WS.

## Description

In 1951, Dr. Petrus Waardenburg reported a syndrome of dystopia canthorum, heterochromia of the irides, and hearing loss. Dystopia canthorum (also called telecanthus) describes a subtle but unusual facial feature in which the inner corners of the eyes (canthi) are spaced farther apart than normal, yet the eyes (pupils) themselves are normally spaced. The result is that the eyes appear to be widely spaced, even though they are not. Heterochromia means different-colored, and irides is the plural form of iris—the colored portion of the eye. Thus, someone with heterochromia of the irides has different-colored eyes, often one brown and one blue. Another feature not originally noted by Dr. Waardenburg, but now considered a major sign of WS is a white forelock (white patch of hair extending back from the front of the scalp). In fact, disturbances in pigmentation (coloring) of various parts of the body are consistent features of WS. Uncommon but serious physical anomalies associated with WS include **Hirschsprung disease** (intestinal malformation), **spina bifida**, cleft lip/palate, and musculoskeletal abnormalities of the arms.

Five types of WS have been defined based on clinical symptoms or genetic linkage. Six different genes are associated with WS. Most families show autosomal dominant **inheritance**, but autosomal recessive inheritance and sporadic (single) cases are also seen. People with WS are not at increased risk for mental retardation, and vision loss is not more common. For the majority of those with WS, hearing loss is the only major medical problem they will have.

WS1 is the "classic" form of WS, and if someone uses just the name Waardenburg syndrome (with no modifying number), they are most likely referring to the group of disorders as a whole or just WS1. WS2 may occasionally be referred to as WS without dystopia canthorum. WS3 is also known as Klein-Waardenburg syndrome, as well as WS with upper limb anomalies. Alternate names for WS4 include Waardenburg-Hirschsprung disease, Waardenburg-Shah syndrome, Shah-Waardenburg syndrome, and Hirschsprung disease with pigmentary anomaly.

## Genetic profile

Since Dr. Waardenburg's original description of his patients in 1951, many more families with the same or similar symptoms have been reported. By 1971, it became clear that a proportion of families have WS without dystopia canthorum. At that point, Waardenburg syndrome was divided into two distinct types, WS1 and WS2. In addition, a few individuals with typical signs of WS1 were found to also have musculoskeletal symptoms. This form of the disorder was named Klein-Waardenburg syndrome, now also known as WS3. Further, some researchers noted yet a different pattern of anomalies involving pigmentation defects and Hirschsprung disease, which eventually became known as WS4. Finally, **genetic testing** of WS2 families has shown at least two subtypes—those that show genetic linkage are designated as WS2A and WS2B.

The four major types of WS have all been studied through **DNA** (genetic) analysis. There is some agreement between the clinical subtypes of WS and mutations in different genes, but genetic analysis has also served to confuse the naming scheme somewhat. The different types of WS, their inheritance patterns, and the genes associated with them, are listed below.

**Waardenburg Syndrome**

| Type | Inheritance | Gene | Chromosome | Demographics | Symptoms |
|------|-------------|------|------------|--------------|----------|
| WS 1 | AD | PAX3 | 2 | 1 in 40,000 for all types; WS 3 and WS 4 are less common than WS 1 and WS 2 | Dystopia canthorum (99%); Medial flare of eyebrow or joining of eyebrows in the middle (70%); Hypopigmentation of skin, hair, and/or irides; Heterochromia of irides (30%); Hearing loss (60%) |
| WS 2A | AD | MITF | 3 | | Same symptoms as WS 1, but without dystopia conthorum; Incidence of symptoms varies from WS 1, e.g. hearing loss (80%), heterochromia of irides (50%), joining of eyebrows (5%) |
| WS 2B | AD | "WS2B" | 1 | | See WS 2A |
| WS 3 | AD or sporadic | Deletions including PAX3 | 2 | | Similar symptoms to WS 1 but also features abnormalities of arm muscles and bones |
| WS 4 | AR | EDNRB | 13 | | Usually dystopia canthorum is absent and incidence of hearing loss is reduced; Hirschsprung disease |
| | AR | EDN3 | 20 | | |
| | AD | SOX10 | 22 | | |

*(Table by GGS Creative Resources. Reproduced by permission of Gale, a part of Cengage Learning.)*

### WS1

A number of different mutations in a single copy of the PAX3 **gene** on **chromosome** 2 are responsible for all cases of WS1, meaning it is always inherited as an autosomal dominant trait. The PAX3 gene plays a role in regulating other genes that have some function in producing melanocytes (pigment-producing cells). PAX3 was formerly known as the HUP2 gene.

### WS2A

People that have typical signs of WS2 are designated as having WS2A only if genetic testing shows them to have a mutation in the MITF gene on chromosome 3. As with WS1, all cases of WS2A appear to be autosomal dominant. There is evidence that MITF is one of the genes regulated by PAX3.

### WS2B

Some individuals with typical WS2 have had normal MITF gene analysis. A search for a different WS2 gene showed that some cases are linked to a gene on chromosome 1. This gene has been tentatively designated WS2B until its exact chromosomal location and protein product are identified. WS2B displays autosomal dominant inheritance.

### WS3

Several people with a severe form of WS1 have been shown by genetic analysis to have a deletion of a small section of chromosome 2. Several genes are located in this section, including the PAX3 gene. Not ·

all patients with WS3 have had the exact same genetic anomaly on chromosome 2, which may explain the variation in symptoms that have been reported. Some families with WS3 have displayed autosomal dominant inheritance, while other individuals with the condition have been sporadic cases.

### WS4

Mutations in three different genes—EDNRB, EDN3, and SOX10 on chromosomes 13, 20, and 22 respectively—have been linked to WS4. Those cases of WS4 associated with the EDNRB and EDN3 show autosomal recessive inheritance, while the SOX10-associated cases are dominantly inherited.

Individuals with one of the autosomal dominant types of WS have a 50% risk of passing on the gene each time they have a child. A couple that has a child with WS4 linked to EDNRB or EDN3 faces a 25% risk for recurrence in each subsequent child. WS is quite variable, even within families. For instance, a parent with minimal pigment disturbance, mild facial features, and no hearing loss may have a child with pronounced physical features and **deafness**, and vice versa. There may be some correlation between specific **gene mutations** and the incidence of certain symptoms, but precise predictions are not possible.

The six genes listed above are those known to be associated with WS. It is expected, however, that more genes will be identified, especially since only a minority of WS2 cases have shown linkage to the MITF and WS2B genes.

## KEY TERMS

**Dystopia canthorum**—A wide spacing between the inner corners of the eyes, with the eyes themselves having normal spacing. Also called telecanthus.

**Heterochromia irides**—A medical term for individuals with different-colored eyes.

**Hirschsprung disease**—A deformation in which the colon becomes enlarged (megacolon), caused by abnormal nerve control of that portion of the large intestine.

**Hypopigmentation**—Decreased or absent color (pigment) in a tissue.

**Neural crest cells**—A group of cells in the early embryo, located on either side of the area that will eventually develop into the spinal cord. The cells migrate (move) away from the area and give rise to various body structures, including melanocytes (pigment producing cells), certain structures of the face and head, and parts of the nervous system.

**Neurocristopathy**—A disorder that results from abnormal development and/or migration of the neural crest cells in the embryo.

**Sensorineural**—Type of hearing loss due to a defect in the inner ear (sensing organ) and/or the acoustic nerve.

**Synophrys**—A feature in which the eyebrows join in the middle. Also called blepharophimosis.

### Demographics

The prevalence of WS is estimated at one in 40,000. About 3% of all children with congenital deafness have WS. WS1 and WS2 occur with approximately the same frequency. WS3 and WS4 are much less common than the other types. The majority of people with WS are Caucasian, but members of other ethnic groups may be affected as well.

### Signs and symptoms

#### WS1

Dystopia canthorum is seen in 99% of people with WS1. Other facial features may include decreased length of the nasal bone, a broad/high nasal root (top of the nose), and increased length of the lower face. Seventy percent of people with WS1 have either a medial flare of the eyebrows or synophrys (joining of the eyebrows in the middle, also called blepharophimosis).

Some type of pigmentary disturbance is nearly always present, and involves hypopigmentation (decreased color) of the skin, hair, and/or irides. However, unlike the more common forms of **albinism** that often involve a generalized lack of pigment in the body, WS is characterized by patches of hypopigmentation—often termed "partial albinism." A white forelock or premature graying is seen in about 70% of people with WS1. The eyelashes and patches of body hair may also be hypopigmented. Heterochromia of the irides may be complete (25% of patients) or partial (5% of patients). In complete heterochromia, each eye is a different color. In partial heterochromia, an individual iris (in one or both eyes) is composed of two colors. Those people with WS1 who do not have iris heterochromia often have brilliant blue coloring of both eyes.

Although estimates vary, hearing loss of some type is present in about 60% of individuals with WS1. The true prevalence is difficult to determine because of the variable nature of the condition. About 80% of those with hearing loss are affected in both ears (bilateral). Profound hearing loss occurs in some 25% of all people diagnosed with WS1.

Spina bifida (open spine) is seen in a very small percentage of newborns with WS1, as is cleft lip/palate. Hirschsprung disease, a deformation in which the colon becomes enlarged (megacolon), is a somewhat more frequent anomaly. Sprengel anomaly (elevated shoulder blade) can also be seen. Overall, about 10% of children with WS1 have one of these anomalies.

#### WS2

The major clinical distinction between WS1 and WS2 is the absence of dystopia canthorum in WS2. Otherwise, the conditions mostly differ by incidences of the various symptoms. The incidence of hearing loss in WS2 is 80%, with about 30% having a profound loss. Heterochromia of the irides occurs in 50% of patients. White forelock, premature graying, and hypopigmented skin patches are each found in about 15–20% of people with WS2. Synophrys occurs in only 5% of patients.

#### WS3

WS3 could be considered a subtype of WS1, since both are associated with the PAX3 gene. The distinction is clinical, with the added feature in WS3 being abnormalities of the muscles and bones of the arms. Some cases of WS3 have been sporadic. Several individuals diagnosed with WS3 have been in families where other members have typical signs of WS1. Thus, in some cases, WS3 can be considered a severe form of PAX3-associated WS, and is a dramatic example of the variability that can occur within families.

### WS4

Individuals with WS4 usually do not have dystopia canthorum, and often do not have hearing loss. Hirschsprung disease is the major distinguishing feature of WS4. In fact, individuals who carry a single abnormal EDNRB or EDN3 gene (as opposed to two abnormal copies of either gene in WS4) have only Hirschsprung disease. A small proportion of people with WS4 have been found to have an abnormal SOX10 gene.

## Diagnosis

In the early 1990s, a group of researchers known as the Waardenburg Consortium established criteria for diagnosing someone with WS1. They considered the major criteria of WS1 to be:

- congenital sensorineural hearing loss (not due to some other obvious cause)
- pigmentary disturbance of the iris
- hair hypopigmentation of some type
- dystopia canthorum
- an affected first-degree relative (parent, sibling, or child)

Minor criteria established by the Waardenburg consortium include:

- several areas of hypopigmented skin
- synophrys or medial flare of the eyebrows
- broad and high nasal root
- hypoplastic alae nasi (cartilage and skin around the nostrils)
- premature graying of hair

In order to be diagnosed with WS1, a person must have two major criteria, or one major plus two minor criteria. A modification of the list for WS2 includes removing dystopia canthorum, and including premature graying as a major criterion. With those modifications, a person with no family history of the condition should have two major criteria to be considered for WS2, and someone with an affected family member need only have one major criterion. Diagnosing WS2 can be more difficult than diagnosing WS1 because of the lack of dystopia canthorum. In addition, some people with a white forelock or premature graying may color their hair, and thus conceal an important sign.

As indicated, the distinction between WS1 and WS3 is clinical, with musculoskeletal anomalies added to the list of criteria for WS1. The criteria for diagnosing WS4 would be similar to those for WS2, with the inclusion of Hirschsprung disease as a major criterion, and the probable exclusion of dystopia canthorum, broad nasal root, and severe hearing loss. In addition, by definition WS4 is not linked to PAX3, MITF, or WS2B, and is linked to one of the established WS4 genes (assuming genetic testing is available and informative).

## Treatment and management

The primary medical consideration for people with WS is hearing loss. The most effective intervention is hearing aids. It is widely accepted that infants at risk for hearing loss, such as those who may inherit WS from a parent, can benefit from screening in the newborn period. An undiagnosed hearing deficit can result in delays in speech and learning. Children with profound hearing loss are eligible for special accommodations in their education, and the entire family can benefit by starting to use sign language very early.

Although spina bifida in WS is uncommon, the potential complications are serious. Infants with spina bifida usually have damage to the spinal cord at the level of the open spine, and consequently have either partial or total paralysis below that point. The opening in the spine can be repaired, but the neurological damage to the spinal cord is permanent. Cleft lip/palate is also uncommon in WS, but is a serious birth defect. Children with cleft lip/palate usually require several surgeries, but the outcome of the repair is generally very good. It would be prudent to screen any infant of a parent with WS for Hirschsprung disease. Surgical removal or repair of the affected segment of colon is often necessary. Depending on the severity of the musculoskeletal anomalies, a child with WS3 might require some sort of orthopedic intervention, such as casting, bracing, or surgery. A few children with WS3 have had only minor joint contractures of the arms and hands.

**Genetic counseling** is indicated for any family with WS. Prenatal diagnosis might be an option if genetic testing in the family is informative, but many couples may not choose invasive testing if they would not terminate a pregnancy for WS.

## Prognosis

The majority of people with WS lead productive lives. In the absence of severe hearing loss, many people with WS would not be noticed as having a condition by anyone in the general population. If hearing loss is present, it usually does not get worse, and is often amenable to treatment. There is little hope for any preventive measures for WS, since all of the features of the syndrome occur early in embryonic development and are present at birth.

### Resources

#### BOOKS

Gorlin, Robert J., Helga V. Toriello, and M. Michael Cohen. *Hereditary Hearing Loss and Its Syndromes.* New York: Oxford University Press, 1995.

#### PERIODICALS

Mishriki, Yehia Y. "Facial Clues to an Inherited Syndrome." *Postgraduate Medicine* (July 2000): 107-110.

#### ORGANIZATIONS

Alexander Graham Bell Association for the Deaf, Inc. 3417 Volta Place NW, Washington, DC 20007-2778. (800) 432-7543. http://www.agbell.org.

FACES: The National Craniofacial Association. PO Box 11082, Chattanooga, TN 37401. (423) 266-1632 or (800) 332-2373. faces@faces-cranio.org. http://www.faces-cranio.org/.

National Association of the Deaf. 814 Thayer, Suite 250, Silver Spring, MD 20910-4500. (301) 587-1788. nadinfo @nad.org. http://www.nad.org.

National Organization for Albinism and Hypopigmentation. 1530 Locust St. #29, Philadelphia, PA 19102-4415. (215) 545-2322 or (800) 473-2310. http://www.albinism.org.

Research Registry for Hereditary Hearing Loss. 555 N. 30th St., Omaha, NE 68131. (800) 320-1171. http://www.boystown.org/btnrh/deafgene.reg/waardsx.htm.

Scott J. Polzin, MS

# Walker-Warburg syndrome

## Definition

Walker-Warburg syndrome is a congenital disorder of the central nervous system involving fatal neurological lesions. Multiple malformations of the brain,

eyes, and muscle tissue distinguish WWS from similar malformation syndromes. It is also known by the acronym HARD +/- E syndrome (hydroencephalus, agyri, retinal **dysplasia**, plus or minus "e" for **encephalocele**).

## Description

Affected individuals typically show a combination of severe brain, eye, and muscle defects. Multiple malformations of the brain include type II **lissencephaly**, a condition in which the brain lacks normal convolutions and is unusually smooth without folds. Eighty-four percent of the infants with WWS have macrocephaly (an enlarged head). In half of these cases, the macrocephaly is apparent at birth, and in a quarter of the cases it develops postnatally. **Hydrocephalus**, or excessive accumulation of cerebrospinal fluid around the brain, occurs in 95% of infants with WWS. This fluid fills abnormally large ventricles or spaces in the brain. Fifty percent of affected infants have an encephalocele, or gap in the skull that does not seal. The meninges or membranes that cover the brain may protrude through this gap. The formation of an encephalocele may be associated with the failure of the neural tube to close during development of the fetus. A malformed cerebellum characterizes the syndrome as well as distinct muscle abnormalities, including congenital **muscular dystrophy**.

Ocular defects occur in 100% of infants with WWS. The most common are abnormally small eyes and retinal abnormalities, which arise from the improper development of the light sensitive area at the back of the eye. Cataracts may also be present and more than three quarters of the infants born with WWS have a defect in the anterior chamber of the eye. WWS syndrome leads to severely retarded mental development and is often lethal in infancy.

### Genetic profile

WWS is inherited in an autosomal recessive pattern. Offspring of parents who have had one affected infant have a 25% chance of having WWS. The locations of the causitive genes remains unknown.

### Demographics

WWS is extremely rare. Cases described in the literature cite siblings with WWS born to consanguineous (closely related) parents as well as cases in families not known to be at risk.

### Signs and symptoms

Clinical signs include a malformed head, small eyes, cataracts, retinal abnormalities, and muscle weakness. An encephalocele may be present as well. Microscopic examination reveals that the cells and tissues of the brain develop in a highly disorganized fashion. Seizures may occur.

### Diagnosis

**Prenatal ultrasound** can reveal some of the brain anomalies associated with WWS, most commonly hydrocephalus and encephalocele. Lissencephaly can not be diagnosed prenatally as normal fetal brains appear smooth. After birth, diagnosis is made on the basis of physical features and ultrasound exams. MRI may be used to confirm the smooth brain feature or type II lissencephaly typical of WWS. Genetic analysis helps distinguish WWS from Fukuyama-type congenital muscular dystrophy (FCMD), which has numerous similar features. WWS can be differentiated from other syndromes that display hydrocephalus or encephalocele by the presence of eye abnormalities including retinal defects, cataracts and anterior chamber defects. **Genetic testing** for Fukuyama-type congenital muscular dystrophy distinguished this from WWS.

### Treatment and management

The severe malformations of the brain defy treatment and many infants with WWS die within the first year of life. Supportive care is required to provide comfort and nursing needs. Seizures may be controlled with medication. Shunting may be required to control the hydrocephalus. A shunt or short plastic tube can be placed to divert the excess cerebral spinal fluid to another area of the body where it can ultimately be absorbed by the body.

---

## QUESTIONS TO ASK YOUR DOCTOR

- What supportive measures do you recommend?
- At what point should seizures be controlled medically?
- What are the risks and benefits of shunting?
- Which family members should undergo genetic testing?

---

**Genetic counseling** is recommended for families at risk.

### Prognosis

Patients have a very limited life expectancy and the syndrome is generally considered lethal. Most patients die before the age of two.

### Resources

#### BOOKS

Menkes, John H., and Harvey B. Sarnat. *Child Neurology.* 6th ed. Philadelphia: Lippincott, Williams & Wilkins, 2000.

Volpe, Joseph J. *Neurology of the Newborn.* 4th ed. Philadelphia: W.B. Saunders, 2001.

#### PERIODICALS

Gasser, B., et al. "Prenatal Diagnosis of Walker-Warburg Syndrome in Three Sibs." *American Journal of Medical Genetics* 76 (March 1998): 107-10.

Hung, N.A., et al. "Gonaddoblastoid Testicular Dysplasia in Walker-Warburg Syndrome." *Pediatric Developmental Pathology* 1 (September-October 1998): 393-404.

Vasconcelos, M.M., et al. "Walker-Warburg Syndrome. Report of Two Cases." *Fetal Diagnostic Therapy* 14 (July-August 1999): 198-200.

#### WEBSITES

"Fukuyama Congenital Muscular Dystrophy." *OMIM– Online Mendelian Inheritance in Man.*http://www.ncbi.nlm.nih.gov/entrez/dispomim.cgi?id = 253800.

"Muscular Dystrophy, Congenital, With Severe Central Nervous System Atrophy and Absence of Large Myelinated Fibers." *OMIM–Online Mendelian Inheritance in Man.*http://www.ncbi.nlm.nih.gov/entrez/dispomim.cgi?id = 601170.

"Walker-Warburg Syndrome." *OMIM–Online Mendelian Inheritance in Man.*http://www.ncbi.nlm.nih.gov/entrez/dispomim.cgi?id = 236670.

#### ORGANIZATIONS

Lissencephaly Network, Inc. 716 Autumn Ridge Lane, Fort Wayne, IN 46804-6402. (219) 432-4310. Fax: (219) 432-

4310. lissennet@lissencephaly.org. http://
www.lissencephaly.org.

National Hydrocephalus Foundation. 12413 Centralia,
Lakewood, CA 90715-1623. (562) 402-3523 or (888)
260-1789. hydrobrat@earthlink.net. http://www.
nhfonline.org.

National Organization for Rare Disorders (NORD). PO
Box 8923, New Fairfield, CT 06812-8923. (203) 746-
6518 or (800) 999-6673. Fax: (203) 746-6481. http://
www.rarediseases.org.

Julianne Remington

Ward-Romano syndrome *see* **Long-QT syndrome**

Weaver-Williams syndrome *see* **Weaver syndrome**

# Weaver syndrome

## Definition

Weaver syndrome is a congenital genetic syndrome associated with rapid growth beginning in the prenatal period as well as with a specific facial appearance and certain skeletal features. It has also been referred to as Weaver-Williams syndrome.

## Description

Weaver syndrome was first described by Dr. David Weaver in 1974. A number of different symptoms occur in Weaver syndrome, however, it primarily results in rapid growth beginning in the prenatal period and continuing through the toddler years and into the elementary school years. It is also strongly associated with the bones developing and maturing more quickly (advanced bone age), a distinctive appearing face, and developmental delay. Babies often have a hoarse low-pitched cry.

## Genetic profile

Weaver syndrome is for the most part a sporadic condition, meaning that a child affected by it did not inherit it from a parent. In a very few families, autosomal dominant **inheritance** has been reported, which means that both a parent and his/her child is affected by Weaver syndrome. The cause of Weaver syndrome is not known and the gene(s) that are involved in it have not been identified.

## Demographics

Weaver syndrome is rare. About 30 to 50 cases have been published in the medical literature. It occurs in both males and females.

## Signs and symptoms

Children with Weaver syndrome tend to have large heads. The faces of children with Weaver syndrome are usually very similar to each other, more so than to other family members, and include a round face, small chin, long philtrum (groove in the midline of the upper lip), large ears, and eyes that are father apart from each other than usual. Other common symptoms include hypertonia (increased muscle tone, tight muscles) as well as hypotonia (decreased muscle tone, "floppy" muscles) and a hoarse low-pitched cry in babies.

The excessive prenatal growth often results in the newborn being large with respect to weight, length and head circumference. The rapid growth continues through the toddler and youth years with the child's length and height often being above the 97th percentile, meaning that out of 100 children of the same age, the child is longer/taller than 97 of the children. There is very limited information on the rate of growth through adolescence and on final height, as most of the patients diagnosed with Weaver syndrome who have been reported in the medical literature have been children. In addition, given that the condition was first described 25 years ago, long-term clinical information is just becoming available.

There are a number of other features that have been associated with Weaver syndrome. The child may have difficulty extending elbows and knees completely, fingers and/or toes may be permanently flexed (camptodactyly) or have other problems such as overlapping fingers/toes or **clubfoot**, and the skin may appear loose. The child may have normal or delayed development; severe mental retardation is rarely seen. Speech may be delayed and when present, may be slurred. A child with Weaver syndrome may also have behavioral problems such as poor concentration, temper tantrums, which may be related to frustrations arising from communication problems, and obsessive and repetitive patterns of play.

### Diagnosis

Diagnosis of Weaver syndrome is based solely upon clinical examination, medical history and x–ray data. There are no laboratory tests that can provide a diagnosis. The clinical criteria that are considered to be diagnostic for Weaver syndrome are excessive growth beginning in the prenatal and infancy period, a characteristic facial appearance, advanced bone age with the bones in the wrist being more advanced than other skeletal bones, metaphyseal flaring in the leg bones (the ends of the bone are wider than normal), and developmental delay.

There are many conditions and genetic syndromes that cause excessive growth, consequently, a baby and/or child who has accelerated growth needs to be thoroughly examined by a physician knowledgeable in overgrowth and genetic syndromes. The evaluation includes asking about health problems in the family as well as asking about the growth patterns of the parents and their final height. In some families, growth patterns are different and thus may account for the child's excessive growth. The child will also undergo a complete physical examination. The child will also be examined in terms of his/her facial appearance with special attention paid to the shape of his/her head, width of the face at the level of the eyes, and appearance of the chin and forehead. Besides measurement of the head circumference, arm length, leg length, and wing span will also be measured. Laboratory testing may also be done. A **chromosome** analysis (**karyotype**) may be performed as well as testing for another genetic syndrome called fragile-X syndrome. The patient's bone age should also be assessed. Bone age is determined by x–rays of the hand. It is known that a child's age can be predicted by the appearance of the wrist bones. In some cases the bones may develop or mature more quickly than normal, or in other words, the child's wrist bones appear to be those of an older child. This is referred to as advanced bone age.

Advanced bone age is present in nearly every child with Weaver syndrome. It does not appear to result in other health problems. If the child begins to lose developmental milestones or appears to stop developing, metabolic testing may be done to evaluate for a metabolic condition called Sanfilippo syndrome. Developmental milestones refer to the skills infants and toddlers acquire as they get older, such as smiling, cooing, grasping toys, rolling over, walking, and talking.

### Treatment and management

There is no cure for Weaver syndrome. However, the symptoms that cause problems can be treated and managed. Surgery may be used to correct any skeletal problems such as clubfoot or finger or toe problems. Physical and occupational therapy may help with muscle tone. Speech therapy may help with speech, and behavioral assessments and treatments may help with behavioral problems.

### Prognosis

With appropriate treatment and management, children with Weaver syndrome appear to do well. Intellectually, most individuals with Weaver syndrome are normal. Weaver syndrome is not associated with a shortened life span.

### Resources

#### BOOKS

Cole, Trevor R.P., N.R. Dennis, and Helen E. Hughes. "Weaver Syndrome: Seven New Cases and a Review of the Literature". In *Congenital Malformation Syndromes*. New York: Chapman and Hall Medical, 1995, pp. 267-280.

#### WEBSITES

Genetic and Rare Conditions Site. http://www.kumc.edu/gec/support/.
Pediatric Database (PEDBASE). http://www.icondata.com/health/pedbase/index.htm.
The Family Village. http://www.familyvillage.wisc.edu/index.htmlx.

## ORGANIZATIONS

Sotos Syndrome Support Group. Three Danda Square East #235, Wheaton, IL 60187. (888) 246-SSSA or (708) 682-8815 http://www.well.com/user/sssa/.

Weaver Syndrome Families Support (WSFS). 4357 153rd Ave. SE, Bellevue, WA 98006 (425) 747-5382.

Cindy L. Hunter, MS, CGC

# Weissenbacher-Zweymuller syndrome

## Definition

Weissenbacher-Zweymuller syndrome (WZS) is a genetic form of dwarfism in which affected individuals are born with small, underdeveloped jaws (micrognathia), **cleft palate**, short arms and legs (rhizomelia), "dumbbell" shaped arm and leg bones, protruding wide spaced eyes (hypertelorism), and incompletely formed back bones (vertebral coronal clefts). Unlike most other forms of dwarfism, individuals affected by Weissebacher-Zweymuller start out being affected by dwarfism and then have a period of gradual growth and bone change that leads to normal physical development by five or six years of age.

## Description

Weissenbacher-Zweymuller syndrome refers to a rare disorder of small underdeveloped jaws (micrognathia), delayed bone growth, and unusual bone formation first described in 1964 by Weissenbacher and Zweymuller. The formation of bones is delayed because an important structural component of bone called cartilage does not form correctly. Since bone development is delayed, early milestones like walking and physical growth are delayed. Due to cleft palate, many individuals affected by WZS have speech and language delays. In most cases, physical, motor, mental, and academic development is normal by five or six years of age. Alternate names sometimes used for WZS include Pierre Robin syndrome with fetal chondrodysplasia and heterozygous otospondylomegaepiphyseal **dysplasia** (OSMED).

## Genetic profile

Weissenbacher-Zweymuller syndrome appears to be caused by a single change or mutation in a **gene** called COL11A2 located on the short arm of **chromosome** 6. The mutation in COL11A2 leads

> ## KEY TERMS
>
> **Autosomal dominant**—A pattern of genetic inheritance where only one abnormal gene is needed to display the trait or disease.
>
> **Autosomal recessive**—A pattern of genetic inheritance where two abnormal genes are needed to display the trait or disease.
>
> **Micrognathia**—A term used to describe small, underdeveloped lower jaw and chin.
>
> **Rhizomelia**—A term used to describe the physical growth difference of short arms and legs.
>
> **Syndrome**—A group of signs and symptoms that collectively characterize a disease or disorder.

to the incorrect formation of collagen. Since collagen is an important structural part of cartilage and bone, a mutation in COL11A2 leads to the signs and symptoms of WZS. The specific mutation that leads to WZS is inherited in an autosomal recessive pattern. An autosomal recessive condition is caused by the **inheritance** of two abnormal copies of a gene.

In the 1970s and 1980s there was some confusion among geneticists who were uncertain if WZS is a separate syndrome or part of another genetic syndrome. Although this confusion is not completely resolved, in 1993 an important study compared WZS to other related genetic syndromes and concluded that WZS is a separate genetic disorder that should not be "lumped" into the category of other genetic syndromes like **Stickler syndrome**. Since that time, a 1998 genetic study found that WZS and another syndrome called otospondylomegaepiphyseal dysplasia (OSMED) appear to be caused by different mutations in the same gene. This finding led the authors to suggest that the term OSMED be used to encompass a broad category that includes WZS as "heterozygous" OSMED while the other syndrome now called OSMED should be called "homozygous" OSMED. Because it has been found that WZS results from both heterozygous and homozygous mutations, researchers have suggested that this disorder follows both autosomal dominant and autosomal recessive inheritance patterns.

## Demographics

WZS is a very rare disorder. The ethnic origin of individuals affected by WZS is varied and is not specific to any one country or ethnic population.

## Signs and symptoms

Signs and symptoms of Weissenbacher-Zweymuller syndrome include: short arms and legs (rhizomelia), short stature at birth, an underdeveloped jaw (micrognathia), cleft palate, widely spaced eyes (hypertelorism), protruding eyes, a "snub" nose (depressed nasal bridge), dumbbell shaped long leg and arm bones (widening of the metaphyses of long bones), and incompletely formed back bones (coronal cleft of the lumbar vertebrae). The most unique sign of WZS is the gradual improvement of these changes.

## Diagnosis

Diagnosis of Weissenbacher-Zweymuller syndrome is usually made from physical examination by a medical geneticist and x–rays of the legs, arms, and back. Careful charts of growth and development over time also help with diagnosis. Most characteristic of WZS is the gradual improvement in bone size, growth, and shape.

Prenatal diagnosis of WZS is difficult, but can sometimes be made through a level II ultrasound examination of bone growth in the late second to third trimester of pregnancy. **Genetic testing** may be available through an **amniocentesis** procedure if the exact mutations running in the family are known. Genetic testing is done on a research basis in most cases.

One of the most important aspects in the diagnosis of WZS is ruling out other diagnoses. Conditions can be eliminated based on features that are not seen in WZS or are missing in other syndromes. For example, other conditions that look like WZS usually have progressively worsening symptoms instead of WZS's characteristic catch-up growth. Additionally, most conditions resembling WZS are inherited in an autosomal dominant pattern through the family. In an autosomal dominant condition, only one copy of the gene for a particular condition is necessary for a person to experience symptoms of the condition. If a parent has an autosomal dominant condition, there is a 50/50 chance for each child to have the same or similar condition.

Conditions to rule out in differential diagnosis include:

- Stickler syndrome, in which affected individuals have eye problems and do not have short arms and legs at birth.
- Kniest dysplasia, in which affected individuals do not have a underdeveloped jaw, but they do have eye abnormalities.

- Marshall syndrome, in which affected individuals have hearing and eye abnormalities but do not have short limbs at birth.
- Isolated Pierre-Robin sequence, in which individuals have an underdeveloped jaw and cleft palate alone without short arms and legs.
- Diastrophic dwarfism, in which affected individuals often have club feet, joint contractures, hypermobile thumbs, and non-bulbous bones.
- Metatropic dwarfism, which is characterized by visible changes of the trunk and short limbs as the spine flattens and the bones become progressively deformed.
- Traditional oto-spondylo-megaepiphyseal dysplasia (OSMED), which includes individuals affected by deafness and abnormal growth and development of the spine and growth plates at the end of the long bones (spondyloepiphyseal dysplasia) with large growth plates at the end of the long bones (epiphyses).

In conclusion, it is important to do a thorough and long-term physical examination, a family history, and test for growth, hearing, and eyesight before making a diagnosis of WZS.

## Treatment and management

The symptoms of WZS can be treated through follow-up and careful evaluation by a pediatric medical geneticist during the first years of life. Especially important to check are eyesight, hearing, and growth. Specific craniofacial clinics can help individuals affected by cleft palate with surgery, speech, and other related issues. Physical, occupational, speech, and language therapy may be suggested to help reduce "catch-up" time and developmental delays. As with any other disorder that includes developmental delays, specialists providing physical and language therapy can assist in the decision on whether special classes may help an individual child develop academically.

## Prognosis

The chance for an individual affected by WZS to have normal physical, motor, mental, and school development by age six or seven is very good. To help in this development, early intervention with physical, occupational, speech, and language therapy and special classes may be helpful. A detailed case report in 1991 notes that the intelligence of children with WZS is generally within normal range, though they may have mild to moderate intellectual delay in the preschool period. The same report notes that physical growth should be normal by age five or six.

## QUESTIONS TO ASK YOUR DOCTOR

- How often should my baby have hearing, vision, and growth monitored?
- Do you recommend physical, occupational, or speech therapy?
- What developmental milestones should I watch for in my child?
- Is there anything we can do during the preschool years in order to monitor intellectual development?

## Resources

### BOOKS

Charles, I., et al. *Dwarfism: The Family & Professional Guide.* Short Stature Foundation Press, 1994.

### PERIODICALS

Gail, A., et al. "Weissenbacher-Zweymuller Syndrome: Long-term Follow-up of Growth and Psychomotor Development." *Developmental Medicine and Child Neurology* 33 (1991): 1101-1109.

Pihlajamaa, T., et al. "Heterozygous Glycine Substitution in the COL11A2 Gene in the Original Patient with Weissenbacher-Zweymuller Syndrome Demonstrates Its Identity with Heterozygous OSMED (Nonocular Stickler Syndrome)." *American Journal of Medical Genetics* 8 (November 1998): 115-20.

### ORGANIZATIONS

Pierre Robin Network. PO Box 3274, Quincy, IL 62305. (217) 224-7480. http://www.pierrerobin.org/index.html.

Stickler Involved People. 15 Angelina, Augusta, KS 67010. (316) 775-2993. http://www.sticklers.org/sip.

### WEBSITES

Cleft Palate Foundation. http://www.cleftline.org/.

Family Village. http://www.familyvillage.wisc.edu/index.html.

LPA (Little People of America) Online. http://www.lpaonline.org/.

Robin, Nathaniel H., and Matthew L. Warman. "Stickler Syndrome." *GeneClinic* http://www.geneclinics.org/profiles/stickler/index.html.

"Weissenbacher-Zweymuller Syndrome." *On-line Mendelian Inheritance in Man* http://www.ncbi.nlm.nih.gov/entrez/dispomim.cgi?id = 277610.

Dawn A. Jacob, MS

# Werner syndrome

## Definition

Werner syndrome is a very rare, inherited disease that resembles premature aging. Since the **gene** responsible was discovered in the mid-1990s, Werner syndrome has greatly interested researchers as a possible model for the study of human aging. It is also being extensively studied for insights it may eventually supply into a number of other diseases including **cancer**, **diabetes** mellitus, and atherosclerosis.

## Description

This syndrome is named for the German physician C. W. Otto Werner (1879-1936). Werner was a medical student in 1903 when he first observed the syndrome in four siblings, all about 30 years of age. The following year, Werner wrote about these observations in his "Inaugural Dissertation."

The clinical signs and symptoms of Werner syndrome start to appear during the teen or early adult years, after which patients appear to age rapidly and have a greater-than-usual chance of developing cancer, cardiovascular disease, or diabetes mellitus. By the time the patient is 30–40 years old, he or she has the look of old age. The most common cause of death is heart attack.

While in many ways the signs and symptoms of Werner syndrome resemble those of premature aging (referred to in adults as progeria), there are also some significant differences. For instance, the tumors commonly seen in Werner syndrome patients are commonly derived from the cells of the mesoderm, a

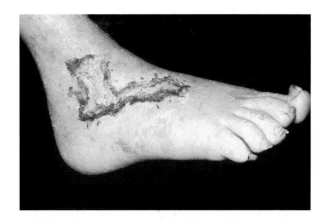

**Individuals with Werner syndrome often have skin abnormalities and may develop severe ulcerations, such as that seen on this foot.** *(Custom Medical Stock Photo, Inc.)*

middle layer of the embryo that gives rise to a variety of tissues including cartilage, muscle, bone, kidneys, and connective tissue. In normal aging, tumors are more likely to be derived from the epithelial cells that cover the body's exterior and line most of its hollow structures. **Osteoporosis** and soft-tissue calcium deposits are found both in Werner syndrome and normal aging, but the distribution of these conditions within the body is different in patients with Werner syndrome. In addition, patients with Werner syndrome do not generally experience symptoms of **Alzheimer disease** or premature cognitive decline, as do their aging counterparts in the general population.

Researchers are uncertain whether the symptoms of Werner syndrome are really a speeding-up of normal aging, or whether the many similarities are coincidental. There is nonetheless considerable optimism that further research into Werner syndrome may lead to a better understanding of aging, cancer, diabetes, systemic sclerosis, atherosclerosis, cataracts, and other conditions.

### Genetic profile

Werner syndrome results from mutation of a single gene. In 1992, the gene responsible (WRN) was mapped to **chromosome** 8p11-12. In 1996, a research group based in Seattle cloned the WRN gene. It was also discovered that the syndrome resulted from an autosomal recessive mutation that affects a member of a family of enzymes known as helicases that unwind **deoxyribonucleic acid** (DNA) and, in some cases, **ribonucleic acid** (RNA).

Despite the discovery that Werner syndrome is caused by a genetic defect, researchers are unable to explain exactly how this defect causes the disease. The purpose of helicases in the body is not fully understood, but they are known to unwind DNA, splitting the double-stranded molecules into separate single-stranded molecules. In this way, the enzymes are involved in the repair, recombination, replication, and transcription of DNA. There appear to be many damaged sites in DNA taken from patients with Werner syndrome. It has therefore been suggested that Werner syndrome may be caused by failure in these DNA-related processes, and that the somatic cells of those with Werner syndrome may be particularly prone to mutations.

The WRN gene is not known to bind to DNA damage, but recent research has suggested it might be able to sense the presence of damaged DNA. Since the discovery of the WRN gene, more than 10 mutations have been uncovered. Many of these mutations were in the Japanese population. It has been suggested that the relatively high incidence of Werner syndrome in that country may be related to traditions of marriages between closely related individuals in some areas of Japan.

As of 2001, researchers were seeking an animal model to allow them to further study Werner syndrome. Specifically, they hoped to create mice with a genetic equivalent of the WRN gene, and to determine whether these mice would age more quickly than normal mice.

### Demographics

Because of the limited number of cases, the demographic distribution of Werner syndrome is difficult to determine. Estimates of the number of people affected range from one in 95,000 to one in 1,000,000 people. Unlike progeria, which can be diagnosed at birth or soon after, Werner syndrome is not usually detected prior to adolescence. It is commonly noticed only after patients have failed to undergo the normal growth spurt associated with their teen years. The full range of symptoms is not usually seen until patients reach their 20s or 30s. Werner syndrome is more common in families in which a close biological relationship exists between parents. It occurs equally in both sexes. There is no evidence of a birth-order effect.

### Signs and symptoms

The cardinal signs and symptoms of Werner syndrome start to appear after the age of 10. They are:

- Cataracts. These occur in both eyes, and usually develop by age 25 or 30.
- Skin problems including tight, shiny, smooth skin, ulceration, general wasting of the skin and localized wasting of the subcutaneous area underneath it, pigmentary changes, a thickening of the horny outer layer of the skin, and a characteristic bird-like facial

appearance, including a beaked or pinched nose and unusually prominent eyes.

- Shortness of stature.
- An affected sibling or a close biological relationship between parents (third cousin or closer).
- Earlier-than-usual graying and/or thinning of scalp hair, usually by age 20.
- Excess amounts of hyaluronic acid (more commonly found in the body's connective tissues and in the fluids of the eyes and joints) in the urine.

Additional signs and symptoms of Werner syndrome include the following:

- Diabetes mellitus. This is usually mild, but can be found in between 44% and 67% of Werner syndrome patients.
- Impaired function of the ovaries or testes, as indicated by small or poorly developed genitalia or reduced fertility.
- Osteoporosis, most commonly in the upper limbs and spine, as well as in the lower limbs, feet, and ankles. In patients with Werner syndrome, osteoporosis is unlikely to be found in the skull or the torso.
- Unusually high bone density in the extremities of the finger and toe bones. This must be established by an x-ray examination.
- Deposits of calcium salts in soft tissues of the body. Common locations are around the Achilles tendon and the tendons of the elbow and the knee.
- Evidence pointing to earlier-than-usual arterial disease, such as a prior heart attack or abnormal electrocardiograms, etc.
- Rare or multiple tumors, or tumors derived from the mesoderm, the middle layer of the embryo. Werner syndrome is not marked by increased occurrence of all forms of tumors, but by selectively higher proportions of certain cancers that are relatively rare.
- Changes to the voice, rendering it squeaky, hoarse, or high-pitched.
- Flat feet.

In addition to the above signs and symptoms used for formal diagnostic purposes, other clinical observations have been reported, including loss of eyelashes and eyebrow hair, nail deformities, as well as the presence of thin limbs with a stocky trunk. A possible link to lung cancer has also been proposed.

In some cases, Werner syndrome can occur in a slower and milder partial form, with only some of the symptoms present.

## QUESTIONS TO ASK YOUR DOCTOR

- What diagnostic criteria did you utilize to arrive at Werner syndrome?
- At what age should my child's heart be evaluated?
- Which family members should undergo genetic testing?
- What screenings for cancer should my child undergo?

## Diagnosis

A definite diagnosis of Werner syndrome is established by the presence of all of the cardinal signs and symptoms listed above, plus at least two of the additional signs and symptoms.

A probable diagnosis is indicated by the presence of all of the first three cardinal signs, plus any two from the additional list.

A possible diagnosis is suggested by the presence of either cataracts or the skin manifestations, plus any four of the other signs or symptoms.

Werner syndrome may be ruled out if the above signs and symptoms appear prior to adolescence. The exception to this rule is shortness of stature, because patterns of pre-adolescent growth are not sufficiently understood.

Diagnosis may involve x–rays to study hormone excretion, skin biopsies, and a blood-sugar test to determine whether diabetes mellitus is present. Werner syndrome can also be diagnosed by mutational analysis of the WRN gene.

## Treatment and management

There is no known cure for Werner syndrome, so treatment is related to the specific symptoms present. For example, cataracts can be corrected by surgery and skin ulcers can be treated with grafts.

## Prognosis

Because it mimics the human aging process, Werner syndrome significantly reduces life expectancy in most patients. Average life expectancy for a Werner symptom patient is somewhere between 40 and 47 years. The most common causes of death are heart attacks, cerebrovascular accidents, and cancers.

## Resources

### BOOKS

Thoene, Jess G., ed. *Physicians' Guide to Rare Diseases*. 2nd ed. Montvale, NJ: Dowden Publishing Company Inc., 1995.

### ORGANIZATIONS

International Progeria Registry. IBR Dept. of Human Genetics, 1050 Forest Hill Rd., Staten Island, NY 10314. (718) 494-5333. wtbibr@aol.com.

International Registry of Werner Syndrome. University of Washington Dept. of Pathology, Health Science Bldg K543, Box 357470, Seattle, WA 98195. (206) 543-5088. http://www.pathology.washington.edu/werner/registry/frame2.html.

March of Dimes Birth Defects Foundation. 1275 Mamaroneck Ave., White Plains, NY 10605. (888) 663-4637. resourcecenter@modimes.org. http://www.modimes.org.

David L. Helwig

Whistling face syndrome *see* **Freeman-Sheldon syndrome**

Williams-Beuren syndrome *see* **Williams syndrome**

# Williams syndrome

## Definition

Williams syndrome is a genetic disorder caused by a deletion of a series of genes on **chromosome** 7q11. Individuals with Williams syndrome have distinctive facial features, mild mental retardation, heart and blood vessel problems, short stature, unique personality traits, and distinct learning abilities and deficits.

## Description

Williams syndrome, also known as Williams Beuren syndrome, was first described in 1961 by Dr. J. C. P. Williams of New Zealand. At that time it was noted that individuals with Williams syndrome had an unusual constellation of physical and mental findings. The physical features include a characteristic facial appearance, heart and cardiovascular problems, high blood calcium levels, low birth weight, short stature, and other connective tissue abnormalities. The intellectual problems associated with Williams include a mild mental retardation and a specific cognitive profile. That is, individuals with Williams syndrome often have the same pattern of learning abilities and disabilities, as well as many similar personality traits.

The findings in Williams syndrome are variable—that is, not all individuals with Williams syndrome will have all of the described findings. In addition to being variable, the physical and mental findings associated with Williams syndrome are progressive—they change over time.

## Genetic profile

Williams syndrome is a genetic disorder due to a deletion of chromosome material on the long arm of chromosome 7. A series of genes are located in this region. Individuals with Williams syndrome may have some or all of these genes deleted. Because of this, Williams syndrome is referred to as a contiguous gene deletion syndrome. Contiguous refers to the fact that these genes are arranged next to each other. The size of the deletion can be large or small, which may explain why some individuals with Williams syndrome are more severely affected than others. If you think of these genes as the letters of the alphabet, some individuals with Williams syndrome are missing A to M, some are missing G to Q and others are missing A to R. While there are differences in the amount of genetic material that can be deleted, there is a region of overlap. Everyone in the above example was missing G to M. It is thought that the missing genes in this region are important causes of the physical and mental findings of Williams syndrome.

Two genes in particular, ELN and LIMK1, have been shown to be important in causing some of the characteristic symptoms of Williams syndrome. The ELN gene codes for a protein called elastin. The job of elastin in the human body is to provide elasticity to the connective tissues such as those in the arteries, joints and tendons. The exact role of the LIMK1 gene is not known. The gene codes for a substance known as lim kinase 1 that is active in the brain. It is thought that the deletion of the LIMK1 gene may be responsible for the visuospatial learning difficulties of individuals with Williams syndrome. Many other genes are known to be in the deleted region of chromosome 7q11 responsible for Williams syndrome and much work is being done to determine the role of these genes in Williams syndrome.

Williams syndrome is an autosomal dominant disorder. Genes always come in pairs and in an autosomal dominant disorder, only one gene need be missing or altered for an individual to have the disorder. Although Williams syndrome is an autosomal disorder, most individuals with Williams syndrome are the only people in their family with this disorder. When this is the case, the chromosome deletion that causes Williams syndrome is called *de novo*. A *de novo* deletion is one that occurs for the first time in the affected individual. The cause of *de novo* chromosome deletions is unknown. Parents of an individual with Williams syndrome due to a *de novo* deletion are very unlikely to have a second child with William syndrome. However, once an individual has a chromosome deletion, there is a 50% chance that they will pass it on to their offspring. Thus individuals with Williams syndrome have a 50% chance of passing this deletion (and Williams syndrome) to their children.

## Demographics

Williams syndrome occurs in one in 20,000 births. Because Williams syndrome is an autosomal dominant disorder, it affects an equal number of males and females. It is thought that Williams syndrome occurs in people of all ethnic backgrounds equally.

## Signs and symptoms

Williams syndrome is a multi-system disorder. In addition to distinct facial features, individuals with Williams syndrome can have cardiovascular, growth, joint and other physical problems. They also share unique personality traits and have intellectual differences.

Infants with Williams syndrome are often born small for their family and 70% are diagnosed with failure to thrive during infancy. These growth problems continue throughout the life of a person with Williams syndrome and most individuals with Williams syndrome have short stature (height below the third percentile). Infants with William syndrome can also be extremely irritable and have "colic-like" behavior. This behavior is thought to be due to excess calcium in the blood (hypercalcemia). Other problems that can occur in the first years include strabismus (crossed eyes), ear infections, chronic constipation, and eating problems.

Individuals with Williams syndrome can have distinct facial features sometimes described as "elfin" or "pixie-like." While none of these individual facial features are abnormal, the combination of the different features is common for Williams syndrome. Individuals with Williams syndrome have a small upturned nose, a small chin, long upper lip with a wide mouth, small widely spaced teeth and puffiness around the eyes. As an individual gets older, these facial features become more pronounced.

People with Williams syndrome often have problems with narrowing of their heart and blood vessels. This is thought to be due to the deletion of the elastin gene and is called elastin arteriopathy. Any artery in the body can be affected but the most common narrowing is seen in the aorta of the heart. This condition is called supravalvar aortic stenosis (SVAS) and occurs in approximately 75% of individuals with Williams syndrome. The degree of narrowing is variable. If left untreated, it can lead to high blood pressure, heart disease and heart failure. The blood vessels that lead to the kidney and other organs can also be affected.

Deletions of the elastin gene are also thought to be responsible for the loose joints of some children with Williams syndrome. As individuals with Williams syndrome age, their heel cords and hamstrings tend to tighten, which can lead to a stiff awkward gait and curving of the spine.

Approximately 75% of individuals with Williams syndrome have mild mental retardation. They also have a unique cognitive profile (unique learning abilities and disabilities). This cognitive profile is independent of their IQ. Individuals with Williams syndrome generally have excellent language and memorization skills. They can have extensive vocabularies and may develop a thorough knowledge of a topic that they are interested in. Many individuals are also gifted musicians. Individuals with Williams syndrome have trouble with concepts that rely on visuospatial ability. Because of this, many people with Williams syndrome have trouble with math, writing and drawing.

People with Williams syndrome also often share personality characteristics. They are noted to be very talkative and friendly—sometimes inappropriately—and they can be hyperactive. Another shared personality trait is a generalized anxiety.

## Diagnosis

The diagnosis of Williams syndrome is usually made by a physician familiar with Williams syndrome and based upon a physical examination of the individual and a review of his or her medical history. It is often made in infants after a heart problem (usually

SVAS) is diagnosed. In children without significant heart problems, the diagnosis may be made after enrollment in school when they are noted to be "slow learners."

While a diagnosis can be made based upon physical examination and medical history, the diagnosis can now be confirmed by a **DNA** test.

Williams syndrome is caused by a deletion of genetic material from the long arm of chromosome 7. A specific technique called **fluorescent in situ hybridization** testing, or FISH testing, can determine whether there is genetic material missing. A FISH test will be positive (detect a deletion) in over 99% of individuals with Williams syndrome. A negative FISH test for Williams syndrome means that no genetic material is missing from the critical region on chromosome 7q11.

Prenatal testing (testing during pregnancy) for Williams syndrome is possible using the FISH test on DNA sample obtained by chorionic villus sampling (CVS) or by **amniocentesis**. Chorionic villus sampling is a prenatal test that is usually done between 10 to 12 weeks of pregnancy and involves removing a small amount of tissue from the placenta. Amniocentesis is a prenatal test that is usually performed at 16–18 weeks of pregnancy and involves removing a small amount of the amniotic fluid that surrounds the fetus. DNA is obtained from these samples and tested to see if the deletion responsible for Williams syndrome is present. While prenatal testing is possible, it is not routinely performed. Typically, the test is only done if there is a family history of Williams syndrome.

### Treatment and management

Because Williams syndrome is a multi-system disorder, the expertise of a number of specialists is required for management of this disorder.

The height and growth of individuals with Williams syndrome should be monitored using special growth curves developed specifically for individuals with Williams syndrome. Individuals who fall off these growth curves should be worked up for possible eating or thyroid disorders.

A cardiologist should evaluate individuals with Williams syndrome yearly. This examination should include measurement of blood pressure in all four limbs and an echocardiogram of the heart. An echocardiogram is a special form of ultrasound that looks at the structure of the heart. Doppler flow studies, which look at how the blood flows into and out of the heart, should also be done. Individuals with supravalvar stenosis may require surgery to fix this

condition. The high blood pressure caused by this condition may be treated with medication. Examinations should take place yearly as some of these conditions are progressive and may worsen over time.

Individuals with Williams syndrome should also have a complete neurological examination. In addition, the blood calcium levels of individuals with Williams syndrome should be monitored every two years. High levels of calcium can cause irritability, vomiting, constipation, and muscle cramps. An individual found to have a high level of calcium should consult a nutritionist to make sure that their intake of calcium is not higher than 100% of the recommended daily allowance (RDA). Because vitamin D can increase calcium levels, individuals with Williams syndrome and high calcium should not take multivitamins containing vitamin D. If calcium levels remain high after limiting vitamin D and decreasing dietary intake of calcium, an individual with hypercalcemia should see a nephrologist for further management and to monitor kidney function.

Strabismus (crossed eyes) can be treated by patching or by surgery. Ear infections can be treated with antibiotics and surgical placement of ear tubes.

The developmental differences of individuals with Williams syndrome should be treated with early intervention and special education classes. Specific learning strategies that capitalize on the strengths of individuals with Williams syndrome should be used. Physical, occupational, and speech therapy should be provided. Behavioral counseling and medication may help with behavioral problems such as hyperactivity and anxiety.

### Prognosis

The prognosis for individuals with Williams syndrome is highly dependent on the medical complications of a particular individual. Individuals with Williams syndrome who have no heart complications, or very minor ones, have a good prognosis. Good medical care and treatment of potential problems allows most individuals with Williams syndrome to lead a long life. The prognosis for individuals with more serious medical complications such as severe heart disease or hypertension is more guarded. Since the medical conditions associated with Williams syndrome are progressive rather than static, it is very important that individuals with Williams syndrome have yearly medical examinations with a health care provider familiar with Williams syndrome.

The range of abilities among individuals with Williams syndrome is very wide and the ultimate functioning of an individual is dependent on his or her abilities. While individuals with Williams syndrome do well in blood are deposited primarily in the brain, liver, kidneys, and the cornea of the eyes.

## Description

Under normal conditions, copper that finds its way into the body through the diet is processed within the liver. This processed form of copper is then passed into the gallbladder, along with the other components of bile (a fluid produced by the liver, which enters the small intestine in order to help in digestive processes). When the gallbladder empties its contents into the first part of the small intestine (duodenum), the copper in the bile enters and passes through the intestine with the waste products of digestion. In healthy individuals, copper is then passed out of the body in stool.

In Wilson disease, copper does not pass from the liver into the bile, but rather begins to accumulate within the liver. As copper levels rise in the liver, the damaged organ begins to allow copper to flow into the bloodstream, where it circulates. Copper is then deposited throughout the body, building up primarily in the kidneys, the brain and nervous system, and the eyes. Wilson disease, then, is a disorder of copper poisoning occurring from birth.

### Genetic profile

Wilson disease is inherited in an autosomal recessive manner. Autosomal recessive refers to the pattern of **inheritance** in which each parent carries a **gene** for the disease on one of his or her **chromosome** pairs. When each parent passes on the chromosome with the gene for Wilson disease, the child will be affected with the disease. Both males and females can be affected with Wilson disease. If an individual is a carrier of the Wilson disease gene they do not have any symptoms of this disease. In order to be affected, an individual must inherit two copies of the gene, one from each parent. Many cases of Wilson disease may not be inherited but occur as a spontaneous mutation in the gene.

The gene for Wilson disease is located on chromosome 13. The name of the gene is called ATP7B and is thought to be involved in transporting copper. Over 70 different mutations of this gene have been identified, making diagnosis by **genetic testing** difficult.

### Demographics

Wilson disease affects approximately 1 in 30,000 to 1 in 100,000 individuals and can affect people from many different populations. Approximately 1 in 90 individuals are carriers of the gene for Wilson disease.

structured environments such as school, their unique abilities and disabilities do not permit them to do as well in unstructured surroundings. Some individuals with Williams syndrome live independently but most live with their parents or in a supervised setting. Many individuals with Williams syndrome can gain employment in supervised settings and do well at tasks that do not require mathematics or visuo-spatial abilities. It is important to encourage individuals with Williams syndrome towards independence but to recognize that their friendly and outgoing personalities may lead them into abusive situations.

## Resources

### BOOKS

Bellugi, Ursula, and Marie St. George. *Journey from Cognition to Brain to Gene: Perspectives from Williams Syndrome.* Cambridge, MA: MIT Press, 2001.

### PERIODICALS

Finn, Robert. "Different Minds." *Discover* (June 1991): 55-58.

### ORGANIZATIONS

Williams Syndrome Association. PO Box 297, Clawson, MI 48017-0297. (248) 541-3630. Fax: (248) 541-3631. TMonkaba@aol.com. http://www.williams-syndrome.org/.

Williams Syndrome Foundation. University of California, Irvine, CA 92679-2310. (949)824-7259. http://www.wsf.org/.

Kathleen Fergus, MS, CGC

# Wilson disease

## Definition

Wilson disease is a rare, inherited disorder that causes excess copper to accumulate in the body. Steadily increasing amounts of copper circulating in the

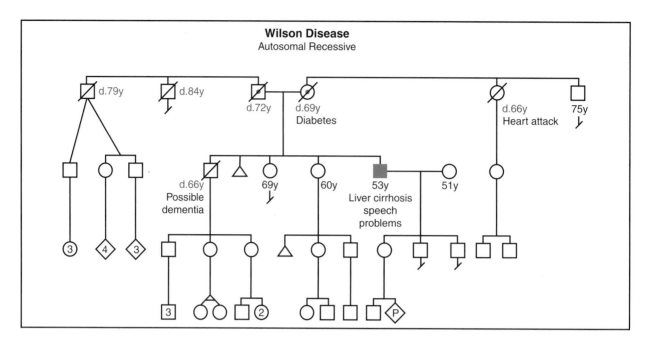

**Wilson Disease**
Autosomal Recessive

(Gale, a part of Cengage Learning.)

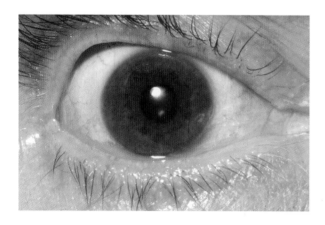

**Copper deposits are visible as a ring around the iris in patients with Wilson disease. Copper deposits in other organs as well and must be removed to avoid severe mental and physical development disorders.** *(Photo Researchers, Inc.)*

### Signs and symptoms

Symptoms typically present between the ages of three and 60, with age 17 considered to be the average age a diagnosis is made. About half of all patients experience their first symptoms in the liver. The illness causes swelling and tenderness of the liver, sometimes with fever, mimicking more common disorders, such as viral hepatitis and infectious mononucleosis. Abnormal levels of circulating liver enzymes reveal that the liver is being seriously damaged. This form of damage is referred to as "fatty degeneration." Without medical intervention, the liver damage will progress to actual cirrhosis. An often-fatal manifestation of liver disease is called fulminant hepatitis. This extremely severe inflammation of the liver (hepatitis) results in jaundice, fluid leaking into the abdomen, low protein circulating in the blood, abnormalities of the blood clotting system, swelling of the brain, and anemia due to the abnormal destruction of red blood cells.

Neurological symptoms are the first to occur in half of all patients due to copper accumulation in the brain and nervous system. The average age of onset for neurological symptoms is 21 years. These symptoms include tremors of the hands, uncontrollable movements of the limbs, stiffness, drooling, difficulty swallowing, difficulty talking, and headache. There is no change in a patient's intelligence.

About one third of all patients with Wilson disease have a variety of psychiatric symptoms as the first signs of the disease. These symptoms include inability to cope, **depression**, irritability, increased anger, and inappropriate behavior. Patients often have trouble completing tasks at work or in school.

Other symptoms that can affect patients with Wilson disease, and may occur before or after a diagnosis has been made, include joint disorders, symptoms of arthritis and skeletal problems such as **osteoporosis**. Patients have occasionally been affected with kidney stones and abnormal handling of glucose in their

**Anemia**—A blood condition in which the level of hemoglobin or the number of red blood cells falls below normal values. Common symptoms include paleness, fatigue, and shortness of breath.

**Bile**—A substance produced by the liver, and concentrated and stored in the gallbladder. Bile contains a number of different substances, including bile salts, cholesterol, and bilirubin.

**Biopsy**—The surgical removal and microscopic examination of living tissue for diagnostic purposes.

**Cell**—The smallest living units of the body which group together to form tissues and help the body perform specific functions.

**Ceruloplasmin**—A protein circulating in the bloodstream that binds with copper and transports it.

**Chromosome**—A microscopic thread-like structure found within each cell of the body and consists of a complex of proteins and DNA. Humans have 46 chromosomes arranged into 23 pairs. Changes in either the total number of chromosomes or their shape and size (structure) may lead to physical or mental abnormalities.

**Cirrhosis**—A chronic degenerative disease of the liver, in which normal cells are replaced by fibrous tissue. Cirrhosis is a major risk factor for the later development of liver cancer.

**Deoxyribonucleic acid (DNA)**—The genetic material in cells that holds the inherited instructions for growth, development, and cellular functioning.

**Gallbladder**—A small, pear-shaped organ in the upper right hand corner of the abdomen. It is connected by a series of ducts (tube-like channels) to the liver, pancreas, and duodenum (first part of the small intestine). The gallbladder receives bile from the liver, and concentrates and stores it. After a meal, bile is squeezed out of the gallbladder into the intestine, where it aids in digestion of food.

**Gene**—A building block of inheritance, which contains the instructions for the production of a particular protein, and is made up of a molecular sequence found on a section of DNA. Each gene is found on a precise location on a chromosome.

**Glucose**—One of the two simple sugars, together with galactose, that makes up the protein lactose, found in milk. Glucose is the form of sugar that is usable by the body to generate energy.

**Hepatitis**—A viral disease characterized by inflammation of the liver cells (hepatocytes). People infected with hepatitis B or hepatitis C virus are at an increased risk for developing liver cancer.

**Jaundice**—Yellowing of the skin or eyes due to excess of bilirubin in the blood.

**Toxic**—Poisonous.

body, and women have menstrual cycle irregularities including temporary stopping of their regular cycle.

### Diagnosis

The diagnosis of Wilson disease can be performed relatively easily through several different tests, however, because Wilson disease is so rare diagnosis is often delayed. The tests used to diagnose Wilson disease can be performed on patients who have or have not already shown symptoms of the disease. It is extremely important to make a diagnosis as soon as possible since liver damage can occur before there are any signs of the disease.

An easy way to diagnose Wilson disease is to measure the amount of a glycoprotein found in the blood called ceruloplasmin. Low levels of ceruloplasmin can diagnose the disease in about 80% of affected patients. This procedure is not as effective for women

taking birth control pills, pregnant women, or infants less than six months of age.

A second test involving an eye examination to detect a characteristic ring of copper deposited in a membrane of the cornea (referred to as Kayser-Fleischer rings) is very easy to perform and is very useful in diagnosing patients who have already exhibited symptoms. This test is not as effective in persons without symptoms. This diagnostic test cannot be used by itself to make a diagnosis because some patients with liver disease but not Wilson disease will test positive.

A third test for diagnosing Wilson disease involves measuring the amount of copper in the liver. This can be accomplished by sampling a portion of the liver in a procedure called a biopsy. This is one of the most effective ways to diagnose Wilson disease, however, the procedure itself is more difficult to perform than the others.

Other tests are also useful, for example, measuring the amount of copper passed into the urine daily (high in Wilson disease). Another lab test measures the ability of a patient's ceruloplasmin to bind with a form of copper (decreased in Wilson disease). And finally, as discussed under genetic profile, some patients can be diagnosed through a **DNA** test to determine whether or not they carry two genes for Wilson disease. This test does not always prove to be useful in certain patients and is used mostly to test the brothers and sisters of affected patients.

### Treatment and management

Treatment involves life-long administration of either D-penicillamine or trientine hydrochloride. Both of these drugs remove copper deposits throughout the body by binding to the copper which is removed from the body in urine. Zinc acetate and a low copper diet are other ways to treat Wilson disease.

Penicillamine has a number of serious side effects:

• joint pain

• neurological problems

• systemic lupus erythematosus

• decreased production of all blood elements

• interference with clotting

• allergic reactions

Careful monitoring is necessary. When patients have side effects from penicillamine, the dose can sometimes be lowered to an effective level that causes fewer difficulties. Alternatively, steroid medications may be required to reduce certain sensitivity reactions. Trientine has fewer potential side effects, but must still be carefully monitored.

Treatment with zinc is also an effective way to remove excess copper from the body. Zinc is a metal that works to block copper absorption and bind copper in the intestinal cells until it is all released into the stool approximately one week later. The benefit of treatment with zinc is that there are no toxic side effects, however, zinc is a slower acting agent than the other drugs. It takes four to eight months for the zinc to be effective in reducing the overall amount of copper in the body.

Finally, patients with Wilson disease are encouraged to follow a diet low in copper, with an average copper intake of 1.0 mg/day. Foods to avoid for their high levels of copper include liver and shellfish. Patients are also instructed to monitor their drinking water for excess levels of copper and drink distilled water instead.

---

## QUESTIONS TO ASK YOUR DOCTOR

• Can you recommend a low copper diet?

• What are the side effects of penicillamine?

• What are the pros and cons of zinc treatment versus medication for removing copper?

• How accurate is the genetic testing for Wilson disease?

### Prognosis

Without treatment, Wilson disease is always fatal. With treatment, symptoms may continue to worsen for the first six to eight weeks. After this time, definite improvement should start to be seen. However, it may take several years (two to five) of treatment to reach maximal benefit to the brain and liver. Even then, many patients are not returned to their original level of functioning. Patients with Wilson disease need to maintain some sort of anti-copper treatment for the rest of their lives in order to prevent copper levels from rising in the body. Interruptions in treatment can result in a relapse of the disease which is not reversible, and can ultimately lead to death.

### Resources

**BOOKS**

Scheinberg, I. Herbert. "Wilson's Disease." *Harrison's Principles of Internal Medicine*. Ed. by Anthony S. Fauci, et al. 14th ed. New York: McGraw-Hill, 1998.

**PERIODICALS**

Gow, P.J., et al. "Diagnosis of Wilson's Disease: An Experience Over Three Decades." *Gut* 46 (March 2000): 415-419.

Hariharan, Ramesh, and L. Fred Herbert. "Wilson's Disease." *Hospital Practice* 31 (August 15, 1996): 556 +.

Robertson, W.M. "Wilson's Disease." *Archives of Neurology* 57, no. 2 (February 2000): 276-7.

**ORGANIZATIONS**

American Liver Foundation. 75 Maiden Lane, Suite 603, New York, NY 10038. (800) 465-4837 or (888) 443-7222. http://www.liverfoundation.org.

National Organization for Rare Disorders (NORD). PO Box 8923, New Fairfield, CT 06812-8923. (203) 746-6518 or (800) 999-6673. Fax: (203) 746-6481. http://www.rarediseases.org.

Wilson's Disease Association. 4 Navaho Dr., Brookfield, CT 06804. (800) 399-0266.

**WEBSITES**

*Wilson's Disease Association*. http://www.medhelp.org/wda/wil.htm.

Katherine S. Hunt, MS

detailed studies, including **fluorescent in situ hybridization**, are warranted and may identify the missing genetic material. WHS may also present as mosaicism. Mosaicism for 4p- syndrome means that the individual has some cells that have normal number 4 chromosomes and other cells that are missing some of the genetic material from 4p.

Approximately 85–90% of cases of WHS occur as the result of a new deletion in the affected individual. This is also known as a *de novo* deletion and simply means that the affected individual's parents did not have any chromosome arrangement that led to the deletion. In this case, the chance for recurrence in future pregnancies of a couple whom has an affected child is not increased. In the remaining 10–15% of cases, one of the parents of the affected individual carries a balanced translocation. A balanced translocation is a rearrangement in the individual's chromosomes that causes that individual no problems since they have all the necessary genetic material that they need. However, when they produce eggs or sperm, the eggs or sperm may end up with an unbalanced arrangement and could lead to the conception of a child who has missing or extra genetic material. This could lead to miscarriage or to the birth of a child with conditions, such as WHS.

When a parent is identified as being a carrier of a balanced translocation, with each pregnancy they have an increased chance for having a child with an unbalanced chromosome arrangement. The chance of this is determined by the individual's specific translocation, how it was identified, and which parent is the carrier of the translocation. **Genetic counseling** should be offered for any family in which a child is diagnosed to have WHS. Other family members should also be offered counseling and chromosome analysis to determine if they are carriers of a balanced translocation.

### Demographics

The incidence of this condition is rare and estimated to be approximately one in 50,000 births. However, as with many genetic conditions, the condition may be misdiagnosed or may not be diagnosed in all individuals who are affected, especially if the condition results in pregnancy loss or loss in the early newborn period. It has been estimated that approximately 35% of individuals who have WHS die within the first two years of life. Also, with the advent of prenatal diagnosis, some fetuses with ultrasound abnormalities may be detected prenatally and the parents may elect to terminate the pregnancy. Approximately two-thirds of reported cases have been females.

### Signs and symptoms

It is important to remember that each individual who may have a particular genetic syndrome is a unique individual. Therefore, all individuals with WHS do not have all of the same signs and symptoms. The most important reason for diagnosing an individual with a syndrome is not to put a label on that person. The reason for a diagnosis is so that predictions can be made to determine the needs of that person, based on the history available from other individuals affected with the same condition.

Signs and symptoms that can be associated with WHS include:

- slow growth before birth
- slow growth after birth (postnatal growth deficiency)
- small head size (microcephaly)
- week cry in infancy
- poor muscle tone (hypotonia)
- seizures
- severe developmental retardation
- severe retardation of motor skills
- crossed eyes (Strabismus)
- widely spaced eyes (hypertelorism)
- droopy eyelids (ptosis)
- skin folds in the corner of the eyes (epicanthal folds)
- cleft lip and/or palate
- short upper lip and philtrum
- small chin (micrognathia)
- asymmetry of the skull (cranial asymmetry)
- skin tag or pit in front of the ear (preauricular tag or pit)
- downturned mouth
- prominent triangular area of the forehead (glabella)
- scalp defects on the center of the back of the head
- underdeveloped fingerprints (dermal ridges)
- a single crease across the palm of the hands (Simian crease)
- misaligned bones in the front part of the foot/clubfoot (talipes equinovarus)
- turned up fingernails
- urinary opening on the underside of the penis (hypospadias)
- undescended testicles (cryptorchidism)
- dimple at the base of the spine
- heart defects
- curvature of the spine (scoliosis)
- underdeveloped bones of the hands and pelvis

## Diagnosis

When WHS is suspected, chromosome analysis should be performed and the laboratory should be informed as to what syndrome is suspected. This ensures that the laboratory carefully looks at chromosome 4 and if the deletion is not visible, then fluorescent in situ hybridization (FISH) can be done specifically for the critical 4p16.3 region of chromosome 4. FISH analysis is a procedure that is used in the laboratory to identify pieces of genetic material that are too small to see by looking at the chromosome under the microscope. Instead, **DNA** that is specific to a particular area of a chromosome is fluorescently labeled, so that it is visible under the microscope. This labeled DNA is then added to the sample and allowed to attach itself to the particular piece of DNA in question. This enables the laboratory technician to then look under the microscope for the fluorescent spot on the chromosome and identify extra or missing pieces of DNA that are too small to see by just looking at the chromosome alone. With this procedure, those individuals who have deletions so small that they cannot be detected by routine chromosome analysis may be able to have the deletion detected by FISH.

Interestingly, there is a syndrome called Pitt-Rogers-Danks syndrome (PRDS) that has been reported to have similar characteristics to WHS. Several individuals who have initially been diagnosed with PRDS subsequently had FISH analysis that detected a deletion of 4p, and thus the individuals were reclassified as having WHS. Some feel that PRDS is actually WHS without obvious deletions of 4p.

When a couple has had a child diagnosed to have WHS, and a member of that couple carries a balanced translocation, genetic counseling should be offered to discuss reproductive options. One option is choosing sperm or egg donation so that the parent who has the translocation does not pass unbalanced genetic material on to his or her child. Another option is preimplantation genetic diagnosis. Preimplantation genetic diagnosis is a very complex process that involves in vitro fertilization and diagnosing the embryos before they are placed into the mother's uterus. Thus, only unaffected embryos are transferred to the uterus. Lastly, the options of CVS and **amniocentesis** for prenatal diagnosis should be discussed. All of these options have allowed couples with balanced translocations to realize the dream of having more children when the fear of having another affected child may have otherwise stopped them from choosing to add to their families.

If ultrasound examination reveals findings consistent with the possibility of WHS in a family with no history of WHS, genetic counseling and prenatal diagnosis should be offered. These ultrasound findings may include heart defects, microcephaly, agenesis of the corpus collosum (missing a specific part of the brain), micrognathia, **cleft lip and palate**, a hole in the diaphragm (diaphragmatic hernia), hypospadius, and clubbed feet. Keep in mind that these findings can also be consistent with other genetic syndromes.

## Treatment and management

There is no treatment for the underlying condition of WHS. Treatment and management for patients who have WHS are specific to each individual. For example, some individuals who have WHS may have heart defects or a cleft lip and/or palate that may require surgery, while others may not. Therefore, there is no specific treatment for individuals who have WHS, rather, the treatment and management is geared toward that particular individual's needs and is likely to include several medical specialists. Information about patients who have WHS has been compiled and provides a comprehensive look into the natural history of this condition. It also allows the following management guidelines to be recommended. The collection of this information has shown that many of these individuals may achieve more development than was previously believed possible.

The following management recommendations have been made by Drs. Battaglia and Carey:

- Feeding problems should be addressed and may require intervention such as placement of a gastrostomy tube.

- Characterization of seizures is important and treatment with antiepileptic medications such as valproic acid should be investigated and may help control the seizure activity in many individuals.

- Skeletal abnormalities such as clubfoot should be addressed and treatment should be considered. It should not be assumed that clubfoot does not need addressed because the child will never walk. Children with WHS have learned to walk unassisted.

- As approximately 30% of individuals may have congenital heart defects, the heart should be examined. Usually, the heart lesions are not severe and may be repaired easily or may not even require surgery.

- Hearing loss may occur and because some children are able to learn to talk in short sentences, they should be screened for hearing problems.

- At what point should my child be evaluated for a heart disorder?
- When should my child's hearing be evaluated?
- When should my child see an ophthalmologist?
- What developmental programs or resources do you recommend?

- Eye abnormalities may be present and thus an ophthalmology exam should be performed to rule out any eye problems, even if no obvious signs are present.

- In regards to the development of patients with WHS, it is suggested that individuals participate in personal development programs to assist with social skills and occupational therapy for motor skills.

### Prognosis

Infants who have WHS may be stillborn or die in the newborn period and prognosis during the newborn period depends upon what birth defects are present. It has been estimated that approximately 35% of individuals who have WHS die within the first two years of life. Many individuals who have WHS survive to adulthood. Universally, children with WHS have severe or profound developmental retardation, however, there are many affected individuals who are able to walk and some that are able to talk in short sentences. It is evident that many patients seem to proceed farther than was previously thought possible. The actual lifespan for individuals who have WHS is unknown, although there are several individuals who have WHS who are in their 20–40s.

### Resources

#### BOOKS

Schaefer, G. Bradley, et al. *Wolf-Hirschhorn Syndrome (4p-): A Handbook for Families.* Munroe-Meyer Media Center, 1996. (1-800-656-3937).

#### PERIODICALS

Battaglia, Agatino, and John C. Carey. "Health Supervision and Anticipatory Guidance of Individuals With Wolf-Hirschhorn Syndrome." *American Journal of Medical Genetics (Semin. Med. Genet.)* 89 (1999): 111-115.

#### WEBSITES

*4p- Support Group.* http://www.4p-supportgroup.org.

#### ORGANIZATIONS

National Organization for Rare Disorders (NORD). PO Box 8923, New Fairfield, CT 06812-8923. (203) 746-6518 or (800) 999-6673. Fax: (203) 746-6481. http://www.rarediseases.org.

Renee A. Laux, MS

# Wolman disease

### Definition

Wolman disease is a rare inherited defect in the body's metabolism of fats (lipids).

### Description

Wolman disease, also known as lysosomal acid lipase disease, is a lethal genetic disorder caused by the lack of the enzyme lysosomal acid lipase. Lysosomal acid lipase is a cellular enzyme widespread throughout the body. It is important in the breakdown of certain body lipids called triglycerides and cholesteryl esters. Individuals without active enzyme accumulate abnormally large amounts of these lipids in their cells. This build-up interferes with the normal metabolic functions of the cells and leads to severe neurological and physical symptoms and early death. A milder disease, cholesteryl ester storage disease (CESD), is caused by mutations in the same gene, but affected individuals may not show symptoms until adulthood.

### Genetic profile

#### Inheritance pattern

Wolman disease is an autosomal recessive disorder affecting both males and females. In individuals with this disorder, both copies of the gene that codes for lysosomal acid lipase are abnormal. Both parents of an affected child have one abnormal copy of the gene, but usually do not show symptoms because they also have one normal copy. The normal copy provides approximately 50% of the usual enzyme activity, a level adequate for the body's needs. Individuals with one abnormal copy of the gene and 50% enzyme activity are said to be carriers or heterozygotes. Because both parents of a child with Wolman disease are carriers, they have a 25% risk in each subsequent pregnancy of having another child who is affected with the same disorder.

# KEY TERMS

**Adrenal gland**—A triangle-shaped endocrine gland, located above each kidney, that synthesizes aldosterone, cortisol, and testosterone from cholesterol. The adrenal glands are responsible for salt and water levels in the body, as well as for protein, fat, and carbohydrate metabolism.

**Amniocentesis**—A procedure performed at 16-18 weeks of pregnancy in which a needle is inserted through a woman's abdomen into her uterus to draw out a small sample of the amniotic fluid from around the baby. Either the fluid itself or cells from the fluid can be used for a variety of tests to obtain information about genetic disorders and other medical conditions in the fetus.

**Autosomal recessive**—A pattern of genetic inheritance where two abnormal genes are needed to display the trait or disease.

**Carrier**—A person who possesses a gene for an abnormal trait without showing signs of the disorder. The person may pass the abnormal gene on to offspring.

**Chorionic villus sampling**—A procedure used for prenatal diagnosis at 10–12 weeks gestation. Under ultrasound guidance a needle is inserted either

through the mother's vagina or abdominal wall and a sample of cells is collected from around the early embryo. These cells are then tested for chromosome abnormalities or other genetic diseases.

**Enzyme**—A protein that catalyzes a biochemical reaction or change without changing its own structure or function.

**Gene**—A building block of inheritance, which contains the instructions for the production of a particular protein, and is made up of a molecular sequence found on a section of DNA. Each gene is found on a precise location on a chromosome.

**Heterozygote**—Having two different versions of the same gene.

**Lysosomal**—Pertaining to the lysosomes, special parts (organelles) of cells that contain a number of enzymes important in the breakdown of large molecules such as proteins and fats.

**Mutation**—A permanent change in the genetic material that may alter a trait or characteristic of an individual, or manifest as disease, and can be transmitted to offspring.

### Gene location

The gene for acid lipase is located on the long arm of **chromosome** 10 at 10q23.2-q23.3. A number of different types of mutations in this gene, all resulting in a lack of enzyme function, have been identified in patients diagnosed with Wolman disease. These include deletions of small portions of the gene, as well as changes in specific nucleotides, the building blocks of the gene. The different mutations may explain why symptoms vary from one individual to another. However, the presence of variability in symptoms even among siblings who have inherited the same mutations from their parents, suggests there may be other, as yet unknown, genetic or environmental factors that affect the severity of the disease. Milder forms, such as the related disorder CESD, appear to be associated with **gene mutations** that result in only partial loss of enzyme function.

### Demographics

In the general population, Wolman disease is exceedingly rare, with approximately 50 or fewer well-described cases to date. CESD is thought to be more common. Individuals with Wolman disease have been reported in

various parts of the world including Western Europe, North America, Iraq, Iran, Israel, China, and Japan.

### Signs and symptoms

Symptoms of Wolman disease appear in the first few weeks of life. Forceful vomiting and distention of the abdomen usually alert parents to a problem. Other general symptoms in the early stages of this disease are watery diarrhea or fat in the stools, fever, and a yellow tint to the skin (jaundice). Medical examination reveals massive enlargement of the liver and spleen (hepatosplenomegaly) due to a build-up of fats that cannot be broken down. Other common findings are severe anemia, calcium deposits in the adrenal glands, and a general decline in mental development.

### Diagnosis

Diagnosis can be difficult because there are no general laboratory tests that point specifically to Wolman disease. Infants with hepatosplenomegaly and evidence of malnutrition should have a careful neurological examination and x–rays of the abdomen to check for calcium deposits in the adrenal glands. If Wolman disease is suspected on the basis of these tests, acid lipase activity can be measured in the laboratory using white blood cells or skin cells. An absence of acid lipase activity confirms the diagnosis.

### Carrier testing

Individuals suspected of being a carrier of Wolman disease can be confirmed by measuring acid lipase activity in their white blood cells. Carriers will typically demonstrate 50% of normal enzyme activity.

### Mutation detection

Specific **DNA** tests that check for changes in the normal sequence of nucleotides in the acid lipase gene can usually detect the particular gene mutation in an affected individual or carrier. This type of test is only available in a few, very specialized DNA laboratories.

### Prenatal diagnosis

Couples who have had one child with Wolman disease may be offered prenatal testing in future pregnancies. Prenatal testing is accomplished by measuring acid lipase activity either in cells from a chorionic villus sampling (CVS) at 10–12 weeks of pregnancy or in amniotic fluid cells obtained by **amniocentesis** between the sixteenth and eighteenth weeks of pregnancy. Alternatively, if specific gene mutations have been identified in parents because they have already had a affected child, fetal DNA from chorionic villus cells or amniotic fluid cells can be studied to look for these same mutations in the fetus. Carrier couples who are considering prenatal diagnosis should discuss the risks and benefits of this type of testing with a geneticist or genetic counselor.

## Treatment and management

There is no specific treatment for Wolman disease. There have been attempts to treat the milder CESD with low-fat diets and cholesterol-lowering drugs, and there has been at least one report of a liver transplant in a patient with CESD. Replacement of the missing enzyme has not been reported.

---

## QUESTIONS TO ASK YOUR DOCTOR

- Do you recommend a low-fat diet?
- What are the risks and expected benefits of cholesterol controlling medication?
- Have you heard reports of enzyme replacement for Wolman disease?
- Do you think liver transplant is a possibility?

---

## Prognosis

Infants diagnosed with Wolman disease usually die by six months of age.

## Resources

### BOOKS

Assmann, G., and U. Seedorf. *The Metabolic & Molecular Bases of Inherited Disease.* Ed. C.R. Scriver, et al. New York: McGraw-Hill, 2001.

### PERIODICALS

Anderson R. A., et al. "Lysosomal Acid Lipase Mutations That Determine Phenotype in Wolman and Cholesterol Ester Storage Disease." *Molecular and Genetic Metabolism* 68, no. 3 (November 1999): 333-45.

Krivit, W., et al. "Wolman Disease Successfully Treated by Bone Marrow Transplantation." *Bone Marrow Transplant* 26, no. 5 (September 2000): 567- 70.

Lohse, P., et al. "Molecular Defects Underlying Wolman Disease Appear To Be More Heterogeneous Than Those Resulting in Cholesteryl Ester Storage Disease." *Journal of Lipid Research* 40, no. 2 (February 1999): 221- 8.

### WEBSITES

"Wolman Disease." *Online Mendelian Inheritance in Man.* http://www.ncbi.nlm.nih.gov/entrez/dispomim.cgi?id = 278000.

### ORGANIZATIONS

National Organization for Rare Disorders (NORD). PO Box 8923, New Fairfield, CT 06812-8923. (203) 746-6518 or (800) 999-6673. Fax: (203) 746-6481. http://www. rarediseases.org.

Sallie Boineau Freeman, PhD

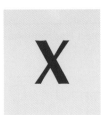

# X-linked hydrocephaly

## Definition

Hydrocephaly refers to the accumulation of cerebrospinal fluid (CSF) in the fluid-filled cavities, called ventricles, that are located deep in the core of the brain. The designation *X-linked* indicates that this form of hydrocephaly results from a mutation in a **gene** that is located on the X **chromosome**, in this case the L1 cell adhesion molecule (L1CAM) gene.

## Description

Cell adhesion molecules (CAMs) provide the traffic signals that guide the cells of developing organs to migrate to their proper places and make the appropriate connections with the cells with which they interact. The L1CAM protein is embedded in the membrane of nerve cell axons. Axons are projections from the nerve cell body that carry impulses to sometimes distant targets. As a developing axon grows toward its target, its leading end is capped by a growth cone similar in function to that of a plant root. The growth cone of a developing axon is rich in L1CAM. The L1CAM protein has a large, complex extracellular domain (portion of the protein outside the nerve cell), a transmembrane domain within the nerve cell membrane, and a small intracellular domain (portion inside the nerve cell). The extracellular domain acts as a feeler, and binds to CAMs that are either on the surface of other cells or floating in the extracellular fluid. The binding of the L1CAM protein to various CAMs in its environment sends signals into the nerve cell that direct the projecting axon to grow to the appropriate length, follow the course required for it to reach its target, and stop when appropriate.

The L1CAM protein is critical for proper development of several long fiber tracts in the forebrain. These include the corpus callosum, which is a thick fiber bridge that connects the left and right cerebral hemispheres, and the cerebrospinal tract, which extends from the motor control region of the cerebral cortex down to the spinal cord.

The developing axon often extends many cell diameters away from the cell body, and must interact with CAMs from many different sources to insure that it follows the correct route to its target. The complex extracellular domain of the L1CAM protein interacts with a variety of CAMs in the environment to serve several important functions. Because of the many functions L1CAM serves, the specific brain changes and functional handicaps that are seen in any individual patient with an L1CAM mutation depend on which of L1CAM's functions are lost and which are spared by the specific mutation that occurs in the L1CAM gene. Most families have their own unique L1CAM mutation. Some mutations abolish all of L1CAM's functions, while others change only a small piece of the L1CAM protein. Therefore, there is marked variability between patients in terms of which brain structures are most affected and what the primary physical and behavioral symptoms will be. Because of this variability, patients with different L1CAM mutations have been given diagnoses such as X-linked hydrocephaly (XLH), X-linked spastic paraplegia type 1 (SPG1), hydrocephaly with stenosis of the aqueduct of Sylvius (HSAS), X-linked agenesis of the corpus callosum (XLACC), and MASA syndrome (mental impairment, aphasia, shuffling gait, adducted thumbs). Because these patients all presented with such different combinations of brain changes and functional handicaps, it was originally thought that these were all distinct disorders, with different biological causes. As of 2001, an effort is being made to unite these disorders under the general heading *L1CAM spectrum*, to reflect the fact that these are not distinct disorders, but merely alternative possible consequences of L1CAM mutations.

## Genetic profile

The L1CAM gene is located close to the end of the long arm of the X chromosome, in the band referred to

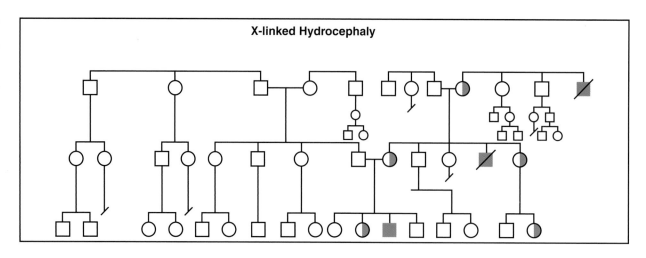

**X-linked Hydrocephaly**

(Gale, a part of Cengage Leaning.)

as Xq28. Since the L1CAM gene is on the X chromosome, usually only males are affected. This is because females have two X chromosomes, while males only have one. In a female, if one X chromosome has an L1CAM mutation on it, the non-mutated L1CAM gene on the other X chromosome can usually provide enough good L1CAM protein to support normal brain development. Males, on the other hand, having only one X chromosome, cannot compensate for an X-linked gene mutation.

The **inheritance** pattern for L1CAM spectrum disorders follows the typical X-linked inheritance pattern. Males are usually the only ones affected, and most females who carry L1CAM mutations are unaffected. There may be several affected brothers in a single family. In addition, in a family where the L1CAM mutation has been passed through several generations, the normally developed mothers of affected males may have affected brothers, or the normally developed sisters of affected males may have affected sons. If a female carries a mutation in L1CAM, she has a 50% chance of passing the mutation to each of her children. Therefore, approximately half her sons will be affected, and approximately half her daughters will be carriers. There is no known case in which an affected male has reproduced.

L1CAM mutations exhibit 100% penetrance, meaning that any male who has the L1CAM mutation will be affected, albeit with varying degrees of severity. This contrasts with some other disorders, in which some family members are unaffected, despite having the same gene mutation that has been seen in other affected family members.

## Demographics

The incidence of hydrocephaly from all causes is approximately one in 2,000 live births in the general population. The X-linked form is thought to account for approximately 5% of the total cases of hydrocephaly, or approximately one in 25,000 to 50,000 males. In very rare cases a female may be affected, usually mildly. There are no systematic data comparing the incidence of L1CAM spectrum disorders in different races.

## Signs and symptoms

Most patients with mutations in L1CAM exhibit mental retardation (MR), the degree of which can vary from mild to severe. The vast majority also exhibit hydrocephaly, which can be mild and not require any medical intervention, or severe enough to be life-threatening. The most severe cases of hydrocephaly are associated with stenosis (narrowing or pinching closed) of the aqueduct of Sylvius. The aqueduct of Sylvius (also called the cerebral aqueduct) is a narrow channel connecting the third ventricle, located deep in the midbrain, to the fourth ventricle, located underneath the cerebellum in the posterior part of the brain. The brain's cerebrospinal fluid (CSF) is made by cells lining the first two ventricles, called the lateral ventricles, which are located in the forebrain. The CSF normally flows from the first two ventricles, through the third ventricle, then into the fourth ventricle, before flowing out of the brain. Stenosis of the aqueduct of Sylvius stops the outflow of CSF, and causes an accumulation of fluid, and pressure, primarily in the first two ventricles. Since there is no mechanism to stop CSF production in the lateral ventricles, this form

**Adducted thumbs**—Thumbs clasped across the palm.

**Aphasia**—Loss of previously acquired ability to speak, or to understand written or spoken language.

**Brain ventricles**—A set of four connected cavities that are located deep in the core of the brain. Cerebrospinal fluid is made by cells lining the walls of the first two ventricles, then flows through the third, then fourth ventricle before flowing out of the brain. The fluid-filled cavities provide mechanical cushion for the brain, and the CSF provides nutrients to, and carries metabolic wastes away from, the cells of the brain.

**Cell adhesion molecule**—Any one of several thousand proteins that together control the cell-to-cell communication that must take place in order for cells to migrate to their proper places, develop into the proper types of cells, and make the appropriate connections with other cells.

**Corpus callosum**—A thick bundle of nerve fibers deep in the center of the forebrain that provides communications between the right and left cerebral hemispheres.

**Corticospinal tract**—A bundle of long nerve fibers that runs from the motor control region of the cerebral cortex to the spinal cord, where it connects to nerves that control movement in the legs.

**Cydrocephaly**—Excessive accumulation of cerebral spinal fluid in the brain ventricles.

**Macrocephaly**—A head that is larger than normal.

**Penetrance**—The degree to which individuals possessing a particular genetic mutation express the trait that this mutation causes. One hundred percent penetrance is expected to be observed in truly dominant traits.

**Spastic paraplegia**—Inability to walk, due to lack of proper neural control over the leg muscles.

**Stenosis**—The constricting or narrowing of an opening or passageway.

**Ventriculoperitoneal shunt**—A tube equipped with a low pressure valve, one end of which is inserted into the lateral ventricles, the other end of which is routed into the peritoneum, or abdominal cavity.

**X-linked**—Located on the X chromosome, one of the sex chromosomes. X-linked genes follow a characteristic pattern of inheritance from one generation to the next.

---

of hydrocephaly is progressive. The pressure can become so great that it stretches the developing skull bones, which are still not fully hardened, resulting in the child having a head that is visibly enlarged (macrocephaly). In the process, the brain tissue is pressed against the skull, with predictably devastating effects on brain function. Many of the more severely hydrocephalic patients are either stillborn or die within one year of birth.

Approximately 80% of patients with L1CAM mutations exhibit adducted thumbs (clasped across the palm). A smaller percentage exhibit aphasia (lack of speech), or problems with leg control that range from walking with a shuffling gait to spastic paraplegia that leaves them unable to walk at all.

The most common finding in brain imaging studies is the absence (agenesis) or underdevelopment (hypoplasia) of the corpus callosum. The corpus callosum is a large fiber tract that projects between the left and right hemispheres of the brain and enables information to be transferred from one hemisphere to the other. It is uncertain whether the abnormalities in the corpus callosum are an important cause of these patients' MR. It is most likely that the pressure exerted on the developing brain tissue by the hydrocephaly is a more consistent and important cause of the MR seen in these patients. Another brain structure seen to be underdeveloped in some patients with L1CAM mutations is the corticospinal tract. The corticospinal tract begins in the motor control region of the cerebral cortex and runs downward to connect with the spinal cord neurons that control the legs. Abnormal development of the corticospinal tract is probably the cause of the shuffling gait/spastic paraplegia seen in some patients with L1CAM mutations.

### Diagnosis

In the more severely hydrocephalic patients, hydrocephaly can be seen by ultrasound at 20 weeks gestation, or approximately half-way through the fetal period. For less severely affected patients, some degree of hydrocephaly is usually noted within a year after birth, along with a general developmental delay. These babies do not roll over, sit up, or reach for objects as early as babies typically do. In rarer cases, some mildly affected patients are not diagnosed until an age at which speech problems or problems with their walking gait can be observed. Adducted thumbs, when present, are noticeable from birth or sometimes upon ultrasound analysis.

**Genetic testing** involves a search for mutations in the L1CAM gene in patients with L1CAM spectrum disorders. The sequence of the L1CAM gene from the affected patient is compared to the normal L1CAM sequence. **DNA** is usually obtained from a blood sample for postnatal diagnosis. For prenatal diagnosis, DNA can be extracted from amniotic fluid cells obtained by **amniocentesis**, or from chorionic villus sampling.

## Treatment and management

In the most severely hydrocephalic cases, the baby must be delivered by Caesarian section, because the head has grown too large by the end of the pregnancy for the baby to be delivered through the vagina. For the more severely affected patients, a ventriculoperitoneal shunt can be used to reduce the pressure inside the brain. The shunt is a tube inserted into the lateral ventricles that allows the CSF to drain into the peritoneum, or abdominal cavity. This provides a means for the CSF to flow out of the brain in cases of HSAS, in which the aqueduct of Sylvius has been closed and the CSF can not flow out of the brain by the usual channel. Shunting markedly reduces the pressure on the brain, and has saved many patients' lives. However, shunting will not prevent these patients from having MR or other L1CAM spectrum features.

Other methods for managing cases of L1CAM spectrum disorders are focused on the specific features the individual patient exhibits. Special education is almost always necessary, with the specific program designed to accommodate the degree of cognitive disability seen in the individual patient. Physical therapy and mechanical aids such as walkers can be used to help patients with milder degrees of spastic paraplegia. Speech therapy has also benefited some of the less severely aphasic patients. There is generally little improvement when these therapies are applied to more severely affected patients.

## Prognosis

The prognosis for patients with L1CAM mutations is highly variable. The most severe cases of L1CAM mutations involve fetal demise, presumably because of the pressure exerted on the developing brain by the hydrocephaly. However, in less severe cases, the life span is determined primarily by general health and care factors. A number of patients with less severe L1CAM spectrum disorders have lived at least into their 50s.

---

## QUESTIONS TO ASK YOUR DOCTOR

- How beneficial will modes of treatment such as physical, occupational or speech therapy be for my child?
- What are the risks and benefits of shunting?
- What is the level of severity of my child's case of x-linked hydrocephaly?
- Which family members should undergo genetic testing?

---

## Resources

### PERIODICALS

Fransen, E., et al. "L1-associated Diseases: Clinical Geneticists Divide, Molecular Geneticists Unite." *Human Molecular Genetics* 6 (1997): 1625-1632.

Kenwrick, S., M. Jouet, and D. Donnai. "X Linked Hydrocephalus and MASA Syndrome." *Journal of Medical Genetics* 33 (1996): 59-65.

Kenwrick, S., A. Watkins, and E. De Angelis. "Neural Cell Recognition Moleculae L1: Relating Biological Complexity to Human Disease Mutations." *Human Molecular Genetics* 9 (2000): 879-886.

### ORGANIZATIONS

Guardians of Hydrocephalus Research Foundation. 2618 Avenue Z, Brooklyn, NY 11235-2023. (718) 743-4473 or (800) 458-865. Fax: (718) 743-1171. guardians1@juno.com.

Hydrocephalus Association. 870 Market St. Suite 705, San Francisco, CA 94102. (415) 732-7040 or (888) 598-3789. Fax: (415) 732-7044. hydroassoc@aol.com. http://neurosurgery.mgh.harvard.edu/ha.

Hydrocephalus Support Group, Inc. PO Box 4236, Chesterfield, MO 63006-4236. (314) 532-8228. hydrobuff@postnet.com.

National Hydrocephalus Foundation. 12413 Centralia, Lakewood, CA 90715-1623. (562) 402-3523 or (888) 260-1789. hydrobrat@earthlink.net. http://www.2nhfonline.org.

National Institute of Neurological Disorders and Stroke. 31 Center Drive, MSC 2540, Bldg. 31, Room 8806, Bethesda, MD 20814. (301) 496-5751 or (800) 352-9424. http://www.ninds.nih.gov.

National Organization for Rare Disorders (NORD). PO Box 8923, New Fairfield, CT 06812-8923. (203) 746-6518 or (800) 999-6673. Fax: (203) 746-6481. http://www.rarediseases.org.

### WEBSITES

L1 Mutation Web Page. http://dnalab-www.uia.ac.be/dnalab/l1/.&gt;

Ron C. Michaelis, PhD, FACMG

# X-linked mental retardation

## Definition

X-linked mental retardation (XLMR) broadly refers to a group of inherited disorders characterized by varying degrees of mental retardation, caused by mutations in various genes present on the X **chromosome**. Mental retardation is defined as the failure to develop cognitive abilities and achieve a level of intelligence and adaptive behavior that is appropriate for a particular age group. XLMR is mostly seen in boys, usually manifests before the age of 18, and is characterized by an overall intelligence quotient (IQ) of less than 70, along with functional deficits in adaptive behavior like daily living, and social and communication skills.

## Description

The X chromosome was so named initially to mean unknown, as the functions of the genes carried on it were not clear. The United States Census of 1890 was the first to collect data that showed that more boys than girls were mentally disabled, and it was suspected that this was due to the difference in the sex chromosomes present in males and females. It was only in 1970 that the most common cause of XLMR, **fragile X syndrome** was described in detail; its mutated gene (FMR1) was not identified until 1991. Mutations in the MECP2 gene are the second most common cause of XLMR, and result in Rett's syndrome. This gene was identified in 1999. Since 2004, about 200 XLMR disease types have been described. With the help of the **Human Genome Project**, of the 150–200 candidate genes on the X chromosome, mutations in about 50 have been identified as being responsible for different XLMR diseases.

XLMR is broadly divided into syndromic and non-syndromic disorders. Syndromic XLMR (S-XLMR) refers to conditions in which mental retardation is accompanied by characteristic and easily recognizable physical and/or neurological features. In non-syndromic XLMR (NS-XLMR), mental retardation is the only key feature without any other distinctive physical or neurological features. Two thirds of XLMR cases are thought to be non-syndromic. In both syndromic and non-syndromic XLMR, affected persons are mostly boys who have developmental delay or mental retardation of variable severity and who usually have another affected male maternal relative (e.g., maternal uncle). With rapid advances in **genetics** afforded by the Human Genome Project, it is now possible to detect some of the mutations known to cause mental retardation even before the child is born, leading to effective counseling and prevention strategies.

## Genetic profile

The complete sequence of the X chromosome was identified in 2005 and it confirmed that an unusually large number of its genes carry information for proteins important for brain functions. Most of the mutated genes in XLMR are thought to be intelligence genes that influence development, cell migration, formation and maintenance of neural networks, and cell-to-cell communication in the brain. The majority of the genes identified so far are linked to syndromic XLMR. It is now recognized that different mutations in the same gene can give rise to either S-XLMR or NS-XLMR.

Females have two X chromosomes and males have one X and one Y chromosome (which determines the male sex). The X chromosome in the male is always derived from the mother. A female uses only one of her two X chromosomes in each cell and randomly inactivates the other X chromosome. Thus, if only one of her X chromosomes has a defective gene, only some of her cells will suffer. The severity of XLMR in the female will consequently depend on the percentage of cells in which the mutated gene is expressed. On the other hand, men have only one X chromosome, so any defective brain genes from that chromosome are invariably expressed.

## Demographics

About 2–3% of the population has mental retardation due to genetic and non-genetic factors (e.g., birth injuries, infections, and developmental anomalies). XLMR is thought to account for approximately 20% of genetic causes of mental retardation and accounts for the 20–30% excess of mental retardation observed in males in comparison to females. Although accurate numbers are difficult to estimate, the prevalence of XLMR may be approximately one in 600 males and one in 400 female carriers.

## Signs and symptoms

About 150 different conditions have been described as of 2005. These can either be malformation syndromes, in which affected patients have mental retardation and multiple birth defects; neuromuscular syndromes, in which patients have mental retardation and abnormalities in various nerves and muscles; metabolic syndromes have a defect in a specific biochemical pathway; or dominant syndromes in which the disorder is inherited in an

## KEY TERMS

**Amniotic fluid**—The liquid that surrounds and cushions the developing fetus inside the mother's womb.

**Anticipation**—The apparent tendency of certain diseases to appear at earlier age and with increasing severity in successive generations.

**Anomaly**—A malformation or abnormality in any part of the body.

**Attention deficit disorder**—Neurological condition that is often evident from childhood, characterized by restlessness, disorganization, hyperactivity, distractibility, and mood swings.

**Autism**—A chronic developmental disorder usually diagnosed between 18 and 30 months of age; symptoms include problems with social interaction and communication, as well as repetitive interests and activities.

**Carrier**—An individual who possesses an unexpressed abnormal gene of a recessive genetic disorder.

**Chorionic villus**—Cells that are present in the placenta that can be used for genetic analysis.

**Chromosome**—A thread-like structure that is present in the nucleus of all cells and contains DNA, which carries genetic information.

**Cognitive**—Brain functions involved in the ability to think, learn, and remember.

**Connective tissue**—Tissue that is the supporting framework of the body and its internal organs; made up of collagen, elastic fibers, and fat.

**Corpus callosum**—Tightly bundled nerve fibers that connect the right and left hemispheres of the brain.

**Deoxyribonucleic acid (DNA)**—A chemical found primarily in the nucleus of cells, which carries the instructions for making all the structures and materials the body needs to function.

**Gene**—The basic unit of heredity; a sequence of DNA nucleotides on a chromosome.

**Human Genome Project**—An international effort begun in 1990 to locate and identify the 100,000 genes on the 46 human chromosomes.

**Lissencephaly**—A developmental disorder where the brain is smooth without the normal surface convolutions.

**Menopause**—The transition in a woman's life whereby menstrual periods stop.

**Microcephaly**—A condition, present at birth, in which the head is much smaller than normal for an infant of that age and gender.

**Mutation**—A spontaneous change in the sequence of nucleotides in a chromosome or gene.

**Neural**—Pertaining to a nerve or the nervous system.

**Nucleotide**—A small molecule composed of three parts: a nitrogen base (a purine or pyrimidine), a sugar (ribose or deoxyribose), and phosphate; they serve as the building blocks of nucleic acids (DNA and RNA).

**Placenta**—A bag-like organ that partially surrounds the fetus during pregnancy; it delivers oxygen and nutrients to, and takes waste away from, the fetus during pregnancy, and is attached to the fetus by the umbilical cord.

**Promoter**—The region of a gene that initiates transcription of the genetic information.

**Psychosis**—A severe mental disorder characterized by loss of contact with reality, causing deterioration of normal social functioning.

**Seizures**—An abnormal electrical discharge from the brain that usually results in convulsion of the body.

**Syndrome**—The group, or recognizable pattern, of symptoms or abnormalities that indicate a particular trait or disease.

---

X-linked dominant fashion with most affected males dying before birth.

The most common known cause of inherited mental retardation is fragile X syndrome, which accounts for 20% of XLMR. It was first described in the late 1970s; the gene was discovered in 1991. Persons from all ethnic and social backgrounds can be affected. It results from a mutation in the fragile X mental retardation (FMR1) gene found on the X chromosome. This gene contains information needed for making

the FMR protein, which is thought to regulate communication between various cells by eliminating unwanted communication neural pathways.

The FMR1 gene contains two distinct regions, one of which is called the promoter region. This region is composed of repeating units or building blocks called nucleotides arranged in a specific sequence. A normal person has 30 such units and can make normal amounts of the FMR protein. When a person has between 55 and 200 units, the gene becomes partially inactivated. They can still make some amount of FMR protein and are said to have a pre-mutation. The pre-mutation occurs in one in 250–300 females and one in 1,000 males. The amount of FMR protein in the body determines the severity of effects due to fragile X. Therefore, patients with a pre-mutation may have few, if any, symptoms and may not even know that they are carrying an abnormal gene. A pre-mutation can be transmitted silently over generations, but with each generation, the number of units increases and there is a higher chance of manifesting the condition (anticipation).

When a person has more than 200 units, the gene itself becomes completely inactivated, making it impossible to produce any FMR protein. The full mutation occurs in one in 3,600 males and one in 4,000–6,000 females. As females have two X chromosomes in each cell, even if one X has the full mutation, the other X carries the normal FMR1 gene, making it possible to produce at least some FMR protein. Therefore, females are less often and less seriously affected than males. Females who do not express the disease, but carry the abnormal gene are called carriers.

If a father carries the FMR1 mutation, he will transmit the mutation to all his daughters but cannot transmit it to his sons, as males receive only the Y chromosome. On the other hand, if a mother carries the mutation on one of her X chromosomes, each of her children (boys or girls) will have a 50% chance of inheriting the FMR1 mutation, depending on which X chromosome they receive.

There is a considerable variability in disease severity of fragile X syndrome in males, with many of the physical symptoms becoming more apparent only after puberty. Prior to puberty, the most common findings include speech delay, developmental delay, and mental retardation. The most noticeable and consistent effect is on intelligence. More than 80% of affected males have an IQ of less than 70, whereas the effect on IQ in an affected female is variable. It is uncommon for persons with fragile X to have severe mental retardation, and most have IQ in the range of 40–85. Females may show normal cognitive development with only mild learning disabilities and a normal IQ. People with fragile X have good memory skills for pictures and visual patterns, but have poor verbal knowledge. They also have poor abstract thinking, organizational skills, and problem-solving capabilities. Despite such limitations, many of them can be trained to acquire jobs and skills to take care of themselves.

Children with fragile X tend to develop certain physical characteristics by the time of puberty. They have a long face or jaw, large protruding ears, and do not grow as tall as other members in the family. Males with fragile X have large testicles, but this does not affect sexual development. They also have problems with connective tissues. They may be flat footed, have loose hyper-extensible joints, and "floppy" heart valves. Later in life, they can manifest hand tremors and difficulty walking. Women with fragile X undergo menopause early due to premature cessation of ovarian function, thus affecting their reproductive capabilities. About 25% of patients have seizures.

Most persons with fragile X syndrome, especially boys, have a lot of anxiety in social situations and become nervous and uncomfortable. They also tend to be easily upset and overwhelmed by sensory stimulation due to sights and sounds and deviance from normal routine. This may emerge as aggression in adolescent boys. Females tend to have less anxiety and are not usually aggressive. Boys have language problems, including speaking, writing, and acquiring social communication skills. Common behavior disturbances include attention deficit disorder, repetitive hand flapping, autistic behaviors, and gaze aversion, and 20% meet full criteria for **autism**.

Rett's syndrome (RS) is the second leading cause of XLMR and the leading cause of mental retardation in girls. It was first described in 1966; the gene was identified in 1999. RS is caused by mutation in the MECP2 gene that causes abnormal truncation of the gene. The MECP2 gene contains information for production of methyl cytosine binding protein 2, which normally helps to turn off other genes appropriately at various points along the process of brain development. If this does not occur, the overactive genes interfere with normal brain maturation and lead to abnormal "wiring" and overload of the brain's electrical system. Other types of mutation in the same MECP2 gene can result in mild mental retardation, tremor, psychosis, or learning disability, both in boys and girls, without producing classic RS.

RS almost exclusively occurs in females with a prevalence of one in 10,000–20,000. In males, the mutation is lethal, and most are severely affected or die before or soon after birth. There is also a phenomenon of preferential inactivation of the normal X chromosome leading to the disease expression even in the female. The affected girl develops normally during the first five months of life. During this period, the child exhibits autistic behaviors. She can be calm and quiet, without making good eye contact, and without showing much interest in toys. After this, head growth slows down and the child loses whatever purposeful hand movements that had already developed. Around three years, the girl child develops repetitive hand washing or hand wringing gestures, loses ability to speak, has trouble sleeping, becomes irritable, and develops an unsteady gait. Varying degrees of mental retardation are present. These children also have seizures.

**WEST SYNDROME.** West syndrome, also known as the infantile spasm-mental retardation syndrome, is caused by mutations in the ARX (aristaless-related homeobox) gene. This is the third most common genetic mutation leading to XLMR. It can occur in both boys and girls and is characterized by developmental delay, mental retardation, and a specific type of seizures called salaam fits or infantile spasms. During the seizures, the children either have a flexion spasm where the body is bent over in a self-hugging position or an extension spasm where the neck and body are arched backwards.

Mutations in the ARX gene can also result in various developmental defects like **lissencephaly** (abnormal accumulation of fluid in the brain, replacing the cerebral hemispheres), absence of the corpus callosum, **microcephaly**, and urinary and genital abnormalities, without causing the classic West syndrome.

Non-syndromic X-linked mental retardation (NS-XLMR) is represented by a heterogeneous group of disorders in which the only recognizable abnormality is mental retardation without other accompanying physical manifestations. As of 2004, about 78 families with NS-XLMR had been described and mutations in 15 genes had been linked with them.

### Diagnosis

The diagnosis of XLMR should be considered in all children with autistic behaviors, mental retardation, developmental delay, or unexplained speech delay; 80–90% of patients with fragile X syndrome are not yet correctly diagnosed. Because the symptoms of fragile X can be quite subtle, especially in young children, and because it is so frequent in the general population, many medical specialists recommend testing for fragile X syndrome. This is, however, not a routine screening test for all children. Testing for FMR1 mutation is possible in people of any age and even before birth.

A variety of diagnostic tests based on **DNA**, chromosomal, or protein analysis is available. Chromosomal tests look for the fragile, or broken, portion of the X chromosome under a microscope, but are generally not very sensitive. Protein tests measure the amount of FMR protein produced by the cells and can determine the severity of the disorder. A DNA-based test to diagnose fragile X was developed in 1992 and is based on detecting an increased number of repeating units. This test is quite accurate, and it can detect both carriers and fully affected individuals. Samples from blood, hair root, or a scraping from inside the cheek can be used to carry out the test. In a pregnant woman, amniotic fluid or cells from the placenta, called chorionic villus, are used to detect the mutation. Similarly, **genetic testing** can be done in specialized laboratories for the other common **gene mutations** associated with XLMR, such as Rett's syndrome.

### Treatment

Currently, there is no cure for any of the conditions associated with XLMR. Best results are obtained when medications are combined with educational, social, and occupational therapy. Early intervention when the child's brain is still developing is advocated in order to maximize its long-term potential. A team comprising of a neurologist, genetic specialist, psychologist, behavioral specialist, physical, occupational, and speech therapists should work with the family and caregivers to ensure that the child receives appropriate therapy based on individual needs. This team can also assess the patient's level of independence and ensure appropriate transition from adolescent to young adult.

The U.S. Food and Drug Administration Agency (FDA) has not approved any specific medication for treatment of fragile X or its symptoms. But several medications have been tried on an empiric basis to ameliorate specific symptoms and problems associated with this disorder. Seizures and mood instability can be treated with drugs used primarily in **epilepsy**, such as carbamazepine, valproate, gabapentin, and topiramate.

The Individuals with Disabilities Act of 1997 ensures free education for children with mental retardation and special cognitive needs until high school or until they reach 21 years. This law also ensures that children are taught in a non-restrictive environment tailored to their special needs. Speech therapists can help in language acquisition and devise innovative ways for nonverbal communication. Occupational therapists can assist the child with adaptive equipment to help overcome physical disabilities. Physical therapists help in designing programs and activities to promote posture, gait, and balance. Behavioral therapists can work with the family and the child in identifying strategies and coping skills to deal with social situations and avoiding aggression.

The Fragile X Research Foundation (FRAXA) funds several endeavors to help find a cure for this disease. Ongoing research is focused on repairing the defective gene, replacing the defective gene, supplying the deficient protein, or substituting the deficient protein with another protein.

### Prognosis

Children with fragile X syndrome have a fairly normal life expectancy. With early diagnosis and treatment, they can grow into independent individuals. Similarly, children with Rett's syndrome usually survive to adulthood and middle age.

### Resources

#### BOOKS

Fenichel, Gerald M. *Clinical Pediatric Neurology*, 4th edition. Philadelphia: W.B. Saunders Company, 2001.

#### PERIODICALS

Check, Erika. "The X Factor." *Nature* 434 (March 2005): 266–267.
Ropers, Hilger H., and Ben C. J. Hamel. "X-linked Mental Retardation." *Nature* 6 (Jan. 2005): 46–57.
Wiesner, Georgia L., Suzanne B. Cassidy, Sarah J. Grimes, Anne L. Matthews, and Louise S. Acheson. "Clinical Consult: Developmental Delay/Fragile X Syndrome." *Primary Care: Clinics in Office Practice* 31 (2004): 621–625.

#### ORGANIZATIONS

International Rett Syndrome Association. 9121 Piscataway Road, Clinton, MD 20735. (800) 818 RETT. (April 24, 2005.) http://www.rettsyndrome.org.
National Fragile X Foundation. P.O. Box 190488, San Francisco, CA 94119. (800) 688 8765. (April 24, 2005.) http://www.nfxf.org.
National Institute of Child Health and Human Development. P.O. Box 3006, Rockville, MD 20847. (800) 370 2943. (April 24, 2005.) http://www.nichd.nih.gov.

#### OTHER

Fragile X Research Foundation (FRAXA). 45 Pleasant Street, Newburyport, MA 01950. (978) 462 1866. (April 24, 2005.) http://www.fraxa.org/.
National Institute of Child Health and Human Development (NICHD). "Families and Fragile X Syndrome." NICHD Publication No. 03-3402. 2004.

Chitra Venkatasubramanian, MBBS, MD

---

# X-linked severe combined immunodeficiency

## Definition

X-linked **severe combined immunodeficiency** (x-linked SCID) is a genetic disorder of the immune system that occurs primarily in boys. It is the most common of the three forms of severe combined immunodeficiency (SCID). Symptoms are present at birth. Males with the disorder are prone to recurrent and persistent infections due to their compromised immune systems.

## Demographics

X-linked SCID occurs almost exclusively in boys. All ethnic groups are affected equally by the disorder. The prevalence is unknown but likely affects at least one in 50,000 to 100,000 newborns in the U.S. and worldwide, according to the National Institutes of Health (NIH). However, since there are no routine screening programs to determine the true incidence, some experts say the NIH estimate may be too small. As of 2009, the number of estimated existing cases was about 6,000 in the U.S., 700 in Canada, 2,100 in Mexico, 4,000 in Brazil, 1,300 in Great Britain, 1,700 in Germany, 3,000 in Russia, 27,000 in China, 2,600 in Japan, 22,000 in India, 3,200 in Pakistan, 3,000 in Bangladesh, 5,000 in Indonesia, 1,300 in France, 1,200 in Italy, 1,000 in South Korea, 800 in Poland, and 85 in Ireland.

## Description

X-linked severe combined immunodeficiency (x-linked SCID) is a hereditary disease, meaning it is passed from parent to child. It is considered a rare disorder by the NIH. It is often called "Bubble Boy" disease based on a Texas boy who spent his entire life inside a germ-free environment or bubble. The boy, David Vetter, died in 1984 at age 12 after a bone marrow transplant failed. Boys with X-linked SCID are susceptible to opportunistic infections that can occur over and over and are resistant to standard antibiotic treatment. The infections are called opportunistic because they do not normally cause sickness in healthy people. In people with the disorder, the body's immune system that normally fights off infections is severely compromised or does not work at all, making any infection serious and potentially life-threatening. Without treatment, infants with the disorder usually die within a year. The primary treatment is a bone marrow transplant.

The disorder is genetic, meaning it is inherited from a parent. Yet more than half of boys with the disease have no family history of early deaths in male relatives on their mother's side, according to the NIH. A woman who is a carrier of the mutated gene that causes the disorder has a 50% chance or transmitting the gene to each child she bears. Her sons that inherit the mutation will get the disorder, but any daughters will become carriers but will not get the disorder. In contrast, men who have the mutated gene will pass it on to their daughters but not their sons. Prenatal testing is available for pregnant women who are known carriers of the gene mutation.

### Risk factors

The primary risk factors include having a mother with the mutated gene and a family history of the disease. The mutated gene that causes the disorder is on the X **chromosome**, one of two chromosomes (Y is the other) that determines sex. Men have one X chromosome and women have two. One unusual characteristic of the disorder is that sons cannot inherit the X-linked mutated gene from their biological father.

## Causes and symptoms

X-linked SCID is caused by mutations in the IL2RG gene that provides information for making a protein that is required for the immune system to function normally. It is the immune system's job to fight infections in the body using a variety of cells, including lymphocytes (a type of white blood cells in the immune system.) Mutations in the IL2RG gene prevent lymphocyte cells from developing normally. With damaged lymphocytes, the immune system cannot fight off infections.

Symptoms can start at birth since the disorder is inherited from parent to child. More commonly, problems are first noticed between three and six months of age. By one year of age, virtually all infants with the disorder express symptoms. They include persistent and frequent infections caused by bacteria, viruses, and fungi that a healthy immune system would fight off. Common infections in infants include influenza and pneumonia, and infections of the ear and urinary tract. Other symptoms include rashes, diarrhea, cough, congestion, fever, other autoimmune conditions, failure to thrive, and short stature. Infants are often born without tonsils and lymph nodes.

## Diagnosis

Diagnosis is usually made when the number of absolute lymphocytes is low, the number of T cells is extremely low, B cells do not work, and the number of natural killer cells is low or zero. T cells are a type of white blood cell involved in rejecting foreign tissue, regulating immunity, and controlling the production of antibodies to fight infection. B cells are a class of lymphocytes, released from the bone marrow, that produce antibodies. Natural killer cells are specialized immune system cells that kill target cells infected with viruses or host cells that have become cancerous.

---

### KEY TERMS

**Bone marrow**—The soft and spongy center of the bones where blood cells are made.

**Chromosomes**—Structures inside cells that carry an individual's genetic information.

**DNA**—Deoxyribonucleic acid, the basic building blocks of all life on Earth. DNA stores genetic information that is passed from parents to their offspring.

**Flow cytometry**—A method of analyzing cells in which cell properties are detected as they flow in a narrow stream through a measuring device.

**Hereditary**—The passing of traits from parents to their offspring.

**Immune system**—The complex group of organs and cells that defends the body against infection and disease.

**Lymphocytes**—White blood cells that fight infection and disease.

**Mutated gene**—A change of DNA sequence that causes a change of the function of the gene and a subsequent disease.

**Opportunistic infections**—Infections that would not usually cause illness in people with a healthy immune system.

---

### Examination

Diagnosis of the disorder is only through specific tests, not physical examination.

### Tests

X-linked SCID can only be diagnosed by measuring the amount of lymphocytes in the body, lymphocyte cell surface staining and counting by flow cytometry, lymphocyte functional tests, and molecular **genetic testing** (used for diagnosis in the womb). Molecular genetic testing allows extra time to search for bone marrow transplant donors. It can also allow treatment to begin shortly after birth rather than waiting a few months for symptoms to appear.

### Procedures

A process called sequence analysis of the IL2RG gene detects a mutation in more than 99% of affected infants. The procedure is available in a clinical setting (a hospital, lab, or doctor's office.) It uses **DNA** usually taken from the blood or a swab of the mouth.

## Treatment

Bone marrow transplant is the primary treatment, although gene therapies have been successfully used since 1990. Since then, several European studies showed that **gene therapy** was a successful treatment, although in a few cases, the side effects included leukemia, a potentially fatal **cancer** of the blood.

### Traditional

Infants and children with X-linked SCID need quick action to restore a healthy or healthier immune system to survive. Untreated infants usually do not live beyond a year, according to the NIH. The primary treatment is usually a bone marrow transplant from a parent or other relative.

### Drugs

Interim treatment while the immune system is being restored includes treating infections with antibiotics and immunoglobulin infusion. Immunoglobulin is a class of proteins that act as antibodies in the immune system. Long-term treatment includes continued infusions of immunoglobulin, and gene therapy using stem cells. Gene therapy is primarily used in children who are either unable to have a bone marrow transplant or in which bone marrow transplantation has failed.

### Alternative

Echinacea, ginger, turmeric, zinc, elderberry, and other herbal supplements can boost the body's immune system, which can help ward off colds and the flu. Alternative treatments work best if used as complementary to traditional therapy once the body's immune function has been restored.

## Prognosis

The survival rate is not clear and the oldest survivors have lived into their 30s, according to the National Center for Biotechnology Information. This may be changing as more research is done and new treatment possibilities are studied. Further advancement in gene therapy, especially stem cell research, may increase life expectancy. Children who have had successful bone marrow transplants should be evaluated by a physician every six to 12 months.

## Prevention

There are no known ways to prevent X-linked SCID.

---

### QUESTIONS TO ASK YOUR DOCTOR

- What are the chances of my children developing this condition?
- Do you know of any recent research or medical breakthroughs concerning my child's condition?
- Would alternative or complementary treatments be useful in treating any of my child's symptoms?
- Are there any current or planned clinical trials or studies of my disorder that my child might be eligible to participate in?

---

## Resources

### BOOKS

Ochs, Hans D., et al. *Primary Immunodeficiency Diseases: A Molecular and Cellular Approach* New York: Oxford University Press, 2006.

Parker, Philip M. *X-Linked Severe Combined Immunodeficiency, Bibliography, and Dictionary for Physicians, Patients, and Genome Researchers* San Diego: ICON Group, 2007.

Rezaei, Nima, et al. *Primary Immunodeficiency Diseases: Definition, Diagnosis, and Management* New York: Springer Publishing, 2008.

Vickers, Peter. *Severe Combined Immune Deficiency: Early Hospitalization and Isolation* Hoboken, NJ: Wiley & Sons, 2009.

### PERIODICALS

Aitui, Alessandro, et al. "Gene Therapy for Immunodeficiency Due to Adenosine Deaminase Deficiency." *New England Journal of Medicine* (Jan. 29, 2009): 447–458.

Associated Press. "Gene Therapy Cures Form of Bubble Boy Disease," *USA Today* (Jan. 28, 2009): N/A.

"FDA Panel Recommends Curtailing Selected Gene Therapy Trials" *Transplant News* (March 17, 2003).

Puck, J.M. and H.L. Malech. "Gene Therapy for Immune Disorders: Good News Tempered by Bad News," *Journal of Allergy and Clinical Immunology* (April 2006): 865–869.

Thrasher, A.J., et al. "Failure of SCID-X1 Gene Therapy in Older Patients." *Blood* (June 1, 2005): 4255–4257.

Zoler, Mitchel L. "Wisconsin Starts SCID Screening in Newborns." *Family Practice News* (April 15, 2008): 15.

### ORGANIZATIONS

American Academy of Allergy, Asthma & Immunology, 555 E. Wells St., Ste 1100, Milwaukee, WI, 53202, (414) 272-6071, info@aaaai.org, http://www.aaaai.org.

American Association of Immunologists, 9650 Rockville Pike, Bethesda, MD, 20814, (301) 634-7178, (301) 634-7887, infoaai@aai.org, http://www.aai.org.

British Society for Immunology, Vintage House, 37 Albert Embankment, London, Great Britain, SE1 7TL, +44 (0) 20 3031 9800, +44 (0)20 7582 2882, online community@immunology.org, http://www.bsi.immunology.org.

Canadian Immunodeficiencies Patient Organization, 362 Concession Rd., Hastings ON, Canada, K0L 1YO, (877) 262-2476, (866) 842-7651, info@cipo.ca, http://www.cipo.ca.

Immune Deficiency Foundation, 40 W. Chesapeake Ave., Ste. 308, Towson, MD, 21204, (800) 296-4433, idf@primaryimmune.org, http://www.primaryimmune.org.

National Institute of Child Health and Human Development, 31 Center Dr., Bldg. 31, Room2A32, MSC 2425, Bethesda, MD, 20892, (800) 370-2943, (866) 760-5947, nichdinformationresourcecenter@mail.nih.gov, http://www.nichhd.nih.gov.

National Organization for Rare Diseases, 55 Kenosha Ave., Danbury, CT, 06813, (203) 744-0100, (800) 999-6673, (203) 798-2291, orphan@rarediseases.org, http://www.rarediseases.org.

Immune Deficiencies Foundation of New Zealand, P.O. Box 75–076, Manurewa, Manukau, New Zealand, 2243, (09) 523-5550, (0508) 300 600, (09) 523 5551, gm@idfnz.org.nz, http://www.idfnz.org.nz.

Primary Immunodeficiency Association, Alliance House, 12 Caxton St., London, Great Britain, SW1H 0QS, +44 (0) 207 976 7640, +44 (0) 207 976 7641, info@pia,org.uk, http://www.pia.org.uk.

Ken R. Wells

# Xeroderma pigmentosum

## Definition

Xeroderma pigmentosum is a rare inherited genetic disease. People with this condition develop skin and eye cancers at young ages because their **DNA** is extremely susceptible to damage caused by ultraviolet radiation. Xeroderma (dry, scaly skin) and pigmentosum (freckling and abnormal skin coloring) refer to changes that occur after exposure to sunlight or other ultraviolet radiation.

## Description

Xeroderma pigmentosum refers to a group of similar conditions. Each subgroup is designated by a letter or a roman numeral. Xeroderma pigmentosum is also often abbreviated XP. XP A and XP I are the same, as are XP B and XP II, XP C and XP III, etc. There are seven types of xeroderma pigmentosum

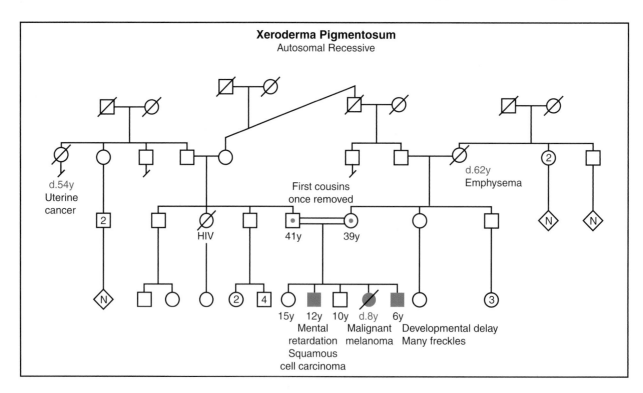

(Gale, a part of Cengage Learning.)

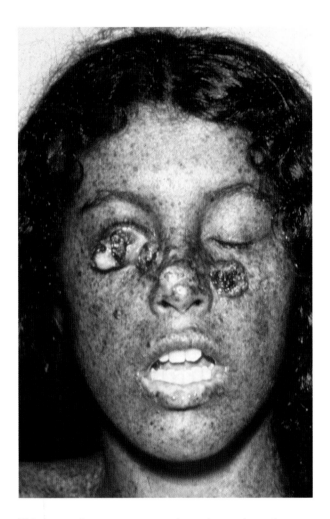

This woman has a severe case of xeroderma pigmentosum. Her right eye is affected, as well as her left cheek. *(Custom Medical Stock Photo, Inc.)*

designated A–G or I–VII. An eighth type of XP is called the "variant" type. XP VIII/XP H was once a separate subgroup; now it known to be part of XP D/ XP IV.

Each of the eight types of xeroderma pigmentosum has its own DNA defect. However, each section of DNA affected is involved in the same process. These defects affect the body's ability to repair DNA damage, especially DNA damage to the skin caused by exposure to ultraviolet radiation. Sunlight is the most common source of ultraviolet radiation. Everyone's DNA is damaged when it is exposed to sunlight. However, the body has complex and very effective methods to repair the DNA damage. This repair mechanism does not work properly in people with xeroderma pigmentosum. They quickly accumulate damage to their DNA if they are exposed to ultraviolet radiation. Cumulative DNA damage leads to **cancer**, especially of the skin and the eyes.

DeSanctis-Cacchione syndrome refers to the combination of xeroderma pigmentosum along with mental retardation, short stature, and other symptoms. Trichothiodystrophy (TTD) is sometimes caused by the same DNA change that causes XP D, and rarely XP B. People with TTD also have brittle hair and nails, and physical and mental retardation.

### Genetic profile

Xeroderma pigmentosum is inherited as an autosomal recessive condition. Everyone inherits one set of genetic material from each parent. People with xeroderma pigmentosum inherited one nonfunctional XP gene from each parent. Their parents have one normal gene and one abnormal gene (of that particular pair); they are called "carriers." Carriers do not have the autosomal recessive conditions because the normal gene in the pair protects them. Two carrier parents have a one in four chance with each pregnancy to have an affected child. A person with xeroderma pigmentosum will have an affected child only if the child's other parent is a carrier or affected with XP.

The **genetics** of xeroderma pigmentosum are a bit complicated. The genetic defect in seven of the subgroups has been identified. Each subgroup (A–G) has its own abnormal gene. Each person with xeroderma pigmentosum has a particular subtype, which is associated with one specific abnormal gene. For example, a person with XP type A has no normal XP A gene but does not have XP type B and does not have the abnormal genes associated with XP type B. The genes for types A, B, C, D, E, F, and G are on chromosomes 9, 2, 3, 19, 11, 16, and 13. If two people with different forms of xeroderma pigmentosum had a child, the child would not have xeroderma pigmentosum. But if two people with the same type of xeroderma pigmentosum mated, all of their children would also have xeroderma pigmentosum.

This discussion involves two different types of DNA changes. The first DNA change is the change that the person with xeroderma pigmentosum inherits from both parents. This change (mutation) affects the repair enzymes and is present in every cell in his or her body. The second type of change discussed is additional DNA mutations that result from exposure to ultraviolet radiation. Since the skin and eyes are commonly exposed to ultraviolet radiation that damages DNA and since the body's repair system is not working, people with this condition have a high rate of mutation in the exposed organs. These mutations often manifest themselves as cancers—abnormal, uncontrolled growths. Thus, it is the combination of genetic defect and environmental exposure that causes the manifestations of this disease. The first DNA change would not be nearly as problematic if it did not predispose the person with it to accumulate many additional DNA mutations.

### Demographics

Xeroderma pigmentosum occurs in every ethnic group. It occurs equally in men and women. Approximately one in 250,000 people in the United States have xeroderma pigmentosum. The most common types are A, C, D, and the variant type.

### Signs and symptoms

People with xeroderma pigmentosum have photosensitive skin. This means that their skin is hypersensitive to the effects of sunlight. Development of cancer at a young age is the most serious consequence. The eyes are also affected. Some people with xeroderma pigmentosum are affected intellectually, but not all. The symptoms a person will have are somewhat predictable based on which mutation he or she has.

#### Cutaneous symptoms

Skin manifestations usually begin in infancy. Early effects of skin exposure to minimal ultraviolet radiation include acute sunburn, blistering, freckles, increased or decreased pigment, birthmark-like spots, inflammation, dryness, and rough spots. The face, hands, neck, and arms are more severely affected because of increased sun exposure. Multiple scars may develop. The skin is normal at birth.

The average age at which people with xeroderma pigmentosum develop the first skin cancer is eight years. The risk to develop skin cancer is increased 1,000 times over the risk of the general population. A cell accumulates multiple abnormalities in its transition from a normal cell to a cancer cell. Cancers that occur frequently in people with xeroderma pigmentosum include squamous cell carcinoma, basal cell carcinoma, and malignant melanoma. Basal cell cancers are malignant and, if untreated, are characterized by relentless local invasion, but not metastasis elsewhere in the body. Squamous cell cancers are also malignant and, like basal cell carcinomas, tend to be local, although they are occasionally capable of metastasis. Malignant melanoma, as the name implies, is also malignant, but it is much more aggressive than either basal cell or squamous cell cancers of the skin. It is especially threatening because, if not diagnosed and treated early, it commonly will spread to internal organs and can be fatal. Cancer may occur on the eyes, lips, and tongue.

#### Ocular symptoms

Most people with xeroderma pigmentosum also have extremely light sensitive eyes. Their eyes easily become irritated, red, and swollen. Abnormal growths may appear. Cataracts may occur at an unusually young age.

#### Other symptoms

The other symptoms associated with xeroderma pigmentosum are variable. Many people who are affected only have eye and skin manifestations. Mental deterioration may occur; when it does, it usually worsens over time. Neurological symptoms are not believed to be associated with sun exposure. Some people have one or a combination of: **deafness**, poor reflexes, lower intelligence, or spasticity (in addition to ocular and cutaneous symptoms).

### Diagnosis

Xeroderma pigmentosum may be suspected based on a person's history of skin changes that occurred after minimal exposure to sunlight. The diagnosis is confirmed by a blood test or a skin test. The skin or blood cells are sent to a specialty laboratory. Studies are performed to determine whether the cells are hypersensitive to ultraviolet radiation. Scientists may examine whether abnormal changes can be seen in the chromosomes. The type of xeroderma pigmentosum may be determined by genetic studies or other specialized studies.

**Genetic testing** for xeroderma pigmentosum is complicated because there are eight different genes involved. Genetic tests are usually very specific, looking for a change in one gene. To confirm a diagnosis of xeroderma pigmentosum by DNA testing, scientists must look for multiple changes in eight different genes.

Prenatal diagnosis may be possible, especially if genetic studies have already been performed on an affected sibling and the parents.

### Treatment and management

The only treatment for xeroderma pigmentosum is avoiding harmful exposure to ultraviolet radiation and treating/removing growths as they occur. The DNA damage caused by exposure to ultraviolet light accumulates over time and the resulting DNA damage is irreversible.

Life is changed dramatically when a family member has xeroderma pigmentosum. Extreme measures must be taken to completely avoid exposure to the sun. Preventative measures include: sunglasses, tightly woven long-sleeved clothing, wide brim hats, sunblock, and protective window coverings (at home, in the car, and at school). Children do not play outside during the day. All sources of ultraviolet radiation are avoided, even exposure to certain light bulbs. These precautions are critical to survival. Levels of ultraviolet radiation at home and at school can be measured with special instruments. Abnormal skin growths and other symptoms are treated/removed as they arise. Regular visits are made to the eye doctor, dermatologist, and neurologist. Often psychosocial support is also helpful.

Treatments that would deliver DNA repair proteins into the skin of affected patients are under investigation. Some people with xeroderma pigmentosum may be offered other types of medication, like isotretinoin. The dermatologist weighs the benefit of prescribing a medication against the side effects associated with that medication.

Because our bodies have different mechanisms for fixing different forms of DNA damage, people with

---

**QUESTIONS TO ASK YOUR DOCTOR**

- How can avoidance of UV light best be accomplished?
- What are the risks and benefits of treatment with medication?
- How often should my child be screened for abnormal growths?
- Which family members should undergo genetic testing?

---

xeroderma pigmentosum are most susceptible to DNA damage by ultraviolet radiation. Some other exposures have been associated with the type of DNA damage caused by ultraviolet radiation. Therefore, people with xeroderma pigmentosum should also avoid exposure to tobacco and certain other drugs.

### Prognosis

Life expectancy is significantly reduced due to morbidity associated with the cancers. Researchers have not determined how effective preventative measures are, e.g. avoidance of ultraviolet radiation.

In the 1990s scientists discovered a great deal about DNA repair mechanisms, and about the genes associated with xeroderma pigmentosum. The range of symptoms associated with each type have been better defined. The media has also been interested in XP, giving it more attention than is typical for such a rare condition. Advocates in the XP community have developed helpful resources for other affected families, such as Camp Sundown.

### Resources

**PERIODICALS**

Cleaver, James. "Stopping DNA Replication in its Tracks." *Science* (July 9, 1999): 212.

McPhee, A.T. "Trapped in Darkness." *Current Science* (September 19, 1997): 10.

Miller, Samantha, and Joseph Tirella. "Into the Night." *People Magazine* (August 24, 1998): 90.

Williams, Monte. "Little Prisoner of the Light." *New York Times* (May 14, 1997): B1.

**WEBSITES**

Horenstein, Marcelo G., and A. Hafeez Diwan. "Xeroderma Pigmentosum." *eMedicine Journal* 2 (February 5, 2001). www.emedicine.com/derm/topic462.htm.

"Understanding Xeroderma Pigmentosum." National Institutes of Health Patient Information Publications.

http://www.cc.nih.gov/ccc/patient_education/pepubs/xeroderma.pdf.

**OTHER**

*Xeroderma Pigmentosum and Cockayne's Syndrome.* Videotape. American Registry of Pathology and Armed Forces Institute of Pathology, 1996. 888-838-1297.

**ORGANIZATIONS**

National Arthritis and Musculoskeletal and Skin Diseases Information Clearinghouse. One AMS Circle, Bethesda, MD 20892-3675. (301) 495-4484.

National Cancer Institute. Office of Communications, 31 Center Dr. MSC 2580, Bldg. 1 Room 10A16, Bethesda, MD 20892-2580. (800) 422-6237. http://www.nci.nih.gov.

Skin Cancer Foundation. 245 Fifth Ave., Suite 1403, New York, NY 10016. (800) 754-6490. info@skincancer.org.

Task Force on Xeroderma Pigmentosum, American Academy of Dermatology. Box 4014, Schaumburg, IL 60168-4014. (708) 330-0230.

Xeroderma Pigmentosum Registry. New Jersey Medical School, Dept. of Pathology, 185 South Orange Ave., Room C-520, Newark, NJ 07103-2714. (201) 982-4405.

Xeroderma Pigmentosum Society, Inc. PO Box 4759, Poughkeepsie, NY 12602. (518) 851-2612. xps@xps.org. http://www.xps.org.

Michelle Queneau Bosworth, MS, CGC

## XO syndrome *see* **Turner syndrome**

# XX male syndrome

## Definition

XX male syndrome occurs when the affected individual appears as a normal male, but has female chromosomes. Two types of XX male syndrome can occur: those with detectable **SRYgene** and those without detectable **SRY (sex determining region Y)**. SRY is the main genetic switch for determining that a developing embryo will become male.

## Description

XX male syndrome is a condition in which the sex chromosomes of an individual do not agree with the physical sex of the affected person. Normally, there are 46 chromosomes, or 23 pairs of chromosomes, in each cell. The first 22 pairs are the same in men and women. The last pair, the sex chromosomes, is two X chromosomes in females (XX) and an X and a Y **chromosome** in males (XY).

In XX male syndrome, the person has female chromosomes but male physical features. The majority of persons with XX male syndrome have the Y chromosome gene SRY attached to one of their X chromosomes. The rest of the individuals with XX male syndrome do not have SRY detectable in their cells. Hence, other genes on other chromosomes in the pathway for determining sex must be responsible for their male physical features.

## Genetic profile

In XX male syndrome caused by the gene SRY, a translocation between the X chromosome and Y chromosome causes the condition. A translocation occurs when part of one chromosome breaks off and switches places with part of another chromosome. In XX male syndrome, the tip of the Y chromosome that includes SRY is translocated to the X chromosome. As a result, an embryo with XX chromosomes with a translocated SRY gene will develop the physical characteristics of a male. Typically, a piece of the Y chromosome in the pseudoautosomal region exchanges with the tip of the X chromosome. In XX male syndrome, this crossover includes the SRY portion of the Y.

In individuals with XX male syndrome who do not have an SRY gene detectable in their cells, the cause of the condition is not known. Scientists believe that one or more genes that are involved in the development of the sex of an embryo are mutated or altered and cause physical male characteristics in a chromosomally female person. These genes could be located on the X chromosome or on one of the 22 pairs of autosomes that males and females have in common. As of 2001, no genes have been found to explain the female to male sex reversal in people affected with XX male syndrome who are SRY negative. Approximately 20% of XX males do not have a known cause and are SRY negative. It is thought that SRY is a switch point, and the protein that is made by SRY regulates the activity of one or more genes (likely on an autosomal chromosome) that contribute to sex development. Also there have been some studies that demonstrate autosomal recessive and autosomal dominant **inheritance** for the XX male.

## Demographics

XX male syndrome occurs in approximately one in 20,000 to one in 25,000 individuals. The vast majority, about 90%, has SRY detectable in their cells. The remaining 10% are SRY negative, although some research indicates that up to 20% can be SRY negative. XX male syndrome can occur in any ethnic

**Disorders associated with multiple X or Y chromosome inheritance**

| Disorder | Chromosome affected | Karotype | Incidence | Symptoms |
|---|---|---|---|---|
| Turner syndrome | X | 45,X (monosomy) | 1in 2,000 | Growth retardation<br>Infertility<br>Cardiovascular malformations<br>Learning disabilities |
| Klinefelter syndrome | X | 47,XXY (trisomy) | 1 in 500–800 | Taller than average<br>Poor upper body strength; clumsiness<br>Mild intention tremor (20–50%)<br>Breast enlargement (33%)<br>Decreased testosterone production<br>Infertility<br>Dyslexia (50%) |
| Triple X | X | 47,XXX (trisomy) | 1 in 1,000 | Mild delays in motor, linguistic and emotional development<br>Learning disabilities<br>Slightly taller than average |
| XYY syndrome | Y | 47,XYY | 1 in 1,000 | Taller than average<br>Lack of coordination<br>Acne<br>Some infertility<br>Learning disabilities (50%)<br>Behavior problems, especially impulse control |
| XX male syndrome | Y | 46,X,t(X,Y) (translocation of the SRY gene [90%] or other gene responsible for male sex determination) | 1 in 20,000–25,000 | Usually normal male physical features but may have ambiguous genitalia, hypospadias or undescended testes<br>Infertility<br>Shorter than average |

(Table by GGS Creative Resources. Reproduced by permission of Gale, a part of Cengage Learning.)

background and usually occurs as a sporadic event, not inherited from the person's mother of father. However, some exceptions of more than one affected family member have been reported.

## Signs and symptoms

### SRY positive XX male syndrome

Males with SRY positive XX male syndrome look like and identify as males. They have normal male physical features including normal male body, genitals, and testicles. All males with XX male syndrome are infertile (cannot have biological children) because they lack the other genes on the Y chromosome involved sperm production. Men with XX male syndrome are usually shorter than an average male, again because they do not have certain genes on the Y chromosome involved in height. A similar syndrome that effects males with two X chromosomes is **Klinefelter syndrome**. Those individuals with 46XX present with a condition similar to Klinefelter, such as small testes and abnormally long legs.

### SRY negative XX male syndrome

People with SRY negative XX male syndrome are more likely to be born with physical features that suggest a condition. Many have **hypospadias**, where the opening of the penis is not at the tip, but further down on the shaft. They may also have undescended testicles, where the testicles remain in the body and do not drop into the scrotal sac. Occasionally, an SRY negative affected male has some female structures such as the uterus and fallopian tubes. Men with SRY negative XX male syndrome can also have gynecomastia, or breast development during puberty, and puberty can be delayed. As with SRY positive XX male syndrome, these men are infertile and shorter than average because they lack other Y specific genes. The physical features can vary within a family, but most affected people are raised as males.

A small portion of people with SRY negative XX male syndrome are true hermaphrodites. This means they have both testicular and ovarian tissue in their gonads. They are usually born with **ambiguous genitalia**, where the genitals of the baby have both male and female characteristics. Individuals with XX male syndrome and true hermaphrodites can occur in the same family, suggesting there is a common genetic cause to both. Research indicates that 15% of 46XX true hermaphrodites have the SRY gene.

### Diagnosis

For people with XX male syndrome who have ambiguous genitalia, hypospadias, and/or undescended testicles, the diagnosis is suspected at birth. For males with XX male syndrome and normal male features, the diagnosis can be suspected during puberty when breast development occurs. Many men do not know they have XX male syndrome until they try to have their own children, are unable to do so, and therefore are evaluated for infertility.

When the condition is suspected in a male, chromosome studies can be done on a small sample of tissue such as blood or skin. The results show normal sex chromosomes, or XX chromosomes. Further **genetic testing** is available and needed to determine if the SRY gene is present.

Some affected individuals have had SRY found in testicular tissue, but not in their blood cells. This is called mosaicism. Most males only have their blood cells tested for SRY and not their testicular tissue. Hence, some men who think they have SRY negative XX male syndrome may actually be mosaic and have SRY in their gonads.

XX male syndrome can be detected before a baby is born. This occurs when a mother-to-be has prenatal testing done that shows female chromosomes but on ultrasound male genitals are found. Often the mother has had prenatal testing for a reason other than XX male syndrome, such as for an increased risk of having a baby with **Down syndrome** due to her age. Genetic testing for the presence of the SRY gene can be done by an **amniocentesis**. An amniocentesis is a procedure in which a needle is inserted through the mother's abdomen into the sac of fluid surrounding the baby. Some of the fluid is removed and used to test for the presence of the SRY gene. Amniocentesis slightly increases the risk of miscarriage.

### Treatment and management

For those with XX male syndrome with normal male genitals and testicles, no treatment is necessary. Affected males with hypospadias or undescended testicles may require one or more surgeries to correct the condition. If gynecomastia is severe enough, breast reduction surgery is possible. The rare person with true hermaphrodism usually requires surgery to remove the gonads, as they can become cancerous.

Parents who learn their child has been diagnosed with XX male syndrome are encouraged to gain both emotional and educational support. Issues such as explaining the condition to their child when they are grown is a topic that can be worked through with the help of both medical professionals, and those whose own children live with the condition.

### Prognosis

The prognosis for males with XX male syndrome is excellent. Surgery can usually correct any physical problems. Men with XX male syndrome have normal intelligence and a normal life span. However, all affected men will be infertile.

## Resources

**BOOKS**

Wilson, J.D., and J.E. Griffin. "Disorders of Sexual Differentiation." In *Harrison's Online*. Ed. Eugene Braunwald, et al. New York: McGraw-Hill, 2001.

**PERIODICALS**

Abramsky, L., et al. "What Parents Are Told After Prenatal Diagnosis of a Sex Chromosome Abnormality: Interview and Questionnaire Study." *British Medical Journal* 322 (2001): 463-466.

Biesecker, B. "Prenatal Diagnoses of Sex Chromosome Conditions: Parents Need More Than Just Accurate Information." *British Medical Journal* 322 (2001): 441-2.

Zenteno, Juan, et al. "Two SRY-negative XX Male Brothers Without Genital Ambiguity." *Human Genetics* 100 (1997): 606-610.

**ORGANIZATIONS**

Intersex Society of North America. PO Box 301, Petaluma, CA 94953-0301. http://www.isna.org.

RESOLVE, The National Infertility Association. 1310 Broadway, Somerville, MA 02144-1779. (617) 623-0744. resolveinc@aol.com.

Carin Lea Beltz, MS, CGC

# XXXX Syndrome

## Definition

XXXX syndrome is a genetic disorder in girls in which they have four X chromosomes rather than two. Also known tetra-X, tetrasomy X syndrome, and 48-X syndrome, the condition may cause lowered intelligence, increased height, speech and language disorders, and infertility.

## Demographics

XXXX syndrome only affects girls, and is extremely rare. It is estimated that there are 100 girls and women in the world with the condition. In 2004, a Penta-Tetra X registry was established in the United Kingdom. Sex **chromosome** disorders in which a baby is born with 47 to 49 chromosomes include a variety of conditions affecting boys and girls, and occur in one out of 400 births. There may be a number of cases of girls with this disorder who have not been diagnosed.

## Description

Humans normally have 46 chromosomes, 23 from each parent. In XXXX syndrome, girls are born with two extra chromosomes, for a total of 48. Symptoms range from mild to severe. Some children with the disorder are never able to lead independent lives although others play sports and attend college. The physical characteristics may be slight and not readily observable. Health problems associated with the syndrome also range from quite mild to more severe. XXXX syndrome was first reported in the medical literature in 1961. Research on XXXX syndrome has been limited, but there has been more interest in the topic in recent years.

Girls with XXXX syndrome generally do not have the obvious appearance of a chromosomal disorder. Their faces appear normal, and if differences are noted they are usually minor. The features that they may possess include epicanthal folds (creases next to the inner corner of the eye), eyes that may slant upward, and extra folds on the back of their neck. Their eyes may be widely spaced apart.

The speech and language disorders associated with XXXX syndrome are believed to be at the root of some of the behavioral problems described with this population. While many of the girls are described as pleasant and easy going, they also may have issues with anger management, mood swings, and shyness. Some girls experience psychiatric problems such as **bipolar disorder** and **depression**. Social difficulties have been reported among this group, although this issue is not consistently found among girls with XXXX syndrome.

Because there are so few cases in the world, studies are based on relatively small numbers. There are reports of four women with XXXX syndrome having a total of seven children. All were normal babies — a mixture of boys and girls — with the exception of one stillbirth and one baby born with **Down syndrome**.

### Risk factors

XXXX syndrome is extremely rare. In a rare number of cases, mothers of XXXX syndrome girls have been found to have an extra X chromosome in some cells.

## Causes and symptoms

### Causes

XXXX syndrome occurs when a girl inherits either three X chromosomes from her mother and one X chromosome from her father or when she inherits both extra chromosomes from her mother. It is believed that, in the formation of the mother's egg, errors in cell division cause the egg to contain multiple X chromosomes rather than only one. In some cases it is believed that the mother's child may first develop five X chromosomes, but one chromosome dies and the baby is left with four. XXXX syndrome can also be caused during conception, if there are errors in cell division at that time or if the mother carries an extra X chromosome in some of her cells.

An environmental cause for XXXX syndrome has not been found, and it is believed that neither environment nor maternal lifestyle cause this condition.

### Symptoms

The clinical symptoms of XXXX syndrome vary from one girl to the next. Some have milder symptoms, while others face more severe issues. The following is a list of symptoms that appear to be more prevalent with this population:

- Delayed physical development (mild)
- Delayed speech development
- Difficulty learning (mild to moderate)
- Tall stature (in some cases)
- Tendency toward stress
- Higher risk of dysfunctioning ovaries
- Higher incidence of respiratory infections (during younger years) than most girls of same age
- High arched palate
- Epicanthal folds, upward slanted eyes, and extra folds in the back of the neck
- Heart conditions of varying levels (affects approximately one-third of the girls)
- Kidney disorders
- Joint problems

As babies, girls with XXXX syndrome exhibit delays in physical development such as sitting and walking. Some of the girls experience weaker muscle tone and abnormally loose ligaments, factors that contribute to such delays. However, it is important to note that when the children gain the ability to walk and run, girls with XXXX syndrome can be quite active. They typically jump and play, and by their teenage years enjoy swimming and other sports.

Kidney disorders range from mild to severe. In some cases, the kidneys are fused together; in others, the girl is born with only one kidney. Because of a defect in valves regulating urine flow that may occur, there may be difficulty with the flow of urine from the kidneys to the bladder.

The palate may be highly arched, leading to a susceptibility toward ear infections as bacteria moves readily from the mouth to the ears. It is important that hearing is monitored to determine if hearing loss occurs, and it is also essential to monitor and treat ear infections promptly. The arch of the palate may also lead to problems with teeth; some girls experience

teeth that erupt too early, while others have a delay in tooth eruption.

Approximately half of the girls experience normal menstruation; the other half lack menstruation (or have irregular menstruation) as well as underdeveloped sexual features.

Approximately one-third of the girls may have varying degrees of heart conditions, ranging from murmurs to holes in either the septum (dividing partition) of the atria (upper chambers) or ventricles (lower chambers).

Problems with joint structure and movement seem to be an issue with this population. Some girls suffer with joints that are stiff or even fused, while others experience joints with hyper-rotation.

At birth, girls with XXXX syndrome are of slightly lower weight, with an average birth weight of 6.2 pounds. The girls tend to eat well and grow at a healthy pace; in fact, they tend to be tall children. Researchers believe it is possible that the extra chromosome adds to height. Another potential rationale for the increase in height among these girls is the lower levels of estrogen secretion. The range in height, although the sample is small because of the rarity of this disorder, is 5 foot 3 inches to 6 foot 2 inches.

In 1979, researchers at the University of California at Los Angeles reported on the first incident of a girl with XXXX syndrome lacking ovaries. The 16-year-old girl had a uterus and fallopian tubes but no ovaries. Consistent with the syndrome, the girl had mental retardation, although mild, as well as other mild characteristics associated with the condition.

The disorder affects intellectual development. A "rule of thumb" is that intelligence decreases 10–15 points for every extra chromosome. The average intelligent quotient (IQ) for the girls ranges from 60 to 80. While some girls attend schools with supportive environments, others go on to college. It has been said that the most representative features of the syndrome are learning disability and delay in speech development. On average, they learn to speak at age three years. Issues with complex speech and vocabulary may persist into the upper grades.

### Diagnosis

#### Examination

The clues that a baby has XXXX syndrome may be subtle at first. Symptoms of a chromosomal disorder, including epicanthal folds, may be present, but slight. In many cases, the baby's low birth weight, failure to meet developmental milestones, and sometimes the lack of

## KEY TERMS

**Epicanthal fold—** A wrinkle in the skin, extending from the nose up to the eyebrow, and sometimes associated with genetic anomalies.

**Renal—**Pertaining to the kidney.

muscle tone, ultimately prompt the pediatrician to suggest **genetic testing**. The diagnosis often comes after parents face an extended period during which their baby does not perform activities that are appropriate for her age.

### Tests

Genetic testing may be performed on body tissues such as blood or skin.

### Procedures

XXXX syndrome may be diagnosed with prenatal chromosome testing such as chorionic villus sampling or **amniocentesis**.

## Treatment

### Traditional

It is important to monitor kidney function because some girls have defects in the renal system. Kidney ultrasounds are recommended, as frequent infections of the kidney may impair kidney function later in life.

Some girls may require ear tubes if they experience recurrent infections.

## Prognosis

Mental retardation of varying degrees limits the chance of an independent life for those who have more severe forms of XXXX syndrome. Girls with mild mental retardation may live independently, but others must live in a setting that offers supervision and support.

Girls who have XXXX syndrome are more likely to have a daughter with the disorder; therefore, **genetic counseling** is strongly suggested if pregnancy is considered.

Infections caused by this syndrome may lead to serious consequences later in life. Infections of the ears, due to the high palate, may lead to **deafness**. Kidney infections may lead to high blood pressure and kidney damage.

## QUESTIONS TO ASK YOUR DOCTOR

- Is my child considered to have a mild or severe case of XXXX syndrome?
- What supportive measures can I take to enhance my daughter's life?

Hormonal problems may also create problems later in life. Low estrogen production can hasten **osteoporosis**, making the girls and women more susceptible to bone fractures.

## Prevention

XXXX syndrome cannot be prevented. Regular medical testing throughout the girl's life, however, plays an important role in preventing complications of the syndrome, such as serious heart or kidney issues.

### Resources

**BOOKS**

Moore, Keith A., and T.V.N. Persaud, *The Developing Human: Clinical Oriented Embryology, 7th Edition*Philadelphia: Saunders, 2003.

Odom, Samuel L. *Handbook of Developmental Disabilities*New York: The Guilford Press, 2007.

**ORGANIZATIONS**

Tetrasomy and Petrasomy X Syndrome Information and Support, tetra-x-list-subscribe@yahoogroups.com, www.tetrasomy.com.

Unique: Rare Chromosome Disorder Support Group, PO Box 2189, CaterhamSurray, United Kingdom, CR3 5GN, 44(0)1883-330766, , , info@rarechromo.org, www.rarechromo.org .

**PERIODICALS**

Blair, Jenny. "From the Beautiful to the Obscure" *Yale Medicine* Winter (2004).

Collin, Robert, et al. "A 48-XXXX Female with Absence of Ovaries" *Journal of Medical Genetics* 6(1980):275–278.

Kim, Yan-Ju, et al. "Parental Decisions of Prenatally Detected Sex Chromosome Abnormality" *Journal of the Korean Medical Society* 17(2002):53–57.

Linden, Mary C., et al. "Sex Chromosome Tetrasomy and Pentasomy " *Pediatrics*96(1996):672–682.

Pena, S.D.J., et al. "A 48-XXXX Female" *Journal of Medical Genetics* 11(1974):211–215.

Rhonda Cloos, RN

# XXXXX syndrome

## Definition

XXXXX syndrome is a rare genetic disorder in girls in which they have five X chromosomes rather than two. The disorder may cause lowered intelligence, physical deformities, and psychological problems.

## Demographics

XXXXX syndrome is very rare. It is estimated that the syndrome is present in one out of 85,000 female births. The condition only affects girls.

## Description

XXXXX syndrome is an extremely rare chromosomal condition affecting only girls. Researchers first described the condition in the *Journal of Pediatrics* in 1963. Seventeen years later there had been only 12 cases noted in professional scientific publications. As of 2005, only 25 cases have been reported in medical journals.

During the 1960s and 1970s, there was a burst of scientific research in XXXXX syndrome and related disorders. After that time period passed, research on the disorder became rare; however, in the early 2000s, scientific interest in XXXXX syndrome grew. In 2009, the National Institutes for Health in Bethesda, Maryland, was accepting participants for a study of XXXXX syndrome and **XXXX syndrome**. The study hoped to determine the effect of the disorders on the development of the brain, and whether brain imaging methods can identify the biological features of the brain that are associated with the disorders.

The most common characteristics of this syndrome are short height, short neck, round face, **microcephaly**, mental retardation, fifth finger clinodactyly, and heart and kidney defects.

Infants with XXXXX syndrome share a number of characteristic features such as a round face, flat nose bridge, deformities of the ears, and upward slanting eyes. The girls also might have mild to severe mental retardation. As a general rule there is a 10 to 15 point reduction in Intelligence Quotient (IQ) for each extra sex **chromosome**. Additionally, the chance of mental retardation and dysmorphism rises with each extra sex chromosome. In the case of XXXXX syndrome, girls have three extra X chromosomes.

### Risk factors

Scientists believe that the presence of one extra X chromosome in a mother creates a slightly higher risk of having a daughter with XXXXX syndrome. Only females are at risk.

## Causes and symptoms

### Cause

XXXXX syndrome is believed to be the result of a nondisjunction error in cell division during the process of chromosome splitting within the mother's ova. As a result of this error, the ovum contains more than 23 chromosomes.

### Symptoms

Girls with XXXXX syndrome may exhibit any number of classic signs, such as:

- Developmental delays: Physical and intellectual delays are possible
- Microcephaly
- Facial features: Round face, upward slanting eyes, wide-set eyes, epicanthal folds, ear and tooth abnormalities, and short neck length
- Musculoskeletal: Deformities in the elbow, foot (club foot may be present), overlapping toes, and larger space between first and second toes, fifth finger clinodactyly, weak muscle tone (hypotonia)
- Heart: Defects in the heart may be present (atrial septal defect, ventricular septal defect, patent ductus arteriosus)
- Kidneys: horseshoe kidneys

Psychiatric symptoms have been described in girls with XXXXX syndrome. It is believed that the psychiatric symptoms are related to the presence of extra chromosomes.

In 1980, one case was reported in which a 3-year-old girl with XXXXX syndrome had one underdeveloped kidney and was missing one ovary. The present ovary was believed to function normally, suggesting to researchers that the girl would be able to reproduce.

In 1999, the first case of XXXXX syndrome along with hyper IgE syndrome (HIE) was reported in a 10-year-old girl. The girl experienced a history of eczema as well as recurrent pneumonia and staphylococcal abscess in addition to the features commonly associated with XXXXX syndrome. This was the first case in which the presence of these two distinct chromosome disorders appeared together in one individual.

## KEY TERMS

**Clinodactyly—** Curving of the finger to the left or right

**Epicanthal folds** —Crease in the skin extending from the nose to the eyebrow.

**Microcephaly**—Abnormal smallness of the head; it often is associated with mental retardation.

The syndrome has also been described in the medical literature as having similar attributes to **Down syndrome**.

### Diagnosis

#### Examination

The symptoms of XXXXX syndrome become more apparent as the girl progresses through early childhood. Ultimately, suspicions lead the parents and health care practitioner to seek testing.

#### Tests

Diagnosis of XXXXX syndrome is usually made during childhood, as the symptoms become more pronounced. Diagnosis is confirmed through chromosome testing, which may include blood or skin tests.

#### Procedures

As of 2005, three cases had been diagnosed through prenatal testing procedures. The syndrome, if present, will appear on chorionic villus sampling or **amniocentesis**.

### Treatment

#### Traditional

Girls with XXXXX syndrome experience medical conditions that range from mild to severe. The level of severity dictates the treatment needed. If medical conditions such as atrial septal defect are present, heart surgery may be needed.

Because the syndrome is associated with poor muscle tone and speech abnormalities, physical, speech, and occupational therapies are recommended.

#### Atrial septal defect

If a child has an atrial septal defect, treatment to close the hole in the septum may be necessary. In the past, open-heart surgery was the only surgical option;

## QUESTIONS TO ASK YOUR DOCTOR

- What are my chances of having another child with XXXXX syndrome?
- How will I know if my daughter's condition is a mild or severe form of XXXXX syndrome?

however, methods of closing certain types of holes without surgery have been developed. Parents will need to discuss the options with their child's physician.

#### Ventricular septal defect

A ventricular septal defect, which may occur, is a hole in the membrane that separates the two ventricles, which are the lower chambers of the heart. Treatment depends on the size of the hole. If it is small, it may not require any treatment. If the hole is large, open heart surgery may be required. If serious symptoms develop in the first months of life, surgery on the baby may be essential. If the symptoms are mild, surgery may be delayed a few years. Surgery involves closing the hole with a patch.

### Prognosis

The long-term prognosis depends on the severity of the syndrome in the individual girl. A more positive prognosis is generally associated with earlier diagnosis, sound treatment for medical conditions, and modalities such as occupational, physical, and speech therapies. If cardiac defects are present, treatment for such defects improves the prognosis.

### Prevention

XXXXX syndrome cannot be prevented.

### Resources

**BOOKS**

Bissonnette, Bruno, and Igor Lugenbuehl. *Syndromes: Rapid Recognition and Perioperative Implications*McGraw-Hill Companies, 2006.

Chen, Harold.*Atlas of Genetic Diagnosis and Counseling*Totowa, NJ: Humana Press, 2006.

Epstein, Charles J.*The Consequences of Chromosome Imbalance (Developmental and Cell Biology Series)* New York: Cambridge University Press, 2007.

Evans, Mark. *Prenatal Diagnosis*McGraw-Hill Companies, 2006.

Long, Toby M., and Holly Lea. *Handbook of Pediatric Physical Therapy*Baltimore: Lippincott, Williams, and Wilkins, 1995.

Odom, Samuel H., and Robert H. Horner. *Handbook of Developmental Disabilities* New York:, The Guilford Press, 2007.

**PERIODICALS**

Boeck, A., et al. "Pentasomy X and Hyper IgE Syndrome: Coexistence of Two Distinct Genetic Disorders." *European Journal of Pediatrics* 158L(1999): 723–7266.

Cho, Y.G., et al. "A Case of 49, XXXXX in Which the Extra Chromosomes Were Maternal in Origin." *Journal of Clinical Pathology* 57(2004):1004–1006.

Kassai, R., et al. "Penta-X syndrome: A Case Report with Review of Literature" *American Journal of Medical Genetics* 1(1991):51–56.

Monheit, A., et al. "The Penta-X Syndrome." *Journal of Medical Genetics* 17(1980):5 394–396.

Thakur, D., et al. "A Case Report of PentaX Syndrome in Association with Isolated Borderline Ventriculomegaly." *Journal of Obstetrics and Gynaecology* 25(2005):208–209.

Toussi, Tahmouresse., et al. "Renal Hypodysplasia and Unilateral Ovarian Agenesis in the Penta-X Syndrome" *American Journal of Medical Genetics* 6(1980):153–162.

Rhonda Cloos, RN

# XYY syndrome

## Definition

XYY syndrome is a **chromosome** disorder that affects males. Males with this disorder have an extra Y chromosome.

## Description

The XYY syndrome was previously considered the *super-male* syndrome, in which men with this condition were thought to be overly aggressive and more likely to become criminals. These original stereotypes came about because several researchers in the 1960s found a high number of men with XYY syndrome in prisons and mental institutes.

These original observations did not consider that the majority of males with XYY syndrome were not in prisons or mental institutes. Since then, broader, less biased studies have been done on males with XYY syndrome. Though males with XYY syndrome may be taller than average and have an increased risk for learning difficulties, especially in reading and speech, they are not overly aggressive. Unfortunately, some text books and many people still believe the inaccurate stereotype of the *super-male* syndrome.

---

## KEY TERMS

**Amniocentesis**—A procedure performed at 16-18 weeks of pregnancy in which a needle is inserted through a woman's abdomen into her uterus to draw out a small sample of the amniotic fluid from around the baby. Either the fluid itself or cells from the fluid can be used for a variety of tests to obtain information about genetic disorders and other medical conditions in the fetus.

**Cell**—The smallest living units of the body which group together to form tissues and help the body perform specific functions.

**Chorionic villus sampling (CVS)**—A procedure used for prenatal diagnosis at 10-12 weeks gestation. Under ultrasound guidance a needle is inserted either through the mother's vagina or abdominal wall and a sample of cells is collected from around the early embryo. These cells are then tested for chromosome abnormalities or other genetic diseases.

**Chromosome**—A microscopic thread-like structure found within each cell of the body and consists of a complex of proteins and DNA. Humans have 46 chromosomes arranged into 23 pairs. Changes in either the total number of chromosomes or their shape and size (structure) may lead to physical or mental abnormalities.

**Embryo**—The earliest stage of development of a human infant, usually used to refer to the first eight weeks of pregnancy. The term *fetus* is used from roughly the third month of pregnancy until delivery.

**Hormone**—A chemical messenger produced by the body that is involved in regulating specific bodily functions such as growth, development, and reproduction.

---

## Genetic profile

Chromosomes are structures in the cells that contain genes. Genes are responsible for instructing our bodies how to grow and develop. Usually, an individual has 46 chromosomes in each cell, or 23 pairs. The first 22 pairs are the same in males and females and the last pair, the sex chromosomes, consist of two X chromosomes in a female, and an X chromosome and an Y chromosome in a male.

XYY syndrome occurs when an extra Y chromosome is present in the cells of an affected individual. People with XYY syndrome are always male. The error that causes the extra Y chromosome can occur in the fertilizing sperm or in the developing embryo.

XYY is not considered an inherited condition. An inherited condition usually is one in which the mother and/or father has an alteration in a **gene** or chromosome that can be passed onto their children. Typically, in an inherited condition, there is an increased chance that the condition will reoccur. The risk of the condition reoccurring in another pregnancy is not increased above the general population incidence.

### Demographics

XYY syndrome has an incidence of one in 1,000 newborn males. However, since many males with XYY syndrome look like other males without XYY syndrome, many males are never identified.

### Signs and symptoms

There are no physical abnormalities in most males with XYY syndrome. However, some males can have one or more of the following characteristics. Males who have XYY syndrome are usually normal in length at birth, but have rapid growth in childhood, typically averaging in the seventy-fifth percentile (taller than 75% of males their same age). Many males with XYY syndrome are not overly muscular, particularly in the chest and shoulders. Individuals with XYY syndrome often have difficulties with their coordination. As a result, they can appear to be awkward or clumsy. During their teenage years, males with XYY syndrome may develop severe acne that may need to be treated by a dermatologist.

Men with XYY syndrome have normal, heterosexual function and most are fertile. However, numerous case reports of men with XYY syndrome presenting with infertility have been reported. Most males with XYY syndrome have normal hormones involved in their sperm production. However, a minority of males with XYY syndrome may have increased amounts of some hormones involved in sperm production. This may result in infertility due to inadequate sperm production. As of 2001, the true incidence of infertility in males with XYY syndrome is unknown.

When XYY men make sperm, the extra Y chromosome is thought to be lost resulting in a normal number of sex chromosomes. As a result, men with XYY syndrome are not at an increased risk for fathering children with chromosome abnormalities. However, some men with XYY syndrome have been found to have more sperm with extra chromosomes than what is found in men without XYY syndrome. Whether these men have an increased risk of fathering a child with a chromosome abnormality is unknown as of 2001.

Men with XYY syndrome usually have normal intelligence, but it can be slightly lower than their brothers and sisters. Approximately 50% of males with XYY syndrome have learning difficulties, usually in language and reading. Speech delay can be noticed in early school years. Males with XYY syndrome may not process information as quickly as their peers and may need additional time for learning.

Males with XYY syndrome have an increased risk of behavior problems. Hyperactivity and temper tantrums can occur more frequently than expected, especially during childhood. As males with XYY syndrome become older, they may have problems with impulse control and appear emotionally immature.

From a psychosocial standpoint, males with XYY syndrome may have low self-esteem due to mild learning disabilities and/or lack of athletic skills due to lack of coordination. Males with XYY syndrome are at risk in stressful environments and have a low ability to deal with frustration.

Men with XYY syndrome are not thought to be excessively aggressive or psychotic. However, because some men with XYY syndrome can have mild learning difficulties and/or have difficulty controlling behavior problems such as lack of impulse control, their actions may lead to criminal behavior if placed in the right environment. It is important to emphasize that this only occurs in a small percentage of men with XYY syndrome. Most men with XYY syndrome are productive members of society with no criminal behavior.

### Diagnosis

Most individuals with 47,XYY go through their entire lives without being diagnosed with this condition. Chromosome studies can be done after birth on a skin or blood sample to confirm the condition. This syndrome can also be diagnosed coincidentally when a pregnant mother undergoes prenatal testing for other reasons, such as being age 35 or older at the time of delivery. Prenatal tests that can determine whether or not an unborn baby will be affected with 47,XXY are the chorionic villi sampling and **amniocentesis** procedures. Both procedures are associated with potential risks of pregnancy loss and therefore are only offered to women who have an increased risk of having a baby born with a chromosome problem or some type of genetic condition.

### Treatment and management

Treatment and management for most men with XYY syndrome is not indicated. However, early identification and intervention of learning disabilities and/or behavior

## QUESTIONS TO ASK YOUR DOCTOR

- When should my son be evaluated for a learning disability?
- Do you recommend physical, occupational, or speech therapy?
- Is genetic testing recommended, and on whom?
- What supportive stress-reducing measures should I implement at home?

difficulties is necessary. Speech therapy, physical therapy, and occupational therapy may be helpful for males with XYY syndrome. Also, because males with XYY syndrome are at risk in stressful environments, a supportive and stimulating home life is important.

### Prognosis

Most males who have learning disabilities and/or behavior problems due to XYY syndrome have an excellent prognosis. Learning disabilities are mild and most affected males learn how to control their impulsiveness and other behavior problems. XYY syndrome does not shorten life span.

### Resources

#### PERIODICALS

Gotz, M.J., et al. "Criminality and Antisocial Behavior in Unselected Men with Sex Chromosome Abnormalities." *Psychological Medicine* 29 (1999): 953-962.

Linden M.G., et al. "Intrauterine Diagnosis of Sex Chromosome Aneuploidy." *Obstetrics and Gynecology* 87 (1996): 469-75.

#### ORGANIZATIONS

Chromosome Deletion Outreach, Inc. PO Box 724, Boca Raton, FL 33429-0724. (561) 391-5098 or (888) 236-6880. Fax: (561) 395-4252. cdo@worldnet.att.net. http://members.aol.com/cdousa/cdo.htm.

Carin Lea Beltz, MS, CGC

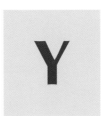

# YY syndrome

## Definition

The YY syndrome is an unusual disorder in the history of pathology. The underlying genetic condition and cause were discovered before any evidence of the syndrome was observed. YY syndrome was discovered through the study of the diversity in the chromosomes of the **chromosome** pair 46. While most males have an X and a Y chromosome, some were observed to have an extra Y chromosome. The question then arose: How does the presence of an extra chromosome influence the normal development of the affected male?

The differences that distinguish the YY male are very subtle and are usually not seen before the age of 10. Many males grow up without even realizing that they have the YY condition. Most of those affected tend to be taller and thinner than age-related norms. There is some evidence of speech delay and learning disabilities. Although the YY male is more aggressive than average, there is no noticeable increase in behavioral problems.

## Demographics

The prevalence rate in the United States is 12 per 10,000 male births with the rate for those of African descent being slightly lower. Studies from Norway and Japan suggest similar rates. The condition only affects males.

## Description

The YY syndrome is a very mild disorder; it is certainly not considered a disease. It is best to know as early as possible if a boy has it, because the mild learning disabilities and the slight language delay can be accommodated better at a young age. However, most boys realize they have the YY condition only after they have grown taller than their peers in late childhood. Many who have it never know they are YY susceptible.

In the usual fertilization of the egg, the father contributes a sperm with either an X chromosome which determines that the resulting **zygote** will be female or with a Y chromosome which determines that the resulting zygote will be male. For an unknown reason, in some cases, the Y chromosome in the sperm splits in two before fertilization. The resulting zygote is male with two Y chromosomes instead of one. The age of either parent is inconsequential in contributing to this disorder. This condition is not considered to be inherited, as the fathers with YY syndrome do not have sons with YY in any greater frequency than the general population.

The studies documenting the severity of the symptoms constantly note how mild and close to average all of the distinctive differences are. The most notable condition is the tendency to grow very tall earlier than peers and the tendency to be thinner than peers. However, the final height and body weight are still within normal range. Most of these boys have a language delay but eventually catch up to peers. Most have a learning disability but also have normal measured intelligence. They tend to be more aggressive than other boys and like physical activities. However, most adapt to the classroom and behavioral problems are no greater than the normal population. As a group they are distinctive but as individuals few are abnormal.

When the condition was first discovered, there was the assumption that such boys would grow up to be infertile. However, longitudinal studies have concluded that as an adult, the YY male is no less fertile than the general population. However, the semen of a YY male is slightly weak because of the presence of more than average dead sperm.

While this is a very mild disorder, it is beneficial to discover its presence in a young boy. The earlier that it

## QUESTIONS TO ASK YOUR DOCTOR

- How can we help our son have a normal life?
- How serious are the conditions?
- What should I watch for in a baby suspected of having the YY syndrome?
- How much should we accept or discourage his aggressive physical activity?
- What kind of problems might be associated with his excessive height?
- What will he need to understand when he wants to start a family?

is detected contributes to the sooner that more serious conditions can be ruled out. Furthermore, with appropriate treatment, the boy can overcome the effects of the language delay and learning disability. If the boy is forewarned, he will not become apprehensive when the rapid growth takes place.

### Causes and symptoms

The condition is caused by an unusual split in the Y chromosome of a pre-insemination human sperm that manages to fertilize a human egg. The resulting zygote evolves over nine months of gestation and is born as a male infant with two Y chromosomes instead of one.

The symptoms as noted above include unusual height and thinness, language delay, learning disability, and aggressive physical activity. Measured intelligence is within normal limits. The cases of behavioral problems within this population of boys are also within normal limits.

### Diagnosis

There are no signs of this disorder at birth. Therefore, there would be no observable sign of this disorder through a **prenatal ultrasound**. This disorder can be detected through a prenatal **amniocentesis**; however, analysis of amniotic fluid does not usually look for the signs of YY syndrome.

Most boys are diagnosed with this disorder as a result of parental concerns for language delay or excessive growth. Diagnosis can take place through noting

evidence for all of the usual symptoms. However, confirmation of this diagnosis must be done through testing blood samples for the presence of the YY chromosome.

The main test for recognizing chromosomal disorders is the fluorescence in-situ hybridization (FISH). This method of analyzing the structures of human **genetics** relies on fluorescent probes designed to link to specific genetic particles such as proteins, genes, or chromosomal material. If the correlating probe cannot link to the material for which it is designed, then the result is accepted as an absence of the material. In testing for YY syndrome, the probes specific to the Y chromosome would be injected into genetic material from the affected person. If examination of the probes detects two Y chromosomes, then the test confirms the person has the YY syndrome.

### Treatment

There is no treatment to cure the YY syndrome. Because of the mildness of the condition, even treatment specific to the symptoms may not be necessary. The most immediate treatment for the boy with YY syndrome may be speech therapy to address the language delay. However, some of the affected boys have been shown to overcome the language problem eventually without therapy. The boy may need special services in the school years to alleviate the learning disorder. Again, this may not be necessary. In one study, almost all boys who were identified early with YY syndrome responded well to preschool as their only treatment for learning disability.

It is important for parents and teachers to be understanding and supportive of the YY syndrome boy. Clear limits should be set regarding the aggression; however, those limits should be made in consideration of the boy's need for physical activity. The boy should be encouraged to take part in organized sports.

## Prognosis

There is no evidence of lower life expectancies for the YY male. There are no increased threats, particularly no increased susceptibility to disease. As noted above, many YY males go through life not even realizing their condition. As an adult, the YY male can expect to father children; the population tends to be within normal expectancies of fertility.

## Resources

### BOOKS

Baum, Andrew, Stanton Newman, John Weinman, and Robert West. *Cambridge Handbook of Psychology, Health, and Medicine*. New York: Cambridge University Press, 1997.

Bissonnette, Bruno, Igor Luginbuehl, Bruno Marciniak, and Bernard Dalens. *Syndromes: Rapid Recognition and Perioperative Implications*. New York: McGraw-Hill Professional, 2006.

### PERIODICALS

Linder, M. G., and B. G. Bender. "Fifty-one Prenatally Diagnosed Children and Adolescents with Sex Chromosome Abnormalities." *American Journal of Medical Genetics*. 2002. 110: 11.

### OTHER

47,XYY syndrome. National Library of Medicine. http://ghr.nlm.nih.gov/condition=47xyysyndrome

### ORGANIZATIONS

Mothers United for Moral Support, 150 Custer Court, Green Bay, WI , 54301, 920-336-5333, http://www.netnet.net/mums.

National Institute of Mental Health, 6001 Executive Blvd., Room 8184, MSC 9663, Rockville, MD, 20892, 301-443-4513, http://www.nimh.nih.gov.

Ray F. Brogan, PHD

# Z

# Zellweger syndrome

## Definition

Zellweger syndrome (ZS) belongs to the Zellweger syndrome spectrum (ZSS), a group of **genetic disorders** resulting from a defective assembly of peroxisomes, the membrane–bound structures within the gel–like fluid (cytoplasm) of cells required to break down certain types of fats, to produce hormones, and to ensure proper nervous system function. The ZSS disorders, also called peroxisome biogenesis disorders (PBDs), are all leukodystrophies, diseases that damage the white matter of the brain and also affect how the body metabolizes substances in the blood and organ tissues. The PBDs have varying degrees of severity, depending on extent of peroxisome defect with ZS considered the most severe condition.

## Description

Individuals born with Zellweger syndrome have consistent clinical characteristics reflecting the impairment of the metabolic processes occuring in normal peroxisomes.

Metabolism includes numerous chemical processes involved in both construction (anabolism) and break down (catabolism) of important components. These processes are catalyzed (or helped along) by enzymes. If any enzymes are missing in the process, a build–up of an initial substance, or a missing end–product, can result. Peroxisomes are filled with enzymes and found in all cells, particularly those of the liver, kidneys, and brain. Substances that are broken down in peroxisomes include very long chain fatty acids, polyunsaturated fatty acids, dicarboxylic fatty acids, prostaglandins, and the side chain of cholesterol. When peroxisomes are absent or defective, very long chain fatty acids, and other substances that peroxisomes normally help to catalyze, begin to build up in the body.

Peroxisomes also play a role in the initial reactions involved in the creation of plasmalogens. Plasmalogens are important components in the structure of myelin, a fatty layer that covers the nerve fibers in the body. This covering helps the transmission of nerve signals. Since plasmalogens require peroxisomes for their formation, a lack of functioning peroxisomes causes a deficiency in plasmalogens. Since the plasmalogens are required for the formation of myelin, the myelin is defective.

Bile acid formation also requires peroxisomes. Bile is secreted by the liver and stored in the gallbladder. It is released when fat enters the intestines. Bile then helps to break down these fats to prepare them for further digestion. Bile acid is produced during the breakdown of cholesterol.

Babies with Zellweger syndrome have severe developmental retardation and impairment of their central nervous system. They lack muscle tone (hypotonia), and are often blind or deaf. They have a distinctive facial appearance, an enlarged liver, jaundice and may have cysts in their kidneys.

## Genetic profile

Zellweger syndrome is an autosomal recessive condition. This means that in order to have the condition, an individual needs to inherit one copy of the **gene** for Zellweger syndrome from each parent. An individual who has only one copy of the gene is called a carrier for the condition and does not have any signs or symptoms of the condition. When two parents are carriers for Zellweger syndrome, they have a 25% chance, with each pregnancy, for having an affected child. They have a 50% chance for having a child who is a carrier for the condition and a 25% chance for having a child who is neither affected nor a carrier for Zellweger syndrome.

The disorders of the Zellweger spectrum are caused by defects in the assembly of the peroxisome, which

## KEY TERMS

**Amniocentesis**—A procedure performed at 16–18 weeks of pregnancy in which a needle is inserted through a woman's abdomen into her uterus to draw out a small sample of the amniotic fluid from around the baby. Either the fluid itself or cells from the fluid can be used for a variety of tests to obtain information about genetic disorders and other medical conditions in the fetus.

**Chorionic villus sampling (CVS)**—A procedure used for prenatal diagnosis at 10–12 weeks gestation. Under ultrasound guidance a needle is inserted either through the mother's vagina or abdominal wall and a sample of cells is collected from around the fetus. These cells are then tested for chromosome abnormalities or other genetic diseases.

**Jaundice**—Yellow discoloration of the skin and eyes caused by too much bilirubin in the blood.

**Metabolism**—Chemical processes that occur in living organisms in order to maintain life.

**Peroxisome**—Membrane–bound structures within the cytoplasm of cells that are needed to break down certain types of fats, to produce hormones, and to help the nervous system work properly.

**Peroxisome biogenesis**—Processes involved in the fabrication of proxisome in cells.

**Zellweger spectrum**—Disorders that result from defects in the assembly of the peroxisome. Also called peroxisome biogenesis disorders (PBD). They include: Zellweger syndrome (ZS), neonatal adrenoleukodystrophy (NALD), rhizomelic chondrodysplasia (RC) and infantile Refsum disease (IRD).

requires at least 12 PEX genes for proper assembly. The PEX genes provide instructions for making peroxins, the proteins required for normal peroxisome assembly. PEX mutations have been identified in all ZSS patients. Mutations in the PEX1 gene are the most common cause of ZSS and are observed in about 68% of affected individuals. It is located on the long arm of **chromosome** 7, at 7q21–q22. When a gene change or mutation occurs in this area that impairs peroxisome assembly, this leads to Zellweger syndrome. Other PEX **gene mutations** have been identified on different chromosomes. These include, but are not limited to, PEX6, PEX26, PEX10, and PEX12, which account for another 26% of all individuals with ZSS. Combined to PEX1 mutations, more than 90% of all affected individuals have a defect in one of these five PEX genes. Other PEX genes are known to be

required for peroxisome assembly, but as of 2009, have not been clearly associated with ZSS.

The cause of Zellweger syndrome is a failure of the peroxisomes to be able to bring newly created peroxisomal proteins into the peroxisomes. Instead, the proteins stay outside of the peroxisomes and are broken down. The peroxisome membranes may be present, but are empty, like the wood frame of an empty house. These empty peroxisomes have been called peroxisome "ghosts."

### Demographics

In the United States, the incidence of ZS is estimated to be 1 in 50,000–100,000. European incidence is reported to be similar. There is no recorded difference in the incidence of ZS for any particular sex or ethnic background.

### Signs and symptoms

The characteristic clinical features of Zellweger syndrome include:

- high forehead
- widely spaced eyes (hypertelorism)
- low, broad, or flat nasal bridge
- "full" cheeks
- small chin (micrognathia)
- forward tilting (anteverted) nostrils
- vertical fold of skin over the inner corner of the eye (epicanthal fold)
- upslanting eyes
- shallow orbital ridges
- minor ear abnormalities

Other characteristics include, but are not limited to:

- breech presentation at birth (feet first)
- extremely weak muscles (hypotonia)
- weak sucking and swallowing reflexes
- high arched palate
- absent deep tendon reflexes
- seizures
- deafness
- enlarged liver (hepatomegaly)
- enlarged spleen
- gastrointestinal bleeding
- slow growth after birth
- severe mental retardation
- abnormal brain findings

- involuntary, rhythmic movements of the eyes (nystagmus)
- large space between the bones of the skull (fontanel)
- flat back part of the head (occiput)
- tiny white or yellow spots on the colored part of the eyes (brushfield spots)
- redundant skin on neck
- congenital cloudy lenses of the eye (cataracts)
- possible heart defects
- a single crease across the palm of the hands (simian creases)
- fixed, immovable joints (contractures)
- misaligned bones in the front part of the foot/club foot (talipes equinovarus)
- undescended testicles (cryptorchidism)
- underdeveloped thymus (thymus hypoplasia)
- hearing impairment
- failure to thrive
- psychomotor retardation
- high levels of iron or copper in the blood

### Diagnosis

Diagnosis is based on clinical characteristics combined with a series of tests to determine the peroxisomal function and structure. Biochemical abnormalities include elevated levels of very long chain fatty acids, a decrease in the levels of a peroxisomal enzyme dihydroxyacetone phosphate acyltransferase (DHAPAT), the presence of abnormal intermediates in bile acid formation, and a lack of plasmalogens in a blood sample. Absence of peroxisomes in liver biopsy specimen is considered essential for the diagnosis of Zellweger syndrome.

Prenatal diagnosis for Zellweger syndrome is possible through chorionic villus sampling (CVS) and **amniocentesis**. Diagnosis may be made by measuring the synthesis of plasmalogens in cultured CVS or amniotic fluid cells or by measuring the amount of very long chain fatty acids. Other tests may be useful, including measuring the amount of the peroxisomal enzyme DHAPAT in the amniotic fluid.

### Treatment and management

There is no cure and no treatment for Zellweger syndrome.

### Prognosis

The prognosis for individuals who have Zellweger syndrome is extremely poor. Those with the disease usually only live for a few months after birth. Rarely do individuals with Zellweger syndrome live longer than one year.

---

## QUESTIONS TO ASK YOUR DOCTOR

- What signs and symptoms are characteristic of Zellweger syndrome?
- What tests or other procedures are used to distinguish Zellweger from other disorders of a similar nature?
- What is the prognosis for a child born with Zellweger syndrome?
- How can I learn about clinical trials that may be ongoing on the causes and/or treatment of Zellweger syndrome?

### Resources

**BOOKS**

Masters, Colin, and Denis Crane. *The Peroxisome: A Vital Organelle*. New York, NY: Cambridge University Press, 2007.

Roels, Frank, et al., editors. *Peroxisomal Disorders and Regulation of Genes*. New York, NY: Springer, 2003.

Woliver, Robbie. *Alphabet Kids —From ADD to Zellweger Syndrome: A Guide to Developmental, Neurobiological and Psychological Disorders for Parents and Professionals*. London, UK: Jessica Kingsley Publishers, 2008.

**PERIODICALS**

Grayer, J. "Recognition of Zellweger syndrome in infancy." *Advances in Neonatal Care* 5 no. 1 (February 2005): 5–13.

Huybrechts, S. J., et al. "Identification of a novel PEX14 mutation in Zellweger syndrome." *Journal of Medical Genetics* 45, no. 6 (June 2008): 376–383.

Krause, C., et al. "Rational diagnostic strategy for Zellweger syndrome spectrum patients." *European Journal of Human Genetics* 17, no. 6 (June 2009): 741–748.

Yik, W. Y., et al. "Identification of novel mutations and sequence variation in the Zellweger syndrome spectrum of peroxisome biogenesis disorders." *Human Mutations* 30, no. 3 (March 2009): E467–E480.

**WEBSITES**

*The Zellweger Spectrum*. Information Page, ULF, August 2, 2007 (May 17, 2009). http://www.ulf.org/types/Zellweger.html.

*What are peroxisomal disorders?* Information Page, Zellweger Baby Support Network, February 7, 2009 (May 17, 2009). http://www.zbsn.org/documents/49.html.

*Zellweger Syndrome*. Information Page, NINDS, December 11, 2007 (May 17, 2009). http://www.ninds.nih.gov/disorders/zellweger/zellweger.htm.

*Zellweger Syndrome.* Information Page, NCBI Genes and Disease (May 17, 2009). http://www.ncbi.nlm.nih.gov/books/bv.fcgi?call = bv.View.ShowSection&rid = gnd.section.240.

**ORGANIZATIONS**

National Institute for Neurological Disorders and Stroke (NINDS). P.O. Box 5801, Bethesda, MD 20824. (800)352-9424 or (301) 496-5751. http://www.ninds.nih.gov.

National Institute of Child Health and Human Development (NICHD). P.O. Box 3006, Rockville, MD 20847. (800)370-2943. Fax : (866)760-5947. Email: NICHD InformationResourceCenter@mail.nih.gov. http://www.nichd.nih.gov.

National Organization for Rare Disorders (NORD). 55 Kenosia Avenue, PO Box 1968, Danbury, CT 06813-1968. (203)744-0100 or (800)999-6673. Fax: (203)798-2291. http://www.rarediseases.org.

United Leukodystrophy Foundation (ULF). 2304 Highland Dr., Sycamore, IL 60178. (800)728-5483. Fax: (815)895-2432. Email: office@ulf.org. http://www.ulf.org.

Zellweger Baby Support Network. 1852 Iron Horse Loop, Spearfish SD 57783. (605)642-2072. Email: pamfreeth@zbsn.org. http://www.zbsn.org.

Renee A. Laux, MS
Monique Laberge, PhD

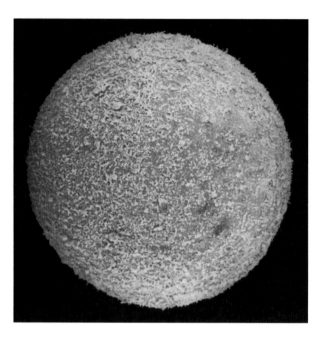

**A human zygote.** *(Photo Researchers, Inc.)*

# Zygote

## Definition

The zygote is the single cell that is formed when the sperm cell fertilizes the egg cell. The zygote divides multiple times, producing identical copies of itself. The cells produced by the division of the zygote form the developing embryo, fetus, and baby. The zygote is the first step in the formation of a new person.

## Description

When the sperm fuses with the egg, a cascade of events begins. Additional sperm are prevented from fertilizing the egg. The membranes of the egg and sperm combine, producing one single cell. The egg and sperm prepare to fuse their genetic material (DNA/chromosomes). Finally, the genetic material combines to produce the zygote with one complete set of chromosomes.

Most cells in the human body have two pairs of 23 chromosomes, i.e. 46 chromosomes total. One set of 23 chromosomes is inherited from the mother, and the complementary set is inherited from the father. When the egg and sperm are formed, the two sets of chromosomes divide evenly, from 46 to 23 chromsomes to produce eggs and sperm with 23 chromosomes each. This ensures that when the egg and sperm fuse during conception, the original number of chromosomes (46) is restored.

The reduction of each parent cell from 46 to 23 chromosomes ensures that each parent contributes half of his or her genetic material to form the zygote and the offspring shares 50% of his or her genes with each parent. Duplication of the single zygote occurs through a complete division of the single ball of cells. This begins the process of forming the fetus and eventually the baby. The first division produces two identical cells, the second produces four cells, the third produces eight cells, etc. After many cell divisions, the cells begin to specialize and differentiate (form particular tissues and organs).

Fertilization usually occurs in the fallopian tube, and the first few cell divisions occur as the developing embryo moves to the uterus. The first division occurs about 30 hours after fertilization. As the zygote divides, some of the cells formed will develop into the placenta. Approximately six days after fertilization, the ball of cells attaches to the uterine wall.

### Sex determination

Men and women each have 22 pairs of non-sex chromosomes and two sex chromosomes. Men's sex chromosomes are X and Y. A mature sperm cell that has undergone the **chromosome** division process from 46 to 23 chromosomes produces a cell that is either

## KEY TERMS

**Chromosome**—A microscopic thread-like structure found within each cell of the body and consists of a complex of proteins and DNA. Humans have 46 chromosomes arranged into 23 pairs. Changes in either the total number of chromosomes or their shape and size (structure) may lead to physical or mental abnormalities.

**Gene**—A building block of inheritance, which contains the instructions for the production of a particular protein, and is made up of a molecular sequence found on a section of DNA. Each gene is found on a precise location on a chromosome.

**Teratogen**—Any drug, chemical, maternal disease, or exposure that can cause physical or functional defects in an exposed embryo or fetus.

X or Y. Women's sex chromosomes are X and X. The eggs that women produce have only X chromosomes. Therefore, the sperm determines whether the zygote is XY or XX, which is the initial step on the biological path to becoming a male or female.

### Developmental periods

The term *embryo* refers to the developing baby between the second week after conception and the eighth week after conception. Doctors use the term *fetus* from the ninth week after conception to birth. A pregnancy is broken down into three trimesters. The first trimester begins with the first day of the woman's last menstrual period and each *trimester* is three calendar months.

### Twins

Twins may arise in two ways. Identical twins are called "monozygotic" because both individuals are formed from the same zygote. As the zygote divides to form the baby, two separate individuals form instead of one. Fraternal twins are called "dizygotic" because each individual develops from a different zygote. Two eggs are ovulated, and a separate sperm fertilizes each egg. Therefore, identical twins have exactly the same **DNA** in each cell and fraternal twins share the same amount of DNA as brothers and sisters. Sometimes it is impossible to tell monozygotic twins from dizygotic twins based on the placenta and the fetal membranes. If a person wants to determine whether twins are monozygotic or dizygotic, DNA studies of blood cells will provide a definitive answer.

### Abnormalities

The zygote normally contains two complete sets of 23 chromosomes, and two copies of every **gene**. If the egg or sperm that fuse to form the zygote is abnormal, the zygote will also be abnormal. For example, **Down syndrome** is caused by an extra chromosome number 21 from the egg or sperm cell. Since the cells formed by division of the zygote are identical to the zygote, any abnormality in the zygote will be in every cell of the baby.

Abnormalities can also arise when the zygote begins to divide. This type of abnormality is usually severe, eventually leading to a miscarriage. If an abnormality occurs after the zygote has divided one or more times, the baby will have some normal cells and some abnormal cells. This situation is referred to as "mosaicism" and may be used to describe the person's condition.

#### Molar pregnancies

Molar pregnancies can occur in one of two ways. Sometimes the original cell that duplicates and divides to form the fetus is completely of paternal origin. The chromosomes in a sperm duplicate themselves, then proceed to divide as if they were a normal zygote. These pregnancies are completely abnormal and miscarry. Another type of molar pregnancy occurs when two sperm fertilize one egg. The zygote is **triploidy** and has 69 chromosomes instead of 46. Although some fetal parts can be seen, these pregnancies normally miscarry in the first or second trimester.

#### Birth defects

The term *birth defect* describes many different types of abnormalities, including physical malformations. Abnormalities of anatomical structures may be significant or insignificant; minor variations in structure are common. Approximately 3% of newborns have major malformations. The causes are: chromosome abnormalities (6–7%), inherited genetic conditions (7-8%), environmental factors (7–10%), and multifactorial causes (20–25%). The cause of the remaining 50–60% of malformations is unknown. *Multifactorial* refers to causes with both genetic and environmental components. Environmental factors include exposures to drugs, chemicals, or other substances that affect the development of the fetus while he/she is in the uterus. Substances that cause birth defects are referred to as teratogens.

### Artificial reproductive technology

Couples may pursue assisted reproductive technologies for a number of reasons. If a couple has *artificial insemination*, the sperm is inserted into the uterus when the woman in ovulating. Fertilization then occurs as it would normally. If a couple has *in vitro fertilization* (IVF), the egg and sperm are mixed outside the body in the laboratory. The zygote forms in a petri dish if fertilization occurs. After a number of cell divisions, the developing embryo is placed in the woman's uterus. If the sperm are incapable of fusing with the egg themselves, the sperm may be injected into the egg. This additional step to the IVF procedure is called *intracytoplasmic sperm injection* (ICSI).

In the year 2001, *preimplantation diagnosis* is possible for a number of genetic diseases. Couples may pursue this if they are at a significant risk for having a child with a disease that could be diagnosed prior to becoming pregnant through preimplantation diagnosis. The procedure is like that of in vitro fertilization, with an additional step. After fertilization occurs and the zygote has begun to divide, a single cell is removed. Removing the cell does not harm the other cells. The cell that is removed is tested for the genetic disease for which the couple is at risk. Multiple developing embryos are tested. Only the embryos that do not have the condition are placed in the woman's uterus to complete development.

The development of a person from the zygote is a fascinating and amazing process. It is a difficult area to study because scientists cannot manipulate human embryos to observe the effects, and the development of the fetus cannot be directly observed. Researchers still have many unanswered questions. Following a doctor's recommendations from prior to the pregnancy throughout pregnancy (such as folic acid intake and avoidance of alcohol and other drugs) increases the chances that the development of a zygote into a full-term infant will be normal. However, there are many babies born with severe birth defects or genetic diseases despite the parents' efforts at doing everything in their power to prevent a problem. Most birth defects and **genetic disorders** occur because of an event out of control of the parents.

## Resources

### BOOKS

Agnew, Connie L. *Twins!: Expert Advice From Two Practicing Physicians on Pregnancy, Birth, and the First Year*. New York: HarperCollins, 1997.

Brasner, Shari E. *Advice From a Pregnant Obstetrician*. New York: Hyperion, 1998.

Nathanielsz, P.W. *Life in the Womb: The Origin of Health and Disease*. Ithaca, NY: Promethean Press, 1999.

Vaughn, Christopher C. *How Life Begins: The Science of Life in the Womb*. New York: Times Books, 1996.

### PERIODICALS

Check, Erika. "What Moms Can Do Now." *Newsweek* (27 September 1999): 57–58.

Christensen, Damaris. "Sobering Work." *Science News* (8 July 2000): 28–29.

Kowalski, Kathiann. "High-tech Conception in the 21st Century." *Current Health* (January 2000): 1–4.

Miller, Annetta, and Joan Raymond. "The Infertility Challenge." *Newsweek* (Spring/Summer 1999 Special Edition): 26–28.

### WEBSITES

The International Council on Infertility Information Dissemination, Inc. http://www.inciid.org.

Maternal and Child Health Bureau. http://www.mchb.hrsa.gov/.

Organization of Teratology Information Services. http://www.otispregnancy.org/index.html.

### ORGANIZATIONS

American College of Obstetricians and Gynecologists. PO Box 96920, 409 12th St. SW, Washington, DC 20090-6920. http://www.acog.org.

American Society for Reproductive Medicine. 1209 Montgomery Highway, Birmingham, AL 35216-2809. (205) 978-5000. asrm@asrm.org. http://www.asrm.org.

RESOLVE, The National Infertility Association. 1310 Broadway, Somerville, MA 02144-1779. (617) 623-0744. resolveinc@aol.com. http://www.resolve.org.

Michelle Queneau Bosworth, MS, CGC

# CHROMOSOME MAP

A chromosome map indicates the relative positions of the genes that code for certain characteristics. The basic format for writing a gene position is the chromosome number, arm, band, sub-band, and sub-sub-band, if known. An example is 3p22.5.

The chromosome number refers to one of the 22 autosomal chromosomes (numbered 1–22) or one of the two sex-determining chromosomes, X and Y. In the example, the gene is on chromosome 3.

Each chromosome has two arms, which are separated by a centromere, the pinched-in area at or above the middle of the chromosome. The short arm, labeled *p,* is above the centromere, and the long arm, *q,* is below it. In the case of the example gene, it is found on the short arm (*p*) of chromosome 3, or 3p.

The arms are further divided into cytogenetic bands (regions) numbered 1, 2, 3, etc. The numbers start at the centromere and increase toward the end of the arm, known as the telomere. These bands can only be seen when stained and viewed under a microscope. Sub-bands, which are numbered the same way as bands, may be visible within bands at greater magnifications. Therefore, the exact location of the example gene is the short arm (*p*) of chromosome 3, band 2, sub-band region 2, and a sub-sub band 5.

The following 24 illustrations demonstrate the approximate gene location for several of the genes relating to disorders mentioned in this encyclopedia. Disorders known to be related to a specific chromosome but not necessarily at an exact location have been placed below the chromosome. These chromosome maps are in no way complete; rather, they provide an introduction to understanding relative size differences of human chromosomes and where geneticists have located the genes associated with the source of certain genetic disorders.

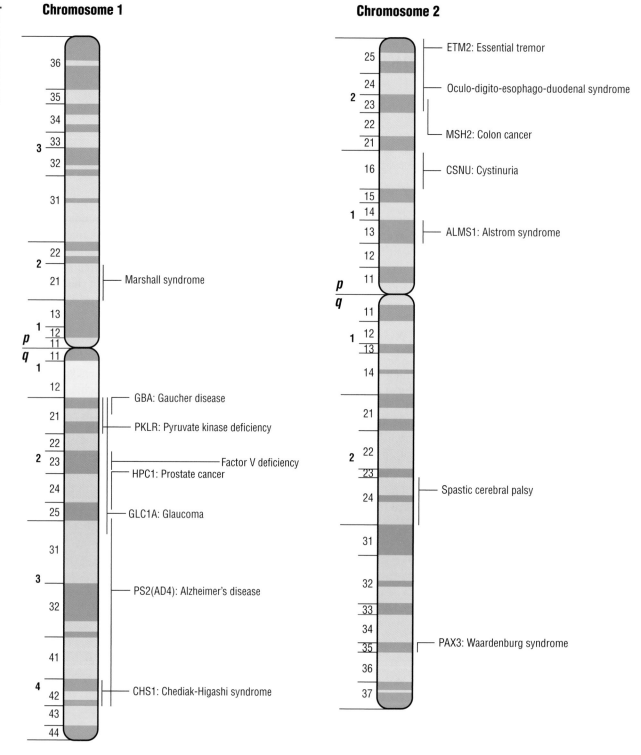

**Chromosome Map**

**Chromosome 1**

**Chromosome 2**

Chromosome 1:
- Marshall syndrome
- GBA: Gaucher disease
- PKLR: Pyruvate kinase deficiency
- Factor V deficiency
- HPC1: Prostate cancer
- GLC1A: Glaucoma
- PS2(AD4): Alzheimer's disease
- CHS1: Chediak-Higashi syndrome

Chromosome 2:
- ETM2: Essential tremor
- Oculo-digito-esophago-duodenal syndrome
- MSH2: Colon cancer
- CSNU: Cystinuria
- ALMS1: Alstrom syndrome
- Spastic cerebral palsy
- PAX3: Waardenburg syndrome

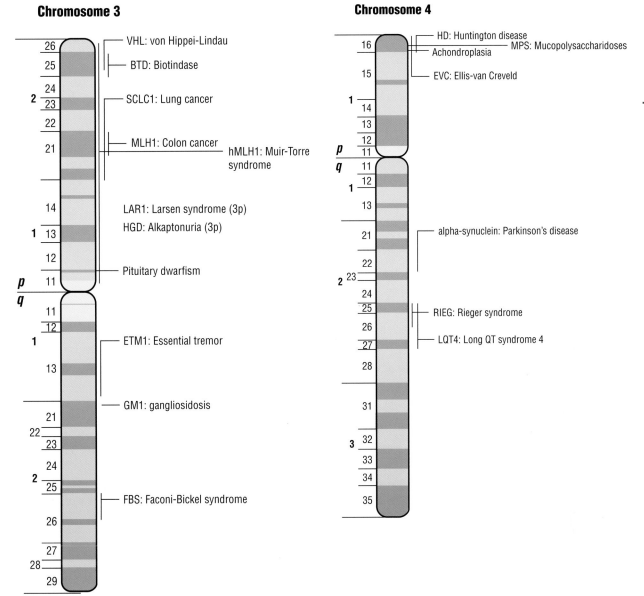

**Chromosome 3**

26 — VHL: von Hippei-Lindau
25 — BTD: Biotindase
24
2 23 — SCLC1: Lung cancer
22
21 — MLH1: Colon cancer — hMLH1: Muir-Torre syndrome

14 — LAR1: Larsen syndrome (3p)
1 13 — HGD: Alkaptonuria (3p)
12
*p* 11 — Pituitary dwarfism
*q*
11
12
1 — ETM1: Essential tremor
13
— GM1: gangliosidosis
21
22
23
24
2 25
— FBS: Faconi-Bickel syndrome
26
27
28
29

**Chromosome 4**

16 — HD: Huntington disease — MPS: Mucopolysaccharidoses
— Achondroplasia
15 — EVC: Ellis-van Creveld
1 14
13
12
*p* 11
*q* 11
12
1 13

21 — alpha-synuclein: Parkinson's disease
22
2 23
24
25 — RIEG: Rieger syndrome
26
27 — LQT4: Long QT syndrome 4
28

31
3 32
33
34
35

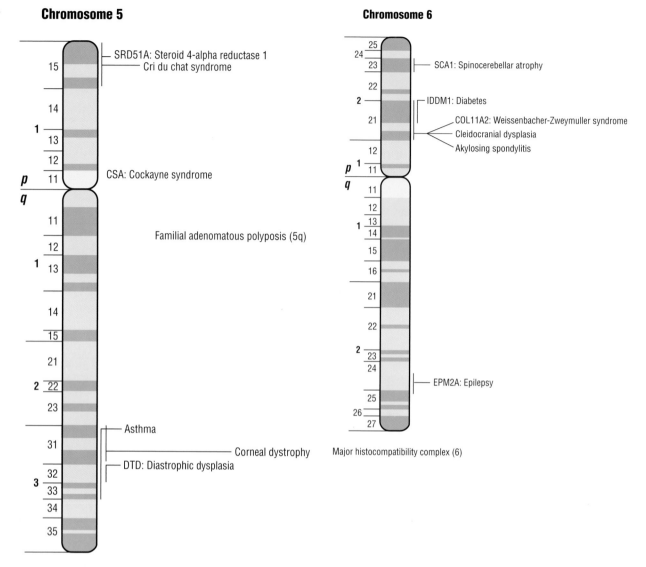

**Chromosome 5**

- SRD51A: Steroid 4-alpha reductase 1
- Cri du chat syndrome

CSA: Cockayne syndrome

Familial adenomatous polyposis (5q)

- Asthma
- Corneal dystrophy
- DTD: Diastrophic dysplasia

**Chromosome 6**

- SCA1: Spinocerebellar atrophy
- IDDM1: Diabetes
- COL11A2: Weissenbacher-Zweymuller syndrome
- Cleidocranial dysplasia
- Akylosing spondylitis

- EPM2A: Epilepsy

Major histocompatibility complex (6)

**Chromosome 7**

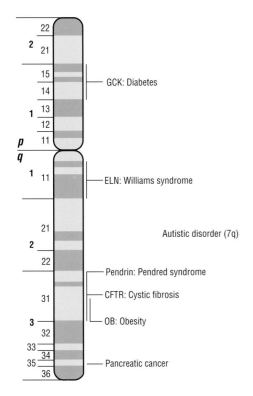

- GCK: Diabetes
- ELN: Williams syndrome
- Autistic disorder (7q)
- Pendrin: Pendred syndrome
- CFTR: Cystic fibrosis
- OB: Obesity
- Pancreatic cancer

**Chromosome 9**

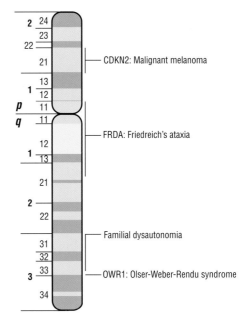

- CDKN2: Malignant melanoma
- FRDA: Friedreich's ataxia
- Familial dysautonomia
- OWR1: Olser-Weber-Rendu syndrome

Distal arthrogryposis syndrome (9)

**Chromosome 8**

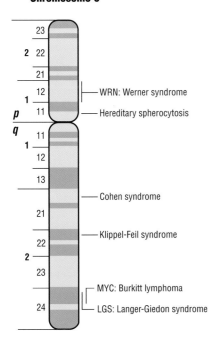

- WRN: Werner syndrome
- Hereditary spherocytosis
- Cohen syndrome
- Klippel-Feil syndrome
- MYC: Burkitt lymphoma
- LGS: Langer-Giedon syndrome

**Chromosome 10**

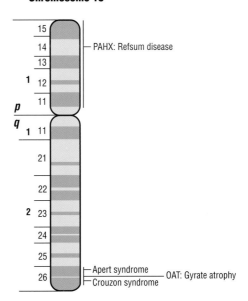

- PAHX: Refsum disease
- Apert syndrome
- Crouzon syndrome
- OAT: Gyrate atrophy

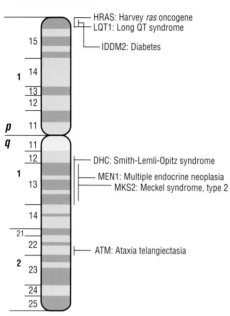

**Chromosome 11**

- HRAS: Harvey *ras* oncogene
- LQT1: Long QT syndrome
- IDDM2: Diabetes
- DHC: Smith-Lemli-Opitz syndrome
- MEN1: Multiple endocrine neoplasia
- MKS2: Meckel syndrome, type 2
- ATM: Ataxia telangiectasia

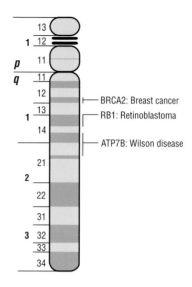

**Chromosome 13**

- BRCA2: Breast cancer
- RB1: Retinoblastoma
- ATP7B: Wilson disease

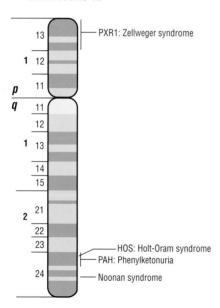

**Chromosome 12**

- PXR1: Zellweger syndrome
- HOS: Holt-Oram syndrome
- PAH: Phenylketonuria
- Noonan syndrome

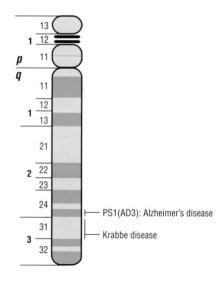

**Chromosome 14**

- PS1(AD3): Alzheimer's disease
- Krabbe disease

## Chromosome 15

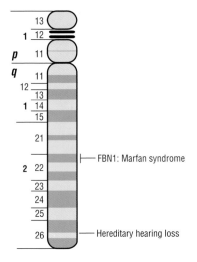

Prader-Willi syndrome (15q)

FBN1: Marfan syndrome

Hereditary hearing loss

## Chromosome 18

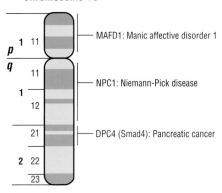

MAFD1: Manic affective disorder 1

NPC1: Niemann-Pick disease

DPC4 (Smad4): Pancreatic cancer

## Chromosome 16

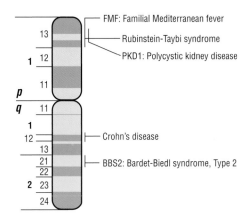

FMF: Familial Mediterranean fever

Rubinstein-Taybi syndrome

PKD1: Polycystic kidney disease

Crohn's disease

BBS2: Bardet-Biedl syndrome, Type 2

ABCC6: Pseudoaxanthoma elasticum (16)

## Chromosome 19

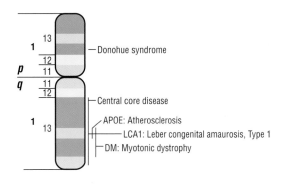

Donohue syndrome

Central core disease

APOE: Atherosclerosis

LCA1: Leber congenital amaurosis, Type 1

DM: Myotonic dystrophy

## Chromosome 17

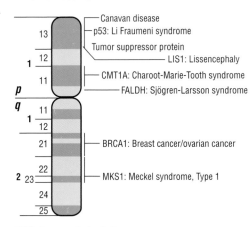

Canavan disease

p53: Li Fraumeni syndrome

Tumor suppressor protein

LIS1: Lissencephaly

CMT1A: Charoot-Marie-Tooth syndrome

FALDH: Sjögren-Larsson syndrome

BRCA1: Breast cancer/ovarian cancer

MKS1: Meckel syndrome, Type 1

SOX9: Campomelic dysplasia

## Chromosome 20

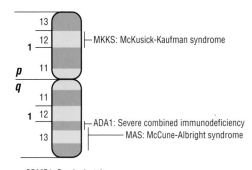

MKKS: McKusick-Kaufman syndrome

ADA1: Severe combined immunodeficiency

MAS: McCune-Albright syndrome

CDMP1: Brachydactyly

## Chromosome 21

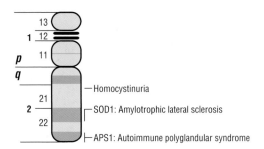

- Homocystinuria
- SOD1: Amylotrophic lateral sclerosis
- APS1: Autoimmune polyglandular syndrome

## Chromosome X

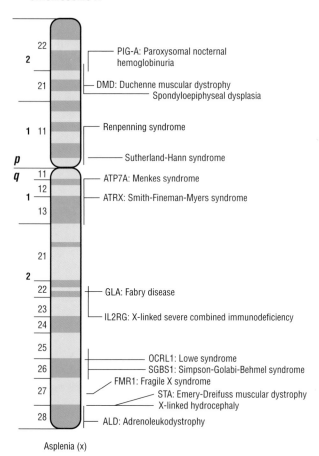

- PIG-A: Paroxysomal nocternal hemoglobinuria
- DMD: Duchenne muscular dystrophy
- Spondyloepiphyseal dysplasia
- Renpenning syndrome
- Sutherland-Hann syndrome
- ATP7A: Menkes syndrome
- ATRX: Smith-Fineman-Myers syndrome
- GLA: Fabry disease
- IL2RG: X-linked severe combined immunodeficiency
- OCRL1: Lowe syndrome
- SGBS1: Simpson-Golabi-Behmel syndrome
- FMR1: Fragile X syndrome
- STA: Emery-Dreifuss muscular dystrophy
- X-linked hydrocephaly
- ALD: Adrenoleukodystrophy

Asplenia (x)

KAL: Kallman syndrome (x)

## Chromosome 22

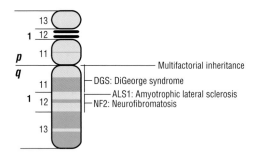

- Multifactorial inheritance
- DGS: DiGeorge syndrome
- ALS1: Amyotrophic lateral sclerosis
- NF2: Neurofibromatosis

## Chromosome Y

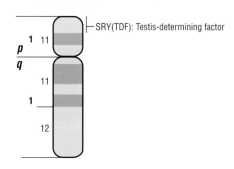

- SRY(TDF): Testis-determining factor

# ORGANIZATIONS

The following is an alphabetical compilation of organizations listed in the *Resources* section of the main body entries. Although the list is comprehensive, it is by no means exhaustive. It is a starting point for gathering further information. Many of the organizations listed provide information for multiple disorders and have links to additional related websites. E-mail addresses and web addresses listed were provided by the associations; Gale, Cengage Learning is not responsible for the accuracy of the addresses or the contents of the web sites.

22q13 Deletion Syndrome Foundation. 250 East Broadway, Maryville, TN 37804. (800) 932-2943. http://www. 22q13.com.

## A

AVENUES National Support Group for Arthrogryposis Multiplex Congenita. PO Box 5192, Sonora, CA 95370. (209) 928-3688. avenues@sonnet.com. http://www. sonnet.com/avenues.

Agenesis of the Corpus Callosum (ACC) Network. Merrill Hall, University of Maine, Room 18, 5749, Orono, ME 04469-5749. (207) 581-3119. um-acc@maine.edu.

Aicardi Syndrome Foundation. 450 Winterwood Dr., Roselle, IL 60172. (800) 373-8518. http://www. aicardi.com.

American Cancer Society. Bone Cancer Resource Center. 1599 Clifton Road, NE, Atlanta, GA 30329. (800) 227-2345 or (404) 320-3333. http://www.cancer.org/.

American Lung Association. 1740 Broadway, New York, NY 10019-4374. (212) 315-8700 or (800) 586-4872. http://www.lungusa.org.

American Medical Association. 515 N. State Street, Chicago, IL 60610. (312) 464-5000. http://www.ama-assn.org/.

American Society of Hypertension. 515 Madison Ave., Suite 1212, New York, 10022. (212) 644-0600. http://www. ash-us.org.

Arc (a National Organization on Mental Retardation). 1010 Wayne Ave., Suite 650, Silver Spring, MD 20910. (800) 433-5255. http://www.thearclink.org.

Arthritis Foundation. 1330 West Peachtree St., Atlanta, GA 30309. (800) 283-7800. http://www.arthritis.org.

Association for Glycogen Storage Disease (United Kingdom). 0131 554 2791. Fax: 0131 244 8926. http:// www.agsd.org.uk.

Association for Neuro-Metabolic Disorders. 5223 Brookfield Lane, Sylvania, OH 43560-1809. (419) 885-1497.

## B

BCCNS Life Support Network. PO Box 321, Burton, OH 44021. (440) 635-0078. http://www.bccns.org.

Breastcancer.org. 7 East Lancaster Avenue, 3rd Floor, Ardmore, PA 19003. http://www.breastcancer.org/.

## C

CHARGE Syndrome Foundation. 2004 Parkade Blvd., Columbia, MO 65202-3121. (800) 442-7604. http:// www.chargesyndrome.org.

Cherub Association of Families & Friends of Limb Disorder Children. 8401 Powers Rd., Batavia, NY 14020. (716) 762-9997.

Chromosome Deletion Outreach, Inc. PO Box 724, Boca Raton, FL 33429-0724. (561) 391-5098 or (888) 236-6880. Fax: (561) 395-4252. cdo@ worldnet.att.net. http://members.aol.com/cdousa/ cdo.htm.

Compassionate Friends. P. O. Box 3696, Oak Brook, IL 60522-3696. (877) 969-0010. E-mail: nationaloffice@ compassionatefriends.org.

Congenital Heart Information Network (C.H.I.N.). 1561 Clark Drive, Yardley, PA 19067. (215) 493-3068. E-mail: mb@tchin.org. (April 10, 2005.) http:// tchin.org/.

Corporation for Menkes Disease. 5720 Buckfield Court, Fort Wayne, IN 46814. (219) 436-0137.

Council of Regional Networks for Genetic Services. Genetic Services Program, Wadsworth Center Labs & Research, PO Box 509, Room E299, Empire State Plaza, Albany, NY 12201-0509. (518) 474-7148. http://www.cc.emory.edu/PEDIATRICS/corn/ corn.htm`.

Craniosynostosis and Parents Support. 2965-A Quarters, Quantico, VA 22134. (877) 686-CAPS or (703) 445-1078. http://www.caps2000.org/.

Crouzon's/Meniere's Parent Support Network. 3757 North Catherine Dr., Prescott Valley, AZ 86314-8320. (800) 842-4681. katy@northlink.com.

Cystic Fibrosis Foundation. 6931 Arlington Rd., Bethesda, MD 20814. (301) 951-4422. http://www.cff.org.

## D

Dubowitz Syndrome Parent Support. PO Box 173, Wheatland, IN 47597. (812) 886-0575.

Dysautonomia Foundation, Inc. 633 Third Ave., 12th Floor, New York, NY 10017-6706. (212) 949-6644. www.med.nyu.edu/fd/fdcenter.html.

## E

EA/TEF Child and Family Support Connection, Inc. 111 West Jackson Blvd., Suite 1145, Chicago, IL 60604-3502. (312) 987-9085. Fax: (312) 987-9086. eatef2@aol.com. http://www.eatef.org/.

Ehlers-Danlos Support Group - UK. PO Box 335, Farnham, Surrey, GU10 1XJ. UK 01252 690 940. http://www.atv.ndirect.co.uk.

Epilepsy and Brain Mapping Program: Huntington Memorial Hospital. 10 Congress Street, Suite 505, Pasadena, California 91105. (800) 621-2102. e-mail: info@epipro.com, http://www.epipro.com/meds.html.

European Chromosome 11q Network. http://www.11q.org.

## F

FACES. The National Craniofacial Assocation. PO Box 11082, Chattanooga, TN 37401. (423) 266-1632 or (800) 332-2373. faces@faces-cranio.org. http://www.faces-cranio.org/.

Families with Moyamoya Support Network. 4900 McGowen St. SE, Cedar Rapids, IA 54203.

Foundation Fighting Blindness–Canada. 60 St. Clair Ave., East Suite 703, Toronto, ON, Canada M4T 1N5. Phone: (416) 360-4200. Toll-free phone: (800) 461-3331. Fax: (416) 360-0060. Email: info@ffb.ca. http://www.ffb.ca/.

Foundation Fighting Blindness. Executive Plaza 1, Suite 800, 11350 McCormick Rd., Hunt Valley, MD 21031-1014. (888) 394-3937. http://www.blindness.org.

Foundation for Blood Research. PO Box 190, 69 US Route One, Scarborough, ME 04070-0190. (207) 883-4131. Fax: (207) 883-1527. http://www.fbr.org.

Foundation for Osteoporosis Research and Education. 300 27th St., Oakland, CA 94612. (888) 266-3015. http://www.fore.org.

Freeman-Sheldon Parent Support Group. 509 East Northmont Way, Salt Lake City, UT 84103-3324. (801) 364-7060.

## G

Genetic Alliance. 4301 Connecticut Ave. NW, #404, Washington, DC 20008. (800) 336-GENE (Helpline) or (202) 966-5557. Fax: (888) 394-3937. info@geneticalliance. http://www.geneticalliance.org.

Glanzmann's Thrombasthenia Support Group. 28 Duke Rd., Newton, Hyde, SK14 4JB. UK 0161-368-0219

Greenberg Center for Skeletal Dysplasias. 600 North Wolfe Street, Blalock 1012C, Baltimore, MD 21287-4922. (410) 614-0977. http://www.med.jhu.edu/Greenberg.Center/Greenbrg.htm.

## H

Hereditary Colon Cancer Association (HCCA). 3601 N 4th Ave., Suite 201, Sioux Falls, SD 57104. (800) 264-6783. http://hereditarycc.org.

HHT Foundation International, Inc. PO Box 8087, New Haven, CT 06530. (800) 448-6389 or (410) 584-7287. Canada: (604) 596-3418. Other countries: (914) 887-5844. Fax: (410) 584-7721 or (604) 596-0138. hhtinfo@hht.org. http://www.hht.org.

Human BSE Foundation (United Kingdom). 0191 389 4157. http://humanbse.foundation@virgin.net.

Human Growth Foundation. 997 Glen Cove Ave., Suite 5, Glen Head, NY, 11545. (800) 451-6434. http://www.hgfound.org.

Hydrocephalus Association. 870 Market St. Suite 705, San Francisco, CA 94102. (415) 732-7040 or (888) 598-3789. Fax: (415) 732-7044. hydroassoc@aol.com. http://www.hydroassoc.org.

## I

Immune Deficiency Foundation. 40 W. Chesapeake Ave., Suite 308, Towson, MD 21204. (800) 296-4433. (410) 321-9165. http://www.primaryimmune.org.

Infantile refsum disease support and information. 6004 NE 108th Avenue, Vancouver, WA, 98662. (360) 891-5878. http://home.pacifier.com/~mstephe/.

International Cohen Syndrome Support Group. 7 Woods Court, Brackley, Northants, NN13-6HP. UK (012) 80-704515.

International Peutz-Jeghers Support Group. Johns Hopkins Hospital, Blalock 1008, 600 North Wolfe St., Baltimore, MD 21287-4922.

International Progeria Registry. IBR Dept. of Human Genetics, 1050 Forest Hill Rd., Staten Island, NY 10314. (718) 494-5333. wtbibr@aol.com.

Intersex Society of North America (ISNA). 979 Golf Course Drive #282, Rohnert Park, CA 97928 http://www.isna.org.

Iron Overload Diseases Association, Inc. 433 Westwind Dr., North Palm Beach, FL 33408. (561) 840-8512. iod@ironoverload.org.

Ivemark Syndrome Association. 52 Keward Ave., Wells, Somerset, BAS-1TS. UK 1-(74)967-2603.

# J

Joubert Syndrome Foundation Corporation. c/o Stephanie Frazer, 384 Devon Drive, Mandeville, LA 70448.

Juvenile Diabetes Foundation International (JDF). 120 Wall St., New York, NY 10005. (212) 785-9500 x708 or (800) 533-2873. http://www.jdf.org.

# K

Kids with Heart. 1578 Careful Dr., Green Bay, WI 54304. (800) 538-5390. http://www.execpc.com/~kdswhrt.

Klinefelter's Organization. PO Box 60, Orpington, BR68ZQ. UK http://hometown.aol.com/KSCUK/index.htm.

Klippel-Trenaunay Syndrome Support Group. Phone: (952) 925-2596. Email: ktnewmembers@yahoo.com. http://www.k-t.org.

# L

Leukaemia Research Fund. 43 Great Ormond St., London, WC1N 3JJ. 020-7405-3139. http://dspace.dial.pipex.com/lrf.

Lissencephaly Network, Inc. 716 Autumn Ridge Lane, Fort Wayne, IN 46804-6402. (219) 432-4310. Fax: (219) 432-4310. lissennet@lissencephaly.org. http://www.lissencephaly.org.

Little People of America, Inc. National Headquarters, PO Box 745, Lubbock, TX 79408. (806) 737-8186 or (888) LPA-2001. lpadatabase@juno.com. http://www.lpaonline.org.

# M

MAGIC Foundation for Children's Growth. 6645 West North Avenue, Oak Park, IL 60302. (708) 383-0808 or (800) 362-4423. E-mail: mary@magicfoundation.org. http://www.magicfoundation.org.

Malignant Hyperthermia Association of the United States. PO Box 1069, 39 East State St., Sherburne, NY 13460. (800) 98-MHAUS. http://www.mhaus.org.

March of Dimes Birth Defects Foundation. 1275 Mamaroneck Ave., White Plains, NY 10605. (888) 663-4637. resourcecenter@modimes.org. http://www.modimes.org.

Meckel-Gruber Syndrome Foundation. http://www.meckel-gruber.org.

Multiple Hereditary Exostoses Family Support Group. 5316 Winter Moss Court, Columbia, MD 21045. (410) 922-5898. http://www.radix.net/~hogue/mhe.htm.

Muscular Dystrophy Association. 3300 East Sunrise Dr., Tucson, AZ 85718. (520) 529-2000 or (800) 572-1717. http://www.mdausa.org.

Muscular Dystrophy Campaign. 7-11 Prescott Place, London, SW4 6BS, United Kingdom. +44(0) 7720 8055. E-mail: info@muscular-dystrophy.org. http://www.muscular-dystrophy.org/.

Myasthenia Gravis Foundation of America. 5841 Cedar Lake Rd., Suite 204, Minneapolis, MN 55416. (800) 541-5454. Fax: (952) 545-6073.

# N

National Adrenal Diseases Foundation. 510 Northern Blvd., Great Neck, NY 11021. (516) 487-4992. http://medhlp.netusa.net/www/nadf.htm.

National Alopecia Areata Foundation (NAAF). PO Box 150760, San Rafael, CA 94915-0760. (415) 456-4644.

National Association of the Deaf. 814 Thayer Avenue, Silver Spring, MD 20910. (301) 587-1788 (voice); (301) 587-1789 (TTY). Fax: (301) 587-1791. E-mail: NADinfo@nad.org. http://www.nad.org.

National Ataxia Foundation. 2600 Fernbrook Lane, Suite 119, Minneapolis, MN 55447. (763) 553-0020. Fax: (763) 553-0167. naf@ataxia.org. http://www.ataxia.org.

National Attention Deficit Disorder Association. P.O. Box 543 Pottstown, PA 19464. (484) 945-2101. http://www.add.org.

National Brain Tumor Foundation. 414 13th St., Suite 700, Oakland, CA 94612-2603. (800) 934-2873. http://www.braintumor.org.

National Cancer Institute. Office of Communications, 31 Center Dr. MSC 2580, Bldg. 1 Room 10A16, Bethesda MD 20892-2580. (800) 422-6237. http://www.nci.nih.gov.

National Center for Health Statistics. Division of Data Services, 6525 Belcrest Rd., Hyattsville, MD 20782-2003. http://www.cdc.gov/nchs.

National Depressive and Manic-Depressive Association. 730 N. Franklin, Suite 501, Chicago, IL 60610-7204. (800) 826-3632 or (312) 642-7243. http://www.ndmda.org.

National Diabetes Information Clearinghouse. 1 Information Way, Bethesda, MD 20892-3560. (800) 860-8747. http://diabetes.niddk.nih.gov/about/index.htm.

National Down Syndrome Society. 666 Broadway, New York, NY 10012-2317. (212) 460-9330 or (800) 221-4602. Fax: (212) 979-2873. http://www.ndss.org info@ndss.org.

National Epidermolysis Bullosa Registry. University of North Carolina at Chapel Hill, Bolin Heights Bldg. #1, CB# 3369, Chapel Hill, NC 27514-3369. (919) 966-2007. Fax: (919) 966-7080. eb_registry@med.unc.edu. http://www.med.unc.edu/derm/nebr_site.

National Eye Institute (NEI). 2020 Vision Place, Bethesda, MD 20892-3655. (301)496-5248. http://www.nei.nih.gov.

National Foundation for Ectodermal Dysplasias (NFED). 410 E. Main St., P.O. Box 114, Mascoutah, IL 62258-0114. (618)566-2020. http://www.nfed.org.

National Foundation for Facial Reconstruction. 317 East 34th St. #901, New York, NY 10016. (800) 422-3223. http://www.nffr.org.

National Fragile X Syndrome Support Group. 206 Sherman Rd., Glenview, IL 60025. (708) 724-8626.

National Hemophilia Foundation. Soho Building, 110 Greene Street, Suite 406, New York, NY 10012. (212) 219-8180. http://www.hemophilia.org/home.htm.

National Human Genome Research Institute (NHGRI). The National Institutes of Health, Building 31, Room 4B09, 31 Center Drive, MSC 2152, 9000 Rockville Pike, Bethesda, MD 20892-2152. (301)402-0911. Fax: (301)402-2218. http://www.nhgri.nih.gov.

National Institute for Neurological Disorders and Stroke (NINDS). P.O. Box 5801, Bethesda, MD 20824. (800)352-9424 or (301)496-5751. http://www.ninds.nih.gov.

National Institute of Allergy and Infectious Diseases (NIAID). 6610 Rockledge Drive, MSC 6612, Bethesda, MD 20892-6612. (301)496-5717 or (866)284-4107. Email: niaidnews@niaid.nih.gov. http://www3.niaid.nih.gov.

National Institute of Arthritis and Musculoskeletal and Skin Diseases (NIAMS). 1 AMS Circle, Bethesda, MD 20892-3675. (301)495-4484 or (877)22-NIAMS (226-4267). Fax: (301)718-6366. Email: NIAMSinfo@mail.nih.gov. http://www.niams.nih.gov.

National Institute of Child Health and Human Development (NICHD). Patient Recruitment and Public Liaison Office, Building 61, 10 Cloister Court, Bethesda, MD 20892-4754. (800) 411-1222, (301) 594-9774 (TTY), (866) 411-1010 (TTY). prpl@mail.cc.nih.gov. http://clinicalstudies.info.nih.gov/detail/A_2000-CH-0141.html.

National Institute of Diabetes and Digestive and Kidney Diseases. Building 31, room 9A04, Bethesda, MD 20892. http://www.niddk.nih.gov.

National Institute of Mental Health (NIMH). 6001 Executive Boulevard, Bethesda, MD 20892-9663. (866)615-6464 or (301)443-4513. Fax: (301)443-4279. Email: nimhinfor@nih.gov. http://www.nimh.nih.gov.

National Institute of Neurological Disorders and Stroke. 31 Center Drive, MSC 2540, Bldg. 31, Room 8806, Bethesda, MD 20814. (301) 496-5751 or (800) 352-9424. http://www.ninds.nih.gov.

National Institute on Deafness and Other Communication Disorders. 31 Center Dr., MSC 2320, Bethesda, MD 20814. (301) 402-0900. nidcdinfo@nidcd.nih.gov. http://www.nidcd.nih.gov.

National Institutes of Health, Osteoporosis and Related Bone Diseases. National Resource Center, 1232 22nd Street NW, Washington, DC 20037-1292. Fax: (202) 223-0344. http://www.osteo.org/hypoph.html.

National Institutes of Health/National Institute of Neurological Disorders and Stroke Brain Resources and Information Network. PO Box 5801, Bethesda, MD 20824. (301) 496 5751. (April 4, 2005.) http://www.ninds.nih.gov.

National Kidney Foundation. 30 East 33rd St., New York, NY 10016. (800) 622-9010. http://www.kidney.org.

National Kidney and Urologic Diseases Information Clearinghouse. 3 Information Way Bethesda, MD 20892-3580. (800) 891-5390. E-mail: nkudic@info.niddk.nih.gov. (April 18, 2005.) http://kidney.niddk.nih.gov/about/index.htm.

National Mental Health Information Center. P.O. Box 2345, Rockville, MD 20847. (800)789-2647. Fax: (240)221-4295. http://mentalhealth.samhsa.gov.

National MPS Society. 102 Aspen Dr., Downingtown, PA 19335. (610) 942-0100. Fax: (610) 942-7188. info@mpssociety.org. http://www.mpssociety.org.

National Multiple Sclerosis Society. 733 Third Avenue 6th Floor, New York, NY 10017-3288. (800) 344-4867. (April 21, 2005.) http://www.nationalmssociety.org.

National Organization for Albinism and Hypopigmentation. 1530 Locust St. #29, Philadelphia, PA 19102-4415. (215) 545-2322 or (800) 473-2310. http://www.albinism.org/infobulletins/hermansky-pudlak-syndrome.html.

National Organization for Rare Disorders (NORD). 55 Kenosia Avenue, PO Box 1968, Danbury, CT 06813-1968. (800) 999-6673. http://www.rarediseases.org/.

National Organization of Disorders of the Corpus Callosum. 18032-C Lemon Drive, PMB 363, Yorba Linda, CA 92886. (April 9, 2005.) http://www.corpuscallosum.org.

National Organization on Fetal Alcohol Syndrome (NOFAS). 900 17th St., NW, Suite 910, Washington, DC 20006. (202)785-4585 or (800) 66NOFAS. Fax: (202)466-6456. http://www.nofas.org.

National Registry for Ichthyosis and Related Disorders. University of Washington Dermatology Department, Box 356524, 1959 N.E. Pacific, Rm. BB1353, Seattle, WA 98195-6524. (800) 595-1265 or (206) 616-3179. http://www.skinregistry.org.

National Sleep Foundation. 1522 K St. NW, Suite 500, Washington, DC 20005. (202)347-3472. Fax: (202)347-3472. Email: nsf@sleepfoundation.org. http://www.sleepfoundation.org.

National Society of Genetic Counselors (NSGC). 401 N. Michigan Ave., Chicago, IL 60611. (312)321-6834. Fax: (312)673-6972. Email: nsgc@nsgc.org. http://www.nsgc.org.

National Tay-Sachs and Allied Diseases Association. 2001 Beacon St., Suite 204, Brighton, MA 02135. (800) 906-8723. ntasd-Boston@worldnet.att.net. http://www.ntsad.org.

National Urea Cycle Disorders Foundation (NUCDF). 4841 Hill Street, La Canada CA 91011. (818)790-2460 or (800)38-NUCDF. Email:info@nucdf.orghttp://www.nucdf.org.

Nephrogenic Diabetes Insipidus Foundation. PO Box 1390, Eastsound, WA 98245. (888) 376-6343. Fax: (888) 376-3842. http://www. Ndi.org.

Neurofibromatosis, Inc. 8855 Annapolis Rd., #110, Lanham, MD 20706-2924. (800) 942-6825. http://www.nfinc.org.

Neurofibromatosis Society of Ontario. 2004 Underhill Court, Pickering, ON L1X 2M6, Canada. (905)683-0811 Or (866)843-6376. http://www.nfon.ca.

Neuropathy Association. 60 East 42nd Street, Suite 942, New York, NY 10165-0999. (212)692-0662

Fax: (212)692-0668. Email: info@neuropathy.org. http://www.neuropathy.org.

Nevus Outreach, Inc. 1616 Alpha St., Lansing, MI 48910. (517) 487-2306. http://www.nevus.org.

Noonan Syndrome Support Group, Inc. c/o Mrs. Wanda Robinson, PO Box 145, Upperco, MD 21155.(888) 686-2224 or (410) 374-5245. andar@bellatlantic.net. http://www.noonansyndrome.org.

Norrie Disease Association. Massachusetts General Hospital, E #6217, 149 13th St., Charlestown, MA 02129. (617) 726-5718. sims@helix.mgh.harvard.edu.

# O

Oculo-Dento-Digital Dysplasia Support Group. 8810 Orchard Road, Pikesville, MD 21208. Phone: (410) 480-0882. Email: jquasneyjr@comcast.net. http://home.comcast.net/~jquasneyjr.

Office of Rare Diseases Research (ORDR). 6100 Executive Blvd., Room 3B01, MSC 7518, Bethesda, MD 20892-7518. (301)402-4336. Fax: (301)480-9655. Email: ordr@od.nih.gov. http://rarediseases.info.nih.gov.

OMIM—Online Mendelian inheritance in Man. http://www.ncbi.nlm.nig.gov.

Online Myotonic & Congenital Dystrophies Support Group International. 185 Unionville Road, Freedom, PA 15042. (724)775-9448 or (724)774-0261. http://www.angelfire. com/pa2/MyotonicDystrophy/index.html.

Organic Acidemia Association. 13210 35th Ave. North, Plymouth, MN 55441. (763) 559-1797. Fax: (863) 694-0017. http://www.oaanews.org.

Organic Acidemias UK. 5 Saxon Rd., Ashford, Middlesex, TW15 1QL. UK (178)424-5989.

Organization of Teratology Services (OTIS). (888) 285-3410. http://www.otispregnancy.org.

Osteogenesis Imperfecta Foundation. 804 W. Diamond Ave., Suite 210, Gaithersburg, MD 20878. (301)947-0083 or (800)981-2663. Fax: (301)947-0456. Email: bonelink@oif.org. http://www.oif.org.

# P

Pallister–Hall Foundation. RFD Box 3000, Fairground Rd., Bradford, VT 05033. (802)222-9683. Email: messer@sover.net.

Pancreatic Cancer UK. 31 Brooklyn Dr., Emmer Green, Reading, Berkshire RG4 8SR, UK. 0118-9472934.

Email: enquiries@pancreaticcancer.org.uk. http://www.pancreaticcancer.org.uk..

Pancreatitis Support Network. http://hometown.aol.com/karynwms/myhomepage/business.html.

Parent Project for Muscular Dystrophy Research. 1012 N. University Blvd., Middletown, OH 45042. (413) 424-0696 or (800) 714-5437. parentproject@aol.com. http://www.parentdmd.org.

Parents of Galactosemic Children Inc. P.O. Box 2401, Mandeville, LA 70470-2401. (866)900-PGC1. http://www.galactosemia.org.

PKS Kids. 123 Carowinds Dr., Greencastle, PA 17225. Email: onebuddy@comcast.net. http://www.pkskids.net.

Polycystic Kidney Disease Foundation. 4901 Main Street, Kansas City, MO 64112-2634. (800) PKD-CURE. http://www.pkdcure.org/home.htm.

Polycystic Ovarian Syndrome Association. PO Box 80517, Portland, OR 97280. (877) 775-PCOS. http://www.pcosupport.org.

Potter's Syndrome Support Group Main Forum. http://forums.delphiforums.com.

Prader-Willi Syndrome Association. 5700 Midnight Pass Rd., Suite 6, Sarasota, FL 34242-3000. (941) 312-0400 or (800) 926-4797. Fax: (941) 312-0142. http://www.pwsausa.org PWSAUSA@aol.com.

Prevent Blindness America. 211 West Wacker Drive, Suite 1700, Chicago, Illinois 60606. (800)331-2020. http://www.preventblindness.org.

Proteus Syndrome Foundation. 6235 Whetstone Dr., Colorado Springs, CO 80918. (719)264-8445. abscit@aol.com. http://www.kumc.edu/gec/support/proteus.html.

Pull–thru Network. 2312 Savoy St., Hoover, AL 35226. (205)978û2930. Email: info@pullthrough.org. http://www.pullthrunetwork.org.

PXE International, Inc. 23 Mountain Street, Sharon, MA 02067. (781) 784-3817. Fax: (781) 784-6672. PXEInter@aol.com. http://www.pxe.org/.

# R

Raynaud & Scleroderma Association (UK). 112 Crewe Road, Alsager, Cheshire, ST7 2JA, UK. (44) (0) 1270 872776. webmaster@raynauds.demon.co.uk. http://www.raynauds.demon.co.uk.

Research Registry for Hereditary Hearing Loss. 555 N. 30th St., Omaha, NE 68131. (800) 320-1171. http://www.boystown.org/btnrh/deafgene.reg/waardsx.htm

RESOLVE, The National Infertility Association. 1310 Broadway, Somerville, MA 02144-1779. (617) 623-0744. resolveinc@aol.com.

Retina International. Ausstellungsstrasse 36, Zürich, CH-8005. Switzerland (+41 1 444 10 77). http://www.retina-international.org.

Retinitis Pigmentosa International. P.O. Box 900, Woodland Hills, CA 91365. Phone: (818) 992-0500. Fax: (818) 992-3265. Email: info@rpinternational.org. http://www.rpinternational.org.

Retinoblastoma International. 4650 Sunset Blvd., MS #88, Los Angeles, CA 90027. (323)669-2299. http://www.retinoblastoma.net.

Rett Syndrome Research Foundation. 4600 Devitt Dr., Cincinnati, OH 45246. http://www.rsfr.org.

Rhizomelic Chondrodysplasia Punctata (RCP) Family Support Group. 137 25th Ave., Monroe, WI 53566.

Robinow Syndrome Foundation. PO Box 1072, Anoka, MN 55303. (612) 434-1152. http://www.robinow.org.

Royal National Institute for the Blind. PO Box 173, Peterborough PE2 6WS. http://www.rnib.org.uk.

Royal National Institute of Blind People. 105 Judd Street, London, WC1H 9NE, UK. +020 7388 1266. http://www.rnib.org.uk.

Rubinstein-Taybi Parent Support Group. c/o Lorrie Baxter, PO Box 146, Smith Center, KS 66967. (888) 447-2989. lbaxter@ruraltelnet. http://www.specialfriends.org.

Russell-Silver Syndrome Support Group. http://groups.yahoo.com/group/RSS-Support.

# S

SADS Foundation. PO Box 58767, 508 East South Temple, Suite 20, Salt Lake City, UT 84102. (800) 786-7723. http://www.sads.org.

Schafer, Frank A. MD. "Achdrogenesis" In *Pediatrics/Genetics and Metabolic Disease, e-medicine* http://www.emedicine.com/ped/topic2.htm.

SHARE-Pregnancy and Infant Loss Support, Inc. St Joseph Health Center, 300 First Capital Dr., St. Charles, MO 63301. (800) 821-6819.

Schepens Eye Research Institute. 20 Staniford St., Boston, MA 02114-2500. (617) 912-0100. http://www.eri.harvard.edu.

Schizophrenics Anonymous. 15920 W. Twelve Mile, Southfield, MI 48076. (248) 477-1983.

Scleroderma Foundation. 12 Kent Way, Suite 101, Byfield, MA 01922. (978) 463-5843 or (800) 722-HOPE. Fax: (978) 463-5809. http://www.scleroderma.org.

Scoliosis Research Society. 6300 N. River Rd., Ste 727, Rosemont, IL 60018-4226. (847)698-1627. Fax: (847) 823-0536. Goulding@aaos.org. http://www.srs.org/.

Shital Parikh, Alvin H. Crawford, and Preeti Batra. Spondyloepiphyseal Dysplasia http://emedicine.medscape.com/article/1260836-overview

Sickle Cell Disease Association of America, Inc. 200 Corporate Point Suite 495, Culver City, CA 90230-8727. (800) 421-8453. Scdaa@sicklecelldisease.org. http://sicklecelldisease.org/.

Smith-Lemli-Opitz Advocacy and Exchange (RSH/SLO). 2650 Valley Forge Dr., Boothwyn, PA 19061. (610) 485-9663. http://members.aol.com/slo97/index. html.

Society for Mucopolysaccharide Diseases. MPS House, Repton Place, White Lion Rd., Amersham, Buckinghamshire HP7 9LP, UK. + 44 0845-389-9901. http://www.mpssociety.co.uk.

Sotos Syndrome Support Group. Three Danda Square East #235, Wheaton, IL 60187. (888) 246-SSSA or (708) 682-8815. http://www.well.com/user/sssa/.

Spina Bifida Association of America. 4590 MacArthur Blvd. NW, Suite 250, Washington, DC 20007-4226. (800) 621-3141 or (202) 944-3285. Fax: (202) 944-3295.

SRPS Family Network. http://www.srps.net.

Stickler Involved People. 15 Angelina, Augusta, KS 67010. (316) 775-2993. http://www.sticklers.org/sip.

Stickler Syndrome Support Group. PO Box 371, Walton-on-Thames, Surrey KT12 2YS, England. 44-01932 267635. http://www.stickler.org.uk.

Sturge-Weber Foundation. PO Box 418, Mount Freedom, NJ 07970. (800) 627-5482 or (973) 895-4445. Fax: (973) 895-4846. swfoffice@aol.com. http://www.sturgeweber.com/.

Sudden Arrhythmia Death Syndrome Foundation. PO Box 58767, 508 East South Temple, Suite 20, Salt Lake City, UT 84102. (800) 786-7723. sads@sads.org. http://www.sads.org.

Sudden Infant Death Syndrome Network. PO Box 520, Ledyard, CT 06339. http://sids-network.org.

Support Groups For MMA Organic Acidemia Association. 13210 35th Avenue Plymouth, MN 55441. (763) 559-1797. http://www.oaanews.

Support Organization for Trisomy 18, 13 and Related Disorders (SOFT). 2982 South Union St., Rochester, NY 14624. (800) 716-SOFT. http://www.trisomy.org.

Support for Parents with Hypospadias Boys. http://clubs.yahoo.com/clubs/mumswithhypospadiaskids.

# T

T.A.R.S.A. Thrombocytopenia Abset Radius Syndrome Association. 212 Sherwood Drive, Linwood, NJ 08324-7658. (609) 927-0418.

Texas Heart Institute Heart Information Service. PO Box 20345, Houston, TX 77225-0345. (800) 292-2221. http://www.tmc.edu/thi/his.html.

Thalassemia Foundation of Canada. 340 Falstaff Ave., North York, ON M6L 2E8, Canada. (416)242-8425. Email: info@thalassemia.ca. http://www.thalassemia.ca.

Thrombophilia Support. http://www.fvleiden.org.

Tourette Syndrome Foundation of Canada. 194 Jarvis Street, #206, Toronto, ONT M5B 2B7. Canada. (800) 361-3120. tsfc.org@sympatico.ca. http://www. tourette.ca.

Treacher Collins Foundation. Box 683, Norwich, VT 05055. (800) 823-2055.

Tuberous Sclerosis Alliance. 801 Roeder Rd., Suite 750, Silver Spring, MD 20910. (800) 225-6872. http://www.tsalliance.org.

Turner Syndrome Society of the United States. 14450 T. C. Jester, Suite 260, Houston, TX 77014. (800) 365-9944 or (832) 249-9988. Fax: (832) 249-9987. tesch@turner-syndrome-us.org. http://www.turner-syndrome-us.org.

Twin Hope, Inc. 2592 West 14th St., Cleveland, OH 44113. (502) 243-2110. http://www.twinhope.com.

Twins Foundation. PO Box 6043, Providence, RI 02940-6043. (401) 751-8946. Twins@twinsfoundation.com.

# U

UNIQUE Rare Chromosome Disorder Group. P.O. Box 2189, Caterham, Surrey CR3 5GN, UK. Phone/Fax: (44)(0)1883 330766. Email: info@rarechromo.org. www.rarechromo.org.

United Cerebral Palsy (UCP) Research & Educational Foundation. 1025 Connecticut Avenue, Suite 701, Washington, DC 20036. (202)496-5060 or (800)USA-5UCP (872-5827). Fax: (202)776-0414. Email: national @ucp.org. http://www.ucpresearch.org.

United Cerebral Palsy Association, Inc. (UCP). 1660 L St. NW, Suite 700, Washington, DC 20036-5602. (202)776-0406 or (800)872-5827. http://www.ucpa.org.

United Leukodystrophy Foundation. 2304 Highland Dr., Sycamore, IL 60178. (815) 895-3211 or (800) 728-5483. Fax: (815) 895-2432. http://www. ulf.org.

United Mitochondrial Disease Foundation. PO Box 1151, Monroeville, PA 15146-1151. (412) 793-8077. Fax: (412) 793-6477. http://www.umdf.org.

University of California–San Francisco. http://itsa.ucsf. edu/~uroweb/Uro/hypospadias/index.html.

University of Texas M.D. Anderson Cancer Center. 1515 Holcombe Blvd., Houston, TX 77030. (800) 392-1611. http://www.mdanderson.org.

University of Washington PKU Clinic. CHDD, Box 357920, University of Washington, Seattle, WA. (206) 685-3015. Within Washington State: (877) 685-3015. Clinic Coordinator: vam@u.washington. edu. http://depts. washington.edu/pku/contact.html..

U.S. National Library of Medicine. 8600 Rockville Pike, Bethesda, MD 20894.

# V

VATER Connection. 1722 Yucca Lane, Emporia, KS 66801. (316) 342-6954. http://www.vaterconnection. org.

Velo-Cardio-Facial Syndrome Research Institute. Albert Einstein College of Medicine, 3311 Bainbridge Ave., Bronx, NY 10467. (718) 430-2568. Fax: (718) 430-8778. rgoldber@aecom.yu.edu. http://www.kumc.edu/gec/ vcfhome.html.

Vestibular Disorders Association. PO Box 4467, Portland, OR 97208-4467. (800) 837-8428. http:// www.vestibular.org.

VHL Family Alliance. 171 Clinton Ave., Brookline, MA 02455-5815. (800) 767-4VHL. http://www.vhl.org.

Vision Community Services. 23 A Elm St., Watertown, MA 02472. (617) 926-4232 or (800) 852-3029. http://www. mablind.org.

# W

We Move. 204 West 84th St., New York, NY 10024. Email: wemove@wemove.org. http://www.wemove.org.

Weaver Syndrome Families Support (WSFS). 4357 153rd Ave. SE, Bellevue, WA 98006 (425) 747-5382.

Williams Syndrome Foundation. University of California, Irvine, CA 92679-2310. (949)824-7259. http:// www.wsf.org/.

Wilson's Disease Association. http://www.medhelp.org/wda/ wil.htm.

World Craniofacial Foundation. PO Box 515838, 7777 Forest Lane, Ste C-621, Dallas, TX 75251-5838. (972) 566-6669 or (800) 533-3315. worldcf@worldnet.att.net. http://www.worldcf.org.

Worldwide Education and Awareness for Movement Disorders (WE MOVE). Mt. Sinai Medical Center, 1 Gustave Levy Place, New York, NY 10029. (800) 437-MOV2. http://www.wemove.org.

# X

Xeroderma Pigmentosum Society, Inc. PO Box 4759, Poughkeepsie, NY 12602. (518) 851-2612. xps@xps.org. http://www.xps.org.

# Y

Yale-LDA Social Learning Disabilities Project. Yale Child Study Center, 230 South Frontage Road, New Haven, CT 06520-7900. (203) 785-3488. http://info.med.Yale. edu/chldstdy/autism.

# Z

Zellweger Baby Support Network. 1852 Iron Horse Loop, Spearfish SD 57783. (605)642-2072. Email: pamfreeth @zbsn.org. http://www.zbsn.org.

# GLOSSARY

## A

**AADC INHIBITORS.** Drugs that block the amino acid decarboxylase; one type of enzyme that breaks down dopamine. Also called DC inhibitors, they include carbidopa and benserazide.

**ATP.** Adenosine triphosphate. The chemical used by the cells of the body for energy.

**ABDOMINAL HERNIA.** Bulging of an organ or tissue through the muscle of the stomach wall.

**ABDUCENS NERVE.** Cranial nerve VI; the nerve that extends from the midbrain to the lateral rectus muscle of the eye and controls movement of the eye toward the ear (abduction).

**ABDUCTION.** Turning away from the body.

**ABSCESS.** A localized collection of pus or infection that is walled off from the rest of the body.

**ABSENCE SEIZURE.** A brief seizure with an accompanying loss of awareness or alertness.

**ACANTHOCYTOSIS.** The presence of acanthocytes in the blood. Acanthocytes are red blood cells that have the appearance of thorns on their outer surface.

**ACANTHOSIS NIGRICANS.** A skin condition distinguished by velvety, dark patches where the skin is folded or creased.

**ACCOMMODATION.** The ability of the lens to change its focus from distant to near objects. It is achieved through the action of the ciliary muscles that change the shape of the lens.

**ACETYLCHOLINE.** A neurotransmitter (chemical messenger) used to certain nerve cells to send messages to adjacent cells.

**ACETYLCHOLINESTERASE (ACHE).** An enzyme found in nerve tissue.

**ACHROMATOPSIA.** The inability to distinguish any colors.

**ACID MALTASE.** The enzyme that regulates the amount of glycogen stored in muscle cells. When too much glycogen is present, acid maltase is released to break it down into waste products.

**ACIDOSIS.** A condition of decreased alkalinity resulting from abnormally high acid levels (low pH) in the blood and tissues. Usually indicated by sickly sweet breath, headaches, nausea, vomiting, and visual impairments.

**ACONDROPLASIA.** An autosomal dominant form of dwarfism caused by a defect in the formation of cartilage at the ends of long bones. Affected individuals typically have short limbs, a large head with a prominent forehead and flattened profile, and a normal-sized trunk.

**ACQUIRED ANGIONEUROTIC EDEMA.** Abbreviated AANE, or AAE, this is a non-hereditary form of angio edema that generally begins to show symptoms in, or after, the fourth decade of life.

**ACQUIRED IMMUNITY.** Also called "specific immunity," refers to immune reaction mediated by B-cells and/or T-cells. Includes humoral and cellular immunity.

**ACROCENTRIC.** A chromosome with the centromere positioned at the top end.

**ACROCEPHALOPOLYSYNDACTYLY SYNDROMES.** A collection of genetic disorders characterized by cone shaped abnormality of the skull and partial fusing of adjacent fingers or toes.

**ACROCEPHALY.** An abnormal cone shape of the head.

**ACROMELIC.** The anatomical term used to denote the end of a limb (arm or leg). In the context of Robinow syndrome, it refers to bones of the hands and feet.

ACROOSTEOLYSIS. Loss of bone tissue at the ends of the fingers and/or toes.

ACROPARESTHESIAS. Painful burning sensation in hands and feet.

ACTION POTENTIAL. The wave-like change in the electrical properties of a cell membrane, resulting from the difference in electrical charge between the inside and outside of the membrane. The action potential acts as a signal for certain activities and processes in the body.

ACUPUNCTURE. An alternative health procedure based on ancient Chinese methods, involving insertion of thin needles at specific pressure points in the body.

ACUTE PHASE REACTANTS. Blood proteins whose concentrations increase or decrease in reaction to the inflammation process.

ACUTE PHASE. The initial phase of LHON where visual blurring begins in both eyes, and central vision is lost.

ADDUCTED THUMBS. Thumbs clasped across the palm.

ADDUCTION. Movement toward the body. In Duane retraction syndrome, turning the eye inward toward the nose.

ADENOCARCINOMA. A type of cancer which is in a gland-like form.

ADENOMATOUS. Derived from glandular structures.

ADJUVANT THERAPY. Adjuvant therapy is treatment given in addition to the primary therapy.

ADRENAL GLAND. A triangle-shaped endocrine gland, located above each kidney, that synthesizes aldosterone, cortisol, and testosterone from cholesterol. The adrenal glands are responsible for salt and water levels in the body, as well as for protein, fat, and carbohydrate metabolism.

ADRENAL INSUFFICIENCY. Problems with the adrenal glands that can be life threatening if not treated. Symptoms include sluggishness, weakness, weight loss, vomiting, darkening of the skin and mental changes.

ADRENAL. A pair of glands located on top of the kidneys that secrete substances or hormones, like steroids and adrenaline, which regulate various functions, such as water balance and stress response.

ADRENOCORTICOTROPIN (CORTICOTROPHIN). A hormone that acts on cells of the adrenal cortex, causing them to produce male sex hormones and hormones that control water and mineral balance in the body.

ADVANCED BONE AGE. The bones, on x ray, appear to be those of an older individual.

ADYSPLASIA. A term referring to the combination of renal agenesis (complete absence of one or both kidneys) and renal dysplasia (developmental anomaly of the kidney).

AFFECTIVE FLATTENING. A loss or lack of emotional expressiveness; sometimes called blunted or restricted affect.

AFLATOXIN. A substance produced by molds that grow on rice and peanuts. Exposure to aflatoxin is thought to explain the high rates of primary liver cancer in Africa and parts of Asia.

AGANGLIONOSIS. Section of bowel in which the normal enteric nerves are absent.

AGE-ASSOCIATED MEMORY IMPAIRMENT (AAMI). A condition in which an older person suffers some memory loss and takes longer to learn new information. AAMI is distinguished from dementia in that it is not progressive and does not represent a serious decline from the person's previous level of functioning.

AGENESIS OF THE CORPUS CALLOSUM. Failure of the corpus callosum to form and develop. The corpus callosum is the band of nerve fibers located between the two sides, or hemispheres, of the brain.

AGENESIS/HYPOPLASIA OF THE CORPUS CALLOSUM. A birth defect in which the two halves of the brain are not properly separated.

AGENESIS. Failure of an organ, tissue, or cell to develop or grow.

AGNOSIA. Loss of the ability to recognize objects by use of the physical senses.

AGYRI. A lack of convolutions or normal folds in the brain tissue.

AKATHISIA. Agitated or restless movement, usually affecting the legs and accompanied by a sense of discomfort; a common side effect of neuroleptic medications.

ALKALINE PHOSPHATASE (ALK PHOS). A body protein, measurable in the blood, that often appears in high amounts in patients with osteosarcoma. However, many other conditions also elevate the level of alkaline phosphatase.

ALKALINE. Having a basic pH; not acidic.

ALKALINIZATION. The process of making a solution more basic, rather than more acidic, by raising the pH.

ALLELE. One of two or more different genes encoding specific and inheritable characteristics that occupy corresponding locations on a pair of chromosomes.

AUTOSOME. One of the 22 chromosomes that are not involved in determining gender (chromosomes 1 through 22 and not the X or Y chromosome).

AXON. Skinny, wire-like extension of nerve cells.

# B

B CELL. Specialized type of white blood cell that is capable of secreting infection-fighting antibodies.

BMPR2. Bone morphogenetic protein receptor 2; it is the gene on which a mutation occurs that is most responsible for cases of familial pulmonary arterial hypertension.

BRCA2. Gene, when altered, known to cause increased risks of breast, ovarian and, possibly, pancreatic cancer.

BALANCED CHROMOSOME TRANSLOCATION. A rearrangement of the chromosomes in which two chromosomes have broken and exchanged pieces without the loss of genetic material.

BAND. A specific region of a chromosome that is identified by its characteristic staining pattern and location within a chromosome, as seen in a karyotype. A band is either part of the short arm (p arm) or the long arm (q arm) of a chromosome and is further defined by a numeric location, such as chromosome band 11q24.1.

BARDET-BIEDL SYNDROME. A human genetic disorder that affects many body systems. It is characterized principally by obesity, retinitis pigmentosa (a type of progressive retinal dystrophy), polydactyly (having additional fingers or toes), mental retardation, hypogonadism (a defect of the gonads that results in underproduction of testosterone), and possibly kidney failure.

BARIUM ENEMA X RAY. A procedure that involves the administration of barium into the intestines by a tube inserted into the rectum. Barium is a chalky substance that enhances the visualization of the gastrointestinal tract on x–ray.

BARIUM. A chemical put into a solution and swallowed to help with outlining the gastrointestinal system during an x ray study.

BASAL CELL CARCINOMA. A cancer originating from skin.

BASAL GANGLIA. A section of the brain responsible for smooth muscle movement.

BASE PAIRS. Building blocks of DNA, the chemical that genes are made of.

BASEMENT MEMBRANE. Part of the epithelium, or outer layer of the cornea.

BECKER MUSCULAR DYSTROPHY (BMD). A type of muscular dystrophy that affects older boys and men, and usually follows a milder course than Duchenne muscular dystrophy.

BECKWITH-WIEDEMANN SYNDROME. A collection of health problems present at birth including an omphalocele, large tongue, and large body size.

BENIGN PROSTATIC HYPERPLASIA (BPH). A noncancerous condition of the prostate that causes growth of the prostate tissue, thus enlarging the prostate and blocking urination.

BENIGN TUMOR. An abnormal proliferation of cells that does not spread to other sites.

BENIGN. A non-cancerous tumor that does not spread and is not life-threatening.

BENZOQUINONE ACETIC ACID. Toxic compound that is formed when oxygen reacts with homogentisic acid.

BETA CELLS. Specialized cells of the pancreas that make insulin.

BETA-2 MICROGLOBULIN. A component protein of class I MHC.

BETA-ADRENERGIC BLOCKER. A drug that works by controlling the nerve impulses along specific nerve pathways.

BIFID UVULA. The uvula is the small, tear drop–shaped piece of flesh hanging in the back of the throat; the uvula is bifid if the bottom area is split in two parts.

BILATERAL BREAST CANCER. Cancer of both breasts, caused by two separate cancer processes.

BILATERAL. Relating to or affecting both sides of the body or both of a pair of organs.

BILE ACIDS. Steroid acids such as cholic acid that occur in bile, an alkaline fluid secreted by the liver and passed into a part of the small intestine where it aids in absorption of fats.

BILE ALCOHOL. A steroid acid with an alcohol group attached.

BILE DUCT. A passageway that carries bile (fluid secreted by the liver involved in fat absorption) from the liver to the gallbladder to the small intestine.

BILE. A substance produced by the liver, and concentrated and stored in the gallbladder. Bile contains a number of different substances, including bile salts, cholesterol, and bilirubin.

**BILIRUBIN.** A yellow pigment that is the end result of hemoglobin breakdown. This pigment is metabolized in the liver and excreted from the body through the bile. Bloodstream levels are normally low; however, extensive red cell destruction leads to excessive bilirubin formation and jaundice.

**BIOCHEMICAL TESTING.** Measuring the amount or activity of a particular enzyme or protein in a sample of blood or urine or other tissue from the body.

**BIOFEEDBACK.** A technique in which patients are trained to gain some voluntary control over certain physiological conditions, such as blood pressure and muscle tension, and to promote relaxation.

**BIOPSY.** The surgical removal and microscopic examination of living tissue for diagnostic purposes.

**BIOPTICS.** Glasses that have small telescopes fitted in the lens.

**BIOSYNTHESIS.** The manufacture of materials in a biological system.

**BIOTIN.** A growth vitamin of the vitamin B complex found naturally in liver, egg yolks, and yeast.

**BIPOLAR DISORDER.** Formerly called "manic depression," this psychological disorder is characterized by periods of mania followed by periods of depression.

**BITEMPORAL CONSTRICTION.** Abnormal narrowing of both sides of the forehead.

**BLACKFAN-DIAMOND SYNDROME (BDS).** A disorder with congenital hypoplastic anemia. Some researchers believe that some or all individuals with Aase syndrome actually have BDS, that Aase syndrome and BDS are not separate disorders.

**BLADDER.** This is the organ that stores urine after it flows out of the kidneys and through the ureters.

**BLEPHAROPHIMOSIS.** A small eye opening without fusion of the upper eyelid with the lower eyelid at the inner and outer corner of the eye.

**BLOOD SERUM.** The clear liquid portion of the blood.

**BLOOD VESSELS.** General term for arteries, veins, and capillaries that transport blood throughout the body.

**BLOOD-BRAIN BARRIER.** A mechanism that acts as a sentry for the brain and only allows certain substances in the circulating blood to pass into the brain.

**BODY ASYMMETRY.** Abnormal development of the body in which the trunk and/or the limbs are not of equal size from one side of the body to the other.

**BODY MASS INDEX (BMI).** Assessment of health related to weight and height.

**BOILS.** Painful areas of inflammation.

**BONE CYSTS.** Fluid- or air-filled space within the bones.

**BONE DYSPLASIA.** Abnormal bone development.

**BONE MARROW TRANSPLANT (BMT).** A medical procedure used to treat some diseases that arise from defective blood cell formation in the bone marrow. Healthy bone marrow is extracted from a donor to replace the marrow in an ailing individual. Proteins on the surface of bone marrow cells must be identical or very closely matched between a donor and the recipient.

**BONE MARROW.** A spongy tissue located in the hollow centers of certain bones, such as the skull and hip bones. Bone marrow is the site of blood cell generation.

**BONE REMODELING.** The process of breaking down old bone and building up new bone.

**BONE SCLEROSIS.** Increased bone density and hardness.

**BOTULINUM TOXIN.** A class of neurotoxins that are produced by a bacteria and that cause paralysis and weakness of muscles.

**BOWMAN'S LAYER.** Transparent sheet of tissue directly below the basement membrane.

**BOY IN THE BUBBLE.** A description for SCID since these children need to be isolated from exposure to germs, until they are treated by bone marrow transplantation or other therapy.

**BRACHYCEPHALY.** An abnormal thickening and widening of the skull.

**BRACHYDACTYLY.** Abnormal shortness of the fingers and toes.

**BRACHYMELIA.** A general medical term used to describe short limbs.

**BRADYKINESIA.** Extremely slow movement.

**BRAILLE.** An alphabet represented by patterns of raised dots which may be felt with the fingertips. It is the main method of reading used by the blind today.

**BRAIN VENTRICLES.** A set of four connected cavities that are located deep in the core of the brain. Cerebrospinal fluid is made by cells lining the walls of the first two ventricles, then flows through the third, then fourth ventricle before flowing out of the brain. The fluid-filled cavities provide mechanical cushion for the brain, and the CSF provides nutrients to, and carries metabolic wastes away from, the cells of the brain.

**BRANCHED-CHAIN.** An open chain of atoms having one or more side chains.

**BRANCHING ENZYME.** Enzyme responsible for building the branched structure of glycogen stores.

**BREAST BIOPSY.** Small sample of tissue taken from the breast and studied, to diagnose and determine the exact type of breast cancer.

**BREAST SELF–EXAM (BSE).** Examination by an individual of their own breasts.

**BREECH DELIVERY.** Birth of an infant feet or buttocks first.

**BROAD LIGAMENT.** The ligament connecting the ovaries to the uterus.

**BRONCHI.** Branching tube–like structures that carry air in and out of the lungs; walls of bronchi contain circular muscles that can constrict (tighten up to make airways narrower) or dilate (relax to make airways wider); bronchi divide into smaller bronchioles within the lung tissue.

**BRONCHIECTASIS.** An abnormal condition of the bronchial tree, characterized by irreversible widening and destruction of the bronchial walls of the lungs.

**BRUCH'S MEMBRANE.** A membrane in the eye between the choroid membrane and the retina.

**BRUTON TYROSINE KINASE (BTK).** An enzyme vital for the maturation of B cells.

**BULBAR MUSCLES.** Muscles that control chewing, swallowing, and speaking.

**BUNDLES OF PROBST.** Abnormally developed nerve fibers in the brain.

**BUNION.** A bulge on the first joint of the big toe, caused by the swelling of a fluid sac under the skin.

**BUPHTHALMOS.** A characteristic enlargement of one or both eyes associated with infantile glaucoma.

# C

**C1 INHIBITOR.** Abbreviated C1-INH, this protein is responsible for preventing the action of the C1 complement molecules in the body. It is this protein that is either deficient or malformed in HANE.

**CA–125 (CARBOHYDRATE ANTIGEN 125).** A protein that is sometimes high when ovarian cancer is present. A blood sample can determine the level of CA–125 present.

**CA-125 (CARBOHYDRATE ANTIGEN 125).** A protein that is sometimes high when ovarian cancer is present. A blood sample can determine the level of CA-125 present.

**CAT (CT) SCAN.** Computerized (axial) tomography. A special x ray technique used to examine various tissues, particularly the brain, in great detail.

**CDKN2A OR P16.** Gene, when altered, known to cause Familial Atypical Multiple Mole Melanoma (FAMMM) syndrome and possibly increased pancreatic cancer risk.

**CFTR.** Cystic fibrosis transmembrane conductance regulator. The protein responsible for regulating chloride movement across cells in some tissues. When a person has two defective copies of the CFTR gene, cystic fibrosis is the result.

**CGG OR CGG SEQUENCE.** Shorthand for the DNA sequence: cytosine-guanine-guanine. Cytosine and guanine are two of the four molecules, otherwise called nucleic acids, that make up DNA.

**COMT INHIBITORS.** Drugs that block catechol-O-methyltransferase, an enzyme that breaks down dopamine. COMT inhibitors include entacapone and tolcapone.

**CAESAREAN SECTION.** Surgical method to deliver a baby that requires making an incision in the mother's abdomen to remove the infant.

**CAFÉ-AU-LAIT SPOTS.** Birthmarks that may appear anywhere on the skin; named after the French coffee drink because of the light-brown color of the marks.

**CALCIFICATION.** The process by which tissue becomes hardened by the depositing of calcium in the tissue.

**CALCITRIOL.** A substance that assists in bone growth by helping to maintain calcium and phosphate levels in the blood. Vitamin D is converted into this substance by the body.

**CALCIUM.** One of the elements that make up the hydroxyapatite crystals found in bone.

**CAMPTODACTYLY.** A condition characterized by the bending of one or more fingers.

**CANCER CELLS.** Have characteristics that distinguish them from normal cells and non-cancerous cells; they are threatening, harmful, and resistant to treatment

**CANCER.** A disease caused by uncontrolled growth of the body's cells.

**CAPILLARY.** Very narrow tube that carries liquid like blood or lymphatic fluid.

**CARBOHYDRATE.** Any of various natural compounds of carbon, hydrogen, and oxygen (as in sugars and starches) that are burned by the body for energy.

**CARCINOGEN.** Any substance capable of causing cancer by mutating the cell's DNA.

**CARCINOMA.** Any cancer that arises in the epithelium, the tissue that lines the external and internal organs of the body.

**CARDIAC CONDUCTION DEFECT.** Abnormality of the electrical system of the heart that regulates the heartbeat.

**CARDIAC MUSCLE.** The muscle of the heart.

**CARDIAC RHABDOMYOMA.** Benign (non-cancerous) tumor of the heart muscle.

**CARDINAL SYMPTOMS.** A group of symptoms that define a disorder or disease.

**CARDIOLIPIN.** A type of lipid (fatty substance) found almost exclusively in the inner mitochondrial membrane where it is essential for the optimal function of numerous enzymes that are involved in mitochondrial energy metabolism.

**CARDIOMYOPATHY.** A thickening of the heart muscle.

**CARNITINE.** An amino acid necessary for metabolism of the long-chain fatty acid portion of lipids. Also called vitamin B7.

**CARPAL TUNNEL SYNDROME.** A condition in which the median nerve is compressed at the wrist, leading to numbness and pain in the hand.

**CARRIER TESTING.** Testing performed to determine if someone possesses one changed copy and one unchanged copy of a particular gene.

**CARRIER.** An individual who possesses an unexpressed abnormal gene of a recessive genetic disorder.

**CARTILAGE OLIGOMERIC MATRIX PROTEIN GENE.** A gene that codes for a specific protein involved in the formation of cartilage.

**CARTILAGE.** A tough elastic tissue that is a building block for bone.

**CASEIN HYDROLYSATE.** A preparation made from the milk protein casein, which is hydrolyzed to break it down into its constituent amino acids. Amino acids are the building blocks of proteins.

**CATABOLISM.** The energy-releasing process of breaking down complex chemical compounds into simpler ones in the body.

**CATAGEN.** The breakdown phase of the hair growth cycle.

**CATALYST.** A substance that changes the rate of a chemical reaction, but is not physically changed by the process.

**CATALYZE.** Facilitate. A catalyst lowers the amount of energy required for a specific chemical reaction to occur. Catalysts are not used up in the chemical reactions they facilitate.

**CATAPLEXY.** A symptom of narcolepsy in which there is a sudden episode of muscle weakness triggered by emotions. The muscle weakness may cause the person's knees to buckle, or the head to drop. In severe cases, the patient may become paralyzed for a few seconds to minutes.

**CATARACT.** A clouding of the eye lens or its surrounding membrane that obstructs the passage of light resulting in blurry vision. Surgery may be performed to remove the cataract.

**CATATONIC BEHAVIOR.** Behavior characterized by muscular tightness or rigidity and lack of response to the environment.

**CATECHOLAMINES.** Biologically active compounds involved in the regulation of the nervous and cardiovascular systems, rate of metabolism, body temperature, and smooth muscle.

**CATHETER.** A narrow, flexible tube used to create a pathway for introducing drugs, nutrients, fluids, or blood products into the body and/or for removing fluid or other substances from the body.

**CATHETERIZATION.** The process of inserting a hollow tube into a body cavity or blood vessel.

**CATIONIC TRYPSINOGEN GENE.** Gene known to cause hereditary pancreatitis when significantly altered.

**CAUDAL.** Pertaining to the tail (bone).

**CAUTERIZATION.** Process of burning tissue either with a laser or electric needle to stop bleeding or destroy damaged tissue.

**CECUM.** The first part of the large bowel.

**CELL ADHESION MOLECULE.** Any one of several thousand proteins that together control the cell-to-cell communication that must take place in order for cells to migrate to their proper places, develop into the proper types of cells, and make the appropriate connections with other cells.

**CELL.** The smallest living units of the body which group together to form tissues and help the body perform specific functions.

**CELLULAR IMMUNITY.** A type of acquired immunity mediated by killer T-cells; important in fighting "hidden" infections, such as those caused by cellular parasites and some viruses.

**CEMENTOMA.** A type of non-cancerous tumor that contains a bony substance known as cementum.

**CENTRAL NERVOUS SYSTEM.** In humans, the central nervous system is composed of the brain, the cranial nerves and the spinal cord. It is responsible for the coordination and control of all body activities.

**CENTRAL POLYDACTYLY.** Occurring between the thumb and little finger or between the big toe and the little toe.

**CENTRAL VISION.** The ability to see objects located directly in front of the eye; necessary for reading and other activities that require people to focus on objects directly in front of them.

**CENTROMERE.** The centromere is the constricted region of a chromosome. It performs certain functions during cell division.

**CEREBELLAR ATAXIA.** Unsteadiness and lack of coordination caused by a progressive degeneration of the part of the brain known as the cerebellum.

**CEREBELLAR.** Involving the part of the brain (cerebellum) that controls walking, balance, and coordination.

**CEREBELLUM.** A portion of the brain consisting of two cerebellar hemispheres connected by a narrow vermis. The cerebellum is involved in control of skeletal muscles and plays an important role in the coordination of voluntary muscle movement. It interrelates with other areas of the brain to facilitate a variety of movements, including maintaining proper posture and balance, walking, running, and fine motor skills, such as writing, dressing, and eating.

**CEREBRAL CORTEX.** The outer surface of the cerebrum made up of gray matter and involved in higher thought processes.

**CEREBRAL PALSY.** Movement disability resulting from nonprogressive brain damage.

**CEREBRAL VENTRICLES.** Spaces in the brain that are located between portions of the brain and filled with cerebrospinal fluid.

**CEREBRAL WHITE MATTER MIGRATION LINES.** Pattern of defects found in the cerebral cortex of the brain probably caused by abnormal migration of neurons during brain formation.

**CEREBRO.** Related to the head or brain.

**CEREBROSIDES.** Fatty carbohydrates that occur in the brain and nervous system.

**CEREBROSPINAL FLUID.** Fluid that bathes and supports the brain and the spinal cord, protecting it from physical impact.

**CEREBRUM.** The largest section of the brain, which is responsible for such higher functions as speech, thought, vision, and memory.

**CEROID.** The byproduct of cell membrane breakdown.

**CERULOPLASMIN.** A copper-containing protein that is involved in iron metabolism.

**CERVICITIS.** Inflammation of the cervix.

**CERVICO–MEDULLARY JUNCTION.** The area where the brain and spine connect.

**CHAPERONIN.** A molecule that captures and refolds misshapen proteins that might interfere with normal cellular functions; also called a protein cage.

**CHEMICAL METHYL GROUP.** One carbon and three hydrogen molecules that can be attached as a signal to DNA in the regulation of gene expression.

**CHEMOTHERAPY.** Treatment of cancer with synthetic drugs that destroy the tumor either by inhibiting the growth of the cancerous cells or by killing the cancer cells.

**CHIARI II ANOMALY.** A structural abnormality of the lower portion of the brain (cerebellum and brainstem) associated with spina bifida; the lower structures of the brain are crowded and may be forced into the foramen magnum, the opening through which the brain and spinal cord are connected.

**CHOANAL ATRESIA.** A bony or membranous blockage of the passageway between the nose and pharynx at birth.

**CHOLESTEROL.** A fatty-like substance that is obtained from the diet and produced by the liver. Cells require cholesterol for their normal daily functions.

**CHOLINESTERASE.** Enzyme whose role is to break down released acetylcholine in the gap between nerve cells.

**CHONDROCYTE.** A specialized type of cell that secretes the material which surrounds the cells in cartilage.

**CHONDROSARCOMA.** A malignant tumor derived from cartilage cells.

**CHOREA.** Involuntary, rapid, jerky movements.

**CHOREOATHETOSIS.** Involuntary rapid, irregular, jerky movements or slow, writhing movements that flow into one another.

**CHORIOCAPILLARIS.** Capillary layer of the choroid.

**CHORION.** The outer membrane of the amniotic sac. Chorionic villi develop from its outer surface early in pregnancy. The villi establish a physical connection with the wall of the uterus and eventually develop into the placenta.

**CHORIONIC VILLUS BIOPSY.** A procedure used for prenatal diagnosis at 10-12 weeks gestation. Under ultrasound guidance a needle is inserted either through the mother's vagina or abdominal wall and a sample of cells is collected from around the early fetus. These cells are then tested for chromosome abnormalities or other genetic diseases.

**CHORIONIC VILLUS SAMPLING (CVS).** A procedure involving removal of a small placenta sample during pregnancy to obtain fetal chromosome results.

**CHORIONIC VILLUS.** Cells that are present in the placenta that can be used for genetic analysis.

**CHOROID PLEXUS.** Specialized cells located in the ventricles of the brain that produce cerebrospinal fluid.

**CHOROID.** A vascular membrane that covers the back of the eye between the retina and the sclera and serves to nourish the retina and absorb scattered light.

**CHROMATID.** Each of the two strands formed by replication of a chromosome. Chromatids are held together by the centromere until the centromere divides and separates the two chromatids into a single chromosome.

**CHROMOSOMAL ANEUPLODIES.** A condition in which the chromosomal number is either increased or decreased.

**CHROMOSOMAL DELETION.** Loss of a segment of DNA from a chromosome.

**CHROMOSOME DELETION.** A missing sequence of DNA or part of a chromosome.

**CHROMOSOME INVERSION.** Rearrangement of a chromosome in which a section of a chromosome breaks off and rejoins the chromosome upside down.

**CHROMOSOME TRANSLOCATION.** The exchange of genetic material between chromosomes, which can lead to extra or missing genetic material.

**CHROMOSOME.** A microscopic thread-like structure found within each cell of the body and consists of a complex of proteins and DNA. Humans have 46 chromosomes arranged into 23 pairs. Changes in either the total number of chromosomes or their shape and size (structure) may lead to physical or mental abnormalities.

**CHROMOSOMES.** The gene-containing structures found in all of the body's cells; in each normal cell, there are 46 chromosomes that come in 23 pairs.

**CHRONIC ATROPHIC GASTRITIS.** Irritation and break down of the stomach wall over a period of time.

**CHYLOMICRON.** A type of lipoprotein made in the small intestine and used for transporting fats to other tissues in the body. MTP is necessary for the production of chylomicrons.

**CILIARY BODY.** A structure within the eye that produces aqueous humor.

**CIRCUMCISION.** The surgical removal of the foreskin of the penis.

**CIRCUMFERENCE.** The length around a circle.

**CIRRHOSIS.** A chronic degenerative disease of the liver, in which normal cells are replaced by fibrous tissue. Cirrhosis is a major risk factor for the later development of liver cancer.

**CLASS I MHC.** Includes HLA-A, HLA-B, and HLA-C. Important in cellular immunity.

**CLASS II MHC.** HLA-DP, HLA-DQ, and HLA-DR. Important in humoral immunity.

**CLASS III MHC.** Includes the complement system.

**CLASSIC CREUTZFELDT-JAKOB DISEASE.** A rare, progressive neurological disease that is believed to be transmitted via an abnormal protein called a prion.

**CLAUDICATION.** Pain in the lower legs after exercise caused by insufficient blood supply.

**CLAVICLE.** Also called the collarbone. Bone that articulates with the shoulder and the breast bone.

**CLEFT LIP.** A separation of the upper lip that is present from birth but originates early in fetal development. A cleft lip may appear on one side (unilateral) or both sides (bilateral) and is occasionally accompanied by a cleft palate. Surgery is needed to completely repair cleft lip.

**CLEFT PALATE.** A congenital malformation in which there is an abnormal opening in the roof of the mouth that allows the nasal passages and the mouth to be improperly connected.

**CLEFT.** An elongated opening or slit in an organ.

**CLINICAL BREAST EXAM (CBE).** Examination of the breasts, performed by a physician or nurse.

**CLINODACTYLY.** An abnormal inward curving of the fingers or toes.

**CLITORIS.** A small mass of erectile tissue in the female genitalia.

**CLONUS.** A sustained series of involuntary rhythmic jerks following quick stretch of a muscle.

**CLOVERLEAF SKULL.** An abnormal, or cloverleaf, appearance to the skull caused by premature fusion of the bones in the skull of an infant.

**CLUBFOOT.** Abnormal permanent bending of the ankle and foot. Also called *talipes equinovarus*.

**CO-DOMINANT.** Describes the state when two alleles of the same gene are both expressed when inherited together.

**CO-ENZYME.** A small molecule such as a vitamin that works together with an enzyme to direct a biochemical reaction within the body.

**COAGULATION.** The solidification or change from a fluid state to a semisolid mass; blood coagulation helps to close open wounds.

**COAGULOPATHY.** A disorder in which blood is either too slow or too quick to coagulate (clot).

**COBB ANGLE.** A measure of the curvature of scoliosis, determined by measurements made on x rays.

**COCHLEA.** A bony structure shaped like a snail shell located in the inner ear. It is responsible for changing sound waves from the environment into electrical messages that the brain can understand, so people can hear.

**COCHLEAR IMPLANTATION.** A surgical procedure in which a small electronic device is placed under the skin behind the ear and is attached to a wire that stimulates the inner ear, allowing people who have hearing loss to hear useful sounds.

**COFACTOR.** A substance that is required by an enzyme to perform its function.

**COGNITION.** The mental activities associated with thinking, learning, and memory.

**COGNITIVE/BEHAVIORAL THERAPIES.** Psychological counseling that focuses on changing the behavior of the patient.

**COLCHICINE.** A compound that blocks the assembly of microtubules, which are protein fibers necessary for cell division and some kinds of cell movements, including neutrophil migration. Side effects may include diarrhea, abdominal bloating, and gas.

**COLECTOMY.** Surgical removal of the colon.

**COLITIS.** Inflammation of the colon.

**COLLAGEN.** The main supportive protein of cartilage, connective tissue, tendon, skin, and bone.

**COLOBOMA OF THE IRIS.** A birth defect leading to missing structures within the eye.

**COLOBOMA.** A birth defect in which part of the eye does not form completely and appears to be cleft or notched.

**COLON.** The large intestine.

**COLONOSCOPY.** Procedure for viewing the large intestine (colon) by inserting an illuminated tube into the rectum and guiding it up the large intestine.

**COLORECTAL.** Of the colon and/or rectum.

**COLOSTOMY.** The creation of an artificial opening into the colon through the skin for the purpose of removing bodily waste. Colostomies are usually required because key portions of the intestine have been removed.

**COMPLEMENT SYSTEM.** Class III MHC (major histocompatobility complex) proteins capable of destroying invading organisms directly via natural immunity, as well as indirectly through an interaction with other components of the immune system.

**COMPLETE SITUS INVERSUS.** A laterality defect resulting in a mirror image of the normal organ formation with heart, spleen, and stomach on the right, and the liver and gallbladder on the left side.

**COMPOUND HETEROZYGOTE.** Having two different mutated versions of a gene.

**COMPUTED TOMOGRAPHY (CT) SCAN; 3D CT SCAN.** A diagnostic imaging procedure in which x-ray and computer technology are used to generate slices or cross-sectional images of the body; 3D CT scan produces three-dimensional images.

**COMPUTED TOMOGRAPHY (CT) SCAN.** An imaging procedure that produces a three-dimensional picture of organs or structures inside the body, such as the brain.

**COMPUTERIZED AXIAL TOMOGRAPHY (CAT) SCAN.** A noninvasive technique to show computerized images of a structure in the body.

**COMPUTERIZED TOMOGRAPHY (CT).** A technique that uses a beam of radiation and a computerized analysis to produce an image of a body structure, often the brain.

**CONCEPTUS.** The products of conception, or the union of a sperm and egg cell at fertilization.

**CONDUCTIVE HEARING LOSS.** Hearing loss that is the result of a dysfunction of the parts of the ear responsible for collecting sound. In this type of hearing loss, the auditory nerve is generally not damaged.

**CONES.** Receptor cells that allow the perception of colors.

**CONFETTI SKIN LESIONS.** Numerous light or white spots seen on the skin that resemble confetti.

**CONGENITAL ANOMALY.** An abnormality that is present at birth.

**CONGENITAL CATARACT.** Clouding of the lens in the eye that is present at birth.

**CONGENITAL DISORDER.** Refers to a disorder which is present at birth.

**CONGENITAL HEART DISEASE.** Structural abnormality of the heart at birth. Examples include a ventricular septal defect and atrial septal defect.

**CONGENITAL HYPOPLASTIC ANEMIA (CHA).** A significant reduction in the number of red blood cells present at birth, usually referring to deficient production of these cells in the bone marrow. Also sometimes called congenital aplastic anemia.

**CONGENITAL.** Refers to a disorder which is present at birth.

**CONNECTIVE TISSUE.** A group of tissues responsible for support throughout the body; includes cartilage, bone, fat, tissue underlying skin, and tissues that support organs, blood vessels, and nerves throughout the body.

**CONOTRUNCAL HEART ABNORMALITY.** Congenital heart defects particularly involving the ventricular (lower chambers) outflow tracts of the heart includes subarterial ventricular septal defect, pulmonic valve atresia and stenosis, tetralogy of Fallot and truncus arteriosus.

**CONSANGUINEOUS.** Sharing a common bloodline or ancestor.

**CONSANGUINITY.** A mating between two people who are related to one another by blood.

**CONTIGUOUS GENE SYNDROME.** A genetic syndrome caused by the deletion of two or more genes located next to each other.

**CONTINENCE.** Normal function of the urinary bladder and urethra, allowing fluid flow during urination and completely stopping flow at other times.

**CONTINGUOUS GENE SYNDROME.** Conditions that occur as a result of microdeletions or microduplications involving several neighboring genes.

**CONTRACTURE.** A tightening of muscles that prevents normal movement of the associated limb or other body part.

**CONVULSION.** Involuntary contractions of body muscles that accompany a seizure episode.

**COPROLALIA.** The involuntary expression of obscene words or phrases.

**COPROPRAXIA.** The involuntary display of unacceptable/obscene gestures.

**CORDOCENTESIS.** A prenatal diagnostic test, usually done between 16-30 weeks of gestation. Using ultrasound guidance, a thin needle is introduced through the abdomen into the amniotic sac. A blood sample is taken directly from the umbilical cord. Tests can then be done on the blood sample.

**CORNEA.** The transparent structure of the eye over the lens that is continous with the sclera in forming the outermost, protective, layer of the eye.

**CORNEAL TRANSPLANT.** Removal of impaired and diseased cornea and replacement with corneal tissue from a recently deceased person.

**CORNEAL.** Pertaining to the cornea of the eye, which is the clear covering that protects the front of the eyeball.

**CORONAL SUTURE.** A fissure between two bony plates in the skull that runs across the top of the head from one ear to the other ear

**CORPUS CALLOSUM.** A band of nerve fibers that connects the right and left hemispheres of the brain.

**CORTICAL TUBER.** Round (nodular) growth found in the cortex of the brain.

**CORTICOSPINAL TRACT.** A bundle of long nerve fibers that runs from the motor control region of the cerebral cortex to the spinal cord, where it connects to nerves that control movement in the legs.

**CORTICOSTEROIDS.** Anti-inflammatory medications. Related to cortisol, a naturally produced hormone that controls many body functions.

COXA VARA. A deformed hip joint in which the neck of the femur is bent downward.

CRANIAL SUTURE. Any one of the seven fibrous joints between the bones of the skull.

CRANIOFACIAL. Relating to or involving both the head and the face.

CRANIOPAGUS. Conjoined twins with separate bodies and one shared head.

CRANIOPHARYNGIOMA. A tumor near the pituitary gland in the craniopharyngeal canal that often results in intracranial pressure.

CRANIOSYNOSTOSIS. Premature, delayed, or otherwise abnormal closure of the sutures of the skull.

CRANIUM. The skeleton of the head, which include all of the bones of the head except the mandible.

CREATINE KINASE (CK). An enzyme that is normally found in the skeletal or voluntary muscle and cardiac muscle; very high levels in the blood usually indicate breakdown of either heart or voluntary muscle.

CREATININE. A normal component of blood kept in low levels in urine by functioning kidneys.

CREUTZFELDT-JAKOB DISEASE. A degenerative disease of the central nervous system caused by a prion, or "slow virus."

CRYPTOORCHIDISM. Failure of descent of the testis from the abdominal cavity into the scrotum.

CRYPTOPHTHALMOS. An abnormal formation of the eye in which the eyelid, or overlaying skin of the eye, is fused shut. Literally, "hidden eye."

CRYPTORCHIDISM. A condition in which one or both testes fail to descend normally.

CURETTAGE. A surgical scraping or cleaning.

CUTANEOUS SYNDACTYLY. Fusion of the soft tissue between fingers or toes resulting in a webbed appearance.

CUTANEOUS. Of, pertaining to, or affecting the skin.

CYANOSIS. A bluish discoloration of the skin and mucous membranes.

CYANOSIS. The bluish color of the skin that occurs when there is very low oxygen in the blood that is being transported throughout the body.

CYCLOOXYGENASE-2 (COX-2) INHIBITORS. Anti-inflammatory drugs that work by blocking the COX-2 enzyme, which plays a role in the inflammatory process, but do not block the COX-1 enzyme, which helps protect the digestive tract.

CYDROCEPHALY. Excessive accumulation of cerebral spinal fluid in the brain ventricles.

CYST. An abnormal sac or closed cavity filled with liquid or semisolid matter.

CYSTIC FIBROSIS. A respiratory disease characterized by chronic lung disease, pancreatic insufficiency and an average age of survival of 20 years. Cystic fibrosis is caused by mutations in a gene on chromosome 7 that encodes a transmembrane receptor.

CYSTIC HYGROMA. Birth defect that appears as a soft bulging under the skin at the neck; the bulging is actually abnormal growths of sac–like structures filled with lymphatic fluid.

CYSTINE. A sulfur-containing amino acid, sometimes found as crystals in the kidneys or urine, that forms when proteins are broken down by digestion.

CYTOKINE. A protein associated with inflammation that, at high levels, may be toxic to nerve cells in the developing brain.

CYTOPLASM. The substance within a cell including the organelles and the fluid surrounding the nucleus.

CYTOSKELETON. The network of proteins underlying and maintaining the integrity of the red blood cell membrane.

# D

DALTON. Indicates a unit of mass equal to one-twelfth the mass of a carbon-12 atom (abbreviated Da).

DANDY-WALKER MALFORMATION. A congenital anomaly of the brain that causes a specific type of hydrocephalus.

DE NOVO. Latin term for new.

DE NOVO MUTATION. Genetic mutations that are seen for the first time in the affected person, not inherited from the parents.

DEBRANCHING ENZYME. Enzyme responsible for breaking down the branched structure of glycogen stores to release glucose into the bloodstream.

DECIDUOUS TEETH. The first set of teeth or "baby teeth".

DECREASED PENETRANCE. Individuals who inherit a changed disease gene, but do not develop symptoms.

**DEFORMATION.** An abnormal form or position of a part of the body caused by extrinsic pressure or mechanical forces.

**DEGENERATIVE DISC DISEASE.** Narrowing of the disc space between the spinal bones (vertebrae).

**DEGENERATIVE DISORDER.** A disorder by which the body or a part of the body gradually loses its ability to function.

**DEGRADATION.** Loss or diminishing.

**DEHYDRATION.** An extreme loss of water in the body which, if untreated, can lead to brain damage and death.

**DELAYED BONE AGE.** An abnormal condition in which the apparent age of the bones, as seen in x rays, is less than the chronological age of the patient.

**DELETION.** The absence of genetic material that is normally found in a chromosome. Often, the genetic material is missing due to an error in replication of an egg or sperm cell.

**DELIRIUM.** A disturbance of consciousness marked by confusion, difficulty paying attention, delusions, hallucinations, or restlessness. It can be distinguished from dementia by its relatively sudden onset and variation in the severity of the symptoms.

**DELUSION.** A fixed, false belief that is resistant to reason or factual disproof.

**DEMENTIA.** A condition of deteriorated mental ability characterized by a marked decline of intellect and often by emotional apathy.

**DENTAL PITS.** Small, shallow holes or crevices in the tooth enamel.

**DENTIN.** A hard, calcareous material that covers the tooth root and, in turn, is covered by cementum and enamel.

**DEOXYRIBONUCLEIC ACID (DNA).** The genetic material in cells that holds the inherited instructions for growth, development, and cellular functioning.

**DEPIGMENTATION.** Loss of pigment or skin color.

**DEPOLARIZATION.** The dissipation of an electrical charge through a membrane.

**DEPOT DOSAGE.** A form of medication that can be stored in the patient's body tissues for several days or weeks, thus minimizing the risk of the patient forgetting daily doses.

**DEPRIVATIONAL DWARFISM.** A condition where emotional disturbances are associated with growth failure and abnormalities of pituitary function.

**DERMABRASION.** Scraping or sanding the epidermal layer of the skin to remove scars and other marks or wrinkles.

**DERMATOLOGIC.** Pertaining to the field of dermatology, the science of the skin and diseases that affect the skin.

**DERMATOLOGIST.** A physician that specializes in disorders of the skin.

**DERMATOSPARAXIS.** Skin fragility caused by abnormal collagen.

**DERMIS.** The layer of skin beneath the epidermis.

**DESCEMET'S MEMBRANE.** Sheet of tissue that lies under the stroma and protects against infection and injuries.

**DESFEROXAMINE.** The primary drug used in iron chelation therapy. It aids in counteracting the life-threatening buildup of iron in the body associated with long-term blood transfusions.

**DESMOID TUMOR.** Benign, firm mass of scar-like connective tissue.

**DESMOPRESSIN (DDAVP).** A drug used in the treatment of von Willebrand's disease.

**DEVELOPMENT.** The process whereby undifferentiated embryonic cells replicate and differentiate into limbs, organ systems, and other body components of the fetus.

**DEVELOPMENTAL DELAY.** When children do not reach certain milestones at appropriate ages. For example, a child should be able to speak by the time he or she is five years old.

**DEVELOPMENTAL MILESTONES.** Infants and toddlers develop skills at certain ages. For example, by nine months, a child should be able to grasp and toss a bottle.

**DEXTROCARDIA.** Defect in which the position of the heart is the mirror image of its normal position.

**DIABETES MELLITUS.** The clinical name for common diabetes. It is a chronic disease characterized by inadequate production or use of insulin.

**DIABETES.** An inability to control the levels of sugar in the blood due to an abnormality in the production of, or response to, the hormone insulin.

**DIAGNOSTIC TESTING.** Testing performed to determine if someone is affected with a particular disease.

**DIALYSIS.** Process by which special equipment purifies the blood of a patient whose kidneys have failed.

**DIAPHRAGMATIC HERNIA.** A defect that occurs when the diaphragm does not close properly, and the intestines are able to be herniated through the diaphragm into the chest cavity.

**DIAPHYSIS.** Primary region of ossification found in the shaft of the long bones.

**DIARRHEA.** Loose, watery stool.

**DIASTOLIC BLOOD PRESSURE.** Blood pressure when the heart is resting between beats.

**DICEPHALUS.** Conjoined twins who share one body but have two separate heads and necks.

**DIFFERENTIATE.** Specialized development to perform a particular function.

**DIGESTIVE ENZYME.** Proteins secreted by the pancreas that enter the small intestine and break down food so it can be absorbed by the body.

**DIGIT.** A finger or a toe.

**DIHYDROTESTOSTERONE (DHT).** A male sex hormone formed from testosterone by the enzyme 5-alpha-reductase. DHT causes hair follicles to shut down, shortening the growth phase of the hair growth cycle and leading to miniaturization.

**DILATED CARDIOMYOPATHY.** A diseased and weakened heart muscle that is unable to pump blood efficiently.

**DIOPTER (D).** A unit of measure for describing refractive power.

**DIPLEGIA.** Paralysis affecting like parts on both sides of the body, such as both arms or both legs.

**DIPLOID.** Two sets of chromosomes; in humans, this is 46 chromosomes.

**DISRUPTION.** A type of anomaly formation in which a breakdown or inhibition of normal tissue development occurs.

**DISTAL ARTHROGRYPOSIS.** A disorder characterized by contractions of the muscles in the hands.

**DISTAL MUSCLES.** Muscles that are furthest away from the center of the body.

**DISTAL MUSCULAR DYSTROPHY (DD).** A form of muscular dystrophy that usually begins in middle age or later, causing weakness in the muscles of the feet and hands.

**DISTAL.** Away from the point of origin.

**DIURETICS.** Medications that increase the excretion of urine.

**DIVERGENT STRABISMUS.** Eyes that point in different directions.

**DIVERTICULAE.** Sacs or pouches in the walls of a canal or organ. They do not normally occur, but may be acquired or present from birth. Plural form of diverticula.

**DIZYGOTIC.** From two zygotes, as in non-identical, or fraternal twins. The zygote is the first cell formed by the union of sperm and egg.

**DNA MUTATION ANALYSIS.** A direct approach to the detection of a specific genetic mutation or mutations using one or more laboratory techniques.

**DNA REPEATS.** A three letter section of DNA, called a triplet, which is normally repeated several times in a row. Too many repeats often cause the gene to not function properly, resulting in disease.

**DNA TESTING.** Analysis of DNA (the genetic component of cells) in order to determine changes in genes that may indicate a specific disorder.

**DNA.** Deoxyribonucleic acid, inheritable material that constitutes the building blocks of life.

**DOLICOCEPHALY.** Elongated and narrow skull shape due to premature closure of the sagittal suture that runs from the forehead to the back of the skull.

**DOMINANT INHERITANCE.** A type of genetic inheritance pattern that results in one form of a gene being dominant over other forms. Therefore, the dominant allele can express itself and cause disease, even if only one copy is present.

**DOMINANT PROGRESSIVE HEARING LOSS.** The main type of nonsyndromic progressive sensorineural hearing loss seen in humans.

**DOMINANT TRAIT.** A genetic trait where one copy of the gene is sufficient to yield an outward display of the trait; dominant genes mask the presence of recessive genes; dominant traits can be inherited from a single parent.

**DOMINANT.** A genetic trait that is expressed when only one copy of the gene is present.

**DOPAMINE RECEPTOR ANTAGONISTS (DAS).** The older class of antipsychotic medications, also called neuroleptics, which primarily block the site on nerve cells that normally receive the brain chemical dopamine.

**DOPAMINE.** A neurochemical made in the brain that is involved in many brain activities, including movement and emotion.

**DORSAL RHIZOTOMY.** A surgical procedure that cuts nerve roots to reduce spasticity in affected muscles.

**DORSAL ROOT GANGLIA.** The subset of neuronal cells controlling impulses in and out of the brain.

**DOWN SYNDROME.** Chromosomal disorder caused by the presence of all or part of an extra 21st chromosome.

**DOWNSHOOT.** Downward movement of the eye.

**DRPLA.** Dentatorubral-pallidoluysian atrophy; also called Haw River syndrome and Natito-Oyanagi disease. DRPLA is a disorder of ataxia, choreoathetosis, and dementia in adults, and ataxia, myoclonus, epilepsy, and mental retardation in children.

**DRUSEN.** Fatty deposits that can accumulate underneath the retina and macula, and sometimes lead to age-related macular degeneration (AMD). Drusen formation can disrupt the photoreceptor cells, which causes central and color vision problems for people with dry AMD.

**DUCHENNE MUSCULAR DYSTROPHY (DMD).** The most severe form of muscular dystrophy, DMD usually affects young boys and causes progressive muscle weakness, usually beginning in the legs.

**DUCT.** Tube-like structure that carries secretions from glands.

**DUCTUS ARTERIOSUS.** The temporary channel or blood vessel between the aorta and pulmonary artery in the fetus.

**DUCTUS.** The blood vessel that joins the pulmonary artery and the aorta. When the ductus does not close at birth, it causes a type of congenital heart disease called patent ductus arteriosus.

**DUODENUM.** Portion of the small intestine nearest the stomach; the first of three parts of the small intestine.

**DUPLICATION.** Production of one or more copies of any piece of DNA, including a base pair, gene, or entire chromosome.

**DWARFISM.** Any condition that results in extremely shortened limbs.

**DYSARTHRIA.** Refers to a group of speech disorders caused by disturbances in the strength or coordination of the muscles of the speech mechanism as a result of damage to the brain or nerves.

**DYSKINESIA.** Impaired ability to make voluntary movements.

**DYSMORPHIC.** An abnormal body structure often associated with a genetic disorder.

**DYSOSTOSIS MULTIPLEX.** A variety of bone and skeletal malformations.

**DYSPHAGIA.** Swallowing problems.

**DYSPHORIA.** Feelings of anxiety, restlessness, and dissatisfaction.

**DYSPLASIA.** The abnormal growth or development of a tissue or organ.

**DYSPLASTIC.** The abnormal growth or development of a tissue or organ.

**DYSTHYMIA.** A psychological condition of chronic depression that is not disabling, but prevents the sufferer from functioning at his or her full capacity.

**DYSTONIA.** Painful involuntary muscle cramps or spasms.

**DYSTOPIA CANTHORUM.** A wide spacing between the inner corners of the eyes, with the eyes themselves having normal spacing. Also called telecanthus.

**DYSTROPHIN.** A protein that helps muscle tissue repair itself. Both Duchenne muscular dystrophy and Becker muscular dystrophy are caused by flaws in the gene that instructs the body how to make this protein.

**DYSTROPHY.** Progressive abnormal changes in a tissue or organ.

# E

**E-CADHERIN/CDH1.** A gene involved in cell-to-cell connection. Alterations in this gene have been found in several families with increased rates of gastric cancer.

**EAR TAGS.** Excess pieces of skin on the outside of the ear.

**ECHOCARDIOGRAM (ECHO).** A diagnostic procedure that uses sound waves to produces images of the heart.

**ECHOCARDIOGRAPH.** A record of the internal structures of the heart obtained from beams of ultrasonic waves directed through the wall of the chest.

**ECHOLALIA.** Involuntary echoing of the last word, phrase, or sentence that is spoken by someone else or by sounds in the environment.

**ECHOPRAXIA.** The imitation of the movement of another individual.

**ECTODERM.** The outermost of the three embryonic cell layers, which later gives rise to the skin, hair, teeth, and nails.

**ECTODERMAL DYSPLASIA.** A hereditary condition that results in the malformation of the skin, teeth, and hair. It is often associated with malfunctioning or absent sweat glands and/or tear ducts.

ECTOPIC. Tissue found in an abnormal location.

ECTRODACTYLY. A birth defect involving a split or cleft appearance of the hands and/or feet, also referred to as a "lobster–claw malformation."

ECZEMA. Inflammation of the skin with redness and other variable signs such as crusts, watery discharge, itching.

EDEMA. Extreme amount of watery fluid that causes swelling of the affected tissue.

EFFLUVIUM. The medical term for massive hair loss or shedding.

ELASTIC FIBER. Fibrous, stretchable connective tissue made primarily from proteins, elastin, collagen, and fibrillin.

ELASTIN. A protein that gives skin the ability to stretch and then return to normal.

ELECTROCARDIOGRAM (ECG, EKG). A test used to measure electrical impulses coming from the heart in order to gain information about its structure or function.

ELECTROCONVULSIVE THERAPY. A psychological treatment in which a series of controlled electrical impulses are delivered to the brain in order to induce a seizure within the brain.

ELECTRODESSICATION AND CURETTAGE. A procedure by which a papula is cut out of the skin (curettage) and bleeding controlled with an electric current (electrodessication).

ELECTROLYTE. A solution or a substance in a solution consisting of various chemicals that can carry electric charges. They exist in the blood as acids, bases, and salts, such as sodium, calcium, potassium, chlorine, and magnesium.

ELECTROMYOGRAPHY. A test that assess the activity of the muscles and the nerves that supply the muscles; one part of the test involves passing electrical current through the nerves and studying the response of the muscles to it, while the other part involves studying muscle activity by inserting a thin needle into it.

ELECTRORETINOGRAPHY (ERG). A diagnostic test that records electrical impulses created by the retina when light strikes it.

EMBOLIZATION THERAPY. Introduction of various substances into the circulation to plug up blood vessels in order to stop bleeding.

EMBRYOGENESIS. The formation and growth of the embryo.

EMOLLIENT. Petroleum or lanolin based skin lubricants.

EMPHYSEMA. A chronic lung disease that begins with breathlessness during exertion and progresses to shortness of breath at all times, caused by destructive changes in the lungs.

ENAMEL. The hard, white coating that covers teeth. Enamel is the hardest material in the body.

ENCAPSULATED. Referring to bacteria that have a thick capsule protecting their cell wall.

ENCEPHALITIS. Inflammation of the brain.

ENCEPHALOCELE. A congenital anomaly in which part of the brain is herniated through the skull.

ENCHONDROMAS. Benign cartilaginous tumors arising in the cavity of bone. They have the possibility of causing lytic destruction within the bone.

END-STAGE RENAL DISEASE. A condition that occurs when the kidneys are no longer able to sustain life.

ENDOCARDITIS. A dangerous infection of the heart valves caused by certain bacteria.

ENDOCRINE GLANDS. A system of ductless glands that regulate and secrete hormones directly into the bloodstream.

ENDOCRINE SYSTEM. A system of ductless glands that regulate and secrete hormones directly into the bloodstream.

ENDOLYMPH. The fluid in the inner ear.

ENDOMETRIUM. Lining of the uterus.

ENDOSCOPIC MUCOSAL RESECTION. Removal of the mucosa during endoscopy.

ENDOSCOPIC RETROGRADE CHOLANGIOPANCREATOGRAPHY (ER. A method of viewing the pancreas by inserting a thin tube down the throat into the pancreatic and bile ducts, injection of dye and performing x rays.

ENDOSCOPY. A slender, tubular optical instrument used as a viewing system for examining an inner part of the body and, with an attached instrument, for biopsy or surgery.

ENDOSTEAL. Relating to the endosteum, which is the lining of the medullary cavity.

ENDOTHELIAL CELLS. The cells lining the inner walls of the blood vessels.

ENDOTHELIUM. Extremely thin innermost layer of the cornea.

ENLARGED VESTIBULAR AQUEDUCT (EVA). An enlargement of a structure inside the inner ear called the vestibular aqueduct, which is a narrow canal that allows fluid to move within the inner ear. EVA is seen in approximately 10% of people who have sensorineural hearing loss.

ENTEROCOLITIS. Severe inflammation of the intestines that affects the intestinal lining, muscle, nerves and blood vessels.

ENTEROSCOPY. A procedure used to examine the small intestine.

ENTHESITIS. Inflammation at the place where the ligaments insert into the bone.

ENTHESOPATHY. Disorder of the ligament attachment to the bone.

ENTRAPMENT. Describes the narrowing of the canals and tunnels through which the nerves travel.

ENZYMATIC REPLACEMENT THERAPY. A treatment method used to replace missing enzymes. It is possible to synthesize enzymes and then inject them intravenously into patients.

ENZYME EFFICIENCY. The rate at which an enzyme can perform the chemical transformation that it is expected to accomplish. This is also called turnover rate. Individuals affected with type A PCD produce an enzyme that is much slower than the normal pyruvate carboxylase enzyme.

ENZYME REPLACEMENT THERAPY (ERT). Class of medications that seek to provide people with sufficient quantities of an important enzyme that they cannot fabricate on their own.

ENZYME. A protein that catalyzes a biochemical reaction or change without changing its own structure or function.

EPENDYMOMA. Tumor of the central nervous system derived from cells that line the central canal of the spinal cord and the ventricles of the brain.

EPI-LASIK. A surgical procedure that uses a blunt, plastic oscillating blade called an epithelial separator to cut a flap in the cornea.

EPIBULBAR DERMOIDS. Cysts on the eyeball.

EPICANTHAL FOLD. A wrinkle in the skin, extending from the nose up to the eyebrow, and sometimes associated with genetic anomalies.

EPIDERMIS. The outermost layer of the skin.

EPIDERMOID CYST. Benign, cystic tumor derived from epithelial cells.

EPIDIDYMIS. Coiled tubules that are the site of sperm storage and maturation for motility and fertility. The epididymis connects the testis to the vas deferens.

EPIGENETIC. Implying a modification outside of actual mutation of the DNA sequence, such as the addition of a methyl group.

EPILEPSY. Disorders associated with the disturbed electrical discharges in the central nervous system that cause convulsions.

EPIPHYSES. Areas at the tip of the long bones that allow them to grow.

EPIPHYSIS. The end of long bones, usually terminating in a joint.

EPITHELIAL CELLS. The layer of cells that cover the open surfaces of the body such as the skin and mucous membranes.

EPITHELIUM. The layer of cells that cover the open surfaces of the body such as the skin and mucous membranes.

ERYTHEMA NODOSUM LEPROSUM. A complication of leprosy characterized by development of painful small swellings due to inflammation of a blood or lymph vessel. It is often accompanied by inflammation of a nerve or nerves, causing decreased function of the affected area.

ERYTHEMA. Redness of the skin due to dilatation of capillaries.

ERYTHROPOIESIS. The process through which new red blood cells are created; it begins in the bone marrow.

ERYTHROPOIETIC. Referring to the creation of new red blood cells.

ESCHARS. Painful patches of dead, blackened tissue.

ESOPHAGUS. The part of the digestive tract which connects the mouth and stomach; the food pipe.

ESOTROPIA. Form of strabismus in which one or both eyes turns inward.

ESTROGEN. A female sex hormone.

ETIOLOGY. The cause of a disease, syndrome, or anomaly.

EVOKED RESPONSE TESTS. Tests that measure the speed of brain connections.

EXCISION. Surgical removal.

EXOCRINE PANCREAS. The secreting part of the pancreas.

EXOMPHALOS. An umbilical protrusion or hernia.

EXON. The expressed portion of a gene. The exons of genes are those portions that actually chemically code for the protein or polypeptide that the gene is responsible for producing.

EXOSTOSE. An abnormal growth (benign tumor) on a bone.

EXOTROPIA. Form of strabismus where the eyes are deviated outward.

EXPANSION. A genetic abnormality caused by a sequence of nucleotides that is repeated too many times in a section of a gene.

EXTERNAL MEATUS. The external opening through which urine and seminal fluid (in males only) leave the body.

EXTRAOCULAR MUSCLE FIBROSIS. Abnormalities in the muscles that control eye movement.

EXTRAPYRAMIDAL SYMPTOMS (EPS). A group of side effects associated with antipsychotic medications, including parkinsonism, akathisia, dystonia, and tardive dyskinesia.

EXTRAPYRAMIDAL. Refers to brain structures located outside the pyramidal tracts of the central nervous system.

EXUDATE. Fluid that accumulates and penetrates the walls of vessels, leaking into the surrounding tissue.

# F

FACIAL ANGIOFIBROMAS. Benign (non-cancerous) tumors of the face.

FACIAL ASYMMETRY. Term used to describe when one side of the face appears different than the other.

FACIOSCAPULOHUMERAL MUSCULAR DYSTROPHY (FSH). This form of muscular dystrophy, also known as Landouzy-Dejerine condition, begins in late childhood to early adulthood and affects both men and women, causing weakness in the muscles of the face, shoulders, and upper arms.

FACTOR VIII. A protein involved in blood clotting that requires vWF for stability and long-term survival in the bloodstream.

FACTORS. Coagulation factors are substances in the blood, such as proteins and minerals, that are necessary for clotting. Each clotting substance is designated with roman numerals I through XIII.

FAILURE TO THRIVE. Significantly reduced or delayed physical growth.

FALLOPIAN TUBE. Either of a pair of tubes that conduct ova from the ovaries to the uterus.

FAMILIAL ADENOMATOUS POLYPOSIS (FAP). Inherited syndrome causing large numbers of polyps and increased risk of colon cancer and other cancers.

FAMILIAL GASTRIC CANCER. Gastric cancer that occurs at a higher rate in some families.

FAMILIAL. Tending to occur in more members of a family than expected by chance alone.

FANCONI SYNDROME. A reabsorbtion disorder in the kidney tubules.

FATAL FAMILIAL INSOMNIA. A rare, progressive neurological disease that is believed to be transmitted via an abnormal protein called a prion.

FATTY ACIDS. The primary component of fats (lipids) in the body. Carnitine palmitoyl transferase (CPT) deficiency involves abnormal metabolism of the long-chain variety of fatty acids.

FECAL BLOOD TESTING. Examination of the stool for any evidence of blood, which may be a sign of cancers in the digestive tract.

FECAL OCCULT BLOOD TEST. Study of stool (feces) to identify loss of blood in the gastrointestinal system.

FERTILE. Able to reproduce.

FETAL ALCOHOL SYNDROME. Syndrome characterized by distinct facial features and varying mental retardation in an infant due to impaired brain development resulting from the mother's consumption of alcohol during pregnancy.

FETAL HYDROPS. A condition in which there is too much fluid in the fetal tissues and/or cavities.

FETOSCOPY. A technique by which a developing fetus can be viewed directly using a thin, flexible optical device (fetoscope) inserted into the mother's uterus.

FETUS IN FETU. In this case, one fetus grows inside the body of the other twin.

FETUS. The term used to describe a developing human infant from approximately the third month of pregnancy until delivery. The term embryo is used prior to the third month.

**FGFR–RELATED CRANIOSYNOSTOSIS.** Group of eight disorders comprising Pfeiffer syndrome, Apert syndrome, Crouzon syndrome, Beare–Stevenson syndrome, FGFR2–related isolated coronal synostosis, Jackson–Weiss syndrome, Crouzon syndrome with acanthosis nigricans (AN), and Muenke syndrome (isolated coronal synostosis) all caused by a mutation of a FGFR gene.

**FIBRILLATION.** A rapid, irregular heartbeat.

**FIBRILLIN-2.** A protein that forms part of the body's connective tissue. The precise function of fibrillin-2 is not known.

**FIBRIN.** The final substance created through the clotting cascade, which provides a strong, reliable plug to prevent further bleeding from the initial injury.

**FIBRINOGEN.** A fibrous protein that circulates in blood and participates in blood clotting by attaching to platelets.

**FIBROBLAST GROWTH FACTOR RECEPTOR GENE.** A type of gene that codes for a cell membrane receptor involved in normal bone growth and development.

**FIBROBLAST GROWTH FACTORS.** Proteins that are important in such functions as the growth of new blood vessels (angiogenesis), in wound healing, and in the growth of embryos.

**FIBROBLAST.** Cells that form connective tissue fibers like skin.

**FIBROFOLLICULOMA.** Small, white or yellow, dome-shaped benign growths on hair follicles.

**FIBROID.** A non-cancerous tumor of connective tissue made of elongated, threadlike structures, or fibers, which usually grow slowly and are contained within an irregular shape. Fibroids are firm in consistency but may become painful if they start to break down or apply pressure to areas within the body. They frequently occur in the uterus and are generally left alone unless growing rapidly or causing other problems. Surgery is needed to remove fibroids.

**FIBROMA.** A non-malignant tumor of connective tissue.

**FIBROSIS.** The abnormal development of fibrous tissue; scarring.

**FINASTERIDE.** An oral medication used to treat male pattern hair loss. Finasteride, sold under the trade names Proscar and Propecia, is an androgen inhibitor.

**FINE NEEDLE ASPIRATION (FNA).** Insertion of a thin needle through the skin to an area of sample tissue.

**FIRST-DEGREE RELATIVE.** A parent, child or sibling is a first degree relative. First-degree relatives have one half of their genes in common.

**FIRST-RANK SYMPTOMS.** A set of symptoms designated by Kurt Schneider in 1959 as the most important diagnostic indicators of schizophrenia: delusions, hallucinations, thought insertion or removal, and thought broadcasting.

**FISH (FLUORESCENCE *IN SITU*.** Technique used to detect small deletions or rearrangements in chromosomes by attempting to attach a fluorescent (glowing) piece of a chromosome to a sample of cells obtained from a patient.

**FISTULA.** An abnormal passage or communication between two different organs or surfaces.

**FLEXION CREASES.** The lines present on the palms of the hands and the soles of the feet from normal bending of these body parts. Some individuals affected with arthrogryposis lack these characteristic lines.

**FLEXION.** The act of bending or condition of being bent.

**FLOW CYTOMETRY.** A method of analyzing cells in which cell properties are detected as they flow in a narrow stream through a measuring device.

**FLUORESCEIN ANGIOGRAPHY.** Procedure to look at the blood vessel system of the eye. Fluorescein, a dye, is injected and photographs are taken as the dye passes through the eye's blood vessels.

**FLUORESCENCE IN-SITU HYBRIDIZATION (FISH).** A method of analyzing the structures of human genetics that uses fluorescent probes designed to link to specific genetic particles such as proteins, genes, or chromosomal material.

**FLUOROCHROME.** A fluorescent compound used for visualization in FISH.

**FMR-1 GENE.** A gene found on the X chromosome. Its exact purpose is unknown, but it is suspected that the gene plays a role in brain development.

**FOCAL SEIZURE.** A seizure that causes a brief and temporary change in movement, sensation, or nerve function.

**FOLATE-SENSITIVE FRAGILE SITE.** A chromosome location which, under folate-deficient conditions, appears as a gap in the chromosome and is susceptible to breakage.

**FOLLICLE-STIMULATING HORMONE (FSH).** A hormone that stimulates estrogen in females and sperm production in males.

**FOLLICLE.** A pouch-like depression.

**FONTANELLE.** One of several "soft spots" on the skull where the developing bones of the skull have yet to fuse.

**FORAMEN.** A small opening or hole in a body part or tissue. Dandy-Walker malformation is characterized by the absence or failure to develop the three foramina in the fourth ventricle of the brain.

**FOREBRAIN.** The anterior of the front section of the brain.

**FOREHEAD PLAQUE.** Flat, fibrous skin growth on the forehead.

**FOUNDER EFFECT.** Increased frequency of a gene mutation in a population that was founded by a small ancestral group of people, at least one of whom was a carrier of the gene mutation.

**FRONTAL BOSSING.** A term used to describe a rounded forehead with a receded hairline.

**FRONTAL PLAGIOCEPHALY.** An abnormal condition of the skull in which the front is more developed on one side than it is on the other side.

**FUNCTIONAL MAGNETIC RESONANCE IMAGING (FMRI).** A form of imaging of the brain that registers blood flow to functioning areas of the brain.

**FUNDUS.** The interior back wall of the eyeball.

# G

**G-TUBE.** A gastrostomy tube, which is inserted surgically into the stomach and used for feeding and for administering medications.

**GAIT DISTURBANCES.** Disturbances that affect the manner of walking.

**GALACTITOL.** An alcohol derivative of galactose that builds up in the lens and causes cataracts.

**GALACTOSEMIA.** Abnormally high levels of galactose in the blood due to an inherited defect in the conversion of galactose to glucose.

**GALACTOSIALIDOSIS.** The inherited disorder known as neuraminidase deficiency with beta-galactosidase deficiency.

**GALACTOSURIA.** High levels of galactose found in the urine that is seen with galactosemia.

**GALLBLADDER.** A small, pear-shaped organ in the upper right hand corner of the abdomen. It is connected by a series of ducts (tube-like channels) to the liver, pancreas, and duodenum (first part of the small intestine). The gallbladder receives bile from the liver, and concentrates and stores it. After a meal, bile is squeezed out of the gallbladder into the intestine, where it aids in digestion of food.

**GAMETE.** A reproductive cell; an ovum or sperm

**GAMMA AMINO BUTYRIC ACID (GABA).** An amino acid that functions as the major inhibitory neurotransmitter in the nervous system.

**GAMMA KNIFE.** Equipment that precisely delivers a concentrated dose of radiation to a predetermined target using gamma rays.

**GANGLIONEUROBLASTOMA.** A tumor of the nerve fibers and ganglion cells.

**GANGLIOSIDE.** A complex membrane lipid made up of a long-chain fatty acid, a long-chain amino alcohol, and an oligosaccharide containing sialic acid.

**GANGRENE.** Death of a tissue, usually caused by insufficient blood supply and followed by bacterial infection of the tissue.

**GASTRIC TUBE.** A tube that is surgically placed though the skin of the abdomen to the stomach so that feeding with nutritional liquid mixtures can be accomplished.

**GASTRIC.** Associated with the stomach.

**GASTROENTEROLOGIST.** A physician who specializes in disorders of the digestive system.

**GASTROESPHAGEAL REFLUX.** The return of the contents of the stomach back up into the esophagus.

**GASTROINTESTINAL (GI) SYSTEM.** Body system involved in digestion, the breaking down and use of food.

**GASTROINTESTINAL REFLUX.** A chronic condition in which acid from the stomach flows back into the lower esophagus, causing pain or tissue damage.

**GASTROINTESTINAL TRACT.** The food intake and waste export system that runs from the mouth, through the esophagus, stomach, and intestines, to the rectum and anus.

**GASTROINTESTINAL.** Concerning the stomach and intestine.

**GASTROSCHISIS.** A small defect in the abdominal wall normally located to the right of the umbilicus, and not covered by a membrane, where intestines and other organs may protrude.

**GASTROSTOMY.** The construction of an artificial opening from the stomach through the abdominal wall to permit the intake of food.

**GAUCHER DISEASE.** Autosomal recessive metabolic disorder caused by dysfunction of the lysosomal enzyme beta–glucosidase.

**GAVAGE.** Feeding tube.

**GENE MUTATION.** A permanent change in genetic material that is transmittable.

**GENE THERAPY.** Replacing a defective gene with the normal copy.

**GENE.** A building block of inheritance, which contains the instructions for the production of a particular protein, and is made up of a molecular sequence found on a section of DNA. Each gene is found on a precise location on a chromosome.

**GENES.** The basic units of heredity that contain the blueprints for the processes crucial to growth and development.

**GENETIC ANTICIPATION.** The tendency for an inherited disease to become more severe in successive generations.

**GENETIC COUNSELING.** Short-term educational counseling process for individuals and families who have a genetic disease or who are at risk for such a disease. Genetic counseling provides patients with information about their condition and helps them make informed decisions.

**GENETIC COUNSELOR.** A health professional with advanced training in genetics and psychology who educates people about genetic conditions and testing.

**GENETIC DISEASE.** A disease that is (partly or completely) the result of the abnormal function or expression of a gene; a disease caused by the inheritance and expression of a genetic mutation.

**GENETIC HETEROGENEITY.** The occurrence of the same or similar disease, caused by different genes among different families.

**GENETIC SEX.** The gender determined by the sex chromosomes; XX is female, XY is male.

**GENETIC TEST.** Testing of chromosomes and genes from an individual or unborn baby for a genetic condition. Genetic testing can only be done if the gene is known.

**GENETIC.** Referring to genes and characteristics inherited from parents.

**GENETICIST.** A specialist (M.D. or Ph.D.) who has training and certification in diagnosing, managing, and counseling individuals/families with genetic disorders. Genetics counselors hold a master's degree in medical genetics, and provide many of the same services as geneticists.

**GENITAL HYPOPLASIA.** Underdeveloped genitals.

**GENITAL TRACT.** The organs involved in reproduction. In a male, they include the penis, testicles, prostate and various tubular structures to transport seminal fluid and sperm. In a female, they include the clitoris, vagina, cervix, uterus, fallopian tubes and ovaries.

**GENITALS.** The internal and external reproductive organs in males and females.

**GENITOURINARY.** Related to the reproductive and urinary systems of the body.

**GENOME.** All of the DNA in one cell.

**GENOTYPE.** The genetic makeup of an organism or a set of organisms.

**GERM LINE MOSAICISM.** A rare event that occurs when one parent carries an altered gene mutation that affects his or her germ line cells (either the egg or sperm cells) but is not found in the somatic (body) cells.

**GERMLINE MUTATION.** A heritable change in the DNA of a germ cell (a cell destined to become an egg or in the sperm). When passed from one generation to the next, a germline mutation is incorporated in every cell of the body.

**GERMLINE.** The cell line from which gametes arise.

**GERSTMANN-STRÄUSSLER-SCHEINKER SYNDROME.** A rare, progressive neurological disease that is believed to be transmitted via an abnormal protein called a prion.

**GESTATIONAL AGE.** An estimation of the age of the pregnancy. The beginning of gestation or pregnancy is counted from the first day of the woman's last menstrual period, although conception usually takes place about two weeks later.

**GINGIVAL FIBROMAS.** Fibrous growths found on the gums.

**GINGIVITIS.** Inflammation of the gums of the mouth, characterized by redness, swelling, and a tendency to bleed.

**GLAUCOMA.** An increase in the fluid eye pressure, eventually leading to damage of the optic nerve and ongoing visual loss.

**GLIAL CELLS.** Supportive cells for nerve cells in the brain and spinal cord.

**GLIOBLASTOMA MULTIFORME.** Tumor of the central nervous system consisting of undifferentiated glial cells.

**GLIOMA.** A tumor of the brain's glial cells.

**GLOBIN.** One of the component protein molecules found in hemoglobin. Normal adult hemoglobin has a pair each of alpha-globin and beta-globin molecules.

**GLOBUS PALLIDUS.** A small paired structure present in the deep portion of the brain, in front of the brainstem, that is considered a part of the basal ganglia and helps in movement control.

**GLOMERULI.** Tiny clusters of capillaries in the kidney.

**GLOMERULUS.** A structure in the kidney composed of blood vessels that are actively involved in the filtration of the blood.

**GLOSSOPTOSIS.** Downward displacement or retraction of the tongue.

**GLUCOCEREBROSIDE.** A cerebroside that contains glucose in the molecule.

**GLUCOSE.** One of the two simple sugars, together with galactose, that makes up the protein, lactose, found in milk. Glucose is the form of sugar that is usable by the body to generate energy.

**GLYCINE.** An amino acid (a building block of proteins) that is important in the transmission of nerve impulses.

**GLYCOGEN.** The chemical substance used by muscles to store sugars and starches for later use. It is composed of repeating units of glucose.

**GLYCOGENESIS.** The metabolic process responsible for the formation of glycogen from many glucose molecules.

**GLYCOGENOLYSIS.** The metabolic process responsible for the break down of glycogen to mobilize glucose.

**GLYCOLYSIS.** The pathway in which a cell breaks down glucose into energy.

**GLYCOPROTEIN IIB/IIIA (GP IIB/IIIA).** Sugar-proteins on the surface of platelets that bind to the fibrous protein, fibrinogin. These sugar-proteins are defective in Glanzmann's thrombasthenia.

**GLYCOPROTEIN.** A protein with at least one carbohydrate group.

**GLYCOSYLPHOSPHATIDYLINOSITOL (GPI).** A fat that attaches proteins to the outside walls of blood cells.

**GOITER.** An enlargement of the thyroid gland, causing tissue swelling that may be seen and/or felt in the front of the neck. May occur in people who have overactive production of thyroid hormones (hyperthyroidism), decreased production of thyroid hormones (hypothyroidism), or among people who have normal production of thyroid hormones.

**GONAD.** The sex gland in males (testes) and females (ovaries).

**GONADOTROPHIN.** Hormones that stimulate the ovary and testicles.

**GONIOSCOPE.** An instrument used to examine the trabecular meshwork; consists of a magnifier and a lens equipped with mirrors.

**GRADE.** As a noun: a classification of the cancerous qualities of an individual tumor. A higher grade indicates a more serious disease than does a lower grade. As a verb: to classify the cancerous qualities of an individual tumor.

**GRAFT-VERSUS-HOST DISEASE.** In bone marrow transplantation, the complication that occurs when the donor's cells attack the recipient's tissues, in part due to non-identical donor-recipient HLA types.

**GRAND MAL SEIZURE.** A seizure that causes a loss of consciousness, a loss of bladder control, generalized muscle contractions, and tongue biting.

**GRANULOCYTOPENIA.** A reduced number of white blood cells in the circulation.

**GRAY MATTER.** Areas of the brain and spinal cord that are comprised mostly of unmyelinated nerves.

**GREAT TOE.** The first and largest toe on the foot.

**GRIEF REACTION.** The normal depression felt after a traumatic major life occurrence such as the loss of a loved one.

**GROWTH FACTORS.** Cellular-signaling components that stimulate cell division or other cell processes.

**GROWTH HORMONE.** A hormone that eventually stimulates growth. Also called somatotropin.

**GUSTATORY LACRIMATION.** Abnormal development of the tear ducts causing tears when chewing.

# H

**HLA TYPE.** Refers to the unique set of proteins called human leukocyte antigens. These proteins are present on each individual's cells and allow the immune system to recognize 'self' from 'foreign'. HLA type is particularly important in organ and tissue transplantation.

**HLA-B27.** Stands for a specific form of human leukocyte antigen, the proteins involved in immune system function. Strongly associated with ankylosing spondylitis.

**HAEMATOPOIETIC STEM CELL TRANSPLANTATION (HSCT).** Transplantation of blood stem cells derived from the bone marrow or blood.

**HAEMATOPOIETIC STEM CELLS.** Stem cells that give rise to all the blood cell types.

**HALLUCAL POLYDACTYLY.** The appearance of an extra great toe.

**HALLUCINATION.** A sensory experience of something that does not exist outside the mind.

**HALLUX.** The great toe.

**HAMARTOMA.** An overgrowth of normal tissue.

**HAMARTOMATOUS RECTAL POLYPS.** Benign (noncancerous) growths found in the rectum.

**HAPLOID.** One single set of chromosomes; in humans, this is 23 chromosomes.

**HAPLOINSUFFICIENCY.** The lack of one of the two normal copies of a gene. Haploinsufficiency can result in a genetic disorder if normal function requires both copies of the gene. Haploinsufficiency is one explanation for a dominant pattern of inheritance.

**HAPLOTYPE.** A set of alleles that are inherited together as a unit on a single chromosome because of their close proximity.

**HARDEROPORPHYRIA.** An especially rare form of hereditary coproporphyria.

**HEAD TURN.** Habitual head position that has been adopted to compensate for abnormal eye movements.

**HEARING THRESHOLD.** The minimum sound level at which a particular individual can hear; also called the hearing level (HL) of that person.

**HEART ARRHYTHMIA.** An abnormal heart rhythm, in which the heartbeats may be too slow, too rapid, too irregular, or too early.

**HEIMLICH MANEUVER.** An action designed to expel an obstructing piece of food from the throat. It is performed by placing the fist on the abdomen, underneath the breastbone, grasping the fist with the other hand (from behind), and thrusting it inward and upward.

**HELLER'S SYNDROME.** Another name for Childhood Disintegrative Disorder (CDD). It is also sometimes called dementia infantilis.

***HELICOBACTER PYLORI.*** Bacterium that infects humans and may be associated with an increased risk of gastric cancer.

**HELPER T-CELL.** Specialized white blood cell that assists in humoral and cellular immunity.

**HEMANGIOBLASTOMA.** A tumor of the brain or spinal cord arising in the blood vessels of the meninges or brain.

**HEMANGIOMA.** Benign tumor made up of clusters of newly formed blood vessels.

**HEMATIN.** A drug administered intravenously to halt an acute porphyria attack. It causes heme biosynthesis to decrease, preventing the further accumulation of heme precursors.

**HEMATOMA.** An accumulation of blood, often clotted, in a body tissue or organ, usually caused by a break or tear in a blood vessel.

**HEMATOPOIETIC GROWTH FACTORS.** Substances that assist in the formation of blood cells.

**HEMATURIA.** The presence of blood in the urine.

**HEME.** The iron-containing molecule in hemoglobin that serves as the site for oxygen binding.

**HEMIHYPERPLASIA.** A condition in which overdevelopment or excessive growth of one half of a specific organ or body part on only one side of the body occurs.

**HEMIHYPERTROPHY.** Asymmetric overgrowth in which there is an increase in size of existing cells.

**HEMIPLEGIA.** Paralysis of one side of the body.

**HEMIVERTEBRA.** A defect in which one side or half of a vertebra fails to form.

**HEMIZYGOUS.** Having only one copy of a gene or chromosome.

**HEMOCHROMATOSIS.** Accumulation of large amounts of iron in the tissues of the body.

**HEMOGLOBIN A (HBA).** Normal adult hemoglobin consists of two alpha globins and two beta globins.

**HEMOGLOBIN F (HBF).** Fetal hemoglobin consists of two alpha and two gamma globins. HbF is produced by the fetus in utero and until about 48 weeks after birth. At this stage, the production of HbA rapidly increases while that of HbF drops off.

**HEMOGLOBIN S.** Hemoglobin produced in association with the sickle cell trait; the beta-globin molecules of hemoglobin S are defective.

**HEMOGLOBIN ELECTROPHORESIS.** A laboratory test that separates molecules based on their size, shape, or electrical charge.

**HEMOGLOBIN.** Protein-iron compound in the blood that carries oxygen to the cells and carries carbon dioxide away from the cells.

**HEMOLYTIC ANEMIA.** Anemia that results from premature destruction and decreased numbers of red blood cells.

**HEMOLYTIC.** Refers to the type of anemia caused by the breakdown of red blood cells, as opposed to anemia due to decreased production, for example.

**HEMORRHAGE.** Very severe, massive bleeding that is difficult to control. Hemorrhage can occur in hemophiliacs after what would be a relatively minor injury to a person with normal clotting factors.

**HEMOSTASIS.** The arrest of bleeding by blood coagulation.

**HEPATIC.** Referring to the liver.

**HEPATITIS.** A viral disease characterized by inflammation of the liver cells (hepatocytes). People infected with hepatitis B or hepatitis C virus are at an increased risk for developing liver cancer.

**HEPATOMEGALY.** An abnormally large liver.

**HEPATOSPLENOMEGALY.** Enlargement of the liver and spleen.

**HEREDITARY ANGIONEUROTIC EDEMA.** Abbreviated HANE, or HAE, this is an inherited kind of angioneurotic edema. Type I HANE is caused by a deficiency of C1-INH. Type II HANE is caused by a malformation of the C1-INH protein.

**HEREDITARY NON–POLYPOSIS COLON CANCER (HNPCC.** A genetic syndrome causing increased cancer risks, most notably colon cancer; also called Lynch syndrome.

**HEREDITARY NON-POLYPOSIS COLON CANCER (HNPCC).** A genetic syndrome causing increased cancer risks, most notably colon cancer. Also called Lynch syndrome.

**HEREDITARY.** The passing of traits from parents to their offspring.

**HERNIA.** A rupture in the wall of a body cavity, through which an organ may protrude.

**HETEROCHROMIA IRIDES.** A medical term for individuals with different-colored eyes.

**HETEROGENEOUS.** A set of symptoms or a disorder caused by several different gene mutations.

**HETEROPLASMY.** When all copies of mitochondrial DNA are not the same, and a mix of normal and mutated mitochondrial DNA is present.

**HETEROTAXY.** Random organ positioning in an individual that can result in multiple malformations with severe heart defects, livers found in the middle of the body, spleen abnormalities, and intestines turned in the opposite direction from normal (gastrointestinal malrotation).

**HETEROTOPIA.** Small nodules of gray matter that are present outside the cortex.

**HETEROZYGOTE.** Having two different versions of the same gene.

**HETEROZYGOUS.** Having two different versions of the same gene.

**HIGH DENSITY LIPOPROTEIN (HDL).** A cholesterol carrying substance that helps remove cholesterol from the cells of the body and deliver it to the liver where it is digested and removed from the body.

**HIGHLY AEROBIC TISSUES.** Tissue that requires the greatest amount of oxygen to thrive.

**HIRSCHSPRUNG DISEASE.** A deformation in which the colon becomes enlarged (megacolon), caused by abnormal nerve control of that portion of the large intestine.

**HIRSUITISM.** The presence of coarse hair on the face, chest, upper back, or abdomen in a female as a result of excessive androgen production.

**HISTAMINE.** A substance released by immune system cells in response to presence of allergen; stimulates widening of blood vessels and increased porousness of blood vessel walls so that fluid and protein leak out from blood to surrounding tissue, causing inflammation of local tissues.

**HISTOLOGIC.** Pertaining to histology, the study of cells and tissues at the microscopic level.

**HISTOLOGICAL STUDIES.** Laboratory tests performed on tissue samples and cells.

**"HITCHHIKER" THUMBS.** A congenital anomaly of the thumb in which it is abnormally positioned at a right angle to the first joint.

**HMLH1 AND HMSH2.** Genes known to control mismatch repair of genes.

**HOLOPROSENCEPHALY.** A malformation of the brain in which the two hemispheres or lobes of the brain do not separate properly.

**HOLT-ORAM SYNDROME.** Inherited disorder characterized by congenital heart defects and abnormalities of the arms and hands; may be associated with Duane retraction syndrome.

**HOMEOPATHIC.** A holistic and natural approach to healthcare.

**HOMEOSTASIS.** A state of physiological balance.

**HOMEOTIC GENES.** Developmental control genes active in the embryo.

**HOMOCYSTEINE.** An amino acid that is not used to produce proteins in the human body.

**HOMOGENTISATE 1,2-DIOXYGENASE (HGD).** Homogentisic acid oxidase, the fourth enzyme in the metabolic pathway for the breakdown of phenylalanine.

**HOMOGENTISIC ACID (HGA).** 2,5-Dihydroxyphenylacetic acid, the third intermediate in the metabolic pathway for the breakdown of phenylalanine.

**HOMOLOGOUS CHROMOSOMES.** Homologous chromosomes are two chromosomes of a doublet set that are identical, particularly for the genes that are on them.

**HOMOLOGUES.** Chromosomes or chromosome parts identical with respect to their construction and genetic content (i.e. the pair of chromosome 1s are homologous, as are the two 2s, 3s, etc...).

**HOMOPLASMY.** When all copies of mitochondrial DNA are the same, or have the same mutation.

**HOMOZYGOTE.** Having two identical copies of a gene or chromosome.

**HOMOZYGOUS.** Having two identical copies of a gene or chromosome.

**HORMONE THERAPY.** Treatment of cancer by changing the hormonal environment, such as testosterone and estrogen.

**HORMONE.** A chemical messenger produced by the body that is involved in regulating specific bodily functions such as growth, development, and reproduction.

**HUMAN GENOME PROJECT.** An international effort begun in 1990 to locate and identify the 100,000 genes on the 46 human chromosomes.

**HUMAN LEUKOCYTE ANTIGENS (HLA).** Proteins that help the immune system function, in part by helping it to distinguish "self" from "non-self."

**HUMORAL IMMUNITY.** A type of acquired immunity mediated by B-cells and their secreted antibodies; important in fighting bacterial and some viral infections.

**HUNTINGTON DISEASE.** A midlife-onset inherited disorder characterized by progressive dementia and loss of control over voluntary movements. It is sometimes called Huntington's chorea.

**HUNTINGTON'S CHOREA.** A hereditary disease that typically appears in midlife, marked by gradual loss of brain function and voluntary movement; some symptoms resemble those of schizophrenia.

**HYALINE.** A clear substance that occurs in cell deterioration.

**HYDRAMNIOS.** A condition in which there is too much amniotic fluid in the womb during pregnancy.

**HYDRANENCEPHALY.** Congenital enlargement of the head and brain.

**HYDROCEPHALUS.** The excess accumulation of cerebrospinal fluid around the brain, often causing enlargement of the head.

**HYDROCEPHALY.** An increase of cerebrospinal fluid in the brain.

**HYDROLASE.** Enzyme that uses water to break down substances.

**HYDROMETROCOLPOS.** An abnormal accumulation of fluids in the uterus and vagina.

**HYDRONEPHROSIS.** Obstruction of the tube that carries urine from the kidney into the bladder causing the pelvis and kidney duct to become swollen with excess urine.

**HYDROPS FETALIS.** A condition characterized by massive edema in a fetus or newborn.

**HYDROXYAPATITE.** A mineral that gives bone its rigid structure and strength. It is primarily composed of calcium and phosphate.

**HYDROXYUREA.** A drug that has been shown to induce production of fetal hemoglobin. HbF has a pair of gamma––globin molecules instead of the beta–globins of HbA. Higher–than–normal levels of HbF can alleviate some of the symptoms of thalassemia.

**HYGROMA.** A condition in which fluid builds up in a sac or cyst.

**HYPERAMMONEMIA.** An excess of ammonia in the blood.

**HYPERCALCEMIA.** High levels of calcium in the blood.

**HYPEREXTENSIBILITY.** The ability to extend a joint beyond the normal range.

**HYPERHIDROSIS.** Excessive perspiration that may be either general or localized to a specific area.

**HYPERLORDOSIS.** An exaggerated curve in the lower (lumbar) portion of the back.

**HYPERMOBILITY.** Unusual flexibility of the joints, allowing them to be bent or moved beyond their normal range of motion.

**HYPEROSTOSIS.** Overgrowth of the bone.

**HYPERPHAGIA.** Over-eating.

**HYPERPIGMENTATION.** An abnormal condition characterized by an excess of melanin in localized areas of the skin, which produces areas that are much darker than the surrounding unaffected skin.

**HYPERPLASIA.** An overgrowth of normal cells within an organ or tissue.

**HYPERSENSITIVITY.** A process or reaction that occurs at above normal levels; overreaction to a stimulus.

**HYPERTELORISM.** A wider-than-normal space between the eyes.

**HYPERTENSION.** Abnormally high blood pressure in an artery.

**HYPERTHERMIA.** Body temperature that is much higher than normal (i.e. higher than 98.6°F).

**HYPERTONIA.** Excessive muscle tone or tension, causing resistance of muscle to being stretched.

**HYPERTRICHOSIS.** Growth of hair in excess of the normal. Also called hirsutism.

**HYPERTROPHIC CARDIOMYOPATHY.** A condition in which the muscle of the heart is abnormally excessively thickened. In microscopic examination, normal alignment of muscle cells is absent (myocardial disarray).

**HYPERTROPHY.** Increase in the size of a tissue or organ brought on by the enlargement of its cells rather than cell multiplication.

**HYPNAGOGIC HALLUCINATIONS.** Dream–like auditory or visual hallucinations that occur while falling asleep.

**HYPOCALCEMIA.** Low calcium concentrations in the body.

**HYPOCHONDROPLASIA.** An autosomal dominant form of dwarfism whose physical features are similar to those of achondroplasia but milder. Affected individuals have mild short stature and a normal facial appearance.

**HYPOGENITALISM.** Retarded development of the external reproductive organs.

**HYPOGLYCEMIA.** An abnormally low glucose (blood sugar) concentration in the blood.

**HYPOGONADISM.** Small testes in men and scarce or irregular menstruation for females.

**HYPOHIDROSIS.** Insufficient perspiration or absent perspiration which may be either general or localized to a specific area.

**HYPOKETOSIS.** Decreased levels of ketone bodies.

**HYPOMELANOTIC MACULES.** Patches of skin lighter than the surrounding skin.

**HYPOMYELINATION.** The death of myelin on a nerve or nerves.

**HYPOPHOSPHATEMIA.** The state of having abnormally low levels of phosphate in the bloodstream.

**HYPOPIGMENTATION.** Decreased or absent color (pigment) in a tissue.

**HYPOPLASIA.** Incomplete or underdevelopment of a tissue or organ.

**HYPOPLASTIC RADIUS.** Underdevelopment of the radius, the outer, shorter bone of the forearm.

**HYPOPLASTIC.** Incomplete or underdevelopment of a tissue or organ. Hypoplastic left heart syndrome is the most serious type of congenital heart disease.

**HYPOSPADIAS.** A birth defect in which the opening to the urinary tract, called the urethra, is located away from the tip of the penis.

**HYPOTHALAMUS.** A part of the forebrain that controls heartbeat, body temperature, thirst, hunger, body temperature and pressure, blood sugar levels, and other functions.

**HYPOTHYROID.** Deficiency in thyroid gland activity or thyroid hormone levels.

**HYPOTONIA.** Low or poor muscle tone, resulting in floppy limbs.

**HYPOXIA.** Lack of oxygen to the cells that may lead to cell injury and ultimately cell death.

# I

**IQ.** Abbreviation for Intelligence Quotient. Compares an individual's mental age to his/her true or chronological age and multiplies that ratio by 100.

**IATROGENIC.** Caused by (-genic) doctor (iatro-). An iatrogenic condition is a condition that is caused by the diagnosis or treatment administered by medical professionals. Iatrogenic conditions may be caused by any number of things, including: unsterile medical instruments or devices, contaminated blood or implantations, or contaminated air within the medical facility.

**ICHTHYOSIS.** Rough, dry, scaly skin that forms as a result of a defect in skin formation.

**IDEOPATHIC.** Of unknown origin.

**IDIOPATHIC.** Of unknown origin.

**IDURONATE SULFATASE.** Enzyme required to metabolize or break down mucopolysaccharides.

**IGE.** An antibody composed of protein; specific forms of IgE produced by cells of immune system in response to different antigens that contact the body; major factor that stimulates the allergic response.

**ILIAC ARTERIES.** Arteries that supply blood to the lower body including the pelvis and legs.

**IMMUNE RESPONSE.** Defense mechanism of the body provided by its immune system in response to the presence of an antigen, such as the production of antibodies.

**IMMUNE SYSTEM.** The complex group of organs and cells that defends the body against infection and disease.

**IMMUNODEFICIENCY.** A defect in the immune system, leaving an individual vulnerable to infection.

**IMMUNOGLOBULIN.** A protein molecule formed by mature B cells in response to foreign proteins in the body; the building blocks for antibodies.

**IMMUNOLOGIC.** Related to immunology, the study of how the body's immune system fights disease.

Many immunologic disorders are characterized by the body's use of antibodies.

**IMMUNOTHERAPY.** Treatment of cancer by stimulating the body's immune defense system.

**IMPERFORATE ANUS.** Also known as anal atresia. A birth defect in which the opening of the anus is absent or obstructed.

**IMPOTENCE.** The inability to have a penile erection, which can be due to tissue damage resulting from sickling within the penis (priapism).

**IMPRINTING.** Process that silences a gene or group of genes. The genes are silenced depending on if they are inherited through the egg or the sperm.

**IN UTERO.** While in the uterus; before birth.

**IN VITRO FERTILIZATION.** Process by which a woman has her eggs surgically removed and fertilized in the laboratory. The developing embryos can then be transferred to her uterus to hopefully achieve a pregnancy.

**INCLUSION BODY.** Abnormal storage compartment inside a cell.

**INCOMPLETE PENETRANCE.** The presence of a gene that is not phenotypically expressed in all members of a family with the gene.

**INDUCTION.** Process where one tissue (the prechordal plate, for example) changes another tissue (for example, changes tissue into neural tissue).

**INFANTILE SPASMS.** The form of grand mal or focal seizures experienced by infants prior to the development of many voluntary muscular controls.

**INFECTIOUS MONONUCLEOSIS.** A common viral infection caused by Epstein-Barr virus with symptoms of sore throat, fever, and fatigue. This infection is not in any way related to cancer.

**INFECTIVE ENDOCARDITIS.** An infection of the endothelium, the tissue lining the walls of the heart.

**INFERIOR OLIVARY NUCLEUS.** A small collection of cells seen in the lower part of the brainstem, which has connections to the cerebellum and is involved in control of movements.

**INFERTILE.** Incapable of reproduction.

**INFERTILITY.** Inability in a woman to become pregnant.

**INFLAMMATION.** Swelling and reddening of tissue; usually caused by immune system's response to the body's contact with an allergen.

**INGUINAL HERNIA.** A condition in which part of the intestines protrudes through a tear in the muscles of the abdomen.

**INHERITANCE PATTERN.** The way in which a genetic disease is passed on in a family.

**INHERITED GIANT PLATELET DISORDER (IGPD).** A group of hereditary conditions that cause abnormal blood clotting and other conditions.

**INSEMINATION.** The process by which sperm is placed into the female reproductive tract for the purpose of impregnation.

**INSOMNIA.** An inability to either fall or stay asleep, particularly at a time of day when sleep is expected. A number of medications are available, and may be used, for treatment.

**INSULIN RECEPTOR GENE.** The gene responsible for the production of insulin receptor sites on cell surfaces. Without properly functioning insulin receptor sites, cells cannot attach insulin from the blood for cellular use.

**INSULIN RESISTANCE.** An inability to respond normally to insulin in the bloodstream.

**INSULIN-LIKE GROWTH FACTOR I.** A hormone released by the liver in response to high levels of growth hormone in the blood. This growth factor is very similar to insulin in chemical composition; and, like insulin, it is able to cause cell growth by causing cells to undergo mitosis (cell division).

**INSULIN.** A hormone produced by the pancreas that is secreted into the bloodstream and regulates blood sugar levels.

**INTERPERSONAL THERAPIES.** Also called "talking therapy," this type of psychological counseling is focused on determining how dysfunctional interpersonal relationships of the affected individual may be causing or influencing symptoms of depression.

**INTRACRANIAL HEMORRHAGE.** Abnormal bleeding within the space of the skull and brain.

**INTRACRANIAL PRESSURE.** The pressure of the fluid between the brain and skull.

**INTRAGENIC.** Occuring within a single gene.

**INTRAUTERINE GROWTH RETARDATION.** A form of growth retardation occurring in the womb that is not caused by premature birth or a shortened gestation time. Individuals affected with this condition are of lower than normal birth weight and lower than normal length after a complete gestation period.

**INTRAVENOUS PYELOGRAM.** An x ray assessment of kidney function.

**INTRAVENOUS.** A route for administration of fluids, nutrients, blood products, or medications. A small flexible plastic tube is inserted into a vein by way of a needle to establish this route.

**INTRON.** That portion of the DNA sequence of a gene that is not directly involved in the formation of the chemical that the gene codes for.

**INTUSSUSCEPTION.** One piece of bowel inside another, causing obstruction.

**INVERSION.** A type of chromosomal defect in which a broken segment of a chromosome attaches to the same chromosome, but in reverse position.

**ION CHANNEL.** Cell membrane proteins that control the movement of ions into and out of the cell.

**ION TRANSPORTER.** A transmembrane protein that transports ions across a plasma membrane against the direction of their concentration (electrochemical) gradient.

**IONIZING RADIATION.** High–energy radiation such as that produced by x rays.

**IRIS.** The colored part of the eye, containing pigment and muscle cells that contract and dilate the pupil.

**IRON DEFICIENCY ANEMIA.** A decrease in the number of red cells in the blood caused by too little iron in the diet, poor absorption of iron by the body, or loss of blood.

**IRON OVERLOAD.** A side effect of frequent blood transfusions in which the body accumulates abnormally high levels of iron. Iron deposits can form in organs, particularly the heart, and cause life–threatening damage.

**ISCHEMIC ATTACK.** A period of decreased or no blood flow.

**ISCHOPAGUS.** Conjoined twins who are attached at the lower half of the body.

**ISOCHROMOSOME.** A chromosome is normally composed of two sections referred to as p and q; instead, an isochromosome is an abnormal chromosome made up of two p sections or two q sections.

**ISOMERISM.** Refers to the organs that typically come in pairs, but where the right organ is structurally different from the left organ. In a condition like asplenia, the organs are identical.

**ISOMERS.** Two chemicals identical in chemical composition (contain the same atoms in the same amounts) that have differing structures. The normal prion protein and the infectious prion protein are conformational isomers of one another. They have the same chemical structures, but for some reason, assume different shapes.

**ISOTOPE.** Any of two or more species of atoms of a chemical element with the same atomic number and nearly identical chemical behavior but with differing atomic mass and physical properties.

**ISOZYME/ISOENZYME.** A group of enzymes that perform the same function, but are different from one another in their structure or how they move.

# J

**JAUNDICE.** Yellowing of the skin or eyes due to excess of bilirubin in the blood.

**JOINT CONTRACTURE.** Inability of the limbs to fully extend.

**JOINT DISLOCATION.** The displacement of a bone from its socket or normal position.

# K

**KALLIKREIN.** A protein necessary for the activation of chemicals that cause dilation of blood vessels to allow increased blood flow to an area that requires more blood than normal. It is also capable of cleaving the complement, C5, into C5a, a much more robust and active form of this complement molecule.

**KANNER'S SYNDROME.** Another name for autism.

**KARYOTYPE.** A standard arrangement of photographic or computer-generated images of chromosome pairs from a cell in ascending numerical order, from largest to smallest.

**KARYOTYPING.** A laboratory procedure in which chromosomes are separated from cells, stained and arranged so that their structure can be studied under the microscope.

**KERATIN.** A tough, nonwater-soluble protein found in the nails, hair, and the outermost layer of skin. Human hair is made up largely of keratin.

**KERATINOCYTES.** Skin cells.

**KERATOACANTHOMA.** A firm nodule on the skin typically found in areas of sun exposure.

**KERATOLYTIC.** An agent that dissolves or breaks down the outer layer of skin (keratins).

**KERATOSIS.** A raised thickening of the outer horny layer of the skin.

**KETOACIDOSIS.** A condition that results when organic compounds (such as propionic acid, ketones, and fatty acids) build up in the blood and urine.

**KETOLACTIC ACIDOSIS.** The overproduction of ketones and lactic acid.

**KETONE BODIES.** Fat breakdown products that can make the blood acidic when present in high levels.

**KETONE BODIES.** Products of fatty acid metabolism in the liver that can be used by the brain and muscles as an energy source.

**KETONURIA.** The presence of excess ketone bodies (organic carbohydrate-related compounds) in the urine.

**KETOSIS.** An abnormal build-up of chemicals called ketones in the blood. This condition usually indicates a problem with blood sugar regulation.

**KIDNEY STONE.** A small, hard crystal of mineral and salts that forms in the kidney.

**KIDNEY TUBULES.** A portion of the kidneys that causes water to be excreted as urine or reabsorbed into the body.

**KIDNEY.** Either of two organs in the lumbar region that filter the blood, excreting the end products of the body's metabolism in the form of urine and regulating the concentrations of hydrogen, sodium, potassium, phosphate and other ions in the body.

**KYPHOSCOLIOSIS.** Abnormal front-to-back and side-to-side curvature of the spine.

**KYPHOSIS.** An abnormal outward curvature of the spine, with a hump at the upper back.

# L

**L-CARNITINE.** A substance made in the body that carries wastes from the body's cells into the urine.

**L1 SYNDROME.** Inherited disorder that primarily affects the nervous system caused by mutations in the L1CAM gene. L1 syndrome involves a variety of features including muscle stiffness (spasticity) of the lower limbs, mental retardation, hydrocephalus, and thumbs bent toward the palm (adducted thumbs).

**LABIA.** The two parts of the vulva (the external female genitalia).

LACRIMAL DUCTS. Tear ducts.

LACTIC ACID. The major by-product of anaerobic (without oxygen) metabolism.

LACTIC ACIDOSIS. A condition characterized by the accumulation of lactic acid in bodily tissues. The cells of the body make lactic acid when they use sugar as energy. If too much of this acid is produced, the person starts feeling ill with symptoms such as stomach pain, vomiting, and rapid breathing.

LACTOSE. A sugar made up of glucose and galactose. It is the primary sugar in milk.

LAPAROSCOPY. A diagnostic procedure in which a small incision is made in the abdomen and a slender, hollow, lighted instrument is passed through it. The doctor can view the ovaries more closely through the laparoscope, and if necessary, obtain tissue samples for biopsy.

LAPAROTOMY. An operation in which the abdominal cavity is opened up.

LARONIDASE. A highly purified protein, also known under its trademark name Aldurazyme, that is identical to a naturally occurring form of the human enzyme alpha–L–iduronidase. It is used in enzyme replacement therapy.

LARYNX. The voice box, or organ that contains the vocal cords.

LASER ABLATION. Removal of a skin papula with a laser beam.

LASER–ASSISTED IN–SITU KERATOMILEUSIS . A surgical procedure that uses a cutting tool and a laser to modify the cornea and correct moderate to high levels of myopia.

LATERAL RECTUS MUSCLE. The muscle that turns the eye outward toward the ear (abduction).

LEARNING DISABILITY. Refers generally to a group of disorders manifested by significant difficulties in the acquisition and use of listening, speaking, reading, writing, reasoning, or math abilities.

LEBERS HEREDITARY OPTIC ATROPHY OR LEBERS HEREDITA. Discovered in 1871 by Theodore Leber, the painless loss of central vision in both eyes, usually occurring in the second or third decade of life, caused by a mutation in mitochondrial DNA. Other neurological problems such as tremors or loss of ankle reflexes, may also be present.

LEFT VENTRICLE. Portion of the heart from which blood is pumped into the system.

LEFT VENTRICULAR ENLARGEMENT. Abnormal enlargement of the left lower chamber of the heart.

LEFT-RIGHT AXIS. The developmental feature in a fetus that determines which side of the body is left and which side is right; it conducts the location and positioning of the fetus' internal organs.

LENS. The transparent, elastic, curved structure behind the iris (colored part of the eye) that helps focus light on the retina.

LENTIGENE. A dark colored spot on the skin.

LEPROSY. A chronic, contagious skin and nervous system disease that leads, in the more serious form, to numbness, muscle weakness, and paralysis. Leprosy is sometimes referred to as Hansen's disease.

LEPTOMENINGEAL ANGIOMA. A swelling of the tissue or membrane surrounding the brain and spinal cord, which can enlarge with time.

LESION. A defective or injured section or region of the brain (or other body organ).

LETHARGY. Fatigue.

LEUCOPENIA. A decrease in white blood cells.

LEUKEMIA. Cancer of the blood forming organs which results in an overproduction of white blood cells.

LEUKOCORIA. Abnormal white reflection from the retina.

LEUKOCYTE. A white blood cell. The neutrophils are a type of leukocyte.

LEUKOCYTOSIS. An increase in the number of leukocytes in the blood.

LEUKODYSTROPHY. A disease that affects the white matter called myelin in the CNS.

LEUKOENCEPHALOPATHY. Any of various diseases, including leukodystrophies, affecting the brain's white matter.

LEVOTHYROXINE. A form of thyroxine (T4) for replacement of thyroid hormones in hypothryoidism.

LEWY BODIES. Areas of injury found on damaged nerve cells in certain parts of the brain associated with dementia.

LHERMITTE-DUCLOS DISEASE. Rare form of benign brain tumor.

LI–FRAUMENI SYNDROME. Inherited syndrome known to cause increased risk of different cancers, most notably sarcomas.

**LI-FRAUMENI SYNDROME.** Inherited syndrome known to cause increased risk of different cancers, most notably sarcomas.

**LIFETIME RISK.** A risk which exists over a person's lifetime; a lifetime risk to develop disease means that the chance is present until the time of death.

**LIGAMENT.** A type of connective tissue that connects bones or cartilage and provides support and strength to joints.

**LIMB GIRDLES.** Areas around the shoulders and hips.

**LIMB-GIRDLE MUSCULAR DYSTROPHY (LGMD).** Form of muscular dystrophy that begins in late childhood to early adulthood and affects both men and women, causing weakness in the muscles around the hips and shoulders.

**LIMITED SCLERODERMA.** A subtype of systemic scleroderma with limited skin involvement. It is sometimes called the CREST form of scleroderma, after the initials of its five major symptoms.

**LINKAGE ANALYSIS.** A method of finding mutations based on their proximity to previously identified genetic landmarks.

**LINKAGE.** The association between separate DNA sequences (genes) located on the same chromosome.

**LIPASE.** A digestive enzyme found in pancreatic fluid that breaks down fats.

**LIPID.** Large, complex biomolecule, such as a fatty acid, that will not dissolve in water. A major constituent of membranes.

**LIPIDS.** A class of organic compounds defined by their tendency to dissolve in organic liquids, such as alcohol and ether, but not in water.

**LIPOMA.** A benign tumor composed of well-differentiated fat cells.

**LIPOPIGMENTS.** Substances made up of fats and proteins found in the body's tissues.

**LIPOPROTEIN.** A complex molecule consisting of a lipid molecule joined with one or more protein molecules.

**LIPOPROTEINS.** Compounds of protein that carry fats and fat-like substances such as cholesterol in the blood.

**LISSENCEPHALY.** A developmental disorder where the brain is smooth without the normal surface convolutions.

**LOCALIZED SCLERODERMA.** Thickening of the skin from overproduction of collagen.

**LOCUS (PLURAL: LOCI).** Position occupied by a gene on a chromosome.

**LONG BONES.** The femur in the leg and the humerus in the arm.

**LORDOSIS.** An abnormal curvature of the spine in which the lumbar, or lower section, is excessively curved.

**LORDOSIS.** An exaggeration of the normal lumbar curve such that the chest is prominent and the small of the back is hollowed.

**LOW DENSITY LIPOPROTEINS (LDL).** A cholesterol carrying substance that can remain in the blood stream for a long period of time.

**LUMBAR LORDOSIS.** Abnormal inward curvature of the spine.

**LUPUS ERYTHEMATOSUS.** A chronic inflammatory disease that affects many tissues and parts of the body including the skin.

**LUTENIZING HORMONE (LH).** A hormone secreted by the pituitary gland that regulates the menstrual cycle and triggers ovulation in females. In males it stimulates the testes to produce testosterone.

**LUTENIZING HORMONE.** A hormone secreted by the pituitary gland that regulates the menstrual cycle and triggers ovulation in females. In males it stimulates the testes to produce testosterone.

**LYMPH NODE.** A bean-sized mass of tissue that is part of the immune system and is found in different areas of the body.

**LYMPHANGIOMYOMATOSIS.** Serious lung disease characterized by the overgrowth of an unusual type of muscle cell resulting in the blockage of air, blood, and lymph vessels to and from the lungs.

**LYMPHATIC SYSTEM.** Lymph nodes and lympatic vessels that transport infection fighting cells to the body.

**LYMPHEDEMA DISTICHIASIS.** Autosomal dominant condition with abnormal or absent lymph vessels. Common signs include a double row of eyelashes (distichiasis) and edema of the limbs beginning around puberty.

**LYMPHOCYTES.** Also called white blood cells, lymphocytes mature in the bone marrow to form B cells, which fight infection.

**LYMPHOMA.** A malignant tumor of the lymph nodes.

**LYMPHOSCINTIGRAPHY.** Procedure that helps to look at the lymph nodes in the body. Requires an injection of radioactive material to help see the lymph nodes and lymphatic system.

**LYNCH SYNDROME.** A genetic syndrome causing increased cancer risks, most notably colon cancer. Also called hereditary non-polyposis colon cancer (HNPCC).

**LYSINE.** A crystalline basic amino acid essential to nutrition.

**LYSIS.** Area of destruction.

**LYSOSOMAL STORAGE DISEASES.** Group of more than forty human genetic disorders that result from defects in lysosomal function.

**LYSOSOMAL.** Pertaining to the lysosomes, special parts (organelles) of cells that contain a number of enzymes important in the breakdown of large molecules such as proteins and fats.

**LYSOSOME.** Membrane-enclosed compartment in cells, containing many hydrolytic enzymes; where large molecules and cellular components are broken down.

# M

**MAO-B INHIBITORS.** Inhibitors of the enzyme monoamine oxidase B. MAO-B helps break down dopamine; inhibiting it prolongs the action of dopamine in the brain. Selegiline is an MAO-B inhibitor.

**MACROCEPHALY.** An unusually large head.

**MACROGLOSSIA.** A large tongue.

**MACROPHAGE.** Specialized white blood cells that play a role in breaking down old or abnormal red blood cells.

**MACROSOMIA.** Overall large size due to overgrowth.

**MACROSTOMIA.** A mouth that is larger or wider than normal.

**MACULA.** A small spot located in the back of the eye that provides central vision and allows people to see colors and fine visual details.

**MACULAR DEGENERATION.** Progressive condition that affects the macula, a small portion of the retina at the back of the eye.

**MACULE.** A flat, discolored spot or patch on the skin.

**MADAROSIS.** The medical term for loss of hair from the eyebrows or eyelashes. Madarosis may be associated with a form of alopecia areata called alopecia totalis. It may also result from such diseases as leprosy and syphilis, or from trauma.

**MADELUNG'S DEFORMITY.** A forearm bone malformation characterize by a short forearm, a arced or bow-shaped radius, and dislocation of the ulna, resulting in wrist abnormalities.

**MAFFUCCI DISEASE.** A manifestation of Ollier disease (multiple enchondromatosis) with hemangiomas, which present as soft tissue masses.

**MAGNETIC RESONANCE IMAGING (MRI).** A diagnostic procedure that uses a combination of high powered magnets, radio frequencies, and computers to generate detailed images of structures within the body.

**MAJOR DEPRESSION.** A psychological condition in which the patient experiences one or more disabling attacks of depression that lasts two or more weeks.

**MAJOR HISTOCOMPATIBILITY COMPLEX (MHC).** Includes HLA, as well as other components of the immune system. Helps the immune system function, in part by helping it to distinguish "self" from "non-self."

**MALABSORPTION.** The inability to adequately or efficiently absorb nutrients from the intestinal tract.

**MALAR HYPOPLASIA.** Small or underdeveloped cheekbones.

**MALFORMATION.** An abnormality in an organ or body structure caused by a dysfunctional developmental process.

**MALIGNANT HYPERTHERMIA.** A condition brought on by anesthesia during surgery.

**MALIGNANT.** A tumor growth that spreads to another part of the body, usually cancerous.

**MALROTATION.** An abnormality that occurs during the normal rotation of an organ or organ system.

**MAMMOGRAM.** A procedure in which both breasts are compressed/flattened and exposed to low doses of x rays, in an attempt to visualize the inner breast tissue.

**MAMMOGRAPHY.** X rays of the breasts; used to screen for breast cancer.

**MANDIBLE.** Lower jaw bone.

**MANDIBULAR HYPOPLASIA.** Underdevelopment of the lower jaw.

**MANNOSE.** A type of sugar that forms long chains in the body.

**MANOMETRY.** A balloon study of internal anal sphincter pressure and relaxation.

MAORI. A native New Zealand ethnic group.

MARFAN SYNDROME. A syndrome characterized by skeletal changes (arachnodactyly, long limbs, lax joints), ectopia lentis, and vascular defects.

MARFANOID HABITUS. An abnormally low weight to height ratio that is sometimes seen in extremely tall and thin people.

MARFANOID. Term for body type which is similar to people with Marfan syndrome. Characterized by tall, lean body with long arms and long fingers.

MASCULINIZATION. Development of excess body and facial hair, deepening of the voice, and increase in muscle bulk in a female due to a hormone disorder.

MASSETER SPASM. Stiffening of the jaw muscles. Often one of the first symptoms of malignant hyperthermia susceptibility that occurs after exposure to a trigger drug.

MATERNAL SERUM SCREENING. A blood test offered to pregnant women usually under the age of 35, which measures analytes in the mother's blood that are present only during pregnancy, to screen for Down syndrome, trisomy 18, and neural tube defects.

MATERNAL UNIPARENTAL DISOMY. Chromosome abnormality in which both chromosomes in a pair are inherited from one's mother.

MATERNAL. Relating to the mother.

MATURITY-ONSET DIABETES OF THE YOUNG (MODY). A rare form of diabetes inherited in an autosomal dominant fashion. It is similar to type II diabetes, but develops before the age of 25.

MAXILLA. The main bone forming the upper jaw and the middle of the face.

MAXILLARY HYPOPLASIA. Underdevelopment of the upper jaw.

MEAN. The average numerical value, such as size, in a set of numbers.

MECONIUM. The first waste products to be discharged from the body in a newborn infant, usually greenish in color and consisting of mucus, bile and so forth.

MEDIAL RECTUS MUSCLE. The muscle that turns the eye inward toward the nose (adduction).

MEDIUM CHAIN ACYL-COA DEHYDROGENASE. Abbreviated MCAD, this is the enzyme responsible for the breakdown of medium chain fatty acids in humans. People affected with MCAD deficiency produce a form of MCAD that is not as efficient as the normal form of MCAD.

MEDIUM CHAIN FATTY ACIDS. Fatty acids containing between four and 14 carbon atoms.

MEDULLARY CAVITY. The marrow-filled cavity inside of a long bone (such as the femur).

MEDULLARY THYROID CANCER (MTC). A slow-growing tumor associated with MEN.

MEDULLOBLASTOMA. Tumor of the central nervous system derived from undifferentiated cells of the primitive medullary tube.

MEGACOLON. Dilation of the colon.

MEGALENCEPHALY. Enlarged brain.

MEIOSIS. The process in which a cell in the testes or ovaries undergoes chromosome separation and cell division to produce sperm or eggs.

MELANIN. Pigments normally produced by the body that give color to the skin and hair.

MELANOCYTE. A cell that can produce melanin.

MELANOMA. Tumor, usually of the skin.

MELANOSOMES. Granules of pigment within melanocytes that synthesize melanin.

MELATONIN. A sleep-inducing hormone secreted by the pineal gland.

MEMORY CELLS. B-cells whose antibodies recognized antigens from a previous infection; able to mount a quick, efficient response upon a second infection by the same organism.

MENDEL, GREGOR. Austrian monk who discovered the basic principals of hereditary.

MENDELIAN GENETICS. A set of parameters describing the traditional method of the transmission of genes from one generation to the next.

MENINGES. The two-layered membrane that covers the brain and spinal cord.

MENINGIOMA. Tumor that grows from the protective brain and spinal cord membrane cells (meninges).

MENINGITIS. An infection of the covering of the brain.

MENOPAUSE. Cessation of menstruation in the human female, usually occurring between the ages of 46 and 50.

MENOPAUSE. The transition in a woman's life whereby menstrual periods stop.

**MENSTRUATION.** Discharge of blood and fragments of the uterine wall from the vagina in a monthly cycle in the absence of pregnancy.

**MENTAL RETARDATION.** Significant impairment in intellectual function and adaptation in society. Usually associated with an intelligence quotient (IQ) below 70.

**MERMAID SYNDROME.** Alternate name for sirenomelia, often used in older references.

**MESENTERY.** Double-layered fold in the peritoneum.

**MESOMELIA.** Shortness of the portion of arm connecting the elbow to the wrist or forearm.

**MESOMELIC.** The anatomical term used to describe the middle of a limb. The bones that constitute the middle of the arm are the radius and ulna, and mesomelic bones of the leg are the tibia and fibula.

**MESONEPHRIC DUCT.** Embryonic structure that in the male becomes the vas deferens, and in both sexes gives rise to the ureters leading to the kidney.

**METABOLIC ACIDOSIS.** High acidity (low pH) in the body due to abnormal metabolism, excessive acid intake, or retention in the kidneys.

**METABOLIC DISORDER.** A disorder that affects the metabolism of the body.

**METABOLIC MYOPATHIES.** A broad group of muscle diseases whose cause is a metabolic disturbance of some type.

**METABOLIC PATHWAY.** A sequence of chemical reactions that lead from some precursor to a product, where the product of each step in the series is the starting material for the next step.

**METABOLISM.** The total combination of all of the chemical processes that occur within cells and tissues of a living body.

**METACARPAL.** A hand bone extending from the wrist to a finger or thumb.

**METACENTRIC.** When a chromosome has the centromere in the middle of the chromosome it is called a metacentric chromosome.

**METACHRONOUS.** Occurring at separate time intervals.

**METAPHYSEAL FLARING.** A characteristic found only by x rays. If present, it means that the ends of the bone are wider than normal.

**METAPHYSIS.** An area of softer bone and cartilage in long bones between the diaphysis (shaft) and epiphysis (end).

**METASTASIS.** The spreading of cancer from the original site to other locations in the body.

**METASTASIZE.** To spread to another part of the body.

**METASTATIC CANCER.** A cancer that has spread to an organ or tissue from a primary cancer located elsewhere in the body.

**METATARSAL.** A foot bone extending from the ankle to a toe.

**METHEMOGLOBINEMIA.** A medical condition of the blood characterized by the presence of an altered form of hemoglobin, known as methemoglobin.

**METHYLATION TESTING.** DNA testing that detects if a gene is active, or if it is imprinted.

**METHYLMALOMIC ACID.** An intermediate product formed when certain substances are broken down in order to create usable energy for the body.

**METHYLMALONIC COA MUTASE (MCM).** The enzyme responsible for converting methylmalonic acid to succinic acid, in the pathway to convert certain substances to usable energy.

**METHYLMALONICACIDEMIA.** The buildup of high levels of methylmalonic acid in the bloodstream due to an inborn defect in an enzyme.

**MICROCEPHALIC PRIMORDIAL DWARFISM SYNDROMES.** A group of disorders characterized by profound growth delay and small head size.

**MICROCEPHALIC.** Having an abnormally small head.

**MICROCEPHALY.** Abnormal smallness of the head; it often is associated with mental retardation.

**MICROCORNEA.** Abnormal smallness of the cornea.

**MICROCYTIC, HYPOCHROMIC ANEMIA.** An anemia marked by deficient hemoglobin and small red blood cells.

**MICRODELETION SYNDROME.** A syndrome caused by the deletion of a very small amount of chromosomal material.

**MICRODELETION.** Loss of a miniscule bit of a chromosome.

**MICRODONTIA.** Small teeth.

**MICROGNATHIA.** A term used to describe small, underdeveloped lower jaw and chin.

**MICROGNATHY.** Having a very small and receding jaw.

**MICROMELIA.** Extremely short arms and legs.

**MICROPHTHALMIA.** Small or underdeveloped eyes.

**MICROTIA.** Small or underdeveloped ears.

**MIDFACIAL HYPOPLASIA.** Subnormal growth of the central face.

**MIDLINE DEFECTS.** Defects involving organs along the center of the body such as the lips, penis, and corpus callosum.

**MIDLINE ORGANS.** Organs found along the center of the body such as the lips, penis, and corpus callosum.

**MIGRAINE.** A condition marked by severe headaches, often on one side of the head and accompanied by nausea, light and sound sensitivity, and other symptoms. Migraines are believed to involve the nerves and blood vessels of parts of the brain and head.

**MINIATURIZATION.** The process of shortening and thinning of the hair shafts that is found in androgenetic alopecia. It is caused by the effects of DHT on the hair follicle.

**MINOXIDIL.** A topical medication sold under the trade name Rogaine for the treatment of male pattern hair loss. It is applied to the scalp as a 2% or 5% solution.

**MISCARRIAGE.** Spontaneous pregnancy loss.

**MISMATCH REPAIR.** Repair of gene alterations due to mismatching.

**MITOCHONDRIA.** Organelles within the cell responsible for energy production.

**MITOCHONDRIAL INHERITANCE.** Inheritance associated with the mitochondrial genome which is inherited exclusively from the mother.

**MITOSIS.** The process by which a somatic cell—a cell not destined to become a sperm or egg—duplicates its chromosomes and divides to produce two new cells.

**MITRAL VALVE PROLAPSE.** A heart defect in which one of the valves of the heart (which normally controls blood flow) becomes floppy. Mitral valve prolapse may be detected as a heart murmur but there are usually no symptoms.

**MITRAL VALVE.** The heart valve that prevents blood from flowing backwards from the left ventricle into the left atrium. Also known as bicuspid valve.

**MIXED-TYPE HEARING LOSS.** Hearing loss that involves both conductive and sensorineural losses.

**MOLECULAR ANALYSIS.** Evaluation of molecules, tests that may identify single gene mutations.

**MONOCLONAL ANTIBODY.** A protein, produced in large quantities in a laboratory, designed to attack a specific target in the body.

**MONOSOMY.** Missing an entire copy of a chromosome or a piece of one copy of a chromosome.

**MONOZYGOTIC.** From one zygote, as in identical twins. The zygote is the first cell formed by the union of sperm and egg.

**MORPHEA.** The most common form of localized scleroderma.

**MORPHOGENESIS.** The normal developmental process of the body's structure and form.

**MOSAIC.** A term referring to a genetic situation in which an individual's cells do not have the exact same composition of chromosomes. In Down syndrome, this may mean that some of the individual's cells have a normal 46 chromosomes, while other cells have an abnormal 47 chromosomes.

**MOSAICISM.** A genetic condition resulting from a mutation, crossing over, or nondisjunction of chromosomes during cell division, causing a variation in the number of chromosomes in the cells.

**MOSAICISM.** A genetic condition resulting from a mutation, crossing over, or nondisjunction of chromosomes during cell division, causing a variation in the number of chromosomes in the cells.

**MOTOR NEURONS.** Class of neurons that specifically control and stimulate voluntary muscles.

**MOTOR SKILLS DISORDER.** A disorder that affects motor coordination or its development, and the control of particular groups of muscles that perform activities.

**MOTOR UNITS.** Functional connection with a single motor neuron and muscle.

**MOTTLED RETINA.** Changes in the retina of the eye causing a loss of visual acuity.

**MUCOCILIARY ESCALATOR.** The coordinated action of tiny projections on the surfaces of cells lining the respiratory tract, which moves mucus up and out of the lungs.

**MUCOLIPID.** Lipid that accumulate in cells in mucolipidosis disorders.

**MUCOLIPIN-1.** Protein in the cell membrane, probably a calcium ion channel, involved in recycling membrane lipids and is deficient in mucolipidosis IV.

MUCOLYTIC. An agent that dissolves or destroys mucin, the chief component of mucus.

MUCOPOLYSACCHARIDE. A complex molecule made of smaller sugar molecules strung together to form a chain. Found in mucous secretions and intercellular spaces.

MUCOPOLYSACCHARIDOSES (MPSS). Inherited lysosomal storage diseases that are caused by the accumulation of mucopolysaccharides, resulting in problems with an individual's development. There are many types of mucopolysaccharidoses. The specific enzyme that is deficient or absent is what distinguishes one type of MPS from another.

MUCOPOLYSACCHARIDOSIS–IH (MPS–IH). Another name for Hurler syndrome.

MUCOSA. Mucus–secreting membrane lining all body cavities or passages that communicate with the exterior.

MUCOUS MEMBRANE. Thin, mucous covered layer of tissue that lines organs such as the intestinal tract.

MULLERIAN DUCT. Two embryo structures that in the female develop into vagina, uterus, and oviducts, and in the male disappear except for the vestigial vagina masculina and the appendix testis.

MULLERIAN DUCTS. Structures in the embryo that develop into the fallopian tubes, the uterus, the cervix and the upper vagina in females.

MULTI-INFARCT DEMENTIA. Dementia caused by damage to brain tissue resulting from a series of blood clots or clogs in the blood vessels. It is also called vascular dementia.

MULTIFACTORIAL INHERITANCE. A type of inheritance pattern where many factors, both genetic and environmental, contribute to the cause.

MULTIFACTORIAL. Describes a disease that is the product of the interaction of multiple genetic and environmental factors.

MULTIFOCAL BREAST CANCER. Multiple primary cancers in the same breast.

MULTIFOCAL. A pathological term meaning that instead of finding one tumor in the tissue multiple tumors are found.

MULTIPLE CARBOXYLASE DEFICIENCY. A type of propionic acidemia characterized by an inability to metabolize biotin.

MULTIPLE SCLEROSIS (MS). A progressive degeneration of nerve cells that causes episodes of muscle weakness, dizziness, and visual disturbances, followed by periods of remission.

MULTIPLEX ASSAY. A procedure that allows the testing of several gene samples simultaneously.

MUSCULAR DYSTROPHY. A group of inherited diseases characterized by progressive wasting of the muscles.

MUTAGEN. An environmental influence that causes changes in DNA.

MUTANT. A change in the genetic material that may alter a trait or characteristic of an individual or manifest as disease.

MUTATED GENE. A change of DNA sequence that causes a change of the function of the gene and a subsequent disease.

MUTATION. A change or alteration that occurs in the DNA that causes alterations in the protein or substance that they were providing the instructions for. Mutations in the PAH gene lead to decreased function of the enzyme phenylalanine hydroxylase.

MYELIN. A fatty sheath surrounding nerves in the peripheral nervous system, which help them conduct impulses more quickly.

MYELINATION. Production and maintenance of the myelin sheath.

MYELODYSPLASIA. A bone marrow disorder that can develop into aplastic anemia requiring bone marrow or stem cell transplantation.

MYELOMENINGOCELE. A sac that protrudes through an abnormal opening in the spinal column.

MYOCLONUS. Twitching or spasms of a muscle or an interrelated group of muscles.

MYOGLOBINURIA. The abnormal presence of myoglobin, a product of muscle disintegration, in the urine. Results in dark-colored urine.

MYOPATHY. Any abnormal condition or disease of the muscle.

MYOPIA. Nearsightedness. Difficulty seeing objects that are far away.

MYOTONIA. The inability to normally relax a muscle after contracting or tightening it.

MYOTONIA. The inability to normally relax a muscle after contracting or tightening it.

MYOTONIC DYSTROPHY. A form of muscular dystrophy, also known as Steinert's condition, characterized by delay in the ability to relax muscles after forceful contraction, wasting of muscles, as well as other abnormalities.

MYOTUBULE. An intermediate stage in muscle fiber development, where the fiber is tubular with a centrally placed nucleus, instead of a peripheral eccentric nucleus.

MYXEDEMA. Swelling of the face, hands, feet, and genitals due to hypothyroidism.

MYXOID. Resembling mucus.

# N

N-ACETYLGLUCOSAMINE-1-PHOSPHOTRANSFERASE (GNPTA). Enzyme that attaches a signal to other enzymes and directs those enzymes to the lysosome; deficient in mucolipidoses II and III.

NANISM. Short stature.

NARCOTICS. Strong, prescription medication that can be effective in treating pain, but have the potential to be habit-forming if their use is not supervised correctly.

NASOGASTRIC TUBE. A long flexible tube inserted through the nasal passageways, down the throat, and into the stomach. Used to drain the contents of the stomach.

NATURAL IMMUNITY. First line immune response that is non-specific. Includes action of phagocytes, natural killer cells, and complement cells.

NATURAL KILLER CELLS. Specialized white blood cells involved in natural immunity. Can kill some viruses and cancer cells.

NECROSIS. Death of a portion of tissue differentially affected by disease or injury.

NECROTIZING ENCEPHALOMYELOPATHY. A progressive degeneration of the brain and central nervous system. This condition is fatal in nearly all individuals affected with type A pyruvate carboxylase deficiency.

NEGATIVE SYMPTOMS. Symptoms of schizophrenia characterized by the absence or elimination of certain behaviors: affective flattening, poverty of speech, and loss of will or initiative.

NEONATAL. Neonatal refers to the first 28 days after birth.

NEONATE. A newborn infant up to six weeks of age.

NEONATOLOGIST. A physician (pediatrician) who has special training in the care of newborns (neonates).

NEOPLASM. An abnormal growth of tissue; for example, a tumor.

NEPHRECTOMY. Surgical removal of a kidney.

NEPHROCALCINOSIS. A disorder in which the concentration of calcium in the kidneys is too high.

NEPHRON. Basic functional filtration unit of the kidney.

NEPHRONS. Microscopic-size tubes that filter the water that flows into the kidneys.

NEPHROPATHY. Kidney disease.

NEPHROSIS. A non-inflammatory disease of the kidneys.

NERVE CONDUCTION TESTING. Procedure that measures the speed at which impulses move through the nerves.

NERVE CONDUCTION. A test that measures the speed of conduction of electrical impulses through nerves using a series of electrical shocks delivered through electrodes placed on the skin surface.

NERVOUS SYSTEM. The complete network of nerves, sense organs, and brain in the body.

NEUCHAL TRANSLUCENCY. A pocket of fluid at the back of an embryo's neck visible via ultrasound that, when thickened, may indicate the infant will be born with a congenital heart defect.

NEURAL CREST CELLS. A group of cells in the early embryo, located on either side of the area that will eventually develop into the spinal cord. The cells migrate (move) away from the area and give rise to various body structures, including melanocytes (pigment producing cells), certain structures of the face and head, and parts of the nervous system.

NEURAL CREST. Embryonic tissue that transforms into more specific tissues later in development.

NEURAL FOLDS AND TUBE. Portions of the developing embryo from which the brain and spinal cord arise.

NEURAL TUBE DEFECT. A defect in closure of the bones of the spine or skull; defects of the brain and skull are called anencephaly, while defects of the spine are called spina bifida.

NEURAL. Regarding any tissue with nerves, including the brain, the spinal cord, and other nerves.

NEUROCRISTOPATHY. A disorder that results from abnormal development and/or migration of the neural crest cells in the embryo.

**NEURODEGENERATIVE.** Relating to degeneration of nerve tissues.

**NEUROFIBROMA.** A soft tumor usually located on a nerve.

**NEUROFIBROMATOSIS.** Progressive genetic condition often including multiple café au lait spots, multiple raised nodules on the skin known as neurofibromas, developmental delays, slightly larger head sizes, and freckling of the armpits, groin area, and iris.

**NEUROIMAGING.** Imaging studies of the brain, such as x ray, computed tomography (CT) scans, or magnetic resonance imaging (MRI) scans.

**NEUROLEPTIC.** Another name for the older type of antipsychotic medications given to schizophrenic patients.

**NEUROLOGIC.** Pertaining the nervous system.

**NEUROLOGICAL.** Relating to the brain and central nervous system.

**NEUROLOGIST.** A physician who specializes in disorders of the nervous system, including the brain, spine, and nerves.

**NEUROMETABOLIC DISORDER.** Any disorder or condition that affects both the central nervous system (CNS) and the metabolism of the body.

**NEUROMUSCULAR JUNCTION.** The site at which nerve impulses are transmitted to muscles.

**NEUROMUSCULAR.** Involving both the muscles and the nerves that control them.

**NEURON.** The fundamental nerve cell that conducts impulses across the cell membrane.

**NEURONAL CEROID LIPOFUSCINOSES.** A family of four progressive neurological disorders.

**NEUROPATHY.** Common term used to denote dysfunction of the nerves in the arms, legs, or face.

**NEUROPROTECTIVE.** Conveying some form of protection to the nervous system from injury.

**NEUROTRANSMITTER.** Chemical in the brain that transmits information from one nerve cell to another.

**NEUTROPENIA.** A condition in which the number of leukocytes (a type of white or colorless blood cell) is abnormally low, mainly in neutrophils (a type of blood cell).

**NEUTROPHIL.** The primary type of white blood cell involved in inflammation. Neutrophils are a type of granulocyte, also known as a polymorphonuclear leukocyte.

**NEVI.** Plural of nevus.

**NEVUS FLAMMEUS.** A flat blood vessel tumor present at birth, also known as a "port wine stain."

**NEVUS.** Any anomaly of the skin present at birth, including moles and various types of birthmarks.

**NEW VARIANT CREUTZFELDT-JAKOB DISEASE.** A more newly identified type of Creutzfeldt-Jakob disease that has been traced to the ingestion of beef from cows infected with bovine spongiform encephalopathy. Known in the popular press as Mad Cow Disease.

**NEWBORN SCREENING.** The act of testing all infants for a specific disease shortly after birth for the purpose of preventing disease progression through prompt medical treatment.

**NITRATES/NITRITES.** Chemical compounds found in certain foods and water that, when consumed, may increase the risk of gastric cancer.

**NONDISJUNCTION.** An error in chromosome separation that occurs during cell division resulting in a woman receiving an extra X chromosome, leading to triple X syndrome.

**NONRENAL HAMARTOMA.** Benign (non-cancerous) tumor-like growths not found in the kidneys that often disrupt the normal function of a particular organ system.

**NONSPHEROCYTIC.** Literally means not sphere–shaped. Refers to the shape of red blood cells in non-spherocytic hemolytic anemia.

**NONSYNDROMIC HEARING LOSS.** Hearing loss that is not accompanied by other symptoms characteristic of a larger genetic syndrome.

**NONTRAUMATIC UNGUAL OR PERIUNGUAL FIBROMA.** Fibrous growth that appears around the fingernails and/or toenails

**NOONAN SYNDROME.** A genetic syndrome that possesses some characteristics similar to cardiofacio-cutanous syndromes. It is unclear whether the two syndrome are different or two manifestations of the same disorder.

**NUCLEAR ISOLATE.** An isolated preparation of the contents of the nucleus of a cell, which contains the DNA.

**NUCLEI.** Plural for nucleus, a special part of the cell that is essential for cell function.

**NUCLEIC ACID.** A type of chemical used as a component for building DNA. The nucleic acids found in DNA are adenine, thymine, guanine, and cytosine.

**NUCLEOTIDE.** A small molecule composed of three parts: a nitrogen base (a purine or pyrimidine), a sugar (ribose or deoxyribose), and phosphate; they serve as the building blocks of nucleic acids (DNA and RNA).

**NUCLEOTIDES.** Building blocks of genes, which are arranged in specific order and quantity.

**NUCLEUS.** The central part of a cell that contains most of its genetic material, including chromosomes and DNA.

**NYSTAGMUS.** Involuntary, rapid, and repetitive movement of the eyes in either a vertical or horizontal direction.

# O

**OBLIGATE CARRIER.** An individual who, based on pedigree analysis, must carry a genetic mutation for a particular genetic disease. Parents of a child with an autosomal recessive disorder are obligate carriers.

**OBSESSIVE COMPULSIVE DISORDER (OCD).** Disorder characterized by persistent, intrusive, and senseless thoughts (obsessions) or compulsions to perform repetitive behaviors that interfere with normal functioning.

**OCCIPITAL LOBE.** An anatomical subdivision, located at the back of the brain, that contains the visual cortex.

**OCHRONOSIS.** A condition marked by pigment deposits in cartilage, ligaments, and tendons.

**OCULAR.** A broad term that refers to structure and function of the eye.

**OCULO-DIGITAL REFLEX.** A reflex causing an individual to press on their eyes with their fingers or fists.

**OCULO.** Related to the eye.

**OCULOCUTANEOUS ALBINISM.** Inherited loss of pigment in the skin, eyes, and hair.

**OCULOMOTOR NERVE.** Cranial nerve III; the nerve that extends from the midbrain to several of the muscles that control eye movement.

**OCULOPHARYNGEAL MUSCULAR DYSTROPHY (OPMD).** Form of muscular dystrophy affecting adults of both sexes, and causing weakness in the eye muscles and throat.

**OKIHIRO SYNDROME.** Inherited disorder characterized by abnormalities of the hands and arms and hearing loss; may be associated with Duane retraction syndrome.

**OLIGODACTYLY.** The absence of one or more fingers or toes.

**OLIGODENDROCYTE.** A cell in the central nervous system that insulates the parts of nerve cells called axons.

**OLIGODONITA.** The absence of one or more teeth.

**OLIGOHYDRAMNIOS.** An abnormally small amount of amniotic fluid.

**OLIGOSACCHARIDE.** Several monosaccharide (sugar) groups joined by glycosidic bonds.

**OLLIER DISEASE.** Also termed multiple enchondromatosis. Excessive cartilage growth within the bone extremities that result in benign cartilaginous tumors arising in the bone cavity.

**OMPHALOCELE.** A birth defect where the bowel and sometimes the liver, protrudes through an opening in the baby's abdomen near the umbilical cord.

**OMPHALOPAGUS.** Conjoined twins who are attached at the abdomen.

**ONCOGENE.** Genes that allow the uncontrolled division and proliferation of cells that lead to tumor formation and usually to cancer.

**ONYCHOGRYPHOSIS.** Overgrowth of the fingernails and toenails.

**OPHTHALMOLOGIST.** A physician specializing in the medical and surgical treatment of eye disorders.

**OPHTHALMOLOGY.** The medical specialty of vision and the eye.

**OPHTHALMOSCOPE.** An instrument, with special lighting, designed to view structures in the back of the eye.

**OPISTHOTONOS.** An arched position of the body in which only the head and feet touch the floor or bed when the patient is lying on their back.

**OPPORTUNISTIC INFECTIONS.** Infections that would not usually cause illness in people with a healthy immune system.

**OPTIC DISC.** Circular area at the back of the eyeball where the optic nerve connects to the retina.

**OPTIC DISC.** The region where the optic nerve joins the eye, also referred to as the blind spot.

**OPTIC NERVE.** A bundle of nerve fibers that carries visual messages from the retina in the form of electrical signals to the brain.

**OPTOMETRIST.** A medical professional who examines and tests the eyes for disease and treats visual disorders by prescribing corrective lenses and/or vision therapy. In many states, optometrists are licensed to use diagnostic and therapeutic drugs to treat certain ocular diseases.

ORAL LOADING TEST. A procedure in which cystine is administered orally to a patient and plasma levels of cystine are measured. Under normal circumstances, amino acids are absorbed by the intestine and result in an increase in plasma amino acid levels. However, in cystinuria, there is a problem in the absorption process and blood levels of amino acids do not rise or rise slowly after eating.

ORBITAL CYSTS. Small fluid-filled sacs that abnormally develop inside the bony cavity of the skull that holds the eyeball.

ORGANELLE. Small, sub-cellular structures that carry out different functions necessary for cellular survival and proper cellular functioning.

ORGANIC ACIDURIA. The condition of having organic acid in the urine.

ORTHODONTIST. Dentist who specializes in the correction of misaligned teeth.

ORTHOKERATOLOGY. A method of reshaping the cornea using a contact lens. It is not considered a permanent method to reduce myopia.

ORTHOPEDIC. Pertaining to the field of orthopedics, the science of the bones and diseases of the bones.

ORTHOSTATIC HYPOTENSION. A sudden decrease in blood pressure upon sitting up or standing. May be a side effect of several types of drugs.

ORTHOSTATIC. Posture that is maintained while standing.

OSMOLARITY. The concentration of an osmotic solution, especially when measured in osmols or milliosmols per liter of solution.

OSMOTICALLY. Referring to the movement of a solvent through a semipermeable membrane (as of a living cell) into a solution of higher solute concentration that tends to equalize the concentrations of solute on the two sides of the membrane.

OSSICLES. Any of the three bones of the middle ear, including the malleus, incus, and stapes.

OSSIFICATION. The process of the formation of bone from its precursor, a cartilage matrix.

OSTEOARTHRITIS. A group of diseases and mechanical abnormalities involving degradation of joints.

OSTEOBLASTS. A bone cell that makes bone.

OSTEOCHONDROMATOSIS. Another name for hereditary multiple exostoses, meaning a growth of bone and cartilage.

OSTEOCLASTS. A bone cell that breaks down and reabsorbs bone.

OSTEOGENIC SARCOMA. Osteosarcoma.

OSTEOGENIC. Creating bone.

OSTEOMA. A benign bone tumor.

OSTEOMALACIA. The adult form of rickets, a lack of proper mineralization of bone.

OSTEOPENIC. Bone density that is somewhat low, but not osteoporotic.

OSTEOPOROSIS. Loss of bone density that can increase the risk of fractures.

OSTEOPOROSIS. Loss of bone density that can increase the risk of fractures.

OTITIS MEDIA. Inflammation of the middle ear, often due to fluid accumulation secondary to an infection.

OTOLARYNGOLOGIST. Physician who specializes in the care of the ear, nose, and throat and their associated structures.

OTOSCLEROSIS. The main type of nonsyndromic progressive conductive hearing loss seen in humans. In very advanced cases, otosclerosis can become of mixed type.

OVA. Another name for the egg cells that are located in the ovaries.

OVARY. The female reproductive organ that produces the reproductive cell (ovum) and female hormones.

OVULATION. The monthly process by which an ovarian follicle or cyst ruptures, releasing a mature egg cell.

OXALATE. A salt that can combine with calcium to produce kidney stones.

OXALOSIS. A condition in which an overload of oxalate begins to gather in the eyes, bones and muscles, circulatory system, and other organs, where it can cause damage.

OXYGENATED BLOOD. Blood carrying oxygen through the body.

OXYTOCIN. A hormone that stimulates the uterus to contract during child birth and the breasts to release milk.

# P

**PACHYDERMA.** An abnormal skin condition in which excess skin is produced that appears similar to that of an elephant (pachyderm).

**PACHYGYRIA.** The presence of a few broad gyri (folds) and shallow sulci (grooves) in the cerebral cortex.

**PAGET'S DISEASE.** A non-cancerous disease marked by excessive growth of abnormal bone material.

**PALATE.** The roof of the mouth.

**PALLIATIVE.** Treatment done for relief of symptoms rather than a cure.

**PALMAR.** Referring to the palms of the hand.

**PALMOPLANTAR KERATODERMA.** Group of mostly hereditary disorders characterized by thickening of the corneous layer of skin (hyperkeratosis) on the palms and soles as a result of excessive keratin formation (protein in the skin, hair and nails).

**PALMOPLANTAR KERATOSIS.** A raised thickening of the outer horny layer of the skin on the palms of the hand and the soles of the feet.

**PALPEBRAL FISSURES.** The opening between the upper and lower eyelids.

**PALPITATION.** An irregular heartbeat.

**PALSY.** Paralysis.

**PALSY.** Uncontrollable tremors.

**PANCREAS.** An organ located in the abdomen that secretes pancreatic juices for digestion and hormones for maintaining blood sugar levels.

**PANCREATIC INSUFFICIENCY.** Reduction or absence of pancreatic secretions into the digestive system due to scarring and blockage of the pancreatic duct.

**PANCREATIC ISLET CELL.** Cells located in the pancreas that serve to make certain types of hormones.

**PANCREATITIS.** Inflammation of the pancreas.

**PANCYTOPENIA.** An abnormal reduction in the number of erythrocytes (red blood cells), leukocytes (a type of white or colorless blood cell), and blood platelets (a type of cell that aids in blood clotting) in the blood.

**PANHYPOPITUITARISM.** Generalized decrease of all of the anterior pituitary hormones.

**PAPILLOMA.** Any benign localized growth of the skin and the linings of the respiratory and digestive tracts. The most common papilloma is the wart.

**PAPILLOMATOUS PAPULES.** Skin-colored, raised bumps (not warts) found on the skin. Most of these growths are benign (non-cancerous) and rarely become malignant (cancerous).

**PAPULA.** A small raised area of the skin that lacks visible fluid.

**PARALYSIS.** Complete loss of muscle function for one or more muscle groups, often with loss of feeling and mobility in the afffected area.

**PARAPAGUS.** Conjoined twins who are joined at the side of their lower bodies.

**PARAPARESIS.** Weakness of the legs without complete paralysis.

**PARAPLEGIA.** Complete paralysis of the legs.

**PARASITIC TWINS.** Occurs when one smaller, malformed twin is dependent on the larger, stronger twin for survival.

**PARASYMPATHETIC GANGLION CELL.** Type of nerve cell normally found in the wall of the colon.

**PARATHYROID GLANDS.** A pair of glands adjacent to the thyroid gland that primarily regulate blood calcium levels.

**PARENCHYMA.** Functional (rather than structural) tissues of an organ.

**PARESTHESIA.** Abnormal subjective sensations like numbness, tingling, pain, burning, or prickling that occur due to neuropathy.

**PARESTHESIA.** Presence of abnormal sensations in the limbs.

**PARKINSON DISEASE.** A disease of the nervous system most common in people over 60, characterized by a shuffling gait, trembling of the fingers and hands, and muscle stiffness. It may be related in some way to Lewy body dementia.

**PARKINSON'S DISEASE.** A progressive disease occurring most often after the age of 50, associated with the destruction of brain cells that produce dopamine and characterized by tremor, slowing of movement, and gait difficulty.

**PARKINSONISM.** A set of symptoms originally associated with Parkinson disease that can occur as side effects of neuroleptic medications: trembling of the fingers or hands, a shuffling gait, and tight or rigid muscles.

**PATELLA.** The kneecap.

**PATENT DUCTUS ARTERIOSUS (PDA).** A congenital anomaly of the heart occurring when the ductus arteriosus (the temporary fetal blood vessel that connects the aorta and the pulmonary artery) does not close at birth.

**PATERNAL.** Relating to one's father.

**PECTORALIS MUSCLES.** Major muscles of the chest wall.

**PECTUS CARINATUM.** An abnormality of the chest in which the sternum (breastbone) is pushed outward. It is sometimes called "pigeon breast."

**PECTUS EXCAVATUM.** An abnormality of the chest in which the sternum (breastbone) sinks inward; sometimes called "funnel chest."

**PEDIGREE ANALYSIS.** Analysis of a family tree, or pedigree, in an attempt to identify the possible inheritance pattern of a trait seen in this family.

**PELVIC EXAMINATION.** Physical examination performed by a physician, often associated with a Pap smear. The physician inserts his/her finger into a woman's vagina, attempting to feel the ovaries directly.

**PENDRIN.** A protein encoded by the PDS (Pendred syndrome) gene located on chromosome 7q31. Pendrin protein is believed to transport iodide and chloride within the thyroid and the inner ear.

**PENETRANCE.** The frequency with which a heritable trait is manifested by individuals carrying the principal gene or genes conditioning it, usually expressed as a percentage.

**PENYLALANINE (PHE).** An essential amino acid. It is considered essential because a body cannot make this amino acid, and it must be obtained through diet (eating protein).

**PEPTIC ULCER.** A wound in the bowel that can be caused by stomach acid or a bacterium called *Helicobacter pylori.*

**PEPTIDE.** A molecular compound made of two or more amino acids.

**PERCHLORATE DISCHARGE TEST.** A test used to check for Pendred syndrome by measuring the amount of iodine stored inside the thyroid gland. Individuals with Pendred syndrome usually have more iodine stored than normal, and thus their thyroid will release

a large amount of iodine into the bloodstream when they are exposed to a chemical called perchlorate.

**PERICARDIAL CAVITY.** Space occupied by the heart.

**PERICARDITIS.** Inflammation of the pericardium, the membrane surrounding the heart.

**PERINATOLOGIST.** A physician (obstetrician) who has special training in managing difficult pregnancies. Some prenatal tests, such as chorionic villus sampling and level II ultrasound, are performed primarily by perinatologists.

**PERIOD OF SUSCEPTIBILITY.** The time when teratogens can cause harm to the developing fetus.

**PERIODONTITIS.** Inflammatory reaction of the tissues surrounding and supporting the teeth that can progress to bone destruction and abscess formation, and eventual tooth loss.

**PERIOSTEAL.** Relating to the periosteum, which is the connective tissue that covers all human bones.

**PERIPHERAL NERVES.** Nerves throughout the body that carry information to and from the spinal cord.

**PERIPHERAL NEUROPATHY.** Any disease of the nerves outside of the spinal cord, usually resulting in weakness and/or numbness.

**PERIPHERAL VISION.** The ability to see objects that are not located directly in front of the eye. Peripheral vision allows people to see objects located on the side or edge of their field of vision.

**PERITONITIS.** Inflammation of the peritoneum, the membrane surrounding the abdominal contents.

**PERNICIOUS ANEMIA.** A blood condition with decreased numbers of red blood cells related to poor vitamin B12 absorption.

**PEROXISOME BIOGENESIS.** Processes involved in the fabrication of proxisome in cells.

**PEROXISOME.** A cellular organelle containing different enzymes responsible for the breakdown of waste or other products.

**PEROXISOMES.** Tiny structures in the cells that break down fats so that the body can use them.

**PERVASIVE DEVELOPMENTAL DISORDER (PDD).** The term used to describe individuals who meet some but not all of the criteria for autism.

**PES PLANUS.** Flat feet.

**PEUTZ-JEGHERS SYNDROME (PJS).** Inherited syndrome causing polyps of the digestive tract and spots on the mouth as well as increased risk of cancer.

**PHAGOCYTE.** White blood cells capable of engulfing and destroying foreign antigen or organisms in the fluids of the body.

**PHALANGES.** Long bones of the fingers and toes, divided by cartilage around the knuckles.

**PHALILALIA.** Involuntary echoing of the last word, phrase, sentence, or sound vocalized by oneself.

**PHENOTYPE.** Observable characteristic or trait of an organism.

**PHENYLALANINE HYDROXYLASE.** The enzyme responsible for converting dietary phenylalanine to tyrosine. If phenylalanine hydroxylase is not working efficiently, phenylalanine levels in the blood increase.

**PHENYLALANINE.** An essential amino acid that must be obtained from food since the human body cannot manufacture it.

**PHENYLKETONURIA (PKU).** An inherited inability to metabolize dietary phenylalanine, resulting in blood phenylalanine levels above 20 mg/dL. If left untreated, elevated blood phenylalanine levels can result in damage to the nervous system, including severe cognitive impairment, often referred to as mental retardation.

**PHEOCHROMOCYTOMA.** A small vascular tumor of the inner region of the adrenal gland. The tumor causes uncontrolled and irregular secretion of certain hormones.

**PHILTRUM.** The center part of the face between the nose and lips that is usually depressed.

**PHLEBOTOMY.** The taking of blood from the body through an incision in the vein, usually in the treatment of disease.

**PHOBIA.** An exaggerated fear.

**PHOSPHATE.** A substance composed of the elements phosphorus and oxygen that contributes to the hydroxyapatite crystals found in normal bones.

**PHOSPHORYLATION.** The addition of phosphoric acid to another compound.

**PHOTOPHOBIA.** An extreme sensitivity to light.

**PHOTOPIGMENT.** Pigment that is most sensitive to a particular wavelength of light.

**PHOTORECEPTOR CELLS.** Specialized cells that convert light into nerve signals that ultimately get transmitted to the brain through the optic nerve.

**PHOTORECEPTOR.** Cells at the back of the eye that process the light that hit them; examples are cone and rod cells.

**PHOTORECEPTORS.** Specialized cells, rod cells and cone cells, lining the innermost layer of the eye that convert light into electrical messages so that the brain can perceive the environment; rod cells allow for peripheral and night vision, while cone cells are responsible for perceiving color and for central vision.

**PHOTOREFRACTIVE KERATECTOMY (PRK).** A procedure that uses an excimer laser to make modifications to the cornea and permanently correct myopia. As of early 1998, only two lasers have been approved by the FDA for this purpose.

**PHOTOSENSITIVITY.** Sensitivity to sunlight.

**PHYTANIC ACID HYDROXYLASE.** A peroxisomal enzyme responsible for processing phytanic acid. It is defective in Refsum disease.

**PHYTANIC ACID.** A substance found in various foods that, if allowed to accumulate, is toxic to various tissues. It is metabolized in the peroxisome by phytanic acid hydroxylase.

**PICK'S DISEASE.** A rare type of primary dementia that affects the frontal lobes of the brain. It is characterized by a progressive loss of social skills, language, and memory, leading to personality changes and sometimes loss of moral judgment.

**PITUITARY GLAND.** A small gland at the base of the brain responsible for releasing many hormones, including luteinizing hormone (LH) and follicle-stimulating hormone (FSH).

**PLACENTA.** A bag-like organ that partially surrounds the fetus during pregnancy; it delivers oxygen and nutrients to, and takes waste away from, the fetus during pregnancy, and is attached to the fetus by the umbilical cord.

**PLANTAR.** Referring to the sole of the foot.

**PLAQUES.** Abnormally deposited proteins that interfere with normal cell growth and functioning and usually progresses to cell death.

**PLASMA CELLS.** Antibody-secreting B-cells.

**PLASMA.** The liquid part of the blood and lymphatic fluid that contains antibodies and other proteins.

**PLASMALOGENS.** Fat molecules that are important components of cells and of the myelin sheath that protects nerve cells.

**PLASMAPHERESIS.** A procedure in which the fluid component of blood is removed from the bloodstream and sometimes replaced with other fluids or plasma.

**PLASMIN.** The blood protein that is responsible for dissolving blood clots.

**PLATELETS.** Small disc-shaped structures that circulate in the blood stream and participate in blood clotting.

**PLETHORA.** An overabundance of blood in the body.

**PLEURAL CAVITY.** Area of the chest occupied by the lungs.

**PLEURITIS.** Inflammation of the pleura, the membrane surrounding the lungs.

**PNEUMONIA.** An infection of the lungs.

**PNEUMOTHORAX.** Abnormal accumulation of air in the chest cavity, outside the lung, often responsible for a collapsed lung.

**POIKILODERMA.** A condition characterized by skin atrophy, widening of the small blood vessels (telangiectasia), and pigment changes giving a mottled appearance.

**POLYDACTYLY.** The presence of extra fingers or toes.

**POLYGENIC.** A trait, characteristic, condition, etc. that depends on the activity of more than one gene for its emergence or expression.

**POLYHADRAMNIOS.** A condition in which there is too much fluid around the fetus in the amniotic sac.

**POLYMER.** A very large molecule, formed from many smaller, identical molecules.

**POLYMERASE CHAIN REACTION (PCR).** A laboratory process used to make a large number of copies of specific genetic information from small amounts of DNA.

**POLYMORPHIC.** Describes a gene for which there exist multiple forms, or alleles.

**POLYMORPHISM.** A change in the base pair sequence of DNA that may or may not be associated with a disease.

**POLYMYOSITIS.** An inflammation of many muscles.

**POLYNEUROPATHY.** A disorder in which a number of nerves in the peripheral nervous system malfunction simultaneously.

**POLYP.** A mass of tissue bulging out from the normal surface of a mucous membrane.

**POLYPECTOMY.** Surgical removal of polyps.

**POLYPOSIS.** A descriptive term indicating that hundreds to thousands of polyps have developed in an organ.

**POLYSACCHARIDE.** Linear or branched macromolecule composed of numerous monosaccharide (sugar) units linked by glycosidic bonds.

**POLYSYNDACTYLY.** Having both extra digits (toes, fingers) as well as webbing (syndactyly) between the digits.

**POOR MUSCLE TONE.** Muscles that are weak and floppy.

**PORENCEPHALY.** A congenital anomaly of the brain in which there are abnormal holes or cavities in the brain.

**PORPHYRIA.** A collection of at least eight disorders in which chemicals known as porphyrins or porphyrin precursors (substances that will become porphyrins) build up to abnormally high levels in the body.

**PORPHYRIN.** An organic compound containing nitrogen.

**PORT-WINE STAIN.** Dark-red birthmarks seen on the skin, named after the color of the dessert wine.

**POSER CRITERIA.** Criteria proposed in 1983 as an update to the Schumacher criteria for diagnosing MS; developed to aid neurologists in determining the existence of lesions and other para-clinical evidence of MS.

**POSITIONAL CLONING.** Cloning a gene simply on the basis of its position in the genome, without having any idea of the function of the gene.

**POSITIVE SYMPTOMS.** Symptoms of schizophrenia that are characterized by the production or presence of behaviors that are grossly abnormal or excessive, including hallucinations and thought-process disorder; DSM-IV subdivides positive symptoms into psychotic and disorganized.

**POSITRON EMISSION TOMOGRAPHY (PET).** A form of nuclear medicine scanning that measures brain activity using low doses of a radioactive substance.

**POST-ICTAL STATE.** A period of lethargy, confusion, and deep breathing following a grand mal seizure that may last from a few minutes to several hours.

**POSTAXIAL POLYDACTYLY.** A condition in which an extra finger or toe is present outside of the normal fifth digit.

**POSTERIOR COLUMN.** Long fiber tracts that run in the spinal cord, carrying vibratory and position sense from the limbs to the brain.

**POSTERIOR FOSSA.** Area at the base of the skull attached to the spinal cord.

**POVERTY OF SPEECH.** A negative symptom of schizophrenia, characterized by brief and empty replies to questions.

**PREAURICULAR PITS.** Small pits in the skin on the outside of the ear.

**PREAXIAL POLYDACTYLY.** An extra finger or toe on the inside of the hand or foot.

**PRECOCIOUS PUBERTY.** An abnormal condition in which a person undergoes puberty at a very young age. This condition causes the growth spurt associated with puberty to occur before the systems of the body are ready, which causes these individuals to not attain normal adult heights.

**PRECURSOR COMPONENTS.** Components in an enzymatic pathway that are formed by previous cellular events.

**PREMUTATION.** A change in a gene that precedes a mutation; this change does not alter the function of the gene.

**PRENATAL DIAGNOSIS.** The determination of whether a fetus possesses a disease or disorder while it is still in the womb.

**PRENATAL TESTING.** Testing for a disease such as a genetic condition in an unborn baby.

**PRENATAL ULTRASOUND.** An imaging test using high-frequency sound waves to create images of internal organs. Prenatal indicates the test is preformed to on fetus while still in the womb.

**PREVALENCE.** The number of individuals living with a particular illness within a particular population at any given time. Prevalence is often expressed in terms of number of individuals per 100 or per 1,000 members of the population.

**PRIMARY ATRIAL SEPTATION.** An improper division of the atria of the heart, or a "hole in the heart," which results in the formation of a common atrium rather than the normal two-chambered atrium.

**PRIMARY CANCER.** The first or original cancer site, before any metastasis.

**PRIMARY CRANIOSYNOSTOSIS.** Abnormal closure of the cranial sutures caused by an abnormality in the sutures themselves.

**PRIMARY IMMUNODEFICIENCY DISEASE (PID).** A group of approximately 70 conditions that affect the normal functioning of the immune system.

**PRIMARY POSITION, PRIMARY GAZE.** When both eyes are looking straight ahead.

**PRIMARY TUMOR.** An original tumor, not a metastatic tumor resulting from cancer's spread.

**PRION.** A term coined to mean "proteinaceous infectious particle." Prior to the 1982 discovery of prions, it was not believed that proteins could serve as infectious agents.

**PROBAND.** The person in the family who is affected by a genetic disorder and who brings the family to the attention of a health care provider.

**PROGERIA.** Genetic abnormality that presents initially as premature aging and failure to thrive in children.

**PROGNATHISM.** A protruding lower jaw.

**PROLACTIN.** A hormone that helps the breast prepare for milk production during pregnancy.

**PROLIFERATION.** The growth or production of cells.

**PROMOTER.** The region of a gene that initiates transcription of the genetic information.

**PROPHYLACTIC.** Preventing disease.

**PROPIONIC ACID.** An organic compound that builds up in the body if the proper enzymes are not present.

**PROPIONYL COA CARBOXYLASE.** An enzyme that breaks down the amino acids isoleucine, valine, threonine, and methionine.

**PROPTOSIS.** Bulging eyeballs.

**PROSTATECTOMY.** The surgical removal of the prostate gland.

**PROTEASE.** An enzyme that acts as a catalyst in the breakdown of peptide bonds.

**PROTEIN.** Important building blocks of the body, composed of amino acids, involved in the formation of body structures and controlling the basic functions of the human body.

**PROTEINURIA.** Excess protein in the urine.

**PROTEOLIPID PROTEIN GENE (PLP).** A gene that makes a protein that is part of the myelin in the central nervous system. Mutations in this gene cause PMD.

**PROTO-ONCOGENE.** A gene involved in stimulating the normal growth and division of cells in a controlled manner.

**PROTOPORPHYRIN.** A precursor molecule to the porphyrin molecule.

**PROXIMAL MUSCLES.** The muscles closest to the center of the body.

**PROXIMAL.** Near the point of origin.

**PSEUDOAUTOSOMAL DOMINANT INHERITANCE.** The pattern of inheritance for a disorder caused by genes in the pseudoautosomal regions of the sex chromosomes. Individuals only require one mutated or nonworking copy of a gene to have signs and symptoms of the disorder. Affected individuals have a 50% chance to have an affected child with each pregnancy.

**PSEUDOAUTOSOMAL REGION.** Genes found on the sex chromosomes that contain the same genetic information whether they are on the X or Y chromosome.

**PSEUDOCAMPTODACTYLY.** A condition in which the fingers curve or bend when the hand is bent back at the wrist.

**PSEUDOCYST.** A fluid-filled space that may arise in the setting of pancreatitis.

**PSEUDODEMENTIA.** A term for a depression with symptoms resembling those of dementia. The term dementia of depression is now preferred.

**PSEUDOTUMOR CEREBRI.** A syndrome of raised pressure within the skull that may cause vomiting, headache, and double vision.

**PSORIASIS.** A common, chronic, scaly skin disease.

**PSYCHODYNAMIC THERAPIES.** A form of psychological counseling that seeks to determine and resolve the internal conflicts that may be causing an individual to be suffering from the symptoms of depression.

**PSYCHOLOGIST.** An individual who specializes in the science of the mind.

**PSYCHOMOTOR.** Movement produced by action of the mind or will.

**PSYCHOSIS.** A severe mental disorder that results in a distorted view of reality.

**PSYCHOTHERAPY.** Psychological counseling that seeks to determine the underlying causes of a patient's depression. The form of this counseling may be cognitive/behavioral, interpersonal, or psychodynamic.

**PSYCHOTIC DISORDER.** A mental disorder characterized by delusions, hallucinations, or other symptoms of lack of contact with reality.

**PTERYGIUM COLLI.** Webbing or broadening of the neck, usually found at birth, and usually on both sides of the neck.

**PTOSIS.** Drooping of the upper eyelid.

**PUBERTY.** Point in development when the gonads begin to function and secondary sexual characteristics begin to appear.

**PULMONARY ARTERY.** An artery that carries blood from the heart to the lungs.

**PULMONARY ATRESIA.** When there is no valve between the right ventricle and the pulmonary artery (the artery leading from the heart to the lungs). In the absence of this valve, the blood does not flow into the lungs well.

**PULMONARY EDEMA.** A problem caused when fluid backs up into the veins of the lungs. Increased pressure in these veins forces fluid out of the vein and into the air spaces (alveoli). This interferes with the exchange of oxygen and carbon dioxide in the alveoli.

**PULMONARY EMBOLISM.** A blood clot in the lungs.

**PULMONARY HYPERTENSION.** A severe form of high blood pressure caused by diseased arteries in the lung.

**PULMONARY HYPOPLASIA.** Underdevelopment of the lungs.

**PULMONARY STENOSIS.** Narrowing of the pulmonary valve of the heart, between the right ventricle and the pulmonary artery, limiting the amount of blood going to the lungs.

**PULMONARY.** Relating to the lungs; the pulmonary artery carries blood from the heart to the lungs.

**PULMONOLOGIST.** A physician who specializes in lung diseases.

**PUNCTATED.** Having a dotted pattern.

**PUPIL.** The opening in the iris through which light enters the eye.

**PURINE.** A nitrogen-containing organic compound whose basic molecular structure consists of two rings joined to each other.

**PURPURA FULMINANS.** Dark, reddish-purple patches of dying tissue that result from clots in small blood vessels that would otherwise feed that tissue.

**PUSTULE.** A pus-filled lesion of the skin that resembles the "pimples" of adolescent acne.

**PYELONEPHRITIS.** Inflammation of the kidney commonly caused by bacterial infections.

**PYGOPAGUS.** Conjoined twins who are joined back to back with fused buttocks.

**PYLORIC SPHINCTER.** Circular smooth muscle found at the outlet of the stomach.

**PYLORIC STENOSIS.** Narrowing of the stomach due to thickening of the pyloris muscle at the end of the stomach.

**PYOGENIC.** Pus forming.

**PYREXIA.** A medical term denoting fevers.

**PYRIDOSTIGMINE BROMIDE (MESTINON).** An anticholinesterase drug used in treating myasthenia gravis.

**PYRUVATE CARBOXYLASE.** The enzyme that is responsible for the first step in the conversion of pyruvate molecules into glucose molecules. Individuals with Type A PCD produce an highly inefficient form of pyruvate carboxylase. Individuals with Type B PCD either completely lack the ability to produce this enzyme, or they cannot produce it in sufficient quantities to sustain life.

**PYRUVATE DEHYDROGENASE COMPLEX.** A series of enzymes and co-factors that allow pyruvate to be converted into a chemical that can enter the TCA cycle.

# Q

**QT INTERVAL.** The section on an electrocardiogram between the start of the QRS complex and the end of the T wave, representing the firing or depolarization of the ventricles and the period of recovery prior to repolarization, or recharging, for the next contraction.

**QUADRIPLEGIA.** Paralysis of all four limbs.

# R

**RNA.** Ribonucleic acid, the intermediate step between DNA and its final expression product. DNA is transcribed into RNA and RNA is translated into protein.

**RACHITIC.** Pertaining to, or affected by, rickets. Examples of rachitic deformities include curved long bones with prominent ends, a prominent middle chest wall, or bony nodules at the inner ends of the ribs.

**RADIAL KERATOTOMY (RK).** A surgical procedure involving the use of a diamond-tipped blade to make several spoke-like slits in the peripheral (non-viewing) portion of the cornea to improve the focus of the eye and correct myopia by flattening the cornea.

**RADIATION THERAPY.** Treatment using high-energy radiation from x-ray machines, cobalt, radium, or other sources.

**RADIATION.** High energy rays used in cancer treatment to kill or shrink cancer cells.

**RADICULOPATHY.** A bulging of disc material often irritating nearby nerve structures resulting in pain and neurologic symptoms. A clinical situation in which the radicular nerves (nerve roots) are inflamed or compressed. This compression by the bulging disc is referred to as a radiculopathy. This problem tends to occur most commonly in the neck (cervical spine) and low back (lumbar spine).

**RADIOGRAPHIC.** Involving an x ray.

**RADIOLUCENT.** Transparent to x ray or radiation. The black area on x-ray film.

**RADIUS.** One of the two bones of the forearm, the one adjacent to the base of the thumb.

**RANSON CRITERIA.** A system of measurements, including age and blood testing, that can be used to predict the outcome of a person who has been hospitalized for an episode of pancreatitis.

**RAYNAUD PHENOMENON/RAYNAUD DISEASE.** A condition in which blood flow to the body's tissues is reduced by a malfunction of the nerves that regulate the constriction of blood vessels. When attacks of Raynaud's occur in the absence of other medical conditions, it is called Raynaud disease. When attacks occur as part of a disease (as in scleroderma), it is called Raynaud phenomenon.

**RECESSIVE GENE.** A type of gene that is not expressed as a trait unless inherited by both parents.

**RECESSIVE.** Genetic trait expressed only when present on both members of a pair of chromosomes, one inherited from each parent.

**RECTAL SUCTION BIOPSY.** The removal and examination of a sample of rectum tissue for diagnostic purposes.

**RECTUM.** The end portion of the intestine that leads to the anus.

**RECURRENCE RISK.** The possibility that the same event will occur again.

RECURRENT. Tendency to repeat.

RED BLOOD CELL. Hemoglobin-containing blood cells that transport oxygen from the lungs to tissues. In the tissues, the red blood cells exchange their oxygen for carbon dioxide, which is brought back to the lungs to be exhaled.

RED BLOOD CELLS. Hemoglobin-containing blood cells that transport oxygen from the lungs to tissues. In the tissues, the red blood cells exchange their oxygen for carbon dioxide, which is brought back to the lungs to be exhaled.

RED NUCLEUS. A small structure present in the brainstem that is involved in the control of movement.

REFRACTION. The bending of light rays as they pass from one medium through another. Used to describe the action of the cornea and lens on light rays as they enter they eye. Also used to describe the determination and measurement of the eye's focusing system by an optometrist or ophthalmologist.

REFRACTIVE EYE SURGERY. A general term for surgical procedures that can improve or correct refractive errors by permanently changing the shape of the cornea.

RENAL AGENESIS. Complete absence of one or both kidneys.

RENAL ANGIOMYOLIPOMA. Benign (non-cancerous) tumors in the kidney that are made up of vascular tissue (angio), smooth muscle (myo), and fat (lipoma).

RENAL CELL CARCINOMA. A cancerous tumor made from kidney cells.

RENAL COLIC. A spasmodic pain, moderate to severe in degree, located in the back, side and/or groin area.

RENAL CYSTS. Fluid- or air-filled spaces within the kidneys.

RENAL DYSPLASIA. A developmental anomaly of the kidney.

RENAL HYPOPLASIA. Abnormally small kidneys.

RENAL SYSTEM. The organs involved with the production and output of urine.

RENAL TUBULAR DISORDER. Various defects in the renal tubular transport processes and their regulation.

RENAL. Pertaining to the kidney.

RENIN. An enzyme produced by the kidneys.

RENPENNING SYNDROME. X-linked mental retardation with short stature and microcephaly not associated with the fragile X chromosome and occurring more frequently in males, although some females may also be affected.

REPLICATE. Produce identical copies of itself.

REPOLARIZATION. Period when the heart cells are at rest, preparing for the next wave of electrical current (depolarization).

RESPIRATORY. Having to do with breathing.

RETICULOCYTE. Immature red blood cells.

RETINA. The light-sensitive layer of tissue in the back of the eye that receives and transmits visual signals to the brain through the optic nerve.

RETINAL ACHROMIC PATCH. Defect in the coloration of the retina.

RETINAL DYSPLASIA. Improper development of the retina that can lead to detachment of the retina.

RETINAL DYSTROPHY. Degeneration of the retina, causing a decline in visual clarity.

RETINAL HAMARTOMAS. Benign (non-cancerous) tumor found on the retina.

RETINAL LACUNAE. Small abnormal cavities or holes in the retina.

RETINAL PIGMENT EPITHELIUM (RPE). The pigmented cell layer that nourishes the retinal cells; located just outside the retina and attached to the choroid.

RETINITIS PIGMENTOSA. Progressive deterioration of the retina, often leading to vision loss and blindness.

RETINOBLASTOMA. A cancerous tumor of the eye.

RETINOIDS. A derivative of synthetic vitamin A.

RETINOPATHY. Any disorder of the retina.

RETINOPATHY. Noninflammatory or degenerative condition involving the retina of the eye.

RHABDOMYOLYSIS. Breakdown or disintegration of muscle tissue.

RHABDOMYOSARCOMA. A malignant tumor of the skeletal muscle.

RHEUMATOID ARTHRITIS. Chronic, autoimmune disease marked by inflammation of the membranes surrounding joints.

RHEUMATOID FACTOR. Antibodies present in the majority of individuals with rheumatoid arthritis. A diagnostic marker for rheumatoid arthritis that is absent from ankylosing spondylitis and other seronegative spondyloarthopathies.

**RHIZOMELIC.** Disproportionate shortening of the upper part of a limb compared to the lower part of the limb.

**RHO/RAC GUANINE EXCHANGE FACTOR.** Member of a class of proteins that appear to convey signals important in the structure and biochemical activity of cells.

**RICKETS.** A childhood disease caused by vitamin D deficiency, resulting in soft and malformed bones.

**RING CHROMOSOME.** An abnormal chromosome in which the terminal ends of the short (p) and long (q) arms have been lost and the remaining p and q arms subsequently join to form a ring.

**ROD.** Photoreceptor that is highly sensitive to low levels of light and transmits images in shades of gray.

**ROSENTHAL FIBERS.** Abnormal and irregularly shaped structures that form in astrocytes.

**RUSSELL SYNDROME.** An alternative term for Russell-Silver syndrome. Many doctors use this term to mean a Russell-Silver syndrome affected individual who does not have body asymmetry.

# S

**SACROILIAC JOINT.** The joint between the triangular bone below the spine (sacrum) and the hip bone (ilium).

**SACROILIITIS.** Inflammation of the sacroiliac joint.

**SACRUM.** Triangular bone at the base of the spinal column.

**SADDLE NOSE.** A sunken nasal bridge.

**SARCOIDOSIS.** A chronic disease characterized by nodules forming in the lymph nodes, lungs, bones, and skin.

**SARCOPLASMIC RETICULUM.** A system of tiny tubes located inside muscle cells that allow muscles to contract and relax by alternatively releasing and storing calcium.

**SATELLITES OF CHROMOSOMES.** Small segments of genetic material at the tips of the short arms of chromosomes 13, 14, 15, 21, and 22.

**SAVANT SKILLS.** Unusual talents, usually in art, math, or music, that some individuals with autism have in addition to the deficits of autism.

**SCAPHOCEPHALY.** An abnormally long and narrow skull.

**SCAPULA.** Shoulder blade.

**SCAPULAR WINGING.** The jutting back of the shoulder blades that can be caused by muscle weakness.

**SCHIZENCEPHALY.** Abnormality of the brain in which there are deep ruts and clefts in the surface of the brain.

**SCHWANNOMA.** Tumor that grows from the cells that line the nerves of the body (Schwann cells).

**SCINTIGRAPHY.** Injection and detection of radioactive substances to create images of body parts.

**SCLERA.** The tough white membrane that forms the outer layer of the eyeball.

**SCLERODERMA.** A relatively rare autoimmune disease affecting blood vessels and connective tissue that makes skin appear thickened.

**SCLEROSIS.** Hardening.

**SCOLIOMETER.** A tool for measuring trunk asymmetry; it includes a bubble level and angle measure.

**SCOLIOSIS.** An abnormal side-to-side curvature of the spine.

**SCREENING.** Process through which carriers of a trait may be identified within a population.

**SEBACEOUS.** Related to the glands of the skin that produce an oily substance.

**SECOND-DEGREE RELATIVE.** Aunts, uncles, nieces, nephews, grandparents, grandchildren and half siblings are second-degree relatives. These individuals have one fourth of their genes in common.

**SECONDARY CRANIOSYNOSTOSIS.** Abnormal closure of the cranial sutures caused by a failure of the brain to grow and expand.

**SEDATIVE.** Medication that has a soothing or tranquilizing effect.

**SEIZURE.** Any unusual body functions or activity that is under the control of the nervous system.

**SEIZURES.** An abnormal electrical discharge from the brain that usually results in convulsion of the body.

**SEMEN.** A whitish, opaque fluid released at ejaculation that contains sperm.

**SEMINAL VESICLES.** The pouches above the prostate that store semen.

**SENSITIVITY.** The proportion of people with a disease who are correctly diagnosed (test positive based on diagnostic criteria). The higher the sensitivity of a test or diagnostic criteria, the lower the rate of 'false negatives,' people who have a disease but are not identified through the test.

**SENSORINEURAL HEARING LOSS (SNHL).** Hearing loss that occurs when parts of the inner ear, such as the cochlea and/or auditory nerve, do not work correctly. It is often defined as mild, moderate, severe, or profound, depending upon how much sound can be heard by the affected individual.

**SENSORINEURAL.** Type of hearing loss due to a defect in the inner ear (sensing organ) and/or the acoustic nerve.

**SENSORY NEURONS.** Class of neurons that specifically regulate and control external stimuli (senses: sight, sound).

**SEPSIS.** An infection of the bloodstream.

**SEPTAL DEFECT.** A hole in the heart.

**SEPTAL.** Relating to the septum, the thin muscle wall dividing the right and left sides of the heart. Holes in the septum are called septal defects.

**SEPTUM PELLUCIDUM.** A membrane made of nerve tissue that separates areas of fluid in the left and right sides of the brain.

**SEQUENCE.** The combination of both a primary structural or functional anomaly, and the secondary anomalies produced by any abnormal forces or processes it generates.

**SERIAL CASTING.** A series of casts designed to gradually move a limb into a more functional position.

**SEROLOGICAL.** Pertaining to serology, the science of testing blood to detect the absence or presence of antibodies (an immune response) to a particular antigen (foreign substance).

**SEROSITIS.** Inflammation of a serosal membrane. Polyserositis refers to the inflammation of two or more serosal membranes.

**SEROTONIN DOPAMINE ANTAGONISTS (SDAS).** The newer second-generation antipsychotic drugs, also called atypical antipsychotics, including clozapine (Clozaril), risperidone (Risperdal), and olanzapine (Zyprexa).

**SEROTYPE.** One form of a bacteria that has unique surface proteins. Each serotype causes a unique antibody response from a person's immune system.

**SERUM CK TEST.** A blood test that determines the amount of the enzyme creatine kinase (CK) in the blood serum. An elevated level of CK in the blood indicates that muscular degeneration has occurred and/or is occurring.

**SERUM CREATININE.** A chemical in the urine of kidney patients used to determine kidney disease and failure. Elevated levels of serum creatinine are an early marker for severe kidney disease or failure.

**SERUM.** The liquid part of blood, from which all the cells have been removed.

**SEVERE COMBINED IMMUNODEFICIENCY (SCID).** A group of rare, life-threatening diseases present at birth, that cause a child to have little or no immune system. As a result, the child's body is unable to fight infections.

**SEX CHROMOSOMES.** The X and Y chromosomes that determine the sex of the individual.

**SEX-LINKED.** A gene located on, and thus a trait linked to, the X or Y chromosomes.

**SHAGREEN PATCH.** Area of tough and dimpled skin.

**SHOCK.** An inability to provide the body with the oxygen it requires, sometimes due to large amounts of bleeding or fluid loss.

**SHORT RIB POLYDACTYLY SYNDROMES.** A collection of genetic disorders characterized by abnormally short ribs and extra fingers or toes. Research is ongoing to determine if these disorders are the result of mutations in a common gene.

**SHORT STATURE.** An abnormally low height.

**SHORT TRUNK.** An abnormally short torso or body.

**SHUNT.** A small tube placed in a ventricle of the brain to direct cerebrospinal fluid away from the blockage into another part of the body.

**SIALIC ACID.** N-acetylneuraminic acid, a sugar that is often at the end of an oligosaccharide on a glycoprotein.

**SIALIDOSIS.** An inherited disorder known as neuraminidase deficiency.

**SICKLE CELL ANEMIA.** A chronic, inherited blood disorder characterized by sickle-shaped red blood cells. It occurs primarily in people of African descent, and produces symptoms including episodic pain in the joints, fever, leg ulcers, and jaundice.

**SICKLE CELL.** A red blood cell that has assumed a elongated shape due to the presence of hemoglobin S.

**SIGMOIDOSCOPY.** The visual examination of the inside of the rectum and sigmoid colon, using a lighted, flexible tube connected to an eyepiece or video screen for viewing.

**SIGN.** An indication of disease, injury, or other physical problem that can be observed by someone other than the person experiencing these conditions.

**SILVER SYNDROME.** An alternative term for Russell-Silver syndrome. Many doctors use this term to mean an individual with Russell-Silver syndrome who also has body asymmetry.

**SITUS SOLITUS.** Normal organ placement in the body with the heart, stomach, and spleen placed towards the left, and the liver and gallbladder on the right.

**SJÖGREN SYNDROME.** A chronic inflammatory disease often associated with rheumatoid arthritis.

**SKELETAL DYSPLASIA.** A group of syndromes consisting of abnormal prenatal bone development and growth.

**SKELETAL MUSCLE.** Muscles under voluntary control that attach to bone and control movement.

**SKEWED INACTIVATION.** Random inactivation of either the paternally or maternally derived X chromosome in the female; also called Lyonization, and occurs early in embryonic development.

**SKIN ERYTHEMA.** Irregular red streaks of skin.

**SKIN HEMATOMA.** Blood from a broken blood vessel that has accumulated under the skin.

**SLEEP APNEA.** A potentially life-threatening condition in which the individual has episodes during sleep in which breathing temporarily stops.

**SLEEP PARALYSIS.** An abnormal episode of sleep in which the patient cannot move for a few minutes, usually occurring on falling asleep or waking up. Often found in patients with narcolepsy.

**SLY DISEASE.** Autosomal recessive metabolic disorder caused by dysfunction of the lysosomal enzyme beta–glucuronidase.

**SMALL INTESTINE.** The part of the digestive tract in-between the stomach and the large intestine.

**SMALL TESTES.** Refers to the size of the male reproductive glands, located in the cavity of the scrotum.

**SOMATIC CELLS.** All the cells of the body except for the egg and sperm cells.

**SOMATIC.** Relating to the nonreproductive parts of the body.

**SOMATOSTATIN.** A body chemical, known as a cyclic peptide, involved in the release of human growth hormone from the pituitary gland.

**SORE.** An open wound or a bruise or lesion on the skin.

**SPASTIC PARAPLEGIA.** Inability to walk, due to lack of proper neural control over the leg muscles.

**SPASTIC QUADRIPARESIS.** Muscle spasms involve both the legs and the arms.

**SPASTIC.** A condition in which the muscles are rigid, posture may be abnormal, and fine motor control is impaired.

**SPASTICITY.** Increased muscle tone, or stiffness, which leads to uncontrolled, awkward movements.

**SPECIFICITY.** The proportion of people without a disease who are correctly classified as healthy or not having the disease (test negative based on diagnostic criteria). The higher the specificity of a test or diagnostic criteria, the lower the number of 'false positives,' people who don't have a disease but who 'test' positive.

**SPEECH THERAPIST.** Person who specializes in teaching simple exercises to improve speech.

**SPHEROCYTES.** Abnormal spherically shaped red blood cells caused by a disorder in the cell membrane; normally, the red blood cell is biconcave in shape.

**SPHINGOMYELIN.** A group of sphingolipids containing phosphorus.

**SPHINGOMYELINASE.** Enzyme required to breakdown sphingomyelin into ceramide.

**SPHYGMOMANOMETER.** An inflatable cuff used to measure blood pressure.

**SPINA BIFIDA OCCULTA.** The failure of vertebrae to close into the neural tube without nerves protruding. This is most often asymptomatic.

**SPINA BIFIDA.** An opening in the spine.

**SPINAL TAP.** A procedure by which a needle is inserted into the space between two lumbar vertebrae to obtain fluid that circulates around the spinal cord.

**SPLAY.** Turned outward or spread apart.

**SPLEEN.** Organ located in the upper abdominal cavity that filters out old red blood cells and helps fight bacterial infections. Responsible for breaking down spherocytes at a rapid rate.

SPLENECTOMY. Removal of the spleen.

SPLENIC FLEXURE. The area of the large intestine at which the transverse colon meets the descending colon.

SPLENOMEGALY. Enlargement of the spleen.

SPONDYLOEPIPHYSEAL DYSPLASIA. Abnormality of the vertebra and epiphyseal centers that causes a short trunk.

SPONDYLOSIS. Arthritis of the spine.

SPONGIFORM ENCEPHALOPATHY. A form of brain disease characterized by a "sponge-like" appearance of the brain either on autopsy or via magnetic resonance imaging (MRI).

SPONTANEOUS. Occurring by chance.

SPONYLOARTHRITIS (SPONDYLITIS). Inflammatory disease of the joints of the spine.

SPORADIC INHERITANCE. A status that occurs when a gene mutates spontaneously to cause the disorder in a person with no family history of the disorder.

SPORADIC. Isolated or appearing occasionally with no apparent pattern.

SPUTUM. A mixture of saliva and mucus from the lungs.

STAGE. As a noun: the extent to which an individual cancer has spread. A higher stage indicates a more serious disease than does a lower stage. As a verb: to determine the extent to which an individual cancer has spread.

STAGING. A method of describing the degree and location of cancer.

STANDARD DEVIATION. A statistical term that refers to the spread of data in a numerical distribution.

STATIC ENCEPHALOPATHY. A disease of the brain that does not get better or worse.

STELLATE. A star-like, lacy white pattern in the iris. Most often seen in light-eyed individuals.

STEM CELLS. Cells found in multi–cellular organisms. They are characterized by the ability to renew themselves through cell division and differentiating into a diverse range of specialized cell types.

STENOSIS. The constricting or narrowing of an opening or passageway.

STENT. A tubular device made of metal or plastic that is inserted into a body duct or tube to prevent collapse, blockage, or overgrowth.

STILLBIRTH. The birth of a baby who has died sometime during the pregnancy or delivery.

STILLBORN. The birth of a baby who has died sometime during the pregnancy or delivery.

STOMACH. An organ that holds and begins digestion of food.

STOMACH. An organ that holds and begins digestion of food.

STRABISMUS. Condition in which the eyes are not properly aligned with each other.

STROKE. A sudden neurological condition related to a block of blood flow in part of the brain, which can lead to a variety of problems, including paralysis, difficulty speaking, difficulty understanding others, or problems with balance.

STROMA. Middle layer of the cornea, representing about 90% of the entire cornea.

SUBARACHNOID SPACE. The space between two membranes surrounding the brain, the arachnoid and pia mater.

SUBCORTICAL BAND HETEROTOPIA. A mild form of lissencephaly type 1 in which abnormal bands of gray and white matter are present beneath the cortex near the ventricles.

SUBCORTICAL INFARCTS. Obstruction of nerve centers below the cerebral cortex of the brain.

SUBEPENDYMAL GIANT CELL ASTROCYTOMA. Benign (non-cancerous) tumor of the brain comprised of star-shaped cells (astrocytes).

SUBEPENDYMAL NODULE. Growth found underneath the lining of the ventricles in the brain.

SUBMETACENTRIC. Positioning of the centromere between the center and the top of the chromosome.

SUBSTANTIA NIGRA. One of the movement control centers of the brain.

SUBSTRATE. A compound on which an enzyme works in a biochemical reaction.

SUDDEN INFANT DEATH SYNDROME (SIDS). The general term given to "crib deaths" of unknown causes.

SULFATE. A chemical compound containing sulfur and oxygen.

SUTURE. "Seam" that joins two surfaces together.

**SYMPHALANGISM.** Fusion of phalanges at their ends.

**SYMPTOM.** An indication of disease, injury, or other physical problem reported by the person experiencing these conditions, but not by some outside observer.

**SYNCHRONOUS.** Occurring simultaneously.

**SYNCOPE.** A brief loss of consciousness caused by insufficient blood flow to the brain.

**SYNDACTYLY.** Webbing or fusion between the fingers or toes.

**SYNDROME.** A group of signs and symptoms that collectively characterize a disease or disorder.

**SYNDROMIC HEARING LOSS.** Hearing loss accompanied by other symptoms that characterize a larger genetic syndrome of which hearing loss is just one of the characteristics.

**SYNKINESIA.** Occurs when part of the body will move involuntarily when another part of the body moves.

**SYNOPHRYS.** A feature in which the eyebrows join in the middle. Also called blepharophimosis.

**SYNOVITIS.** Inflammation of the synovium, a membrane found inside joints.

**SYRINGOMYELIA.** Excessive fluid in the spinal cord.

**SYSTEMIC SCLEROSIS.** A rare disorder that causes thickening and scarring of multiple organ systems.

**SYSTOLIC BLOOD PRESSURE.** Blood pressure when the heart contracts (beats).

# T

**TCA CYCLE.** Formerly know as the Kreb's cycle, this is the process by which glucose and other chemicals are broken down into forms that are directly useable as energy in the cells.

**TACHYCARDIA.** An excessively rapid heartbeat; a heart rate above 100 beats per minute.

**TAFAZZIN GENE.** A human gene that encodes the enzyme tafazzin, which is expressed at high levels in cardiac and skeletal muscle. Mutations in this gene have been associated with a number of disorders, including Barth syndrome and dilated cardiomyopathy.

**TAFAZZIN.** An enzyme involved in the biosynthesis of cardiolipin.

**TAI-CHI.** A Chinese system of physical exercises that uses slow, smooth body movements to help with posture control and relaxation.

**TALIPES EQUINOVARUS.** A type of club-foot characterized by a downward and inward pointing foot.

**TAY-SACHS DISEASE.** An inherited biochemical disease caused by lack of a specific enzyme in the body. In classical Tay-Sachs disease, previously normal children become blind and mentally handicapped, develop seizures, and decline rapidly. Death often occurs between the ages of three to five years. Tay-Sachs disease is common among individuals of eastern European Jewish background but has been reported in other ethnic groups.

**TELANGIECTASIA.** An abnormal widening of groups of small blood vessels in the skin.

**TELANGIECTASIS.** Very small arteriovenous malformations, or connections between the arteries and veins. The result is small red spots on the skin known as "spider veins."

**TELANGIECTATIC.** A localized collection of distended blood capillary vessels.

**TELOGEN.** The resting phase of the hair growth cycle.

**TENDON REFLEX.** Reflex contraction of the muscle that is observed by tapping on its tendon.

**TENDON.** A strong connective tissue that connects muscle to bone.

**TENOTOMY.** A surgical procedure that cuts the tendon of a contracted muscle to allow lengthening.

**TENSILON TEST.** A test for diagnosing myasthenia gravis. Tensilon is injected into a vein and, if the person has MG, their muscle strength will improve for about five minutes.

**TERATOGEN.** Any drug, chemical, maternal disease, or exposure that can cause physical or functional defects in an exposed embryo or fetus.

**TERATOGENIC FACTOR.** Any factor that can produce congenital abnormalities.

**TERATOGENIC.** Any agent that can cause birth defects or mental retardation in a developing fetus. Common teratogens are medications or other chemicals but they also include infections, radiation, maternal medical condition, and other agents.

**TERMINAL DELETION.** The abnormal early termination of a chromosome caused by the deletion of one of its ends.

**TESTES.** The male reproductive organs that produce male reproductive cells (sperm) and male hormones.

**TESTICLES.** Two egg-shaped glands that produce sperm and sex hormones.

**TESTOSTERONE.** Hormone produced in the testicles that is involved in male secondary sex characteristics.

**TETRALOGY OF FALLOT.** A heart defect involving a ventricular septal defect, enlarged right ventricle, malformed aorta, and pulmonary stenosis.

**TETRAMER.** Protein that consists of four amino acid chains.

**TETRAPHOCOMELIA.** Absence of all, or a portion of, all four limbs. The hands or feet may be attached directly to the trunk.

**TETRAPLEGIA.** Paralysis of all four limbs. Also called quadriplegia.

**TETRASOMY.** Referring to the presence of four parts or copies of a chromosome or part of a chromosome.

**THALAMUS.** A pair of large egg-shaped structures near the brainstem that act as the main sensory relay station and help with control of movement.

**THALIDOMIDE.** A mild sedative that is teratogenic, causing limb, neurologic, and other birth defects in infants exposed during pregnancy. Women used thalidomide (early in pregnancy) in Europe and in other countries between 1957 and 1961. It is still available in many places, including the United States, for specific medical uses (leprosy, AIDS, cancer).

**THERMOLABILE.** Heat-sensitive. A thermolabile protein is a protein that easily loses its shape when heated even only slightly.

**THORACIC CAVITY.** The chest.

**THORACOPAGUS.** Conjoined twins joined at the upper body who share a heart.

**THORAX.** Chest cavity.

**THROMBOCYTOPENIA.** A persistent decrease in the number of blood platelets usually associated with hemorrhaging.

**THROMBOEMBOLISM.** A condition in which a blood vessel is blocked by a free-floating blood clot carried in the blood stream.

**THROMBOPHILIA.** A disorder in which there is a greater tendency for thrombosis (clot in blood vessel).

**THROMBOPHLEBITIS.** Inflammation of veins due to blood clots.

**THYMUS GLAND.** An endocrine gland located in the front of the neck that houses and transports T cells, which help to fight infection.

**THYROID STIMULATING HORMONE (THYROTROPIN).** A hormone that stimulates the thyroid gland to produce hormones that regulate metabolism.

**THYROXINE (T4).** Thyroid hormone.

**TIC.** Brief and intermittent involuntary movement or sound.

**TINNITUS.** Noises in the ear that can include ringing, whistling or booming.

**TISSUE.** Group of similar cells that work together to perform a particular function. The four basic types of tissue include muscle, nerve, epithelial, and connective tissues.

**TITUBATION.** Tremor of the head.

**TONE.** A term used to describe the tension of muscles. Increased tone is increased tension in the muscles.

**TONOMETER.** A device used to measure fluid pressures of the eye.

**TORSADE DE POINTES.** Term that means turning of the points; a type of fast heart beat or tachycardia of the ventricles that is characteristic of long QT syndrome.

**TORTICOLLIS.** Twisting of the neck to one side that results in abnormal carriage of the head and is usually caused by muscle spasms. Also called wryneck.

**TORTUOUS.** Having many twists or turns.

**TOXIC.** Poisonous.

**TRABECULAR MESHWORK.** A sponge–like tissue that drains the aqueous humor from the eye.

**TRACHEA.** Long tube connecting from the larynx down into the lungs, responsible for passing air.

**TRACHEO-ESOPHAGEAL FISTULA.** Abnormal connection between the trachea and esophagus, frequently associated with the esophagus ending in a blind pouch.

**TRACHEOSTOMY.** An opening surgically created in the trachea (windpipe) through the neck to improve breathing.

**TRACTION ALOPECIA.** Hair loss caused by pressure or tension on the scalp related to certain types of hair styles or equipment worn on the head.

**TRANS-RECTAL ULTRASOUND.** A procedure where a probe is placed in the rectum. High-frequency sound waves that cannot be heard by humans are sent out from the probe and reflected by the prostate. These sound waves produce a pattern of echoes that are then used by the computer to create sonograms or pictures of areas inside the body.

**TRANSCRIPTION FACTOR.** A factor that activates the transformation of DNA to RNA (the next step is translation, where RNA is changed into protein).

**TRANSCRIPTION FACTORS.** Cellular-signaling components that cause the transcription of a gene.

**TRANSCRIPTION.** The process by which genetic information on a strand of DNA is used to synthesize a strand of complementary RNA.

**TRANSFUSION.** The injection of a component of the blood from a healthy person into the circulation of a person who is lacking or deficient in that same component of the blood.

**TRANSIENT ISCHEMIC ATTACK (TIA).** A neurologic dysfunction that comes and goes quickly and is similar to a stroke.

**TRANSLATION.** The process by which RNA is changed into protein.

**TRANSLOCATION.** The transfer of one part of a chromosome to another chromosome during cell division. A balanced translocation occurs when pieces from two different chromosomes exchange places without loss or gain of any chromosome material. An unbalanced translocation involves the unequal loss or gain of genetic information between two chromosomes.

**TRANSMEMBRANE.** Anything that spans the width of a membrane.

**TRANSMISSIBLE SPONGIFORM ENCEPHALOPATHY.** A term that refers to a group of diseases, including kuru, Creutzfeldt-Jakob disease, Gerstmann-StrSussler-Scheinker syndrome, fatal familial insomnia, and new variant Creutzfeldt-Jakob disease. These diseases share a common origin as prion diseases, caused by abnormal proteins that accumulate within the brain and destroy brain tissue, leaving spongy holes.

**TRANSPLANTATION.** The implanting of an organ from either a deceased person (cadaver) or from a live donor to a person whose organ has failed.

**TRANSPOSITION OF THE GREAT ARTERIES.** A reversal of the two great arteries of the heart, causing blood containing oxygen to be carried back to the lungs and blood that is lacking in oxygen to be transported throughout the body.

**TRANSPOSITION OF THE GREAT VESSELS (TGV).** A congenital heart defect in which the major vessels of the heart are attached to the wrong chambers of the heart.

**TRANSVAGINAL ULTRASOUND.** A way to view the ovaries using sound waves. A probe is inserted into the vagina and the ovaries can be seen. Color doppler imaging measures the amount of blood flow, as tumors sometimes have high levels of blood flow.

**TRANSVERSION.** A genetic term referring to a specific substitution of one base pair for another. There are only four possible tranversions: guanine for cytosine, cytosine for guanine, adenine for thymine, or thymine for adenine.

**TRAUMA.** Injury.

**TRICHOTILLOMANIA.** A psychiatric disorder characterized by hair loss resulting from compulsive pulling or tugging on one's hair.

**TRIGGER DRUGS.** Specific drugs used for muscle relaxation and anesthesia that can trigger an episode of malignant hyperthermia in a susceptible person. The trigger drugs include halothane, enflurane, isoflurane, sevoflurane, desflurane, methoxyflurane, ether, and succinylcholine.

**TRIGLYCERIDE.** A type of lipid consisting of a molecule of glycerol and three fatty acid fragments.

**TRIGLYCERIDES.** Certain combinations of fatty acids (types of lipids) and glycerol.

**TRIGONOCEPHALY.** An abnormal development of the skull characterized by a triangular shaped forehead.

**TRIIODOTHYRONINE (T3).** Thyroid hormone.

**TRIMESTER.** A three-month period. Human pregnancies are normally divided into three trimesters: first (conception to week 12), second (week 13 to week 24), and third (week 25 until delivery).

**TRINUCLEOTIDE REPEAT EXPANSION.** A sequence of three nucleotides that is repeated too many times in a section of a gene.

**TRINUCLEOTIDE.** A sequence of three nucleotides.

**TRIOSE PHOSPHATE ISOMERASE.** Abbreviated TPI, this is the enzyme responsible for the conversion of dihydroxyacetone phosphate (DHAP) into D-glyceraldehyde-3-phosphate (GAP). DHAP and GAP are the two major products of a step in the multi-step process that converts glucose into ATP to supply the body with the energy it needs to sustain itself. Only GAP can continue in this process, but DHAP is produced in much higher quantities. People with TPI deficiency cannot change DHAP into GAP as efficiently as unaffected people, resulting in insufficient amounts of ATP from glucose to maintain normal cell function.

**TRIPHALANGEAL THUMB (TPT).** A thumb that has three bones rather than two.

**TRIPLOID.** Three sets of chromosomes; in humans, this is 69 chromosomes.

**TRISMUS.** Inability to open the mouth completely.

**TRISOMY 18.** A chromosomal alteration where a child is born with three copies of chromosome number 18 and as a result is affected with multiple birth defects and mental retardation.

**TRISOMY.** The condition of having three identical chromosomes, instead of the normal two, in a cell.

**TRUNCUS ARTERIOSUS.** Having only one artery coming from the heart instead of two. Often there is a ventricular septal defect (VSD) present.

**TRYPSIN.** A digestive enzyme found in pancreatic fluid that breaks down proteins. This enzyme is abnormal in hereditary pancreatitis.

**TRYPTOPHAN.** A crystalline amino acid widely distributed in proteins and essential to human life.

**TUBULE.** A small tube lined with glandular epithelium in the kidney.

**TUMOR NECROSIS FACTOR.** A protein that plays an early and major role in the rheumatic disease process.

**TUMOR SUPPRESSOR GENE.** Genes involved in controlling normal cell growth and preventing cancer.

**TUMOR.** An abnormal growth of cells. Tumors may be benign (noncancerous) or malignant (cancerous).

**TURNER SYNDROME.** Chromosome abnormality characterized by short stature and ovarian failure, caused by an absent X chromosome. Occurs only in females.

**TYMPANOPLASTY.** Any of several operations on the eardrum or small bones of the middle ear, to restore or improve hearing in patients with conductive hearing loss.

**TYPE I INCONTINENTIA PIGMENTI.** Sporadic IP. This disorder is caused by mutations in the gene at Xp11. These mutations are not inherited from the parents, they are *de novo* mutations. This type of IP probably represents a different disease than type II IP.

**TYPE II INCONTINENTIA PIGMENTI.** Familial, male-lethal type IP. This type of IP is the "classic" case of IP. It is caused by mutations in the NEMO gene located at Xq28. Inheritance is sex-linked recessive.

**TYPE XI COLLAGEN.** A type of collagen that produces an organic gel which helps cartilage to convert into bone and helps bone growth in the developing fetus.

**TYROSINE.** An aromatic amino acid that is made from phenylalanine.

# U

**ULNA.** One of the two bones of the forearm, the one opposite the thumb.

**ULTRASONOGRAM.** The image produced by the use of inaudible sound of high frequency called ultrasound to photograph a tissue, organ, or infant.

**ULTRASOUND EVALUATION.** A procedure which examines the tissue and bone structures of an individual or a developing baby.

**ULTRASOUND EXAMINATION.** Visualizing the unborn baby while it is still inside the uterus.

**ULTRASOUND.** An imaging technique that uses sound waves to help visualize internal structures in the body.

**UMBILICAL HERNIA.** Protrusion of the bowels through the abdominal wall, underneath the navel.

**UNDESCENDED TESTICLES.** Testicles that failed to move from the abdomen to the scrotum during the development of the fetus.

**UNILATERAL.** Refers to one side of the body or only one organ in a pair.

**UNIPARENTAL DISOMY.** Chromosome abnormality in which both chromosomes in a pair are inherited from the same parent.

**UPSHOOT.** Upward movement of the eye.

**UREA CYCLE DISORDER.** A disease that is caused by a lack of an enzyme that cleans the blood of ammonia.

**UREA CYCLE.** A series of complex biochemical reactions that remove nitrogen from the blood so ammonia does not accumulate.

**UREA.** A nitrogen-containing compound that can be excreted through the kidney.

**UREMIC POISONING.** Accumulation of waste products in the body.

URETERS. Tubes through which urine is transported from the kidneys to the bladder.

URETHRA. The tubular portion of the urinary tract connecting the bladder and external meatus through which urine passes. In males, seminal fluid and sperm also pass through the urethra.

URETHRITIS. Inflammation of the urethra.

URINARY URGENCY. An exaggerated or increased sense of needing to urinate.

URTICARIA. Also known as hives. Usually associated with an allergic reaction.

UTERUS. A muscular, hollow organ of the female reproductive tract. The uterus contains and nourishes the embryo and fetus from the time the fertilized egg is implanted until birth.

UVEITIS. Inflammation of all or part of the uvea, which consists of the middle vascular portion of the eye including the iris, ciliary body, and choroid.

# V

VACCINE. An injection, usually derived from a microorganism, that can be injected into an individual to provoke an immune response and prevent future occurrence of an infection by that microorganism.

VACUOLATION. The formation of multiple vesicles, or vacuoles, within the cytosol of cells.

VARIABLE EXPRESSION. Ability of the same gene to cause different symptoms in different people (with the same disorder).

VARIABLE EXPRESSIVITY. Differences in the symptoms of a disorder between family members with the same genetic disease.

VARIABLE PENETRANCE. A term describing the way in which the same mutated gene can cause symptoms of different severity and type within the same family.

VARIABLE PENETRANCE. A term describing the way in which the same mutated gene can cause symptoms of different severity and type within the same family.

VAS DEFERENS. The long, muscular tube that connects the epididymis to the urethra through which sperm are transported during ejaculation.

VASCULAR MALFORMATION. Abnormality of the blood vessels that often appears as a red or pink patch on the surface of the skin.

VASCULAR. Having to do with blood vessels.

VASODILATOR. A drug that relaxes blood vessel walls.

VELLUS HAIRS. The fine lighter-colored hairs that result from miniaturization.

VELO. Derived from the Latin word *velum*, meaning palate and back of the throat.

VENOUS THROMBOEMBOLISM. A blood clot that breaks free of its location in a vein and moves elsewhere in the body.

VENOUS THROMBOSIS. A condition caused by the presence of a clot in the vein.

VENOUS. Term used to describe a vein or the entire system of veins.

VENTILATOR. Mechanical breathing machine.

VENTRAL WALL DEFECT. An opening in the abdomen (ventral wall). Examples include omphalocele and gastroschisis.

VENTRICLE. The fluid filled spaces in the center of the brain that hold cerebral spinal fluid.

VENTRICLES. One of the chambers (small cavities) of the heart through which blood circulates. The heart is divided into the right and left ventricles.

VENTRICULAR SEPTAL DEFECT (VSD). An opening between the right and left ventricles of the heart.

VENTRICULOPERITONEAL SHUNT. A tube equipped with a low pressure valve, one end of which is inserted into the lateral ventricles, the other end of which is routed into the peritoneum, or abdominal cavity.

VERMIS. The central portion of the cerebellum, which divides the two hemispheres. It functions to monitor and control movement of the limbs, trunk, head, and eyes.

VERTEBRA. One of the 23 bones which comprise the spine. *Vertebrae* is the plural form.

VERTEBRAE. Boney structures of the spine.

VERTEBRAL DIVISIONS. The human vertebral regions are divided into cervical, thoracic, lumbar, and sacral from the neck to the tailbone.

VERTEBRAL. Related to the vertebrae.

VERTICAL GAZE PALSY. Uncontrolled up and down motions of the eye.

VERY LONG CHAIN FATTY ACIDS (VLCFA). A type of fat that is normally broken down by the peroxisomes into other fats that can be used by the body.

**VERY-LOW-DENSITY LIPOPROTEINS (VLDLS).** Lipoproteins located in the blood that transport fats and cholesterol from the liver to other places in the body.

**VESTIBULAR NERVE.** The nerve that transmits the electrical signals collected in the inner ear to the brain. These signals, and the responses to them, help maintain balance.

**VESTIBULAR SYSTEM.** A complex organ located inside the inner ear that sends messages to the brain about movement and body position. Allows people to maintain their balance when moving by sensing changes in their direction and speed.

**VISUAL ACUITY.** The ability to distinguish details and shapes of objects.

**VISUAL CORTEX.** The area of the brain responsible for receiving visual stimuli from the eyes and integrating it to form a composite picture of an object.

**VITAMIN K.** A vital substance that is obtained by eating certain foods, such as leafy greens, but mainly through bacterial manufacture in the large intestine.

**VITAMIN DEFICIENCY.** Abnormally low levels of a vitamin in the body.

**VITREOUS HUMOR OF THE EYE.** The clear gel inside the eyeball.

**VITREOUS.** The jelly-like substance that fills the inner eyeball.

**VOLTAGE-GATED CALCIUM CHANNEL.** A type of voltage-gated (voltage-dependent) ion channel found in excitable cells (such as muscles, neurons) that are permeable to the calcium ion.

**VOLUNTARY MUSCLE.** A muscle under conscious control, such as arm and leg muscles.

**VOLVULUS.** A twisted loop of bowel, causing obstruction.

**VON WILLEBRAND FACTOR (VWF).** A protein found in the blood that is involved in the process of blood clotting.

# W

**WEYERS ACROFACIAL DYSOSTOSIS.** The condition resulting from a mutation of the same gene that shows mutation in Ellis-van Creveld syndrome. As is usually the case when comparing expressions of the same gene mutation, the single dose Weyers acrofacial dysostosis presents milder symptoms than the double dose Ellis-van Creveld syndrome.

**WHIPPLE PROCEDURE.** Surgical removal of the pancreas and surrounding areas, including a portion of the small intestine, the duodenum.

**WHITE BLOOD CELL.** A cell in the blood that helps fight infections.

**WHITE MATTER.** A substance found in the brain and nervous system that protects nerves and allows messages to be sent to and from to brain to the various parts of the body.

**WILSON DISEASE.** A rare hereditary disease marked by high levels of copper deposits in the brain and liver.

**WOLFFIAN DUCTS.** Structures in the embryo that develop into epididymides, vasa deferentia, and seminal vesicles in males.

**WOOD'S LIGHT.** An ultraviolet light used in medical settings because of its ability to create fluorescence in the presence of substances such as porphyrins.

**WORD SALAD.** Speech that is so disorganized that it makes no linguistic or grammatical sense.

**WORMIAN BONES.** A condition of the bones and cartilage in which growing bones are abnormally connected by thin string-like structures.

# X

**X CHROMOSOME.** One of the two sex chromosomes (the other is Y) containing genetic material that, among other things, determine a person's gender.

**X INACTIVATION.** Sometimes called "dosage compensation". A normal process in which one X chromosome in every cell of every female is permanently inactivated.

**X RAY.** An imaging test that uses beams of energy to create images of structures within the body.

**X–LINKED GENE.** A gene carried on the X chromosome, one of the two sex chromosomes.

**X-LINKED DISORDER.** Any disorder caused by genes located on the X chromosome.

**X-LINKED DOMINANT INHERITANCE.** The inheritance of a trait by the presence of a single gene on the X chromosome in a male or female, passed from an affected female who has the gene on one of her X chromosomes.

**X-LINKED MENTAL RETARDATION.** Subaverage general intellectual functioning that originates during the developmental period and is associated with impairment in adaptive behavior. Pertains to genes on the X chromosome.

X-LINKED MUTATION. An abnormal gene transmitted on the X chromosome.

X-LINKED RECESSIVE INHERITANCE. The inheritance of a trait by the presence of a single gene on the X chromosome in a male, passed from a female who has the gene on one of her X chromosomes. She is referred to as an unaffected carrier.

X-LINKED TRAITS. Genetic conditions associated with mutations in genes on the X chromosome. A male carrying such a mutation will contract the disorder associated with it because he carries only one X chromosome. A female carrying a mutation on just one X chromosome, with a normal gene on the other chromosome, will not be affected by the disease.

X-LINKED. A genetic trait that is carried on the X chromosome.

XANTHOMAS. Small, yellow fat deposits that appear in the skin.

YOGA. An exercise that combines relaxation and breathing techniques to combat stress and help circulation and movement of the joints; yoga has its origin in ancient Indian medicine.

# Z

ZELLWEGER SPECTRUM. Disorders that result from defects in the assembly of the peroxisome. Also called peroxisome biogenesis disorders (PBD). They include: Zellweger syndrome (ZS), neonatal adrenoleukodystrophy (NALD), rhizomelic chondrodysplasia (RC) and infantile Refsum disease (IRD).

ZYGOTE. The sperm and egg combined to form the initial cell when a new organism is produced by means of sexual reproduction.

# INDEX

In the index, references to individual volumes are listed before colons; numbers following a colon refer to specific page numbers within that particular volume. **Boldface** page numbers indicate main topical essays. Photographs and illustration references are highlighted with an *italicized* page number; and tables are also indicated with the page number followed by a lowercase, italicized *t*.

1-deamino-8-D-arginine vasopressin. *See* Desmopressin

3-methylcrotonylglycemia, 2:1129, 1131, 1132

3-methylglutaconic acid, 1:181

3-methylglutaconic aciduria type II. *See* Barth syndrome

3,4-DAP, for congenital myasthenic syndromes, 1:291

3B hydroxysteroid dehydrogenase deficiency, 1:765

3GUCY2D gene mutations, 1:350

4-Maleylacetoacetic acid, 1:70

4-phenylbutyrate, for ALD, 1:47

4p-syndrome. *See* Wolf-Hirschhorn syndrome

5-alpha reductase, hair loss and, 1:691, 694

5-OH-indole-3-acetic acid, Cornelia de Lange syndrome and, 1:376

5p minus Society, 1:393

5p minus syndrome. *See* Cri du chat syndrome

6RIM1 gene mutations, 1:350

7-dehydrocholesterol, Smith-Lemli-Optiz syndrome and, 2:1418, 1419

7Pipherin/RDS gene mutations, 1:350

11B-hydroxlase deficiency, 1:765

11q deletion syndrome. *See* Jacobsen syndrome

13GUCA1A,18 gene mutations, 1:350

17-beta-hydroxysteroid dehydrogenase, 2:1232

17-hydroxyprogesterone, congenital adrenal hyperplasia and, 1:352, 354

18p deletion syndrome. *See* De Grouchy syndrome

18q deletion syndrome. *See* De Grouchy syndrome

21-hydroxylase deficiency, 1:765

21-hydroxylase deficiency (CAH21), 1:351, 352, 353, 657

22q11 deletion syndrome. *See* Deletion 22q11 syndrome

22q11.2 deletion syndromes, 1:272, 273

22q13 deletion syndrome, 1:**1–3**

22q13 Deletion Syndrome Foundation, 1:1, 2

47,XXX syndrome. *See* Triple X syndrome

47,XXY syndrome. *See* Klinefelter syndrome

47,XYY syndrome. *See* XYY syndrome

48-X syndrome. *See* XXXX syndrome

69,XXX/69,XXY/69,XYY karyotype, 2:1502, 1503

# A

A-beta amyloid neuritic plaques, 1:89

A-beta amyloid protein, 1:87, 88, 89

A-DNA, 1:462

A-T. *See* Ataxia-telangiectasia

A-T gene mutations, 1:159, 160

AACAP (American Academy of Child and Adolescent Psychiatry), 1:164

AAD (American Academy of Dermatology), 1:18

AAO (American Academy of Ophthalmology), 2:1051

AAP (American Academy of Pediatrics), 1:25, 27, 2:1217

Aarskog, Dagfinn, 1:3

Aarskog syndrome, 1:**3–5**, *4*

Aase syndrome, 1:**5–7**

ABCA1 gene mutations, 2:1459–1460, 1461

ABCA4 gene mutations, 2:1448, 1449

ABCC6 gene mutations, 2:1288, 1289

ABCC8 gene mutations, 1:447

ABCR gene mutations. *See* ABCA4 gene mutations

Abdominal mass, with pyloric stenosis, 2:1291

Abdominal pain
   familial Mediterranean fever, 1:558, 559
   hereditary coproporphyria, 1:731, 732, 733
   hereditary pancreatitis, 1:751–752, 753
   lipoprotein lipase deficiency, 1:905, 906
   ovarian cancer, 2:1157
   pancreatic cancer, 2:1172
   porphyrias, 2:1245

Abdominal wall abnormalities
   amelia, 1:91, 94
   amyoplasia, 1:104
   Beckwith-Wiedemann syndrome, 1:192, 194
   gastroschisis, 1:*619*, 619–622
   prune-belly syndrome, 2:1280, 1281
   triploidy, 2:1504
   trisomy 18, 2:1517
   *See also* Omphaloceles

Abducens nerve abnormalities, 1:473, 2:988

Abduction, Duane retraction syndrome and, 1:473, 476

Aberfeld syndrome. *See* Schwartz-Jampel syndrome

Abetalipoproteinemia (ABL), 1:**7–9**

ABGC (American Board of Genetic Counseling), 1:636

ABL. *See* Abetalipoproteinemia

Ablation of tumors, for liver cancer, 1:720

Abnormal *vs.* normal conditions, 1:652–653

Abortion. *See* Termination of pregnancy

Abortive cryptophthalmos, 1:589, 590

Absence of vas deferens, 1:**10–12**

Absence seizures, with Aicardi syndrome, 1:50

Absent corpous callosum. *See* Agenesis of the corpus callosum

Alopecia areata
    celiac disease and, 1:275
    as hair loss syndrome, 1:692, 693,
        694, 695
ALP. *See* Alkaline phosphatase
Alpers disease *vs.* Leigh syndrome,
    1:890
Alpha-1 antitrypsin, 1:**75–79**, 717
Alpha-1 microglobulin, Dent's
    disease and, 1:435
Alpha agonists, for glaucoma, 1:665
Alpha/beta blockers, for essential
    hypertension, 1:535
Alpha-blockers, for essential
    hypertension, 1:535
Alpha-fetoprotein (AFP) testing
    for amelia, 1:93
    amniocentesis and, 1:100
    for anencephaly, 1:117
    for ataxia-telangiectasia, 1:160
    for Beckwith-Wiedemann
        syndrome, 1:195
    for encephaloceles, 1:516
    for liver cancer, 1:719
    for Meckel-Gruber syndrome,
        2:962, 963
    for neural tube defects, 2:1077
    for oligohydramnios sequence,
        2:1115
    for omphaloceles, 2:1116
    as screening test, 1:97
    for spina bifida, 2:1430
    *See also* Maternal serum alpha-
        fetoprotein testing
Alpha-galactosidase A, 1:541, 542, 543
Alpha globin, 1:196, 2:1469, 1472
Alpha globin gene mutations, 1:363,
    2:1472, 1473
Alpha-glucosidase, 1:672
Alpha-glucosidase inhibitors, 1:451
Alpha-L-iduronidase, 2:1002,
    1005–1006, 1007, 1008
Alpha-mannosidosis, 2:939, 940
Alpha-N-acetylneuraminidase.
    *See* Neuraminidase
Alpha-sarcoglycan protein, 2:1038
Alpha-synuclein, 2:1181
Alpha thalassemia major, 2:1469,
    1473, 1474–1475, 1476
Alpha thalassemia mental retardation
    syndrome, 2:1473
Alpha thalassemia minor, 2:1469
Alpha thalassemia silent carriers,
    2:1469, 1473
Alpha thalassemia trait, 2:1471, 1473
Alpha-thalassemia X-linked mental
    retardation syndrome, 1:**79–82,** 2:1473
Alpha thalassemias
    as anemia, 1:79, 81
    demographics, 2:1471
    description, 2:1468–1469
    genetics, 2:1472–1473
    hydrops fetalis and, 1:790, 791

ALPL gene mutations, 2:1413
Alport's syndrome, 1:561–564, 565,
    736, 737, 740
ALS. *See* Amyotrophic lateral sclerosis
ALS Society, 1:108
Alstrom, Carl-Henry, 1:82
Alstrom syndrome, 1:**82–85**
ALT (Alanine aminotransferase)
    tests, 1:78
Alternative treatments
    ALS, 1:108
    arthrogryposis multiplex
        congenital, 1:136–137
    Asperger syndrome, 1:141
    asthma, 1:152
    cancer, 1:254
    cystic fibrosis, 1:406
    dystonia, 1:493
    Ehlers-Danlos syndrome, 1:507
    familial pulmonary arterial
        hypertension, 1:568–569
    multiple sclerosis, 2:1032
    osteogenesis imperfecta, 2:1146
    Parkinson disease, 2:1184
    porphyrias, 2:1247
    X-linked severe combined
        immunodeficiency, 2:1601
Altmann, Richard, 1:461
Alzheimer, Alois, 1:85, 599
Alzheimer's disease, 1:**85–90**, *86*
    as dementia, 1:425–426, 429
    Down syndrome and, 1:87, 88, 89,
        426, 470
    *vs.* frontotemporal dementia, 1:602
    genetic testing and, 1:88, 648
Amantadine
    for Friedreich ataxia, 1:596
    for Parkinson disease, 2:1184
Amastia, 1:495, 497
Ambiguous genitalia, 1:**656–659**
    androgen insensitivity syndrome,
        1:112
    hermaphroditism, 1:765
    trisomy 13, 2:1513
    XX male syndrome, 2:1607, 1608
AMC (Arthrogryposis multiplex
    congenital), 1:102
Amelia, 1:**90–94**
Ameloblastin production, 1:95
Amelogenesis imperfecta, 1:**94–96,**
    349, 350
Amelogenin, 1:95
AMELX gene mutations, 1:95
AMELY gene mutations, 1:95
Amenorrhea, 1:352, 353, 2:1531
American Academy of Child and
    Adolescent Psychiatry (AACAP),
    1:164
American Academy of Dermatology
    (AAD), 1:18
American Academy of Neurology,
    1:602, 2:980

American Academy of
    Ophthalmology (AAO), 2:1051
American Academy of Pediatrics
    (AAP), 1:25, 27, 2:1217
American Board of Genetic
    Counseling (ABGC), 1:636
American Cancer Society (ACS)
    breast cancer, 1:228
    cancer signs and symptoms, 1:252
    Cowden syndrome, 1:386
    gastric cancer, 1:617
    mammogram recommendations,
        1:253
    ovarian cancer, 2:1157
    pancreatic cancer, 2:1172
    Pap smear recommendations, 1:488
    prostate cancer, 2:1270, 1271
American College of Medical
    Genetics, 1:244
American College of Obstetricians
    and Gynecologists (ACOG), 1:97,
    244, 2:1254
American Diabetes Association, 1:448
American Heart Association, 1:359
American Institute of Ultrasound
    Medicine, 2:1253
*American Journal of Medical Genetics*,
    2:1424
*American Journal of the Diseases of
    Children*, 2:1070
American Optical/Hardy, Rand and
    Ritter Pseudoisochromatic test, 1:344
American Porphyria Foundation,
    1:733
Americans with Disabilities Act of
    1990, 1:165
AMH (Anti-mullerian hormone).
    *See* Mullerian-inhibiting substance
Amiloride
    Dent's disease, 1:435
    nephrogenic diabetes insipidus,
        2:1071
Amine precursor and uptake
    decarboxylase system (APUD),
    2:1018
Amino acid decarboxylase inhibitors,
    for Parkinson disease, 2:1183
Amino acid therapy
    ALS, 1:108
    arginase deficiency, 1:130
    metabolism disorders,
        2:1129–1133
    Osler-Weber-Rendu syndrome,
        2:1139
Amino-levulinic acid, hereditary
    coproporphyria and, 1:732, 733
Amino-levulinic acid dehydratase,
    1:51, 2:1242, 1243, 1245
Aminoaciduria, 1:433, 434, 435
Aminocaproic acid, for Osler-Weber-
    Rendu syndrome, 2:1139
Aminoglycoside antibiotics, 1:406, 740

Antibiotics *(continued)*
  for polycystic kidney disease, 2:1230
  for propionic acidemia, 2:1266
Antibodies, 1:232, 233, 234
  *See also* Immune system
Anticholinergics, 1:493, 2:1184
Anticipation
  Azorean disease, 1:174
  dentatorubral-pallidoluysian atrophy, 1:431
  fragile X syndrome, 1:586
  hereditary spastic paraplegia, 1:755
  Machado-Joseph disease, 2:922
  myotonic dystrophy, 2:1054
  oculodentodigital syndrome, 2:1110
  spinocerebellar ataxias, 2:1435
Anticoagulants
  Factor V Leiden thrombophilia, 1:548
  familial pulmonary arterial hypertension, 1:568
  moyamoya, 2:997
  protein C deficiency, 2:1274
  protein S deficiency, 2:1276, 1277
Anticodons, 2:1340
Anticonvulsants
  acardia, 1:13
  acrocallosal syndrome, 1:33
  Aicardi syndrome, 1:50
  Angelman syndrome, 1:120–121
  arginase deficiency, 1:130
  Batten disease, 1:186
  bipolar disorder, 1:210–211
  cerebral palsy, 1:288
  congenital heart disease, 1:358
  epilepsy, 1:527
  Kabuki syndrome, 1:848
  Machado-Joseph disease, 2:924
  Paine syndrome, 2:1162
  Sturge-Weber syndrome, 2:1455
  tuberous sclerosis complex, 2:1523
  Wolf-Hirschhorn syndrome, 2:1585
  X-linked mental retardation, 2:1598
Anti-craving medications, for alcoholism, 1:64
Antidepressants
  ADHD, 1:165
  Alzheimer's disease, 1:89
  bipolar disorder, 1:210, 211
  depression, 1:440–441, 2:1331
Antidiuretic hormone (ADH)
  diabetes insipidus and, 1:445
  nephrogenic diabetes insipidus and, 2:1068, 1069–1070, 1071
Anti-endomysium, celiac disease and, 1:276
Antifungal agents, for hair loss, 1:694

Antigen-presenting cells (APCs), 2:931, 932
Antigens, asthma and, 1:148
Antigliadin, celiac disease and, 1:276
Antihypertensive agents
  essential hypertension, 1:535
  familial nephritis, 1:565
Anti-inflammatory agents, 1:137
  *See also* Nonsteroidal anti-inflammatory drugs
Anti-itch agents, for ichthyosis, 1:820
Anti-mullerian hormone (AMH).
  *See* Mullerian-inhibiting substance
Antinuclear antibody tests, for scleroderma, 2:1371
Antioxidants
  age-related macular degeneration, 2:929
  ataxia-telangiectasia, 1:160
  familial pulmonary arterial hypertension, 1:568
  frontotemporal dementia, 1:603
  multiple sclerosis, 2:1032
  Stargardt disease, 2:1449
Antipruritics, for ichthyosis, 1:820
Antipsychotics
  Asperger syndrome, 1:141
  autism, 1:171
  bipolar disorder, 1:210
  schizophrenia, 2:1363–1364
Antireticulin, celiac disease and, 1:276
Anti-Rh antibodies, for Rh incompatibility, 1:790, 791, 792
Antirheumatic agents, for rheumatoid arthritis, 2:1331
Antiseizure medications.
  *See* Anticonvulsants
Antitrypsin. *See* Alpha-1 antitrypsin
Anti-tuberculosis agents, acquired sideroblastic anemia from, 1:115
Antley-Bixler syndrome, 2:1394
Anxiety
  ADHD, 1:164
  amniocentesis, 1:99
  Asperger syndrome, 1:141
  panic disorder, 2:1174, 1175, 1177
  Tourette syndrome, 2:1489, 1491
Anxiety neurosis. *See* Panic disorder
AOII (Atelosteogenesis type II), 1:453
AOIII (Atelosteogenesis type III), 1:876
Aortic aneurysms, 1:201, 202
Aortic arch abnormalities, 1:421
Aortic dissection, 1:201, 202, 2:1526
Aortic enlargement, 2:943, 945
Aortic-pulmonary shunts, 2:1187–1188
Aortic regurgitation
  bicuspid aortic valves, 1:201, 202
  Marfan syndrome, 2:943
Aortic valve calcifications, with pseudo-Gaucher disease, 2:1282

Aortic valve stenosis
  bicuspid aortic valves, 1:201, 202, 203
  description, 1:357
  surgery for, 1:359
  Williams syndrome, 2:1575, 1576
Aortic valves, bicuspid. *See* Bicuspid aortic valves
AP gene mutations, 1:227
AP3B1 gene mutations, 1:762–763
APC (Activated protein C), 1:546, 547–548
APC (Adenomatous polyposis of the colon). *See* Familial adenomatous polyposis
APC gene mutations
  familial adenomatous polyposis, 1:551–552, 553
  gastric cancer, 1:616
  genetic testing for, 1:648
  hereditary colorectal cancer, 1:729
  hereditary desmoid disease, 1:734, 735
Apert, Eugene, 1:125
Apert syndrome, 1:**124–128**, *125*
  craniosynostosis and, 1:389, 390, 391
  as fibroblast growth factor receptor mutation, 1:583
  *vs.* Pfeiffer syndrome, 2:1209, 1210, 1211
Apgar scores, cerebral palsy and, 1:288
Aphasia
  dementia, 1:427
  X-linked hydrocephaly, 2:1593, 1594
Aplasia cutis congenita, 1:38, 39
Aplastic anemia
  Fanconi anemia and, 1:571, 573
  hereditary spherocytosis and, 1:760
  paroxysmal nocturnal hemoglobinuria and, 2:1186
  sickle cell disease and, 2:1399
Apnea
  Joubert syndrome, 1:844, 845
  lissencephaly, 1:910
  MCAD deficiency, 2:954
  *See also* Sleep apnea
APOB gene mutations, 1:183
ApoE (Apolipoprotein E) gene mutations, 1:87, 88, 426
Apoenzymes, 2:973, 974
Apolipoprotein B deficiency.
  *See* Bassen-Kornzweig syndrome
Apolipoprotein B gene mutations, 1:183, 184
Apolipoprotein C-II, 1:906
Apolipoprotein E (ApoE) gene mutations, 1:87, 88, 426

# C

CMT1 (Charcot-Marie-Tooth syndrome type 1), 1:292, 293

CMT2 (Charcot-Marie-Tooth syndrome type 2), 1:292, 293–294, 346, 348

CMT4 (Charcot-Marie-Tooth syndrome type 4), 1:292, 293, 294

CNGA3 gene mutations, 1:343

CNGB3 gene mutations, 1:343

CNM (Centronuclear myopathy). *See* Myotubular myopathy

Coagulation disorders
cerebral palsy and, 1:285, 289
Factor V Leiden thrombophilia as, 1:546–548
hemophilia as, 1:713

Coagulation problems
hereditary angioneurotic edema, 1:725
Noonan syndrome, 2:1102, 1103
paroxysmal nocturnal hemoglobinuria, 2:1185, 1186
protein C deficiency, 2:1272, 1273
protein S deficiency, 2:1275, 1276
Sebastian syndrome, 2:1381, 1382
TAR syndrome, 2:1463
thrombasthenia of Glanzmann and Naegeli, 2:1484
von Willebrand disease, 2:1554–1555, 1557

Coarctation of the aorta, 1:357

Cobalamin. *See* Vitamin B/s112/s0

Cobb angle, 2:1380

Cobblestone dysplasia.
*See* Lissencephaly

Cobblestone lissencephaly, 1:909, 910, 911

Cobblestone lissencephaly without other birth defects (CLO), 1:909

Cochin Jewish disorder. *See* Haim-Munk syndrome

Cochlea abnormalities
Pendred syndrome, 2:1198
Usher syndrome, 2:1533

Cochlear implants
Jervell and Lange-Nielsen syndrome, 1:842
Pendred syndrome, 2:1199, 1200
Usher syndrome, 2:1534, 1537

Cockayne, Edward A., 1:327

Cockayne syndrome, 1:**327–329**

Codons, 1:317, 645

Coenzyme A, 2:1178, 1179

Coenzyme Q10, 1:295

Coffin, Grange S., 1:331

Coffin-Lowry syndrome, 1:**329–331**, *330*

Coffin-Siris syndrome, 1:**331–333**

Cogan's map-dot-fingerprint dystrophy. *See* Epithelial basement membrane dystrophy

Cogentin. *See* Benztropine

Cognitive-behavioral therapy
alcoholism, 1:64
Asperger syndrome, 1:141
depression, 1:441
hair loss, 1:694
panic disorder, 2:1176, 1177

Cognitive impairment
Apert syndrome, 1:127
autism, 1:171
Bardet-Biedl syndrome, 1:178, 179
Batten disease, 1:185, 186
Bloom syndrome, 1:215–216
CADASIL, 1:281, 282
Cowden syndrome, 1:385
deletion 22q11 syndrome, 1:423
dementia, 1:424
with dementia, 1:427
ectodermal dysplasias, 1:495
frontotemporal dementia, 1:601, 602
Hallermann-Streiff syndrome, 1:697, 698
Huntington disease, 1:783, 784
hyperphenylalaninemia and, 1:800
Jacobsen syndrome, 1:838, 839
Joubert syndrome, 1:843, 845
Kabuki syndrome, 1:848, 849
Krabbe disease, 1:870
leukodystrophy, 1:895
Marshall-Smith syndrome, 2:950, 951
Menkes syndrome, 2:966
mucopolysaccharidoses, 2:1002, 1005, 1006, 1007
Niemann-Pick syndrome, 2:1092
Nijmegen breakage syndrome, 2:1096
otopalatodigital syndrome, 2:1154
Pallister-Hall syndrome, 2:1164
pervasive development disorders, 2:1203
phenylketonuria, 2:1216, 1217
prion diseases, 2:1260, 1261
pyruvate dehydrogenase complex deficiency, 2:1297
Rett syndrome, 2:1326
Rieger syndrome, 2:1338
Sturge-Weber syndrome, 2:1454
triple X syndrome, 2:1500
trisomy 8 mosaicism syndrome, 2:1508, 1509, 1510
tuberous sclerosis complex, 2:1520, 1522
Williams syndrome, 2:1574, 1575
Wolman disease, 2:1588
*See also* Mental retardation

COH1 gene region mutations, 1:333, 334

Cohen, Michael, 2:1277

Cohen, M.M., Jr., 1:333

Cohen syndrome, 1:**333–336**

COL1A1 gene mutations, 2:1144, 1149

COL1A2 gene mutations, 2:1144

COL2A1 gene mutations
collagenopathy, types II and X, 1:337, 338, 2:1413
hypochondrogenesis, 1:800, 801, 802
Kniest dysplasia, 1:868
Langer-Saldino achondrogenesis, 1:874
osteoarthritis, 2:1142
spondyloepiphyseal dysplasia, 2:1439, 1443
Stickler syndrome, 2:948, 1450, 1451, 1453

COL3A1 gene mutations, 1:505

COL4A3 gene mutations, 1:563

COL4A4 gene mutations, 1:563

COL4A5 gene mutations, 1:563

COL6A1 gene mutations, 2:1038

COL6A2 gene mutations, 2:1038

COL6A3 gene mutations, 2:1038

COL8A2 gene mutations, 1:370

COL9A1 gene mutations, 1:338, 2:1142

COL9A2 gene mutations, 2:1023, 1025

COL9A3 gene mutations, 2:1023, 1025

COL10A1 gene mutations, 2:1413

COL11A1 gene mutations
collagenopathy, types II and X, 1:338, 2:1413
Marshall syndrome, 2:948
Stickler syndrome, 2:1450, 1451, 1453

COL11A2 gene mutations
collagenopathy, types II and X, 1:337, 338, 2:1413
Nance-Insley syndrome, 2:1064, 1065
Stickler syndrome, 2:1450, 1451, 1453
Weissenbacher-Zweymuller syndrome, 2:1569

Colchicine, for familial Mediterranean fever, 1:558, 559, 560

Cold exposure, Raynaud disease and, 2:1301–1302

Cold stimulation tests, 2:1303

Colectomy
familial adenomatous polyposis, 1:553–554
hereditary nonpolyposis colon cancer, 1:749
Muir-Torre syndrome, 2:1015

Colesevelan, for hyperlipoproteinemia, 1:795

Colestipol (Colestid), for hyperlipoproteinemia, 1:795

Collagen abnormalities
alkaptonuria, 1:71
Ehlers-Danlos syndrome, 1:503, 505, 506
Marshall syndrome, 2:947, 948

Crouzon syndrome, 1:**394–397**
craniosynostosis and, 1:389, 390,
394, 396, 397
as fibroblast growth factor receptor mutation, 1:583
*vs.* Pfeiffer syndrome, 2:1209,
1210, 1211
*vs.* Saethre-Chotzen syndrome,
2:1356
Crouzon syndrome with acanthosis
nigricans.
*See* Crouzonodermoskeletal
syndrome
Crouzonodermoskeletal syndrome,
1:**397–400**
CRTAP gene mutations, 2:1144
CRX gene mutations, 1:350
Cry, cat-like, 1:392, 393
Cryoprecipitates, for von Willebrand
disease, 2:1558
Cryosurgery, for liver cancer, 1:720
Cryotherapy, for retinoblastomas,
2:1323
Cryptophthalmos, with Fraser
syndrome, 1:589, 590, 591
Cryptophthalmos syndactyly
syndrome. *See* Fraser syndrome
Cryptorchidism
ambiguous genitalia, 1:657
Carpenter syndrome, 1:268
CHARGE syndrome, 1:299
Ellis-van Creveld syndrome, 1:509
Fraser syndrome, 1:591
Jacobsen syndrome, 1:839, 840
Kallmann syndrome, 1:851
McKusick-Kaufman syndrome,
2:959, 960
multiple lentigines syndrome, 2:1027
Noonan syndrome, 2:1101,
1102–1103
Opitz syndrome, 2:1124, 1125
Pallister-Hall syndrome, 2:1164
prune-belly syndrome, 2:1280, 1281
Robinow syndrome, 2:1344
Russell-Silver syndrome, 2:1351,
1352
Simpson-Golabi-Behmel syn-
drome, 2:1404, 1405
trisomy 8 mosaicism syndrome,
2:1508, 1510
trisomy 13, 2:1513
Wolf-Hirschhorn syndrome, 2:1585
XX male syndrome, 2:1607, 1608
Crystal, Ronald, 1:77
CSF. *See* Cerebrospinal fluid
CST (Christ-Siemens-Touraine
syndrome), 1:489
CT scans. *See* Computed tomography
CTAFS, 1:367
CTG repeats
myotonic dystrophy, 2:1053–1054,
1053*t*
spinocerebellar ataxias, 2:1435

CTMX. *See* X-linked Charcot-Marie-
Tooth syndrome
CTNS gene mutations, 1:408
CTSK gene mutations, 2:1373, 1413
CTX (Cerebrotendinous
xanthomatosis), 1:895, 896
Curcumin, for Charcot-Marie-Tooth
syndrome, 1:295
Curvature of the spine. *See* Scoliosis
Cushing, Harvey, 1:34
Cutaneous abnormalities. *See* Skin
abnormalities
Cutaneous syndactyly
Adams-Oliver syndrome, 1:39
Carpenter syndrome, 1:268
Fraser syndrome, 1:590
Cutis gyrata, 1:189, 190
Cutis gyrata syndrome of Beare and
Stevenson. *See* Beare-Stevenson
cutis gyrata syndrome
CVS. *See* Chorionic villus sampling
Cx32 gene mutations, 1:291, 293,
294, 295
Cyanide-nitroprusside tests, 1:412
Cyanosis, 1:358
Cyanotic congenital heart defects,
1:357
Cyclic AMP regulated enhancer
binding protein (CREBBP), 2:1348
Cyclooxygenase 2 (COX2) gene
mutations. *See* COX2 gene
mutations
Cyclopamine, holoprosencephaly
and, 1:771–772
Cyclophosphamide, for rheumatoid
arthritis, 2:1331
Cycloplegics, for ankylosing
spondylitis, 1:124
Cyclosporine
Alport's syndrome, 1:565
myasthenia gravis, 2:1046
rheumatoid arthritis, 2:1331
Cynanosis, 1:363
CYP1B1 gene mutations, 1:663–664
CYP2D6, pharmacogenetics and,
2:1214
CYP4V2 gene mutations, 1:370
CYP21 gene mutations, 1:353, 354
Cyprostat, for polycystic ovary
syndrome, 2:1233
Cyproterone, for polycystic ovary
syndrome, 2:1233
Cystathionine b-synthase, 1:776, 777
Cystathionine b-synthase deficiency
(CBS deficiency), 1:776–779
Cystathionine beta-synthetase.
*See* Homocystinuria
Cysteamine bitartrate, 1:409, 410
Cysteine metabolism, 1:777, 778

Cysteine-rich with EGF-like domains
gene mutations. *See* CRELD1 gene
mutations
Cystic fibrosis (CF), 1:**400–407**, *401, 402*
absence of vas deferens and,
1:10–11
gene therapy for, 1:406, 633
genetic testing and, 1:647–648
*vs.* Kartagener syndrome, 1:854
pedigree analysis and, 2:1191, *1192*
Cystic fibrosis transmembrane
conductance regulator (CFTR) gene
mutations, 1:400, 401, 404
Cystic fibrosis transmembrane
conductance regulator (CFTR)
protein
absence of vas deferens and, 1:10
cystic fibrosis and, 1:400, 404
Cystic kidneys. *See* Kidney cysts
Cystine
cystinosis and, 1:407, 408, 409
cystinuria and, 1:410–411, 412
Cystine-lysine-arginine-ornithinuria.
*See* Cystinuria
Cystine-lysinuria. *See* Cystinuria
Cystinosis, 1:**407–410**
Cystinuria, 1:**410–413**
Cystinuria dibasic amnioaciduria.
*See* Cystinuria
Cysts
Birt-Hogg-Dubé syndrome, 1:212,
213
branchiootorenal syndrome,
1:222, 224
Dandy-Walker malformation,
1:415, 416
nevoid basal cell carcinoma syndrome, 2:1090, 1091, 1092
polycystic kidney disease, 2:1227,
1228, 1230
short-rib polydactyly, 2:1392
trisomy 13, 2:1513
Von Hippel-Lindau syndrome,
2:1547–1548
*See also* Kidney cysts
Cytochrome P450
glaucoma and, 1:663
heme biosynthesis and, 2:1241
pharmacogenetic testing and,
1:649, 2:1214
polycystic ovary syndrome and,
2:1232
Cytogenetic bands, 1:318
Cytogenetic mapping. *See* Genetic
mapping
Cytokines
cerebral palsy and, 1:286
major histocompatibility complex
and, 2:931
Cytomegalovirus
cerebral palsy and, 1:285
holoprosencephaly and, 1:771
Cytoreductive surgery, 1:253

Cytosine, 1:174, 317, 459–460, 461

Cytoskeletons, hereditary spherocytosis and, 1:759–760

Cytoxan, for rheumatoid arthritis, 2:1331

Czech dysplasia, 1:336, 337

# D

D-glyceraldehyde-3-phosphate (GAP), 2:1498

D-penicillamine
cystinuria, 1:413
scleroderma, 2:1371
Wilson disease, 2:1580

Dactylitis, with sickle cell disease, 2:1399

Dairy-free diet, 1:612

Damus-Kay-Stansel procedure, 1:359

Dandy-Walker malformation, 1:**415–417,** 591

Dantrolene
cerebral palsy, 1:288
malignant hyperthermia, 1:291, 2:936, 938

DAO gene mutations, 2:1362

DAOA gene mutations, 2:1362

Dark adaptation curve testing, 2:1319

DAs (Dopamine receptor antagonists), for schizophrenia, 2:1364

Daughter cells, 1:312, 313

David-O'Callaghan VACTERL-H subtype, 2:1543

Day, Richard, 1:555

Daytime sleepiness, 2:*1066,* 1066–1068

DBS. *See* Deep brain stimulation

DCC gene mutations, 1:729

DCO. *See* Dyschondrosteosis

DCX gene mutations. *See* XLIS gene mutations

DD (Distal muscular dystrophy), 2:1036, 1040

DDAVP. *See* Desmopressin

De Grouchy syndrome, 1:**417–419**

De novo deletions
Williams syndrome, 2:1575
Wolf-Hirschhorn syndrome, 2:1585

De novo mutations
achondroplasia, 1:26
Adelaide-type craniosynostosis, 1:41
Aicardi syndrome, 1:49–50
Alexander disease, 1:66, 67
alpha-thalassemia X-linked mental retardation syndrome, 1:80
amelogenesis imperfecta, 1:95
Bloom syndrome, 1:214

deletion 22q11 syndrome, 1:420–421
Duchenne muscular dystrophy, 1:480–481
dyschondrosteosis, 1:485
ectrodactyly-ectodermal dysplasia-clefting syndrome, 1:500
Goltz syndrome, 1:679
Hallermann-Streiff syndrome, 1:696
hemophilia, 1:714, 715
Holt-Oram syndrome, 1:773
hypochondrogenesis, 1:801
incontinentia pigmenti, 1:823
Jacobsen syndrome, 1:839
Langer-Saldino achondrogenesis, 1:873, 874
lissencephaly, 1:908
Marfan syndrome, 2:946
microphthalmia with linear skin defects, 2:983
Miller-Dieker syndrome, 2:985
multiple epiphyseal dysplasia, 2:1024
myotubular myopathy, 2:1056, 1058
nail-patella syndrome, 2:1061
neurofibromatosis, 2:1087, 1088
osteogenesis imperfecta, 2:1144–1145
Pfeiffer syndrome, 2:1210
progeria syndrome, 2:1263
pseudoachondroplasia, 2:1285
severe combined immunodeficiency, 2:1389
spinal muscular atrophy, 2:1433
spinocerebellar ataxias, 2:1435
trisomy 18, 2:1516
tuberous sclerosis complex, 2:1520

De Vries, Hugo, 1:626

Deafness
black locks albinism deafness syndrome, 1:57
CHARGE syndrome, 1:298
choroideremia, 1:308
hereditary, 1:736–743, *737*
Jervell and Lange-Nielsen syndrome, 1:841
Norrie disease, 2:1104
trisomy 13, 2:1513
Usher syndrome, 1:739, 2:1533
Zellweger syndrome, 2:1621
*See also* Hearing loss

Deafness, congenital, and functional heart disease. *See* Jervell and Lange-Nielsen syndrome

Deafness-functional heart disease. *See* Jervell and Lange-Nielsen syndrome

Death rates. *See* Mortality

Debulking surgery, for cancer, 1:253

Decadron therapy. *See* Dexamethasone therapy

Deciduous teeth, cleidocranial dysplasia and, 1:323

Decompression craniectomy, for sclerosing bone dysplasias, 2:1377

Deep brain stimulation (DBS)
essential tremor, 1:540
Tourette syndrome, 2:1493

Deep vein thrombosis
cystathionine b-synthase deficiency, 1:778
Factor V Leiden thrombophilia, 1:547
protein C deficiency, 2:1273
protein S deficiency, 2:1276

Deferasirox
beta thalassemia, 1:200
porphyria cutanea tarda, 2:1247

Deficiency of cathepsin A. *See* Neuraminidase deficiency with beta-galactoside deficiency

Deficiency of lysosomal protective protein. *See* Neuraminidase deficiency with beta-galactoside deficiency

Deformations. *See specific types*

Degenerative myopia, 2:1047

Degenerative scoliosis, 2:1379

Degree of curvature, with scoliosis, 2:1380

Dehydration
cystinosis, 1:407, 408
Dent's disease, 1:434
methylmalonic acidemia, 2:974
nephrogenic diabetes insipidus, 2:1069, 1071
organic acidemias, 2:1131

Dehydrogenase deficiency. *See* MCAD deficiency

Dejerine-Sottas syndrome, 1:292, 293

Del(18p) syndrome. *See* De Grouchy syndrome

Del(18q) syndrome. *See* De Grouchy syndrome

Delayed growth. *See* Growth and developmental delay

Deleted in colon cancer (DCC) gene mutations. *See* DCC gene mutations

Deletion 4p syndrome. *See* Wolf-Hirschhorn syndrome

Deletion 22q11 syndrome, 1:**420–424**
CHARGE syndrome and, 1:299
conotruncal anomaly face syndrome and, 1:367, 368
as deletion syndrome, 1:272, 314

Deletion syndromes
description, 1:314–315
fluorescence in situ hybridization testing and, 1:585
Hirschsprung disease and, 1:767
*See also specific syndromes*

Deletions
Alagille syndrome, 1:54
amelia, 1:92
Angelman syndrome, 1:118

Dermatan sulfate, 2:1005, 1006, 1007, 1008, 1009, 1010, 1011

Dermatitis herpetiformis, 1:276

Dermatologic and Ophthalmic Drug Advisory Commmittee, 1:16, 18

Dermatomes, spina bifida and, 2:1429

Dermatophytes, hair loss and, 1:692, 694

Dermatosparaxis Ehlers-Danlos syndrome, 1:506

Dermis layer, Goltz syndrome and, 1:679

DeSanctis-Cacchione syndrome, 2:1603

Descemet's membrane, and corneal dystrophy, 1:370

Desferrioxamine treatment
aceruloplasminemia, 1:21
beta thalassemia, 1:199, 2:1475
hemochromatosis, 1:709
sickle cell disease, 2:1401
sideroblastic X-linked anemia, 1:115
thalassemias, 2:1475

Desflurane, malignant hyperthermia and, 2:935

Desipramine
depression, 1:441
panic disorder, 2:1176

Desmoid tumors
familial adenomatous polyposis, 1:552–553, 554, 728
hereditary desmoid disease, 1:734, 735

Desmopressin
Hermansky-Pudlak syndrome, 1:764
nephrogenic diabetes insipidus, 2:1071
thrombasthenia of Glanzmann and Naegeli, 2:1486
von Willebrand disease, 2:1557–1558

Desyrel, for rheumatoid arthritis, 2:1331

Detection rates, 1:641

Determination stage of sexual development, 2:1447

Developmental delay. See Growth and developmental delay

DEXA, for osteoporosis, 2:1149

Dexamethasone therapy
congenital adrenal hyperplasia and, 1:354, 355
for multiple sclerosis, 2:1032

Dextroamphetamine
ADHD, 1:164
Paine syndrome, 2:1162

Dextrocardia
laterality sequence, 1:878, 879, 880, 881
microphthalmia with linear skin defects, 2:984

Dextromethorphan, for nonketotic hyperglycemia, 2:1099

DFNA loci, for hearing loss, 1:739

DFNB loci, for hearing loss, 1:739, 2:1536

DGSX (Dysplasia gigantism syndrome X-linked). See Simpson-Golabi-Behmel syndrome

DHAP (Dihydroxyacetone phosphate), 2:1498

DHAPAT. See Dihydroxyacetone phosphate acyltransferase

DHCR7 gene mutations, 2:1417

DHOF (Focal dermal hypoplasia). See Goltz syndrome

DHPR protein, malignant hyperthermia and, 2:936

DHT. See Dihydrotestosterone

Diabetes, 1:443, **443–453**, 444
Donohue syndrome and, 1:464
as teratogen, 2:1466
See also specific types

Diabetes bronze, 1:445

Diabetes insipidus
Alstrom syndrome, 1:83
description, 1:445
nephrogenic, 2:1068–1072
pituitary, 2:1071

Diabetes mellitus
aceruloplasminemia and, 1:19, 20–21
Bloom syndrome and, 1:215
cystic fibrosis and, 1:403
description, 1:443–445
gestational, 1:444, 448, 450
hemolytic-uremic syndrome and, 1:712
multifactorial inheritance and, 2:1017
from pancreatic beta cell agenesis, 2:1168–1169
pancreatic cancer and, 2:1170, 1172
polycystic ovary syndrome and, 2:1233
Turner syndrome and, 2:1525
Werner syndrome and, 2:1573
See also Maternal diabetes mellitus; Type I diabetes mellitus; Type II diabetes mellitus

Diabetic embryopathy, 1:771

Diabetic ketoacidosis, 1:449, 451, 452

Diabetic nephropathy, 1:450

Diabetic neuropathy, 1:448

Diabetic retinopathy, 1:448, 450

Diacyclothrombopathia IIb-IIIa. See Thrombasthenia of Glanzmann and Naegeli

Diagnostic and Statistical Manual of Mental Disorders, 4th ed. (DSM-IV)
ADHD, 1:164
alcoholism, 1:61

Asperger syndrome, 1:139, 140
autism, 1:170–171
bipolar disorder, 1:210
dementia, 1:424, 427
depression, 1:437, 440
pervasive development disorders, 2:1201
schizophrenia, 2:1360, 1363
Tourette syndrome, 2:1492

Diagnostic genetic testing, 1:649

Dialysis
familial nephritis, 1:565
hemolytic-uremic syndrome, 1:712
hyperoxaluria, 1:797
ornithine transcarbamylase deficiency, 2:1136
polycystic kidney disease, 2:1230
renal agenesis, 2:1311
renal failure due to hypertension, 2:1313, 1314

Diaphragm abnormalities
amelia, 1:91, 94
Duchenne muscular dystrophy, 2:1039

Diaphragmatic hernias
Fryns syndrome, 1:603–604
microphthalmia with linear skin defects, 2:984

Diaphyseal aclasis. See Hereditary multiple exostoses

Diarrhea
Bruton agammaglobulinemia, 1:234
celiac disease, 1:276
Dubowitz syndrome, 1:479
hemolytic-uremic syndrome, 1:711, 712
Wolman disease, 2:1588

Diastasis recti, 1:192

Diastolic pressure, 1:533, 534

Diastrophic dysplasia, 1:**453–457,** 2:1413, 1570

Diastrophic dysplasia sulfate transporter (DTDST) gene mutations. See DTDST gene mutations

Diazepam
cerebral palsy, 1:288
essential tremor, 1:539
hereditary spastic paraplegia, 1:758
panic disorder, 2:1176
porphyrias, 2:1246

Dibasic amino acids, 1:410–411, 412

Dicephalus conjoined twins, 1:366

Diclofenac, for rheumatoid arthritis, 2:1330

Diet and nutrition therapy
alkaptonuria, 1:74
ALS, 1:108
asthma, 1:150
autism, 1:172
Bassen-Kornzweig syndrome, 1:184

# E

Fused cervical vertebrae, 1:862, 863, 864

Fusiform bones, with Engelmann disease, 1:518

Fusion of digits. *See* Syndactyly

Fusion of skull bones. *See* Craniosynostosis

Fusion oncogenes, 2:1121

# G

G-6-PD deficiency. *See* Glucose-6-phosphate dehydrogenase deficiency

G proteins, 2:955–956, 1335

G4.5 gene mutations, 1:180

G6PD deficiency. *See* Glucose-6-phosphate dehydrogenase deficiency

G236V gene mutations, 1:529

G985A mutations, 2:952, 953, 954

G3460A mutations, 1:886, 887

G11778A mutations, 1:886, 887

GAA repeats, 1:595, 596

GABA (Gamma amino butyric acid), essential tremor and, 1:537

Gabapentin
    bipolar disorder, 1:211
    entrapment neuropathy, 1:521
    essential tremor, 1:539
    hereditary spastic paraplegia, 1:758

GAGs (Glycosaminoglycans). *See* Mucopolysaccharides

Gait abnormalities. *See* Walking problems

Gait ataxia
    Angelman syndrome, 1:118
    Cockayne syndrome, 1:328
    Machado-Joseph disease, 2:922

Galactokinase, 1:607

Galactokinase deficiency, 1:**607–610,** 611, 612

Galactorrhea, 2:957

Galactosamine-6-sulfatase, 2:1003

Galactose, Fanconi-Bickel syndrome and, 1:570

Galactose-1-phosphate, 1:612

Galactose-1-phosphate-uridyl transferase, 1:376, 607

Galactose-1-phosphate-uridyl transferase (GALT) gene mutations, 1:607

Galactose-free diet, 1:609, 612

Galactose metabolism, 1:610–611

Galactosemia, 1:607, *610,* **610–614**

Galactosemia type I. *See* Classic galactosemia

Galactosemia type II. *See* Galactokinase deficiency

Galactosemia type III, 1:611, 612

Galactosialidosis. *See* Neuraminidase deficiency with beta-galactoside deficiency

Galactosuria, 1:609

Galactosylceramidase, 1:870

Galactosylceramide, 1:870

GALC gene mutations, 1:870, 871

GALE gene mutations, 1:611, 612

GALK deficiency. *See* Galactokinase deficiency

GALK1 gene mutations, 1:607, 611, 612

Gallbladder abnormalities
    asplenia, 1:145
    laterality sequence, 1:880

Gallstones
    beta thalassemia, 1:198
    cystic fibrosis, 1:403
    erythropoietic photoporphyria, 1:532
    hereditary spherocytosis and, 1:760
    pyruvate kinase deficiency, 2:1299
    sickle cell disease, 2:1400

GALNS. *See* N-acetylgalactosamine-6-sulfate sulfatase

GALT gene mutations, 1:611, 612

Gametogenesis
    defined, 1:830
    imprinting and, 1:821, 833

Gamma amino butyric acid (GABA), essential tremor and, 1:537

Gamma globin chains, 1:196, 2:1472

Gamma globin gene mutations, 2:1472

Gamma-sarcoglycan protein, limb-girdle muscular dystrophy and, 2:1038

Gammaglobulins, 1:233

Ganglion cell development, 1:766, 767

Gangliosides
    neuraminidase deficiency with beta-galactoside deficiency and, 2:1084
    Tay-Sachs disease and, 2:1464

Gangliosidosis-GM1. *See* GM1-gangliosidosis

GAP (D-glyceraldehyde-3-phosphate), 2:1498

Gardner syndrome, 1:551, 728, 729, 734
    *See also* Familial adenomatous polyposis

Garrod, Archibald, 1:69–70, 411

GARS gene mutations, 1:292, 293, 346

Gas chromatography-mass spectrometry
    alkaptonuria, 1:73
    organic acidemias, 2:1132

Gascoyen, G.G., 1:217

Gastric cancer, 1:*614,* **614–619,** *615,* 746

Gastric ulcers, 1:375, 376

Gastrinomas, with multiple endocrine neoplasias, 2:1018

Gastroesophageal reflux
    Cornelia de Lange syndrome, 1:375, 376
    deletion 22q11 syndrome, 1:422

Gastrointestinal polyps, with Peutz-Jeghers syndrome, 2:1204, 1205, 1207, 1208

Gastrointestinal tract abnormalities
    asplenia, 1:145
    blue rubber bleb nevus syndrome, 1:217–218
    caudal dysplasia, 1:269, 271
    Cornelia de Lange syndrome, 1:374, 375
    cystic fibrosis, 1:400, 402–403
    Down syndrome, 1:469
    FG syndrome, 1:578, 579
    Fraser syndrome, 1:591
    laterality sequence, 1:879, 880
    McKusick-Kaufman syndrome, 2:960
    Niemann-Pick syndrome, 2:1093
    organic acidemias, 2:1131
    trisomy 13, 2:1513
    trisomy 18, 2:1517
    Wolman disease, 2:1588
    *See also* Digestive problems

Gastroschisis, 1:104, *619,* **619–622**

Gastrostomy
    Pierre-Robin sequence, 2:1221
    Russell-Silver syndrome, 2:1352
    trisomy 13, 2:1514
    Wolf-Hirschhorn syndrome, 2:1585
    *See also* Tube feeding

Gaucher, Philippe, 1:622

Gaucher disease, 1:**622–624**
    compression neuropathy and, 1:346
    gene therapy for, 1:633, 634
    hydrops fetalis and, 1:791
    *vs.* Niemann-Pick syndrome, 2:1094

Gaucher disease type I, 1:622, 623–624

Gaucher disease type II, 1:622, 623–624

Gaucher disease type III, 1:622, 623–624

Gaucher disease type IIIC. *See* Pseudo-Gaucher disease

Gaucher-like disease. *See* Pseudo-Gaucher disease

GBA gene mutations, 1:346, 2:1282, 1283

GCGR gene mutations, 1:447

GCK gene mutations, 1:447

# H

De Grouchy syndrome, 1:419
deletion 22q11 syndrome, 1:423
Down syndrome, 1:469, 472
Ellis-van Creveld syndrome, 1:508
Emery-Dreifuss muscular dystrophy, 1:511, 513–514
Fanconi anemia, 1:571, 573
Friedreich ataxia, 1:595–596
Holt-Oram syndrome, 1:773, 774,
775
hydrolethalus syndrome, 1:788,
789
hydrops fetalis and, 1:790
Jacobsen syndrome, 1:838
Kabuki syndrome, 1:848
laterality sequence, 1:880, 881
Marfan syndrome, 2:943, 945
monosomy 1p36 syndrome, 2:991
Mowat-Wilson syndrome, 2:994
mucopolysaccharidoses, 2:1002,
1007, 1008
multiple lentigines syndrome,
2:1027
Opitz syndrome, 2:1124, 1125,
1126
oral-facial-digital syndrome,
2:1128
polycystic kidney disease, 2:1229
Smith-Lemli-Optiz syndrome,
2:1418
thalidomide embryopathy, 2:1478,
1479, 1480
triploidy, 2:1504
trisomy 8 mosaicism syndrome,
2:1508, 1510
trisomy 13, 2:1511, 1513
trisomy 18, 2:1515, 1517
tuberous sclerosis complex, 2:1520
Turner syndrome, 2:1526
VATER association, 2:1541, 1542,
1543, 1544
Williams syndrome, 2:1574, 1575,
1576
Wolf-Hirschhorn syndrome,
2:1584, 1585
XXXX syndrome, 2:1610
XXXXX syndrome, 2:1612, 1613
See also Cardiovascular abnormalities; specific types
Heart arrhythmias. See Arrhythmias
Heart block, with Emery-Dreifuss
muscular dystrophy, 1:513
Heart conduction defects
Emery-Dreifuss muscular
dystrophy, 2:1035
multiple lentigenes syndrome,
2:1027
Heart disease
Barth syndrome, 1:181, 182
cystathionine b-synthase
deficiency, 1:777
diabetes, 1:443, 448, 452
Fabry disease, 1:541, 542
Herceptin and, 1:722, 723

hydrops fetalis, 1:790
Jervell and Lange-Nielsen
syndrome, 1:841, 842
mucolipidosis, 2:999
mucopolysaccharidoses, 2:1005,
1006, 1007, 1008, 1010
neuraminidase deficiency, 2:1081
neuraminidase deficiency with
beta-galactoside deficiency,
2:1082, 1085
pseudoxanthoma elasticum,
2:1287, 1289
scleroderma, 2:1371
Shprintzen-Goldberg craniosynostosis syndrome, 2:1394
Simpson-Golabi-Behmel syndrome, 2:1405
Tangier disease, 2:1459, 1461
TAR syndrome, 2:1463
Turner syndrome and, 2:1525
See also Congenital heart disease
Heart failure
acardiac pump twin, 1:14
Alstrom syndrome, 1:83
Barth syndrome, 1:182
beta thalassemia, 2:1474
bicuspid aortic valves, 1:202
hydrops fetalis, 1:790
mucopolysaccharidoses, 2:1006
triose phosphate isomerase deficiency, 2:1499
Heart-hands syndrome. See Holt-
Oram syndrome
Heart murmur, with patent ductus
arteriosus, 2:1189, 1190
Heart transplantation, for congenital
heart disease, 1:359
Heat treatment, arthrogryposis
multiplex congenital, 1:137
Heavy metal exposure
dementia from, 1:425
dystonia and, 1:492
hair loss and, 1:694
vs. prion diseases, 2:1261
Hebephrenic schizophrenia.
See Disorganized schizophrenia
Hecht, Frederick, 2:1506
Hecht-Beals-Wilson syndrome.
See Trismus-pseudocamptodactyly
syndrome
Hecht syndrome. See Trismus-
pseudocamptodactyly syndrome
Height abnormalities. See Short
stature; Tall stature
Heinz bodies, asplenia and, 1:145
Helicases, Werner syndrome and,
2:1572
Helicobacter pylori infections, 1:615
Helix structure of DNA, 1:459, 460,
461–462, 584
Heller, Theodore, 2:1201
Heller's syndrome. See Childhood
disintegrative disorder

Helper T cells, 1:149, 2:931, 932
Hemangioblastomas, with Von
Hippel-Lindau syndrome, 2:1545,
1547, 1548, 1549
Hemangiomas, with blue rubber bleb
nevus syndrome, 1:217–218
Hematin, for porphyrias, 2:1246
Hematopoietic growth factors, 1:574
Hematopoietic stem cell
transplantation. See Stem cell
transplantation
Hematuria
Dent's disease, 1:433
erythropoietic porphyria, 1:529
familial nephritis, 1:561, 562, 563
porphyrias, 2:1245–1246
Heme
ALA dehydratase deficiency and,
1:51, 52
hereditary coproporphyria and,
1:731, 732
porphyrias and, 2:1241–1243,
1244, 1246
Heme therapy
acute intermittent porphyria,
2:1247
ALA dehydratase deficiency, 1:52
hereditary coproporphyria, 1:733
Hemifacial hyperplasia, 1:705
Hemifacial microsomia, 1:702–705,
2:1495
Hemifacial microsomia with radial
defects. See Goldenhar syndrome
Hemihyperplasia.
See Hemihypertrophy
Hemihypertrophy, 1:705–708, 706
Beckwith-Wiedemann syndrome,
1:193, 194
Proteus syndrome, 2:1279
Hemiplegia, 1:284
Hemizygosity, 1:831
Hemochromatosis, 1:708–710
beta thalassemia, 1:198, 199,
2:1471, 1475
hereditary spherocytosis, 1:760,
761
liver cancer, 1:717, 719
sideroblastic X-linked anemia,
1:115, 116
Hemodialysis, 2:1314
See also Dialysis
Hemoglobin
alpha-thalassemias and, 2:1469
congenital methemoglobinemia
and, 1:363
sideroblastic X-linked anemia and,
1:113, 115
thalassemias and, 2:1472
See also specific types
Hemoglobin A (HbA), 1:196, 197,
2:1472
Hemoglobin A1c testing, 1:450–451

Hermaphroditism, true, 1:657–658, 765, 2:1607–1608
Hernias
  Donohue syndrome, 1:465
  mucopolysaccharidoses, 2:1005, 1007
  neuraminidase deficiency, 2:1080
  otopalatodigital syndrome, 2:1155
  Pallister-Killian syndrome, 2:1167
  polycystic kidney disease, 2:1229
  Schwartz-Jampel syndrome, 2:1367
  Simpson-Golabi-Behmel syndrome, 2:1405
  trisomy 13, 2:1512
  *See also* Diaphragmatic hernias; Umbilical hernias
Herniation of the cerebellar tonsils. *See* Arnold-Chiari malformation
Hers' disease, 1:670, 671, 672, 673, 674
HESX1 gene mutations, 2:1384–1385
Heterochromatin repulsion (HR), 1:92, 93
Heterochromia of the irides, 2:1561, 1563, 1564
Heterogeneous nuclear RNA (hnRNA), 2:1340
Heteroplasmic mitochondrial DNA mutations, 1:885
Heterotaxy, 1:143, 144, 879, 880
Heterozygosity
  defined, 1:831
  double, 2:1285, 1286
  Factor V Leiden thrombophilia, 1:547
  prion diseases and, 2:1260
  propionic acidemia, 2:1265–1266
  *See also* Carrier status; Compound heterozygosity
Heterozygote advantage
  cystic fibrosis, 1:402
  defined, 1:641
  sickle cell anemia, 1:641
Heterozygous beta thalassemia. *See* Beta thalassemia minor
Heterozygous otospondylomegaepiphyseal dysplasia. *See* Weissenbacher-Zweymuller syndrome
HEXA gene mutations, 2:1464
Hexosaminidase A, Tay-Sachs disease and, 2:1464, 1465
HF. *See* Harlequin fetus; Hydrops fetalis
HFE gene mutations, 1:708–709
HFN4A gene mutations, 1:447
HFU (Hand-foot-uterus syndrome), 1:698–699
HGA (Homogentisic acid), 1:69, 70–71, 72, 73
HGD (Homogentisate 1,2-dioxygenase), 1:70, 73

HGD (Homogentisate 1,2-dioxygenase) gene mutations, 1:71–72
HGDP (Human Genome Diversity Project), 1:630
HGH. *See* Human growth hormone
HGPS (Hutchinson-Gilford progeria syndrome). *See* Progeria syndrome
HH. *See* Hypogonadotropic hypogonadism
HHT (Hereditary hemorrhagic telangiectasia). *See* Osler-Weber-Rendu syndrome
Hidrotic ectodermal dysplasias, 1:489, 495, 497
HIE (Hyper IgE syndrome), 2:1612
Hierarchical shotgun sequencing, 1:780
High blood pressure. *See* Hypertension
High-calorie diet
  ALA dehydratase deficiency, 1:52
  cystic fibrosis, 1:405
High-density hypoprotein deficiency. *See* Tangier disease
High-density lipoproteins (HDLs), 1:793, 794, 2:1459
High-fat diet
  epilepsy, 1:528
  pyruvate dehydrogenase complex deficiency, 2:1297
High-functioning autism *vs.* Asperger syndrome, 1:140
High molecular weight RNA, 2:1340
High myopia, 2:1048, 1049
High-performance liquid chromatography
  sickle cell disease, 2:1400
  thalassemias, 2:1473
Hip abnormalities
  central core disease, 1:279
  distal arthrogryposis syndrome, 1:458
  Marfan syndrome, 2:944
  metaphyseal dysplasia, 2:971
  multiple epiphyseal dysplasia, 2:1025
  nail-patella syndrome, 2:1061, 1062, 1063
  progeria syndrome, 2:1263
  spondyloepiphyseal dysplasia, 2:1440, 1443, 1444
Hip coring surgery, for sickle cell disease, 2:1402
Hip dislocations
  campomelic dysplasia, 1:240
  Ehlers-Danlos syndrome, 1:506
  Larsen syndrome, 1:875
  oculodentodigital syndrome, 2:1111
  Pallister-Hall syndrome, 2:1164
  Schwartz-Jampel syndrome, 2:1367
Hippocampus, schizophrenia and, 2:1362

Hirschsprung disease, 1:**766–769**
  McKusick type metaphyseal dysplasia, 2:971
  Mowat-Wilson syndrome, 2:993, 994, 995
  Smith-Lemli-Optiz syndrome, 2:1419
  Waardenburg syndrome, 2:1561, 1563, 1564
Hirschsprung disease-mental retardation syndrome. *See* Mowat-Wilson syndrome
Hirschsprung disease with pigmentary anomaly. *See* Waardenburg syndrome 4
Hirsutism
  Coffin-Siris syndrome, 1:331, 332
  Donohue syndrome, 1:465
  mucopolysaccharidoses, 2:1005
  polycystic ovary syndrome, 2:*1231,* 1233, 1234
Histamine
  asthma and, 1:148
  Cornelia de Lange syndrome and, 1:376
  familial dysautonomia and, 1:556
Histological examination. *See* Microscopic examination
Histones, 1:310, 316
Histrelin, for Russell-Silver syndrome, 2:1352
Hitchhiker thumb
  diastrophic dysplasia, 1:455
  skeletal dysplasia, 2:1411
HIV (Human immunodeficiency virus), 1:633–634, 716
HL (Hearing level), 1:741
HLA-A genes, 2:932
HLA-B genes, 2:932
HLA-B27, 1:121–122, 124
HLA-B60, 1:122
HLA-C genes, 2:932
HLA-DP gene mutations, 1:445, 2:932
HLA-DQ gene mutations
  diabetes insipidus and, 1:445, 446
  major histocompatibility complex and, 2:932
  narcolepsy and, 2:1066
HLA-DR gene mutations
  diabetes insipidus and, 1:445–446
  major histocompatibility complex and, 2:932
  narcolepsy and, 2:1066
HLA-DR2 haplotype, multiple sclerosis and, 2:1030
HLA-DR4 markers, rheumatoid arthritis and, 2:1328
HLA genes
  diabetes and, 1:445–446
  major histocompatibility complex and, 2:931–932
  rheumatoid arthritis and, 2:1328

Huntington chorea. *See* Huntington disease

Huntington disease, 1:**781–784,** *782*
dystonia and, 1:492, 782
genetic testing and, 1:648
paternal *vs.* maternal inheritance and, 1:315

HUP2 gene mutations. *See* PAX3 gene mutations

Hurler-Scheie syndrome.
*See* Mucopolysaccharidosis type I H/S

Hurler syndrome.
*See* Mucopolysaccharidosis type I H

Hurler-variant. *See* GM1-gangliosidosis

HUS. *See* Hemolytic-uremic syndrome

Hutchinson, Jonathan, 2:1262

Hutchinson-Gilford progeria syndrome (HGPS). *See* Progeria syndrome

Hyaline cartilage abnormalities, 1:336

Hyaline panneuropathy.
*See* Alexander disease

Hyaluronic acid, 2:1573

Hyaluronidase, 2:1004

Hyaluronidase deficiency.
*See* Mucopolysaccharidosis type IX

Hybridization, defined, 2:1034

Hydramnios. *See* Polyhydramnios

Hydratiform moles, 2:1502

Hydration therapy
cystic fibrosis, 1:406
cystinuria, 1:413
nephrogenic diabetes insipidus, 2:1071

Hydrocephalus, 1:**784–788,** *785*
Accutane embryopathy, 1:17
achondroplasia, 1:28
agenesis of the corpus callosum with, 1:381
Alexander disease, 1:68
Beare-Stevenson cutis gyrata syndrome, 1:190
Carpenter syndrome, 1:267
craniosynostosis, 1:388, 390
Crouzon syndrome, 1:395–396, 397
Dandy-Walker malformation, 1:415, 416–417
encephaloceles and, 1:516
Fraser syndrome, 1:591
hydrolethalus syndrome, 1:789
mucopolysaccharidoses, 2:1003, 1010, 1011
myotubular myopathy, 2:1058
neural tube defects, 2:1076, 1077
neurofibromatosis, 2:1088
Pfeiffer syndrome, 2:1211
Shprintzen-Goldberg craniosynostosis syndrome, 2:1393, 1394
spina bifida, 2:1430
VATER association, 2:1543, 1544

von Recklinghausen's neurofibromatosis, 2:1551
Walker-Warburg syndrome, 2:1565, 1566
X-linked, 2:1591–1594, *1592*

Hydrocephalus ex-vacuo, 1:785

Hydrocephaly with stenosis of the aqueduct of Sylvius (HSAS), 2:1591, 1594

Hydrochlorothiazide
Dent's disease, 1:435
nephrogenic diabetes insipidus, 2:1071

Hydrodiuril.
*See* Hydrochlorothiazide

Hydrogen bonds, 1:317

Hydrolases, mucolipidosis and, 2:1000

Hydrolethalus syndrome, 1:**788–789**

Hydrometrocolpos, with McKusick-Kaufman syndrome, 2:959, 960

Hydrometrocolpos syndrome.
*See* McKusick-Kaufman syndrome

Hydronephrosis
Schinzel-Giedion syndrome, 2:1358
trisomy 8 mosaicism syndrome, 2:1508, 1510

Hydrops fetalis (HF), 1:**789–792**
achondrogenesis, 1:23
conjoined twins, 1:366
Langer-Saldino achondrogenesis, 1:874
Langer-Saldino achondrogenesis and, 1:873
McKusick-Kaufman syndrome, 2:960

Hydroquinone, acquired ochronosis from, 1:74

Hydroxyapatite, hypophosphatemia and, 1:811, 812

Hydroxychloroquine, for rheumatoid arthritis, 2:1331

Hydroxycholestanoic acids, infantile Refsum disease and, 1:826, 827

Hydroxylysl pyridinoline, Ehlers-Danlos syndrome and, 1:506

Hydroxymethylglutaric acidemia, 2:1129, 1131, 1132

Hydroxyurea
beta thalassemia, 1:199, 200, 2:1475
erythropoietic porphyria, 1:530
sickle cell disease, 2:1401

Hyper IgE syndrome (HIE), 2:1612

Hyperactivity
ADHD, 1:162, 163–164, 165
Angelman syndrome, 1:120

Hyperammonemia
arginase deficiency, 1:129
MCAD deficiency, 2:953
ornithine transcarbamylase deficiency, 2:1133, 1134

Hyperammonemia type II.
*See* Ornithine transcarbamylase deficiency

Hyperbaric oxygen, for cerebral palsy, 1:289

Hyperbilirubinemia
beta thalassemia, 1:198
hereditary spherocytosis, 1:760

Hypercalcemia, with Williams syndrome, 2:1575

Hypercalciuria, with Dent's disease, 1:433, 435
Dent's disease, 1:434

Hyperchylomicronemia. *See* Bürger-Grütz syndrome

Hyperglycemia
diabetes and, 1:443
nonketotic, 2:1097–1100
organic acidemias, 2:1131

Hyperglycinemia with ketoacidosis and lactic acidosis (propionic type).
*See* Propionic acidemia

Hyperhidrosis, with Apert syndrome, 1:126

Hyperkalemic periodic paralysis, 1:291

Hyperkeratosis
ectodermal dysplasias, 1:497
harlequin fetus, 1:700, 701
Sjögren-Larsson syndrome, 2:1409, 1410

Hyperlipoproteinemia, 1:**793–795**

Hyperlipoproteinemia type I.
*See* Lipoprotein lipase deficiency

Hyperlipoproteinemia type II, 1:793, 795

Hyperlipoproteinemia type III, 1:793–794, 795

Hyperlipoproteinemia type IV, 1:794, 795

Hyperlipoproteinemia type V, 1:794, 795

Hypermobility
Ehlers-Danlos syndrome, 1:*503, 505*, 506, 507
Larsen syndrome, 1:875, 877
Marfan syndrome, 2:941
pseudoachondroplasia, 2:1284, 1285
Shprintzen-Goldberg craniosynostosis syndrome, 2:1393
Stickler syndrome, 2:1452

Hypermobility-type Ehlers-Danlos syndrome, 1:505

Hyperostosis, with sclerosing bone dysplasias, 2:1372, 1375–1376, 1377

Hyperostosis corticalis familiaris.
*See* Van Buchem disease

Hyperoxaluria, 1:**795–798**

Hyperparathyroidism, 2:1018, 1020, 1021–1022

Hyperphenylalaninemia, 1:**798–800**

Immunodeficiency *(continued)*
   biotinidase deficiency, 1:205
   Bloom syndrome, 1:214, 215, 216
   Bruton agammaglobulinemia,
      1:232–234
   Chediak-Higashi syndrome,
      1:300–301
   deletion 22q11 syndrome, 1:420,
      421, 423
   diabetes and, 1:449–450
   Donohue syndrome, 1:465
   Down syndrome, 1:469
   Dubowitz syndrome, 1:478
   Griscelli syndrome, 1:683, 684
   hemolytic-uremic syndrome and,
      1:711
   metaphyseal dysplasia, 2:971
   Nijmegen breakage syndrome,
      2:1095, 1096
   paroxysmal nocturnal hemoglobi-
      nuria, 2:1186
   severe combined immunodefi-
      ciency, 2:971, *1387,* 1387–1390,
      1599–1602
   triose phosphate isomerase defi-
      ciency, 2:1499
   Wiskott-Aldrich syndrome,
      2:1582, 1583
   X-linked severe combined
      immunodeficiency, 2:1599–1602
Immunoelectrophoresis, for Bruton
   agammaglobulinemia, 1:234
Immunofluorescence
   epidermolysis bullosa, 1:524
   thrombasthenia of Glanzmann
      and Naegeli, 2:1486
Immunoglobulin A (IgA), ataxia-
   telangiectasia and, 1:158, 160
Immunoglobulin E (IgE)
   asthma and, 1:148, 149
   ataxia-telangiectasia and, 1:158, 160
Immunoglobulin therapy
   Bruton agammaglobulinemia,
      1:234, 235
   myasthenia gravis, 2:1046
   Wiskott-Aldrich syndrome, 2:1583
   X-linked severe combined
      immunodeficiency, 2:1601
Immunosuppression
   myasthenia gravis and, 2:1046
   ornithine transcarbamylase
      deficiency and, 2:1135
   rheumatoid arthritis and, 2:1331
Immunotherapy
   cancer, 1:254
   multiple sclerosis, 2:1032
Impaired fasting glucose, 1:444–445
Impaired glucose tolerance, 1:444, 445
Imprinting, 1:**820–822**
   Angelman syndrome, 1:118, 119,
      120, 315
   Beckwith-Wiedemann syndrome,
      1:195

description, 1:833
   Prader-Willi syndrome, 1:315,
      2:1250, 1251
Impulsivity, attention deficit
   hyperactivity disorder and, 1:162,
   163–164, 165
Imuran. *See* Azathioprine
In vitro fertilization
   absence of vas deferens and, 1:11–12
   acardia risk, 1:13
   Beckwith-Wiedemann syndrome
      and, 1:194
   description, 2:1626
   imprinting and, 1:822
   monosomy 1p36 syndrome
      prevention, 2:993
   *See also* Intracytoplasmic sperm
      injection
In vivo gene therapy, 1:633
Inability-to-open-the-mouth-fully
   syndrome. *See* Trismus-
   pseudocamptodactyly syndrome
Inattention, with attention deficit
   hyperactivity disorder, 1:162,
   163–164, 165
Inborn errors of metabolism
   biotinidase deficiency, 1:205–206
   cystinuria, 1:411
   mannosidosis as, 2:939
   origin of term, 1:69
   phenylketonuria, 1:169
   propionic acidemia, 2:1265
   urea cycle disorders, 2:1529
Incisors, prominent, with Cohen
   syndrome, 1:334
Inclusion (education), for Down
   syndrome, 1:472
Incomitant strabismus, 1:473
Incomplete cleft lip, 1:319
Incomplete cryptophthalmos, 1:589
Incontinence
   epispadias, 1:814
   hypospadias, 1:814
   multiple sclerosis, 2:1031
   Parkinson disease, 2:1182
Incontinentia pigmenti (IP), 1:495,
   496, 497, **822–826**, *823,* 2:1106
Increased bone density without
   modification of bone shape, 2:1413
Inderal. *See* Propranolol
Indeterminate sex. *See* Ambiguous
   genitalia
Indirect DNA testing, 1:646
   *See also* Linkage analysis
Individuals with Disabilities Act of
   1997, 2:1598
Indomethacin
   nephrogenic diabetes insipidus,
      2:1071
   patent ductus arteriosus, 2:1190
   rheumatoid arthritis, 2:1330

Inducible nitric oxide synthase
   (iNOS), 1:148–149
Infantile Alexander disease, 1:67, 68
Infantile alpha-mannosidosis, 2:939,
   940
Infantile autism. *See* Autism
Infantile dwarfism, 1:22
Infantile GM1-gangliosidosis,
   1:676–677, 678
Infantile hypertrophic pyloric
   stenosis. *See* Pyloric stenosis
Infantile hypophosphatasia, 1:808
Infantile nephropathic cystinosis,
   1:407
Infantile-onset pyruvate carboxylase
   deficiency, 2:1292, 1294
Infantile polycystic kidney disease,
   2:1227, 1228, 1230
Infantile Pompe disease, 1:669,
   2:1238, 1239, 1240
Infantile Refsum disease (IRD),
   1:**826–829**
   *See also* Refsum disease
Infantile scoliosis, 2:1379
Infantile spasm-mental retardation
   syndrome. *See* West syndrome
Infantile spasms
   Aicardi syndrome, 1:50
   lissencephaly, 1:910
   West syndrome, 2:1598
Infantile spongy degeneration.
   *See* Canavan disease
Infections
   Barth syndrome and, 1:181, 182
   Bruton agammaglobulinemia and,
      1:233–234
   cerebral palsy and, 1:285
   Chediak-Higashi syndrome and,
      1:301
   dementia from, 1:425
   diabetes and, 1:449–450
   Haim-Munk syndrome and, 1:687,
      688
   hemolytic-uremic syndrome and,
      1:711
   ichthyosis and, 1:820
   Jacobsen syndrome and, 1:838,
      839
   Kabuki syndrome and, 1:848
   maternal-fetal, 1:285
   microcephaly and, 2:981, 982
   myasthenia gravis and, 2:1044
   opportunistic, 2:1599
   severe combined immunodefi-
      ciency and, 2:1388–1389
   sickle cell disease and, 2:1397
   as teratogen, 2:1466–1467, 1468
   Wiskott-Aldrich syndrome and,
      2:1582, 1583
   X-linked severe combined
      immunodeficiency and, 2:1599,
      1600
   *See also specific types*

Infective endocarditis, with Marfan syndrome, 2:943, 945
Infertility
androgen insensitivity syndrome, 1:111, 112
Bardet-Biedl syndrome, 1:178
Bloom syndrome, 1:215
cystic fibrosis, 1:404, 406
polycystic ovary syndrome, 2:1233, 1234
urogenital adysplasia syndrome, 2:1532
See also Female infertility; In vitro fertilization; Male infertility
Inflammation
ankylosing spondylitis, 1:121, 123, 124
asthma, 1:147, 148
celiac disease, 1:275
cystic fibrosis, 1:403, 404, 406
familial Mediterranean fever, 1:557, 558, 559
Meckel's diverticulum, 2:964
multiple epiphyseal dysplasia, 2:1023
osteoarthritis, 2:1142
rheumatoid arthritis, 2:1327–1328, 1329, 1330
Rothmund-Thomson syndrome, 2:1346
Inflammatory nonscarring hair loss, 1:692, 695
Inflammatory scarring hair loss, 1:692, 695
Infliximab
depression, 1:441
rheumatoid arthritis, 2:1331
Inguinal hernias, with Donohue syndrome, 1:465
Inheritance, 1:829, **829–834**
ADHD, 1:162–163
autism, 1:168–169
cancer, 1:246, 250–251, 252, 255–259, 256t
cerebral palsy, 1:284
Charcot-Marie-Tooth syndrome, 1:292–293
cleft lip and palate, 1:320
clubfoot, 1:325
description, 1:629
epilepsy, 1:526–527
erythropoietic photoporphyria, 1:531
frontonasal dysplasia, 1:597
gastric cancer, 1:615–617
Gerstmann-Straussler-Scheinker disease, 1:660, 661
hereditary colorectal cancer, 1:728
hereditary desmoid disease, 1:734
multiple sclerosis, 2:1029–1030
myopia, 2:1047–1049
Nance-Insley syndrome, 2:1064
omphaloceles, 2:1116
osteoarthritis, 2:1142

osteoporosis, 2:1148–1149
ovarian cancer, 2:1156–1157
pancreatic cancer, 2:1170–1172
panic disorder, 2:1174
Pierre-Robin sequence, 2:1220
polycystic ovary syndrome, 2:1232
polydactyly, 2:1236
prostate cancer, 2:1268
retinitis pigmentosa, 2:1335–1336
rheumatoid arthritis, 2:1328–1329
Russell-Silver syndrome, 2:1351
Schinzel-Giedion syndrome, 2:1358
See also specific types
Inherited giant platelet disorders (IGPDs), 2:1381
Inherited nephrogenic diabetes insipidus, 2:1069
Injuries
cerebral palsy and, 1:286
hair loss and, 1:692
hemophilia and, 1:716
See also Self-injury
Inorganic pyrophosphate, hypophosphatasia and, 1:809
iNOS (Inducible nitric oxide synthase), 1:148–149
INS gene mutations, 1:446
INSERM (France), 1:139
Insertions
nonketotic hyperglycemia, 2:1098
prion diseases, 2:1260
pyruvate dehydrogenase complex deficiency, 2:1296
INSR gene mutations, 1:446, 464
Institute of Medicine, 1:575, 576
Insulin
diabetes and, 1:443, *443*, 446, 447, 449, 451
Donohue syndrome and, 1:464
pancreatic beta cell agenesis and, 2:1168, 1169
Insulin-dependent diabetes mellitus. See Type I diabetes mellitus
Insulin gene (INS) mutations, 1:446
Insulin-like growth factor-1
for amyotrophic lateral sclerosis, 1:108
pituitary dwarfism and, 2:1222
Insulin-like growth factor-2 gene mutations. See IGF-2 gene mutations
Insulin receptor (INSR) gene mutations, 1:446, 464
Insulin resistance
Alstrom syndrome, 1:83
diabetes, 1:444
Donohue syndrome, 1:464, 466
polycystic ovary syndrome, 2:1231, 1232, 1233, 1234
type A, 1:464
Insulinomas, with multiple endocrine neoplasias, 2:1018

Insurance considerations
breast cancer genetic testing, 1:230
cancer genetic testing, 1:253
genetic testing, 1:646, 650
Human Genome Project and, 1:635
Integrin, congenital muscular dystrophy and, 2:1039
Intellectual impairment. See Cognitive impairment
Intention tremors. See Kinetic tremors
Intercostal muscle weakness, 2:1432
Interdigital neuropathy, 1:520
Interferon
liver cancer and, 1:721
for multiple sclerosis, 2:1032
Interferon regulatory factor 6 gene mutations, 2:1539
Interleukin-1 receptor antagonists, for rheumatoid arthritis, 2:1331
Interleukin-6 gene mutations, 2:1149
Interleukin receptor gamma chain gene mutations. See IL2RG gene mutations
Intermedia Cooley's anemia. See Beta thalassemia intermedia
Intermediate Charcot-Marie-Tooth syndrome, 1:292
Intermediate-density lipoproteins, 1:793
Intermediate metabolizers, 2:1214
Intermittent acute porphyria. See Acute intermittent porphyria
Internal radiation therapy, 1:254
Internal tremors, with essential tremor, 1:537
International Gastric Cancer Linkage Consortium, 1:616, 618
International Incontinentia Pigmenti Consortium, 1:823
International Registry for Calcium Stone Diseases, 1:436
International Registry for LQTS, 1:914
International System on Cytogenetic Nomenclature (ISCN), 1:585, 856
Interpersonal therapy, for depression, 1:441
Interphase, oncogenes and, 2:1118
Interrupted aortic arch, with deletion 22q11 syndrome, 1:421
Intersexuality. See Ambiguous genitalia
Interstitial deletions, with Jacobsen syndrome, 1:839
Interstitial radiation, for glioblastoma multiforme, 1:156
Intestinal abnormalities
gastroschisis, 1:620, 621
Hermansky-Pudlak syndrome, 1:58

Intestinal abnormalities *(continued)*
laterality sequence, 1:879, 880
oculo-digito-esophago-duodenal
syndrome, 2:1107, 1108
Pallister-Killian syndrome, 2:1167
sirenomelia, 2:1407, 1408
Tangier disease, 2:1461
thalidomide embryopathy, 2:1478,
1479
VATER association, 2:1544
Intestinal lymphoma, celiac disease
and, 1:275, 278
Intestinal malrotation, with Cornelia
de Lange syndrome, 1:375
Intestinal obstructions, with
Hirschsprung disease, 1:767, 768
Intestinal villi, 1:275, *275, 277*
Intracerebral hemorrhage, cerebral
palsy and, 1:285, 286
Intracranial pressure
astrocytomas, 1:154, 155
sclerosing bone dysplasias, 2:1377
Intracytoplasmic sperm injection (ICSI)
absence of vas deferens, 1:11–12
description, 2:1626
Kartagener syndrome-related
infertility, 1:855
Intragenic mutations, with spinal
muscular atrophy, 2:1433
Intraneuronal neurofibrillary tangles,
1:89
Intraocular lens implants (IOLs),
2:1051
Intraocular surgery, for myopia,
2:1051
Intrauterine exposure
clubfoot and, 1:325
genetic counseling and, 1:639
Moebius syndrome and, 2:989
teratogens and, 2:1466–1468
VATER association and, 2:1543
Intrauterine growth restriction
(IUGR)
clubfoot, 1:325
deformations and, 1:653–654
Neu-Laxova syndrome, 2:1074
oligohydramnios sequence, 2:1114
renal agenesis, 2:1308
Russell-Silver syndrome, 2:1350,
1351
Seckel syndrome, 2:1383
Sutherland-Haan syndrome,
2:1456, 1457
triploidy, 2:1502, 1503, 1504
trisomy 18, 2:1517
Wolf-Hirschhorn syndrome,
2:1584, 1585
Intravenous pyelograms (IVPs)
Bardet-Biedl syndrome, 1:179
ectrodactyly-ectodermal dysplasia-clefting syndrome, 1:502
Introns, 1:626, 823, 2:1340

Intussusceptions, with Meckel's
diverticulum, 2:964
Inversions
Angelman syndrome, 1:119
defined, 1:626
description, 1:314, 627
Miller-Dieker syndrome, 2:986
Nijmegen breakage syndrome,
2:1095
non-Mendelian inheritance and,
1:832
Involuntary movement.
*See* Choreoathetotis; Dystonia;
Tremors
Iodine, Pendred syndrome and,
2:1196
IOLs (Intraocular lens implants),
2:1051
Ion channels
channelopathies, 1:290–292
long QT syndrome and, 1:911
Ionizing radiation
ataxia-telangiectasia and, 1:158,
159
as carcinogen, 1:157
as teratogen/mutagen, 2:1466,
1468
IP. *See* Incontinentia pigmenti
IRD. *See* Infantile refsum disease
IRF6 gene mutations, 2:1539
Iridogoniodysgenesis with somatic
anomalies. *See* Rieger syndrome
Iris abnormalities
colobomas, 1:340, 342
von Recklinghausen's neurofibromatosis, 2:1551
Waardenburg syndrome, 2:1561,
1563, 1564
Iron
aceruloplasminemia and, 1:19–20
for aceruloplasminemia contraindication, 1:21–22
beta thalassemia and, 1:199
diabetes bronze and, 1:445
Friedreich ataxia and, 1:595
hemochromatosis and, 1:708, 709,
710
for Osler-Weber-Rendu syndrome, 2:1140
pantothenate kinase-associated
neurodegeneration and, 2:1178,
1179
for thrombasthenia of Glanzmann
and Naegeli, 2:1486
Iron chelation therapy
aceruloplasminemia, 1:21
beta thalassemia, 1:199
Iron-deficiency anemia. *See* Anemia
Iron level monitoring, 1:199
Iron overload. *See* Hemochromatosis
Iron overload anemia.
*See* Sideroblastic anemia
Irregular heartbeat. *See* Arrhythmias

Irritability
Canavan disease, 1:242, 244
hydrocephalus, 1:786
leukodystrophy, 1:895
IRT tests, for cystic fibrosis, 1:405
Ischopagus conjoined twins, 1:365
ISCN (International System on
Cytogenetic Nomenclature), 1:585
Ishihara test, 1:344
IsK gene mutations. *See* KCNE1 gene
mutations
Islets of Langerhans, 1:192
Isochromosome 12p syndrome.
*See* Pallister-Killian syndrome
Isochromosomes, with Pallister-
Killian syndrome, 2:1166, 1167
Isoelectric focusing tests, for sickle
cell disease, 2:1400
Isoflurane, malignant hyperthermia
and, 2:935
Isolated cerebral palsy, 1:284
Isolated choroideremia, 1:308
Isolated hemihypertrophy, 1:705, 706
Isolated lissencephaly sequence (ILS),
1:908–909, 910, 911
Isolated nonketotic hyperglycinemia.
*See* Nonketotic hyperglycemia
Isolated polydactyly, 2:1235, 1236,
1237
Isomerism sequence, 1:879
Isoniazid, acquired sideroblastic
anemia from, 1:115
Isosorbide, for hydrocephalus, 1:787
Isotretinoin
lipoprotein lipase deficiency and,
1:907
for Muir-Torre syndrome, 2:1015
Isotretinoin embryopathy.
*See* Accutane embryopathy
Isovaleric acidemia (IA), 2:1129,
1130–1131
Isselbacher, K. J., 1:607
Italian populations, galactose
deficiency in, 1:608
Itching, with ichthyosis, 1:818, 820
IUGR. *See* Intrauterine growth
restriction
Ivemark syndrome. *See* Asplenia
IVPs. *See* Intravenous pyelograms

# J

Jackson-Weiss syndrome, 1:**835–837**
as fibroblast growth factor receptor mutation, 1:583
*vs.* Pfeiffer syndrome, 2:1209,
1210, 1211
Jacobsen, Petra, 1:838
Jacobsen syndrome, 1:**837–840**

# K

mucopolysaccharidoses, 2:1001, 1006

neuraminidase deficiency, 2:1078–1079

neuraminidase deficiency with beta-galactoside deficiency, 2:1083

Lysosomal trafficking regulator. *See* Chediak-Higashi syndrome

Lysosomes
Batten disease and, 1:185
Chediak-Higashi syndrome and, 1:300, 301
cystinosis and, 1:407, 408, 409
GM1-gangliosidosis and, 1:675
mannosidosis and, 2:939

Lysyl hydroxylase, Ehlers-Danlos syndrome and, 1:506

# M

M cones, 1:343

M hemoglobin. *See* Hemoglobin M

Maceration of skin, for ichthyosis, 1:819–820

Machado, William, 1:173, 2:922

Machado-Joseph disease, 2:**922–925,** 1434
*See also* Azorean disease

Machado-Joseph disease type I, 2:922

Machado-Joseph disease type II, 2:922

Machado-Joseph disease type III, 2:922

Macrocephaly
achondroplasia, 1:27
acrocallosal syndrome, 1:31, 32
Adelaide-type craniosynostosis, 1:40
Alexander disease, 1:68
campomelic dysplasia, 1:240
Canavan disease, 1:242, 243
cardiofaciocutaneous syndrome, 1:260
Cowden syndrome, 1:385
Crane-Heise syndrome, 1:387
Dandy-Walker malformation, 1:415, 416
FG syndrome, 1:578, 579
holoprosencephaly, 1:772
hypochondrogenesis, 1:801
Joubert syndrome, 1:845
Langer-Saldino achondrogenesis, 1:874
nevoid basal cell carcinoma syndrome, 2:1091
nevoid basal cell carcinoma syndrome and, 2:1090
Tay-Sachs disease, 2:1465
thanatophoric dysplasia, 2:1483
triploidy, 2:1503

Walker-Warburg syndrome, 2:1565, 1566
Weaver syndrome, 2:1567
X-linked hydrocephaly, 2:1593

Macroglossia
Beckwith-Wiedemann syndrome, 1:192, 194
Coffin-Siris syndrome, 1:331, 332
congenital hypothyroid syndrome, 1:361
hepatoblastomas, 1:195
mucolipidosis, 2:999
mucopolysaccharidoses, 2:1003
Pompe disease, 2:1239
Simpson-Golabi-Behmel syndrome, 2:1404, 1405

Macrophages, Gaucher disease and, 1:622–623

Macrosomia, with Beckwith-Wiedemann syndrome, 1:192, 194

Macugen, for age-related macular degeneration, 2:929

Macular corneal dystrophy, 1:370, 371, 372

Macular degeneration, with Stargardt disease, 2:1448–1450

Macular degeneration - age-related (AMD), 2:*925,* **925–930,** 1449

Macular dystrophy with flecks. *See* Stargardt disease

Macules. *See* Cherry-red macules; Lentigines

Mad cow disease. *See* New variant Creutzfeld-Jakob disease

Madarosis, 1:689

Madelung's deformity, 1:485, 486

Madisson, H., 2:1530

Madopar, for Parkinson disease, 2:1183

Maffuci disease, 1:305, 306
*See also* Chondrosarcomas

Magenis, Ellen, 2:1420

Magnani, M., 1:608

Magnesium sulfate, cerebral palsy and, 1:289

Magnetic resonance imaging (MRI)
ADHD, 1:163
agenesis of the corpus callosum, 1:381
Aicardi syndrome, 1:50
ALD, 1:46–47
Alzheimer's disease, 1:85, 87, 89
ankylosing spondylitis, 1:124
asplenia, 1:145
astrocytomas, 1:155
Beckwith-Wiedemann syndrome, 1:194
bicuspid aortic valves, 1:203
breast cancer, 1:228–229
CADASIL, 1:282
Canavan disease, 1:243
cancer, 1:252
cerebral palsy, 1:288

congenital heart disease, 1:358
conjoined twins, 1:366
Crouzonodermoskeletal syndrome, 1:399
Dandy-Walker malformation, 1:416
De Grouchy syndrome, 1:419
dementia, 1:429
dystonia, 1:493
epilepsy, 1:527
essential tremor, 1:537
familial pulmonary arterial hypertension, 1:568
frontotemporal dementia, 1:602
Gerstmann-Straussler-Scheinker disease, 1:661
hemochromatosis, 1:709
holoprosencephaly, 1:*770*
hydrocephalus, 1:786
Larsen syndrome, 1:877
laterality sequence, 1:881
Leigh syndrome, 1:890
lissencephaly, 1:910
Marfan syndrome, 2:944
microcephaly, 2:981
Miller-Dieker syndrome, 2:987
moyamoya, 2:997
multiple sclerosis, 2:1031
neurofibromatosis, 2:1088
Osler-Weber-Rendu syndrome, 2:1139
Pallister-Hall syndrome, 2:1164
pantothenate kinase-associated neurodegeneration, 2:1179
Pelizaeus-Merzbacher disease, 2:1194
Pendred syndrome, 2:1198, 1199
Pfeiffer syndrome, 2:1211
pituitary dwarfism, 2:1223–1224
prion diseases, 2:1261
Schinzel-Giedion syndrome, 2:1359
skeletal dysplasia, 2:1414
spinocerebellar ataxias, 2:1436
Sturge-Weber syndrome, 2:*1454*
tuberous sclerosis complex, 2:1523
Von Hippel-Lindau syndrome, 2:1548
von Recklinghausen's neurofibromatosis, 2:1552

Mainstreaming, for Down syndrome, 1:472

Maintenance phase of schizophrenia, 2:1360, 1364

MAIS (Mild androgen insensitivity syndrome), 1:110*t,* 111, 112, 113

Majewski syndrome, 2:1391, 1392

Major anomalies, 1:652, 653, 654

Major depressive episodes, 1:437, 438
*See also* Depression

Major groove (DNA), 1:462

Major hereditary leptocytosis. *See* Beta thalassemia major

Major histocompatibility complex (MHC), 2:**930–934**, 930*t*
  diabetes and, 1:445
  multiple sclerosis and, 2:1030
  myasthenia gravis and, 2:1044
Malarial resistance
  heterozygote advantage and, 1:641
  sickle cell trait and, 2:1395
  thalassemia and, 2:1471
Male hormones. *See* Androgens
Male hypogenitalism, with Alstrom syndrome, 1:84
Male infertility
  absence of vas deferens, 1:11, 12
  androgen insensitivity syndrome, 1:111, 112
  Kartagener syndrome, 1:852, 853, 854
  Kennedy disease, 1:857, 858
  Klinefelter syndrome, 1:860, 861
  XX male syndrome, 2:1607
  XYY syndrome, 2:1615
Male pattern hair loss (MPHL), 1:691, 692–693, 694, 695
Male Turner syndrome. *See* Noonan syndrome
Males
  Aarskog syndrome, 1:3, 4
  ADHD, 1:163
  albinism, 1:58
  alpha-thalassemia X-linked mental retardation syndrome, 1:79, 80
  ambiguous genitalia, 1:656–659
  amelia, 1:92–93
  Asperger syndrome, 1:139
  asplenia, 1:144
  asthma, 1:149
  autism, 1:169
  Bassen-Kornzweig syndrome, 1:183
  breast cancer, 1:225, 227, 228, 229
  campomelic dysplasia, 1:239
  carnitine palmitoyltransferase deficiency, 1:263
  chondrosarcomas, 1:306
  Coffin-Lowry syndrome, 1:329
  color blindness, 1:343
  Emery-Dreifuss muscular dystrophy, 1:511, 512, 513
  Fabry disease, 1:541
  fragile X syndrome, 1:586, 587
  karyotype, 1:857
  Kennedy disease, 1:857, 858
  Lesch-Nyhan syndrome, 1:891
  liver cancer, 1:719
  liver disease, 1:77
  Lowe oculocerebrorenal syndrome, 1:918, 919
  mucopolysaccharidoses, 2:1011
  muscular dystrophy, 1:479, 480
  osteoporosis, 2:1148
  otopalatodigital syndrome, 2:1153, 1154

  prune-belly syndrome, 2:1281
  pseudohermaphroditism, 1:764–765
  Renpenning syndrome, 2:1315
  sex determination, 1:110
  sex determining region Y, 2:*1446*, 1446–1447
  Smith-Fineman-Myers syndrome, 2:1415–1416
  Sutherland-Haan syndrome, 2:1456–1457
  Wiskott-Aldrich syndrome, 2:1581
  X-linked hydrocephaly, 2:1592
  X-linked inheritance and, 1:641
  X-linked mental retardation, 2:1595, 1597
  X-linked recessive inheritance and, 1:832
  XX male syndrome, 2:1606–1609, 1607*t*
  XYY syndrome, 2:1614
  YY syndrome, 2:1617
Malformations, 1:653, 654, 655
  *See also specific types*
Malignant fever. *See* Malignant hyperthermia
Malignant hyperpyrexia. *See* Malignant hyperthermia
Malignant Hyperthermia Association of the United States, 2:938
Malignant hyperthermia (MH), 2:**934–939**
  central core disease and, 1:280
  as channelopathy, 1:291
  Freeman-Sheldon syndrome and, 1:594
  pharmacogenetics and, 2:1213
  Schwartz-Jampel syndrome and, 2:1368
Malignant infantile osteopetrosis (MIOP), 2:1373, 1375
Malignant keratosis. *See* Harlequin fetus
Malignant melanoma, 2:1604
Malignant tumors, 1:245
  *See also* Tumors
Malnutrition. *See* Nutritional deficiency
Mammography
  ACS recommendations, 1:253
  breast cancer and, 1:225, 228, 230
  Li-Fraumeni syndrome and, 1:899
  ovarian cancer and, 2:1158
  Peutz-Jeghers syndrome and, 2:1208
MANB gene mutations, 2:939
MANB1 gene mutations, 2:939
Mandibulofacial dysostosis. *See* Treacher Collins syndrome
Manic-depressive psychosis. *See* Bipolar disorder
Manic episodes, with bipolar disorder, 1:207, 209, 210, 211, 440

Manipulative treatment, for clubfoot, 1:325, 326
Mannosidosis, 2:**939–941**
MAOIs. *See* Monoamine oxidase inhibitors
Map-dot-fingerprint dystrophy, 1:370, 371
Map units (m.u.), 1:642
Mapping. *See* Genetic mapping
MAPT gene mutations, 1:600
Marchiafava-Micheli syndrome. *See* Paroxysmal nocturnal hemoglobinuria
Marden-Walker syndrome, 2:1368
Marfan, Antoine, 2:941
Marfan syndrome, 2:**941–947**, *942*
  *vs.* cystathionine b-synthase deficiency, 1:778
  description, 1:358
Marfanoid body type, 2:1392, 1393, 1394
Marfanoid craniosynostosis syndrome. *See* Shprintzen-Goldberg craniosynostosis syndrome
Marfanoid syndromes, 2:944
Marie, Pierre, 1:34
Marie-Strumpell spondylitis Bechterew syndrome. *See* Ankylosing spondylitis
Marie's ataxia. *See* Spinocerebellar ataxias
Marker chromosomes, VATER association and, 2:1542
Marker X syndrome. *See* Fragile X syndrome
Markers of aneuploidy, prenatal ultrasound and, 2:1255–1257
Maroteaux-Lamy syndrome. *See* Mucopolysaccharidosis type VI
Marshall-Smith syndrome, 2:**949–952**
Marshall syndrome, 2:**947–949**
  *vs.* Stickler syndrome, 2:1451
  *vs.* Weissenbacher-Zweymuller syndrome, 2:1570
Martin-Bell syndrome. *See* Fragile X syndrome
Martin syndrome, 1:771
MAS. *See* McCune-Albright syndrome
MASA syndrome, 2:1591
  *See also* X-linked hydrocephaly
Masculinized external genitals, 1:351, 352, 353, 355
Mason, H. H., 1:607
Massachusetts General Hospital, 1:166
Massage therapy, for arthrogryposis multiplex congenital, 1:136, 137
Masseter spasm, 2:935, 937
Mast cells, 1:148

mucopolysaccharidoses, 2:1003, 1006, 1007, 1008
neuraminidase deficiency with beta-galactoside deficiency, 2:1082
nonketotic hyperglycemia, 2:1098, 1099
Norrie disease, 2:1104, 1105, 1106
oculo-digito-esophago-duodenal syndrome, 2:1108
oral-facial-digital syndrome, 2:1128
ornithine transcarbamylase deficiency, 2:1134, 1136
Paine syndrome, 2:1161
Pallister-Killian syndrome, 2:1165, 1166, 1167
Pelizaeus-Merzbacher disease, 2:1194
pervasive development disorders, 2:1203
phenylketonuria, 2:1215, 1216, 1217
Prader-Willi syndrome, 2:1251
for propionic acidemia, 2:1266
Renpenning syndrome, 2:1314, 1315
rhizomelic chondrodysplasia punctata, 2:1332, 1333, 1334
Roberts SC phocomelia, 2:1341
Rubinstein-Taybi syndrome, 2:1348, 1349, 1350
Saethre-Chotzen syndrome, 2:1355, 1357
Schinzel-Giedion syndrome, 2:1358
Seckel syndrome, 2:1383
Shprintzen-Goldberg craniosynostosis syndrome, 2:1393
Sjögren-Larsson syndrome, 2:1408, 1409, 1410
Smith-Fineman-Myers syndrome, 2:1415, 1416
Smith-Lemli-Optiz syndrome, 2:1417, 1418
Smith-Magenis syndrome, 2:1420, 1421
Sutherland-Haan syndrome, 2:1456, 1457
trichorhinophalangeal syndrome, 2:1496, 1497
trisomy 8 mosaicism syndrome, 2:1509, 1510
trisomy 13, 2:1512, 1513
trisomy 18, 2:1515
Usher syndrome, 2:1535, 1536
Walker-Warburg syndrome, 2:1566
X-linked hydrocephaly, 2:1592, 1593
XXXX syndrome, 2:1610, 1611
XXXXX syndrome, 2:1612
*See also specific types*
Mental retardation X-linked, syndrome 3 (MRXS3).
*See* Sutherland-Haan syndrome

Mental status examination
dementia, 1:428
depression, 1:440
frontotemporal dementia, 1:602
Meralgia paresthetica, 1:520
Mercaptopropionylglycine (MPG), 1:413
Merck Pharmaceuticals, 2:1330
Merlin, neurofibromatosis and, 2:1087
Mermaid syndrome. *See* Sirenomelia
Meroanencephaly, 1:117, 2:1076
Meromelia, 1:90
Merosin, congenital muscular dystrophy and, 2:1039
MERRF syndrome, hearing loss and, 1:740
Merrick, Joseph (John), 2:1277
Merzbacher, L., 2:1193
MESA (Microsurgical epididymal sperm aspiration), 1:11
Mesobrachyphalangy, 2:1107, 1108
Mesoderm
caudal dysplasia and, 1:270
description, 1:270, 500
Meckel-Gruber syndrome and, 2:961
VATER association and, 2:1542
Werner syndrome and, 2:1571–1572, 1573
Mesoectodermal dysplasia. *See* Ellis-van Creveld syndrome
Mesomelia, with dyschondrosteosis, 1:485, 486
Mesonephric duct, 1:10
Messenger RNA (mRNA), 1:462, 626, 2:1339–1340
Mestinon
congenital myasthenic syndromes, 1:291
myasthenia gravis, 2:1046
Metabolic acidosis, 1:796, 2:972
Metabolic disorders
microcephaly and, 2:981
as teratogen, 2:1466, 1468
Metabolism
description, 1:776–777
malignant hyperthermia and, 2:935, 936
Zellweger syndrome and, 2:1621
*See also* Inborn errors of metabolism
Metacarpals, 1:219, 220
Metacarpophalangeal profiles, 1:221
Metacentric chromosomes, 1:318
Metachromatic leukodystrophy, 1:895, 896
Metalloporphyrins, 1:52
Metaphase, 1:318
Metaphyseal acroscyphodysplasia, 2:970, 972

Metaphyseal anadysplasia, 2:970, 971
Metaphyseal dysostosis. *See* Jansen type metaphyseal dysplasia; Spahr-type metaphyseal chondrodysplasia
Metaphyseal dysplasia, 2:**970–972,** 1413
Metarhodopsin II, 2:1335
Metastatic liver cancer, 1:717, *718,* 719, 721
Metatarsals, 1:219–220
Metatropic dwarfism, 2:1570
Metformin
diabetes, 1:451
polycystic ovary syndrome, 2:1234
Methemoglobin, congenital methemoglobinemia and, 1:363
Methemoglobinemia, beta-globin type. *See* Congenital methemoglobinemia
Methionine
metabolism of, 1:*776, 777, 778*
prion diseases and, 2:1260
Methotrexate
for ankylosing spondylitis, 1:124
for rheumatoid arthritis, 2:1331
as teratogen, 1:92
Methoxyflurane, malignant hyperthermia and, 2:935
Methyl CpG-binding protein 2 gene mutations. *See* MECP2 gene mutations
Methylation testing, 2:1251
Methylene blue, for congenital methemoglobinemia, 1:364
Methylene H4-folate (MTHFR), 1:779
Methylmalonic acidemia (MMA), 2:**972–975**
methylmalonicaciduria and, 2:976, 977
as organic acidemia, 2:1129, 1131, 1132
pancreatic beta cell agenesis and, 2:1168, 1169
Methylmalonic CoA mutase (MCM), 2:975
Methylmalonicaciduria due to methylmalonic CoA mutase deficiency, 2:**975–978**
Methylmalonyl-CoA, 2:973, 974, 975–976
Methylphenidate
ADHD, 1:164
Asperger syndrome, 1:141
autism, 1:171
depression, 1:441
Methylprednisone
multiple sclerosis, 2:1032
rheumatoid arthritis, 2:1330
Metopic craniosynostosis, 1:388, 391

Multiple endocrine neoplasia 2A (MEN2A), 1:648, 2:1018, 1019, 1020, 1021, 1022

Multiple endocrine neoplasia 2B (MEN2B), 2:1018, 1019, 1020, 1021, 1022

Multiple endocrine neoplasia 3 (MEN3). *See* Multiple endocrine neoplasia 2B

Multiple endocrine neoplasias (MEN), 2:**1018–1023,** 1019*t*

Multiple epiphyseal dysplasia (MED), 1:453, 2:**1023–1026,** 1413

Multiple hereditary exostoses (MHE). *See* Hereditary multiple exostoses

Multiple lentigines syndrome, 2:**1027–1028,** 1103

Multiple sclerosis (MS), 2:**1028–1033,** *1029*

Multiple Sleep Latency Tests, 2:1066–1067

Multiplex infantilis. *See* Engelmann disease

Multiplex ligation-dependent probe amplification (MLPA), 2:**1033–1035**

Muscle atrophy
abetalipoproteinemia, 1:8
ALS, 1:105, 106, 107
amyoplasia, 1:102, 103
ASL deficiency, 1:43
Azorean disease, 1:174, 175
Duchenne muscular dystrophy, 1:479
Emery-Dreifuss muscular dystrophy, 1:511, 513
hereditary spastic paraplegia, 1:756
Kennedy disease, 1:857
leukodystrophy, 1:895
limb-girdle muscular dystrophy, 1:900, 902
spinal muscular atrophy, 2:1431, 1432, 1434

Muscle biopsy
limb-girdle muscular dystrophy, 1:904
malignant hyperthermia, 2:937, 938
muscular dystrophy, 2:1041
myotonic dystrophy, 2:1055
myotubular myopathy, 2:1059
Schwartz-Jampel syndrome, 2:1367
spinal muscular atrophy, 2:1433

Muscle CPT deficiency, 1:264, 265

Muscle cramps, glycogen storage diseases and, 1:668

Muscle degeneration. *See* Muscle atrophy

Muscle diseases. *See* Myopathies

Muscle-eye-brain disease (MEB), 1:909

Muscle pain. *See* Myalgia

Muscle relaxants
for cerebral palsy, 1:288
malignant hyperthermia and, 1:291, 2:935, 936, 938

Muscle spasms
Alexander disease, 1:68
Canavan disease, 1:242
hereditary spastic paraplegia, 1:754, 757
malignant hyperthermia, 2:936, 937
micro syndrome, 2:979
Niemann-Pick syndrome, 2:1093, 1094
nonketotic hyperglycemia, 2:1099
oral-facial-digital syndrome, 2:1128
pantothenate kinase-associated neurodegeneration, 2:1179
pyloric stenosis, 2:1291

Muscle stiffness
Canavan disease, 1:242
malignant hyperthermia, 2:935, 936, 937, 938
oculodentodigital syndrome, 2:1110, 1111
Paine syndrome, 2:1161
Parkinson disease, 2:1182
*See also* Spasticity

Muscle tone, poor. *See* Hypotonia

Muscle transfer surgery, for amyoplasia, 1:104

Muscle twitching. *See* Fasciculations

Muscle weakness
ALS, 1:106, 107
Azorean disease, 1:174
Barth syndrome, 1:180
Canavan disease, 1:242
central core disease, 1:279, 280
cerebral palsy, 1:287, 288
channelopathies, 1:291–292
Charcot-Marie-Tooth syndrome, 1:294
Chediak-Higashi syndrome, 1:301
Duchenne muscular dystrophy, 1:479, 481–482
Emery-Dreifuss muscular dystrophy, 1:511, 512, 513
Engelmann disease, 1:518, 519
facioscapulohumeral muscular dystrophy, 1:544
familial dysautonomia, 1:556
Freeman-Sheldon syndrome, 1:593
glycogen storage diseases, 1:669, 670, 671, 672, 674
Joubert syndrome, 1:843, 845
Kennedy disease, 1:857, 858
limb-girdle muscular dystrophy, 1:900, 902, 903
lissencephaly, 1:910
Lowe oculocerebrorenal syndrome, 1:919
metaphyseal dysplasia, 2:970

muscular dystrophy, 2:1035, 1036, 1039
myasthenia gravis, 2:1043
myasthenic crises, 2:1045
myotonic dystrophy, 2:1054
myotubular myopathy, 2:1058, 1059, 1060
Niemann-Pick syndrome, 2:1093, 1094
nonketotic hyperglycemia, 2:1099
Noonan syndrome, 2:1102, 1103
Pallister-Killian syndrome, 2:1165, 1166
Pompe disease, 2:1239–1240
porphyrias, 2:1245
scleroderma, 2:1370
spinal muscular atrophy, 2:1432, 1434
spondyloepiphyseal dysplasia, 2:1440

Muscular dystrophy, 2:**1035–1043,** *1036*
*vs.* leukodystrophy, 1:895
*vs.* Pompe disease, 2:1237
types of, 1:479
with Walker-Warburg syndrome, 2:1565, 1566
*See also specific types*

Muscular Dystrophy Association, 1:108, 279, 280

Musculoskeletal abnormalities
Cornelia de Lange syndrome, 1:374–375
glycogen storage diseases, 1:668
Niemann-Pick syndrome, 2:1093, 1094
Waardenburg syndrome, 2:1561, 1563, 1564
*See also* Skeletal abnormalities

Mutagens, 1:627, 2:1466

Mutated in colon cancer (MCC) gene mutations. *See* MCC gene mutations

Mutation analysis
diastrophic dysplasia, 1:455
Menkes syndrome, 2:968, 969
multiple epiphyseal dysplasia, 2:1025
phenylketonuria, 2:1217
thanatophoric dysplasia, 2:1483

Mutations. *See* Gene mutations

Mutons, 1:625

Myalgia
familial Mediterranean fever, 1:558
limb-girdle muscular dystrophy, 1:904
lipoprotein lipase deficiency, 1:906

Myasthenia. *See* Muscle weakness

Myasthenia gravis, 2:**1043–1047,** *1044*

Myasthenic crises, 2:1045

*Mycoplasma* infections, 1:233

Index

GALE ENCYCLOPEDIA OF GENETIC DISORDERS 3

1795

cystic fibrosis, 1:403, 405
Donohue syndrome, 1:465, 466
galactose deficiency, 1:609
*See also specific deficiencies*
NVC (Neurovision correction),
2:1051
Nystagmus
albinism, 1:58, 59
Alstrom syndrome, 1:83
cone-rod dystrophy, 1:349
Cornelia de Lange syndrome,
1:376
Dandy-Walker malformation,
1:416
Hermansky-Pudlak syndrome,
1:763
infantile Refsum disease, 1:827
Joubert syndrome, 1:843, 845
Kallmann syndrome, 1:851
Pelizaeus-Merzbacher disease,
2:1194
Refsum disease, 2:1306

# O

OA (ocular albinism), 1:56, 57, 58
Oates, Robert, 1:10
Obesity
Alstrom syndrome, 1:82, 83
Bardet-Biedl syndrome, 1:178, 179
as cancer risk factor, 1:251
Cohen syndrome, 1:333, 334
diabetes, 1:447, 448
polycystic ovary syndrome,
2:1233, 1234
Prader-Willi syndrome, 2:1250,
1251, 1252
skeletal dysplasia, 2:1414
*See also* Weight issues
Obesity-hypotonia syndrome.
*See* Cohen syndrome
Obligate carrier status, defined, 1:832
Obsessive-compulsive disorder,
Tourette syndrome and, 2:1489,
1491, 1493
Obstruction congenital heart defects,
1:357
Obstructive azoospermia, 1:11
Obstructive hydrocephaus. *See* Non-
communicating hydrocephalus
Obstructive sleep apnea
Hallermann-Streiff syndrome,
1:697
hypochondroplasia, 1:805
Marfan syndrome, 2:944
OCA (oculocutaneous albinism),
1:56, 57, 58
OCA2 gene mutations, 1:58
Occipital encephaloceles, 1:515,
516–517

Occipital horn syndrome (OHS),
2:966
Occupational factors
astrocytomas, 1:154, 157
cancer, 1:252
clubfoot, 1:325
color blindness, 1:344
dementia, 1:428
pancreatic cancer, 2:1170
Occupational therapy
ALS, 1:108
Angelman syndrome, 1:121
campomelic dysplasia, 1:241
cardiofaciocutaneous syndrome,
1:261
cerebral palsy, 1:288
Charcot-Marie-Tooth syndrome,
1:295
Cohen syndrome, 1:336
compression neuropathy, 1:348
diastrophic dysplasia, 1:456
ectodermal dysplasias, 1:498
Emery-Dreifuss muscular dystrophy, 1:514
entrapment neuropathy, 1:521
familial dysautonomia, 1:556
Friedreich ataxia, 1:596
Huntington disease, 1:783
Larsen syndrome, 1:877
muscular dystrophy, 2:1042
myotonic dystrophy, 2:1055
myotubular myopathy, 2:1060
Pelizaeus-Merzbacher disease,
2:1195
spinocerebellar ataxias, 2:1437
trismus-pseudocamptodactyly
syndrome, 2:1507
X-linked mental retardation,
2:1598
Ochronosis
alkaptonuria, 1:69, 71, 72, 73, 74
spondyloepiphyseal dysplasia,
2:1441
Ochronotic arthritis, 1:69, 72, 74, 75
Ochronotic arthropathy, 1:72
OCRL1 gene mutations
Dent's disease, 1:433, 434, 435
Lowe oculocerebrorenal
syndrome, 1:918, 920
Octanol, for essential tremor, 1:540
Octreotide, for acromegaly, 1:36, 37
Ocular albinism (OA), 1:56, 57, 58
Ocular fundus, Sjögren-Larsson
syndrome and, 2:1409
Ocular hypertelorism
acrocallosal syndrome, 1:31, 32
Adelaide-type craniosynostosis,
1:40, 41
Alagille syndrome, 1:55
arthrogryposis multiplex
congenital, 1:135
Fraser syndrome, 1:590
frontonasal dysplasia, 1:597, 598

Greig cephalopolysyndactyly,
1:681, 682
hypochondrogenesis, 1:801
Jacobsen syndrome, 1:839
Larsen syndrome, 1:875, 877
laterality sequence, 1:881
Marshall syndrome, 2:947, 948
multiple lentigines syndrome,
2:1027
Nance-Insley syndrome, 2:1064
Neu-Laxova syndrome, 2:1073
Opitz syndrome, 2:1124, 1126
otopalatodigital syndrome,
2:1153, 1154
Pallister-Killian syndrome, 2:1166
Robinow syndrome, 2:1344
Saethre-Chotzen syndrome,
2:1355, 1357
Shprintzen-Goldberg craniosynos-
tosis syndrome, 2:1393
Simpson-Golabi-Behmel syndrome,
2:1404, 1405
triploidy, 2:1505
Weaver syndrome, 2:1567
Weissenbacher-Zweymuller
syndrome, 2:1569, 1570
Wolf-Hirschhorn syndrome,
2:1584, 1585
XXXX syndrome, 2:1609
Zellweger syndrome, 2:1622
Oculo-auriculo-vertebral spectrum.
*See* Goldenhar syndrome
Oculo-digital reflex, Leber congenital
amaurosis and, 1:883
Oculo-digito-esophago-duodenal
syndrome (ODED), 2:**1107–1109**
Oculoauriculovertebral spectrum.
*See* Hemifacial microsomia
Oculocerebrorenal syndrome of
Lowe. *See* Lowe oculocerebrorenal
syndrome
Oculocutaneous albinism (OCA),
1:56, 57, 58, 762, 764
Oculodentodigital syndrome
(ODDS), 2:**1109–1112**
Oculomandibulodyscephaly with
hypotrichosis. *See* Hallermann-
Streiff syndrome
Oculomotor nerve, Duane retraction
syndrome and, 1:473
Oculopharyngeal muscular dystrophy
(OPMD), 2:1036, 1039, 1040, 1042
ODDS. *See* Oculodentodigital
syndrome
ODED. *See* Oculo-digito-esophago-
duodenal syndrome
Odontohypophosphatasia, 1:809
OFD. *See* Oral-facial-digital
syndrome
Office of Rare Diseases (ORD), 1:116,
180, 2:1540
Ohio State University, 2:1203

Palmoplantar keratoderma disorders, 1:687, 688

Palpebral fissures
 oculo-digito-esophago-duodenal syndrome, 2:1107, 1108
 otopalatodigital syndrome, 2:1153, 1154

Pamelor. *See* Nortriptyline

Pancreas, description of, 1:750

Pancreas abnormalities
 Bürger-Grütz syndrome, 1:236
 diabetes, 1:443–444
 Donohue syndrome, 1:464
 Shwachman-Diamond syndrome, 2:971
 trisomy 18, 2:1517
 Von Hippel-Lindau syndrome, 2:1548

Pancreatic beta cell agenesis, 2:**1168–1169**

Pancreatic beta cells, diabetes and, 1:445, 446, 447

Pancreatic cancer, 2:**1169–1174,** *1170*
 breast cancer and, 1:227, 228, 229
 as common cancer, 1:250
 hereditary pancreatitis and, 1:752, 753
 ovarian cancer and, 2:1157, 1158

Pancreatic carcinoma. *See* Pancreatic cancer

Pancreatic enzymes
 cystic fibrosis, 1:405, 406
 hereditary pancreatitis and, 1:753

Pancreatic insufficiency, with cystic fibrosis, 1:402, 405

Pancreatic insufficiency and bone marrow dysfunction.
 *See* Shwachman-Diamond syndrome

Pancreatic tumors
 Beckwith-Wiedemann syndrome, 1:192
 multiple endocrine neoplasias and, 2:1018–1019, 1022
 Von Hippel-Lindau syndrome, 2:1548

Pancreatitis
 defined, 1:750
 hemorrhagic, 1:752
 hereditary, 1:750–754, *751*
 with lipoprotein lipase deficiency, 1:906–907
 pancreatic cancer and, 2:1170, 1171

Panhypopituitarism, 2:1222, 1224

Panic attacks, 2:1174, 1175, 1176, 1177

Panic disorder, 2:**1174–1178**

PANK2 gene mutations, 2:1178–1179

Pansinusitis, 1:403

Pantothenate kinase-associated neurodegeneration (PKAN), 2:**1178–1180**

PAP-A (Postaxial polydactyly type A). *See* Postaxial polydactyly

Pap smears, 1:487

Papillomatous papules
 Costello syndrome, 1:382, 384
 Goltz syndrome, 1:*678,* 679, 680

Papillon-Leage syndrome, 2:1127

Papillon-Lefevre syndrome, 1:687–688

PAPP-A (Pregnancy-associated plasma protein-A), 1:376

Paralysis
 ALS, 1:107
 cerebral palsy, 2:1426
 compression neuropathy, 1:348
 leukodystrophy, 1:895
 neural tube defects, 2:1076, 1077
 periodic, 1:291
 spina bifida, 2:1429–1430
 Tay-Sachs disease, 2:1465
 thalidomide embryopathy, 2:1479
 tomaculous neuropathy, 2:1488

Paranoid schizophrenia, 2:1360

Parapagus conjoined twins, 1:366

Paraplegin gene mutations, 1:755

Parasitic conjoined twins, 1:366

Parathyroid gland
 deletion 22q11 syndrome and, 1:422
 Dent's disease and, 1:434, 435
 multiple endocrine neoplasias and, 2:1018, 1019

Parathyroid hormone (PTH), multiple endocrine neoplasias and, 2:1021

Parentage testing, HLA typing and, 2:934

Parental age
 progeria syndrome and, 2:1263
 Smith-Magenis syndrome and, 2:1421
 *See also* Maternal age; Paternal age

Paresis, with cerebral palsy, 1:284, 287

Paresthesia
 micro syndrome, 2:979
 multiple sclerosis, 2:1031
 prion diseases, 2:1261

Parietal encephaloceles, 1:515, 516

Parkes-Weber syndrome, 1:866

Parkinson, James, 1:536, 2:1181

Parkinson disease, 2:*1181,* **1181–1185**
 *vs.* Alzheimer's disease, 1:87
 dystonia and, 1:492
 *vs.* essential tremor, 1:536, 537
 *vs.* frontotemporal dementia, 1:602

Parkinsonism, 2:1182

Parkinsonism plus disorders, 2:1182

Parlodel. *See* Bromocriptine

Parnate, for depression, 1:441

Paroxetine
 depression, 1:441
 panic disorder, 2:1176
 Tourette syndrome, 2:1493

Paroxysmal nocturnal hemoglobinuria (PNH), 2:**1185–1187**

Paroxysmal polyserositis. *See* Familial Mediterranean fever

Partial 11q monosomy syndrome. *See* Jacobsen syndrome

Partial albinism, 1:683, 684, 2:1563

Partial androgen insensitivity syndrome (PAIS), 1:110*t,* 111, 112

Partial biotinidase deficiency, 1:205, 206

Partial dysgenesis of the corpus callosum, 1:378

Partial hepatectomy, 1:720

Partial molar pregnancies, 2:1502

Partial paralysis, 2:1031

Partial seizures, 1:50, 526

Partial situs inversus, 1:853

Partial trisomy
 trisomy 13, 2:1512, 1513
 trisomy 18, 2:1515, 1516, 1519

Parvovirus infections, 2:1399

Passive motion therapy, for trismus-pseudocamptodactyly syndrome, 2:1507

Passive smoking, cancer and, 1:251

Patau, Klaus, 2:1511

Patau syndrome. *See* Trisomy 13

Patella abnormalities
 multiple epiphyseal dysplasia, 2:1025, 1026
 nail-patella syndrome, 2:1061, 1062, 1063

Patent ductus arteriosus (PDA), 2:**1187–1190,** *1188*
 achondrogenesis and, 1:23
 as congenital heart defect, 1:356
 Cornelia de Lange syndrome and, 1:375, 377
 Costello syndrome and, 1:382
 deletion 22q11 syndrome and, 1:421
 monosomy 1p36 syndrome and, 2:991
 trisomy 13 and, 2:1513
 XXXXX syndrome and, 2:1612

Paternal age
 Beare-Stevenson cutis gyrata syndrome and, 1:190
 cardiofaciocutaneous syndrome and, 1:260
 CHARGE syndrome and, 1:297
 Crouzon syndrome and, 1:395
 Marfan syndrome and, 2:946
 Shprintzen-Goldberg craniosynostosis syndrome and, 2:1393
 spondyloepiphyseal dysplasia and, 2:1445

Paternal inheritance
 Angelman syndrome, 1:119, 120
 Apert syndrome, 1:125

Selective estrogen receptor modulators (SERMs), for osteoporosis, 2:1150

Selective serotonin reuptake inhibitors (SSRIs)
Alzheimer's disease, 1:89
Asperger syndrome, 1:141
autism, 1:171
depression, 1:441
frontotemporal dementia, 1:603

Selegiline, for Parkinson disease, 2:1183

Self-examination, for cancer, 1:253
*See also* Breast self-examination

Self-injury
Lesch-Nyhan syndrome, 1:891, 892, 893
Smith-Magenis syndrome, 2:1422
Tourette syndrome, 2:1489, 1491

Self-stimulating behavior, with autism, 1:168

Semantic dementia, 1:600

Semen, absence of vas deferens and, 1:11

Semilobar holoprosencephaly, 1:770, 772

Seminal vesicle cysts, with urogenital adysplasia syndrome, 2:1531

Senile osteoporosis, 2:1148

Senile plaques, 1:89

Senility. *See* Dementia

Sense of smell abnormalities. *See* Anosmia

Sensitivity of diagnosis, 1:124, 641

Sensorineural hearing loss
hereditary, 1:736, 737, 741, 742
Pendred syndrome, 2:1196–1197, 1198, 1199, 1200
Stickler syndrome, 2:1450, 1452
Usher syndrome, 2:1533, 1534, 1535, 1536
Waardenburg syndrome, 2:1564

Sensory nervous system
Charcot-Marie-Tooth syndrome and, 1:292, 294
compression neuropathy and, 1:346
entrapment neuropathy and, 1:519
familial dysautonomia and, 1:555, 556

Sensory neurons
Charcot-Marie-Tooth syndrome and, 1:292
Kennedy disease and, 1:857

Sensory tricks, 1:493

Septal defects
Cayler cardiofacial syndrome, 1:272, 273
description, 1:357
Holt-Oram syndrome, 1:774, 775
trisomy 13, 2:1513
trisomy 18, 2:1517

XXXXX syndrome, 2:1612, 1613
*See also* Atrial septal defects; Ventricular septal defects

Septal dermoplasty, 2:1139

Septo-optic dysplasia (SOD), 2:**1384–1387**

Septum pellucidum
microphthalmia with linear skin defects and, 2:984
septo-optic dysplasia and, 2:1384, 1385, 1386

Sequence tagged sites (STSs), 1:643

Sequencing, 1:*637*
Alagille syndrome, 1:55
alpha-thalassemia X-linked mental retardation syndrome, 1:81
direct, 1:646
ectodermal dysplasias, 1:498
familial Mediterranean fever, 1:559
Human Genome Project, 1:780
multiple epiphyseal dysplasia, 2:1025
X chromosome, 2:1595
X-linked severe combined immunodeficiency, 2:1600

SERMs (Selective estrogen receptor modulators), for osteoporosis, 2:1150

Seronegative spondyloarthropathies, 1:121
*See also* Ankylosing spondylitis

Serositis, with familial Mediterranean fever, 1:557, 559, 560

Serotonin
alcoholism and, 1:64
depression and, 1:438, 439
panic disorder and, 2:1174
schizophrenia and, 2:1364
Tourette syndrome and, 2:1490

Sertraline
depression, 1:441
lipoprotein lipase deficiency, 1:907
panic disorder, 2:1176
Tourette syndrome, 2:1493

Serum amyloid A (SAA), familial Mediterranean fever and, 1:559

Serum ceruloplasmin, 1:20, 21

Serum ferritin tests, 1:199

Serum glutamic oxaloacetic transaminase (SGOT) tests, 1:78

Serum glutamic pyruvic transaminase (SGPT) tests, 1:78

Severe achondroplasia with developmental delay and acanthosis nigricans (SADDAN) dysplasia, 1:582

Severe asthma, 1:150–151

Severe atypical sperocytosis due to ankyrine defect, 1:758–762

Severe combined immunodeficiency (SCID), 2:971, *1387*, **1387–1390**, 1599–1602

Severe hearing loss, 1:741, 2:1197, 1533

Severe hemophilia, 1:713

Sevoflurane, malignant hyperthermia and, 2:935

Sex assignment. *See* Gender assignment

Sex cells, 1:312

Sex chromosomes
aneuploidy of, 1:*312, 313*
centromeres and, 1:318
defined, 1:317
zygote formation and, 2:1624–1625
*See also* X chromosome; Y chromosome

Sex determining region Y (SRY), 2:**1445–1448,** *1446*

Sex hormone-binding globulin, polycystic ovary syndrome and, 2:1233

Sex hormones
androgen insensitivity syndrome and, 1:110–111
campomelic dysplasia and, 1:239
*See also specific hormones*

Sex-influenced inheritance, 1:830

Sex-linked genes, 1:625

Sex-linked inheritance, 1:830

Sex reversal
campomelic dysplasia, 1:239
short-rib polydactyly, 2:1392
Smith-Lemli-Optiz syndrome, 2:1418

Sexual behavior, as cancer risk factor, 1:251

Sexual development abnormalities
androgen insensitivity syndrome, 1:110–111, 112
campomelic dysplasia, 1:239, 240
Donohue syndrome, 1:464, 465
Prader-Willi syndrome, 2:1248
progeria syndrome, 2:1263
sex determining region Y and, 2:1447
XX male syndrome, 2:1606

Sexual orientation, androgen insensitivity syndrome and, 1:113

SFMS. *See* Smith-Fineman-Myers syndrome

SGBS. *See* Simpson-Golabi-Behmel syndrome

SGOT (Serum glutamic oxaloacetic transaminase) tests, 1:78

SGPT (Serum glutamic pyruvic transaminase) tests, 1:78

SGS. *See* Shprintzen-Goldberg craniosynostosis syndrome

SH3TC2 gene mutations, 1:293

Shagreen patches, with tuberous sclerosis complex, 2:1522, 1523

amelia from, 1:92
cerebral palsy and, 1:285
holoprosencephaly from,
1:771–772
thalidomide as, 1:92, 93, 2:1467,
1478
Teratology Society, 2:1479
Teriparatide, for osteogenesis
imperfecta, 2:1146
Terminal deletions
Jacobsen syndrome, 1:839
microphthalmia with linear skin
defects, 2:983
monosomy 1p36 syndrome, 2:990,
991
Terminal phalanges, 1:219, 220
Termination codons, 2:1340
Termination of pregancy
alpha thalassemia major and, 2:1476
amniocentesis results and, 1:99
genetic counseling and, 1:639
hypochondrogenesis and,
1:802–803
prenatal ultrasound and,
2:1254–1255
triploidy and, 2:1505
Terminology, importance of, 1:653
Teschler-Nicola/Killian syndrome.
*See* Pallister-Killian syndrome
Testalactone, for McCune-Albright
syndrome, 2:957
Testicle abnormalities
campomelic dysplasia, 1:239
hormone secretion and, 1:110–111
Kennedy disease, 1:857, 858
Klinefelter syndrome, 1:859, 860
Renpenning syndrome,
2:1314–1315
sex determination and, 2:1447
Sutherland-Haan syndrome,
2:1456, 1457
*See also* Cryptorchidism
Testicle sperm extraction (TSE), 1:11
Testicular feminization syndrome.
*See* Androgen insensitivity
syndrome
Testis-determining factor (TDF),
1:657, 2:1446
Testosterone
ambiguous genitalia and, 1:657,
658
androgen insensitivity syndrome
and, 1:110–111
congenital adrenal hyperplasia
and, 1:351, 352
hair loss and, 1:691, 694
Klinefelter syndrome and, 1:861
McCune-Albright syndrome and,
2:956
prostate cancer and, 2:1271
Tetra-amelia, 1:91
Tetra-X. *See* XXXX syndrome
Tetralinoleoyl-cardiolipin, 1:181

Tetralogy of Fallot
Cayler cardiofacial syndrome,
1:272, 273, 274
Cornelia de Lange syndrome,
1:375, 377
deletion 22q11 syndrome, 1:421
description, 1:357
frontonasal dysplasia, 1:598
surgery for, 1:359
TAR syndrome, 2:1463
Tetraphocomelia, with Roberts SC
phocomelia, 2:1341
Tetraploidy, 1:313
Tetrasomy, 2:1166, 1609
Tetrasomy 12p mosaicism.
*See* Pallister-Killian syndrome
Tetrasomy X syndrome. *See* XXXX
syndrome
TGFB1 gene mutations
corneal dystrophy, 1:370
Engelmann disease, 1:518
osteoporosis, 2:1149
sclerosing bone dysplasias, 2:1373
TGM1 gene mutations, 1:819
Thalamic stimulation. *See* Deep brain
stimulation
Thalamotomy, for essential tremor,
1:540
Thalassemia intermedia. *See* Beta
thalassemia intermedia
Thalassemia major. *See* Beta
thalassemia major
Thalassemia minor. *See* Beta
thalassemia minor
Thalassemias, 2:**1468–1477**, *1469*
*See also specific types*
Thalidomide, as teratogen, 1:92, 93,
2:1467, 1478
Thalidomide embryopathy (TE),
2:*1477*, **1477–1481**
THAM (Tris-hydroxy-methyl
aminomethane), for Leigh
syndrome, 1:890
Thanatophoric dysplasia, 1:582,
2:1391, *1481*, **1481–1484**
Thermotherapy, for retinoblastomas,
2:1323
Thiamine treatment, for Leigh
syndrome, 1:890
Thiazide diuretics
Dent's disease, 1:435
nephrogenic diabetes insipidus,
2:1071
Thiazolidinediones, for diabetes, 1:451
Third-degree relatives, defined, 2:1191
Third-trimester ultrasound, 2:1257
Thirst
Dent's disease, 1:434
infantile nephropathic cystinosis,
1:407
nephrogenic diabetes insipidus,
2:1070–1071

Thomson, Matthew S., 2:1346
Thoracopagus conjoined twins, 1:365
Thorazine, for schizophrenia, 2:1364
Thorium dioxide, liver cancer and,
1:718
Thought insertion/withdrawal, with
schizophrenia, 2:1363
Throat abnormalities. *See* Pharynx
abnormalities
Thrombasthenia of Glanzmann and
Naegeli, 2:**1484–1487**
Thrombin
protein C deficiency and, 2:1272,
1273
protein S deficiency and, 2:1275
Thrombocytopenia
Chediak-Higashi syndrome, 1:301
hemolytic-uremic syndrome,
1:710, 712
Niemann-Pick syndrome, 2:1094
Noonan syndrome, 2:1101
TAR syndrome, 2:1462,
1463–1464
Wiskott-Aldrich syndrome, 2:1582
X-linked, 2:1581, 1582
Thrombocytopenia-absent radius
syndrome. *See* TAR syndrome
Thromboembolism
cystathionine b-synthase deficiency, 1:778, 779
Factor V Leiden thrombophilia,
1:547, 548
protein C deficiency, 2:*1272*, 1273
Thrombophlebitis, 2:1276
Thrombosis. *See* Blood clots
Thumb abnormalities
arthrogryposis multiplex
congenital, 1:135
diastrophic dysplasia, 1:455
distal arthrogryposis syndrome,
1:458
hand-foot-uterus syndrome,
1:698
Holt-Oram syndrome, 1:774
Okihiro syndrome, 1:474, 476
Pfeiffer syndrome, 2:1210
Rubinstein-Taybi syndrome,
2:1348, 1349
Saethre-Chotzen syndrome,
2:1357
skeletal dysplasia, 2:1411
thalidomide embryopathy, 2:1479
X-linked hydrocephaly,
2:1593–1594
Thurston syndrome, 2:1127, 1128
Thymectomy, for myasthenia gravis,
2:1046
Thymine
Azorean disease and, 1:174
in chromosomes, 1:317
description, 1:459–460, 461
Thymomas, with myasthenia gravis,
2:1045

multifactorial inheritance and, 2:1017
symptoms, 1:449
Type I fiber hypotrophy with central nuclei. *See* Myotubular myopathy
Type I lissencephaly. *See* Classical lissencephaly
Type II alpha-mannosidosis. *See* Adult-onset alpha-mannosidosis
Type II Cornelia de Lange syndrome, 1:374
Type II diabetes mellitus
Alstrom syndrome and, 1:82, 83, 84
demographics, 1:448–449
description, 1:444, *444*
diagnosis of, 1:450–451
genetics, 1:446–447
INSR gene mutations and, 1:464
multifactorial inheritance and, 2:1017
symptoms, 1:449
Type II lissencephaly. *See* Cobblestone lissencephaly
Type III Cornelia de Lange syndrome, 1:374
Typical distal arthrogryposis syndrome, 1:457
*See also* Distal arthrogryposis syndrome
TYR gene mutations, 1:58
Tyrosinase-related oculocutaneous albinism, 1:57
Tyrosine
albinism and, 1:58
alkaptonuria and, 1:70
phenylketonuria and, 2:1215, 1216, 1217
Tyrosine kinases, as proto-oncogene, 2:1120
Tyrosinemia, 1:717
TYRP1 gene mutations, 1:58
Tysabri, for multiple sclerosis, 2:1032

# U

UBE3A gene mutations, 1:119, 120
UCE. *See* Ornithine transcarbamylase deficiency
UGT 1A1 gene mutations, 1:760
Ulcerations, with Werner syndrome, 2:*1571*, 1572
Ulcers, 1:375, 376
Ulnar neuropathy, 1:346, 519–520
Ultra metabolizers, 2:1214
Ultrasonic flow sensors, for hydrocephalus, 1:787
Ultrasound imaging
asplenia, 1:145
Bardet-Biedl syndrome, 1:179

breast cancer, 1:228
craniosynostosis, 1:391
Dandy-Walker malformation, 1:416
glycogen storage diseases, 1:672, 673
hemifacial microsomia, 1:704–705
liver cancer, 1:719
Osler-Weber-Rendu syndrome, 2:1139
ovarian cancer, 2:1157–1158
pancreatic cancer, 2:1172, 1173
Peutz-Jeghers syndrome, 2:1207
polycystic kidney disease, 2:1229
polycystic ovary syndrome, 2:1233
prostate cancer, 2:1270
pyloric stenosis, 2:1291
retinoblastomas, 2:1323
urogenital adysplasia syndrome, 2:1532
Von Hippel-Lindau syndrome, 2:1548–1549
*See also* Prenatal ultrasound
Ultrasound markers, 2:1255–1257
Ultraviolet irradiation sensitivity
cancer, 1:252
Cockayne syndrome, 1:327
xeroderma pigmentosum, 2:1602, 1603, 1604–1605
Umbilical abnormalities
cerebral palsy, 1:286
Rieger syndrome, 2:1336, 1337
sirenomelia, 2:1406
trisomy 18, 2:1517
Umbilical cord blood stem cell transplantation, for sickle cell disease, 2:1401
Umbilical cord blood transplantation
mucopolysaccharidoses, 2:1008
thalassemias, 2:1475
Wiskott-Aldrich syndrome, 2:1583
*See also* Cord blood testing
Umbilical hernias
Beckwith-Wiedemann syndrome, 1:192
Carpenter syndrome, 1:268
Donohue syndrome, 1:465
fetal development and, 1:620
Fraser syndrome, 1:591
neuraminidase deficiency, 2:1080
Rieger syndrome, 2:1337, 1339
Unbalanced translocations
defined, 1:832
Jacobsen syndrome, 1:839
trisomy 18, 2:1516
Uncomplicated hereditary spastic paraplegia, 1:754, 756
Unconsciousness episodes. *See* Fainting
Underdeveloped genitals, 1:418
Undescended testicles. *See* Cryptorchidism

Undifferentiated schizophrenia, 2:1361–1362
Unicoronomal craniosynostosis, 1:388, 390, 391
Unilateral absence of vas deferens, 1:10
Unilateral clefts, 1:319
Unilateral hearing loss, 1:736
*See also* Hearing loss
Unilateral renal agenesis, 2:1307, 1308, 1309–1310
Uniparental disomy
Angelman syndrome, 1:119, 120, 314–315
Beckwith-Wiedemann syndrome, 1:193
description, 1:833
imprinting and, 1:821
pancreatic beta cell agenesis, 2:1168
Prader-Willi syndrome, 1:314–315, 2:1249, 1250, 1251, 1252
Uniparental heterodisomy, 1:833
Uniparental isodisomy, 1:833
United Cerebral Palsy Association, 1:287, 289
United States Renal Data Service (USRDS), 2:1313
University of California-Los Angeles, 2:1203, 1610
University of Indiana, 2:1203
University of Kentucky, 1:426
University of Michigan Neurogenetic Disorders Clinic, 1:757
University of Pittsburgh, 1:426
University of Utah, 2:1138
University of Washington, 1:780
Unknown conditional probabilities, 1:641
Upshoot, Duane retraction syndrome and, 1:474, 476
Uracil, 1:461, 2:1339
Urea cycle, 1:128–129, 2:1293
Urea cycle disorder, OTC type. *See* Ornithine transcarbamylase deficiency
Urea cycle disorders, 1:128–131, 2:1133–1136, **1529–1530**
Uremia, polycystic kidney disease and, 2:1229, 1230
Urethra abnormalities. *See* Epispadias; Hypospadias
Uric acid, excess. *See* Hyperuricemia
Uridine-diphosphate-galactose-4-epimerase deficiency, 1:607
Urinalysis
ALA dehydratase deficiency, 1:52
alkaptonuria, 1:73
Alstrom syndrome, 1:84
Barth syndrome, 1:181
Canavan disease, 1:243
cancer, 1:252

# V

# X